*Whole Body
Computed
Tomography*

Second Edition, Revised and Extended

Whole Body Computed Tomography

Otto H. Wegener

Department of Radiology and Nuclear Medicine
Altona General Hospital, Hamburg, Germany

WITH THE COLLABORATION OF

Regine Fassel and Doris Welger

Department of Radiology and Nuclear Medicine
Altona General Hospital, Hamburg, Germany

ENGLISH TRANSLATION BY

Suzyon O'Neal Wandrey

ENGLISH LANGUAGE EDITION
WITH THE ADVICE AND EXPERTISE OF

Adrian K. Dixon

Consultant Radiologist, Addenbrooke's Hospital
Cambridge, UK

AND

Udo Schumacher

Professor of Anatomy and Head of Human Morphology
University of Southampton, UK

BOSTON

Blackwell Scientific Publications

OXFORD LONDON EDINBURGH
MELBOURNE PARIS BERLIN VIENNA

© 1992 by
Blackwell Wissenschafts-Verlag
English language edition
© 1993 by
Blackwell Scientific Publications, Inc.
Editorial Offices:
238 Main Street, Cambridge
Massachusetts 02142, USA
Osney Mead, Oxford OX2 0EL, England
25 John Street, London WC1N 2BL, England
23 Ainslie Place, Edinburgh EH3 6AJ, Scotland
54 University Street, Carlton, Victoria 3053
Australia

Other Editorial Offices:
Librairie Arnette SA
1, rue de Lille
75007 Paris
France

Blackwell Wissenschafts-Verlag GmbH
Kurfürstendamm 57
10707 Berlin
Germany

Blackwell MZV
Feldgasse 13
A-1238 Wien
Austria

First published 1981
(*Ganzkörpercomputertomographie*)
English translation 1983
Second edition 1992
This translation published 1993
Reprinted 1994

Editorial assistance:
Dr. med. S. Weber, Berlin
Graphics: P. Hamann, Elmshorn

Set by Satz- und Reprotechnik GmbH,
69494 Hemsbach; Printed in Germany by
Druckhaus Beltz, 69494 Hemsbach
and bound by Buchbinderei Spinner,
77833 Ottersweier

94 95 96 97 5 4 3 2

DISTRIBUTORS

USA
    Blackwell Scientific Publications, Inc.
    238 Main Street
    Cambridge, MA 02142
    (*Orders*: Tel: 800 759-6102
                  617 876-7000)

Canada
    Times Mirror Professional Publishing, Ltd
    130 Flaska Drive
    Markham, Ontario L6G 1B8
    (*Orders*: Tel: 800 268-4178
                  416 470-6739)

Australia
    Blackwell Scientific Publications Pty Ltd
    54 University Street
    Carlton, Victoria 3053
    (*Orders*: Tel: 03 347-5552)

Outside North America and Australia
    Marston Book Services Ltd
    PO Box 87
    Oxford OX2 0DT
    (*Orders*: Tel: 0865 791155
                  Fax: 0865 791927
                  Telex: 837515)

**Library of Congress Cataloging-in-
Publication Data**

Wegener, O. H.:
Whole body computed tomography.
Reve. ed. of: Whole body computerized
tomography. c. 1983.
Includes bibliographical references and index.
1. Tomography. I. Fassel, Regine. II. Welger,
Doris. III. Wegener, O. H. Whole body
computerized tomography. IV. Title [DNLM:
1. Anatomy, Regional. 2. Tomography, X-Ray
Computed. WN 160 W411g]
RC78.7.T6W44   1993   616.07′572   92-35853
ISBN 0-86542-223-0

Preface to the second German edition

Since the first edition of this book was published eleven years ago, computed tomography (CT) has come to play an important role in the field of radiology. The technique now has a wider range of applications and is well documented in the current literature.

The aim of this book is to provide a practical introduction to computer tomographic imaging and image analysis. The revised text is based on personal experience and the large data base that has been built up since publication of the first edition. All the artwork has been revised and benefits from the addition of many new CT images which in turn are supported by computerised graphics enabling the reader to analyse the most abstract morphological processes. An extensive bibliography, published as a supplement, complements this volume, allowing the reader access to a broad range of original literature.

Most of the CT images appearing in the book originate from the archives of the Altona General Hospital in Hamburg and were processed with the Somatom DRH (Siemens). The helpful cooperation of several colleagues from other departments of the hospital made it possible to provide a broad range of diagnostic images. The chapters on the lung and liver were particularly enriched by contributions from my colleagues *H.-J. Triebel, M.D., P. Uhrmeister, M.D.,* and *C. Zwicker, M.D.* The accompanying anatomical diagrams were made with the Somatom Plus, provided by the *Siemens Corporation*. Other rare and interesting images were supplied by *Prof. E. Gerstenberg, M.D, D. Rehnitz, M.D., A. Rieber, M.D.,* and *Prof. H.-D. Weiß, M.D.*

This book would not have been possible without the initiative and active support of *Mrs. B. Behrends-Steins, Ph.D.,* of Schering AG and my publisher *A. Bedürftig, M.D.* For their constant readiness to provide me the necessary assistance and their support of my ideas and the entire concept of the book, I am immensely grateful.

An English edition will be published later this year. The Italian and French versions are scheduled for publication in the summer of 1993.

I would be delighted if this second edition enjoys the same popularity as its predecessor. Suggestions for improvement are always welcome.

Hamburg, July 1992   O. H. Wegener

Preface to the second English edition

As this English translation was completed while the original German edition was still in production its publication is possible just a few months after the German edition appeared.

The English version has the added bonus of more than 4,000 references, a comprehensive keyword index and an author index.

Most of the references come from the following journals:

Journal of Computer Assisted Tomography (JCAT)

Radiology

American Journal of Roentgenology (AJR)

Neuroradiology

American Journal of Neuroradiology (AJNR)

Fortschritte auf dem Gebiet der Röntgenstrahlen (RöFo)

Der Radiologe

and include all relevant articles from 1980 onwards.

Some readers may wish to check which articles deal with a particular organ, a region of the body or a disease: the keyword index allows for this. Each of the approx. 250 keywords is followed by the corresponding numbers listed in the literature section.

Quite often, the name of the author rather than the article itself is known. Therefore, the author index gives an alphabetical list of *all* (and not just first-mentioned) authors appearing in the literature section.

Although the literature section does not claim to be complete it should prove a useful tool for quick reference.

Contributors of Photographic Material

Prof. Dr. Claus Claussen
  Direktor der Radiologischen Abteilung
  Universitätsklinik Tübingen
  Hoppe-Seyler-Straße 3

  7400 Tübingen 1, Germany

Prof. Dr. Ekkardt Gerstenberg
  Chefarzt der Strahlenabteilung
  Auguste-Viktoria-Krankenhaus
  Rubensstraße 125

  1000 Berlin 41, Germany

Prof. Dr. Michael Haertel
  Chefarzt des Instituts für Diagnostische
  Radiologie
  Kantonsspital

  9007 St. Gallen, Switzerland

Prof. Dr. H.H. Jend
  Ltd. Arzt des Radiologischen Instituts
  Zentralkrankenhaus Bremen-Ost
  Züricher Straße 40

  2800 Bremen 44, Germany

Dr. Bernd Lochner
  Radiologische Gemeinschaftspraxis
  Mainzer Landstraße 191

  6000 Frankfurt 1, Germany

Dr. Detlev Rehnitz
  Chefarzt der Radiologischen Abteilung
  Diakonie Kreiskrankenhaus Schwäbisch Hall
  Diakoniestraße

  7170 Schwäbisch Hall, Germany

Dr. Andrea Rieber
  Abt. Radiologische Diagnostik
  (Direktor Prof. Dr. C. Claussen)
  Univ.-Klinik Tübingen
  Hoppe-Seyler-Straße 3

  7400 Tübingen 1, Germany

Dr. Hans-Jörg Triebel
  Abt. Strahlendiagnostik
  der Radiologischen Klinik
  (Direktor Prof. Dr. E. Buecheler)
  Univ.-Krankenhaus Eppendorf
  Martinistraße 52

  2000 Hamburg 20, Germany

Dr. Peter Uhrmeister
  Strahlenklinik und Poliklinik
  (Direktor Prof. Dr. R. Felix)
  Klinikum Rudolf Virchow
  Spandauer Damm 130

  1000 Berlin 19, Germany

Prof. Hans-Dieter Weiß
  Direktor des Instituts für Radiologie
  Med. Universität zu Lübeck
  Ratzeburger Allee 160

  2400 Lübeck, Germany

Dr. Christian Zwicker
  Strahlenklinik und Poliklinik
  (Direktor Prof. Dr. R. Felix)
  Klinikum Rudolf Virchow
  Spandauer Damm 130

  1000 Berlin 19, Germany

Table of Contents

Preface to the second German edition . V

Preface to the second English edition . VII

Chapter 1
Techniques of Computed Tomography

Mathematical Principles 3
Technical Realization 4
  Single Detector Rotate-Translate
  Systems 4
  Multiple Detector Rotate-Translate
  Systems 4
  Rotation Scanner with Movable
  Detectorts 4
  Rotation Scanner with Stationary
  Detectors 4
Image Reconstruction 5
  Picture Elements 5
Density Value 7
  Hounsfield Density Scale 7
  Densitometry 7
Image Variation 8

Chapter 2
Anatomy 11

Chapter 3
Image Analysis

Structural Image Analysis 81
  Interpretation of Images 81
  Window Settings 81
Morphological Image Analysis 83
  Tubular and Nodular Structures . . . 83
  Evaluation of Boundary Surfaces . . 83
  Space-occupying Processes 84
  Infiltrating Processes 84

Quantitative Image Analysis
(Densitometry) 85
  The Individual Attenuation Value . . 85
  Falsification of Density
  Measurements 85
  Attenuation Value of Boundary
  Surfaces 87
  Pathomorphological Variation 87
  Bone Densitometry 91
Intravenous Bolus Injection of Contrast
Medium 93
  Intravascular Enhancement 93
  Parenchymatous Enhancement . . . 93
  Differential Diagnosis of Contrast
  Enhanced Images 95

Chapter 4
Contrast Media

Intravascular Administration 99
Basic Principles of Contrast
Enhancement 99
Urographic Contrast Media 100
  Pharmacokinetics 100
  Intravenous Bolus Injection
  (CM Bolus) 102
  Intravenous Infusion 104
  Intra-arterial Injection 105
Biliary Contrast Media 105
  Pharmacokinetics 105
Intracavitary Opacification 106
  Intestinal Opacification 106
  CT-Assisted Peritoneography 109
  CT-Assisted Myelography 110

Chapter 5
Techniques and Strategies of Examination

Diagnostic Procedures 113
  Patient Preparation 113

Technical Parameters 113
Administration of Contrast Medium 114
Selection of Technical Parameters for
Scans with and without Contrast
Medium Enhancement 114
Examination Strategies 115
Interventional Computed Tomography 116
CT-Guided Biopsy 116
Abscess Drainage 117
Examination Schemes 118

Chapter 6
The Mediastinum

Anatomy and Imaging 137
Mediastinal Spaces 137
Mediastinal Vessels 137
Trachea 141
Thyroid Gland 141
Esophagus 141
Fasciae 141
Lymph Nodes 143
Thymus Gland 144
Lymph Node Enlargement 145
Malignant Lymphoma 145
Lymph Node Metastases 150
Involvement of Lymph Nodes in
Granulomatous Diseases 151
Primary Tumors of the Anterior
Mediastinum 153
Mesenchymal Tumors 153
Tumors of the Thymus 154
Teratoid Blastomas 155
Goiter 157
Parathyroid Tumors 158
Primary Tumors of the Middle
Mediastinum 159
Tumors of the Trachea 159
Bronchogenic Cysts 159
Pleuropericardial (Mesothelial) Cysts 160
Primary Tumors of the Posterior
Mediastinum 160
Solid Neurogenic Tumors 160
Cystic Lesions 161
Vascular Processes 162
Aorta 162
Aneurysms of the Thoracic Aorta . . 162
Dissecting Aneurysms 165
Ectasia of the Brachiocephalic Trunk 166
Ectasia of Pulmonary Arteries . . . 167
Ectasia of the Azygos Vein 167

Mediastinal Inflammation 168
Acute Mediastinitis 168
Chronic Mediastinitis 168
Mediastinal Lesions 169
Pneumomediastinum
(Mediastinal Emphysema) 169
Mediastinal Hematoma 169

Chapter 7
The Heart

Anatomy and Imaging 173
Functional Conditions of the Heart . . 174
Volume Stress 174
Pressure Stress 174
Cardiomyopathy 175
Coronary Heart Disease 175
Valvular Defects 176
Intracavitary Masses 176
Pericardium 177
Anatomy and Imaging 177
Pericardial Anomalies 178
Pericardial Fluid Collection 178
Chronic Constrictive Pericarditis . . 180
Tumors 180

Chapter 8
The Lungs

Anatomy and Imaging 183
Bronchial Tree 183
Septa 183
Bronchovascular Structures –
Hilum of the Lung 185
Bronchopulmonary Segments . . . 185
Lobules of the Lung
(Secondary Lobules) 186
Pulmonary Nodules 186
Lung Density 187
Respiration Defects of the Lungs . . . 188
Partial Loss of Volume 188
Atelectasis 189
Round Atelectasis 192
Parenchymal Lung Abnormalities . . . 192
Infiltrations 192
Emphysema 195
Bronchopulmonary Anomalies 197
Pulmonary Sequestration 197
Bronchiectasis 197

Pulmonary Inflammation 199
  Pneumonia 199
  Pulmonary Abscess 200
Interstitial Lung Diseases 203
  Idiopathic Pulmonary Fibrosis 203
  Sarcoidosis 203
  Histiocytosis X
  (Eosinophilic Granuloma) 206
  Pulmonary Lymphangiomyomatosis . 206
  Asbestosis 207
  Silicosis 208
  Carcinomatous Lymphangitis 209
  Interstitial Tumor Infiltration 210
Pulmonary Embolism and Infarction . 210
Lung Injuries 211
Pulmonary Neoplasms 212
  Benign Tumors 212
  Bronchial Adenoma 212
  Bronchial Carcinoma 213
  Pulmonary Metastases 221
  Solitary Nodules 222

Chapter 9
The Pleura

Anatomy and Imaging 225
Pleural Effusion 225
Empyema 227
Pleural Thickening 229
Asbestosis 230
Primary Neoplasms of the Pleura . . . 231
  Benign Neoplasms 231
  Malignant Mesothelioma 232
Pleural Metastases 233

Chapter 10
The Chest Wall

Anatomy and Imaging 237
Tumors 237
Inflammations 241
Trauma 242

Chapter 11
The Liver

Anatomy and Imaging 245
  Contrast Enhancement of Hepatic
  Structures 248
Cystic Liver Diseases 249
  Dysontogenetic Cysts 249
  Solitary Hepatic Cysts 249

Solid Tumors of the Liver 251
  Adenomas and Focal Nodular
  Hyperplasia (FNH) 252
  Hepatic Lipoma 254
  Hemangioma 254
  Mesenchymal Hamartoma 256
  Hepatocellular Carcinoma (HCC) . . 256
  Cholangiocarcinoma 258
  Fibrolamellar Hepatocellular
  Carcinoma 260
  Secondary Tumors of the Liver
  (Metastases) 263
  Lymphoma Manifestation in the
  Liver 264
Inflammatory Regressive Changes in
the Liver 266
  Fatty Infiltration of the Liver 266
  Hepatitis 266
  Cirrhosis 267
  Hemochromatosis 268
  Abscesses 269
  Echinococcosis (Hydatid Disease) . . 271
Trauma 272
Vascular Processes 275
  Portal Venous Thrombosis 275
  Budd-Chiari Syndrome 275

Chapter 12
The Biliary System

Anatomy and Imaging 279
  Gallbladder Enlargement 279
Inflammatory Changes of the
Gallbladder 279
  Cholecystitis 279
  Cholelithiasis 281
Gallbladder Tumors 282
Biliary Obstruction 283
Biliary Tract Infections 284
Tumors of the Biliary Tract 286
Choledochal Cysts 286
Caroli's Disease 287

Chapter 13
The Pancreas

Anatomy and Imaging 291
Cystic Pancreatic Diseases 294
  Dysontogenetic Cyst 294
  Retention Cysts and Pseudocysts . . 294
Pancreatic Tumors 296
  Microcystic Adenoma 296

Macrocystic Adenoma 296
Pancreatic Carcinoma 297
Cystadenocarcinoma 301
Islet Cell Tumors 302
Secondary Tumors 303
Pancreatitis 304
Acute Pancreatitis 304
Chronic Pancreatitis 307
Pancreatic Abscess 310
Pancreatic Trauma 311
Lipomatosis and Atrophy 312

Chapter 14
The Gastrointestinal Tract

Anatomy and Imaging 315
The Esophagus 317
Esophageal Tumors 317
Inflammatory Esophageal
Abnormalities 319
Esophageal Varices 320
The Stomach 321
Tumors of the Stomach 321
Gastric Carcinoma 321
Gastric Sarcomas 324
Benign Gastric Tumors 325
Gastric Inflammation 326
Small Intestine and Colon 326
Cysts 326
Solid Tumors 327
Benign and malignant Tumors 327
Malignant Lymphomas and
Myosarcomas 327
Small Intestine Carcinoids 327
Colorectal Carcinoma 328
Tumor Recurrence after Proctectomy 331
Inflammatory Diseases 332
Crohn's Disease 332
Ulcerative Colitis 334
Appendicitis 335
Diverticulitis 336
Functional Diseases of Intestine 338
Mesenteric Ischemia 338

Chapter 15
The Peritoneal Cavity

Anatomy and Imaging 341
Supramesocolic Compartment 341
Inframesocolic Compartment 341
Mesentery 342
Ascites 346
Peritonitis – Intraperitoneal Abscess . . 347
Hemorrhage in the Abdominal Cavity . 349
Biliary Ascites 350
Pseudomyxoma Peritonei 350
Primary and Metastatic Peritoneal
Neoplasms 351

Chapter 16
The Spleen

Anatomy and Imaging 357
Cystic Splenic Diseases 359
Solid Tumors of the Spleen 359
Malignant Lymphomas 361
Inflammatory Splenic Diseases 362
Trauma 363
Splenic Hematoma 363
Vascular Processes 364
Splenic Infarction 364
Splenic Vein Thrombosis 365
Splenic Anomalies 366

Chapter 17
The Kidney

Anatomy and Imaging 369
Cystic Renal Diseases 369
Renal Cysts 369
Polycystic Renal Disease in Children
(Cystic Kidney) 371
Polycystic Renal Disease in Adults
(Cystic Kidney) 371
Multicystic Renal Dysplasia 372
Multilocular Cystic Nephroma . . . 373
Solid Tumors 374
Renal Cell Carcinoma 374
Nephradenoma 379
Oncocytoma 380
Mesenchymal Tumors 380
Tumors of the Renal Pelvis 381
Renal Lymphoma 384
Renal Metastases 385
Nephroblastoma 386
Inflammatory Renal Diseases 387
Acute Pyelonephritis –
Local Bacterial Nephritis 387
Renal Abscess 389
Emphysematous Pyelonephritis . . . 390
Xanthogranulomatous Pyelonephritis 390
Chronic Pyelonephritis 391

Renal Tuberculosis 391
Renal Transplants 392
Fibrolipomatosis 393
Renal Trauma 393
Renal Contusion 394
Renal Pedicle Injuries 394
Renal Hematoma 394
Obstructive Uropathies 395
Hydronephrosis 395
Pyonephrosis 396
Urolithiasis 397
Vascular Processes 398
Arteriosclerosis 398
Renal Artery Stenosis 398
Renal Infarction 398
Renal Vein Thrombosis 399
Congenital Variations, Anomalies . . . 399

Chapter 18
The Adrenal Glands

Anatomy and Imaging 403
Hyperplasia and Tumors of the Adrenal
Cortex 404
Adrenocortical Hyperplasia 404
Adrenocortical Adenoma 404
Adrenocortical Carcinoma 405
Nonfunctioning Adenoma 406
Adrenal Medullary Tumors 407
Myelolipoma 407
Pheochromocytoma 407
Pheochromoblastoma
(Malignant Pheochromocytoma) . . 408
Neuroblastoma 408
Metastases into the Adrenals 409
Adrenal Cysts 410
Hemorrhage 410
Inflammations 411
Hypoplastic Atrophy 412

Chapter 19
The Urinary Bladder

Anatomy and Imaging 415
Displacement 415
Anomalies 416
Infections 416
Tumors of the Urinary Bladder 417
Papillomas, Carcinomas 417
Mesenchymal Tumors 420

Chapter 20
The Prostate and Seminal Vesicles

Anatomy and Imaging 425
Prostatic Cysts 426
Prostatic Adenoma
(Benign Prostatic Hyperplasia) 426
Prostatic Tumors 427
Prostatic Infections 429
Seminal Vesicles 430

Chapter 21
The Female Genital Organs

Anatomy and Imaging 433
Uterine Tumors 436
Myomas (Uterine Leiomyoma) . . . 436
Cervical Carcinoma 437
Carcinoma of the Body of the Uterus 439
Recurrent Malignant Uterine Tumors 441
Ovarian Tumors 442
Cysts 442
Cystic Solid and Solid Tumors of the
Ovary 444
Inflammatory Processes 448
Uterine Inflammations 448
Adnexal Inflammations 448
Parametrial Inflammations 449

Chapter 22
The Retroperitoneal Cavity

Anatomy and Imaging 453
Retroperitoneal Vessels 453
Retrocrural Space 455
Diaphragm 455
Fascial Spaces of the
Retroperitoneum 457
Subperitoneal Fascial Spaces 459
Lymph Nodes 459
Peri- and Pararenal Lesions 462
Exudative Hemorrhagic Lesions of
the Perirenal Space 462
Urinomas (Perirenal Pseudocysts) . . 463
Perirenal Hematoma 464
Solid Perirenal Lesions 464
Lesions in the Anterior Pararenal
Space 465
Lesions in the Posterior Pararenal
Space 465
Iliopsoas Muscle 466
Lesions in the Subperitoneal Space . . 467

Lesions not Bound by Compartmental
Fascia 467
    Primary Retroperitoneal Fibrosis . . 467
    Secondary Retroperitoneal Fibrosis . 469
    Pelvic Fibrolipomatosis 470
    Malignant Lymphoma 470
    Lymph Node Metastases 474
    Benign Lymphadenopathies 477
    Primary Retroperitoneal Tumors . . 478
Vascular Lesions 481
    Aneurysms 481
    Aortic Trauma 485
    Anomalies of the Inferior Vena Cava 485
    Thrombosis of the Inferior Vena
    Cava (Including the Pelvic Veins) . . 486

Chapter 23
Muscle Tissue

Atrophy 491
Progressive Muscular Dystrophy 491
Inflammatory Muscular Diseases . . . 492
    Pyogenic Myositis
    (Muscular Abscess) 492
    Sarcoidosis 493
    Polymyositis 493
Muscular Hematoma 493
Myositis Ossificans 494

Chapter 24
Soft-Tissue Tumors 497

Chapter 25
Bone Tumors

Chondrogenous Tumors 503
Osteogenic Tumors 504
Fibrous Tumors 505
Myelogenic Tumors 505

Chapter 26
The Spine

Anatomy and Imaging 513
Degenerative Spinal Diseases 518
    Degenerative Processes in
    Intervertebral Discs 518

Disc Herniation and Prolapse 519
The Disc after Surgery –
    Recurrent Herniation 524
    Spondylarthrosis 526
    Spondylosis – True Spondylolisthesis 527
Spinal Stenosis 527
Spinal Injuries 530
    Impacted Compression Fracture . . . 533
    Incomplete Burst Fracture 533
    Complete Burst Fracture 535
    Chance Fracture –
    Distraction Trauma 535
    Flexion – Distraction Trauma 536
    Translation Injuries 536
    Atlanto-Occipital Dislocation 537
    Atlanto-Odontoid Subluxation . . . 537
    Rotatory Atlantoaxial Dislocation . . 537
    Fractures of the Atlas 539
    Dens Fractures 539
    Fractures of the Arch of the Axis . . 541
    Fractures of the Cervical Arches and
    Articular Processes of the Middle
    and Lower Cervical Spine (C3–7) . . 541
Vertebral Tumors and Tumor-Like
Lesions 542
Intraspinal Masses 544
    Congenital Masses 544
    Acquired Masses 544
Spondylitis – Spondylodiscitis 549

Chapter 27
The Bony Pelvis

Anatomy and Imaging 553
Pelvic Trauma 555
    Fractures of the Posterior Pelvic
    Girdle 556
    Acetabular Fractures 557
Coxitis 559
Sacroiliitis 560

Chapter 28
CT-Terminology 563

Literature 581

Subject Index 683

Chapter 1
Techniques of Computed Tomography

Techniques of Computed Tomography

Tomography was introduced to radiology during the Thirties. Whereas conventional radiological techniques produce summed images of an object, tomographic scanners rotate to divide the object and organize it into spatially consecutive, parallel image sections. The process, which was originally totally mechanical, has been improved upon by new technology. In computed tomography (CT), a computer stores a large amount of data (attenuation values) from a selected region of the body, making it possible to determine the spatial relationship of the radiation-absorbing structures within it. The computed tomogram consists of a matrix of attenuation values depicted in various shades of grey, thereby creating a spatial image of the scanned object. Since the attenuation values measured by CT are reproducible, important diagnostic information about tissues in the scanned regions of interest is thereby obtained.

Mathematical Principles

Fig. 1–1b represents a square cross-section of an object divided into 8 x 8 square picture elements with different attenuation values. The attenuation measurements from rows I_0 and I_x alone do not provide sufficient information to reliably calculate individual absorption by mathematical equations. Additional measurements from different spatial levels are needed to accurately determine the individual absorption values (total of n x n, i. e., 8 x 8 projections in this example). For technical realization of computed tomograms, the number and quality of data from individual picture elements, i.e. the degree of spatial resolution, increases in proportion with the number of attenuation measurements taken from different angles.

Fig. 1-1a. Scanning. Bundled X-ray beams perpendicular to the long axis of the body penetrate a slice of the body from different angles. Attenuation is registered by an array of detectors.

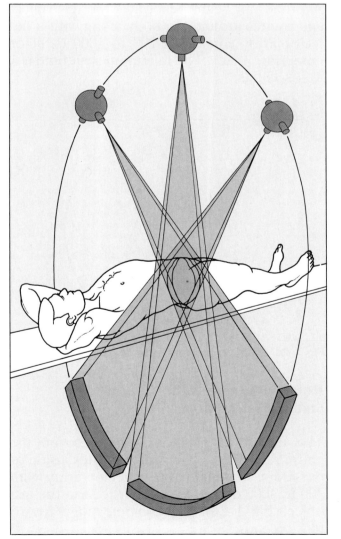

Fig. 1-1b. Mathematic principles (see text).

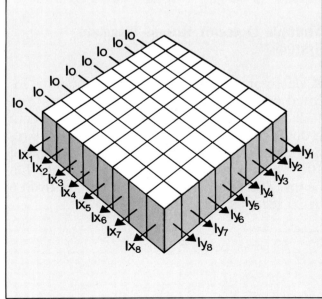

Technical Realization

Attenuation is measured by detectors which are aligned behind the patient, opposite to the X-ray source. There are basically four different types of CT scanning systems:

Single Detector Rotate-Translate Systems*

A fine X-ray beam scans the body through 180 steps of 1°. The intensity of the beam is measured by individual contralateral detector elements. After each angular increment, a (linear) translation is made as the beam traverses the body (Fig. 1–2a). A minimum of several minutes is required for scanning.

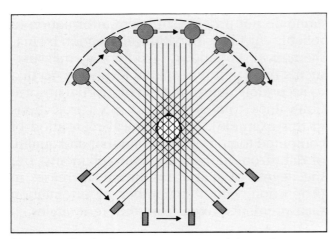

Fig. 1-2a. Single detector rotate-translate system.

Multiple Detector Rotate-Translate Systems**

A detector array with 5 to 50 elements is located contralateral to the X-ray source (Fig. 1–2b). A pencil X-ray beam or a fan beam reduces the number of angular increments required for scanning. Scans are made at steps of 10°, which corresponds to the angle of the fan beam. The minimum scan time ranges from 6 to 20 seconds.

---

*	1st generation
**	2nd generation
***	3rd generation
****	4th generation

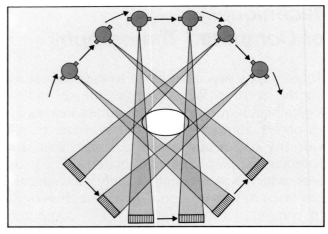

Fig. 1-2b. Multiple detector rotate-translate system.

Rotation Scanner with Movable Detectors***

A broad fan beam penetrates the test object and rotates around the body along with a detector array containing 200 to 1000 detector units (Fig. 1–2c). The minimum scan time is 1 to 4 seconds.

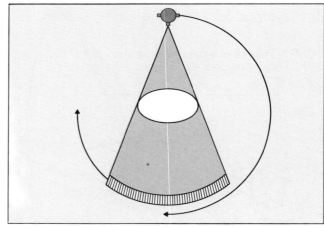

Fig. 1-2c. Rotation scanner with movable detectors.

Rotation Scanner with Stationary Detectors****

The angle of the fan X-ray beam covers the entire test object. The source rotates inside or outside a stationary ring detector array with 300 to 4000 detectors in order to scan the test object (Fig. 1–2d). The scan time ranges from 3 to 8 seconds.

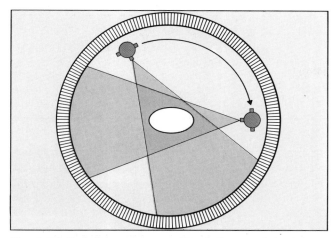

Fig. 1-2d. Rotation scanner with stationary detectors.

registered in the computer, and the CT image is reconstructed by means of a complex computational process. The finite number of attenuation values corresponding with the scanned object are organized in matrix form. The translation of these numbers into various analogous grey levels creates a visual image of the scanned cross-sectional area. Due to their different absorptive capacities, different internal structures will be identifiable on the picture image. The size of the image matrix, i.e. the number of calculated picture elements, is dependent on the number of individual projections. Matrix size, therefore, also influences the quality of image resolution.

Image Reconstruction

Short scanning times are desirable in whole-body computed tomography, since motion artifacts caused by breathing, peristalsis and the beat of the heart can thereby be eliminated. Slow scanning systems with alternating, contra-rotating movements are therefore being replaced by continuously rotating systems with faster scanning times. The attenuation values for each set of projections are

Picture Elements

The smallest unit of a computed tomogram is the individual picture point or *picture element* (pixel). Depending on the size of the scanning field and the image matrix, the pixel represents a certain proportion of the total cross-sectional area. Based on the slice thickness, the pixel also represents a tissue element the volume of which is determined by slice thickness, matrix

Fig. 1-3. Volume of a volume element (voxel). The area of the picture element as well as slice thickness (d) determine the volume of the volume element (a). (b) = edge length of the picture element (pixel), (D) = diameter of the scanning field or field of measurement.

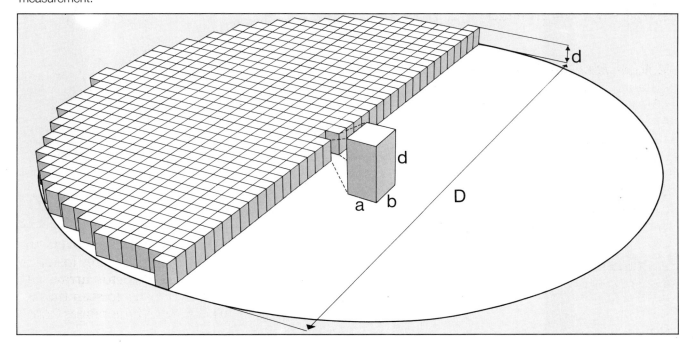

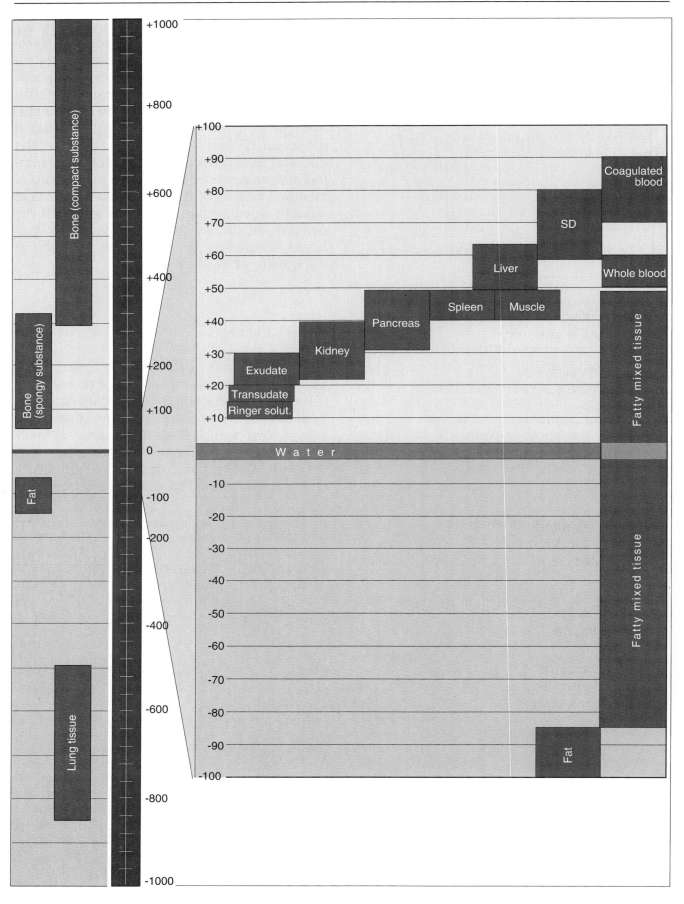

Table 1-1. Attenuation values for various body tissues and fluids.

Tissue Type	Standard Value (HU)	Scatter (HU)
Bone (compact)	> 250	
Bone (spongy)	130 ± 100	
Thyroid	70 ± 10	
Liver	65 ± 5	45–75
Muscle	45 ± 5	35–50
Spleen	45 ± 5	35–55
Lymphoma	45 ± 10	40–60
Pancreas	40 ± 10	25–55
Kidney	30 ± 10	20–40
Fat	−65 ± 10	−80–(−100)

Fluids	Standard Value (HU)
Blood (coagulated)	80 ± 10
Blood (venous whole blood)	55 ± 5
Plasma	27 ± 2
Exudate (>30 g protein/l)	>18 ± 2
Transudate (<30 g protein/l)	<18 ± 2
Ringer solution	12 ± 2

size and diameter of the scanning field (Fig. 1–3). Under these conditions, a picture element also represents a *volume element* (voxel).

Density Value

Each volume element is given a numerical value, i.e. attenuation value, which corresponds with the average amount of radiation absorbed by the tissue in that picture element. CT density is directly proportional (linear proportion) to the attenuation coefficient, a tissue constant influenced by many factors. The attenuation coefficient quantifies the absorption of x-irradiation. After internal calibration of the scanner, the CT density of water is set at 0, and that of air at −1000 Hounsfield units (HU). The various types of body tissue are assigned values relative to the Hounsfield scale (Fig. 1–4). CT numbers are therefore arbitrary but relative values that abide by the laws of attenuation.

Hounsfield Density Scale

In CT, attenuation values are measured in Hounsfield units (HU). The attenuation value of air and water (defined as −1000 HU and 0 HU, resp.) represent fixed points on the CT density scale that remain unaffected by tube voltage. Depending on the effective radiation of the scanning device, the relationship of different tissue types to water attenuation will vary. Density values listed in the literature must therefore be considered as mere guidelines.

Densitometry

The arrangement of detectors on a scanning gantry facilitates quantitative density measurements in freely selectable areas on the test object (regions of interest). The CT number represents the arithmetic mean of all attenuation values measured in an individual volume element. The gray-scale display of a scanned object alone provides some information on the relative density (radiodensity) of a structure on the image. Upon comparison with the surrounding tissue, the structure may be described as *isodense* (same density), *hypodense* (low-density) or *hyperdense* (high-density). In parenchymatous organs like the brain, liver, kidney and pancreas, the attenuation value of healthy surrounding tissue is normally used for comparison. CT numbers in the water range are henceforth described as *water-dense*, those in the fat range as *fat-dense*, and those in the muscle range as *muscle-dense*.

Fig. 1-4. Hounsfield scale. Its lower limit is −1000 HU, corresponding with air density. Very dense bone structures exceed the value of 1000 HU. The attenuation values of most types of tissue and bodily fluids overlap in the range of −100 to +100 HU (see Table 1–1.).

Image Variation

The attenuation values for image reconstruction, ranging from −1000 HU to +1000 HU, are conventionally depicted in numerous corresponding shades of grey. However, the human eye can distinguish only ca. 15 to 20 of these shades. If the entire density scale of ca. 2000 HU were to be displayed in a single image, the evaluator would be able to distinguish only a single shade of grey in the diagnostically important soft-tissue range. He or she could not visualize all densitometric nuances measurable by the computer, and important diagnostic information would be lost.

The *image window* was therefore developed as a means of producing vivid contrasts of even slight densitometric differences. The concept

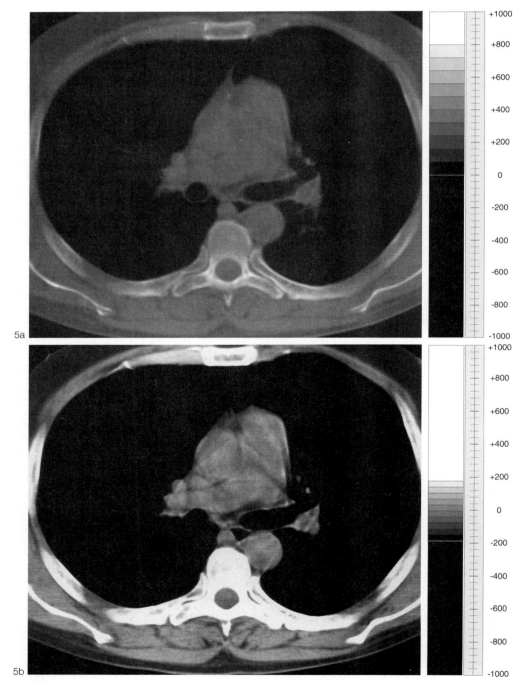

5a

5b

Fig. 1-5. Window settings. The full range of CT densities, represented as a matrix of attenuation values, can be usefully demonstrated only if limited by different window settings. By selecting a specific window level and window width, a limited range of grey values (see grey-scale column beside density scale) are assigned to a specific light range of the CT scanner. Any structures with attenuation values above that range appear white, and those with CT numbers below the window range appear black.

Fig. 1-5a. Bone window. Bone structures in higher density ranges should be scanned at a higher and broader window level for more vivid images.

Fig. 1–5b. Soft-tissue window. Tissues in the usual diagnostically significant soft-tissue range are best demonstrated at this window level and width. The grey scale representation of fat and soft-tissue structure is adequate for diagnosis.

of the window makes it possible to "expand" the grey scale (*window width*) according to an arbitrarily set density range (25 to 1000 HU). Attenuation values above the upper window limit appear white, and those below the lower limit are black on the image. The *window level* (center of the density scale) determines which attenuation values, i.e. which organ structures, are represented in the medium shades of grey.

The window adjustments must be set in accordance with the structures to be diagnosed. Narrow window widths provide high-contrast images, however, there is a danger that structures outside that window range may be inadequately demonstrated or overlooked. With broad window settings, minor density differences appear homogeneous and are thus masked. Resolution is thereby reduced.

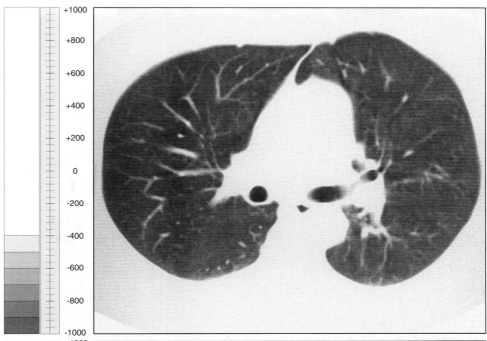

Fig. 1-5c. Lung window. Since it contains air, lung tissue has a wide range of densities. Satisfactory images can be obtained with a negative window level and a broad window width.

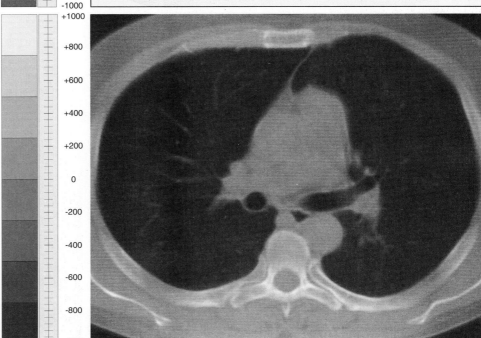

Fig. 1-5d. Pleural window (special window). This window is very wide (2000 HU) in order to demonstrate all structures, albeit less vividly. Pleural and hilar transitional zones are thus better demonstrated.

Chapter 2
Anatomy

Key to Symbols

A   Artery

A*   Arterial branch

AV   Vessels (arteries and accompanying veins)

AV*   Branches of these vessels

V   Vein

V*   Venous branch

M   Muscle

M*   Muscle tendon

O   Organs

O1   Heart

O2   Lung

O3   Liver

O4   Pancreas, spleen

O5   Urogenital tract

O6   Reproductive organs

O7   Gastrointestinal tract

O8   Glands

O9   Larynx

S   Skeleton

S1   Vertebra

S2   Rib

S3   Scapula

S4   Pelvis

S5   Femur

S6   Sacrum, coccyx

S7   Humerus

S8   Crus

SC   Cranial bone

N   Nerves

C*   Miscellaneous

All anatomical structures retain these symbols in the various sectional levels (except **C** = miscellaneous)

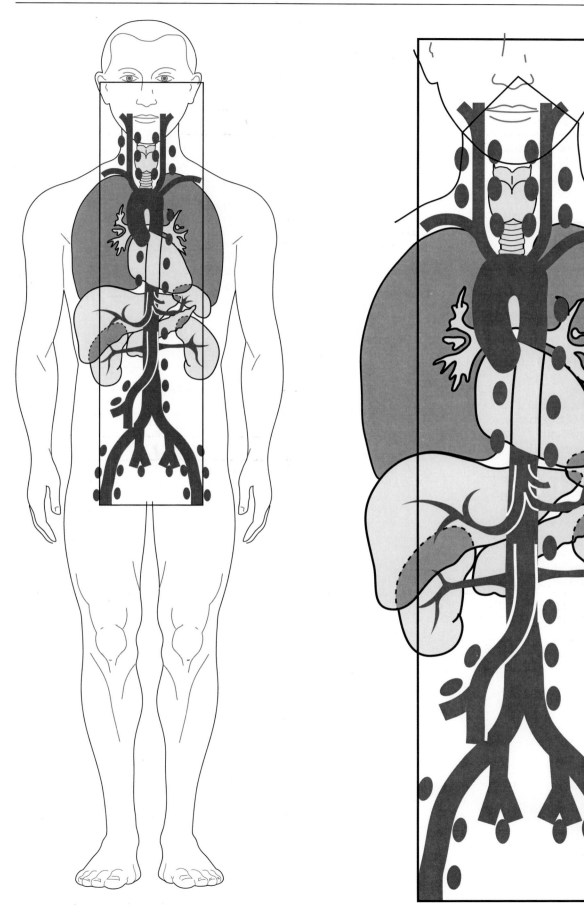

	1/2
A31	Internal carotid artery
V5	Internal jugular vein
V31	Posterior facial vein
M4	Splenius capitis muscle
M84	Muscles of the tongue
M85	Medial pterygoid muscle
M86	Lateral pterygoid muscle
M87	Temporal muscle
M88	Masseter muscle
M89	Buccinator/Orbicularis oris muscles
M95	Tensor palati muscle
M96	Levator palati muscle
M97	Longus capitis muscle
M98	Soft palate muscle
O84	Paratoid gland
SC1	Mandible
SC5	Occipital bone
SC13	Ramus of the mandible
SC20	Maxillary sinus
SC23	Hard palate
SC24	Medial pterygoid plate
SC25	Lateral pterygoid plate
SC26	Anterior nasal process
SC40	Mastoid air cells
SC41	Styloid process
SC42	Mastoid process
C*1	Tubal elevation

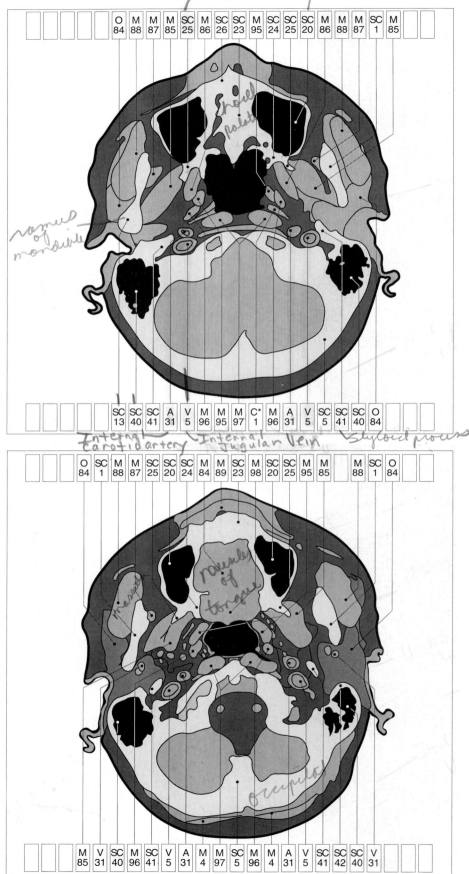

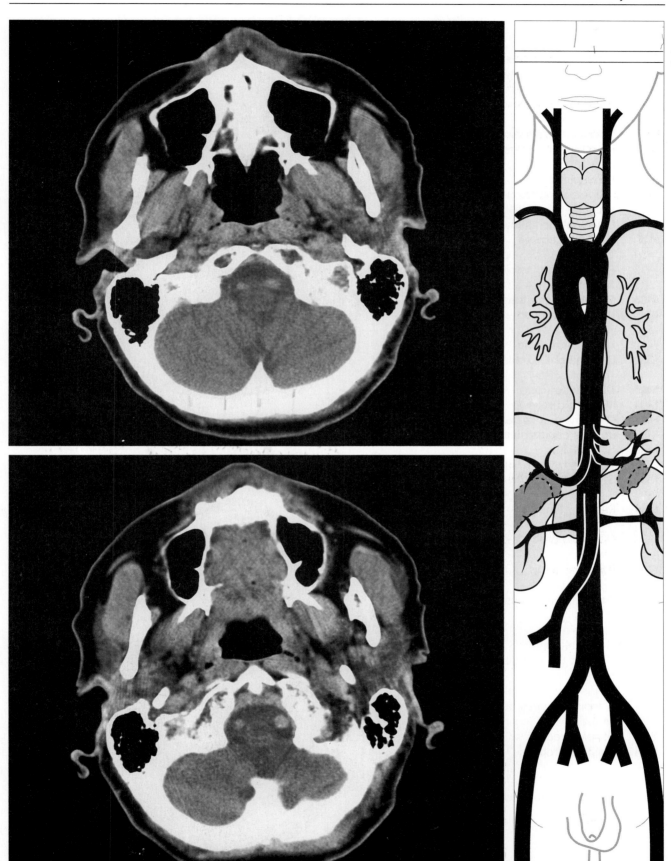

3/4

A8	Vertebral artery
A31	Internal carotid artery
A*33	Lingual artery (branches)
V5	Internal jugular vein
V31	Retromandibular vein
M3	Semispinalis capitis/Longissimus cervicis muscles
M4	Splenius capitis muscle
M5	Levator scapulae muscle
M17	Sternocleidomastoid muscle
M84	Muscles of the tongue
M85	Medial pterygoid muscle
M88	Masseter muscle
M89	Buccinator/Orbicularis oris muscles
M91	Digastric muscle
M92	Mylohyoid muscle
M93	Geniohyoid muscle
M97	Longus capitis muscle
M98	Soft palate
M*98	Uvula
M99	Stylohyoid muscle
O84	Parotid gland
S*1	Odontoid process of the axis
S11	Vertebral body
S14	Spinous process
S15	Transverse process
SC1	Mandible
SC5	Occipital bone
SC14	Body of the mandible
SC20	Maxillary sinus
SC24	Medial pterygoid plate
SC27	Alveolar process of the maxilla
SC41	Styloid process
SC42	Mastoid process
C*1	Tonsils
C*2	Vestibule of the mouth

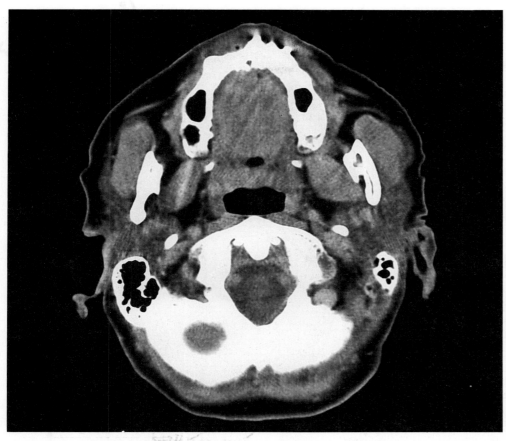

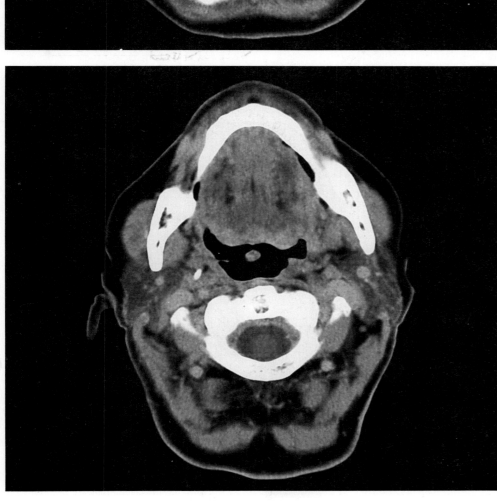

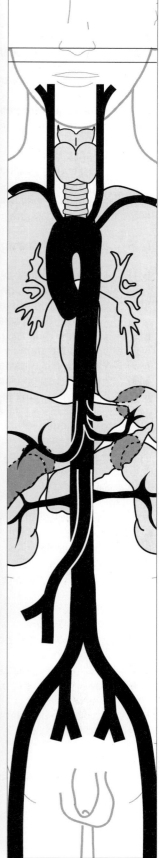

	5/6
A8	Vertebral artery
A31	Internal carotid artery
A33	Lingual artery
A*33	Lingual artery (branch)
V5	Internal jugular vein
V31	Retromandibular vein
M3	Semispinalis capitis/Longissimus cervicis muscles
M4	Splenius capitis muscle
M5	Levator scapulae muscle
M17	Sternocleidomastoid muscle
M18	Longus cervicis muscle
M84	Muscles of the tongue
M90	Superior constrictor muscle of the pharynx
M91	Digastric muscle
M92	Mylohyoid muscle
M93	Geniohyoid muscle
M97	Longus capitis muscle
M99	Stylohyoid muscle
O83	Submandibular gland
O84	Parotid gland
S11	Vertebral body
S14	Spinous process
SC14	Body of the mandible
C*1	Oropharynx

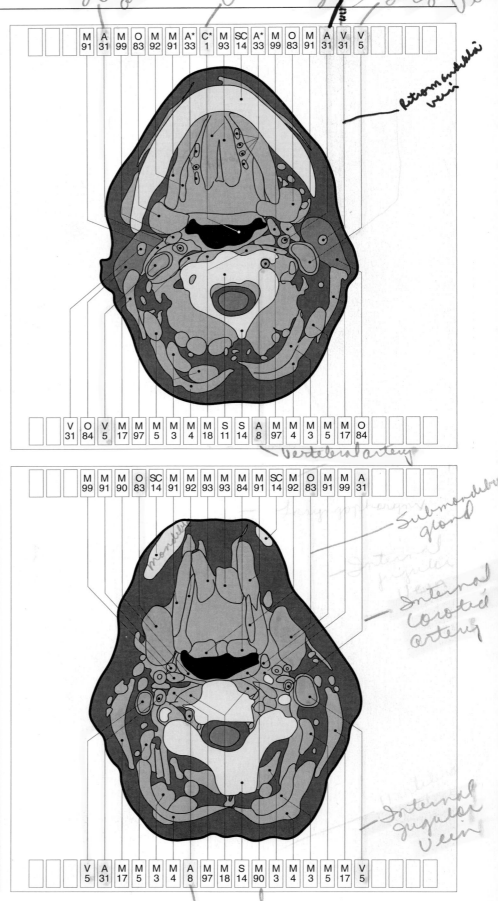

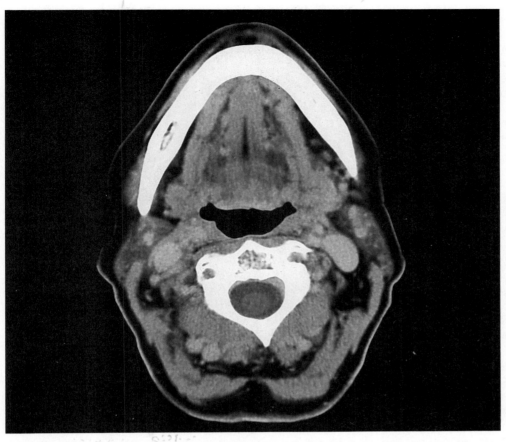

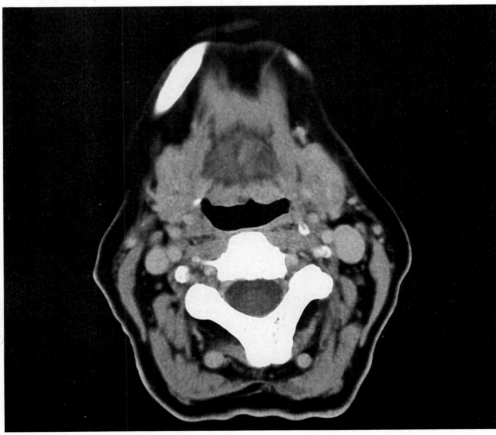

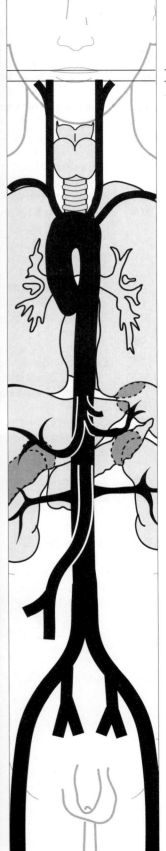

	7/8
A5	Common carotid artery
A8	Vertebral artery
A31	Internal carotid artery
A32	External carotid artery
V5	Internal jugular vein
V8	External jugular vein
V23	Deep cervical vein
M3	Semispinalis capitis/Longissimus cervicis muscles
M4	Splenius capitis muscle
M5	Levator scapulae muscle
M13	Scalenus anterior muscle
M14	Scalenus medius muscle
M17	Sternocleidomastoid muscle
M18	Longus cervicis muscle
M82	Sternothyroid muscle
M90	Superior constrictor muscle of the pharynx
M91	Digastric muscle
M93	Geniohyoid muscle
M97	Longus capitis muscle
M99	Stylohyoid muscle
O83	Submandibular gland
O91	Epiglottis
S11	Vertebral body
S14	Spinous process
SC6	Hyoid bone
SC61	Body of the hyoid bone
SC62	Greater cornu of the hyoid bone
SC63	Lesser cornu of the hyoid bone
C*1	Laryngopharynx

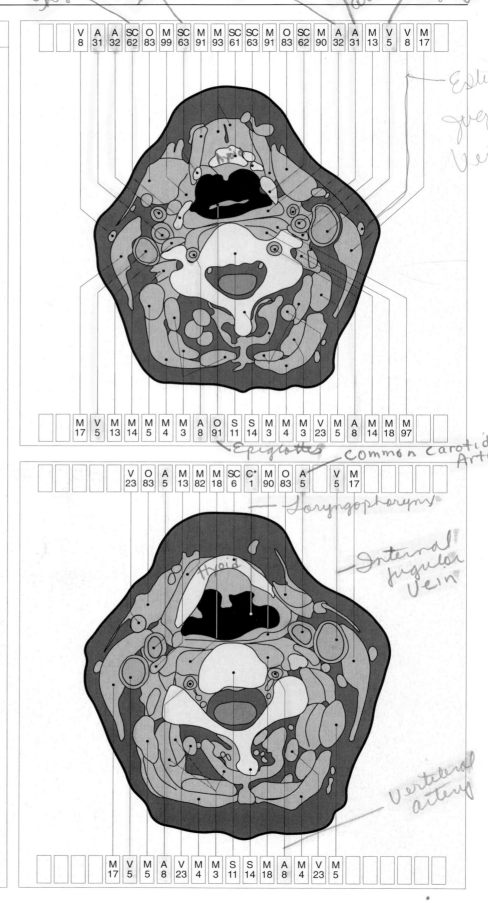

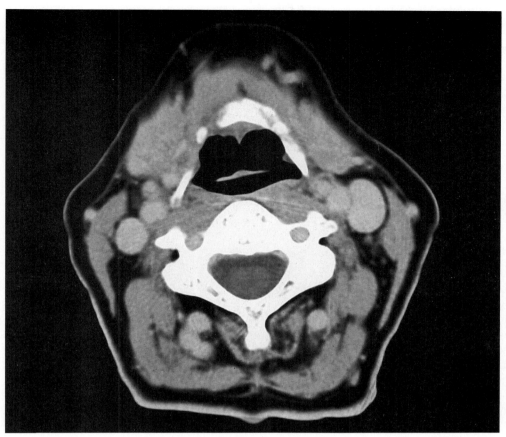

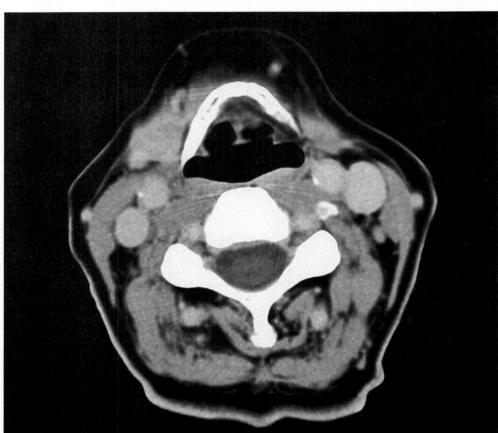

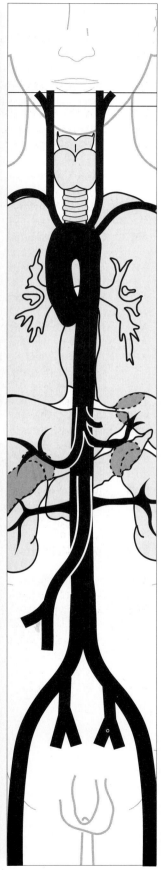

9/10

A5	Common carotid artery
A8	Vertebral artery
V5	Internal jugular vein
V8	External jugular vein
M1	Trapeziusa muscle
M3	Semispinalis capitis/Longissimus cervicis muscles
M4	Splenius capitis muscle
M5	Levator scapulae muscle
M13	Scalenus anterior muscle
M14	Scalenus medius muscle
M17	Sternocleidomastoid muscle
M18	Longus colli muscle
M82	Sternothyroid muscle
M90	Superior constrictor muscle of the pharynx
O9	Larynx
O92	Aryepiglottic fold
O96	Thyroid cartilage
O97	Superior cornu
S11	Vertebral body
S14	Spinous process
S15	Transverse process
S18	Vertebral canal
N11	Brachial plexus
C*1	Laryngopharynx

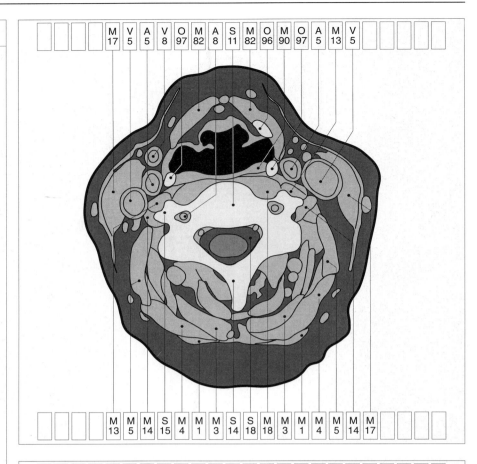

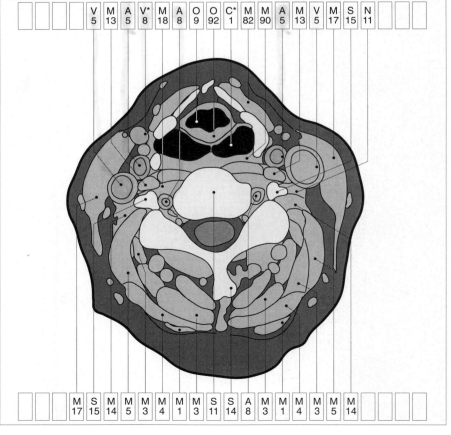

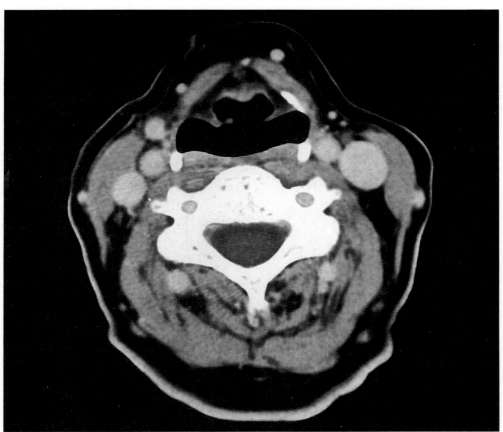

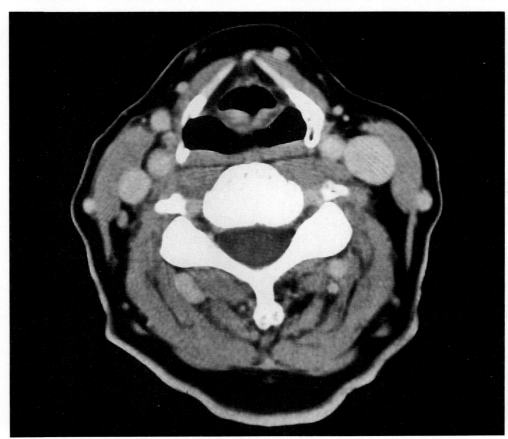

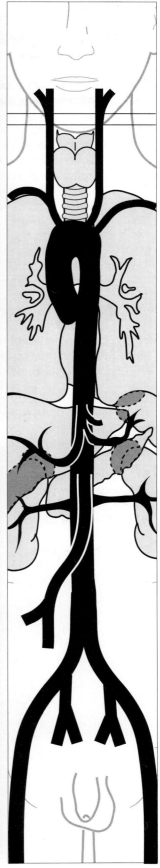

11/12

A5	Common carotid artery
A8	Vertebral artery
V5	Internal jugular vein
V8	External jugular vein
V23	Anterior jugular vein
M1	Trapezius muscle
M3	Semispinalis capitis/Longissimus cervicis muscles
M4	Splenius capitis muscle
M5	Levator scapulae muscle
M13	Scalenus anterior muscle
M14	Scalenus medius muscle
M17	Sternocleidomastoid muscle
M18	Longus cervicis muscle
M82	Sternothyroid muscle
M90	Superior constrictor muscle of the pharynx
O93	Arytenoid cartilage
O95	Vocal fold
O96	Thyroid cartilage
S11	Vertebral body
S14	Spinous process
N11	Brachial plexus
C*1	Piriform sinus

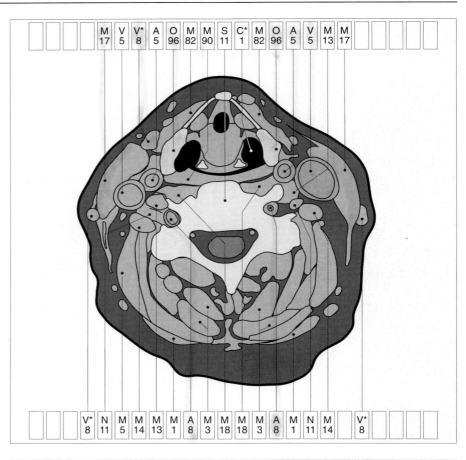

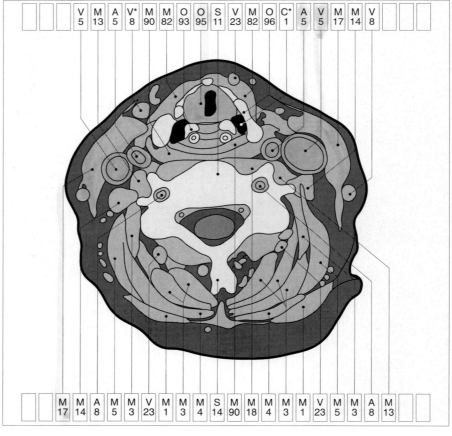

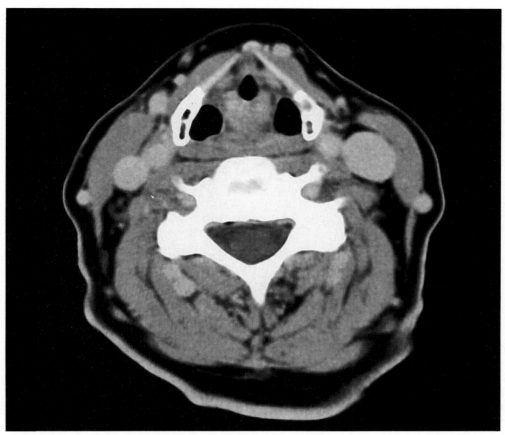

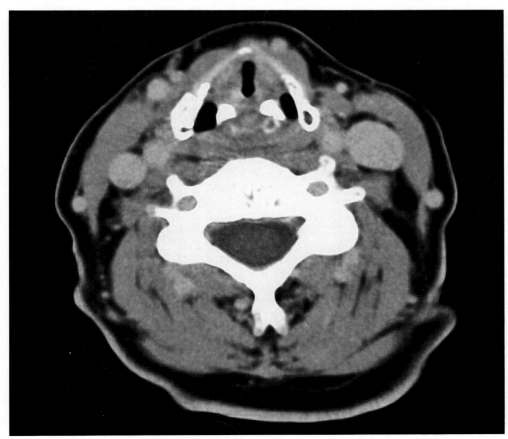

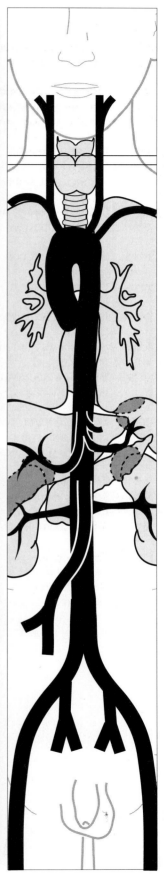

13/14

A5	Common carotid artery
A8	Vertebral artery
V5	Internal jugular vein
V8	External jugular vein
V23	Anterior jugular vein
M1	Trapezius muscle
M3	Semispinalis capitis/ Longissimus cervicis muscles
M4	Splenius capitis muscle
M5	Levator scapulae muscle
M13	Scalenus anterior muscle
M14	Scalenus medius muscle
M15	Scalenus posterior muscle
M16	Sternohyoid, omohyoid muscles
M17	Sternocleidomastoid muscle
M18	Longus cervicis muscle
M82	Sternothyroid muscle
M90	Superior constrictor muscle of the pharynx
O21	Trachea
O81	Thyroid gland
O98	Cricoid cartilage
O99	Inferior cornu
S11	Vertebral body
S14	Spinous process
S15	Transverse process
N11	Brachial plexus

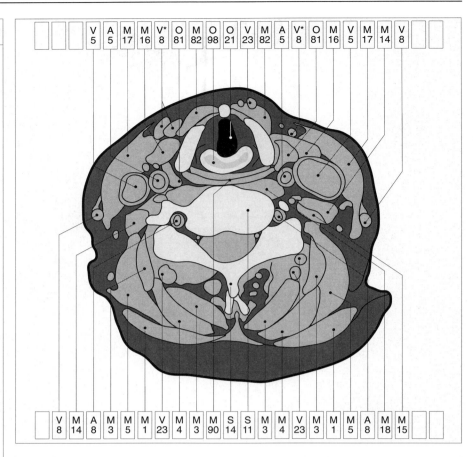

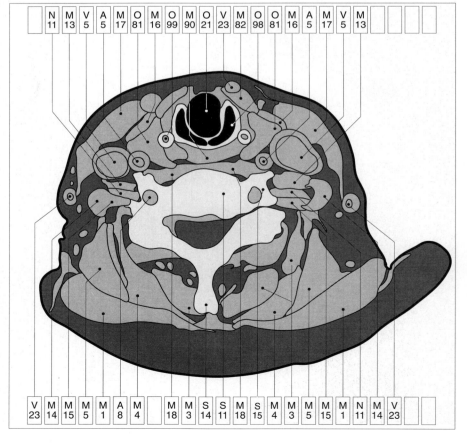

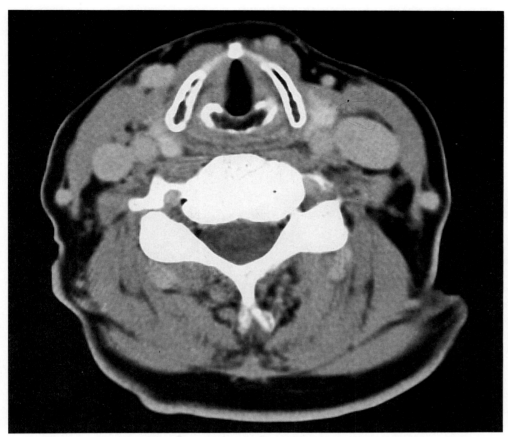

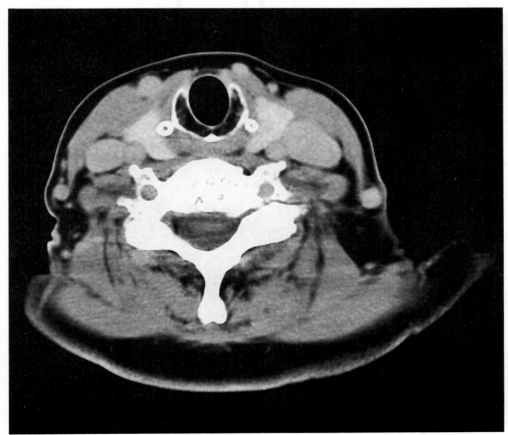

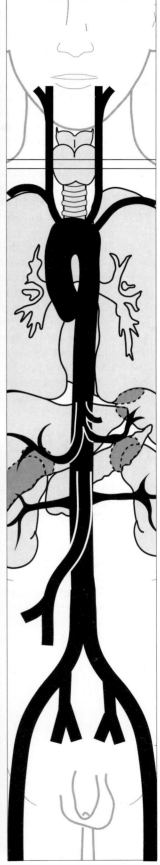

15/16

A4	Brachiocephalic trunk
A5	Common carotid artery
A6	Subclavian artery
A7	Axillary artery
V5	Internal jugular vein
V6	Subclavian vein ●
V7	Axillary vein
M1	Trapezius muscle
M2	Deltoid muscle
M4	Splenius capitis muscle
M5	Levator scapulae muscle
M7	Supraspinatus muscle
M8	Infraspinatus muscle
M9	Teres major muscle
M11	Subscapularis muscle
M12	Latissimus dorsi muscle
M19	Pectoralis major muscle
M20	Pectoralis minor muscle
M40	Obturator internus muscle
M55	Serratus posterior superior muscle
O2	Lung
O21	Trachea
O71	Esophagus
O81	Thyroid gland
S2	Rib (shaft)
S11	Vertebral body
S14	Spinous process
S15	Transverse process
S21	Head of the rib
S29	Clavicle
S31	Spine of the scapula
S32	Acromion
S33	Coracoid process
S71	Head of the humerus

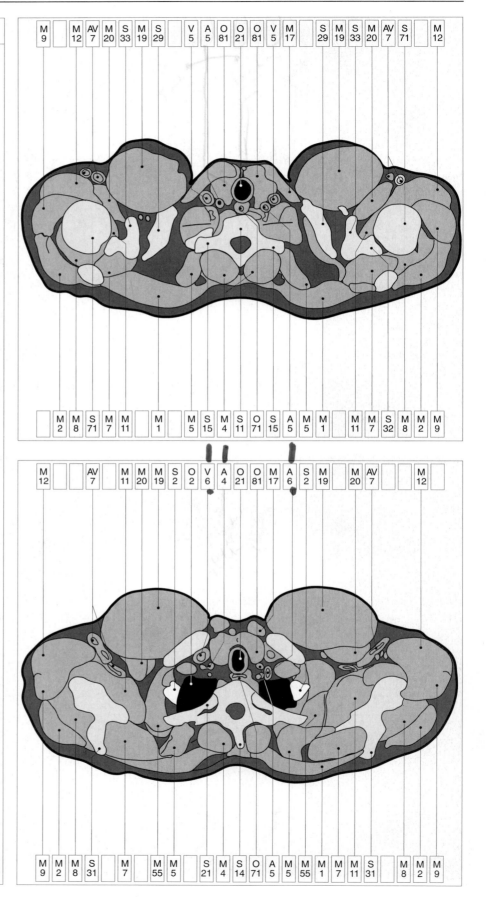

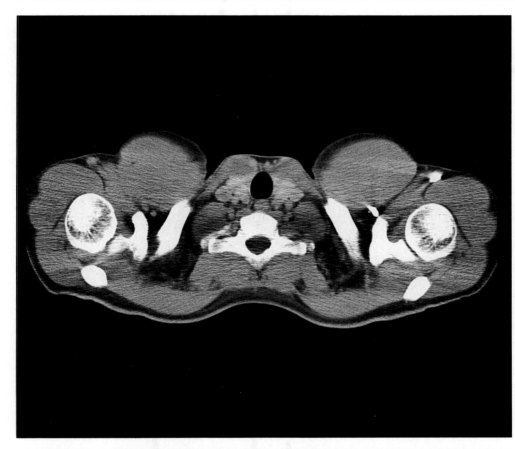

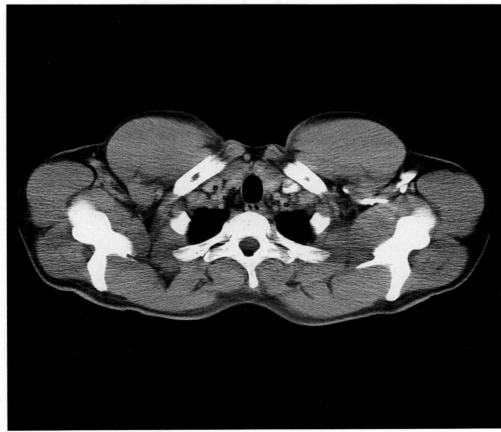

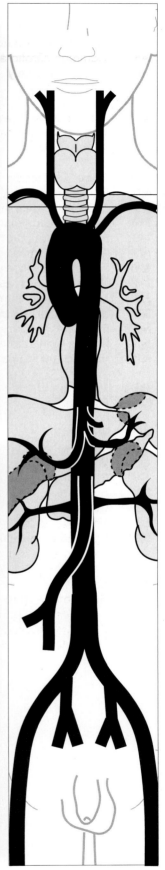

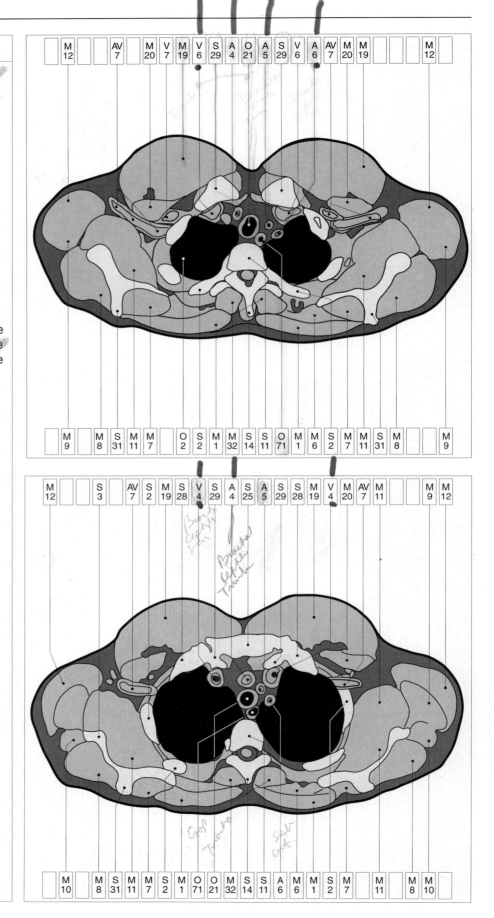

17/18

A4	Brachiocephalic trunk
A5	Common carotid artery
A6	Subclavian artery
A7	Axillary artery
V4	Brachiocephalic vein
V6	Subclavian vein
V7	Axillary vein
M1	Trapezius muscle
M6	Rhomboid (major, minor) muscles
M7	Supraspinatus muscle
M8	Infraspinatus muscle
M9	Teres major muscle
M10	Teres minor muscle
M11	Subscapularis muscle
M12	Latissimus dorsi muscle
M19	Pectoralis major muscle
M20	Pectoralis minor muscle
M32	Erector spinae muscle
M37	Gluteus medius muscle
O21	Trachea
O71	Esophagus
S2	Rib (shaft)
S3	Scapula
S11	Vertebral body
S14	Spinous process
S25	Sternum
S28	Costal cartilage
S29	Clavicle
S31	Spine of the scapula

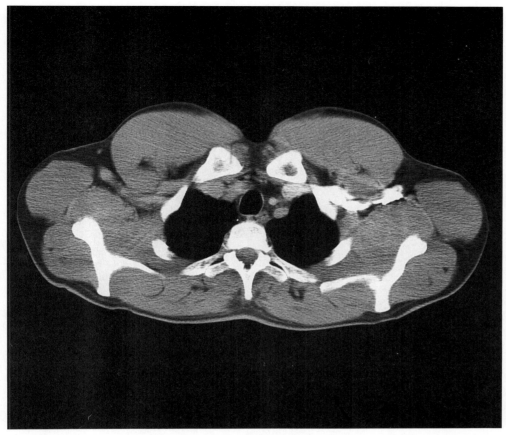

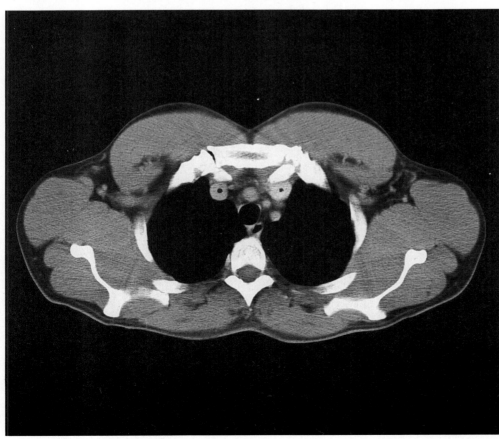

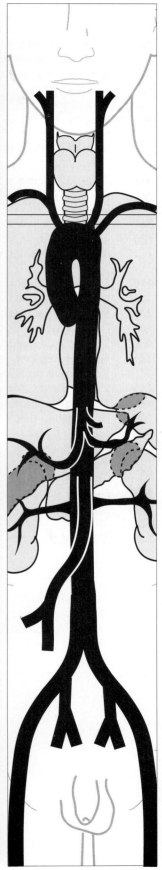

19/20

A1	Thoracic aorta
A3	Pulmonary artery
A4	Brachiocephalic trunk
A5	Common carotid artery
A6	Subclavian artery
A9	Internal thoracic artery
V1	Superior vena cava
V3	Pulmonary vein
V4	Brachiocephalic vein
V9	Internal thoracic vein
M1	Trapezius muscle
M3	Semispinalis capitis/ Longissimus cervicis muscles
M6	Rhomboid (major, minor) muscles
M8	Infraspinatus muscle
M9	Teres major muscle
M10	Teres minor muscle
M11	Subscapularis muscle
M12	Latissimus dorsi muscle
M19	Pectoralis major muscle
M20	Pectoralis minor muscle
M21	Intercostal muscles (internal, middle, external)
M22	Serratus anterior muscle
M32	Erector spinae muscle
O21	Trachea
O71	Esophagus
S2	Rib (shaft)
S3	Scapula
S11	Vertebral body
S14	Spinous process
S15	Transverse process
S21	Head of the rib
S25	Sternum
S28	Costal cartilage

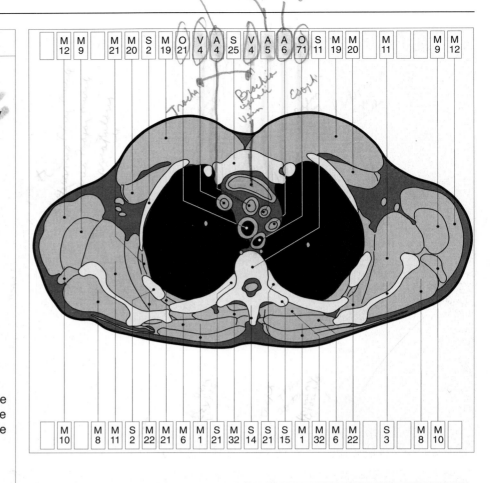

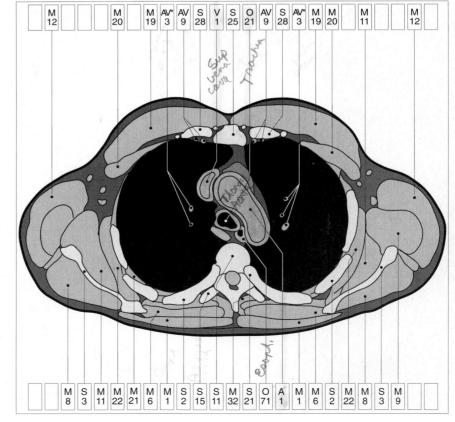

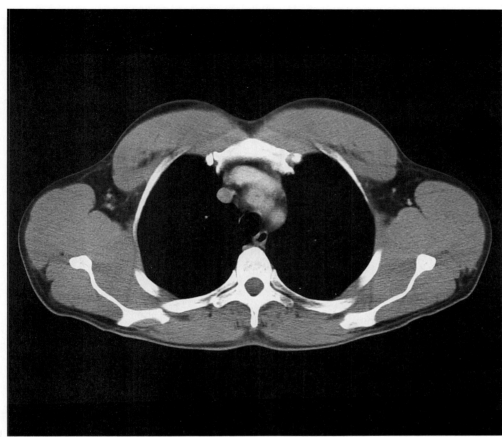

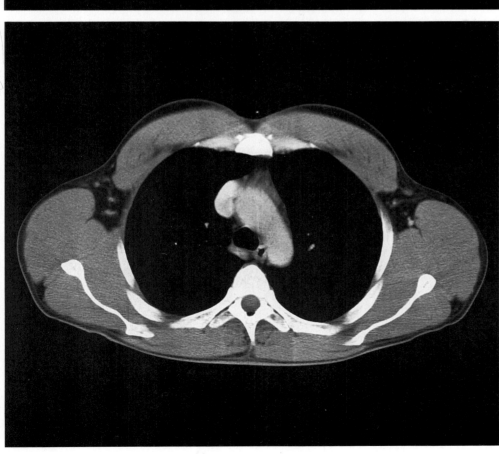

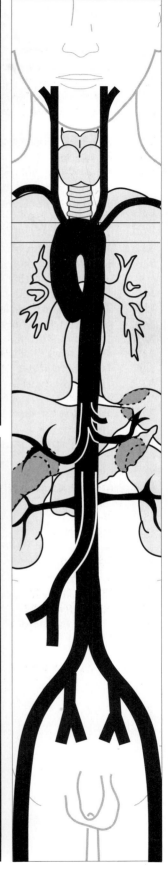

21/22

A1	Thoracic aorta
A2	Pulmonary trunk
A3	pulmonary artery
A*3	Branch of the pulmonary artery
A9	Internal thoracic artery
V1	Superior vena cava
V3	Pulmonary vein
V*3	Branch of a pulmonary vein
V9	Internal thoracic vein
V10	Azygos vein
M1	Trapezius muscle
M6	Rhomboid (major, minor) muscles
M8	Infraspinatus muscle
M9	Teres major muscle
M11	Subscapularis muscle
M12	Latissimus dorsi muscle
M19	Pectoralis major muscle
M21	Intercostal muscles (internal, middle, external)
M22	Serratus anterior muscle
M32	Erector spinae muscle
O22	Primary bronchus
O23	Lobar bronchus
O71	Esophagus
S2	Rib (shift)
S3	Scapula
S11	Vertebral body
S14	Spinous process
S*15	Costotransverse joint
S25	Sternum
S28	Costal cartilage

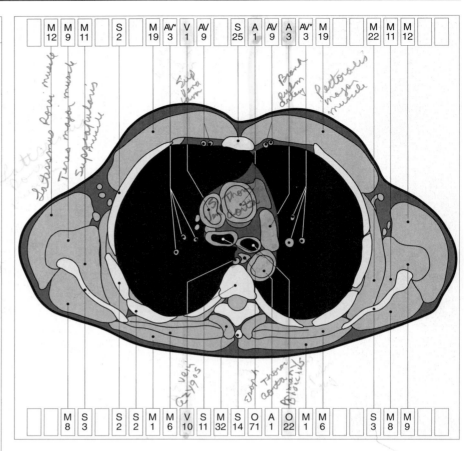

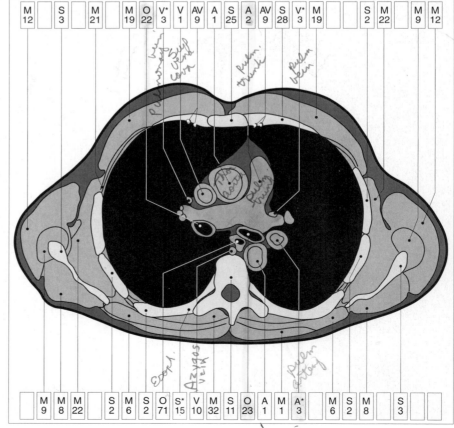

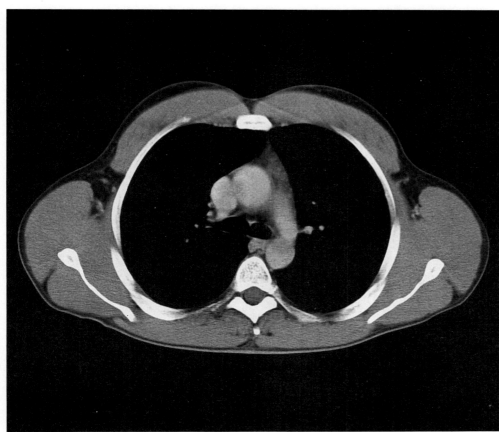

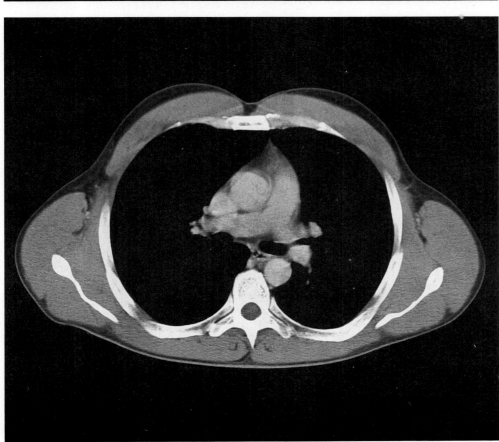

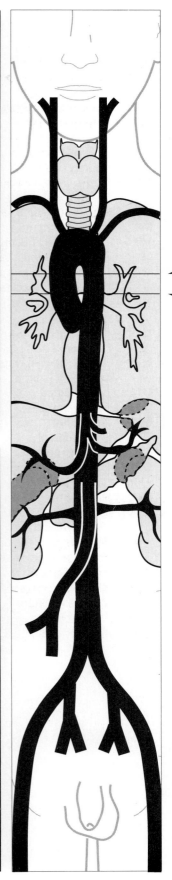

23/24

A1   Thoracic aorta
A3   Pulmonary artery
A9   Internal thoracic artery

V1   Superior vena cava
V3   Pulmonary vein
V9   Internal thoracic vein
V10   Azygos vein

M1   Trapezius muscle
M6   Rhomboid (major, minor) muscles
M8   Infraspinatus muscle
M9   Teres major muscle
M12   Latissimus dorsi muscle
M19   Pectoralis major muscle
M21   Intercostal muscles (internal, middle, external)
M22   Serratus anterior muscle
M32   Erector spinae muscle

O11   Left ventricle
O12   Right ventricle
O13   Left atrium
O14   Right atrium
O23   Lobar bronchus
O71   Esophagus

S2   Rib (shaft)
S3   Scapula
S11   Vertebral body
S14   Spinous process
S15   Transverse process
S21   Head of the rib
S25   Sternum
S28   Costal cartilage

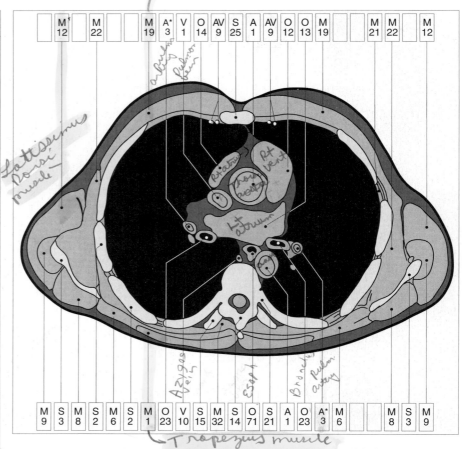

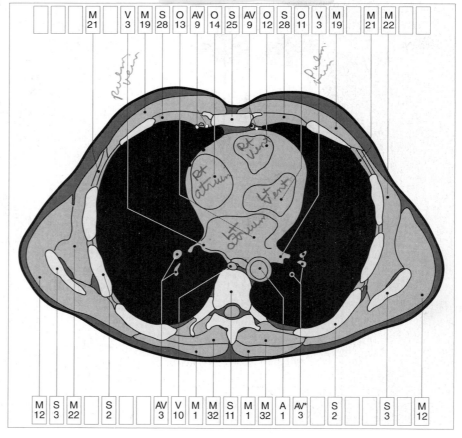

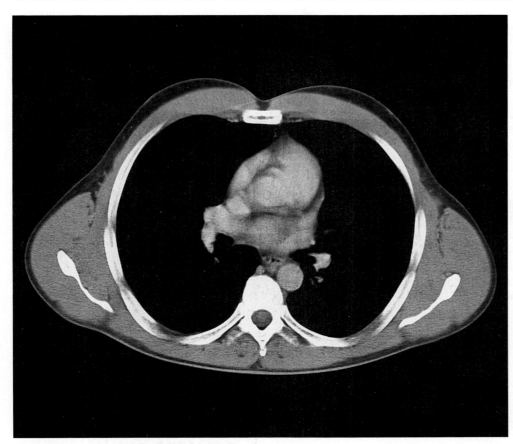

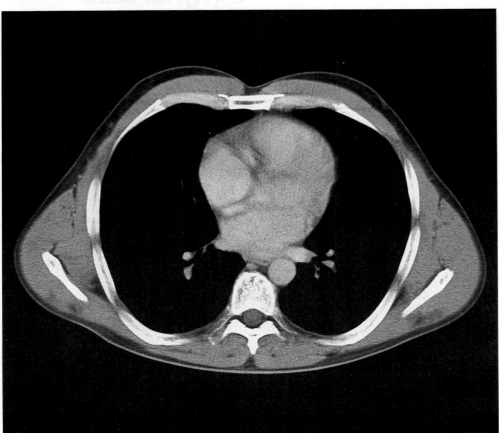

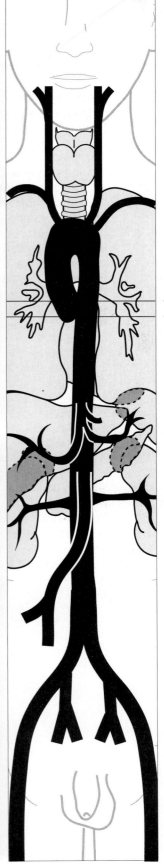

25/26

A1	Thoracic aorta
A3	Pulmonary artery
A9	Internal thoracic artery
V3	Pulmonary vein
V9	Internal thoracic vein
V10	Azygos vein
M1	Trapezius muscle
M12	Latissimus dorsi muscle
M19	Pectoralis major muscle
M21	Intercostal muscles (internal, middle, external)
M22	Serratus anterior muscle
M32	Erector spinae muscle
O11	Left ventricle
O12	Right ventricle
O13	Left atrium
O14	Right atrium
O15	Intraventricular septum
O71	Esophagus
S2	Rib (shaft)
S3	Scapula
S11	Vertebral body
S15	Transverse process
S25	Sternum
S28	Costal cartilage
N6	Phrenic nerve

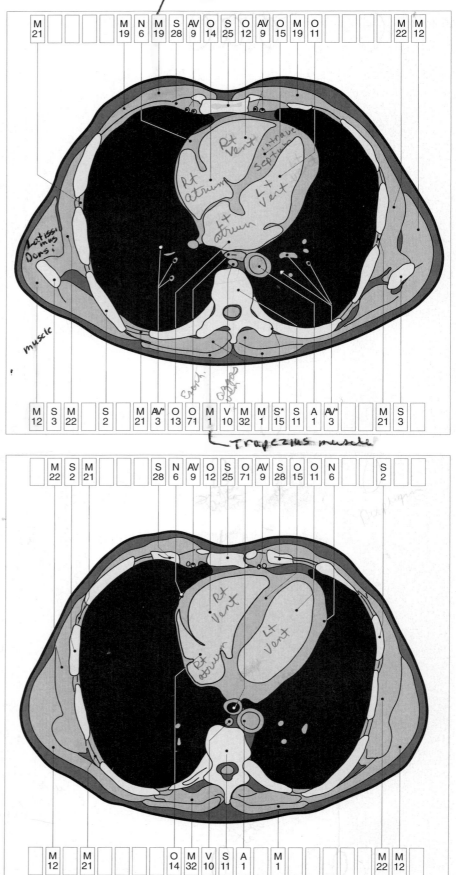

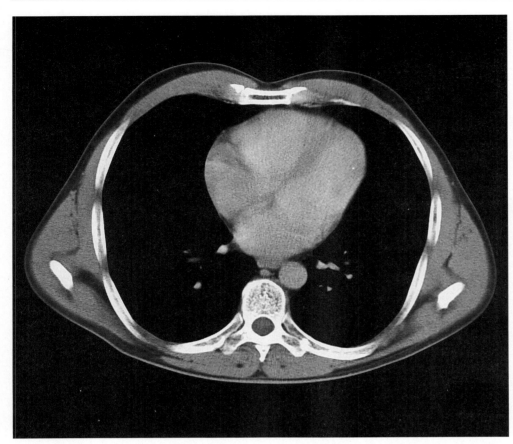

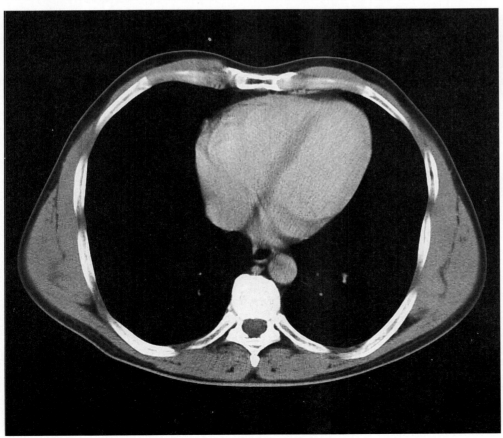

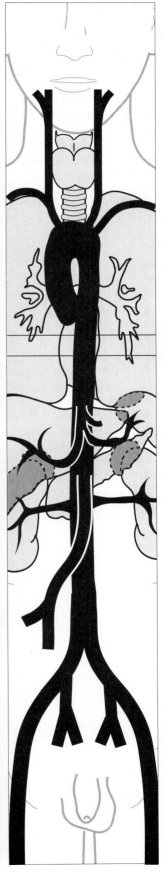

27/28

A1	Thoracic aorta
V1	Inferior vena cava
V10	Azygos vein
M1	Trapezius muscle
M12	Latissimus dorsi muscle
M21	Intercostal muscles (internal, middle, external)
M22	Serratus anterior muscle
M32	Erector spinae muscle
M51	Diaphragm
O3	Liver
O11	Left ventricle
O12	Right ventricle
O17	Coronary sinus
O26	Costophrenic recess
O45	Spleen
O71	Esophagus
O*71	Esophageal opening
O72	Stomach
S2	Rib (shaft)
S11	Vertebral body
S21	Head of the rib
S25	Sternum
S28	Costal cartilage

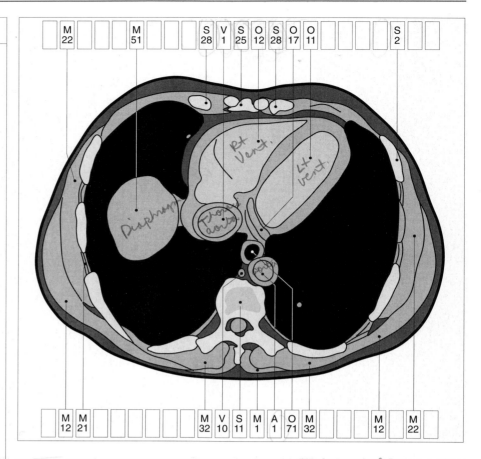

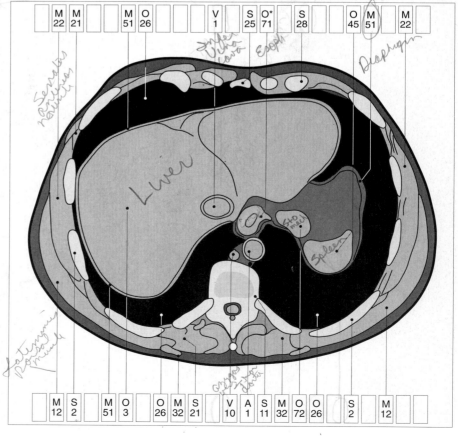

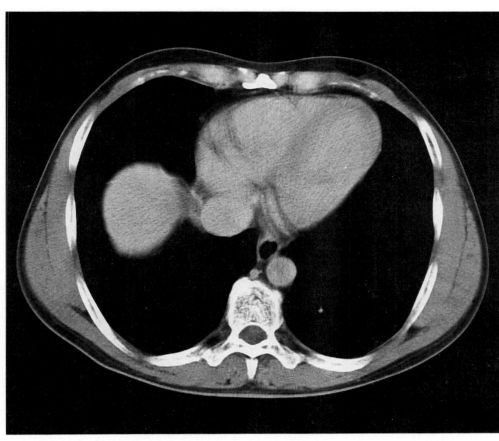

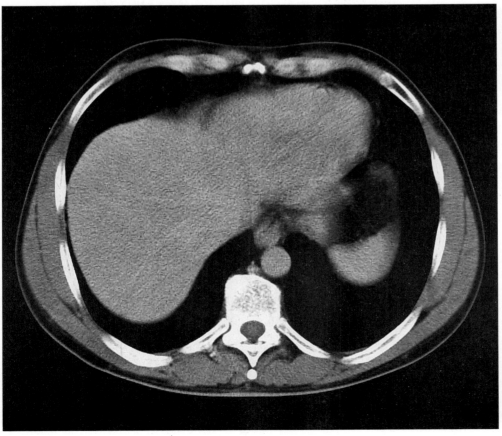

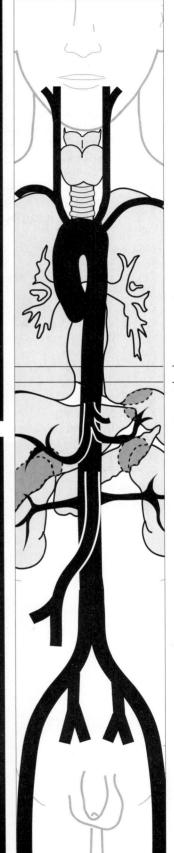

29/30

A1	Abdominal aorta
A12	Splenic artery
A13	Left gastric artery
V1	Inferior vena cava
V10	Azygos vein
V11	Inferior hemiazygos vein
V12	Splenic vein
V33	Hepatic vein
M12	Latissimus dorsi muscle
M21	Intercostal muscles (internal, middle, external)
M22	Serratus anterior muscle
M32	Erector spinae muscle
M51	Diaphragm
O3	Liver
O26	Costophrenic recess
O45	Spleen
O72	Stomach
S1	Vertebra
S2	Rib (shaft)
S14	Spinous process
S15	Transverse process

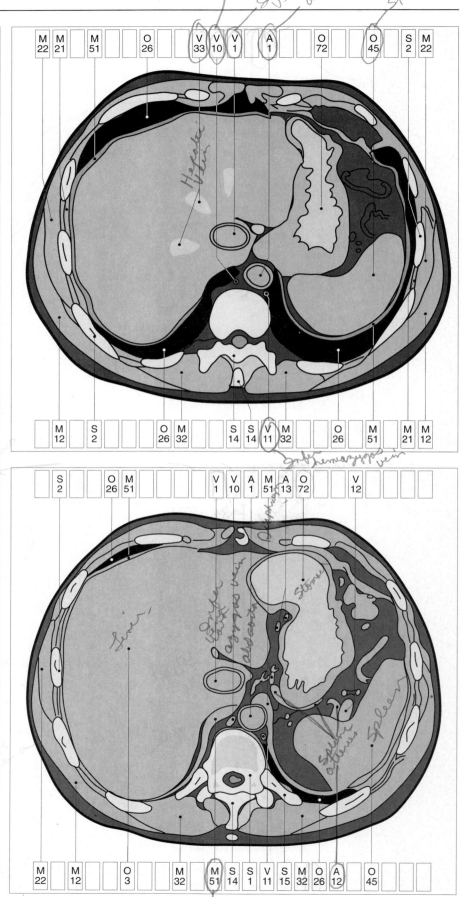

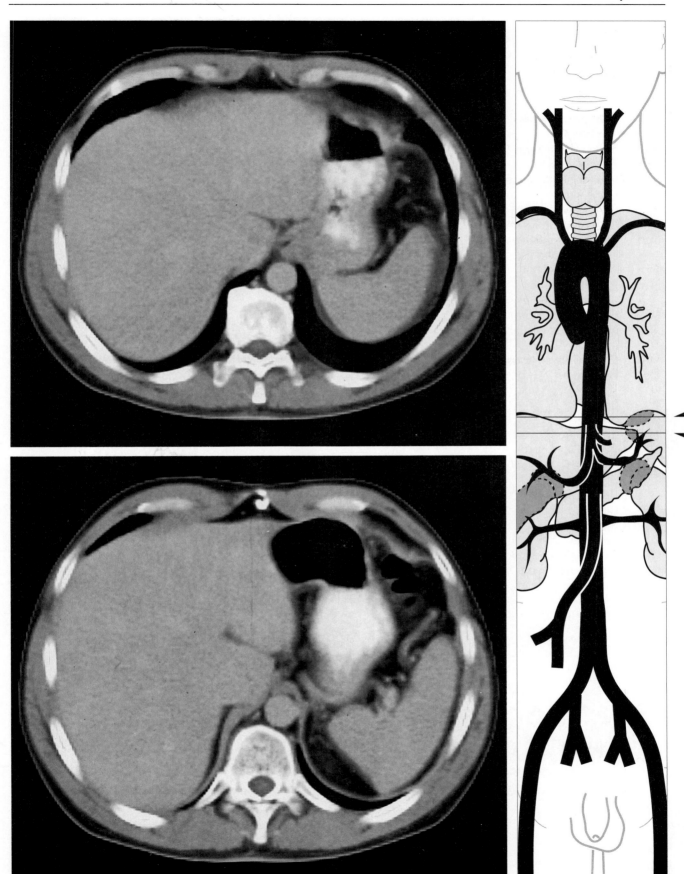

31/32

A1	Abdominal aorta
A10	Coeliac trunk
A11	Hepatic artery
A12	Splenic artery
A13	Left gastric artery
V1	Inferior vena cava
V10	Azygos vein
V11	Inferior hemiazygos vein
V13	Portal vein
M12	Latissimus dorsi muscle
M21	Intercostal muscles (internal, middle, external)
M24	Rectus abdominis muscle
M25	External oblique muscle
M27	Transversus abdominis muscle
M32	Erector spinae muscle
M51	Diaphragm
O3	Liver
O5	Kidney
O35	Ligamentum teres of the liver
O43	Pancreas
O45	Spleen
O54	Renal calyces
O55	Cortex, renal
O72	Stomach
O74	Jejunum
O77	Flexures of the colon
O82	Suprarenal gland
S1	Vertebra
S2	Rib (shaft)

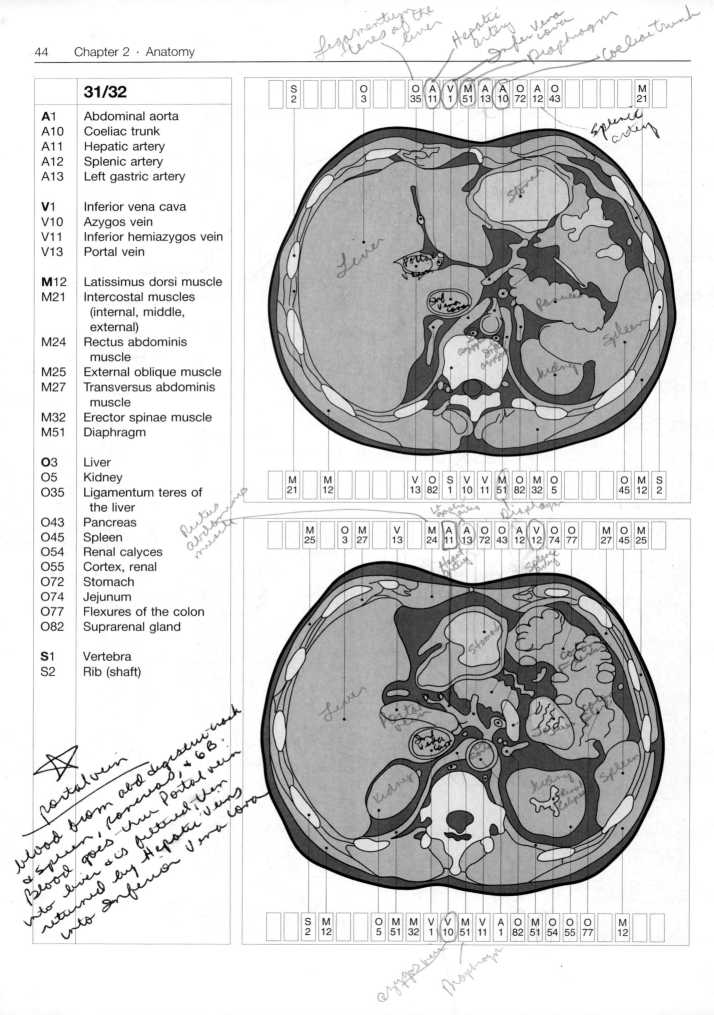

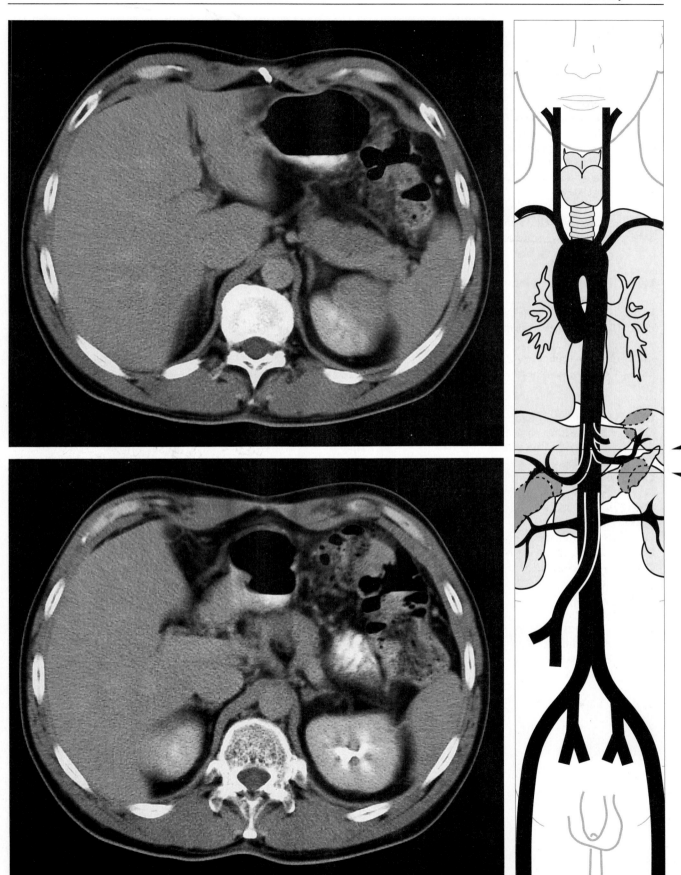

33/34

A1	Abdominal aorta
A14	Superior mesenteric artery
A15	Renal artery
V1	Inferior vena cava
V12	Splenic vein
V14	Superior mesenteric vein
V15	Renal vein
M12	Latissimus dorsi muscle
M21	Intercostal muscles (internal, middle, external)
M24	Rectus abdominis muscle
M25	External oblique muscle
M27	Transversus abdominis muscle
M29	Psoas muscle
M32	Erector spinae muscle
M51	Diaphragm
O31	Right lobe of liver
O37	Gallbladder
O41	Head of the pancreas
O42	Uncinate process
O43	Pancreas
O45	Spleen
O52	Renal sinus
O53	Renal pelvis
O54	Renal calyces
O55	Cortex, renal
O73	Duodenum
O74	Jejunum
O76	Colon
S1	Vertebra
S2	Rib (shaft)
S14	Spinous process
S27	Costal arch

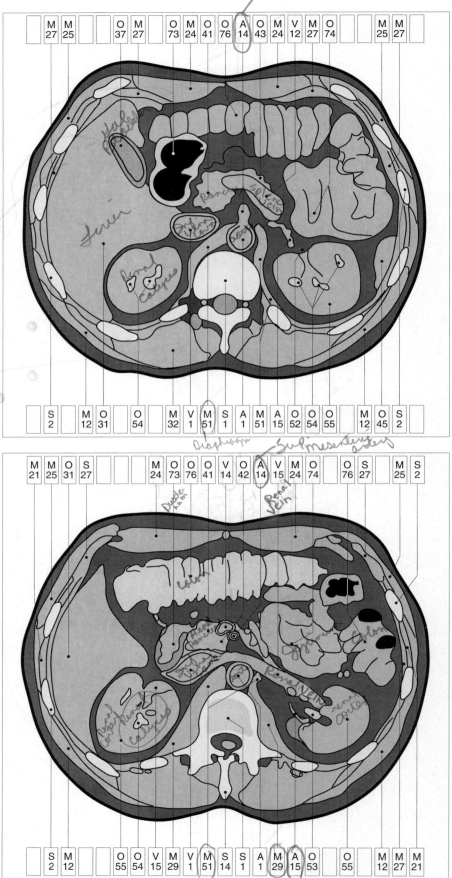

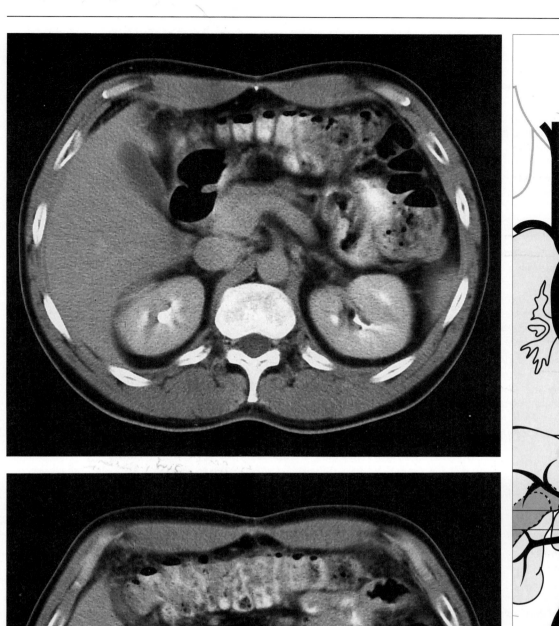

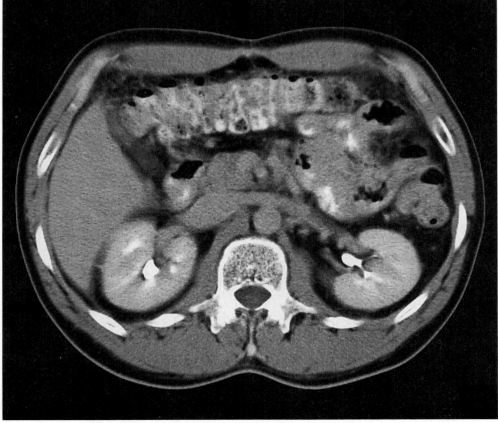

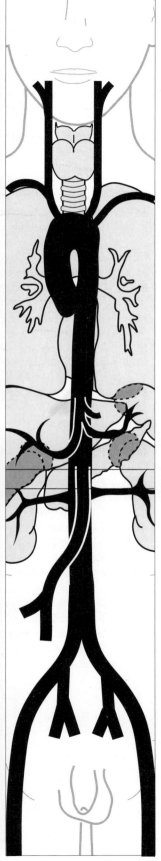

35/36

A1 Abdominal aorta
A14 Superior mesenteric artery
A15 Renal artery
A*14 Mesenteric vessels (branches)

V1 Inferior vena cava
V14 Superior mesenteric vein
V15 Renal vein

M12 Latissimus dorsi muscle
M24 Rectus abdominis muscle
M25 External oblique muscle
M26 Internal oblique muscle
M27 Transversus abdominis muscle
M28 Quadratus lumborum muscle
M29 Psoas muscle
M33 Iliocostalis lumborum muscle
M34 Longissimus dorsi muscle
M51 Diaphragm

O31 Right lobe of the liver
O42 Uncinate process
O53 Renal pelvis
O54 Renal calyces
O55 Cortex, renal
O73 Duodenum
O74 Jejunum
O76 Colon
O77 Flexures of the colon

S1 Vertebra
S2 Rib (shaft)
S14 Spinous process
S15 Transverse process
S27 Costal arch

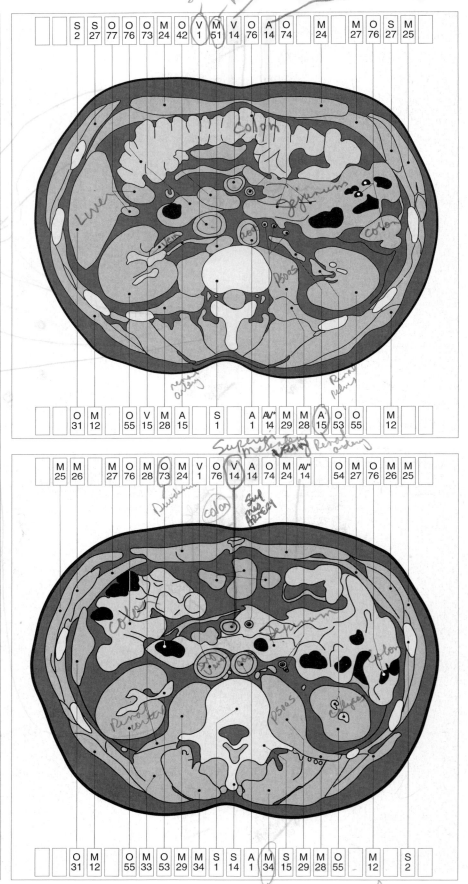

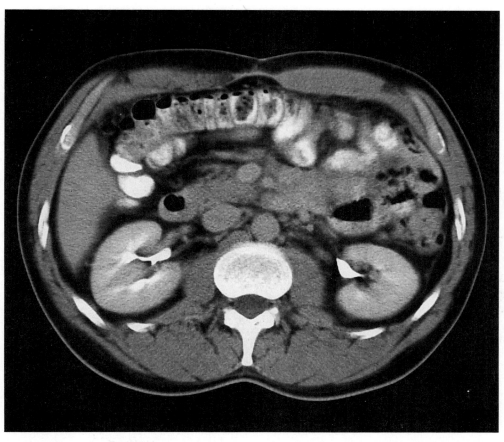

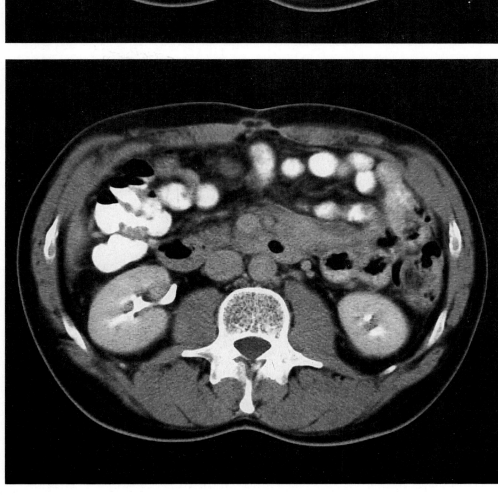

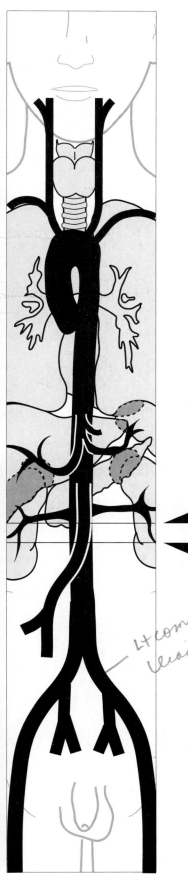

Lt commo
iliac

37/38

A1	Abdominal aorta
A14	Superior mesenteric artery
AV*14	Mesenteric vessels (branches)
V1	Inferior vena cava
V14	Superior mesenteric vein
M24	Rectus abdominis muscle
M25	External oblique muscle
M26	Internal oblique muscle
M27	Transversus abdominis muscle
M28	Quadratus lumborum muscle
M29	Psoas muscle
M33	Iliocostalis lumborum muscle
M34	Longissimus dorsi muscle
O54	Renal calyces
O55	Cortex, renal
O56	Ureter
O73	Duodenum
O74	Jejunum
O75	Ileum
O76	Colon
S1	Vertebra
S14	Spinous process
S15	Transverse process

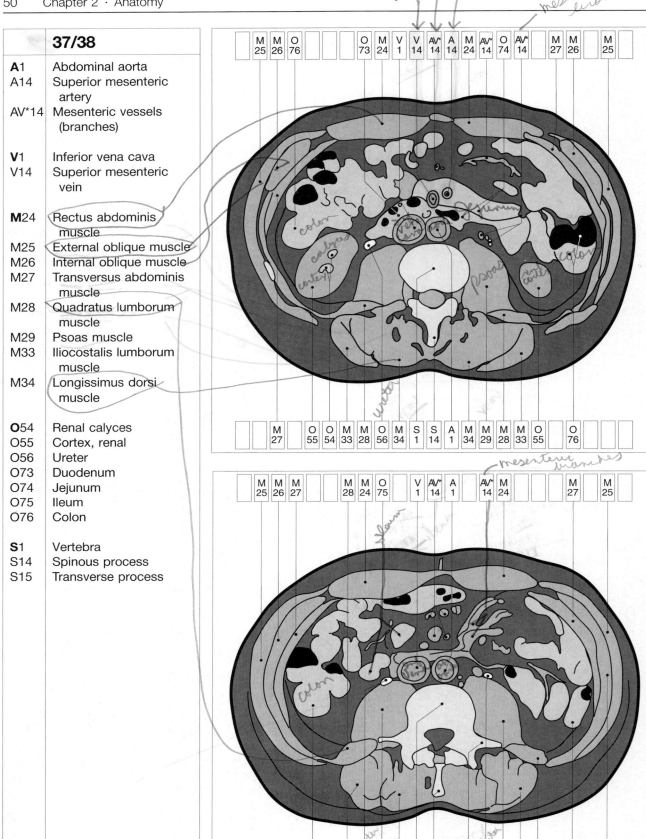

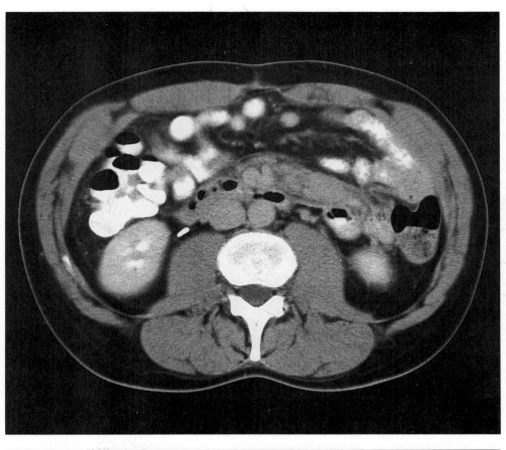

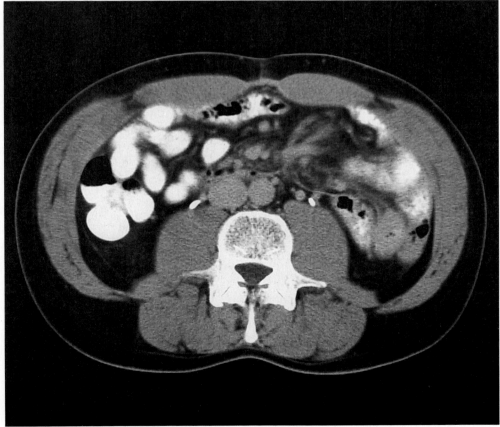

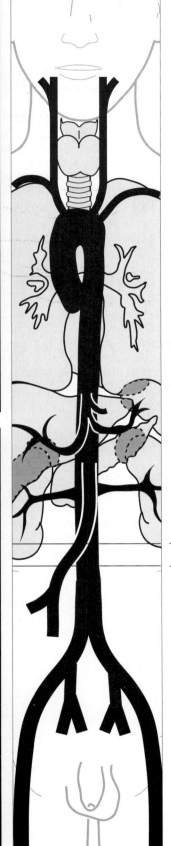

39/40	
A1	Abdominal aorta
AV*14	Mesenteric vessels (branches)
V1	Inferior vena cava
M24	Rectus abdominis muscle
M25	External oblique muscle
M26	Internal oblique muscle
M27	Transversus abdominis muscle
M28	Quadratus lumborum muscle
M29	Psoas muscle
M33	Iliocostalis lumborum muscle
M34	Longissimus dorsi muscle
O56	Ureter
O74	Jejunum
O75	Ileum
O*75	Ileocaecal valve
O76	Colon
S1	Vertebra
S14	Spinous process
S15	Transverse process

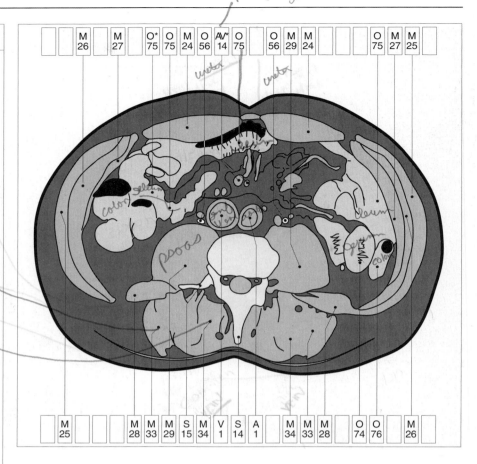

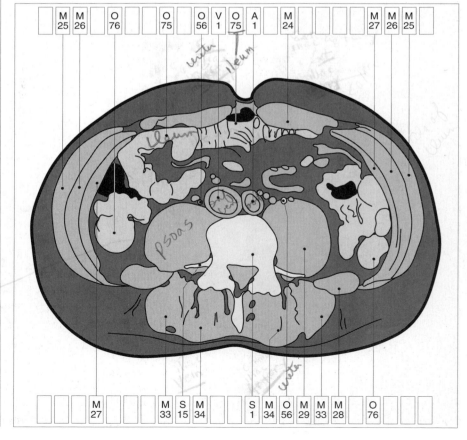

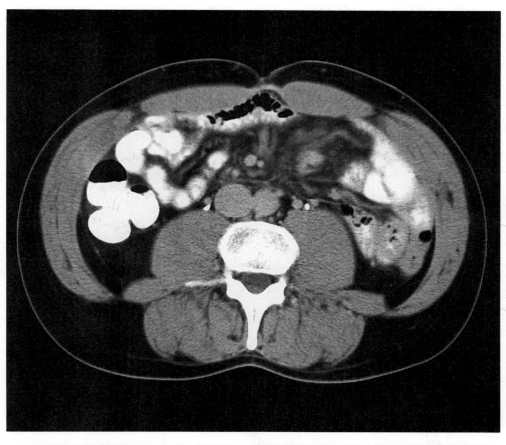

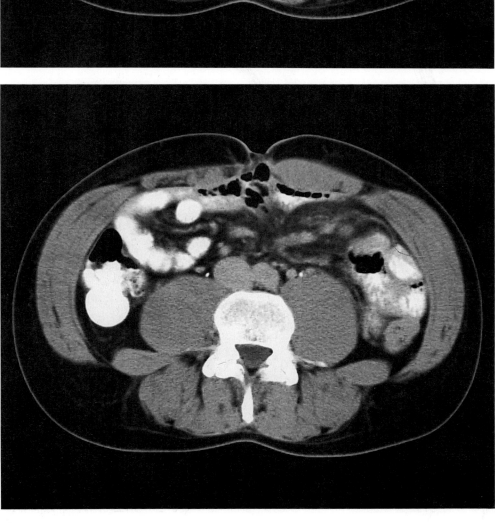

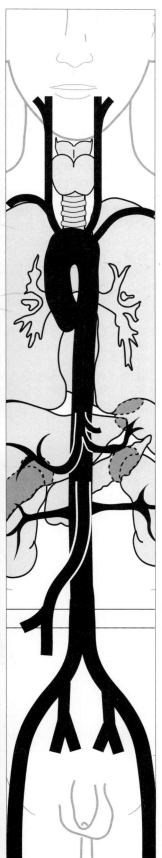

41/42

A18	Common iliac artery
V1	Inferior vena cava
V18	Common iliac vein
M24	Rectus abdominis muscle
M25	External oblique muscle
M26	Internal oblique muscle
M27	Transversus abdominis muscle
M28	Quadratus lumborum muscle
M29	Psoas muscle
M30	Iliacus muscle
M33	Iliocostalis lumborum muscle
M34	Longissimus dorsi muscle
M35	Multifidus muscle
M36	Gluteus maximus muscle
M37	Gluteus medius muscle
O75	Ileum
O76	Colon
S1	Vertebra
S14	Spinous muscle
S41	Ala of the ilium

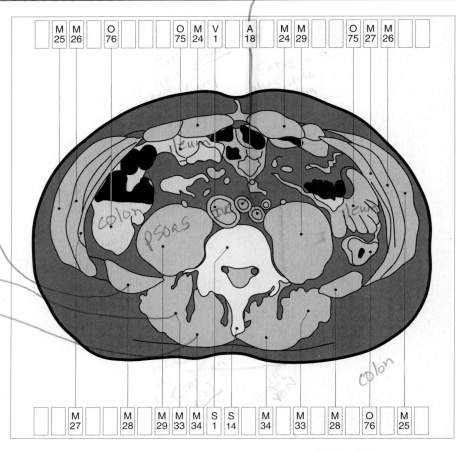

R & L Common Illiac Artery → Int. > Iliac arteris
Ext.

Int - supplies blood to pelvic organs

Ext - supplies blood to lower limb

-ower limb starts c̄ External iliac Artery & ends at veins of foot. Next artery is Common Femoral Artery, then it divides into femoral & deep femoral arteries. At the knee the popliteal artery begins. Then anterior Tibial artery, then Dorsalis Pedis artery for C & foot.

43/44	
A19	Internal iliac artery
A*19	Internal iliac artery (branch)
A20	External iliac artery
V18	Common iliac vein
V19	Internal iliac vein
V20	External iliac vein
M24	Rectus abdominis muscle
M26	Internal oblique muscle
M27	Transversus abdominis muscle
M29	Psoas muscle
M30	Iliacus muscle
M31	Iliopsoas muscle
M35	Multifidus muscle
M36	Gluteus maximus muscle
M37	Gluteus medius muscle
M38	Gluteus minimus muscle
O56	Ureter
O75	Ileum
O76	Colon
S41	Ala of the ilium
S61	Anterior sacral foramina
S62	Articular tubercle of the sacrum
S64	Promontory
S65	Sacroiliac joint

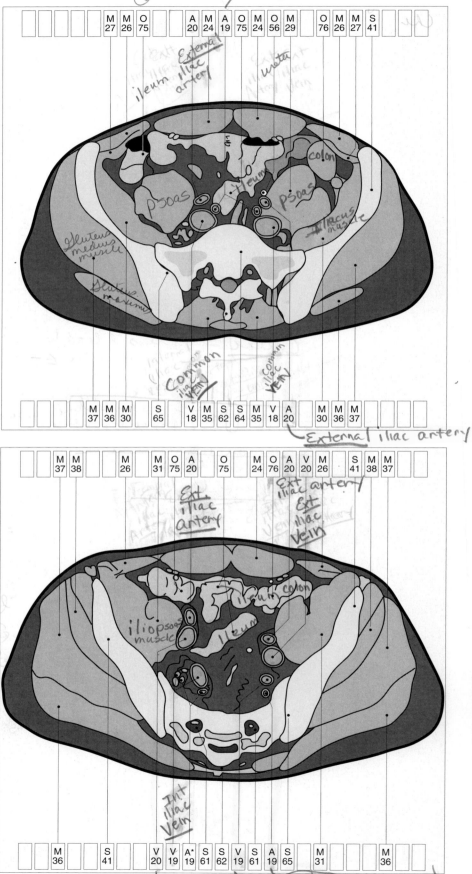

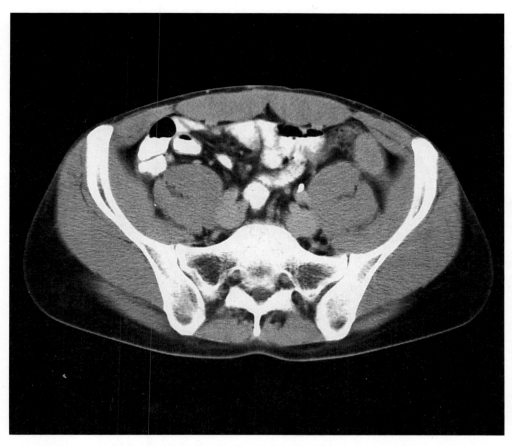

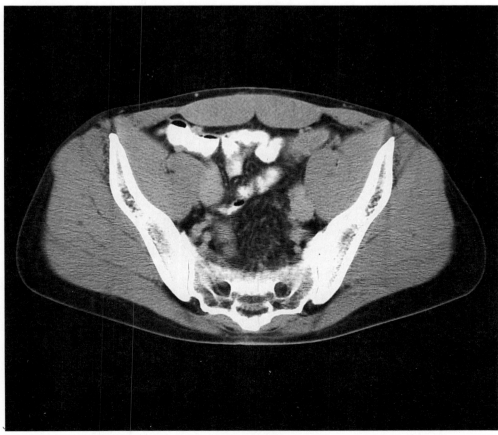

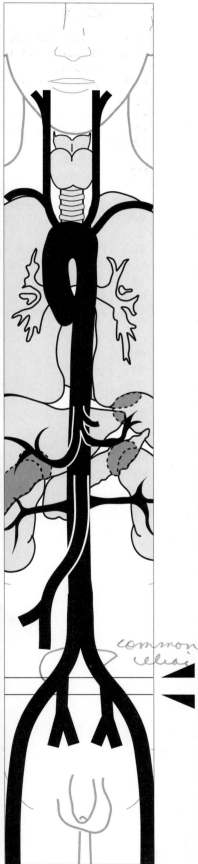

common
iliac

45/46

A19	Internal iliac artery
A20	External iliac artery
AV*19	Internal iliac vessels (branches)
V19	Internal iliac vein
V20	External iliac vein
M24	Rectus abdominis muscle
M26	Internal oblique muscle
M31	Iliopsoas muscle
M36	Gluteus maximus muscle
M37	Gluteus medius muscle
M38	Gluteus minimus muscle
M39	Piriformis muscle
M40	Obturator internus muscle
O56	Ureter
O75	Ileum
O78	Sigmoid colon
S6	Sacrum, coccyx
S41	Ala of the ilium
S42	Acetabulum
N1	Sciatic nerve

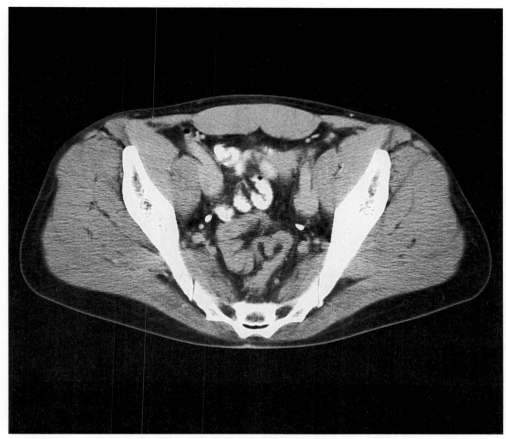

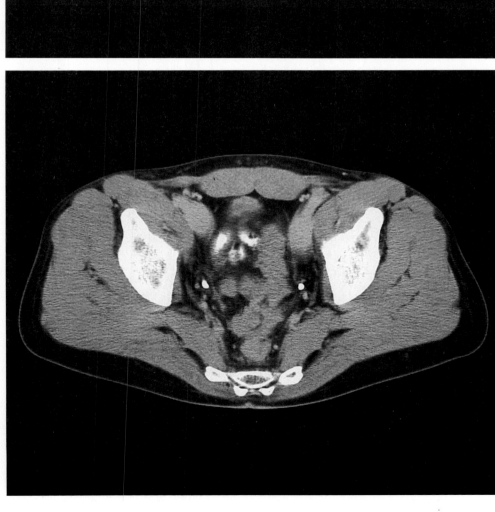

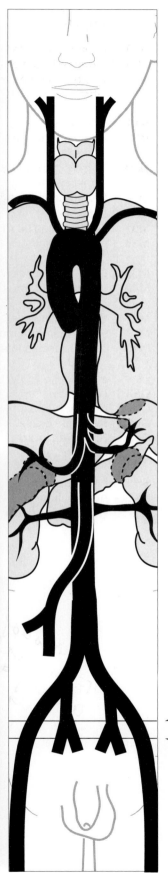

47/48

A20	External iliac artery
A21	Femoral artery
V20	External iliac vein
V21	Femoral vein
M24	Rectus abdominis muscle
M26	Internal oblique muscle
M31	Iliopsoas muscle
M36	Gluteus maximus muscle
M37	Gluteus medius muscle
M38	Gluteus minimus muscle
M39	Piriformis muscle
M40	Obturator internus muscle
M46	Sartorius muscle
M47	Rectus femoris muscle
M48	Tensor fasciae latae muscle
O56	Ureter
O57	Urinary bladder
O62	Seminal vesicle
O63	Spermatic cord
O79	Rectum
S6	Sacrum, coccyx
S42	Acetabulum
S51	Head of the femur
N1	Sciatic nerve

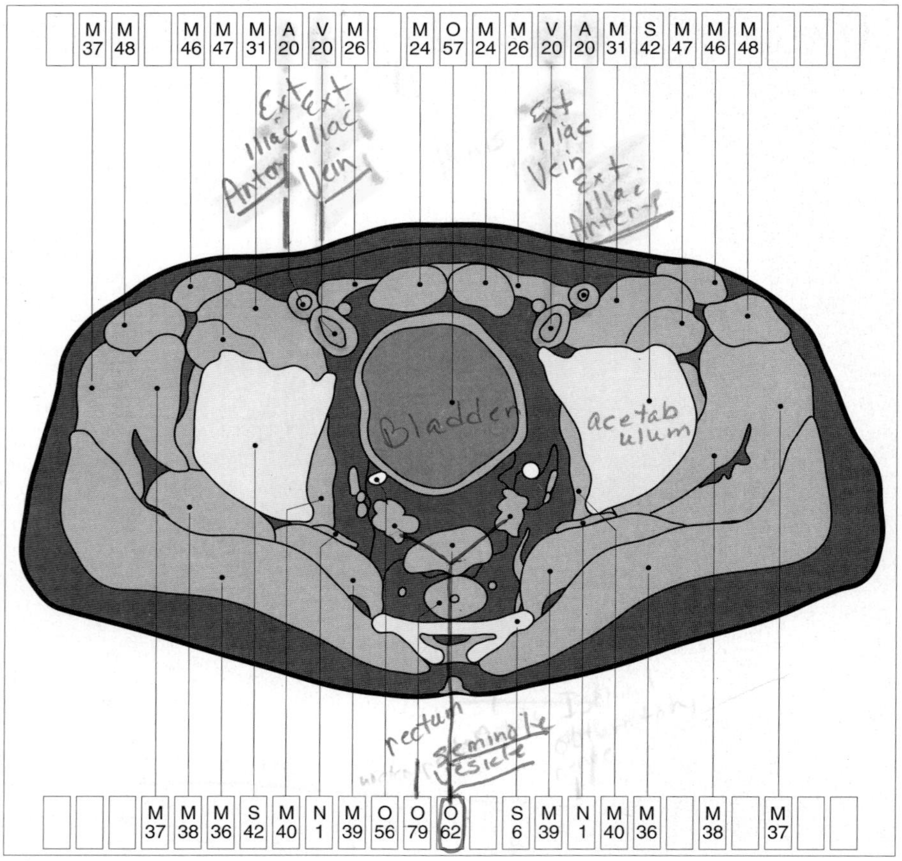

Top section box labels (top row): M37 M48 | M46 M47 M31 A20 V20 M26 | M24 O57 M24 M26 V20 A20 M31 S42 M47 M46 M48

Top section box labels (bottom row): M37 M38 M36 S42 M40 N1 M39 O56 O79 O62 | S6 M39 N1 M40 M36 M38 M37

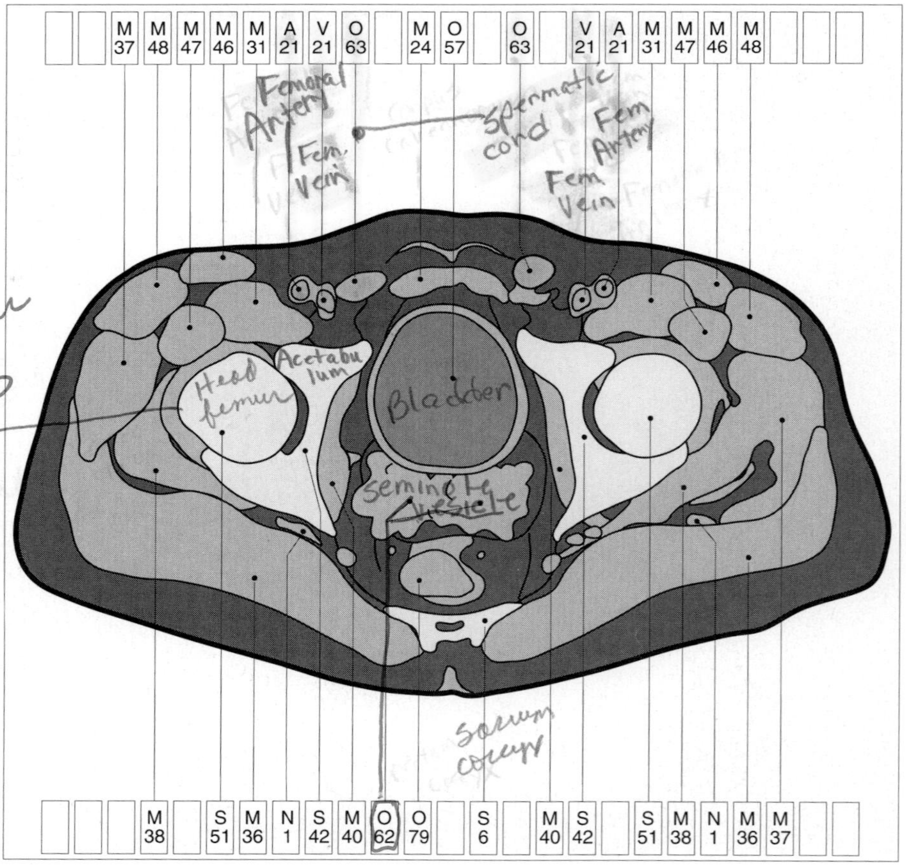

Handwritten annotations: Ext Iliac Artery, Ext Iliac Vein; Ext Iliac Vein, Ext Iliac Artery; Bladder; Acetabulum; rectum, seminal vesicle

Bottom section box labels (top row): M37 M48 M47 M46 M31 A21 V21 O63 | M24 O57 | O63 V21 A21 M31 M47 M46 M48

Bottom section box labels (bottom row): M38 | S51 M36 N1 S42 M40 O62 O79 | S6 | M40 S42 | S51 M38 N1 M36 M37

Handwritten annotations: Femoral Artery, Fem Vein; Spermatic cord, Fem Artery, Fem Vein; Head of femur, Femoral artery + vein starts; Head femur, Acetabulum; Bladder; seminal vesicle; Sacrum coccyx

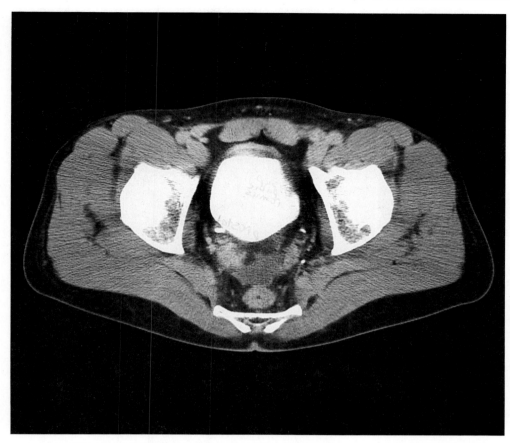

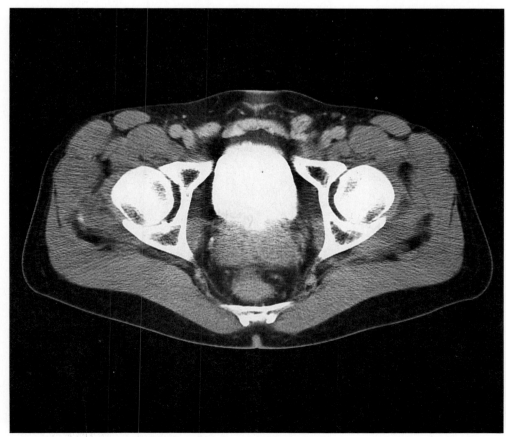

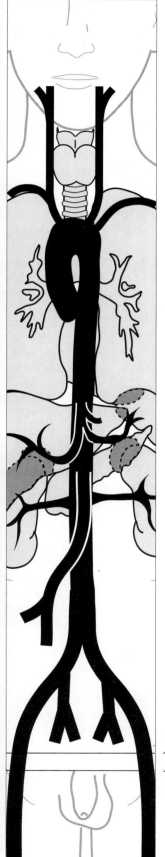

	49/50
A21	Femoral artery
A22	Pudendal artery
A23	Dorsal a. of the penis
A24	Obturator artery
V21	Femoral vein
V22	Pudendal vein
V24	Obturator vein
M31	Iliopsoas muscle
M36	Gluteus maximus muscle
M37	Gluteus medius muscle
M40	Obturator internus muscle
M41	Gemellus (superior, inferior) muscle
M42	Obturator externus muscle
M43	Pectineus muscle
M46	Sartorius muscle
M47	Rectus femoris muscle
M48	Tensor fasciae latae muscle
M49	Vastus lateralis muscle
M50	Levator ani muscle
O61	Prostate
O63	Spermatic cord (Vas deferens and vessels)
O64	Penis
O65	Corpus cavernorum
O79	Rectum
S44	Body of the ischium
S46	Public symphysis
S47	Superior pubic ramus
S48	Inferior pubic ramus
S51	Head of the femur
S53	Greater trochanter
S54	Hip joint
S55	Neck of the femur
S66	Coccyx
N3	Obturator nerve
N4	Femoral nerve

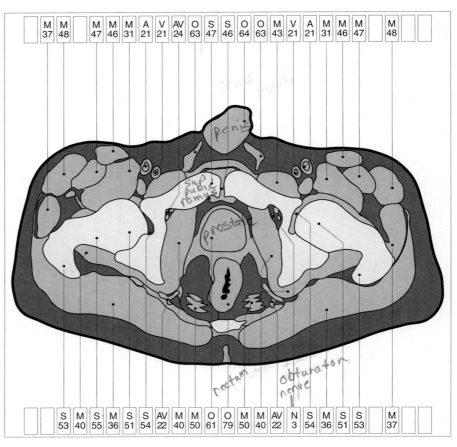

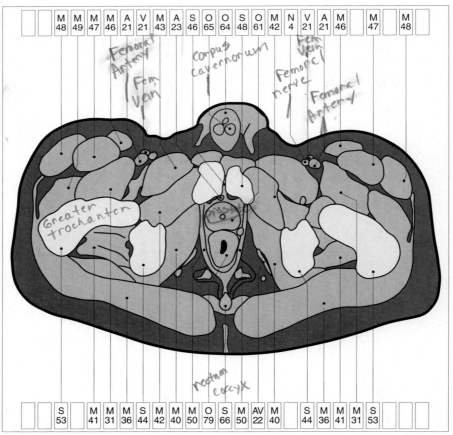

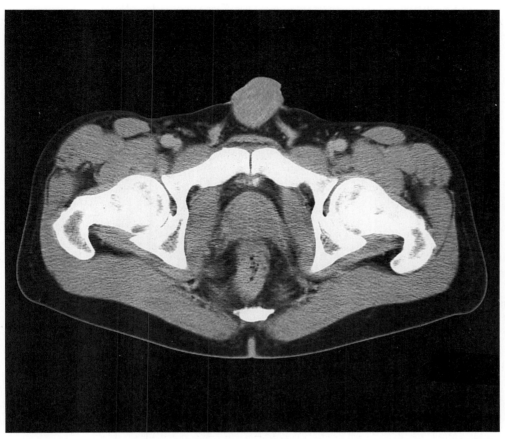

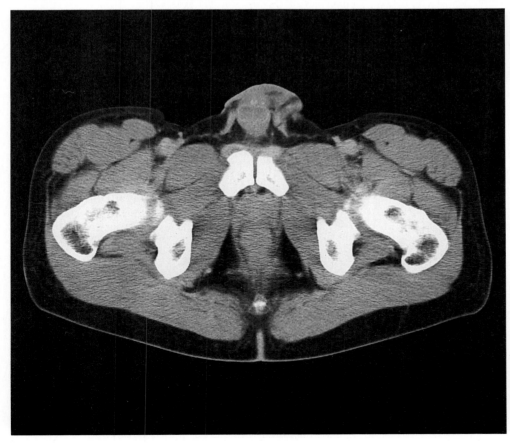

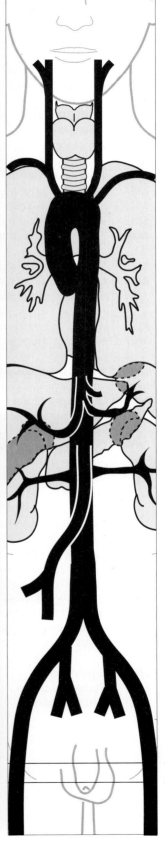

51/52

A22	Pudendal artery
V22	Pudendal vein
M31	Iliopsoas muscle
M36	Gluteus maximus muscle
M40	Obturator internus muscle
M42	Obturator externus muscle
M43	Pectineus muscle
M44	Adductor longus muscle
M46	Sartorius muscle
M47	Rectus femoris muscle
M48	Tensor fasciae latae muscle
M49	Vastus lateralis muscle
M50	Levator ani muscle
M54	Quadratus femoris muscle
M56	Adductor brevis muscle
M57	Adductor magnus muscle
M58	Ischiocavernosus muscle
M59	Bulbospongious muscle
M60	Sphincter ani externus muscle
M61	Superficial transversus perinei muscle
M*64	Semitendinosus muscle (tendon)
O61	Prostate
O64	Penis
O66	Testicle
S5	Femur
S43	Ischial tuberosity
S44	Body of the ischium
S48	Inferior pubic ramus
S56	Shaft of the femur
N1	Sciatic nerve
N2	Pudendal nerve
N4	Femoral nerve

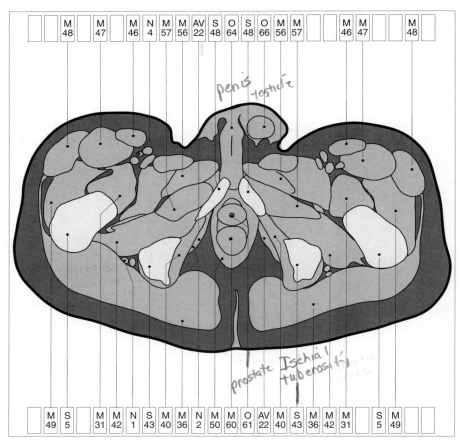

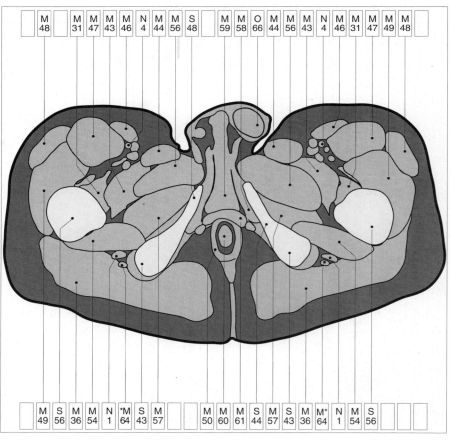

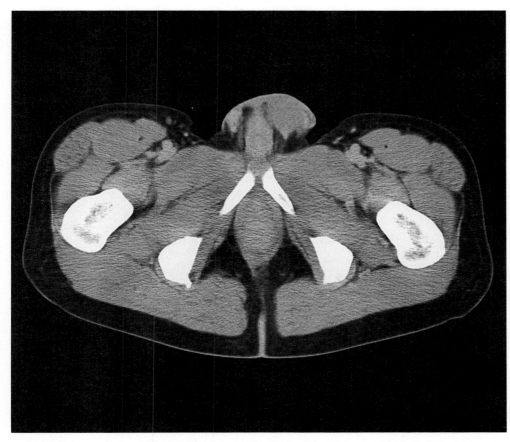

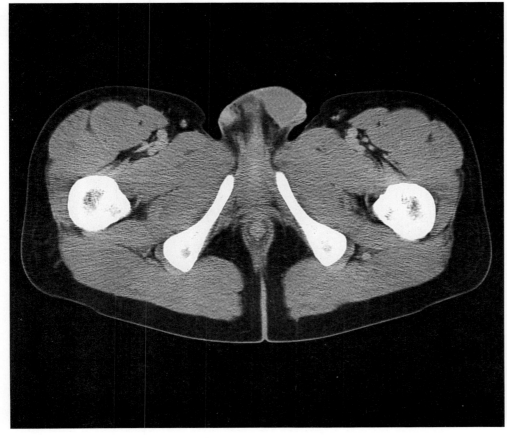

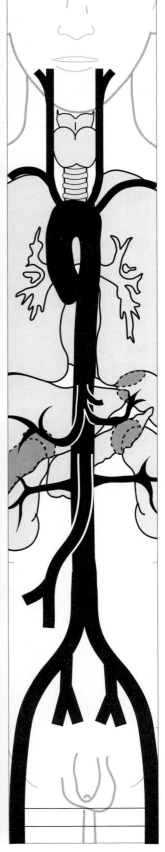

	53
M36	Gluteus maximus muscle
M43	Pectineus muscle
M44	Adductor longus muscle
M45	Gracilis muscle
M46	Sartorius muscle
M47	Rectus femoris muscle
M48	Tensor fasciae latae muscle
M49	Vastus lateralis muscle
M54	Quadratus femoris muscle
M56	Adductor brevis muscle
M57	Adductor magnus muscle
M62	Vastus intermedius muscle
M*64	Semitendinosus muscle (tendon)
M*65	Semimembranosus muscle (tendon)
O67	Scrotum
S43	Ischial tuberosity
S56	Shaft of the femur
N1	Sciatic nerve
N4	Femoral nerve

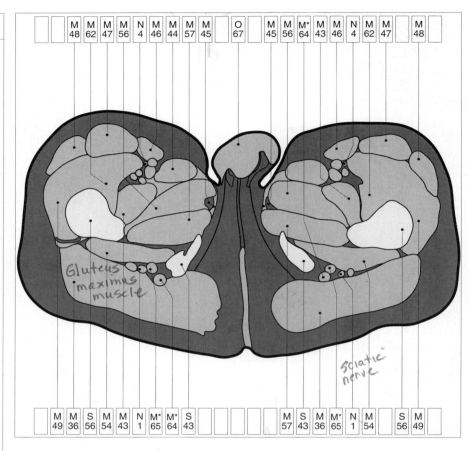

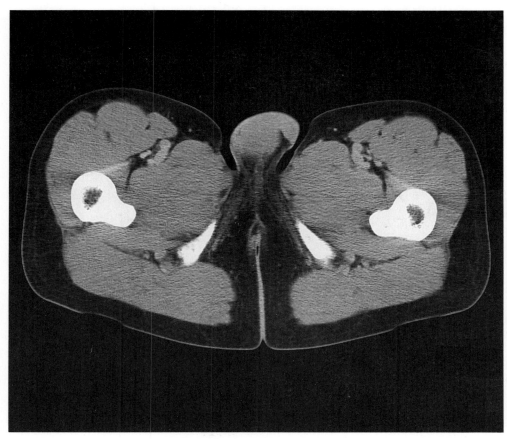

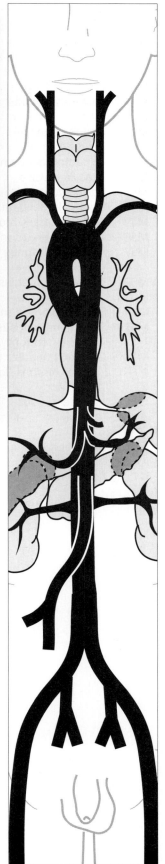

60/61

A21	Femoral artery
A25	Profunda femoris artery
V21	Femoral vein
V25	Profunda femoris
M36	Gluteus maximus muscle
M44	Adductor longus muscle
M45	Gracilis muscle
M46	Sartorius muscle
M47	Rectus femoris muscle
M49	Vastus lateralis muscle
M56	Adductor brevis muscle
M57	Adductor magnus muscle
M62	Vastus intermedius muscle
M64	Semitendinosus muscle
M*65	Semimembranosus muscle (tendon)
M*67	Common head of the biceps femoris (long head) and semitendinous muscles
S56	Shaft of the femur
N1	Sciatic nerve

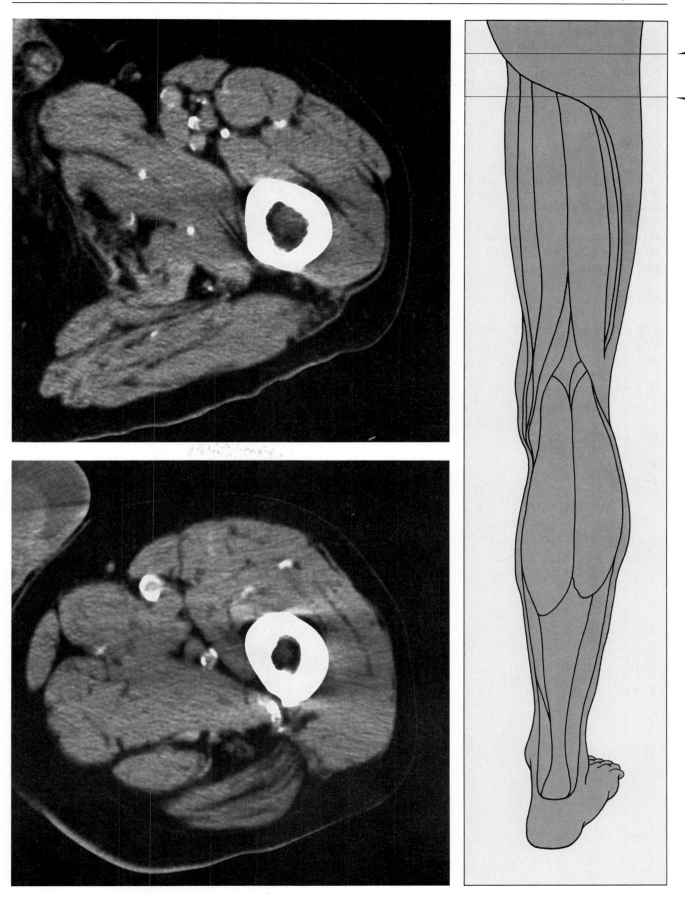

62/63

A21	Femoral artery
A25	Profunda femoris artery
A*25	Ramus of the profunda femoris artery
V21	Femoral vein
V25	Profunda femoris vein
V34	Great saphenous vein
M44	Adductor longus muscle
M45	Gracilis muscle
M46	Sartorius muscle
M47	Rectus femoris muscle
M49	Vastus lateralis muscle
M57	Adductor magnus muscle
M62	Vastus intermedius muscle
M63	Vastus medialis muscle
M64	Semitendinosus muscle
M65	Semimembranosus muscle
M67	Long head of the biceps femoris muscle
S56	Shaft of the femur
N1	Sciatic nerve

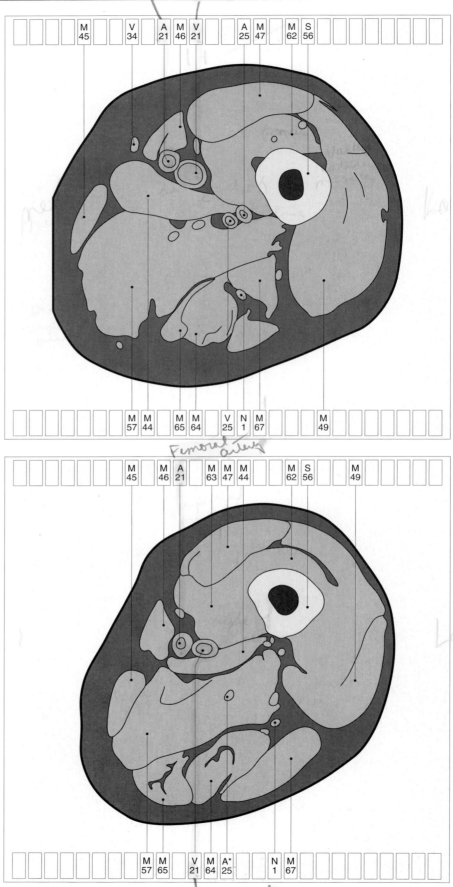

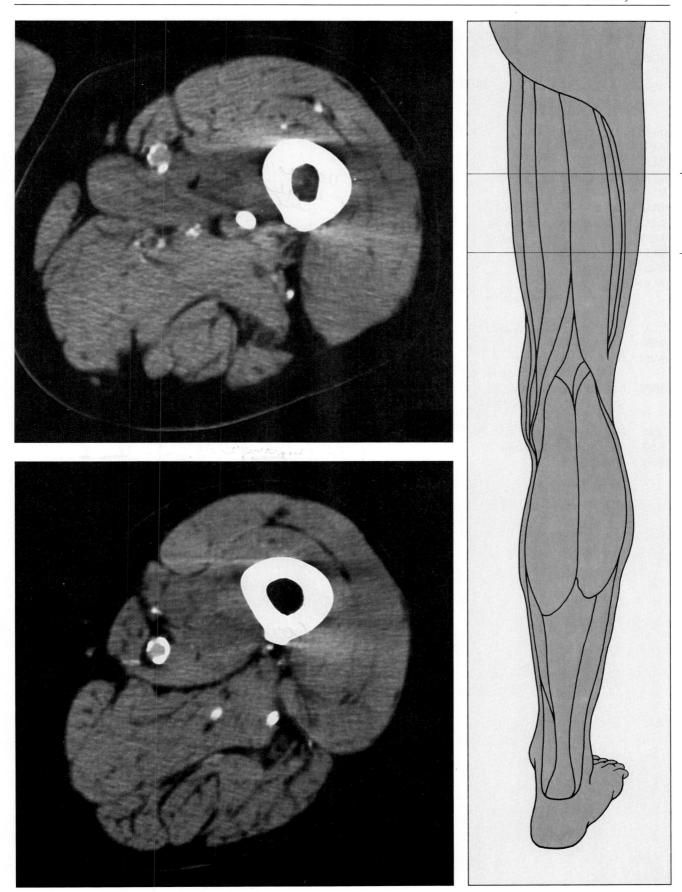

	64/65
A26	Popliteal artery
V26	Popliteal vein
V34	Great saphenous vein
M45	Gracilis muscle
M*45	Gracilis muscle (tendon)
M46	Sartorius muscle
M*47	Rectus femoris muscle (tendon)
M49	Vastus lateralis muscle
M63	Vastus medialis muscle
M64	Semitendinosus muscle
M65	Semimembranosus muscle
M66	Short head of the biceps femoris muscle
M67	Long head of the biceps femoris muscle
M68	Plantaris muscle
M69	Medial head of the gastrocnemius muscle
M70	Lateral head of the gastrocnemius muscle
S56	Shaft of the femur
S57	Condyle of the femur
S59	Patella

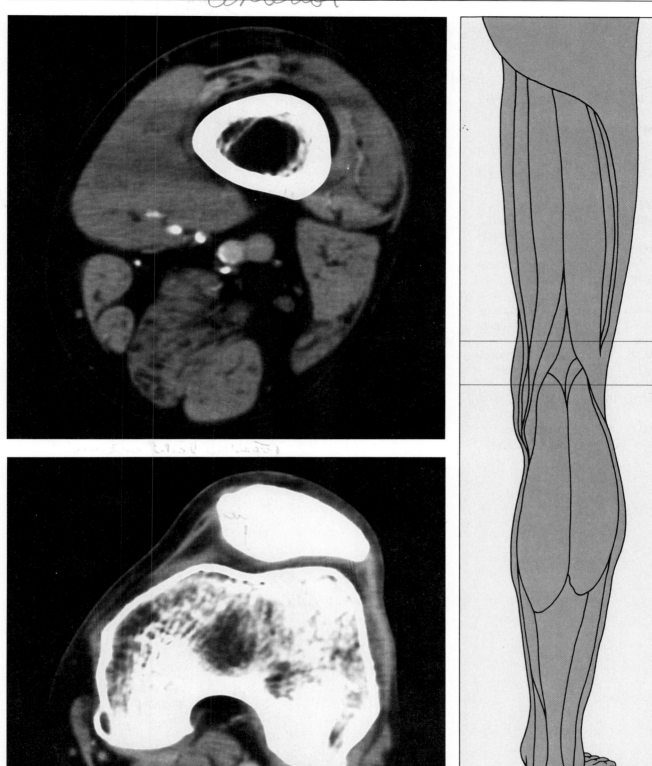

66/67	
A26	Popliteal artery
V26	Popliteal vein
V34	Great saphenous vein
M*46	Sartorius muscle (tendon)
M*67	Long head of the biceps femoris muscle (tendon)
M68	Plantaris muscle
M69	Medial head of the gastrocnemius muscle
M70	Lateral head of the gastrocnemius muscle
M71	Popliteus muscle
M72	Soleus muscle
M73	Tibialis anterior muscle
M*73	Tibialis anterior muscle (tendon)
M74	Tibialis posterior muscle
M75	Extensor digitorum longus muscle
M76	Peroneus longus muscle
M81	Patellar ligament or ligamentum patellae
S81	Head of the tibia
S82	Shaft of the tibia
S83	Fibula

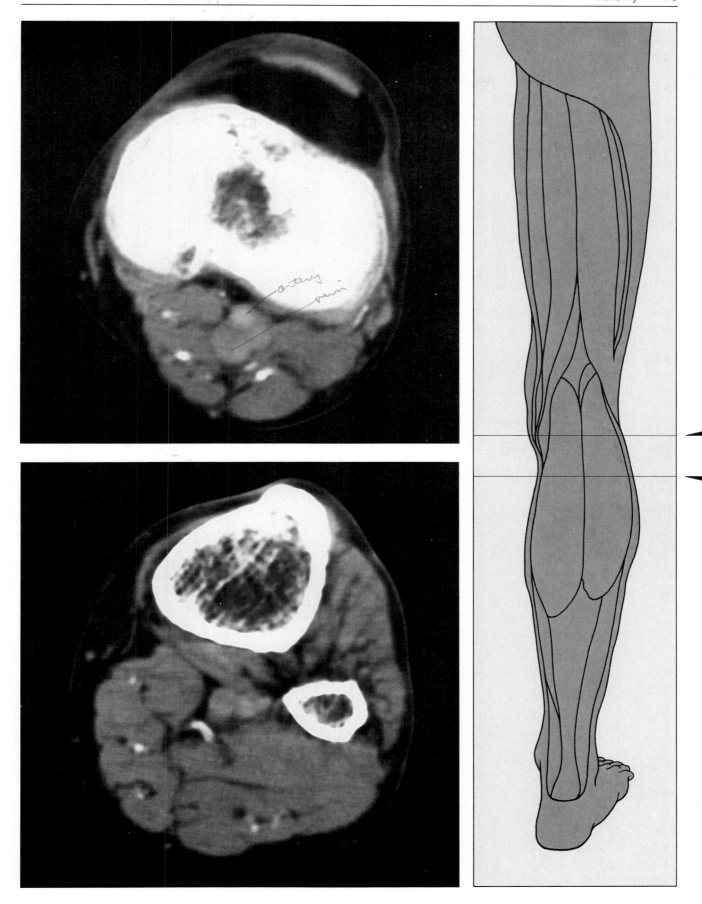

68/69

A27	Posterior tibial artery
A28	Anterior tibial artery
A29	Peroneal artery
V27	Posterior tibial vein
V28	Anterior tibial vein
V29	Peroneal vein
V34	Great saphenous vein
M69	Medial head of the gastrocnemius muscle
M70	Lateral head of the gastrocnemius muscle
M72	Soleus muscle
M73	Tibialis anterior muscle
M*73	Tibialis anterior muscle (tendon)
M74	Tibialis posterior muscle
M75	Extensor digitorum longus muscle
M76	Peroneus longus muscle
M77	Flexor digitorum longus muscle
M*77	Flexor digitorum longus muscle (tendon)
M78	Extensor hallucis longus muscle
M79	Flexor hallucis longus muscle
M80	Achilles tendon
S82	Shaft of the tibia
S83	Fibula

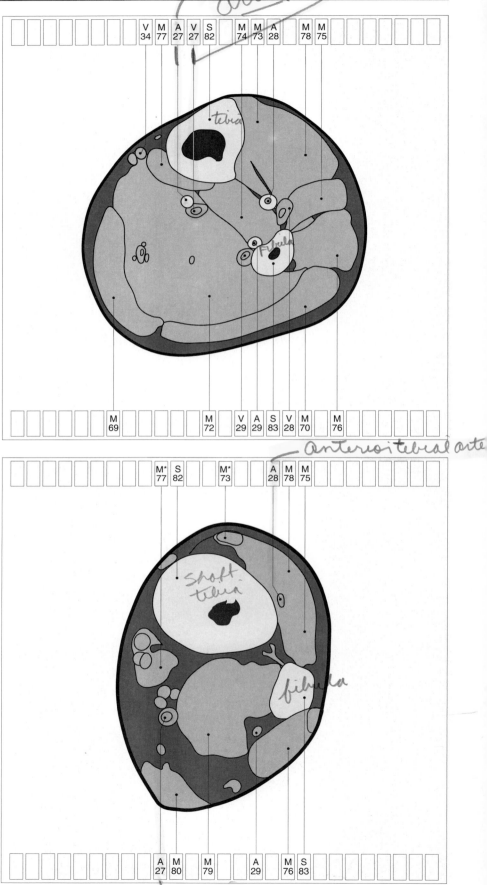

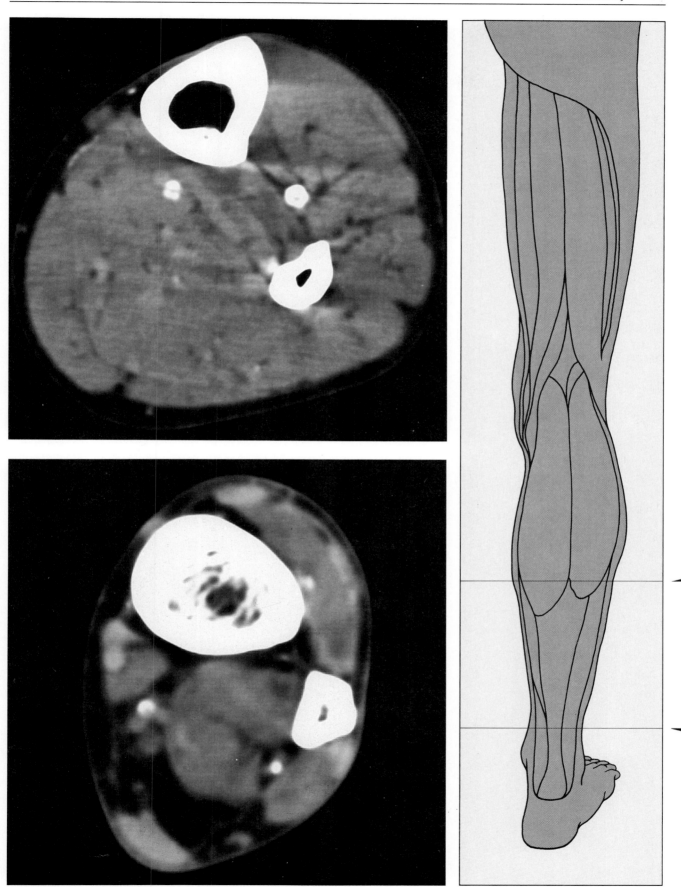

Chapter 3
Image Analysis

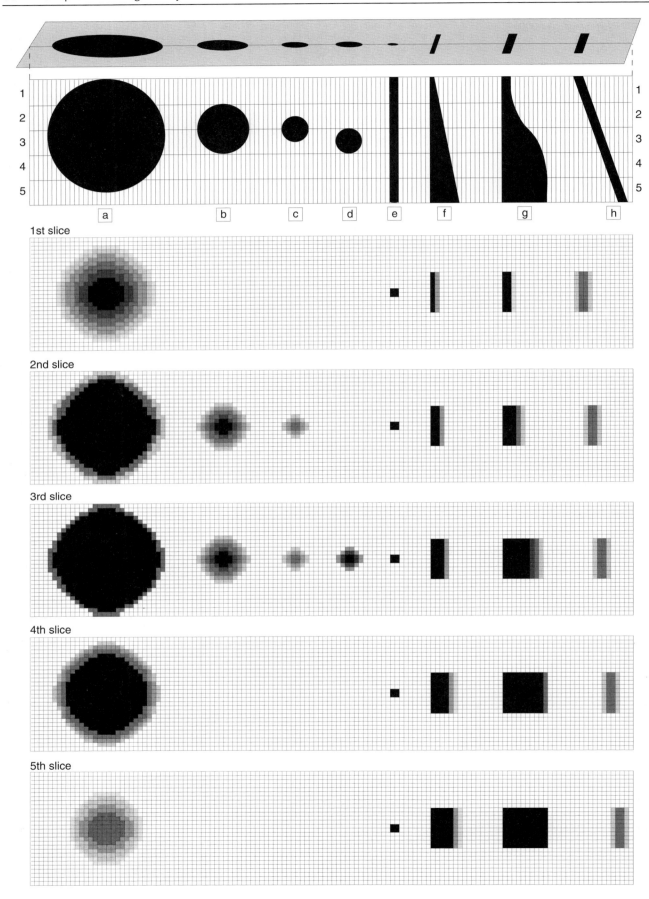

Image Analysis

Characteristic imaging features of CT must be known before proper image interpretation and *structural analysis* can be made. The *attenuation value* and *enhancement with contrast media* are two features that help to determine the final diagnosis.

Structural Image Analysis

Interpretation of Images

In computed tomography, the mean volume of an inhomogeneously dense area is calculated by dividing the area into multiple sections of equal thickness with a fixed number of individual picture or volume elements. Characteristic image disturbances, particularly those due to *partial volume* averaging, may therefore occur. These artifacts become more severe as the size of volume elements increases. In normal practice, sections of 8 to 10 mm thickness are scanned with an image matrix of 512×512 image points. Volume elements are then more rod-shaped (base to height ratio = ca. 1:8), which results in *horizontal masking* and *vertical tangential scanning phenomena*.

The attenuation value represents the average density of all tissue included in a volume element (voxel). When the density of structures within the volume element is not homogeneous, the individual structures exert a partial effect on the mean attenuation value, which is equal to the ratio of their size to the total size of the volume element. This means that the radiodensity of a boundary surface that passes through the volume element will not be directly demonstrated on CT scans. It is averaged in the attenuation value, which represents the mean density of all tissue included in that volume element. Because of the orthogonal structure of stacked volume elements (volume elements running vertical to the plane of the slice) boundary surfaces are represented as oblique or curved, stepped structures. When the slice thickness is 8 to 10 mm (which is the case in normal practice), interstices running horizontal to the sectional plane are identifiable only if a sharp difference in density clearly alters the attenuation value of the investigated volume elements. Such interstitial structures are frequently *masked*.

Normal scanning parameters usually provide better horizontal resolution (finely gridded image matrix, small field of measurement) than vertical resolution, and the latter diminishes in proportion to slice thickness. This also explains *tangential scanning phenomena:* narrow vertical structures (septa, vessels) are better represented in the mean volume of the normally axial, oblong volume elements, which makes them more easily detectable than oblique or horizontal structures. These effects can be minimized by reducing the slice thickness, which shortens the rectangular volume elements to small cubes.

Window Settings

Partial volume averaging makes the attenuation value of a boundary surface fall somewhere between that of contiguous structures. This creates the optical impression of half-shadows on the grey-scale image of boundary surfaces. The spatial resolution of morphological structures is frequently improved by adjusting the width of the window, which makes certain structures (e. g. lesions in the pleural recess) more readily visible. Very narrow window widths minimize the penumbral effects

Fig. 3-1. Characteristics of various structures as seen in CT scans. The first four structures (a-d) are round objects of various sizes placed in different locations; (e) is a tubular structure extending through the slice; (f) is an expanding, wedge- shaped structure; (g) is a bell-shaped structure; (h) passes diagonally through the slices. The configuration of these structures varies from slice to slice. The true attenuation value (black) is measured only in positions where the more dense part of the medium completely fills the volume element in the slice. Mixed attenuation values arise when this condition is not fulfilled, and optical half-shadows (penumbras) appear on the CT image. In cross- sectional images, sharpness of contour exists only in areas where more dense parts of the medium run perpendicular to the plane of the slice while completely filling the area of the volume element (e-g). Penumbras and mixed attenuation values will also arise when boundary surfaces extend diagonal to the slice plane.

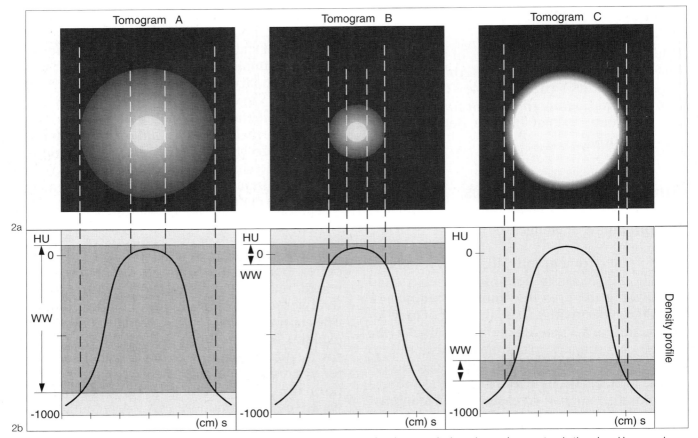

Fig. 3-2a, b. Object size vs. image window. The level and width of an image window determines not only the visual impression, but also the size of an object in the CT image (a). At a wide window setting, the object appears at its true size, but with a low level of contrast (A). Tomograms B and C display the object size only in a limited density range (core shadow). The lower section (2b) demonstrates the effects of window variation in a pulmonary nodule with a density profile curve.

Fig. 3-3. The appropriate window settings have been selected for imaging of a pulmonary process. Only at a wide window setting (a) can the exact size of the imaged structure be determined.

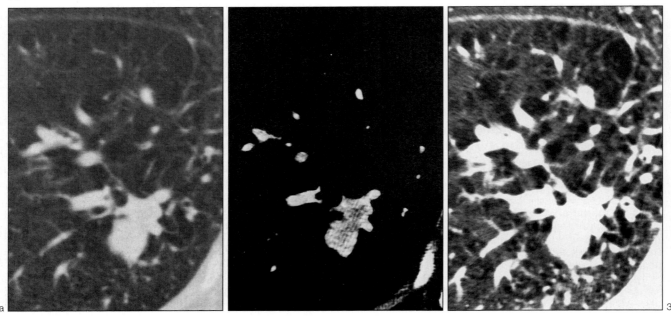

and optically enlarge the investigated structure. Both the window level and width should therefore be adjusted to fit the diagnostic problems of the patient and the expected density (density differences) of the investigated structures.

Morphological Image Analysis

Since computed tomographic images of an organ are divided into multiple sections, morphological analysis can be made only by compiling the individual sections. In doing so, one should carefully evaluate any masking of boundary layers caused by partial volume averaging.

Tubular and Nodular Structures

The classification of round structures at CT is of great practical significance. Contiguous slices must be carefully evaluated in order to determine whether an axial tubular structure (e.g. a vessel) or a nodular structure (e.g. lymph nodes) has been scanned. Craniocaudad continuation of the figure as a sharply demarcated, round figure of constant caliber is characteristic of tubular structures. Nodular structures tend to disappear on adjacent slices. In some cases, a broad window width can facilitate the classification of scanned structures by creating penumbra along their boundary surfaces. This may be of special diagnostic significance when curved tubular structures (vessel, bronchus) appear to be constricted or dilated.

Evaluation of Boundary Surfaces

Organs enclosed in a *capsule* or fascia have smooth outer margins that can be assessed only on tangential scans. The poles of the kidney, the dome of the liver, and the roof of the bladder may, therefore, be poorly demonstrated. Poor image definition can, in part, be overcome by scanning thinner sections. The *septa* and *fasciae* can be identified as fine fibrous boundary surfaces only in places where they are tangentially intersected, i.e. where their axial alignment is greatest (e.g. the costoparietal, but not the diaphragmatic pleura).

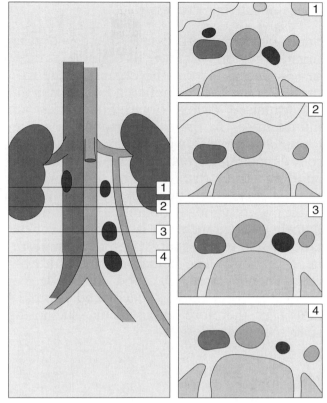

Fig. 3-4. Tubular and nodular structures seen in CT sections can be distinguished on the basis of the structure's appearance in contiguous slices.

Fig. 3-5a, b. Boundary surfaces. The lung structure is indistinct in 8 mm slices (a); the main septum is only discretely visible. After reducing the size of the slice to 2 mm, this structure can be clearly seen (b).

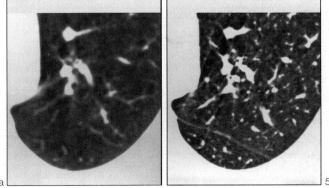

5a   5b

Space-occupying Processes

Space-occupying processes expand within an organ or region, but leave its boundaries more or less intact. Hence, the organ capsule may protrude, but the surrounding fat remains uncompromised (when organ boundaries are unimpaired). In the same manner, a space-occupying process will merely displace surrounding parenchyma, contiguous organs and adjacent structures. Take, for example, the *capsule sign:* when intraparenchymal hemorrhage occurs within an organ, the surrounding, deformable parenchyma is flattened, yet the taut capsule remains intact despite hemato-related pressure. The hematoma therefore becomes lenticulated. A good knowledge of anatomical boundaries, spaces and compartments is therefore essential in diagnosing space-occupying lesions.

Infiltrating Processes

Unlike space-occupying lesions, infiltrating lesions do not respect organ or fascia borders. Masking of surrounding fat is indicative of organ invasion. It is relatively easy to identify whether the fasciae of contiguous structures have been penetrated if one has a good knowledge of the usual paths of spreading.

Boundary surfaces that run oblique or horizontal to the sectional plane cannot always be optimally demonstrated by computed tomography. Partial volume averaging must therefore be considered when diagnosing infiltration. It is even more difficult to make a final diagnosis if there is not a sufficient amount of fat positioned between adjacent organs. Then,

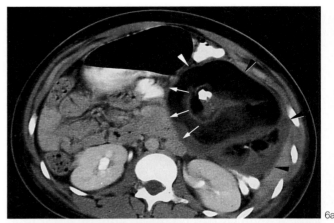
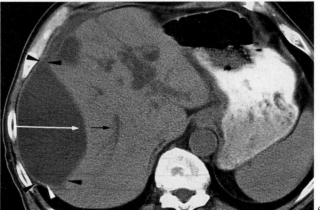
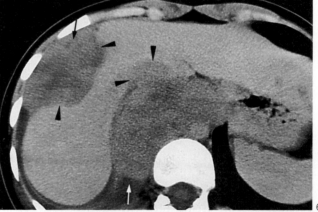
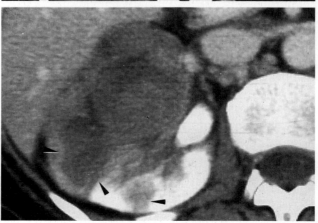

Fig. 3-6a. Space-occupying lesions. This dermoid cyst demonstrates smooth borders and capsule formation (►). Displacement of surrounding organs is seen (→).

Fig. 3-6b. Space-occupying process. Biloma. Subcapsular fluid (►) has accumulated. This causes medial displacement of the hepatic parenchyma (→).

Fig. 3-6c. Infiltrating process. Metastasizing osteosarcoma (→). Metastases have penetrated the borders of the liver and are indistinctly demarcated from the hepatic parenchyma (►).

Fig. 3-6d. Infiltrating process. Renal cell carcinoma. Non-uniform infiltration is seen in the renal parenchyma with ill-defined tumor borders (►).

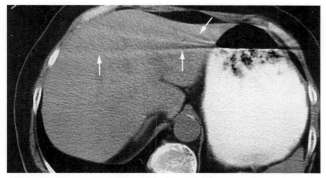

Fig. 3-7a. Motion artifact. Movement of stomach fluid during scanning leads to the formation of streaklike artifacts that falsify the attenuation values of the liver.

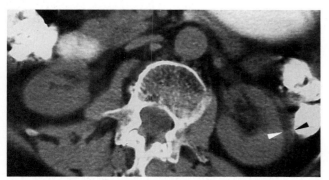

Fig. 3-7b. Motion artifact. Longitudinal displacement of the kidney due to breathing motion leads to the appearance of a double contour simulating a subcapsular hematoma (►).

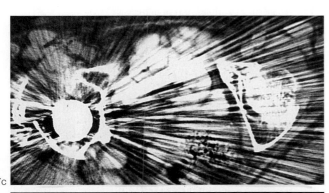

7c

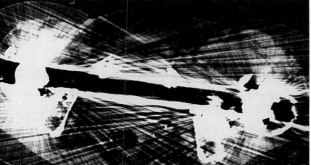

7d

diagnosis of organ infiltration is possible only when contour defects and density variation are clearly seen.

Intravenous *contrast media* will often improve image clarity. Additional boundary structures become visible after contrast enhancement, and one can judge whether the organ boundaries are intact or have been infiltrated.

Quantitative Image Analysis (Densitometry)

The Individual Attenuation Value

The attenuation value of a given volume element is subject to statistical variance, which is expressed as graininess (image noise). The degree of statistical variance is proportional to the dose of irradiation and is numerically expressed as a standard deviation from a mean value. The investigated regions of interest (ROI) must be large enough to increase the accuracy of the mean value. Localized spot measurements are therefore not advisable.

Falsification of Density Measurements

Object-related falsification of density measurements must be differentiated from errors caused by measurement-related, statistical inaccuracy. The former are referred to as *artifacts*.

Most *motion artifacts* are caused by excursions of the diaphragm and heart. In computed tomography, a fan beam must make multiple tangential scans of moving organs that are constantly changing their position. The projections, therefore, can no longer be precisely

Fig. 3-7c. High-contrast artifacts. A metal prosthesis in the right hip leads to the development of radial image disturbance that completely falsifies attenuation value measurement. Only sketchy images of morphological structures are visible.

Fig. 3-7d. High-contrast artifacts. The two high-contrast objects located in this cross-sectional scan lead to radial image disturbance in several projections in areas located between the objects.

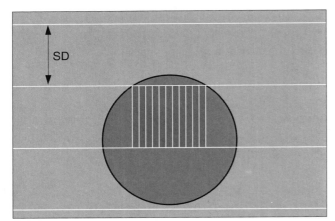

Fig. 3-8. Attenuation value vs. diameter of an object. Only when the slice thickness is less than half the object diameter one can safely assume that the volume elements of at least one layer of the object will be filled completely for accurate measurement of attenuation value.

reconstructed to an exact position. Organ motion can falsify an entire projection, and the resulting motion artifacts may extend across an entire scan as streaks of density disturbance. These areas of falsification show positive and negative amplitudes of density variation. Variation of attenuation values in the heart can mimic calcification. Motion artifacts can usually be identified by the fact that they remain visible throughout several different window levels. The contour of the moving organ can usually be identified, because it is tangentially intersected by the streak of the artifact (vertical to the direction of motion).

High-contrast artifacts (dental crowns, metal implants) cause severe image disturbances, because projections passing through these objects will falsify the attenuation measurements.

Beam-hardening artifacts occur in more dense organ structures (or with contrast media). They are caused by non-uniform hardening of

---

Fig. 3-9a. Attenuation value of blood and its fractions with respect to the hematocrit level. The increased CT number of a fresh hematoma (▲) corresponds with a higher hemoconcentration, i.e., raised hematocrit (HCT).

Fig. 3-9b. Attenuation value of hemoglobin and serum iron with respect to concentration (g%, mg%).

Fig. 3-9c. Attenuation value of body fluids. This increases linearly in proportion to the protein concentration.

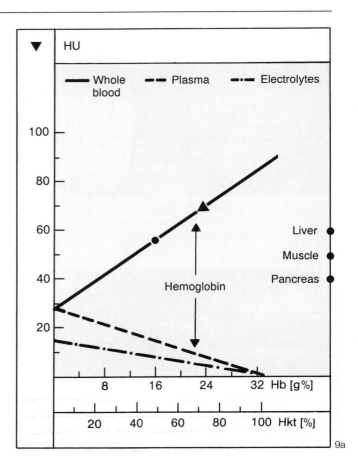

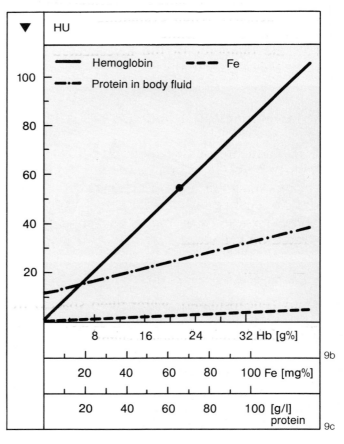

the X-ray beam within an object. The hardening corrections in the computer's reconstruction program covers many, but not all, morphological possibilities. Hardening artifacts normally cause only minor (shadowy or patchy) density falsifications, but they must be taken into consideration when evaluating low-grade density enhancement (e.g. accumulation of contrast medium in a lesion near the contrasted renal pelvis).

Attenuation Value of Boundary Surfaces

Since the CT numbers reflect the average radiodensity of all tissue within the volume element, the density of a specific tissue type can be reliably determined if the slice contains only that one tissue type. Density measurements should therefore be painstakingly made along structural borders in order to ensure that each slice contains only that single tissue type. Generally, partial volume artifacts arise when the diameter of an investigated structure is smaller than the slice thickness. When that is indeed the case, it is impossible to accurately measure tissue density. When evaluating round structures, the slice thickness should be less than half the diameter of the investigated lesion (e.g. pulmonary nodule).

Pathomorphological Variation

Body tissue inside a living organism cannot be regarded as a static parameter. It undergoes various reactions after trauma, infection, metabolic change, and neoplastic infiltration. Some of these tissue reactions can be demonstrated on CT scans.

• Fluid-Filled Formations

Cysts (encapsulated, water-filled spaces) frequently develop. The contents of a cyst have a CT number that is typically slightly higher than that of water. In addition to measurement inaccuracies and electrolytes, an increase in attenuation value may also be attributable to changes in protein content, which may be caused by inflammation or by decomposition

of hemoglobin. In that case, the CT numbers rise and may even approximate soft-tissue density. Since they are avascular, cysts do not become enhanced by contrast medium and can therefore be easily distinguished from other structures.

The protein content of *exudates* is different from that of *transudates* ($\geq$ 30 g/l), and their attenuation values can range from 20 to 30 Hounsfield units.

• Blood/Hematoma

The attenuation value of blood is mainly determined by the protein content of the blood cells. Blood from healthy individuals with normal hematocrit and hemoglobulin levels has a CT density of 55 ± 5 HU. Around 40 HU is attributable to hemoglobin, and ca. 15 HU to

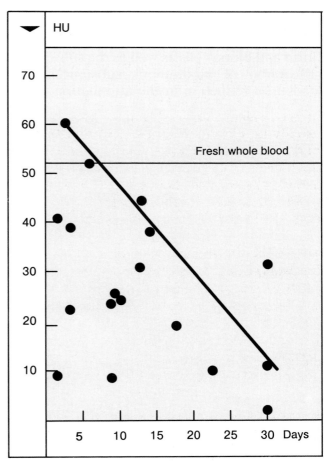

Fig. 3-10. Attenuation value of hematomas. This is dependent on the age of the hematoma. The line drawn through the points corresponds with data by Bergström. Data points underneath the curve are attenuation values for hematomas of known age, as measured by the author, as well as data by Gürtler.

plasma. Plasma protein and electrolytes both contribute equally to the radiodensity of plasma. The CT density of blood is thus directly dependent on the hemoglobin content and the hematocrit level. The amount of iron in hemoglobin has hardly any effect on the radiodensity of blood. Except in the liver and thyroid, the attenuation value of blood is normally slightly higher than that of the organ parenchyma. When the hemoglobin or hematocrit levels decrease, vessels and internal cardiac spaces can be distinguished from organ parenchyma on plain scans because of the noticeable reduction in density.

When blood coagulates, hemoconcentration due to retraction of fibrin occurs with a corresponding increase in hematocrit levels. When still fresh, a compact hematoma is therefore hyperdense as compared with fresh venous blood. This hyperdensity lasts up to seven days after the onset of bleeding. The degradation of fibrin and blood cells as well as the subsequent absorption of albuminous substances then leads to a reduction in the attenuation value.

The attenuation value of larger hematomas with a capsule of granular tissue can drop to the water range, depending on the protein content of the hematoma (posttraumatic cyst).

In whole-body CT, there is not such a generally applicable, fixed relationship of the attenuation value to the maturity of a hemorrhage, as is observed in cerebral lesions. Although hyperdensity is characteristic of fresh hemorrhage, hypodensity is a nonspecific sign, which indicates that a broad range of fluid collections must be considered in the diagnosis.

• Abscesses

The body's response to infection is inflammation with local hyperemia, exudation and leukocyte migration. The process is reversible as long as tissue destruction has not occurred. The pathological substrate of pus contains necrotic tissue, exudates and dead leukocytes. The consistency of pus varies according to the relative percentage of these components in the substrate. From the 3rd to 5th day after pus development, cells in the granulation tissue be-

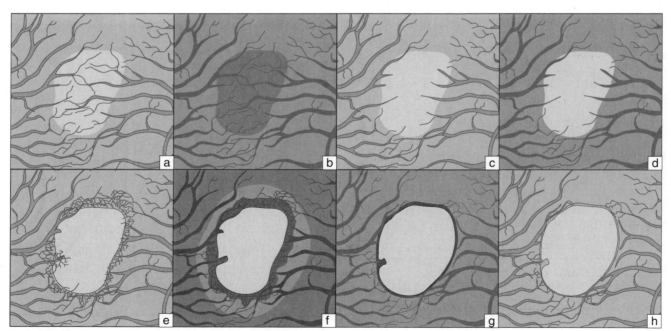

Fig. 3-11. Development and healing of an abscess. Local inflammation leads to circumscribed hypodensity due to accompanying edema formation (a). An area of discrete hyperdensity is sometimes seen after contrast medium (CM) administration (b). After liquefaction has begun, persistent hypodensity is seen, even after contrast medium administration (c). This becomes more intense as development continues (d). Sprouting granulation tissue appears as an area of a ringlike enhancement around the indistinctly delineated area of hypodensity, as can be demonstrated after contrast medium administration (e). Granulation tissue thickens to form a pyogenic membrane, thus sharply delineating the area. The abscess is usually surrounded by a hypodense halo attributable to an accompanying edema (f). After the symptoms of inflammation have subsided, the demarcated tissue zone, which still enhances after contrast medium administration, becomes thinner and sharply delineated (g) until a cystlike wall ultimately develops (h).

gin to proliferate and ultimately form the walls of an abscess. In successful antibiotic treatment, sterile pus is absorbed; otherwise, a (protein-rich) cyst develops. Regardless of whether drained via incision or spontaneously, scar tissue then develops and gradually replaces the granulation tissue.

These processes produce variability in the CT numbers of abscesses. In early stages of leukocytic immigration, the accompanying edema may show with low hypodensity. CT numbers are significantly reduced after liquefaction of pus has occurred. The attenuation values then stabilize at around 30 HU. Depending on the method of treatment, pus drainage will result in the formation of scar tissue or the development of a protein-rich cyst. Scar tissue is connective tissue-dense, while cysts approximate water density.

The administration of contrast media can provide additional diagnostic information. The characteristically opacified, hyperdense ring around the hypodense abscess makes it easier to distinguish well-vascularized granular tissue. Zones of liquefaction do not become enhanced, but fresh inflammations (hypodense zones) are enhanced because of hyperemia.

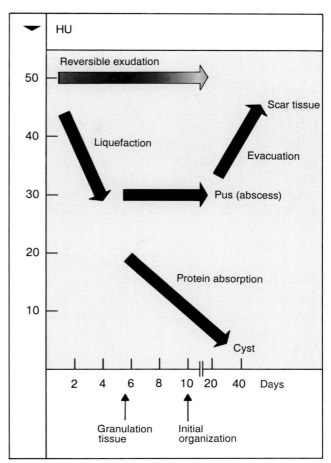

Fig. 3-12. Attenuation values for abscesses with respect to various pathophysiological processes.

• *Solid Tissue*

The attenuation value of *bone* is dependent on its mineral content. The radiodensity of all other forms of solid tissue is dependent on their variable content of protein, water and fat. The protein-rich parenchyma of the liver, muscles and spleen, for example, have higher attenuation values than the better hydrated renal parenchyma. *Fatty tissue* has an attenuation value of -80 to -120 HU. For practical reasons, the term *soft-tissue* will be used to describe various tissue types, the CT number of which is clearly higher than that of fat.

The attenuation value of *mixed tissue* is determined by the volume ratio of the different tissue components. When there are only two density components, the volume ratio can be easily deduced from the attenuation value (directly proportional). Tissue zones with a certain proportion of fat and connective tissue may have the attenuation value of water

(0 HU). Homogeneous water-dense structures may therefore correlate with solid tissue.

The degree of fatty infiltration in the liver can similarly be directly calculated from the attenuation value (10% fatty infiltration corresponds with a 14 HU decrease in attenuation). Accumulations of water (edema) can also cause a drop in radiodensity in renal and muscle tissue.

The CT numbers of *lung and bone tissue* are widely scattered due to the inclusion of a highly contrasting elements (air, compact substance) in the soft tissue.

• *Regressive Change*

Calcification within necrotic material or denatured proteins is a well-known diagnostic sign

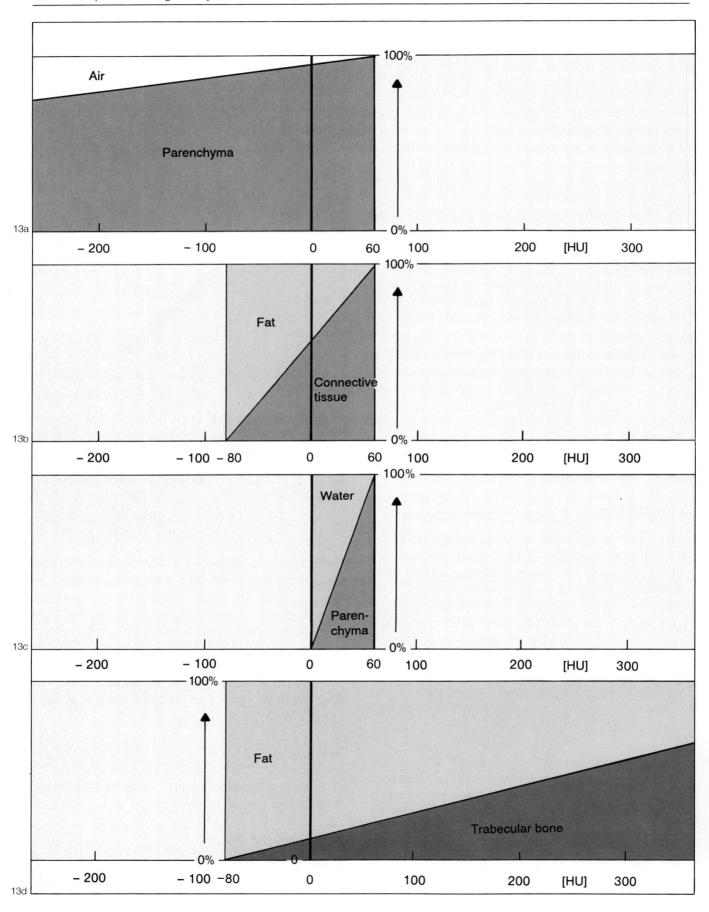

that can be more sensitively detected by computed tomography than by conventional radiography.

Amyloidosis frequently leads to organ enlargement and is characterized by the accumulation of interstitial and intercellular protein deposits. It can also lead to a reduction in parenchymal density.

Liquefactive necrosis causes a clear but variable reduction in attenuation value, which may drop to water density. Liquefactive necrosis frequently develops in inflamed tissue as well as rapidly growing tumors. It develops in tumors as a result of hypoxia or hemorrhage and can be rather smoothly demarcated ("cystic degeneration"). In aseptic necrosis, e. g. after the embolization of an organ artery, *gas* not attributable to bacteria frequently accumulates. Gas within cystic formations is generally considered to be a pathognomonic sign of an abscess (gas formation by anaerobic bacteria).

Bone Densitometry

Bone is made stable by a collagen-rich, organic matrix which contains hydroxyapatite, a calcium-rich mineral salt. The content of mineral salts, which is dependent on the packing density of the trabecula of the bone, is an indicator of the mechanical load capacity of a given bone. In order to diagnose osseous mineralization disturbances, one normally measures the density of trabecular bone of the medullary space of a vertebral body, which is sensitive to metabolic changes.

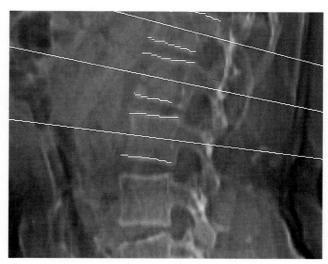

Fig. 3-14. The center of a vertebral body can be determined precisely by means of a lateral topogram. In some cases, the line of intersect between the upper and lower plates of two vertebral bodies must be used.

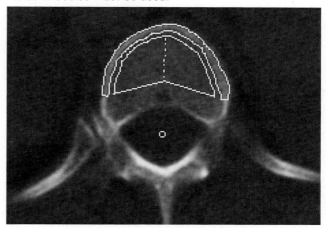

Fig. 3-15. In trabecular (spongy) and cortical vertebra, the attenuation value is determined on the basis of elliptical or contour-adjusted regions of interest (ROI).

Fig. 3-16. A calibration curve is made by scanning a reference phantom placed underneath the patient. This is used to transform the CT number into values of bone mineral density (BMD; mg/cm³).

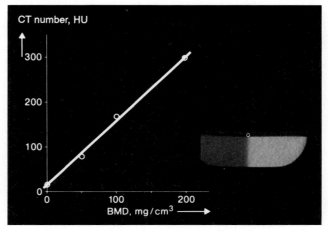

Fig. 3-13. Attenuation value of mixed tissues. In a mixed tissue consisting of two different components, the percentage content of each component can be calculated on the basis of the attenuation value. Thus, it is possible to calculate the air content in lung tissue (a), the fat content in fatty parenchymal tissue (b), the water content of an edema (c), and the content of mineralized bone substances in osseous tissue, provided that the attenuation value of both components is known.

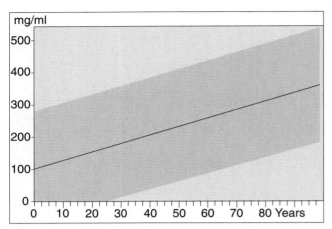

Fig. 3-17. Fat content of trabecular bone according to age (based on ref. 34).

Fig. 3-18. Bone mineral density in women, for cortical (a) and trabecular bone (b), according to age (ref. 2891). (±2 SD). .... SEQCT ——— DEQCT

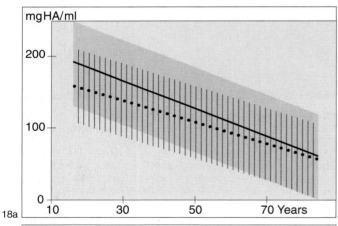

18a

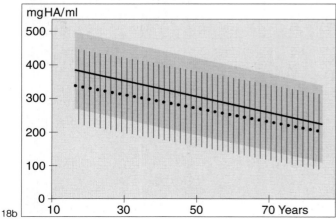

18b

In order to obtain representative reference values upon which adequate correlations can be made, the following measurement conditions must be properly maintained:
- The slice must be reproducible, contain a section of the upper plate, and be free of partial volume artifacts.
- An 8 mm slice must pass exactly through the middle of the upper plates of the vertebral bodies (or precisely intersect the angle of wedge-shaped vertebral bodies).
- The regions of interest (ROI) should be standardized as either elliptical regions or be located at a fixed distance from the contours of vertebral bodies (individualized measurement is therefore preferable to automated measurement).
- The mean attenuation value of each ROI (measured in Hounsfield units) should be calculated as bone mineral density (mg $Ca_5(PO_4)_3OH/cm^3$) in order to prevent the potentially great effects of tube voltage on measurement results. A water hydroxyapatite phantom (or its equivalent) should therefore used to calibrate the scanner.

The calculated bone mineral attenuation values are equivalent values that normally underestimate the actual mineral content by as much as 30%, because bone tissue is composed of three densitometrically different tissue components: the calcium-rich bone matrix, hematogenic soft-tissue, and substitutional fatty tissue. Deposits of the latter increase with age, thus displacing the calibrated ratio of the three components. Age-related correction tables can significantly reduce "fat error".

The level of measurement accuracy in standard single-energy quantitative CT (SEQCT) was significantly improved by dual-energy quantitative CT (DEQCT), which scans a section of a vertebral body with two different tube voltages. Quantitative comparison of the pair of images allows selective calculation of the calcium content. This is especially important, since the attenuation value of calcium is greatly affected by the amount of irradiation energy used, which is not the case with soft-tissue and fat.

Intravenous Bolus Injection of Contrast Medium

Contrast media provide additional evidence to prove or, in some cases, exclude or further differentiate pathogenic processes. Contrast-enhanced scans usually supplement plain scans.

Intravascular Enhancement

An intravascular injection of contrast medium improves visualization of the lumen of vessels by opacifying the blood. Vessel patency, intraluminal pathologies, occlusions, dissections and ruptures can then be assessed. In many diagnostic examinations (staging), enhancement of arterial and venous beds is essential for distinguishing lymph nodes from surrounding vessels. In such cases, venous return (e.g. in the pelvis) is also an important diagnostic sign.

Temporary artifacts caused by laminar flow are frequently observed in the part of the inferior vena cava above the renal veins. These artifacts can be differentiated from thrombi by rescanning after a time lapse. Thrombi, which normally appear as sharp and constant structures, are demarcated from the enhanced blood.

Parenchymatous Enhancement

After a bolus injection of contrast medium, lesions that remain isodense on plain scans can be identified after enhancement of the parenchyma when the *vascularity* of the lesions differs from that of surrounding parenchyma. Hypervascularized lesions appear *hyperdense* (briefly), and hypovascularized lesions are *hypodense*. Lesions frequently display a very irregular pattern of vascularization, resulting in a density difference that makes them distinguishable from the surrounding parenchyma. Avascular lesions can be identified as such, because they remain unopacified by contrast medium.

Internal organ structures must also be evaluated in order to make some subtle diagnoses. On plain CT scans, diagnosis of the structure of

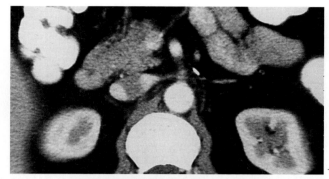
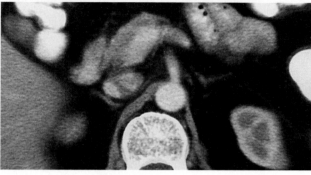
19a
19b

Fig. 3-19. Flow phenomena after bolus contrast medium administration. Signs of a filling defect are detected in the inferior vena cava due to inflow of blood from the renal veins. This filling defect disappears within one minute (b), and can then be differentiated from a potential thrombus.

Fig. 3-20. Internal structures. Atypical thickening of the renal parenchyma (a→) can be precisely analyzed after contrast medium administration. The normal myelocortical markings are absent, i.e., a clearly pathological process exists (contralateral metastases of a renal cell carcinoma).

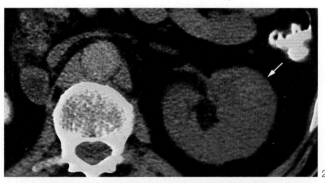
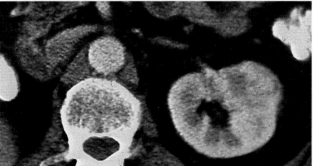
20a
20b

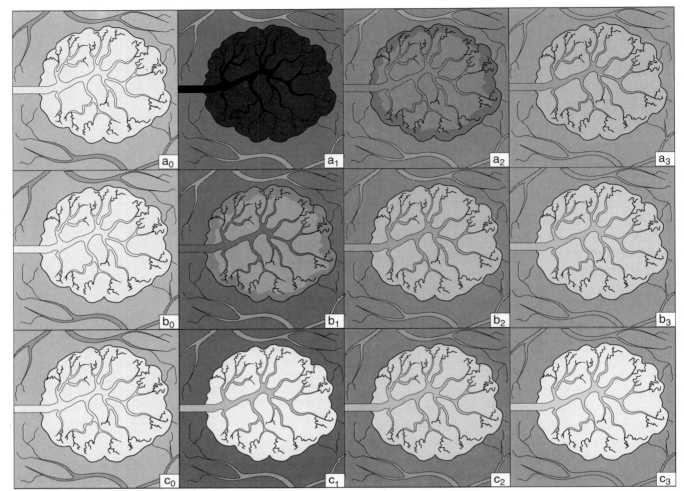

Fig. 3-21. Effects of vascularization on the CT appearance of lesions. Depending on their degree of vascularization (as compared with healthy organ tissue), lesions that appear hypodense in plain scans present a variable appearance in different phases of organ contrast enhancement. A hypervascularized lesion is best demonstrated in the arterial phase (a_1). Peripheral enhancement is frequently seen in the parenchymal phase (30 – 120 s) (a_2), and it is more difficult to visualize the lesion in the compensatory phase (a_3). A hypovascularized lesion is best delineated in the arterial phase (c_1) when the surrounding organ tissue shows the most intense enhancement. Contrast-enhanced scans of isovascularized lesions often provide no more essential evidence than plain scans (b_0). However, neovascularization in the peripheral region often serves to improve demarcation of the lesion.

parenchymal organs is limited by the presence of large vessels and fatty deposits. The internal structures of the organ (e.g. the renal medulla and cortex) can be evaluated only in certain phases of enhancement.

Since the organ contours may remain unchanged, changes in parencyhmal structure may be indicative of parenchymal lesions, even when no abnormality was found on plain scans. A loss of pulp trabeculation of the spleen can be seen in the early bolus phase and can be interpreted as a sign of diffuse organ infiltration.

When there is a localized area of density reduction in the liver, the absence of displacement or distortion contraindicates the presence of a mass and is suggestive of focal fatty degeneration of the liver.

Knowledge of normal internal structures is therefore essential and can increase the sensitivity of contrast-enhanced CT in detecting pathological lesions. The walls and boundaries (fasciae) of hollow organs must frequently be evaluated. In these cases, homogeneous, lamellar enhancement is indicative of intact structure.

Differential Diagnosis of Contrast Enhanced Images

The body responds to an injury or inflammatory process by forming *granulation tissue.* Capillaries develop in these areas, so the granulation tissue is well vascularized and has many functions. It promotes leukocytic defense, absorbs retained fluids, and serves as filling and demarcating tissue before it ultimately transforms into scar tissue (fibrosis).

In chronic disorders (e.g. absorption of a hematoma, abscess or false cyst), a variably thick (non-epithelialized) wall will ultimately develop. Thanks to its high vascularity, granulation tissue can be readily demonstrated on CT scans after a bolus of contrast medium has been injected. The tissue is demonstrated as a thin rim of hyperdensity with a frequently stratified wall structure. Granulation tissue accumulates in the presence of absorbing or organizing processes.

Neoplastic tumor growths normally have a nodular appearance, and the degree of vascularity can vary greatly. Avascular neoplastic areas on CT scans suggest necrosis or hemorrhage. These regions usually are not outlined by enhanced, demarcating tissue.

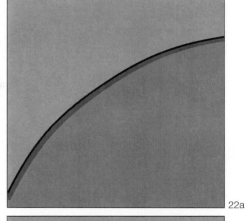

22a

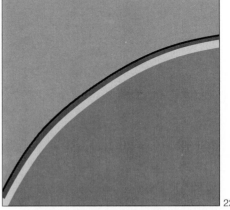

22b

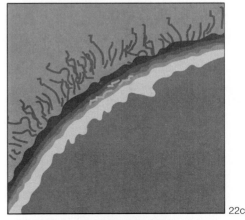

22c

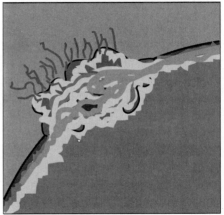

22d

Fig. 3-22. Contrast-enhancement of boundary surfaces. Contrast enhancement of healthy bladder and intestinal walls is, at best, very discrete (a). Inflammatory processes lead to the development of a rimlike area of enhancement due to mucosal or submucosal inflammation. A similar picture is seen in absorbing boundary surfaces of an inflamed connective tissue apparatus (e.g. fascia) (b). Chronic and subacute processes often lead to reinforcement and thickening of border structures and/or irregularities in the mucosal surface. However, discrete, uniform stratification of mural structures can usually be seen after enhancement with contrast medium (c). In contrast to these frequently chronic processes, neoplastic processes are characterized by the loss or dissolution of their stratified structure (d), which is best demonstrated after administration of contrast medium.

Chapter 4
Contrast Media

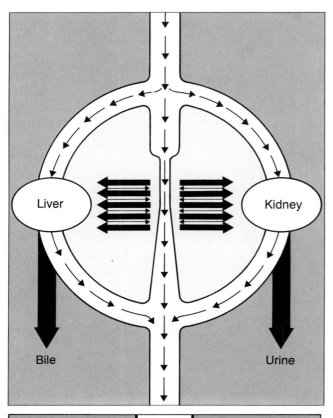

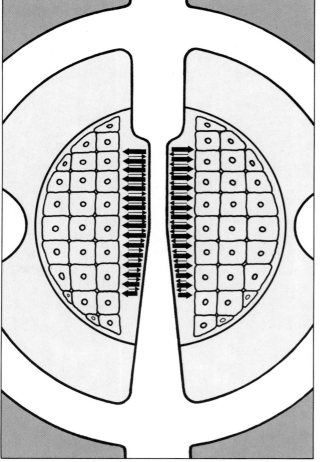

Fig. 4-1. Distribution of intravascular contrast medium.
a) Contrast medium injected into the blood stream disperses into the extracellular space. At the same time, contrast medium is excreted by the kidney (and, possibly, the liver).

b) Components of contrast medium that are not bound to protein diffuse through the capillaries into the interstitial space (large arrows) and do not enter the cells. This process of elimination decreases the concentration of contrast medium in blood. The contrast medium is redistributed to the blood stream when the blood concentration becomes lower than the concentration in interstitial tissues (small arrows).

Contrast Media

Contrast media for computed tomography are administered primarily by intravascular and intracavitary methods.

Intravascular Administration

Basic Principles of Contrast Enhancement

Intravascular administration of contrast medium (CM) leads to time-dependent distribution of contrast medium in different tissue compartments. Contrast enhancement is dose-dependent on the one hand and, on the other hand, dependent on different pharmacokinetic factors (e.g. hemodynamics, hydrophilia, lipophilia, osmolality, protein binding, etc.). Nonionic radiologic contrast media in wide use today are well tolerated, display high renal clearance and low protein binding ($< 1\%$); contrast medium is distributed almost exclusively in the extracellular space. Most unbound contrast medium diffuses from the vessel lumina via the capillary walls to the interstitial space. The contrast medium is then eliminated from the blood in the kidney by means of glomerular filtration. Osmosis-related tubular reabsorption of water into the kidney leads to an increase in the contrast medium concentration in the renal tubules and collecting tubules (urography), which facilitates the diagnosis. High protein binding would prevent rapid glomerular filtration and lead to active intake of contrast medium in the liver cells. Finally, contrast medium is secreted into the bile ducts (choledochography). The plasma concentration of contrast medium drops as a result of this process of elimination. Contrast medium then passes from the interstitial space to the intravascular space until elimination is complete.

• Angiography

As in conventional angiography, CT also makes use of the fact that intravascular contrast medium only gradually enters the inter-

stitial tissues, thereby providing a longer period of positive vascular contrast. First the veins, then (after heart-lung passage) the arteries are opacified by intravenously administered contrast medium. As in intravenous digital subtraction angiography, the contrast medium reaches the target organ after a certain preliminary circulation period.

• Parenchymal Contrast Enhancement

The supplying arteries are briefly opacified during the infusion phase. The contrast medium then reaches the parenchyma of the organ via the capillaries. The subsequent brief contrast enhancement of the entire capillary bed associated with partial passage of contrast medium into the extracellular space comprises parenchymal contrast enhancement.

• Renography

After reaching the renal parenchyma, contrast medium is excreted via glomerular filtration. As in conventional urography, the resulting contrast enhancement of the renal medulla and cortex can be diagnostically evaluated. High density resolution is, however, essential for CT analysis.

• Choledochography

After it reaches the liver, contrast medium is excreted by liver cells into the bile ducts. The amount of contrast medium excreted depends on the degree of protein binding. High protein binding ($> 45\%$) will lead to contrast enhancement of the bile ducts and gallbladder. Although well proven in conventional radiography, choledochographic contrast techniques are only seldom utilized in computed tomography.

• Blood-Brain Barrier

If the blood-brain barrier is intact, contrast medium will remain within the vessel lumina of the brain, creating highly contrasted images of intracranial vessels. Healthy brain parenchyma then remains relatively nonenhanced. Pathological processes render the blood-brain barrier partially permeable, causing *local* parenchymatous contrast enhancement. The lesion is *selectively* opacified.

Different characteristics of contrast media are used to achieve different diagnostic goals. The contrast phase opacifying the target organ or pathological process must be long enough for scanning purposes. Since contrast media can be given in restricted doses only, the scanning time is also limited. A good knowledge of physiological and pharmacokinetic principles can significantly improve the efficacy of contrast-enhanced CT examinations.

Fig. 4-2. Bolus injection. Iodine concentration in the external iliac artery after a rapid intravenous injection of urographic contrast medium (5 ml in 1 s). Maximum concentration is achieved 16 seconds later. Second and third peaks indicate recirculation.

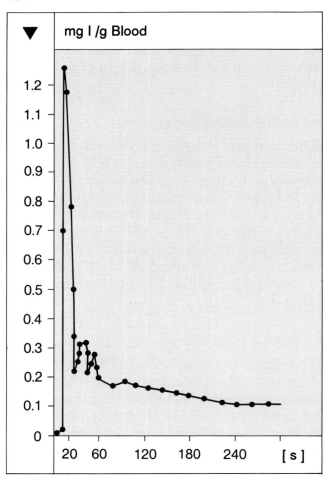

Urographic Contrast Media

Pharmacokinetics

Intravenous *bolus injection* of urographic contrast media leads to time-dependent contrast enhancement of blood; the time-density curve is best illustrated via the abdominal aorta (Fig. 4-2). Contrast enhancement reaches a maximum approx. 15 seconds after injection, but quickly drops to around 1/7th of the maximum value (20 s). A few small rises in concentration occur afterwards; they are due to recirculation effects. The time span from the start of injection to maximum vessel concentration of contrast medium is termed "peak time". While dose level and rate of injection determine the duration of the injection, they only slightly affect the peak time.

In the right atrium, the column of contrasted blood is mixed and distributed in fractionated portions with each heart beat to pulmonary circulation channels. Because the pulmonary capillary bed is so broad, the contrast medium passage time is extended, thereby delaying the transport of contrast medium through the lung. The contrast enhanced blood, which is further modulated by each heart beat, subsequently enters the aorta. These hemodynamic factors create a typical time-density curve (bolus geometry, Fig. 4-3) with a much broader base than the rectangular configuration characteristic of the primary bolus time-density curve.

The capacitive properties of the pulmonary veins as well as restricted cardiac output prevent proportional maximum contrast enhancement of the aorta, even when the injection rate is raised. No significant increase in maximum contrast enhancement of the aorta can be achieved by raising the injection rate to more than 8 ml/s.

This dynamic, intravascular phase of bolus injection is followed by a compensatory phase during which contrasted and noncontrasted blood mix. The contrast medium is, at the same time, refluxed from intravascular to the extravascular compartment, i.e., the density of contrast (radiodensity) of the aortic lumina slowly and steadily decreases.

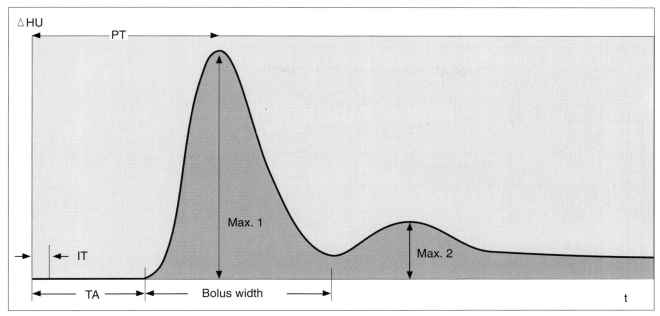

Fig. 4-3. Bolus geometry. Density curve for the aorta after injection of 50 to 70 ml of contrast medium (based on Claussen et al., ref. 138, 139). IT = injection time; TA = time of appearance; PT = peak time; Max. 1 = maximum contrast enhancement (CE) after first peak; Max. 2 = maximum CE after second peak (first recirculation).

Fig. 4-4. Bolus injection. Relative distribution of contrast medium (% dose) in intravascular spaces (V) and in easily accessible extracellular compartments (EC). The contrast medium concentration in both compartments equalizes within three minutes. A predominantly intravascular (A) contrast enhancement can be differentiated from parenchymal contrast enhancement (B) (analogue computer simulation, Schering AG).

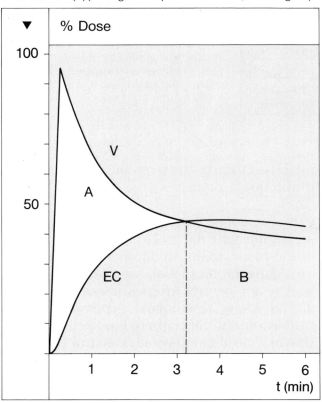

The above-mentioned pharmacodynamic and pharmacokinetic principles determine the behavior of contrast medium within *parenchymatous* organs:

The arteries of an organ and their branches are demonstrated as opaque-laden structures during the infusion phase.

Subsequent parenchymal enhancement homogeneously opacifies the parenchyma, and stromal structures within the parenchyma become visible.

Contrast enhancement is reduced by the influx of new blood, which eventually leaves the veins only weakly enhanced.

Even as contrast medium passes through the organ, it is being distributed from the capillaries to the interstitial tissues, so persistent residual enhancement occurs. When contrast medium is administered in a rapid high-dose bolus, a much weakened second peak occurs due to recirculation of the wave of contrast medium that was already widely distributed. Finally, generalized enhancement of the organ is seen. The attenuation of blood and the parenchyma is broadly equalized. The remaining vascular structures or lymph nodes outside the parenchymatous organs remain contrasted for a time span of approx. 10 minutes.

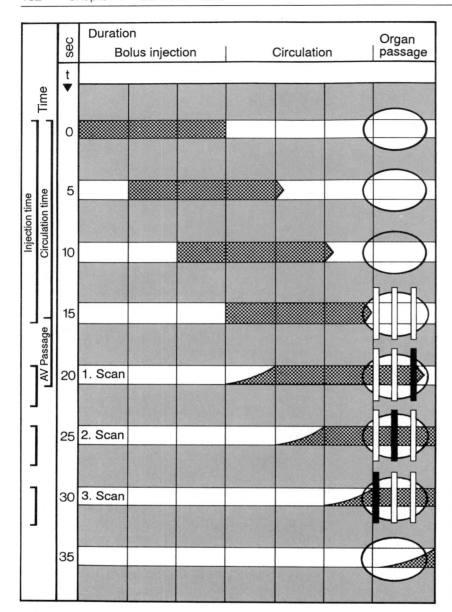

Fig. 4-5. Time sequence of targeted bo-lus injection. With an injection time of 15 seconds, it is possible to scan a series of 3 slices (scan intervals = 5 s) during the phase of maximum organ contrast enhancement. By lengthening the injection time, the dura-tion of contrast enhancement of the target organ is increased, and a larger number of slices can be scanned in the bolus phase (protracted bolus injection).

Intravenous Bolus Injection (CM Bolus)

An intravenous bolus injection of a sufficiently high dose of contrast medium will provide the high degree of contrast enhancement required for CT diagnosis. Various circulatory parameters must be maintained when this short-term contrast enhancement is to be utilized for diagnostic purposes. The actual CT examination should begin just after the wave of contrast medium has reached the target organ (Fig. 4-5). The time between the start of infusion and the start of scanning is termed the *preliminary circulation time*, and reflects the time it takes the blood to circulate from the site of injection to the target organ.

Circulation time is defined as the time required for the injected material to flow from one point in the bloodstream to another. In healthy individuals, the circulation time from the cubital vein to the central arteries (carotid, abdominal) is 13 to 22 seconds, depending on the cardiac output. Since there is a linear relationship of central blood volume to stroke volume, Schad's equation can be used to calculate the circulation time in terms of pulse beats when the heart rate is known (Table 4-1).

Table 4-1. Circulation time (t) in seconds. Pulse beats (n), according to Schad.

Arm – Right ventricle	4
Arm – Left ventricle	11
Arm – Thoracic aorta	12
Arm – Abdominal aorta	13
Arm – Brain	13
Arm – Iliac artery	15

with $t = n \frac{60}{f}$ [s]

f = heart rate [min^{-1}]

The overall *duration of the injection* determines the duration of the primary bolus phase, which is significantly lengthened by slow heart-lung passage, as described above. The bolus injection time (extended and sloped off) determines how long the target organ will be contrasted and thus determines the effective scanning time.

The *scan sequence time* is the time required to perform the bolus sequence. It must be at least as long as the injection time. The number of slices to be scanned should be determined beforehand. In patients with circulatory insufficiency, the bolus phase should be sloped off to create extended but weakened contrast enhancement.

● *Protracted Bolus Injection*[*]

The targeted bolus injection was originally designed to contrast single CT scans, each with scan times of 5 to 12 seconds that were separated by intervals of 20 to 40 seconds. Modern scanners have much shorter scan times (ca. 1 to 2 s) separated by intervals of 5 to 7 seconds or less. The protracted bolus injection (PBI) has therefore become widely accepted. In a PBI, contrast medium is injected at a steady rate of ca. 2 ml/s (1–3 ml/s). A scan sequence time of up to two minutes is therefore possible with a total dose of 100 to 150 ml. This method can

achieve intra-arterial enhancement of 120 to 180 HU, depending on the rate of injection. The more slices that can be scanned in this time period, the better the time-restricted enhancement of the bolus injection can be utilized. Rapid scanning programs (e.g. spiral CT) are, logically, the best means of utilizing bolus geometry and reducing the need for administering additional contrast medium.

● *Controlled Bolus Injection*

In scanners with instant image reconstruction, the intra-arterial enhancement can be checked on the monitor while the contrast medium is being injected. The injection rate can thus be interactively adjusted to achieve optimum contrast enhancement, thereby improving diagnostically important details about the investigated organ or region. Adjustments can be made for various circulatory parameters, and it is possible to immediately repeat bad slices (breathing errors, etc.).

● *Bolus Injection during Sequential CT*[*]

If the contrast behavior of an organ or organ lesion is to be assessed, a scan sequence should be made of that particular region. Scanning must be started quickly to secure at least one good plain scan as a reference scan (fixed table position). This means shortening the preliminary circulation period.

The slice sequence should be timed so that arterial contrast medium flooding, parenchymal contrast enhancement, wash-out, and venous contrast enhancement can be imaged in a single scan sequence. Most consoles also allow graphic representation of contrast behaviour as a time-density curve. It is recommended that contrast medium be injected by means of an automated, flow-controlled pressure pump to improve the reproducibility of measurements.

● *Methods of Administration*

It is essential that the patient understands the instructions of the radiology technician. Proper performance of breathing instructions is espe-

---

* dynamic incremental scan, extended bolus injection

* dynamic sequential scanning

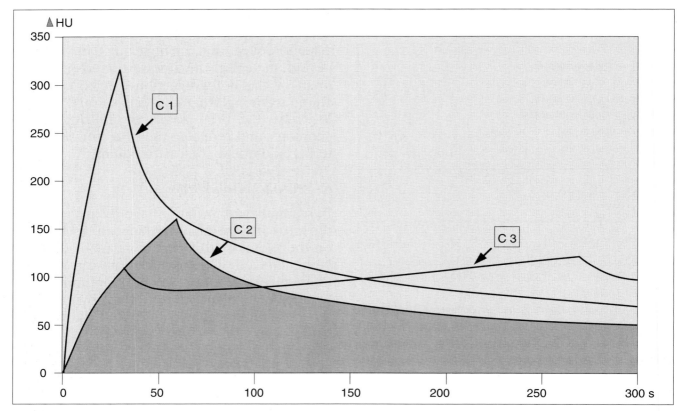

Fig. 4-6. Contrast enhancement of the aorta with different rates of injection.

C 1: Forced bolus injection at rate of 6 ml/s in 30 seconds (= 900 mg I/kg body weight).

C 2: Conventional protracted bolus injection at rate of 2 ml/s (= 600 mg I/kg body weight).

C 3: Bolus injection at rate of 2 ml/s within 30 seconds, followed by a rapid infusion at rate of 30 ml/min for 4 minutes (= 900 mg I/kg body weight).

A comparison of the curves shows that the forced bolus injection (C 1) improves vessel and organ contrast enhancement only in the first minute. The bolus-infusion technique (C 3) using an equally high dose of iodine (54 g) shows contrast enhancement, but this does not reach the maximum level achieved by means of the conventional bolus injection with a total of 36 g of iodine.

cially important. One may wish to practice them with the patient several times prior to the examination, because the success of a rapid scanning sequence depends on good cooperation between the patient and the radiologist. The region of interest (ROI) and number of slices to be scanned should be determined beforehand.

Rate of injection: 1 to 8 ml/s.

Duration of injection: approx. equal to the scan sequence time, i.e., the number of scans plus number of intervals between scans.

Dosage of contrast medium: 1.5 to 2 ml/kg body weight.

Intravenous Infusion

Infusions lack the dynamic component of bolus injections. The time required for sufficient contrast enhancement of vessels is primarily dependent upon the rate of infusion. With normal infusion rates of 25 ml/min, an adequate level of enhancement (ca. 75 HU) is achieved in 10 minutes. During this slow infusion of contrast medium, the distribution of contrast medium into the extracellular compartment and renal excretion of contrast medium counteract the increased blood concentration of contrast medium. Since modern CT scanners function with short scan times and intervals, the short enhancement phase provided by bolus injection can be better utilized. Therefore, more and more radiologists have abandoned the exclusive use of contrast medium infusions.

Infusion of contrast medium can only provide sufficient contrast enhancement of the organ parenchyma. Adjusting the infusion rate intensifies the difference in attenuation of the blood and the organ parenchyma only slightly. The excretory capacity of the kidney leads to stronger opacification of renal parenchyma, so this infusion technique is sufficient for identifying pathological processes there. The infusion technique is normally inadequate for a detailed analysis of internal structures of the kidney, such as the renal medulla and cortex. It is often advisable to administer an infusion of 30 ml CM/min after an initial bolus injection (see Fig. 4-6).

Intra-arterial Injection

CT examinations requiring intra-arterial contrast media are infrequent and reserved for special cases. The indications for CT hepatography are somewhat less infrequent.

• CT Hepatography

Arterial hepatographic CT (AHCT) is sometimes indicated for preoperative diagnosis of liver tumors. Contrast medium is selectively injected in the superior mesenteric artery and the splenic artery, which results in homogeneous and especially vivid contrast enhancement of liver tissue via the branches of the portal vein.

• Methods of Administration

An angiography catheter is inserted in the superior mesenteric artery and splenic artery before or after liver arteriography. A steady (automated) dose of 0.7 to 1 ml/s of contrast medium is administered during automated table movement. Depending on the time available for scanning, a total dose of 70 to 100 ml of contrast medium is administered for imaging the entire liver.

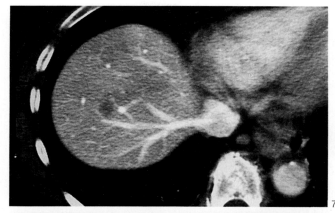
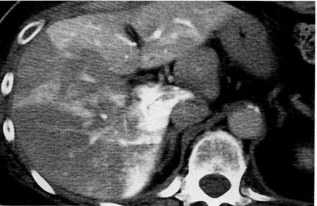

Fig. 4-7. CT portography. a) When portovenous contrast enhancement is uniform, even very small lesions (< 1 cm) can be detected. They appear hypodense.
b) Irregular, maplike contrast enhancement of the liver frequently occurs when contrast medium is injected into only one of the two vessels (splenic artery or superior mesenteric artery). This is due to laminar flow in the portal vein.

Biliary Contrast Media

Pharmacokinetics

Biliary contrast media are absorbed by liver cells and excreted into the bile ducts by active transport mechanisms. Factors that affect contrast enhancement of liver tissue include intracellular contrast media accumulation, intraluminal cholangiographic contrast media concentration, and the level of contrast media in blood in the interstitial compartment. Maximum enhancement is achieved 30 to 60 minutes after infusion or slow intravenous injection. The difference in attenuation value is only

10 to 15 HU and is thus insufficient; however, the attenuation contrast can be improved by additional urographic contrast media. Biliary contrast media are therefore used only in special cases to demonstrate the bile ducts.

● *Methods of Administration*

30 ml Biliscopin® (i.v.) is injected slowly (> 5 min; iodine dose: 5.4 g) or 100 ml is infused (iodine dose: 5.0 g). Rapid bolus injections are not performed because of severe side effects.

Intracavitary Opacification

The rules for intracavitary opacification are quite simple. Basically, the lumen of the bladder, subarachnoid space and digestive tract are considered to be closed compartments where contrast medium mixes with the corresponding fluids. Contrast medium normally does not pass through the intestinal wall or bladder wall. The dose and volume of distribution therefore determine the degree of opacification.
Urographic contrast media which contain *iodine* are predominantly used for intracavitary contrast opacification. Diluted *barium suspensions* or *water* (negative CM) may also be used to opacify the intestines.

Intestinal Opacification

The configuration and position of most sections of the digestive tract can be demonstrated on plain scans. However, the soft-tissue density of intestinal contents may render plain scans quite difficult to interpret. The duodenum, for example, may simulate an enlarged

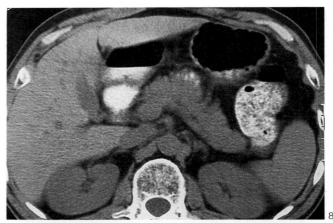

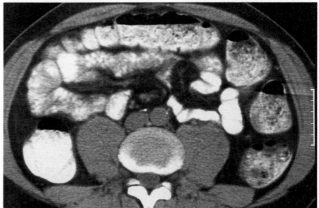

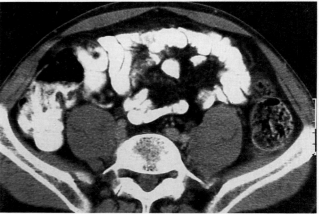

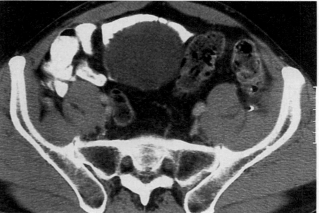

Fig. 4-8a-d. Contrast enhancement of the bowel after oral administration of diluted Gastrografin®. All sections of the small intestine show clear, detailed contrast enhancement after uniform, protracted contrast medium ingestion. The greater portion of the paracolic gutter is also filled with contrast medium.

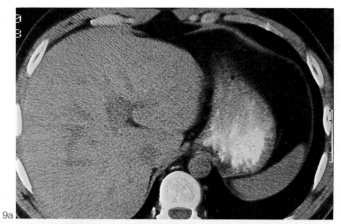

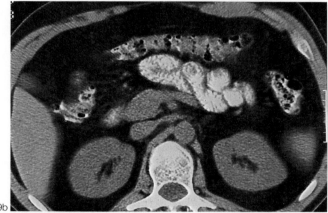

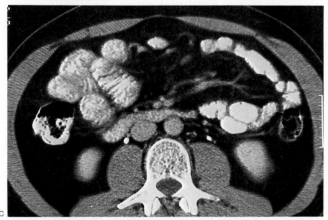

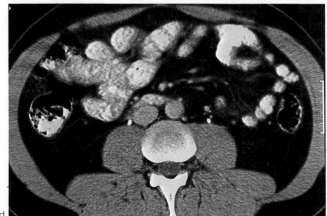

head of the pancreas, and the intestinal loops may mimic a mass in the tail of the pancreas or a lymphoma. Detailed evaluation of pelvic organs frequently becomes problematic. The use of oral intestinal contrast media was therefore quickly adopted as routine procedure. For epigastric diagnosis, especially for evaluation of the position of the pancreas, it is normally sufficient to opacify only the upper gastrointestinal tract to the proximal ileum with contrast medium. However, both the small and large bowel must also be opacified for precise diagnosis of the retroperitoneal space and pelvic organs.

Opacification of the intestinal lumen should be restricted to a certain range to avoid artifacts. Because of partial volume artifacts, a density of contrast of 150 to 200 HU is recommended for clear evaluation of the intestine. Since different scanners are variably sensitive in detecting iodine, it is not possible to make a general rule for contrast medium dilution. In practice, 2 to 4% Gastrografin® solutions have proven effective; the dilution can be adjusted according to individual experience. Density enhancement of more than 200 HU should be avoided, because excessive opacification could result. Especially in air-containing organs such as the stomach and intestine, slight movements might then cause severe artifacts.

The absorption physiology of the intestine determines how much opacification can be achieved. It is important that the patient drinks the contrast medium in small portions until just prior to the examination. When further doses of contrast medium are evenly distributed and ingested, uniform transport of contrast medium can be achieved throughout the gut. The patient should be turned to a right lateral position for better emptying of the stomach. Since intestinal passage of contrast medium is ex-

Fig. 4-9a-d. Contrast enhancement of the bowel after oral administration of diluted barium suspension. As compared to contrast enhancement with Gastrografin, there is no clear qualitative difference.

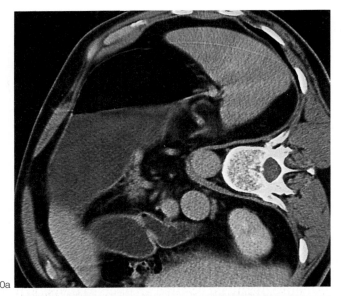

10a

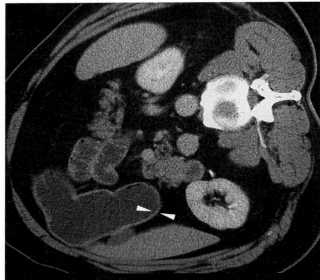

10b

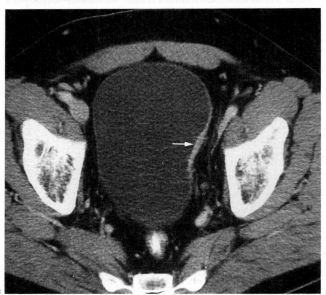

10c

tremely variable, the time required for optimum opacification (also of the rectum) cannot be reliably predicted. Especially for gynecological diagnosis of the true pelvis, it is advisable to administer an additional rectal dose of contrast medium. The rectal contrast medium should be of the same concentration as the oral Gastrografin®.

Barium suspensions are subject to the same physiological laws as oral iodine solutions. The usual contra-indications for barium opacification of the gastrointestinal tract apply.
For specific problems, some parts of the intestine (stomach, rectum, sigmoid) should be filled with *water* to achieve a negative contrast image. After a subsequent, intravenous bolus of contrast medium, a highly detailed, hyperdense image of the intestinal wall is seen.

• *Methods of Administration*

Partial Bowel Contrast (small bowel)

Approximately 500 ml of diluted Gastrografin® solution (3–5 vol.%) is ingested orally in equal portions until just prior to the examination. It is recommended that the patient be briefly turned to a right lateral position to improve the transport of contrast medium. For special diagnostic evaluation of the area near the head of the pancreas, the patient should be given an additional 100 ml of contrast medium solution while lying in the right lateral position on the CT table.

Fig. 4-10a, b. The gastric wall in CT scans after the stomach has been filled with water and enhanced with intravenous contrast medium. As compared with the gastric lumen and surrounding structures, it appears as a well-defined, homogeneous contrasted structure.

Fig. 4-10c. The wall of the urinary bladder after retrograde filling of the urinary bladder with saline solution and bolus contrast medium administration. When fully distended, delicate wall contours should be seen from a tangential view. Thickening of the bladder wall towards the lumen or surrounding organs should be easily detected.

Complete Bowel Contrast

The patient is given an oral dose of up to 1500 ml of diluted Gastrografin® solution (3–5 vol. %). Starting 60 minutes prior to the examination, the patient must slowly drink the solution in evenly distributed portions up until the beginning of the examination.

In patients with a colostomy, the small bowel should be partially opacified with a maximum of 1000 ml of diluted Gastrografin® solution.

Colon Contrast

Rectal administration: The patient receives an enema of 500 ml diluted Gastrografin® solution immediately prior to the examination.

Oral administration: The patient receives 3 × 2 doses of freshly prepared, diluted Gastrografin® with bulk-forming material 24 hours before the examination. Preparation: One half teaspoon of Gastrografin® and one tablespoon of bulk-forming material are mixed with ca. 250 ml water in a cup.

CT-Assisted Peritoneography

The method described by Dunnick can be used to evaluate intraperitoneal fluid distribution by adding contrast medium to hemodialysis solution (chemotherapeutic agents can be added for patients with peritoneal carcinomatosis).

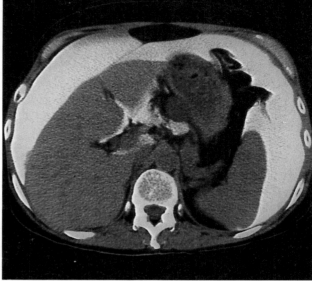

11a

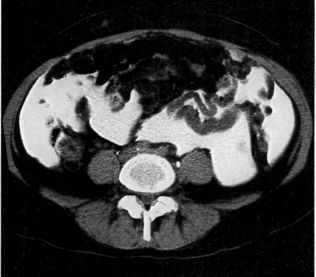

11b

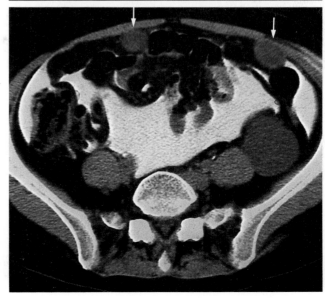

Fig. 4-11a-c. Peritoneography. The peritoneal cavity is brightly contrasted after contrast medium instillation. Communicating compartments are therefore visible. Encapsulated structures that are not reached by contrast medium and chemotherapeutic agents show absence of contrast enhancement (→).

11c

The diagnostic value of CT peritoneography is limited, however, so this examination technique is only seldom used. Approx. 40 ml of a 60% urographic contrast medium are added to each liter of instillation solution.

CT-Assisted Myelography

CT-assisted myelography is normally performed as a secondary examination subsequent to conventional myelography. Computed tomography of the questionable section of the vertebral column is performed 1 hour or, at most, 6 hours after the patient receives a normal dose of ca. 10 ml (7 to 15 ml) of myelographic agent containing 250 mgI/ml. A wide window setting can normally correct the high level of opacification observed in early postmyelographic CT scans without causing artifacts. This adjustment results in high image detail.

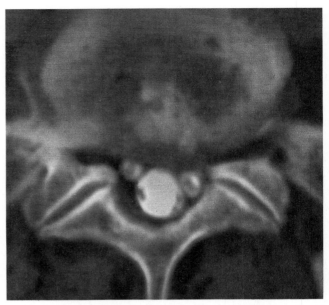

Fig. 4-12. CT myelography. After myelography, the thecal sac and its contents show contrast enhancement. The pockets of the nerves are also contrasted, so the nerve roots extending here are also visible as punctiform, hypodense structures.

Chapter 5
Techniques and Strategies of Examination

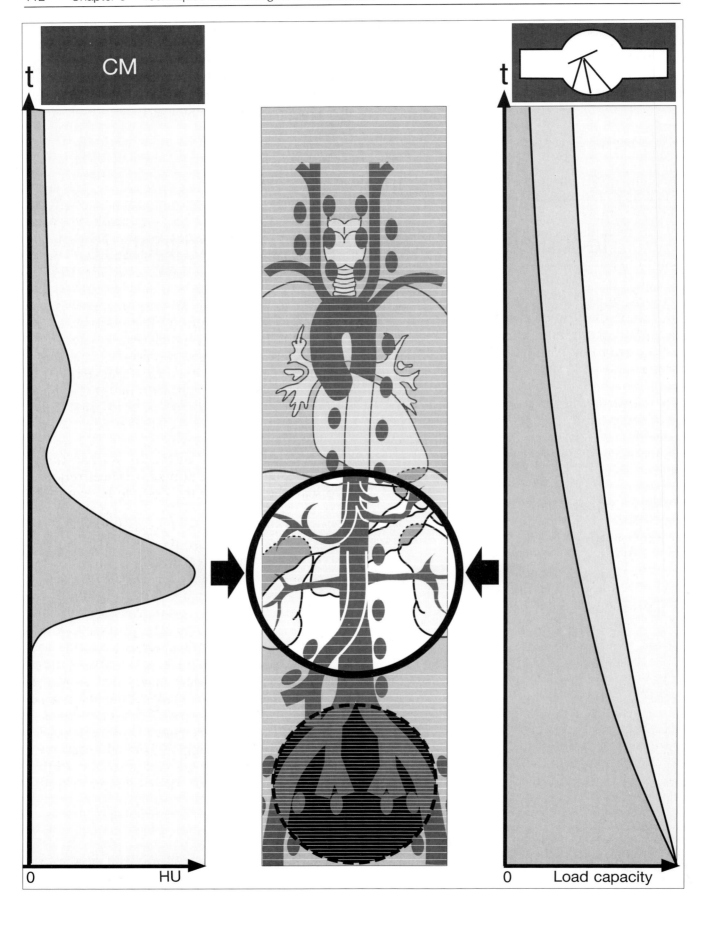

CM

t

0   HU

t

0   Load capacity

Techniques and Strategies of Examination

Diagnostic Procedures

The diagnostic strategy should be designed to answer all clinical questions as precisely as possible. For this purpose, all technical capabilities of the scanning system and pharmacokinetics of the contrast medium must be used intelligently. Any pathomorphologic signs should be demonstrated as precisely as possible. The pathomorphology of a disease process as well as the nature of its progress, routes of spread, and potential accompaniments must be anticipated if they are to be correctly identified and interpreted.

The *diagnostic methodology* is part of diagnostic strategy and includes patient *preparation*, selection of *examination parameters*, and *administration of contrast medium*.

Patient Preparation

Before starting an abdominal examination, preparation of the bowel with *oral contrast medium* is an essential prerequisite for exact diagnosis. Non-opaque loops of the bowel can simulate a mass or lymph node enlargement. Prior contrast medium preparation of the large intestine is also vitally important for the success of pelvic examinations, especially when attempting to diagnose gynecological problems.

Because new generation scanners now have very short scan times, it is no longer necessary to always administer intravenous *antiperistaltic agents* (e.g. Buscopan®, Glucagon®) for reduc-

---

Fig. 5-1. The kinetics of contrast medium as well as the load capacity of the X-ray tube determine the time course of a CT examination.

tion of motion artifacts due to peristalsis. However, if the scan time is long (> 2 s), antiperistaltic agents may improve the image quality. Such agents are still recommended for distension of hollow organs in which mural abnormalities are to be diagnosed.

Technical Parameters

• Slice Thickness

This determines the vertical resolution and, thus, the extent of partial volume averaging in the imaged organ structures. Border surfaces which pass diagonally through the slice (e.g. in the floor of the mouth or in the throat) become more sharply defined on CT images when the slice thickness is reduced. Structures that pass horizontally through the slice (e.g. the upper pole of the kidney near the capsule of the liver) can frequently be demonstrated only when thin sections are scanned, depending on the width of these spaces. The question of whether organ infiltration has occurred can often be answered only when thin-section scanning techniques are used. The selected slice thickness determines, at the same time, the number of slices required to scan the region of the body to be examined (scan sequence) as well as the total scan time. By making the intervals between the slices (table increment) larger than the slices themselves, the total scan time can be reduced, but pathological processes may remain hidden in the non-imaged regions. The slice thickness and interval must, therefore, correspond to the diagnostic expectations and problems which determine the overall examination strategy. Contiguous sections must be scanned when secondary image reconstruction (reformatting) is to be performed. On the other hand, a reduction in slice thickness will lead to increased noise if the radiation dose per slice is not increased correspondingly. The tube capacity determines whether the dose increase will increase the duration of stops (interscan times) between scans.

• Gantry Angulation

The gantry can be tilted for better demonstration of morphological border layers that lie at an angle to the axis of the body. Spaces (e.g. those of the intervertebral disc) can then be demonstrated without partial volume effects, and other border surfaces are intersected tangentially, yielding sharper images.

• *Scan Time*

Short scan times minimize motion artifacts, which can lead to considerable falsification of imaged structures and attenuation values in computed tomography. Short scan times additionally reduce the radiation dose but increase image noise. Since motion artifacts usually cause worse effects than noise (e.g. in the upper part of the liver), a reduction in contrast resolution is the more acceptable alternative. Good patient preparation (e.g. antiperistaltic agents) is also an important factor in reducing motion artifacts. The number of slices to be scanned determines the total scan (and interscan) time, which must be taken into consideration when planning intravenous bolus administration of contrast medium. This information is essential for optimum utilization of the bolus phase.

• *Radiation Dose*

The capacity of the X-ray tube limits the number of slices that can be scanned per unit time at the selected dose level. In other words, it determines the period in which the desired number of slices and spatial or contrast resolution must be coordinated. Depending on the slice thickness and size of the computer matrix, the selected dose per slice determines the degree of spatial and contrast resolution.

Administration of Contrast Medium

Sequential computed tomography (Serio-CT) can be performed only if the location of a lesion is known. This is usually performed as a supplemental examination and is a special type of parenchymal contrast enhancement. The sequential effects of contrast enhancement are demonstrated on a single slice (without table advance).

Parenchymatous contrast enhancement also requires prior knowledge of the target organ, because only a limited number of sections can be scanned in this method of time-restricted, bolus contrast enhancement. The target region is determined during a previously performed plain scan sequence.

The (subsequent) *persistent phase of intravascular contrast medium* is less critical, because its effects persist in the entire body for a long period of time if an adequate dose of contrast medium was administered. This technique is used to diagnose aneurysms as well as to differentiate vessels from lymph nodes of the same diameter.

Selection of Technical Parameters for Scans with and without Contrast Medium Enhancement

Determined by factors related to the individual diagnostic problem, whereby the following questions must be answered:

– Which region of the body is to be scanned? (Larger regions usually require larger slice intervals and thicknesses.)
– Which organ or lesion needs to be demonstrated particularly well? (Focusing.)
– Which border surfaces are diagnostically significant? (Selection of slice thickness, gantry angulation.)
– How much spatial resolution is needed to make a diagnosis, and how much is desirable? (High-contrast structures like the bone and lungs can be demonstrated well with thin sections, an appropriate matrix size, and short scan times.)
– How much contrast resolution is needed to demonstrate the suspected lesion? (The contrast resolution is improved with thicker slices, smaller matrices, and a higher radiation dose per slice.)
– Where is the overshadowing of artifacts so critical that they must be countered by reducing the scan time?

Technical parameters can be freely adjusted, as long as the necessary variation of scan time and scan interval can be supported by the scanner capacity. However, this freedom of selection is considerably limited with *bolus injections of contrast media*. In bolus administration of contrast medium, multiple organ sections must be scanned during parenchymatous contrast enhancement, i.e., in a relatively short period. The selection of technical parameters for contrast-enhanced scans must therefore fit in a tight time frame. These parameters can be set after the following questions have been answered:

– Which organ structures are of special diagnostic significance for optimum parenchymal contrast enhancement? (Plain scan images should be used to make this decision.)

– Which regions of the body can be demonstrated adequately with less complicated intravascular contrast enhancement? (It is of utmost importance that regions with poor scanning topography be determined beforehand on the basis of plain scan images.)

The answers to these question make up a list of desirable examination parameters which must be mutually compatible and fit within the given time frame. Several examination techniques have been developed from everyday practice.

Examination Strategies

• *Organ-Oriented Scanning*

This technique is used in cases with clearly organ-related problems (e.g. vertebral fracture, sternoclavicular dislocation). In most cases, computed tomography is performed as a supplement to other examinations. Plain scans alone will often suffice for diagnosis of high-contrast structures (e.g. classical objects of conventional tomography such as lungs and bones).

• *Organ-Oriented Scanning with Contrast Medium Bolus*

In most cases, especially in soft-tissues, intravenous contrast administration is required for more precise evaluation of an underlying pathological process. The diagnostically critical sections are selected on the basis of plain scan images. Scanning parameters such as slice thickness, intervals, and radiation dose can then be appropriately selected. Examples: soft-tissue tumors in the extremities, renal abscesses, adrenal tumors.

• *Evaluation of Spread*

When a pathological process is not restricted to one organ, the scan sequence must be extended to include an evaluation of spread (extent). The determination of extent is an important part of tumor evaluation (staging). The typical paths of spread, preferred organs of metastases, and the frequency of metastatic involvement must be considered in the diagnosis. This means that some parts of the body will be examined cursorily while others are investigated in detail. Continuous scanning is usually necessary for demonstration of inflammatory processes, due to the nature of spreading. A plain scan sequence can be used for localization purposes before a bolus series. When the presence of a tumor is known (lymphoma, testicular tumor), it may be possible to make the diagnosis on the basis of plain scan images when the paths of spread are then clearly visible.

• *Evaluation of Spread in Sequence with Contrast Medium Enhancement*

In most cases, an enhanced sequence (CM sequence) must be performed as a supplement to plain scans. Critical areas that are otherwise poorly demonstrated can be scanned in greater detail and sharpness. Contrast medium also makes it possible to distinguish lymph nodes from vascular structures (vessel contrast) and to identify infiltration (enhancement of border surfaces). In regions that are generally difficult to demonstrate (e.g. the neck), a primary contrast medium sequence with a protracted bolus injection of contrast medium can make plain scans superfluous.

• *Evaluation of Adjacent Structures*

An evaluation of adjacent structures can be called an extended organ-oriented examination or an abbreviated evaluation of spread. Spreading is evaluated in the immediate vicinity of the process, and is demonstrated in plain and/or an enhanced sequence.

• *Screening (orientational scans)*

Screening may be necessary as a non-targeted examination in a particular region of the body when ultrasound examinations provide poor results due to poor access (air) or when the transducer could not be used because of post-operative wound dressings etc., or when the patient has severe pain on pressure. Screening may also be performed when the results of ultrasound were negative, but general clinical symptoms are still indicative of a pathological (consumptive) process. When the screening examination reveals abnormalities, scanning can be continued as an organ-oriented examination or for evaluation of spread.

Interventional Computed Tomography

CT-Guided Biopsy

This provides highly detailed images of organ structures in the CT section and allows for precise localization of a lesion in its surroundings. The access route can be set on a transverse plane in such a way that critical structures such as vessels, nerves and intestine will not be injured.

All biopsy procedures are basically the same. After localization of the structure to be punctured, the approach is determined and the

Fig. 5-2. CT-guided lung biopsy. With the patient lying in the prone position, the pulmonary nodule is localized, the angle and length of the access route are determined, and the puncture needle is inserted. Small-caliber cut-biopsy needles and tru-cut systems may be used.

Fig. 5-3. CT-guided biopsy in vertebral and paravertebral spaces. Here, also, one uses the same basic procedure:
1. Localization of the lesion.
2. Determination of the approach.
3. Insertion of the puncture needle parallel to the selected sectional plane.
a) Biopsy of a tumor of the erector spinae muscle.
b) Puncture of a paravertebral (tuberculous) abscess for bacteriological testing.

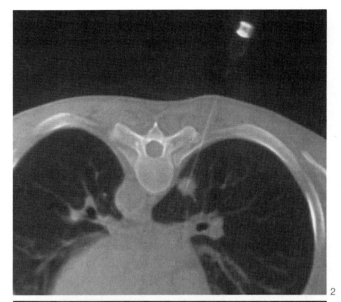
2

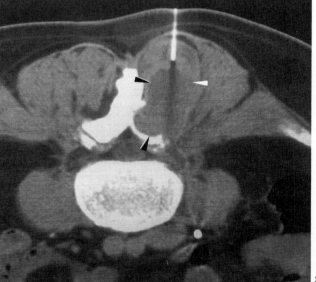
3a

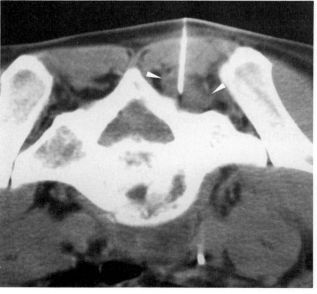
3b

puncture spot is marked on the skin. This can be verified on the CT monitor (e.g. with a Plexiglas rod). Distance and angle measurements from CT images provide precise information about the puncture depth and angle of the needle. Local anesthesia is administered, and the puncture needle (which should have a scale) is inserted in the direction of the focus. The direction of the needle is checked by CT. Tissue samples are removed after the needle has reached the lesion.

Exact position control is possible only if the direction of puncture is parallel to the plane of the section. Combined computed tomographic and X-ray techniques can be used to perform craniocaudal, angular punctures.

Contraindications to CT-guided biopsy are blood-clotting disorders (e.g. anticoagulant therapy) in patients with Quick test results of under 50 percent. Complications such are hematomas and nerve injuries rarely develop if conventional biopsy needles in sizes of 16 to 20 G are used. Pneumothorax (after lung biopsy) or damage in the costophrenic recess develops in 10 to 15% of all cases, so proper caution should be used.

Abscess Drainage

The advantages of CT-guided puncture can also be implemented for abscess drainage. Drainage sets available today facilitate the positioning of the drainage catheter by means of the Seldinger technique.

For further information, see Seibel, R.M.M., Grönemeyer, D.H.W. (eds.): Interventional Computed Tomography, Blackwell Scientific Publications, 1990.

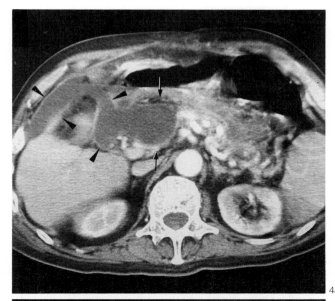
4a

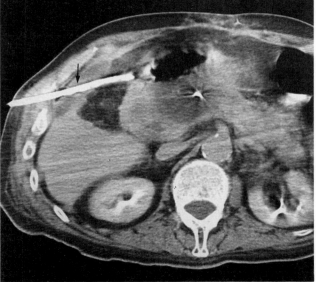
4b

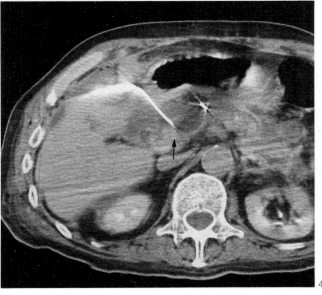
4c

Fig. 5-4. CT-guided abscess drainage. Here, a subhepatic abscess (►) is found to be infiltrating the bed of the pancreas (→) after cholecystectomy (a). After a trocar (b→) has been guided to the abscess, a wide-caliber pigtail catheter is inserted via the trocar into the bed of the pancreas (c→). Cachetic patients will recover quickly if the wound is irrigated daily. After 14 days of treatment, the abscess should no longer be demonstrable.

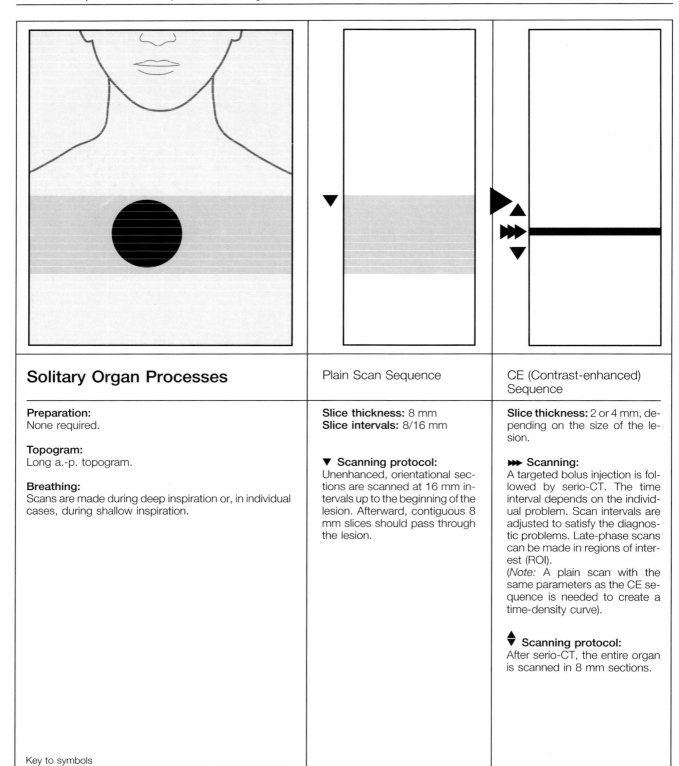

Solitary Organ Processes

Preparation:
None required.

Topogram:
Long a.-p. topogram.

Breathing:
Scans are made during deep inspiration or, in individual cases, during shallow inspiration.

Key to symbols

▼	Obligatory scanning protocol Scanning begins in direction of arrow
▽	Optional scanning protocol Scanning begins in direction of arrow
▶▶	Sequential CT (Serio-CT)
▶	Obligatory scanning protocol (slice level); determined by findings in plain scans

Plain Scan Sequence

Slice thickness: 8 mm
Slice intervals: 8/16 mm

▼ Scanning protocol:
Unenhanced, orientational sections are scanned at 16 mm intervals up to the beginning of the lesion. Afterward, contiguous 8 mm slices should pass through the lesion.

CE (Contrast-enhanced) Sequence

Slice thickness: 2 or 4 mm, depending on the size of the lesion.

▶▶ Scanning:
A targeted bolus injection is followed by serio-CT. The time interval depends on the individual problem. Scan intervals are adjusted to satisfy the diagnostic problems. Late-phase scans can be made in regions of interest (ROI).
(*Note:* A plain scan with the same parameters as the CE sequence is needed to create a time-density curve).

▼ Scanning protocol:
After serio-CT, the entire organ is scanned in 8 mm sections.

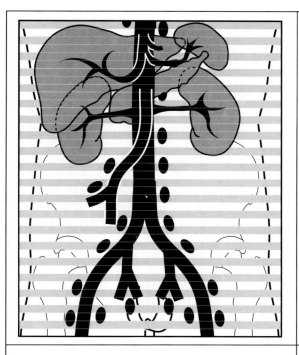

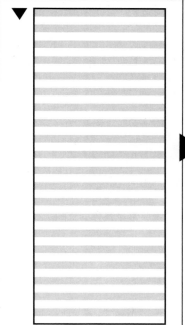

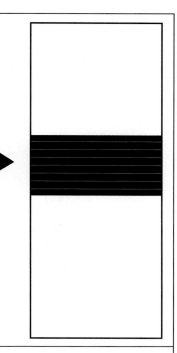

Orientational (Scout) Examination

Oral contrast medium administration:
If possible, 1000–1500 ml of diluted Gastrografin® should be administered for complete contrast enhancement of the bowel.

Antiperistaltic agents:
30 mg Buscopan® i.v. or 1–2 mg Glucagon® i.v. to counteract artifacts due to peristalsis.

Breathing:
Scans should be made during deep inspiration or, if not otherwise possible, during shallow inspiration.

Topogram:
Long a.-p. topogram.

An orientational CT examination should be performed when clinical tests or sonographic findings were not helpful. Plain scan findings are only as definitive as the condition of the patient and the quality of patient preparation allows. These findings determine whether and in which regions of the body a contrast-enhanced sequence (contrast medium bolus) should be performed.

Key to symbols

▼ Obligatory scanning protocol
Scanning begins in direction of arrow
▽ Optional scanning protocol
Scanning begins in direction of arrow
▸▸▸ Sequential CT (Serio-CT)
▶ Obligatory scanning protocol (slice level);
determined by findings in plain scans

Plain Scan Sequence

Slice thickness: 8 mm
Slice intervals: 16 mm

▼ **Scanning protocol:**
Beginning in the abdomen, from the diaphragm to the symphysis.

CE Sequence

Slice thickness: 8 mm
Slice intervals: 8 mm

▶ **Scanning protocol:**
Determined by findings in plain scans.

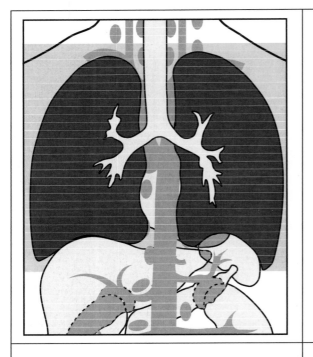

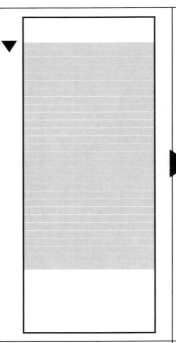

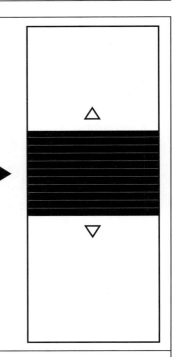

Chest-CT

Preparation:
None required.

Topogram:
Long a.-p. topogram (from base of skull to liver).

Breathing:
Scans are made during deep inspiration.

Window settings:
Soft tissue window 35 ± 175 HU
Lung window -900 ± 400 HU
Pleural window -50 ±1000 HU

Plain Scan Sequence

Slice thickness: 8 mm
Slice intervals: 8 mm

▼ **Scanning protocol:**
Scanning proceeds from the attachment of the diaphragm to 2 cm above the jugular vein.

If demonstration of the central bronchial tree or hilum is poor, the **slice thickness** should be reduced to 4 mm.

CE Sequence

Slice thickness: 8 mm
Slice intervals: 8 mm

▶ **Scanning protocol:**

Scanning proceeds mostly caudocranial. For better differentiation of structures, the hilar region as well as localized pathological processes in the thorax should be scanned in the relatively early bolus phase.

Structural Lung Disease

Fibrosis, Asbestosis, Sarcoidosis etc.

Additional scanning techniques include

High-resolution CT (HRCT):

5 – 10 thin sections
Slice thickness: 1 mm, in representative areas of the lung (e.g. 2 in upper fields, 5 in the hilar region, 3 in lower fields).

Image reconstruction with "bony" algorithm and zooming.

CE sequence is not advisable.

Key to symbols

▼	Obligatory scanning protocol Scanning begins in direction of arrow
▽	Optional scanning protocol Scanning begins in direction of arrow
▶▶▶	Sequential CT (Serio-CT)
▶	Obligatory scanning protocol (slice level); determined by findings in plain scans

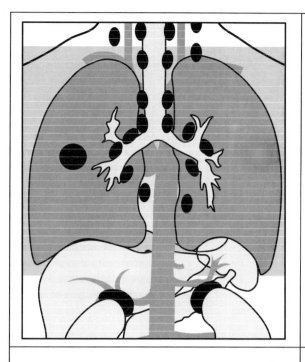 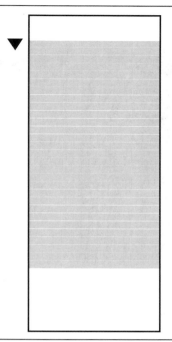 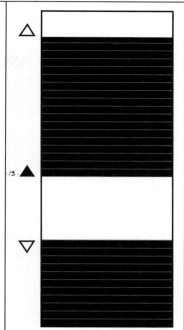

	Plain Scan Sequence	CE Sequence

Bronchial Carcinoma

Plain scans are used to determine local spread of peripheral bronchial carcinoma (BC) and for evaluation of the overall situation in centralized BC (lung collapse, effusion, enlarged lymph nodes). A bolus of contrast medium will provide further differentiation; the paths of mediastinal lymphatics must be demonstrated in detail.

Plain Scan Sequence

Slice thickness: 8 mm
Slice intervals: 8 mm

▼ **Scanning protocol:**
Scanning proceeds from the attachment of the diaphragm to 2 cm above the jugulum.

For peripheral BC, thin sections should be scanned for better evaluation of pleural invasion. For central BC, for precise demonstration of the bronchial tree and hilium:
Slice thickness: 4 mm.

CE Sequence

Slice thickness: 8 mm
Slice intervals: 8 mm

Scanning protocol:
▲ Scanning proceeds craniocaudal, from below the hilum to the jugulum (if retrocardial findings are normal).

▽ To be performed for confirmation of tentative diagnosis of BC via CT demonstration of the adrenals (typical location of blood-borne metastases).

Evaluation of Tumor Spread in the Cervical Region (Combined Chest and Neck Examination):

Examination is continued after the arms have been taken from behind the head (crossed) and placed at the sides of the body.

Slice thickness: 8 mm
Slice intervals: 8 mm

△ **Scanning protocol:**
Extended scanning, proceeding from the jugular vein to the base of the skull. Performed after additional administration of ca. 100 ml contrast medium.

Key to symbols

▼	Obligatory scanning protocol Scanning begins in direction of arrow
▽	Optional scanning protocol Scanning begins in direction of arrow
▶▶▶	Sequential CT (Serio-CT)
▶	Obligatory scanning protocol (slice level); determined by findings in plain scans

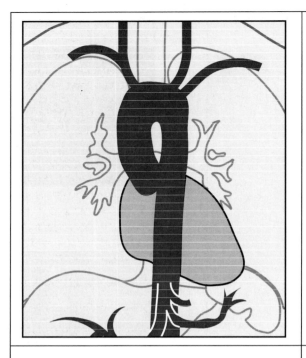

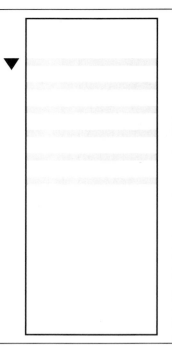

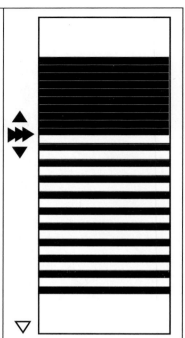

Thoracic Aorta

Preparation:
None required.

Breathing:
Scans are made during deep inspiration.

Plain Scan Sequence

Slice thickness: 8 mm
Slice intervals: 8/16 mm

▼ Scanning protocol:
Scanning proceeds from the arch to the root of the aorta for detection of hyperdense regions indicative of hemorrhage.

CE Sequence

Slice thickness: 8 mm
Slice intervals: 0/8/16 mm

Scanning:
▶▶▶ First, several images of the root of the aorta and descending aorta are obtained without table increment (serio-CT) for detection of a double lumen in the early contrast medium phase.

▲ Scanning then proceeds craniocaudal, covering the aorta in contiguous slices up to the origins of vessels branching from the aortic arch.

▼ Next, sections of the descending aorta are scanned proceeding craniocaudal below in serio-CT scan level at intervals of 16 mm.

▽ The abdominal aorta may also be scanned for detection of caudal spread.

Key to symbols

▼	Obligatory scanning protocol Scanning begins in direction of arrow
▽	Optional scanning protocol Scanning begins in direction of arrow
▶▶▶	Sequential CT (Serio-CT)
▶	Obligatory scanning protocol (slice level); determined by findings in plain scans

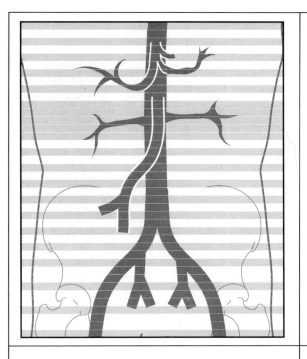

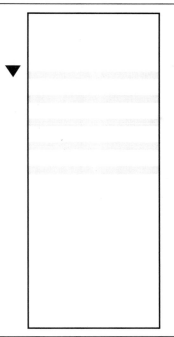

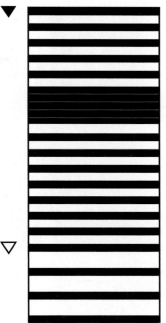

Abdominal Aorta

Preparation:
None required.

Antiperistaltic agents:
30 mg Buscopan® i.v. or 1–2 mg Glucagon® i.v. to prevent artifacts due to peristalsis.

Breathig:
Scans are made during deep inspiration.

Topogram:
Long a.-p. topogram.

Plain Scan Sequence

Slice thickness: 8 mm
Slice intervals: 8/16 mm

▼ **Scanning protocol:**
Scanning begins in the middle of the liver. Branches of the renal arteries should be evaluated in contiguous sections. Further caudal, intervals should be increased to 16 mm, proceeding down to the aortic bifurcation.

CE Sequence

Slice thickness: 8 mm
Slice intervals: 8/16 mm

▼ **Scanning protocol:**
A bolus of contrast medium is administered to demonstrate any aneurysms, also in branches of the renal artery.

▽ The examination may be extended for detection of aneurysms in pelvic arteries.

Key to symbols

▼	Obligatory scanning protocol Scanning begins in direction of arrow
▽	Optional scanning protocol Scanning begins in direction of arrow
▶▶▶	Sequential CT (Serio-CT)
▶	Obligatory scanning protocol (slice level); determined by findings in plain scans

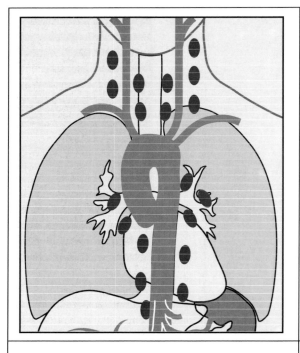

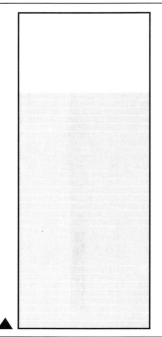

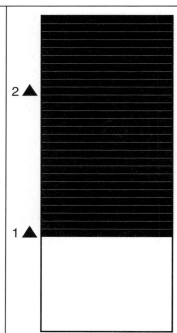

Staging of Thoracic (and Cervical) Lymph Nodes

Preparation:
None required.

Topogram:
Long a.-p. topogram (from base of skull to liver).

Breathing:
Scans are made during deep inspiration.

Window settings:
Soft tissue window 35 ± 175 HU
Lung window −900 ± 400 HU
Pleural window −50 ± 2000 HU

Key to symbols

▼   Obligatory scanning protocol
     Scanning begins in direction of arrow
▽   Optional scanning protocol
     Scanning begins in direction of arrow
▶▶▶ Sequential CT (Serio-CT)
▶   Obligatory scanning protocol (slice level);
     determined by findings in plain scans

Plain Scan Sequence

Slice thickness: 8 mm
Slice intervals: 8 mm

▲ **Scanning protocol:**
Scanning proceeds from attachment of the diaphragm to 2 cm above the jugulum.

CE Sequence

Slice thickness: 8 mm
Slice intervals: 8 mm

Scanning protocol:
1▲ Mostly caudocranial scanning direction. For better differentiation, the hilar region should be scanned in the relatively early bolus phase, as should a localized pathological process in the chest.

2▲ After repositioning the arms from behind the head to the sides of the body, the cervical region is scanned after an additional, protracted bolus injection of 100 ml contrast medium.

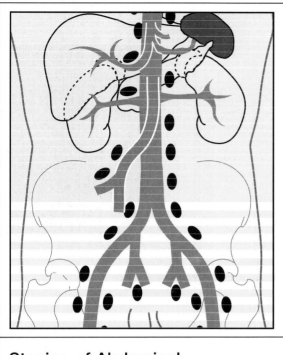

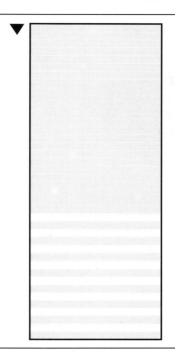

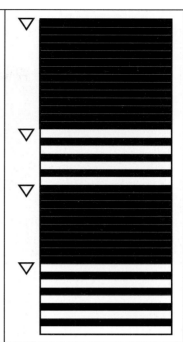

Staging of Abdominal Lymph Nodes	Plain Scan Sequence	CE Sequence
The bowel should be completely and uniformly enhanced. **Oral contrast medium administration:** 1000–1500 ml of diluted Gastrografin® is administered for complete enhancement of the bowel. **Rectal contrast medium administration:** 1000 ml diluted Gastrografin® solution may be administered in an enema directly prior to the examination only as required. **Antiperistaltic agents:** 30 mg Buscopan® i.v. or 1–2 mg Glucagon® i.v. to prevent artifacts due to peristalsis. **Topogram:** Long a.-p. topogram.	**Slice thickness:** 8 mm **Slice intervals:** 8/16 mm ▼ **Scanning protocol:** Sections are scanned with 8 mm intervals, from the diaphragm to the pelvic inlet. In more caudal locations, intervals are increased to 16 mm; scans extend to the symphysis. However, contiguous slices should also be scanned if abnormalities are found.	**Slice thickness:** 8 mm **Slice intervals:** 8/16/24 mm ▽ **Scanning protocol:** A bolus injection of contrast medium is administered primarily for better differentiation of lymph node structures, especially against vessels. Critical regions include the aortic bifurcation, internal iliac structures, mesenteric attachment, pancreatic region, and porta hepatis. The CE scanning protocol must be adjusted accordingly.
Malignant Lymphoma	Same as above.	The spleen should be evaluated in the early bolus phase for more sensitive detection of parenchymal lesions.
Testicular Tumors	**Slice thickness:** 8 mm **Slice intervals:** 8/16 mm ▼ **Scanning protocol:** The entire region from the diaphragm to the bottom of the aortic bifurcation should be demonstrated in contiguous slices. Larger intervals can be made in the pelvis.	Same as above. ▽ **Scanning protocol:** When investigating testicular tumors, the renal pedicles, retropancreatic region and aortic bifurcation must be examined carefully. Intrapelvic lymph node involvement in early tumor stages is improbable.

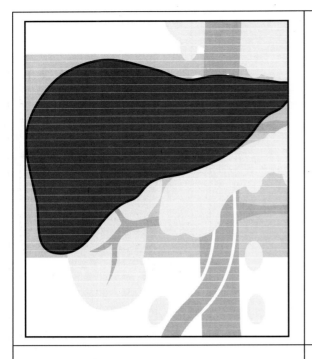

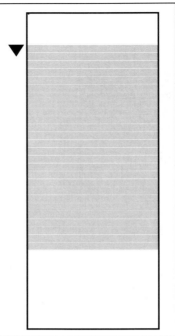

Liver CT

Preparation:
None required. When pathological processes are found in the left lobe of the liver, it is advisable to give the patient one cup of water and scan in 30° RAO to minimize artifacts.

Patient instruction:
In order to prevent motion artifacts around the dome of the liver, the patient must fully understand the breathing instructions.

Antiperistaltic agents:
30 mg Buscopan® i.v. or 1–2 mg Glucagon® i.v. to prevent artifacts due to peristalsis.

Evaluation:
Plain scans should be made at narrow window settings (35 ± 75 HU).

Key to symbols

▼   Obligatory scanning protocol
     Scanning begins in direction of arrow
▽   Optional scanning protocol
     Scanning begins in direction of arrow
▶▶▶ Sequential CT (Serio-CT)
▶   Obligatory scanning protocol (slice level);
     determined by findings in plain scans

Plain Scan Sequence

Slice thickness: 8 mm
Slice intervals: 8 mm

▼ **Scanning protocol:**
Scanning proceeds craniocaudal, from the dome of the liver to the bottom of the right lobe of the liver.

CE Sequence

Slice thickness: 8 mm
Slice intervals: 8 mm

▼ **Scanning protocol:**
The bolus scanning sequence is started in suspicious areas that were detected on plain scans. The sequence should be finished as quickly as possible (e.g. spiral CT; table increment).

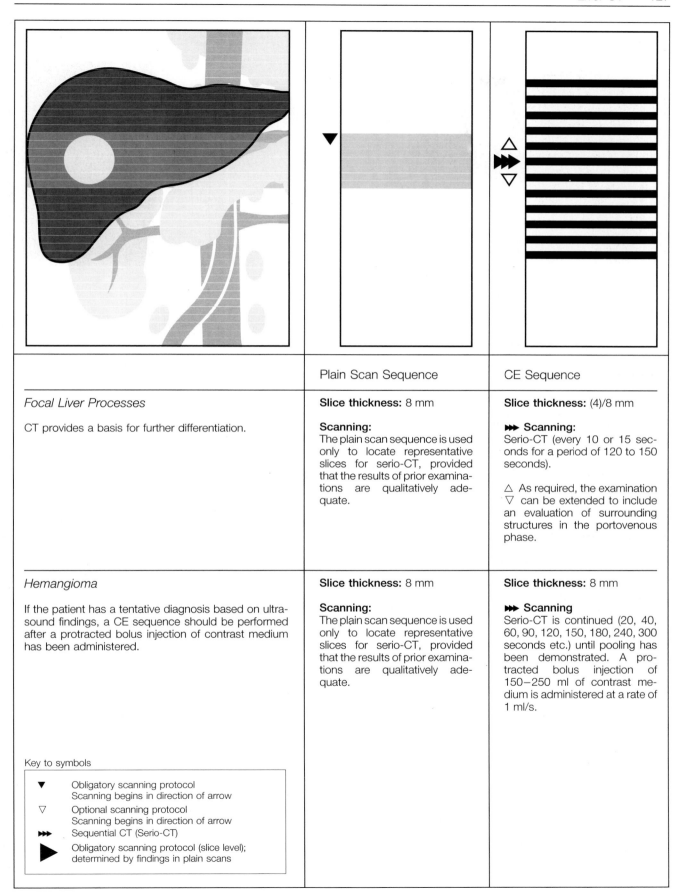

	Plain Scan Sequence	CE Sequence
Focal Liver Processes CT provides a basis for further differentiation.	**Slice thickness:** 8 mm **Scanning:** The plain scan sequence is used only to locate representative slices for serio-CT, provided that the results of prior examinations are qualitatively adequate.	**Slice thickness:** (4)/8 mm ▶▶ **Scanning:** Serio-CT (every 10 or 15 seconds for a period of 120 to 150 seconds). △ As required, the examination ▽ can be extended to include an evaluation of surrounding structures in the portovenous phase.
Hemangioma If the patient has a tentative diagnosis based on ultrasound findings, a CE sequence should be performed after a protracted bolus injection of contrast medium has been administered.	**Slice thickness:** 8 mm **Scanning:** The plain scan sequence is used only to locate representative slices for serio-CT, provided that the results of prior examinations are qualitatively adequate.	**Slice thickness:** 8 mm ▶▶ **Scanning** Serio-CT is continued (20, 40, 60, 90, 120, 150, 180, 240, 300 seconds etc.) until pooling has been demonstrated. A protracted bolus injection of 150–250 ml of contrast medium is administered at a rate of 1 ml/s.

Key to symbols

▼	Obligatory scanning protocol Scanning begins in direction of arrow
▽	Optional scanning protocol Scanning begins in direction of arrow
▶▶	Sequential CT (Serio-CT)
▶	Obligatory scanning protocol (slice level); determined by findings in plain scans

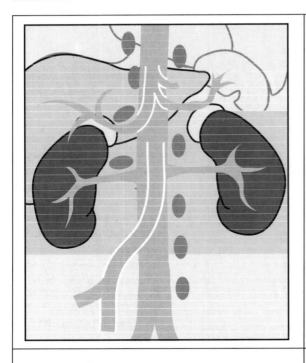
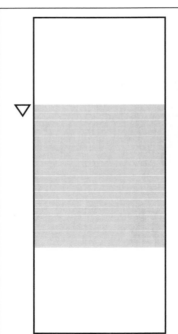
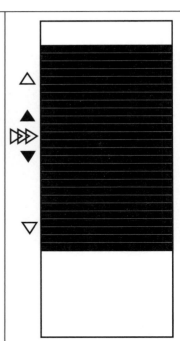

Kidney CT

Oral contrast medium administration:
500 ml diluted Gastrografin® is administered for partial opacification of the bowel, especially in nephrectomized patients.

Antiperistaltic agents:
30 mg Buscopan® i.v. or 1–2 mg Glucagon® i.v. to prevent artifacts due to peristalsis.

Breathing:
Scans are made during deep inspiration.

Plain scans:
Required for demonstration of calcareous structures, calculi and fresh hematomas.

Plain Scan Sequence

Slice thickness: 8 mm
Slice intervals: 8 mm

▽ **Scanning protocol:**
Contiguous slices proceeding craniocaudal are scanned through both kidneys. If necessary, scout sections can be scanned to evaluate neighboring structures.

CE Sequence

Slice thickness: 8 mm
Slice intervals: 8 mm

Scanning protocol:
▷▷▷ Scanning of localized lesions identified on plain scans begins with serio-CT.

▼ One minute later, the remaining sections of the kidney are scanned in contiguous slices.

△ Depending on the pathologi-
▽ cal process, the examination may be extended to include adjacent structures, e. g. extended craniocaudal to diagnose involvement of the liver. Post-contrast scans of the renal collecting system can be obtained later, if necessary, for better demonstration of intrapelvic masses.

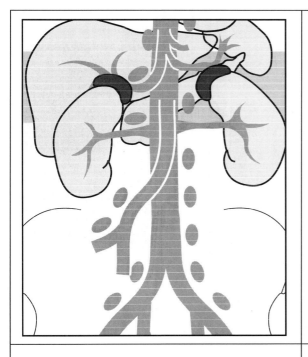

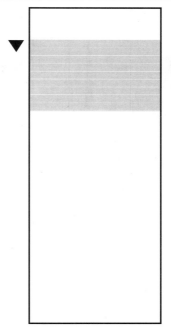

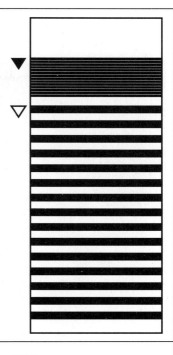

Adrenals

Preparation:
None required.

Antiperistaltic agents:
30 mg Buscopan® i.v. or 1–2 mg Glucagon® i.v. to prevent artifacts due to peristalsis.

Breathing:
Scans are made during deep inspiration.

Pheochromocytoma

When scanning to confirm a tentative diagnosis, 500 ml of diluted Gastrografin® should administered orally for partial bowel contrast.

Plain Scan Sequence

Slice thickness: 8 mm
Slice intervals: 8 mm

▼ **Scanning protocol:**
Scanning proceeds craniocaudal, from the attachment of the diaphragm to the middle of the left kidney.

CE Sequence

Slice thickness: 4 mm
Slice intervals: 4 mm

▼ **Scanning protocol:**
A targeted bolus injection of contrast medium is administered to the adrenals. The kidneys are then demonstrated in contiguous 8 mm sections.

Same as above.

▽ **Scanning protocol:**
When adrenal findings are negative, the para-aortic region is scanned down to the aortic bifurcation to find any phenochromocytomas in possibly extra-adrenal locations.

Key to symbols

▼	Obligatory scanning protocol Scanning begins in direction of arrow
▽	Optional scanning protocol Scanning begins in direction of arrow
▶▶▶	Sequential CT (Serio-CT)
▶	Obligatory scanning protocol (slice level); determined by findings in plain scans

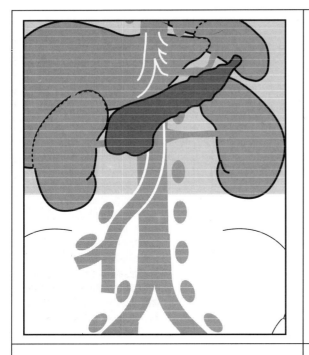

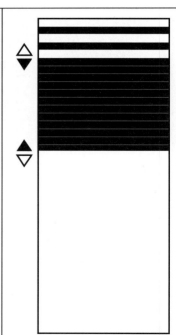

Pancreas-CT

Oral contrast medium administration:
500 ml diluted Gastrografin® is administered for partial opacification of the bowel. Directly prior to the examination, the patient should drink the solution while lying in a right lateral position (on the CT table).

Antiperistaltic agents:
30 mg Buscopan® i.v. or 1–2 mg Glucagon® i.v.

Breathing:
Scans are made during deep inspiration.

Patient positioning:
It may help to place the patient in a right lateral position when dealing with problematic processes in the head of the pancreas.

Evaluation:
Zooming is recommended for focal processes in the head of the pancreas.

Pancreatitis

Oral contrast medium administration can be omitted in severe cases.

Plain Scan Sequence

Slice thickness: 8 mm
Slice intervals: 8 mm

▼ **Scanning protocol:**
Scanning proceeds craniocaudal, from the attachment of the diaphragm to the bottom of the right renal pedicle. For problematic processes in the head of the pancreas, the patient may be placed in a right lateral position.

Slice thickness: 8 mm
Slice intervals: 16 mm

Scanning protocol:
An orientational (scout) scan sequence is performed to determine the extent of spread.

CE Sequence

Slice thickness: 8 mm
Slice intervals: 4/8 mm

Scanning protocol:
▲ After the extend of spread has been determined with plain scans, the corresponding sections of the pancreas are scanned during the early bolus phase. As required, localized pathological changes may be scanned in 4 mm sections.

△ In order to determine its involvement, the liver (including the porta hepatis) is scanned during the late bolus phase.

Slice thickness: 8 mm
Slice intervals: 8/16/24 mm

Scanning protocols:
▼ After the bolus injection of contrast medium has arrived in the bed of the pancreas, vital pancreatic tissue is demonstrated in contiguous scan slices.

▽ Depending on the degree of exudative spread, the slice intervals can be broadened for demonstration of the borders of the pathological process.

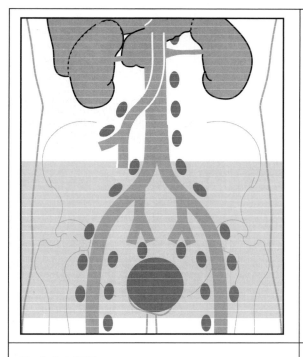
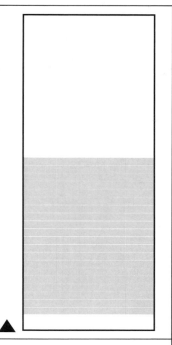
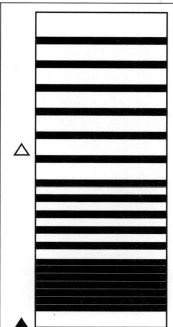

Pelvic CT

	Plain Scan Sequence	CE Sequence

Oral contrast medium administration:
1000–1500 ml diluted Gastrografin® solution for complete bowel enhancement.

Rectal contrast medium administration:
(Especially important for gynecological problems). 1000 ml diluted Gastrografin® solution is administered directly prior to the CT examination.

Breathing:
Scans are obtained during shallow inspiration.

Antiperistaltic agents:
30 mg Buscopan® i.v. or 1–2 mg Glucagon® i.v. to prevent artifacts due to peristalsis.

Plain Scan Sequence

Slice thickness: 8 mm
Slice intervals: 8 mm

▲ **Scanning protocol:**
Scanning proceeds caudocranial, from the symphysis to the aortic bifurcation.

CE Sequence

Slices thickness: 8 mm
Slices intervals: 8/16 mm

Scanning protocol:
▲ The target organ is scanned in contiguous sections, subsequently in 16 mm intervals, up to the aortic bifurcation. When the veins of the pelvis show poor contrast enhancement, an additional dose of contrast medium should be administered for evaluation of critical structures.

△ When there is extensive malignant growth in the pelvis, the region from the retroperitoneal space to the upper pole of the kidney should also be scanned.

Urinary Bladder:

The bladder should be fully distended. A catheter is inserted and physiological saline solution is infused (retrograde filling) until the patient reports bladder pressure.

Same as above.

Slice thickness: 4 mm
Slice intervals: 4/8 mm

▲ **Scanning protocol:**
When the borders of the bladder are curved and cannot be intersected tangentially, thin sections should be scanned.

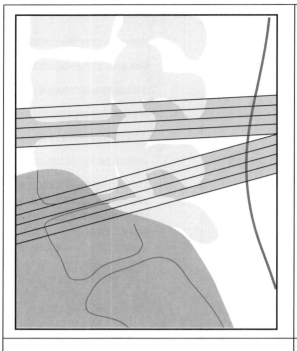

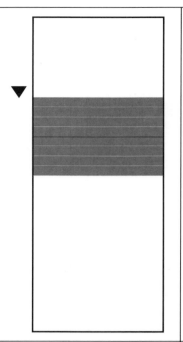

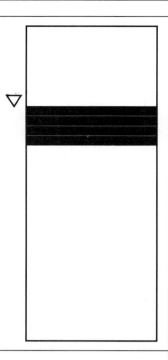

Spinal CT	Plain Scan Sequence	CE Sequence

Spinal CT

Preparation:
Patient preparation is not necessary. X-rays of the lumbar spine are required for correct evaluation of the lumbar spine and evaluation of segmental anomalies.

Patient positioning:
The patient should be placed in a dorsal position. To compensate for lumbar spine lordosis and to minimize muscle strain, the calves are elevated with cushions.

Topogram:
Long lateral topogram.

Scanning plane:
As a rule, the scanning plane is parallel to the space of the disk. If it becomes clear in the topogram that the angle of the space of the disk (e. g. L5/S1) is more than 25°, the patient's buttocks should be elevated accordingly.
The number of disk spaces to be examined is determined by the clinical findings. Clinically suspicious, adjacent segments should also be routinely evaluated.

Plain Scan Sequence

Lumbar spine:
Slice thickness: 4 mm
Slice intervals: 4 mm

Cervical spine:
Slice thickness: 2 (1) mm
Slice intervals: 2 mm

▼ Scanning protocol:
After tilting the gantry parallel to the space of the disk, contiguous slices are scanned from the middle of one to the middle of the next body of the vertebra.

If the contours of the intervertebral disk are difficult to visualize, it is advisable to make additional 2 mm slices.

CE Sequence

In suspected cervical disk prolapse:
Slice thickness: 2 (1) mm
Slice intervals: 2 mm

▽ Scanning protocol:
Scanning proceeds parallel to intervertebral disk, from the middle of one to the middle of the next body of the vertebra. Serio-CT may be performed, if necessary.

Contrast medium administration: 100–150 ml of contrast medium may be administered to provide evidence of venous stasis.

Recurring Prolapse and Spondylodiscitis

Same as above.

For demonstration of subtle bone arrosion, a high-resolution reconstruction filter should be used.

Slice thickness 4 (2) mm
Slice intervals: 4 (2) mm

▼ Scanning protocol:
Parallel to the intervertebral disk, from the middle of one to the middle of the next body of the vertebra. Serio-CT may be performed, as necessary.

Contrast medium administration: 150–200 ml contrast medium. Maximum contrast enhancement usually occurs only after 2 to 3 minutes. Therefore, a slow scan sequence is required.

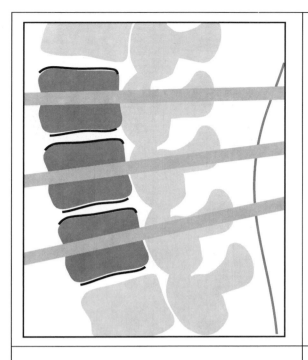

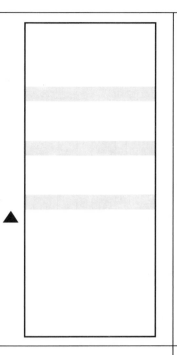

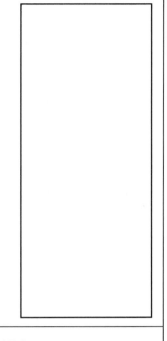

Osteo-CT

Preparation:
None required.

Reference phantom:
Placed underneath the patient at the site of measurement, or mat with reference phantom is placed in position.

Topogram:
Lateral, from the lower thoracic spine to the pelvis.

Evaluation:
Made with standardized regions of interest (ROI) or with an automated contour-finding program (see manufacturer's instructions).

Plain Scan Sequence

Scan thickness: 8 mm

▲ **Scanning:**
Mid-vertebral slices are made through the 12th thoracic vertebra to the 3rd lumbar vertebra. The plane of the slice must correspond exactly with the angle intersect between the upper plates of the vertebra, as can be determined in the topogram. If desired, this can be done via an automated contour-finding program.

If available, Dual Energy System should be used.

CE Sequence

Not required.

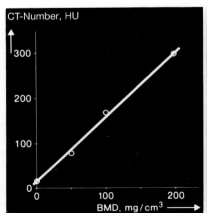

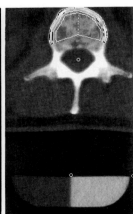

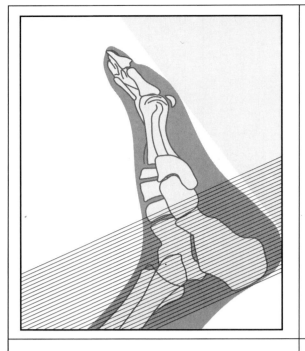

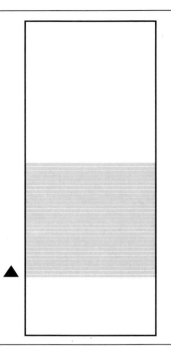

Calcaneum

Preparation:
None required.

Patient positioning:
The patient is placed with his feet towards the gantry. The knees should be bent at a 30° angle. The feet are then placed on the patient couch and are secured with a foam wedge and adhesive strapping. Both feet are examined to provide a comparison.

Topogram:
Short lateral topogram.

Gantry angulation:
Perpendicular to the heel-bone or couch.

Plain Scan Sequence

Slice thickness: 4 mm
Slice intervals: 4 mm

▲ **Scanning protocol:**
Contiguous slices are scanned craniocaudal, to include the entire calcaneum and cuboid.

The set of raw data should also be entered for reconstruction in high-resolution (HR) and normal resolution scans.
Zoom factor 3.0 to 3.5.

CE Sequence

Not required.

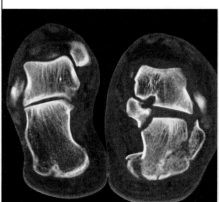

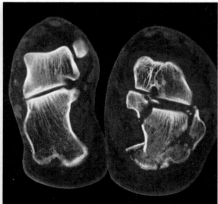

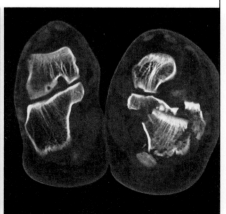

Chapter 6
The Mediastinum

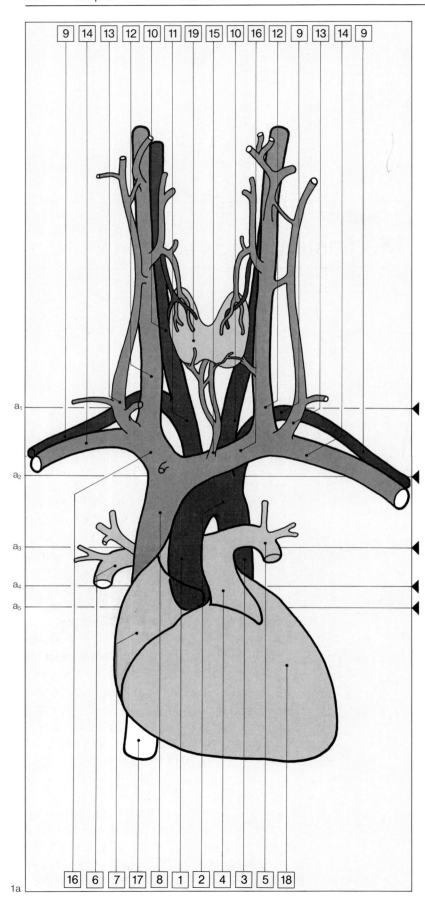

Fig. 6-1. Mediastinal Vessels.

a) Situs.
b) Transverse sections (for level, see a).

Key to symbols:

 1 Ascending aorta
 2 Arch of the aorta
 3 Descending aorta
 4 Pulmonary trunk
 5 Left pulmonary artery
 6 Right pulmonary artery
 7 Right auricle of the heart
 8 Superior vena cava
 9 Subclavian artery
10 Common carotid artery
11 Brachiocephalic trunk
12 Internal jugular vein
13 External jugular vein
14 Subclavian vein
15 Thyroid vein
16 Brachiocephalic vein
17 Inferior vena cava
18 Heart
19 Thyroid gland
20 Azygos vein

1a

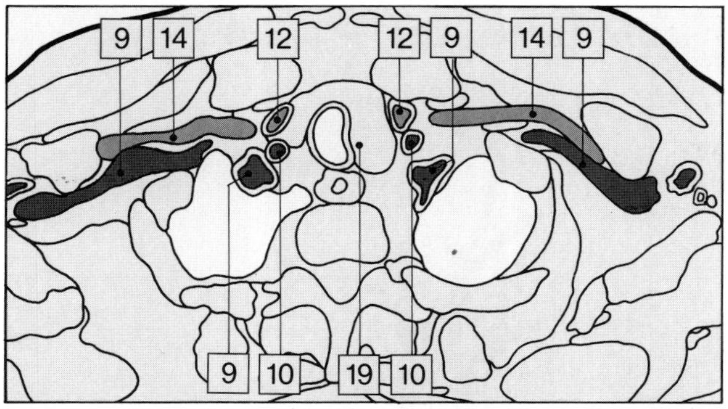

1b₁

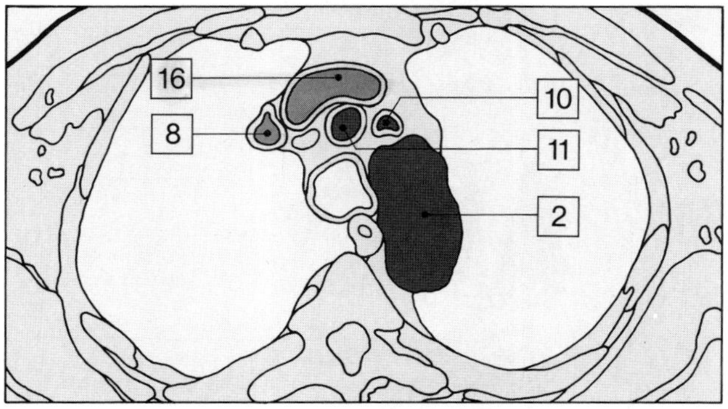

1b₂

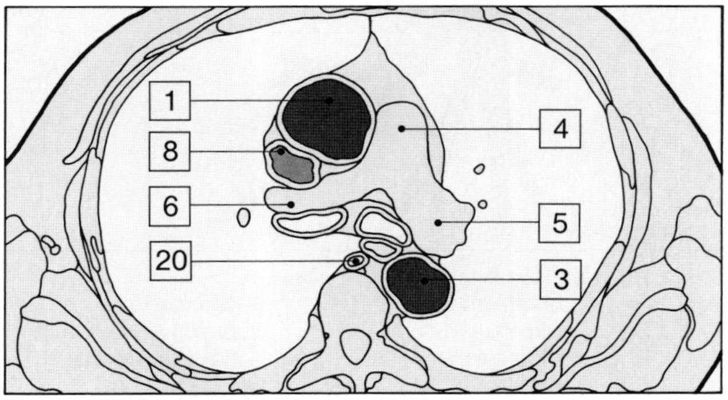

1b₃

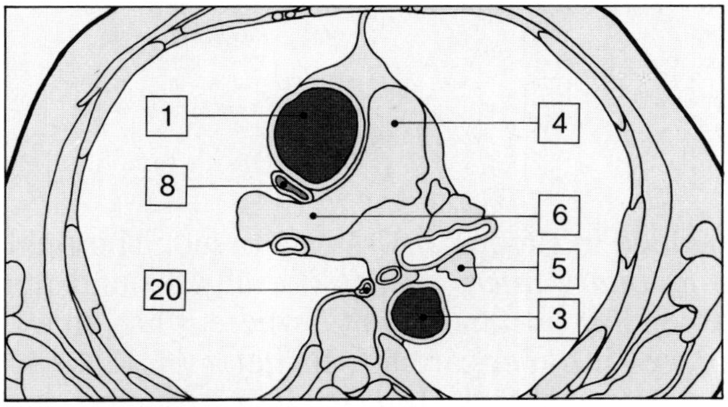

1b₄

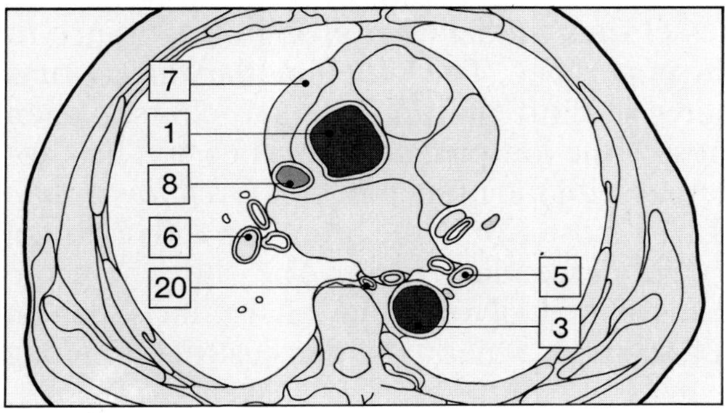

1b₅

The Mediastinum

Anatomy and Imaging

Mediastinal Spaces

Various authors will divide the mediastinum into different compartments based on various anatomical, pathological or diagnostic criteria. Computed tomography can provide highly sophisticated images for morphological assessment of the mediastinum. In the present volume, a subdivision of the mediastinum into *anterior*, *middle* and *posterior* compartments has been selected for optimum tumor imaging.

Mediastinal Vessels

The large vessels form distinctive structures in the mediastinum. The more longitudinal the course of a vessel, the better it can be demonstrated on transverse CT scans. Some vessel segments fulfil this criterion better than others. As a rule, image analysis should start at the *aorta*, which is always readily identifiable. The brachiocephalic branches of the aorta, which run a craniocaudal course, are easily identifiable. The left *subclavian artery* originates most dorsal and arches slightly and characteristically forward to meet the left apex of the lung. On CT scans, the left (innominate) *brachiocephalic vein* is located obliquely above and in front of the aortic arch. Its caliber and course can vary greatly. The right brachiocephalic vein arches slightly to outline the right mediastinal contours. The site where these two vessels join to form the *superior vena cava* (SVC) is usually clearly demonstrated on plain scans. Along an axial course, the SVC can be reliably traced laterodorsal to the ascending aorta to the point where it enters the right atrium. In contrast, the subclavian vein and the internal and external jugular veins cannot always be clearly demonstrated in their confluence at the level of the *inlet of the thorax*. This often makes

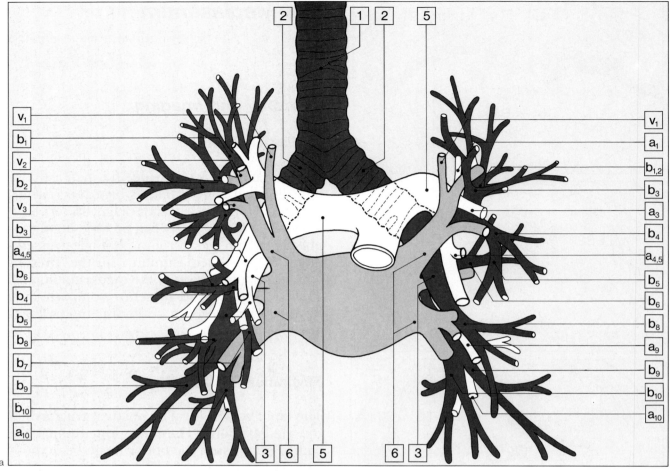

2a

Fig. 6-2. Bronchovascular structures of the pulmonary hilum.
a) Situs, as seen ventrally.
b) Transverse sections
cranial (b₁)
caudal (b₅).
c) CT scans
after contrast medium bolus, cranial (c₁);
caudal (c₅) in double window.

Key to symbols:
Bronchi:
1   Trachea
2   Main bronchus
3   Lobar bronchus
B_ul   Bronchus, lower lobe
B_ol   Bronchus, upper lobe
b₁₋₁₀   Segmental bronchus 1–10

Heart and Arteries:
4   Left atrium
5   Pulmonary artery
A_l   Left pulmonary artery
A_R   Right pulmonary artery
a₁₋₁₀   Segmental arteries 1–10

Veins:
6   Pulmonary vein
7   Superior vena cava
v₁₋₁₀   Segmental veins 1–10
V_ol   Collecting veins, upper lobe
V_ul   Collecting veins, lower lobe

it necessary to administer intravascular contrast medium to differentiate these vascular structures from enlarged lymph nodes, especially in cases of age-related ectasia. The subclavian vein and the axillary vein are found in front of the corresponding arteries, and it is usually not difficult to trace their course from below the pectoralis minor muscle to the axilla. The accompanying nerve structures of the brachial plexus normally cannot be seen on CT scans, not even at high-resolution.

The pulmonary outflow tract and branches of the *pulmonary trunk* can usually be readily demonstrated on CT scans, since they are embedded in subepicardial fatty tissue. The right *pulmonary artery* swings dorsally around the ascending aorta and SVC, where it has an average (intrapericardial) diameter of 12 to 15 mm. Ventral to the intermediate bronchus, the vessel runs caudal after giving off a branch to the upper lobe. The left pulmonary artery runs only a short intrapericardial course, then crosses the left primary bronchus and lies, together with the branch from the *left lower lobe* (LLL), posterior to the bronchus and proximal to the descending aorta. The site where the veins of the LLL enter the left atrium is seen on CT scans as a markedly dense structure along

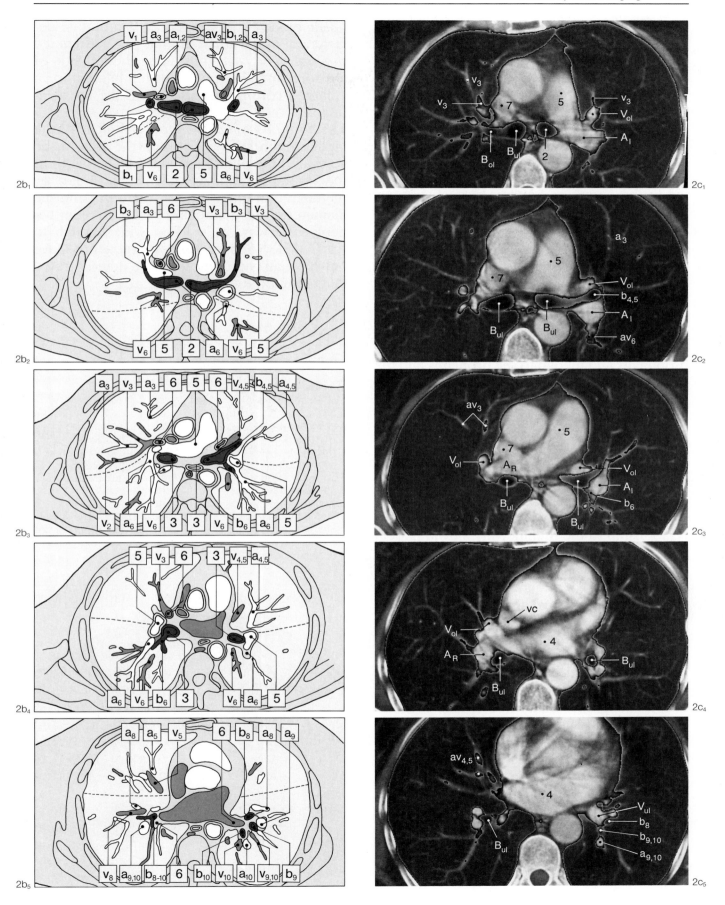

the lateral border of the heart. The veins of the upper lobe course in front of the arteries and bronchi towards the heart.

The *hilum of the lung*, a rather complex structure, is best scanned through a broad window setting, because the formation of half-shadows (penumbra) will increase spatial resolution. The starting point is the branching structure of the bronchial tree. The bronchi are accompanied to the periphery by their respective arteries. The pulmonary veins course along the lobe borders and segmental borders to the hilum. The *azygos vein* ascends paravertebrally behind the heart on the right. Depending on the amount of fat, the azygos vein can be demonstrated in the posterior mediastinum when its diameter is at least 3 to 5 mm. At the level of the 4th and 6th thoracic vertebrae, the azygos vein courses on the right, running lateral to the esophagus and medial to the bronchus and the artery of the right upper lobe and extending to the right tracheobronchial angle. This vessel is seen as a lateroconvex arch on transverse CT scans. Above the azygos arch, the pleura folds inward behind the trachea at different medial depths, creating the *supraazygeal recess*. Below the azygos arch at the level of the hilum and the heart, there is a similar pulmonary protrusion called the *azygo-esophageal recess*. Its relationship to the midline varies from patient to patient. Especially in cases of pulmonary emphysema, it can extend from behind the esophagus, across the midline to the opposite side. In young patients, a lateroconvex configuration due to forward esophageal protrusion may even be observed.

Drainage of the right *internal thoracic vein* into the SVC can be demonstrated well, especially when collateral vascular channels have been found along the right mediastinal contour. After emerging through the diaphragm, the *inferior hemiazygos vein* lies behind the descending aorta, anterior to the thoracic vertebrae. Like the accessory hemiazygos vein, it is not visible on scans of healthy individuals. The left superior *intercostal vein*, which communicates with the superior vena hemiazygos, is of diagnostic importance. Since the left superior intercostal vein can align with the left side of the aortic arch before flowing into the brachioce-

phalic brachiocephalic vein, it can imitate detachment of the aortic intima. A persistent *left superior vena cava* runs along the left side of the aortic arch in front of the left hilum into an enlarged coronary sinus behind the left ventricle.

The *aortopulmonary window* is a niche of the mediastinum located between the arch of the aorta and the pulmonary trunk. The width of the aortic-pulmonic window is determined by the degree of elongation of the aorta and the diameter of the pulmonary vessel. In older patients, the window is often wide enough to scan, while younger patients frequently have only a small gap that cannot be demonstrated by computed tomography.

Fig. 6-3. Normal thyroid gland.

a) Situs.
b) CT scan.

Key to symbols:
1 Thyroid gland
2 Trachea
3 Esophagus
4 Cervical vertebra
5 Sternocleidomastoid
  muscle
6 Sternothyroid muscle
7 Sternohyoid muscle
8 Longus cervicis muscle
9 Scalenus anterior
  muscle
10 Scalenus medius and
   posterior muscles
11 Common carotid artery
12 Internal jugular vein
13 Anterior jugular vein
14 Vertebral artery
15 Vertebral vein
16 Middle thyroid veins
17 Deep cervical lymph nodes
18 Inferior parathyroid gland
19 Vagus nerve
20 Cervical plexus

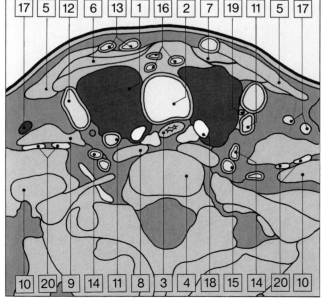

3a

Trachea

The mediastinal pleura is situated on the right, directly lateral and dorsal to the trachea. The layer of soft-tissue between the tracheal lumen and the lungs is normally 4 mm thick. Any abnormal accumulation of fat or constitutional variations that can lead to an increase in tracheal caliber is readily demonstrated by CT. In the infraglottis, the lumen appears on CT scans as a round structure that flattens out after passing the membranous part. Cartilaginous structures of soft-tissue density may contain calcified deposits.

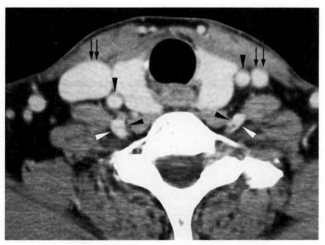

Fig. 6-3b. Thyroid gland. Appears hyperdense after contrast medium administration. The juxtaposition of the jugular vein frequently varies (⇒). Common carotid artery (►), vertebral artery (► ◄).

Thyroid Gland

The thyroid gland forms a convexoconcave structure ventral to the trachea and thyroid cartilage. It normally appears on CT scans as a smooth, homogeneous soft-tissue structure. The diameter of the internal jugular vein can vary, and the radiodensity of this vessel is often not distinctly different from that of thyroid tissue. The carotid artery mediodorsal to the internal jugular vein is more clearly demarcated. Due to its iodine content, normal thyroid tissue will have an attenuation value of 70 ± 10 HU, which is higher than the CT number of muscle tissue. Due to its high degree of vascularisation, thyroid tissue becomes strongly enhanced after the administration of contrast medium.

Esophagus

The esophagus can often be identified by the air contained within it. When esophageal fat is insufficient, it may be necessary to give an oral dose of diluted Gastrografin® to opacify the lumen. In the upper mediastinum, the esophagus lies close to the dorsal wall of the trachea. The esophagus is virtually midline at the level of the tracheal bifurcation. It then deviates slightly to the left and crosses the descending aorta ventrally behind the heart. Wall thicknesses of up to 3 mm are considered normal.

Esophageal nerves and the *thoracic duct* cannot be demonstrated directly on a CT scan. Their position must be estimated with respect to the adjacent organs. Only the phrenic nerve can sometimes be identified as a punctiform structure along the outer margins of the heart.

Fasciae

As in the retroperitoneal space, the borders of the fascia of the mediastinum also determine the paths of spreading of hemorrhagic and exudative processes. The esophagus and trachea are both surrounded by a narrow, common layer of loose connective tissue enclosed in *perivisceral fascia*. This perivisceral space is a continuation of the cervical compartment. It is formed by the pretracheal and buccopharyngeal fascia and includes the larynx, trachea and pharynx. The perivisceral space extends from the bronchi to the periphery of the lung and communicates with the subepicardial fatty tissue of the heart. The periaortic adventitia is bound to the perivisceral fascia by connective tissue.

The *prevertebral fascia* surrounds the paravertebral connective tissue and extends from the base of the skull to the sacrum. It comprises the first barrier against vertebral and paravertebral inflammations, which explains the tendency for craniocaudal spreading of inflammation.

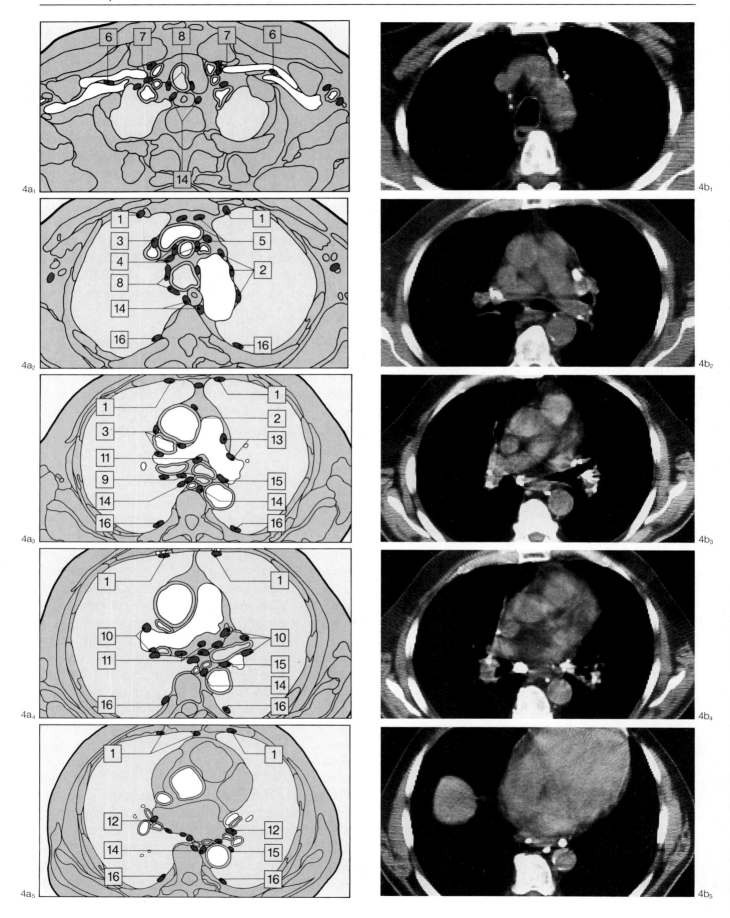

Lymph Nodes

The lymph nodes of the anterior mediastinum can be divided into two groups: the sternal (anterior parietal or internal mammary) and the anterior mediastinal (prevascular) lymph nodes. The sternal lymph nodes are located bilateral and posterior to the costal cartilage. Although the anterior mediastinal lymph nodes do have some retrosternal (pericardial) locations, they are normally located beside large vessels like the SVC, the innominate vein, and the ascending aorta. The posterior mediastinum contains the *intercostal* lymph nodes, which are located proximal to the heads of the ribs. They communicate with the *posterior mediastinal* lymph nodes, which extend alongside the lower esophagus and the descending aorta. In the middle mediastinum, the *parietal* lymph nodes, which extend along the lower circumference of the pericardium and pulmonary ligaments, are greatly outnumbered by *visceral* lymph nodes. Corresponding with their location, some visceral lymph nodes can be further classified as tracheobronchial: they include tracheal, bronchial, bronchopulmonary, and pulmonary lymph nodes. Only a few tracheal lymph nodes are found in front of the trachea; most are paratracheal and located

---

Fig. 6-4. Mediastinal lymph nodes.

a) Topography in transverse section (see 6-1b).
b) Calcified lymph nodes in CT scan.

Key to symbols:
Anterior Mediastinum
  1   Sternal (mammary) lymph nodes
  2–7 Prevascular lymph nodes
  2   Preaortic lymph nodes
  3   Precaval lymph nodes
  4   Bronchomediastinal lymph nodes
  5   Brachiocephalic vein lymph nodes
  6   Subclavian lymph nodes
  7   Internal jugular lymph nodes

Middle Mediastinum
8 Paratracheal lymph nodes
9 Tracheobronchial lymph nodes
10 Bronchopulmonary lymph nodes
11 Bifurcal (subcarinal) lymph nodes
12 Pulmonary vein lymph nodes
13 Arterial duct lymph nodes

Posterior Mediastinum
14 Paraesophageal lymph nodes
15 Paraaortic lymph nodes
16 Intercostal lymph nodes

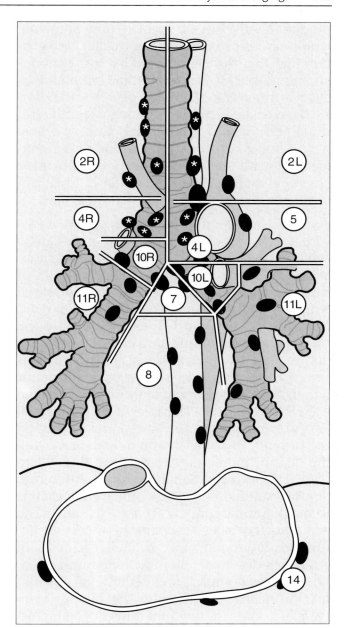

Fig. 6-5. Classification of mediastinal lymph nodes (as suggested by the American Thoracic Society).
  2R Right upper paratracheal lymph nodes
  2L Left upper paratracheal lymph nodes
  4R Right lower paratracheal lymph nodes
  4L Left lower paratracheal lymph nodes
  5   Aortopulmonary lymph nodes
  6   Anterior mediastinal (prevascular) lymph nodes
  7   Subcarinal lymph nodes
  8   Paraesophageal lymph nodes
  9   Lymph nodes of the right and left pulmonary ligament
10R Right tracheobronchial lymph nodes
10L Left peribronchial lymph nodes
11   Intrapulmonary lymph nodes
14   Upper diaphragmatic lymph nodes

An asterisk (*) indicates lymph nodes demonstrable by mediastinoscopy; nodes 5, 6 and 2L can be demonstrated via anterior parasternal thoracotomy.

predominantly on the right. They drain the lymph nodes proximal to the tracheal bifurcation and the bronchopulmonary lymph nodes via this path. Normal mediastinal lymph nodes have a transverse diameter of 0.3 to 0.6 cm. Because of the increased drainage near the tracheal bifurcation (bronchial and tracheal lymph nodes, especially at the site of communication with the azygos vein), lymph node enlargement must be greater than 11 to 12 mm to be considered pathologically abnormal.

As in the retroperitoneal space, lymph nodes with a diameter of ca. 0.5 cm and more can be can be assessed under favorable scanning conditions, i.e, if there is an adequate amount of surrounding fat. This means that mediastinal lymph nodes of normal size (0.3 to 0.6 cm) are just barely visible on CT scans. Because the trachea, ascending and descending aorta, superior vena cava, esophagus, and the azygos vein form clear axial boundaries, even minor lymph node enlargement in those locations can be readily detected. Because of their diagonal or horizontal course, the boundaries formed by the primary bronchi, the pulmonary cone and the central pulmonary vessels are difficult to scan. The aortopulmonary window is therefore demonstrated on CT scans only if the distance to the pulmonic trunk is great (> 1.5 cm). The acute-angled azygo-esophageal recess is deformed lateroconvexly by enlargement of lymph nodes near the tracheal bifurcation. Due to the complex architecture of vascular and bronchial structures in the hilum, intravascular contrast medium must be administered to reliably demonstrate slight lymph node enlargements on CT scans.

Thymus

The thymus also belongs to the lymphatic system. It weighs ca. 20 g in newborns and increases to over 30 g by puberty. It is a bilobed organ that is situated in front of the large vessels at the root of the aorta. Its left lobe is usually larger than the right lobe and extends into the aortopulmonary window. Although the thymus extends up to the jugular vein in toddlers, it recedes in the further course of mediastinal growth and retains it position in front

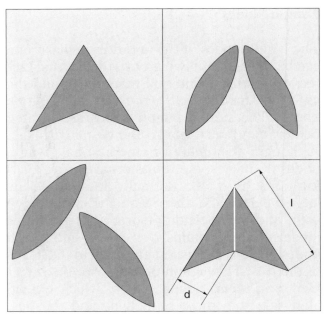

Fig. 6-6a. Configuration of the thymus. The lobes may be fused into an arrow-shaped configuration (62 %) or are visible as two individual structures (32 %). Sometimes, only one lobe is present (6 %). To determine the size of the thymus, the length (l) and thickness (d) of the lobes are measured.

of the root of the aorta in the anterior part of the mediastinal fold.

Like the adrenal gland, it is better to measure the thickness rather than the length of a thymic fold. In patients up to age 20, the thickness should not exceed 1.8 cm. The normal thickness in older patients is a maximum of 1.3 cm.

Fig. 6-6b. The thymus of a 25-year-old male. This normally sized organ (→) is clearly involuted with fat. This makes it difficult to evaluate the lobar borders. (Main finding: aortic aneurysm (▸).

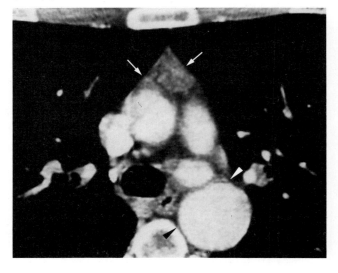

In small children and adolescents, thymic tissue is muscle-dense. The tissue density of the thymus gradually decreases after age 20 and, with the increasing involution of fat, it has usually become fat-dense in individuals over age 50. Uniform or irregular permeation of fat can be observed during various stages of fat involution. Frequently, a delicate, fibrous organ matrix can still be seen in the final stage.

The shape of the thymus varies from patient to patient. Its lobes can be fused or divided by a sagittal (usually left paramedian) boundary, which is demonstrated on CT scans. The contour of the lobes is usually smooth, and the degree of lateroconvex bulging varies from patient to patient.

Lymph Node Enlargement

Malignant Lymphoma

Hodgkin's disease comprises the largest group of malignant lymphomas (53% of all cases diagnosed by biopsy). The distribution of the disease according to age is bimodal, with a first peak in the 3rd decade and a second peak in the 6th to 8th decade of life. Spread from one lymph node chain to another adjacent one is typical. Extranodal invasion of adjacent tissue was found in up to 15% of all reported cases, and later hematogenous spreading has been seen in 5 to 10% of all patients.

Non-Hodgkin's lymphomas (NHL) comprise a histologically heterogeneous group of lymphomas that are subdivided into different types. It is assumed that the genesis of NHL is multifocal. Lukes considers malignant lymphoma and leukemia to be different manifestations of the same disease. While lymphatic lymphoblastomas usually occur in childhood, other NHL's usually occur in the 6th or 7th decade of life. In contrast to Hodgkin's lymphomas, one finds different patterns of invasion, a larger percent of extranodal tumor growth, and different patterns of dissemination at the onset of disease.

Intrathoracic spread is found at the initial presentation in two-thirds of all patients with Hodgkin's lymphomas and in one-third of all patients with NHL's. There is seldom dissemination in the mediastinum (mediastinal skip). Mediastinal and hilar lymphomas are found in one quarter of all patients with leukemic forms of the disease, especially with lymphocytic types. There are no major differences between patterns of involvement of the mediastinum in Hodgkin's lymphomas and NHL that might be

Fig. 6-7. Pattern of involvement of malignant lymphomas.

Morbus Hodgkin's Disease	Non-Hodgkin's Lymphomas
Centripetal involvement: predominantly in lymph nodes along the longitudinal axis of the body	Centrifugal involvement and multicentric, non-contiguous spreading
Neither epitrochlear, gastrointestinal, testicular regions nor Waldeyer's tonsillar ring are commonly affected	Frequently with involvement of the epitrochlear, testicular and gastrointestinal lymph nodes, including Waldeyer's tonsillar ring
Mediastinal manifestation occurs in over 50% of all cases	Mediastinal involvement is infrequent (20%)
Abdominal lymph node involvement occurs infrequently in asymptomatic patients. Is common in elderly patients, appearing with a raised temperature or night sweat	Abdominal lymph nodes are frequently affected
Regional (localized) involvement with contiguous spread is common	Regional (localized) involvement is rare
Bone marrow involvement is rarely observed	Bone marrow is frequently affected
Hepatic manifestations are rare but, if found, concomitant involvement of the spleen is almost always observed, these manifestations only rarely occur without raised temperature and night sweat	Involvement of the liver is often observed with follicular lymphomas, but seldom with diffuse lymphomas

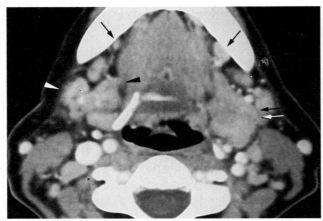

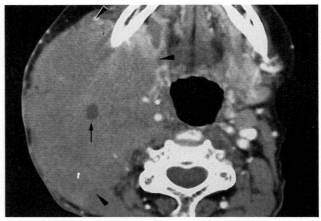

Fig. 6-8. Non-Hodgkin's lymphoma. Sharply delineated, moderately enlarged lymph nodes can be seen near the floor of the mouth (→) and cervical perivascular sheath (internal jugular nodes ⇒). They absorb a moderate amount of contrast medium and therefore appear isodense as compared with the submandibular gland (►).

Fig. 6-9. Non-Hodgkin's lymphoma. Diffusely distributed, sharply delineated lymph nodes near the floor of the mouth, the cervical perivascular sheath, and sternocleidomastoid muscle.

Fig. 6-10. Non-Hodgkin's lymphoma. The lymph nodes posterior to the internal jugular vein (→) must be differentiated from the scalenus muscles (►). Brachiocervical plexus (⇒).

Fig. 6-11. Non-Hodgkin's lymphoma. Diffuse, extensive mass in right angle of the mandible; infiltrates floor of the mouth as well as the dorsal muscles (►). Moderate contrast enhancement (ca. 20 HU) after contrast medium administration; cystoid, regressive changes are demarcated (→).

Fig. 6-12. Non-Hodgkin's lymphoma. Evidence of an extensive axillary lymphoma (→) that is mostly isodense as compared with the surrounding muscles.

Fig. 6-13. Anaplastic plasmocytoma. Evidence of a lymph node conglomerate in the right cardiodiaphragmatic angle (→).

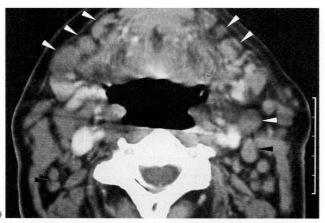

9

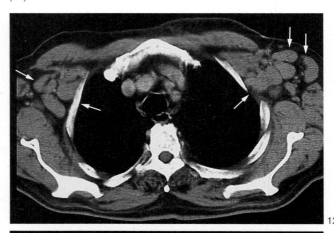

12

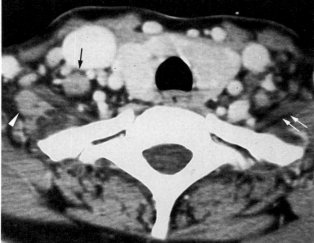

10

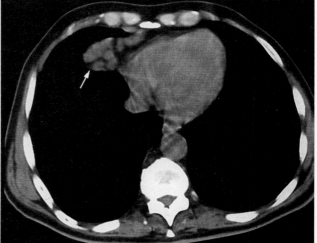

13

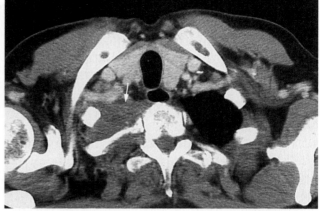

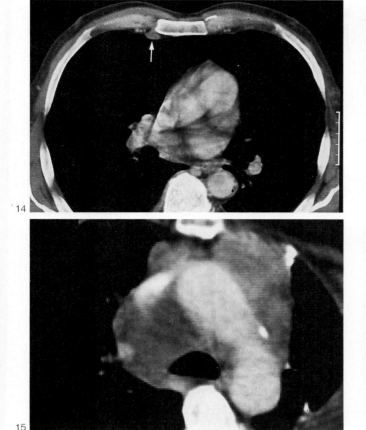

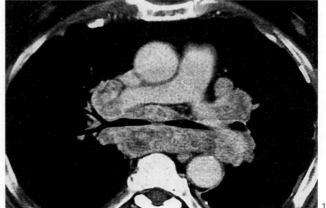

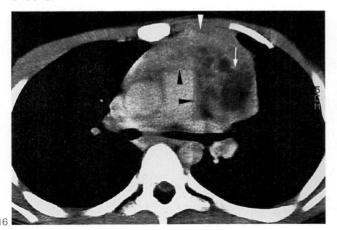

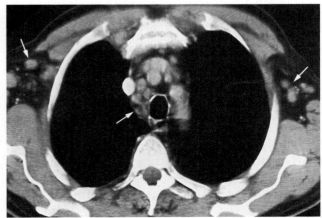

Fig. 6-14. Non-Hodgkin's lymphoma. Very subtle lymph node enlargement in the region of the internal mammarian nodes (→).

Fig. 6-15. Non-Hodgkin's lymphoma. Diffuse permeation of the upper mediastinum by soft-tissue masses. These show slight inhomogeneity after contrast medium administration. The superior vena cava is moderately compressed.

Fig. 6-16. Hon-Hodgkin's lymphoma. Extensive mass in the upper anterior mediastinum (►) with clear regressive changes seen as a delineated, indistinctly hypodense zone after contrast medium administration (→). A teratoma must be considered in the differential diagnosis when an isolated mass is found.

Fig. 6-17. Plasmocytoma. A soft-tissue structure is found near the 2nd right rib; it is located on the lung (→). This mass cannot be differentiated from Pancoast's tumor, especially in view of the fact that it also displays slight bone erosion.

Fig. 6-18. Immunocytoma. Evidence of a nodular, sometimes confluent mass filling the entire middle mediastinum, including the hila. After contrast medium administration, there is clear, non-uniform contrast enhancement.

Fig. 6-19. Hodgkin's lymphoma with moderately enlarged, well delineated mediastinal and axillary lymph nodes (→).

used for differential diagnosis. In Hodgkin's disease, primary involvement of the cervical lymph nodes is more frequent, and it leads to preferential spreading to the upper anterior mediastinum and the paratracheal lymph nodes due to the contagious nature of the disease. In contrast to NHL, the paracardiac lymph nodes and lymph nodes of the lower posterior mediastinum are almost always skipped. Hilar lymphomas, which have been reported in isolated cases, are rare.

• CT

Lymphomas appear as nodular or unstructured soft-tissue zones. They can be most sensitively detected in paratracheal, paravertebral and retrocrural locations as well as in pericaval, preaortic and retrosternal lymph nodes. Ectatic (venous) vessels and sections of the thyroid lobes in the inlet of the thorax must be enhanced with contrast medium. *Calcification* of lymphomas is very rare and occurs only in chronic cases, usually as a result of irradiation. Displacement of the trachea, bronchi or vessels is not a rare occurrence in extensive processes; the condition may cause pulmonary metastases.

The *attenuation value* of lymphomas is within or slightly below the soft-tissue range. Cystic or necrotic areas are constellations of special pathological interest. As a rule, one should thoroughly search the pleura, retrosternal space and the pericardium for nodular structures. Direct infiltration of a lymphoma into the lungs, pleura or the thoracic wall is not unusual in patients with large tumor masses. When evaluating the residual tumor during or after therapy, the same criteria as for infradiaphragmatic manifestations (→ retroperitoneum) apply.

Contrast-enhanced scans: A bolus injection of contrast medium only slightly enhances attenuation differences (up to 20 HU); cystic and necrotic zones can be identified.

Differential diagnosis: If a solitary soft-tissue mass is detected, the entire spectrum of solid mediastinal neoplasms must be considered in the diagnosis.

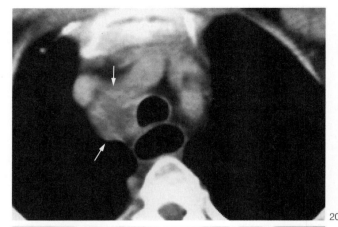

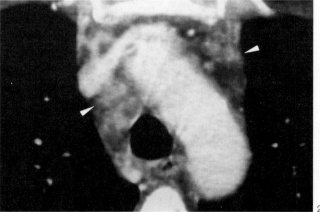

Fig. 6-20. Paratracheal metastases of a bronchial carcinoma (→).

Fig. 6-21. Metastases of a muciferous adenocarcinoma. The pattern of spread is reticular with fine nodules (▸).

Fig. 6-22. Metastasizing melanoma. A compact, confluent soft-tissue structure is located right paratracheal; there is rim-like contrast enhancement (▸). This structure cannot be differentiated from a bronchial carcinoma that invades the mediastinum.

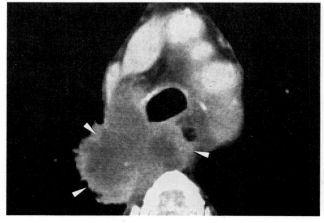

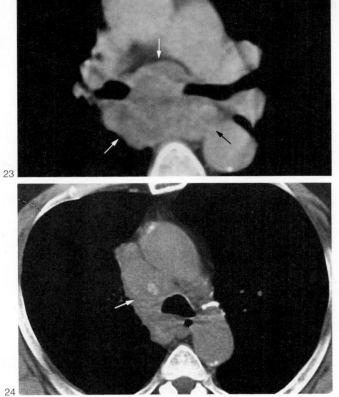

23

24

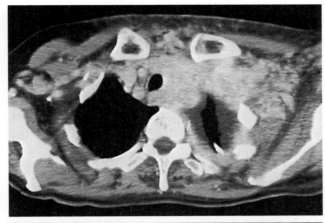

26a

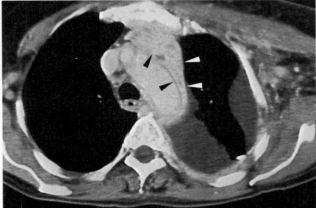

26b

Fig. 6-23. Infracarinal metastases of a bronchial carcinoma. After contrast medium administration, this mass can be reliably differentiated from the left atrium.

Fig. 6-24. Metastasizing, small-cell bronchial carcinoma. Evidence of very fine, punctiform calcification within these compact, confluent lymph node metastases.

Fig. 6-25. Metastasizing, small-cell bronchial carcinoma (oat cell carcinoma). Confluent metastases in the upper mediastinum. In addition to subtle calcification, clearly regressive changes are also demarcated after contrast medium administration. There is considerable compression of the superior vena cava (→). Evidence of collateral circulation via the azygos vein (►) and internal mammarian vein (⊫).

Fig. 6-26. Metastasizing carcinoma of the breast. This spreads from the left axilla through the inlet of the thorax via confluent lymph node conglomerates, which can be seen near the arch of the aorta (►), where they appear as a compact soft-tissue conglomerate. An unusual feature is the high degree of contrast enhancement, indicating strong vascularization of tumor tissue.

Fig. 6-27. Metastasizing pheochromoblastoma. After bolus injection of contrast medium, the highly vascularized mass of 3 mm diameter (→) can be seen. With its central necrotic zone, it resembles the primary tumor.

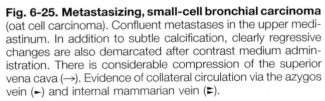

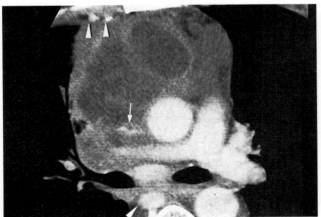

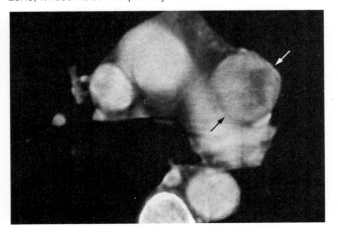

Lymph Node Metastases

Most mediastinal lymph node metastases arise from primary intrathoracic tumors, mainly bronchial and esophageal carcinoma. The rest arise, in decreasing order of frequency, from malignant tumors of the stomach, pancreas, breast, kidneys, testes, prostate, thyroid gland, and larynx. Extrathoracic tumors often spread via lymphatics to the mediastinal lymph nodes. As compared with carcinomas, lymphatic spread of sarcomas to the mediastinum is relatively rare.

• CT

Plain scans: Like malignant lymphomas, lymph nodes enlarged by metastases appear on CT scans as soft-tissue structures, but they do not become as extensive as malignant lymphomas. Since they affect nerves and vessels (e.g. recurrent paresis), even minor lymph node enlargement quickly causes noticeable clinical symptoms. According to the drainage zones, the ipsilateral hilum should be thoroughly investigated in patients with bronchial carcinoma, whereas retrosternal lymph nodes are the primary targets of carcinoma of the breast. If a tumor is found in the gastrointestinal tract, kidney, scrotum or prostate, or if a carcinoma is found in the larynx and thyroid gland, the lymph nodes of the superior mediastinum must also be examined.

A transverse diameter of 10 mm or more is generally assumed to indicate pathological enlargement of a lymph node. Smaller nodes, however, may contain micrometastases, and larger lymph nodes may simply be enlarged due to inflammation. It is easier to properly diagnose lymph node enlargement when the primary tumor site and lymphatic drainage zones are considered in the evaluation. Large lymph node conglomerates can mask some parts of mediastinal structures. Most enlarged lymph nodes in the paracardiac and cardiophrenic angles prove to be malignant.

Calcification is rare, but sometimes occurs in metastasizing mucinous tumors (ovarian carcinomas) and bronchio-alveolar carcinomas, or after radiotherapy.

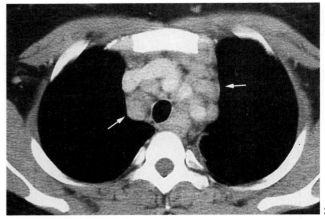

28a

Fig. 6-28a. Sarcoidosis. In the upper mediastinum, there are sharply demarcated nodular structures which do not seriously compromise the vessels.

Fig. 6-28b,c. Caudally, at the level of the carina tracheae, the soft-tissue structure becomes more confluent, thereby displacing the arch of the azygos vein. In retrocardial areas as well as in the hilar region, one finds compact, confluent lymph node masses.

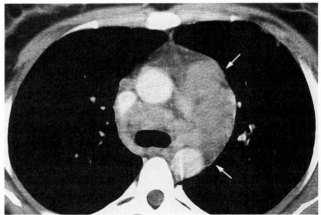

28b

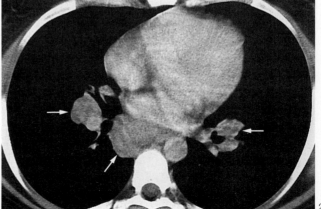

28c

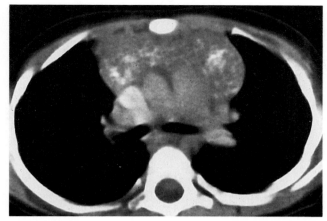

Fig. 6-29. Histiocytosis X. Retrosternal soft-tissue structures dorsally displace large vessels. Lymph node structures are confluent and display cloudy, amorphous calcification.

Fig. 6-30. Silicosis. Compact calcification of lymph nodes in the mediastinum; subtle "egg-shell" calcification. The lymph nodes in the right hilar region are not calcified.

Fig. 6-31. Pneumocystis carinii lymphadenopathy. Considerably enlarged, sometimes confluent lymph nodes with ringlike calcification and a hypodense center.

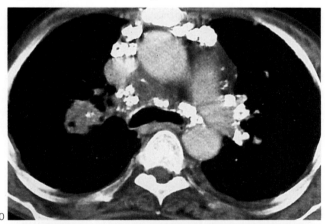

30

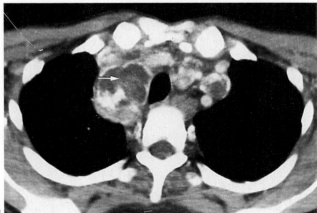

31

Contrast-enhanced scans: A bolus injection of contrast medium normally causes only slight enhancement of the margins of lymph node structures. Hypervascularized metastases of a renal, thyroid or a small-celled pulmonary carcinoma are found infrequently on CT scans with consecutive, additional contrast enhancement. Contrast medium is normally required to distinguish lymph nodes from vessels, especially near the inlet of the thorax and the hila.

Involvement of Lymph Nodes in Granulomatous Diseases

Sarcoidosis usually leads to enlargement of the paratracheal and pre-aortic lymph nodes in the upper mediastinum as well as symmetrical lymphadenopathy in hilar regions. The enlarged lymph nodes are usually readily distinguishable. Mediastinal involvement that does not lead to enlargement of the hilar lymph nodes is atypical. If pulmonary changes are absent, malignant lymphoma must be considered in the differential diagnosis, because lymph nodes may merge to form larger conglomerates in sarcoidosis. *Calcification* in the healing stage has been observed in isolated cases.

Florid *lymph node tuberculosis* causes enlargement of lymph nodes (paratracheal, tracheobronchial). On CT scans, they demonstrate peripheral enhancement and central areas of necrosis-related hypodensity. These normally asymmetrically affected lymph nodes can merge, conglomerate and assume the nature of a mass lesion. *Calcification* is often seen during healing stages.

In *pneumoconiosis*, ringlike *calcification* frequently occurs in addition to minor enlargement of hilar and mediastinal lymph nodes. Typical pulmonary changes occur, so it normally is not difficult to diagnose pneumoconiosis.

In *angiofollicular hyperplasia*, there is highly vascularized lymphatic tissue that, after a bolus injection of contrast medium, becomes intensely enhanced. Enlarged lymph nodes can

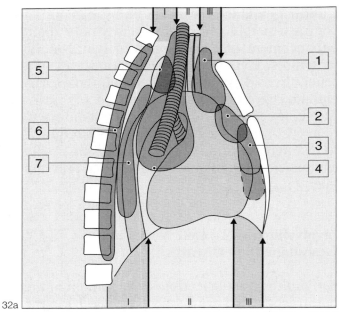

32a

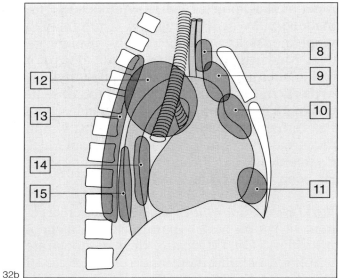

32b

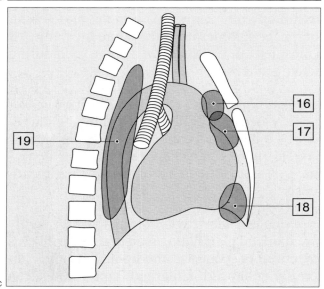

32c

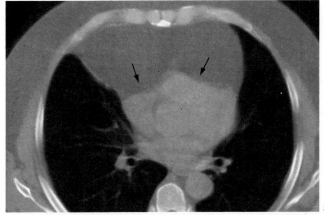

33

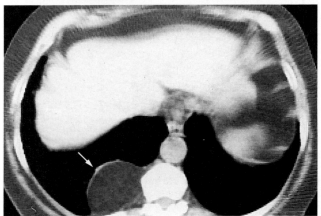

34

Fig. 6-33. Mediastinal lipoma. This mass with homogeneous attenuation values in the fat range rests on the heart and ventrally displaces the ventricles of the heart due to its expanding growth (→).

Fig. 6-34. Lipoferous mass. Dorsal herniation of retroperitoneal fat through the diaphragm in the right paracardial region (→). "Diaphragmatic lipoma".

Fig. 6-32. Primary lesions of the mediastinum.

Key to symbols:

a) Solid masses
1 Retrosternal goiter
2 Thymoma, thyroid adenoma, hemangioma (lymph granuloma)
3 Teratoma, fibroma (dysgerminoma)
4 Primary malignant lymphomas
5 Retrotracheal goiter
6 Neurogenic tumors
7 Esophageal tumors, fibrosarcomas

b) Cystic masses
8 Thyroid cysts
9 Thymic cysts

10 Cystic teratomas
11 Mesothelioma (lymphangioma)
12 Bronchogenic cysts
13 Meningoceles
14 Neuroenteral cysts
15 Lymphangioma

c) Lipoferous masses
16 Thymic lipoma
17 Dermoid cysts
18 Lipoma
19 Liposarcoma

then be seen. Rare hypervascularized metastases arising from thyroid and renal cell carcinomas, hemangiomas, intrathoracic goiter and parathyroid adenomas must also be considered in the diagnosis.

In *non-specific hyperplasia*, the lymph nodes normally appear only slightly enlarged and sharply marginated. Calcification frequently occurs in patients with pneumocystis carinii infections who have received pentamidine prophylaxis.

Neither infectious nor granulomatous enlargement of lymph nodes has a specific morphological appearance pattern of distribution which might serve as a diagnostic criterion to safely distinguish them from malignant disease. In many cases, however, the history, clinical findings and CT examination of the lungs, throat and abdomen may clarify the situation, thus eliminating the need for mediastinoscopy.

Primary Tumors of the Anterior Mediastinum

Mesenchymal Tumors

Mesenchymal tumors can be found in all three portions of the mediastinum, however, they are most often located in the anterior compartment.

The overall occurrence of *lipomas* is rare, and they are most often unilateral. Lipomas may spread outside the mediastinal space in a caudad and cranial direction, thereby assuming an hourglass configuration, similar to the one seen when omental fat herniates into the lower posterior mediastinum. Because of their soft consistency, lipomas do not displace adjacent organs and are often discovered incidentally. A possible iatrogenic cause of *lipomatosis* is corticosteroid treatment.

Lipo-fibrosarcomas are extremely rare. They are usually found in the posterior mediastinum and can lead to significant displacement of adjacent organs.

Fibromas evoke clinical complaints only after they have reached a substantial size. Pleural

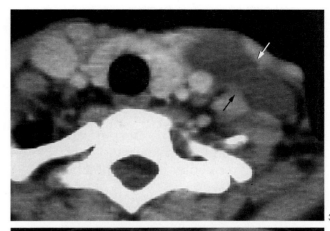
35

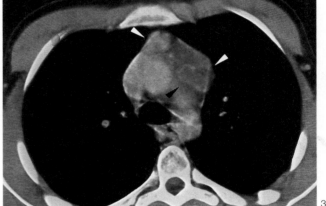
36

Fig. 6-35. Lymphangioma. Evidence of a cystic structure in the left inlet of the thorax (→); there is moderate displacement of adjacent organs.

Fig. 6-36. Thymic hyperplasia. After chemotherapy for Hodgkin's disease, clear enlargement of the thymus was found. This later resided without treatment.

Fig. 6-37. Cystic thymoma. Evidence of a smoothly marginated, water dense mass of 3 cm diameter (→). It is contiguous with the left pulmonary trunk and has a ventrally located area of calcification (►).

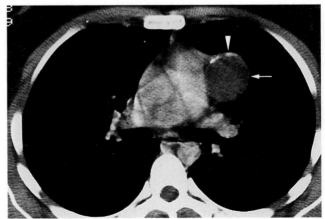

effusion occasionally accompanies fibromas and *fibrosarcomas*, the latter being located predominantly in the posterior mediastinum. *Hemangiomas (cavernous hemangiomas, hemangio-endotheliomas, hemangiosarcomas)* are rare neoplasms. Approximately 65% of them are found in the anterior mediastinum. They are surrounded by a fibrous capsule, are extremely variable in shape, and may be multiple. They frequently contain phleboliths.

Lymphangiomas (hygromas) occur primarily in children. They may extend as far as the cervical region and cause considerable displacement. A distinction is made between cavernous and cystic types. In adults, lymphangiomas usually appear as smooth, multichambered soft masses in the lower anterior mediastinum. They cause no problems if chylothorax does not develop.

● **CT**

Lipomas and *lipomatoses* are clearly identifiable due to their homogeneous CT numbers in the fatty tissue range (-80 to -120 HU). If the density of a fatty neoplasm in the posterior mediastinum is significantly greater than that of normal fatty tissue, malignancy *(liposarcoma)* must be suspected, even if lymph node metastases and bone destruction are not apparent.

Fibromas are difficult to differentiate from other non-cystic masses, but they are distinguishable from more common thymomas, teratomas and parathyroid tumors. The presence of phleboliths within a fibroma could be due to a focal *hemangioma*. A targeted, protracted bolus injection of contrast medium makes it possible to visualize the high vascularity of fibromas. *Lymphangiomas* and *hygromas* have the appearance of a water-filled mass. On the basis of their location, they can be differentiated from brachial cysts.

Tumors of the Thymus

The most common thymic tumor is the *thymoma*. It can occur in patients of all ages, but usually appears in the 4th decade. Thymomas

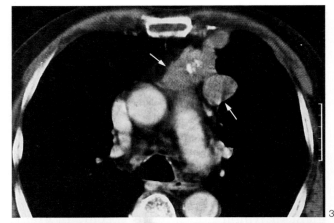
38a

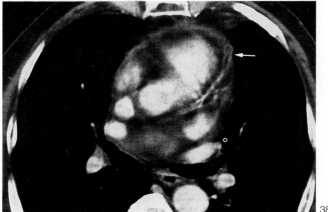
38b

Fig. 6-38. Malignant thymoma. Soft-tissue dense, nodular mass (a→) superior to the left pulmonary trunk; its borders with the mediastinal pleura are irregular. Evidence of central calcification. Pericardial thickening (b→) is found 3 cm caudal. This is a sign of pericardial effusion which, in turn, is indicative of pericardial infiltration.

Fig. 6-39. Malignant thymoma. Nodular metastases permeate the anterior and posterior mediastinum (►) and infiltrate the liver. These signs of effusion are indicative of pleural invasion (→).

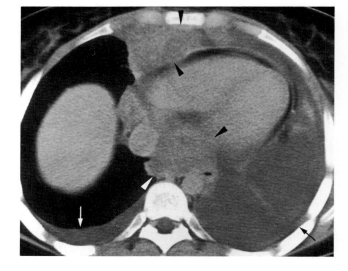

normally do not become as large as teratomas. Malignancy or degeneration occurs in ca. 30% of all thymomas. Highly aggressive invasion of adjacent tissue is characteristic. Pleuropericardial spread frequently occurs, whereas hematogenous and lymphatic metastases are rare. The thymoma is often an accompanying finding in thymic hyperplasia (65%) and myasthenia gravis (15%). *Thymic lipomas* and *thymic cysts* are rare and are characterized by very well-differentiated thymic tissue.

• CT

Plain scans: Thymomas appear on CT scans as round to oval masses, either smoothly marginated or lobulated. They normally lie asymmetrically along the cardiac junction to large vessels or directly in front of the ascending aorta. Regardless of tumor status, peripheral plaques of calcification or diffuse intratumoral calcification is often found. Attenuation values lie in the solid tissue range. The cystic components have lower attenuation values, but the CT numbers seldom drop to the water range. Since the tumor capsule can be fused to the pericardium and pleura, the absence of a demarcating rind of fat does not necessarily imply tumor invasion. Tumor invasion must be assumed when tumor definition is poor as compared to adjacent fatty tissue, when solid components cause pleural or pericardial thickening, and when effusion fluid collects in the serous cavities. A malignant thymoma may also spread to the posterior mediastinum, through the diaphragm, and into the abdominal cavity.

A *thymic lipoma* may contain obvious connective tissue components, leading to raised CT numbers as compared with normal adipose tissue.

True thin-walled *thymic cysts* are very rare, and can be diagnosed as such only on the basis of their mediastinal position.

Contrast-enhanced scans: A bolus injection of contrast medium helps to demarcate cystic tissue components and organ boundaries. The invasion of vascular structures appears as a contour defect only after a sufficient dose of contrast medium has been administered.

Differential diagnosis: *Physiological enlargement of the thymus* is usually seen in children and adolescents and may accompany hyperthyroidism. The thymus expands bilaterally in the upper anterior mediastinum, although the shape of the thymic lobes may remain unchanged. *Thymic hyperplasia* (lymphoid follicular hyperplasia) sometimes occurs with organ enlargement. It frequently occurs after combined steroid treatment and chemotherapy (rebound phenomenon). Since the condition is only temporary, follow-up examinations are recommended to identify recurring tumors. *Persistent thymic enlargement*, usually with mostly small, nodular, retrosternal structures, some of which are permeated with fat, seldom leads to the formation of larger masses. The thymus is occasionally the primary

Fig. 6-40. Teratoma. This extensive growth is located at the typical site above the vessels; it rests against the heart. After contrast medium administration, sharply marginated cystoid structures are demarcated (→); they show parietal contrast enhancement (a ►). Encapsulated fatty tissue (b ⇛), an important criterium for diagnosis of the tumor type, is also found.

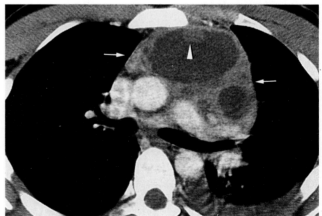

40a

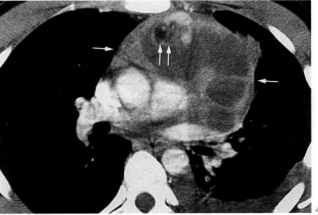

40b

site of other neoplasms, e.g. Hodgkin's lymphomas. It then is not unusual to find large cysts contained within the mass.

Teratoid Blastomas

Teratoblastomas, which account for 11 to 17% of all masses at this site, occur at approximately the same frequency as thymomas. They arise from primitive germ cells and contain various tissue types. Teratomas have ectodermal, mesodermal and endodermal tissue elements. Dermoid cysts, on the other hand, are epidermal in origin. They are divided into cystic and solid types. Seminomas, teratocarcinomas and chorionepitheliomas are much more infrequent. Teratoblastomas occur more frequently in men between the 2nd and 4th decade, and approx. 25% of these tumors are malignant. Cystic tumors normally tend to be benign. Calcified structures are found in 50%.

• CT

Teratomas and *dermoid cysts* usually develop in the anterior mediastinum at the point where the large vessels leave the heart. They are only rarely found in the posterior mediastinum. Lobular contours and solid tissue are normally indicative of a malignant growth, while round, smoothly marginated cystic masses suggest a benign lesion. Teratomas and dermoid cysts may have *calcification* (mostly plaques). Some calcified lesions of the skin (bone, teeth) are pathognomonic characteristics of dermoid cysts. As the size of the cysts increases, symptoms of displacement become more severe (compression of the bronchi and SVC). Although rapid growth is usually a sign of malignancy, a cystic lesion may also show an increase in size due to hemorrhage. Local invasion and pulmonary or regional metastases are, however, unequivocal criteria of malignancy.

The *attenuation* of a tumor is dependent on its tissue composition. Cystic components usually display attenuation values in the water range. The attenuation value of hemorrhage can be similar to that of tumor tissue, so *contrast medium* must be administered to unmask solid, vascularized tumor components and to clearly

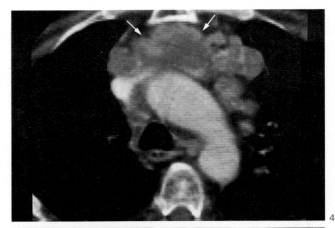

41a

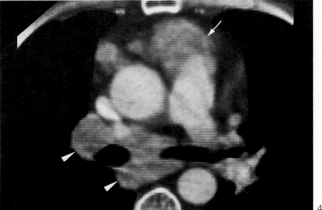

41b

Fig. 6-41. Metastasizing teratoma. The compact mass located superior to the aorta in the anterior mediastinum displays parietal contrast enhancement after contrast medium administration; the center, however, is slightly inhomogeneous (→). Near the mass, there is evidence of small, similarly vascularized nodular structures which also extend posterior to the superior vena cava (►).

demarcate avascular zones. Teratomas may contain adipose tissue with a negative CT numbers but do not, however, drop to the range of pure fatty tissue (-100 HU). Dermoid cysts frequently contain sebaceous material with a negative attenuation value. Fat-containing teratomas and thymic lipomas are indistinguishable on CT scans.

Most *seminomas* appear as a lobulated mass of homogeneously dense tissue. *Teratocarcinomas* and *chorionepitheliomas* are characterized by invasive growth, early necrosis and hemorrhage which, after the administration of contrast medium, can be seen as hypodense areas in well vascularized tumor tissue. If clinical signs of feminization exist, a *chorionepithelioma* must be considered.

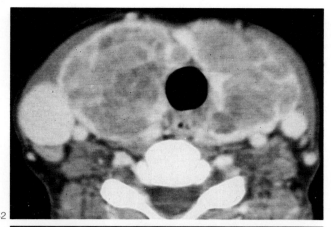

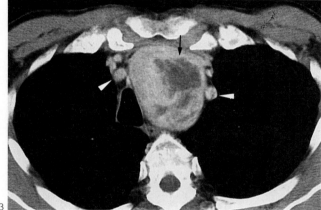

Fig. 6-42. Colloid goiter. After contrast medium administration, colloidal thyroid tissue becomes structured by fine, clearly contrast enhanced septa.

Fig. 6-43. Retrosternal goiter. In the typical manner, the brachiocephalic vessels are laterally displaced in a "basket-like" fashion by the goiter (►). Normal, well vascularized thyroid tissue delineates regressive changes and hemorrhage as hypodense zones (→).

Fig. 6-44. Substernal goiter. In plain scans, the attenuation value of this substernal (endothoracic) goiter (75 HU) was slightly elevated as compared with the adjacent arch of the aorta. The calcification is indicative of regressive tissue changes (►).

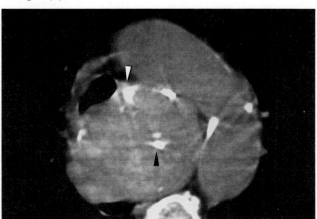

Since teratoblastomas frequently invade the thymic region or the thymus itself, they must be considered in the diagnosis. The diagnosis must be considered within the clinical setting.

Goiter

Hyperplasia (iodine deficiency, hyperthyroidism) and inflammation (Riedel, Hashimoto) lead to a generalized enlargement of the thyroid gland, i.e., goiter.

75 to 80% of all substernal goiters arise from the lower poles of the thyroid lobes or isthmus. They may extend retrosternally in front of the trachea. The remaining goiters originate in the dorsal thyroid gland and spread from retrotracheal or retro-esophageal areas, including the brachiocephalic vessels, to the posterior (preferentially right) mediastinum. These lesions are surrounded by a firm capsule. They receive their blood supply from vessels communicating with the thyroid.

Ectopic mediastinal goiter is rare. Displacement phenomena occur in the early stages of disease. The diagnosis of goiter is confirmed when radionuclides accumulate near the mass but not in the thyroid tissue of the cervical region.

• CT

Plain scans: The severity of displacement and distortion of the trachea depends on the location of the thyroid mass. Brachiocephalic vessels are displaced laterally. The veins may appear dilated due to compression of the SVC. Regressive changes, including plaque-like calcification, are common. While cystic changes do not occur as frequently, they are not unusual. Since radionuclides do not usually accumulate in intrathoracic thyroid tissue, computed tomography must especially define the morphological relationship between the thyroid gland and the mass. If a typical communicating branch is found, the presence of a substernal or cervicothoracic goiter is very probable. Slightly raised tissue density (70 HU) on plain scans is a further sign of thyroid tissue and is attributable to its increased iodine concentration. One can assume the lesion has transformed to a malignant goiter if infiltration of surrounding structures or regional lymph node enlargement has been found.

Contrast-enhanced scans: After a bolus injection of contrast medium, the well vascularized thyroid tissue becomes clearly enhanced. Regressive hypodense components, adenomas and carcinomas are well demarcated, while cysts remain unenhanced. Contrast administration also helps to define the relationship of the organs to contiguous intrathoracic structures (vessels, trachea, esophagus) for preoperative evaluation.

Differential diagnosis: It is not possible to differentiate malignant lesions from adenomas and inflammation in the absence of secondary malignancy criteria.

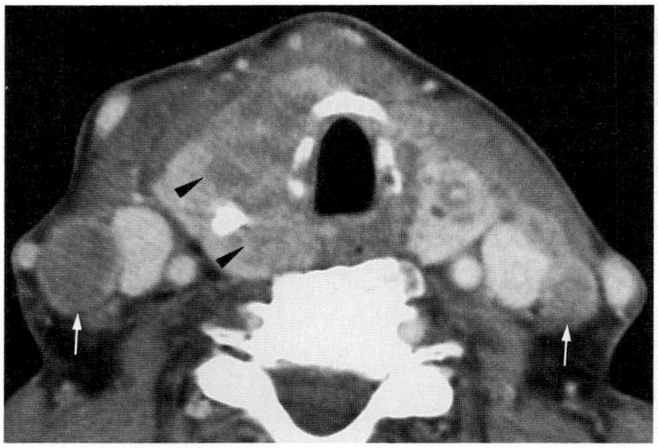

Fig. 6-45. Thyroid carcinoma. Especially in the right thyroid lobe, the areas of tumor infiltration (►) appear hypodense as compared with the well contrasted surrounding thyroid tissue. Furthermore, there is evidence of regional lymph node enlargement (→); the tissue structure in these areas is similar to that of the primary tumor.

Parathyroid Tumors

Approximately 90% of all epithelial bodies are found behind the thyroid gland. If ectopia has occurred, they are found predominantly in the anterior superior mediastinum (especially in the bed of the thymus), but rarely in the posterior superior mediastinum along the tracheo-esophageal angle. Approximately 90% of all cases with hyperfunction are caused by adenomas, and 10% by hyperplasia. Most adenomas are hormonally active. The diameter of parathyroid tumors usually ranges from 0.5 to 3 cm, but diameters of over 10 cm have been observed.

• CT

Plain scans: These circumscribed masses with muscle-dense attenuation values are found behind and along the lower poles of the thyroid gland. Because of their small diameter, they are best demonstrated by thin-section scanning (sections < 4 mm). When searching for ectopic

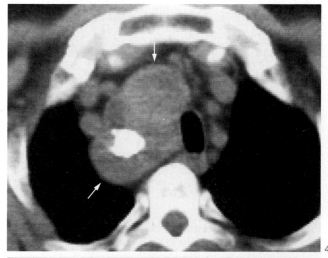

46

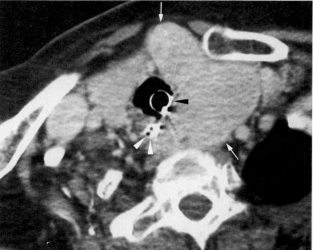

47

Fig. 6-46. Episternal goiter with regressive changes. In plain scans, one finds glandular tissue and calcification with contrasting CT numbers.

Fig. 6-47. Episternal goiter showing retrotracheal growth (→). After contrast medium administration, there is clear contrast enhancement. Regressive changes can be excluded. Tracheal tube (►); esophageal probe (▶).

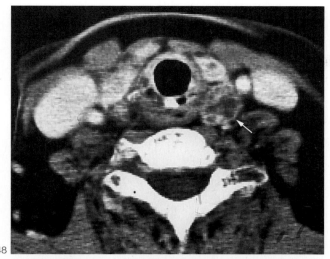

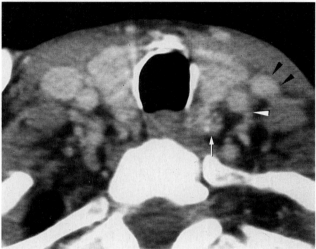

Fig. 6-48. Adenoma of the parathyroid. At the upper pole of the left thyroid lobe, a 1.2 cm diameter, lightly lobular mass is seen. Peripheral enhancement is seen with hypodense, relatively sharply demarcated areas indicative of hemorrhage or necrosis (→).

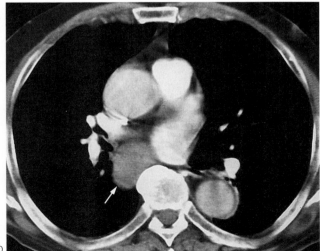

adenomas, thin sections should be scanned up to the level of the carina. The bed of the thymus and the tracheo-esophageal angle should be given special attention. Calcification and cysts are rare findings.

Contrast-enhanced scans: The majority of adenomas homogenously absorb contrast medium, which makes them distinguishable from mediastinal lymph node structures. Hypodense areas indicate either hemorrhage into the tumor or necrosis.

Primary Tumors of the Middle Mediastinum

Tumors of the Trachea

Tracheal myelomas and *carcinomas* are rare. The carcinoma spreads in the paratracheal space and invades the lymph nodes of that region. The degree of restriction and displacement of the trachea depends on how far the tumor has extended and is readily demonstrated on CT scans. These tumors can be distinguished from metastasizing bronchial carcinomas only in the early stages of development.

Bronchogenic Cysts

Most bronchogenic cysts are found proximal to the tracheobronchial angle. They seldom protrude into the posterior mediastinum. Some cysts (even small ones) may cause tracheobronchial obstruction, especially in children. However, even large bronchogenic cysts usually cause no major clinical complaints, and they frequently are discovered incidentally.

Fig. 6-49. Adenoma of the parathyroid. Evidence of a small, 0.8 cm diameter mass (→) posterior to the left lobe of the thyroid gland; it absorbs a slight amount of contrast medium. Common carotid artery (►); internal jugular vein (►).

Fig. 6-50. Bronchogenic cyst. There is a slightly lobular, hypodense lesion in a typical location directly beneath the carina. Its attenuation value of 55 HU remains constant after contrast medium administration, making it impossible to diagnose the nature of the lesion.

The secretory product of bronchogenic cysts may vary in consistency from serous to highly viscous.

• CT

Around half of all bronchogenic cysts have a CT number close to that of water. The attenuation value can rise due to a change in protein or calcium content. In the latter case, contrast medium must be administered to confirm the avascularity and cystic nature of the mass.

Pleuropericardial (Mesothelial) Cysts

Most of these cysts are found in the right anterior pericardiophrenic angle, but they may also develop on the left side in the hilar region and in the anterior mediastinum. Pleuropericardial cysts are usually 3 to 8 cm large, and their size rarely exceeds 13 cm.

• CT

The mass is demonstrated on CT scans as a thin-walled cystoid structure of variable shape. The attenuation value ranges from -5 to 25 HU.

Primary Tumors of the Posterior Mediastinum

Approximately 30% of all tumors of the posterior mediastinum are malignant.

Solid Neurogenic Tumors

Sympathetic blastomas occur in early childhood. Neurofibromas and neurinomas, on the

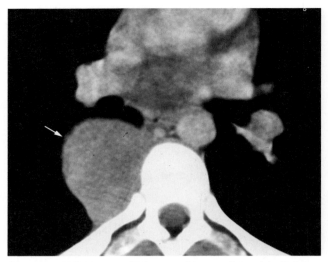

Fig. 6-51. Neurinoma. This smoothly marginated, soft-tissue dense paravertebral lesion shows no signs of bone erosion or intraspinal spread. Slight contrast enhancement (ca. 30 HU) develops after contrast medium administration.

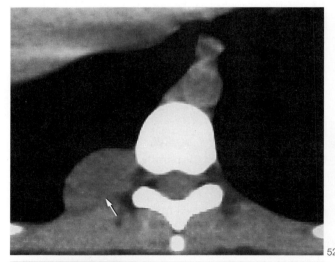

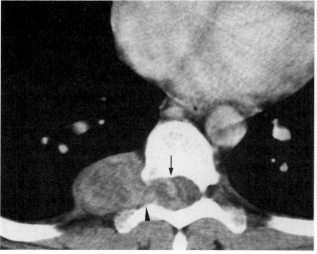

Fig. 6-52. Neurinoma. This smoothly marginated, round lesion adjacent to the head of the rib is slightly hypodense in the area facing the muscle (→). There was no evidence of a dilated intervertebral foramen or intraspinal spread.

Fig. 6-53. Neurinoma. The tumor spreads in an hourglass fashion, extending through the dilated foramen (►) into the spinal canal (→). Inhomogeneous contrast enhancement is seen after contrast medium administration.

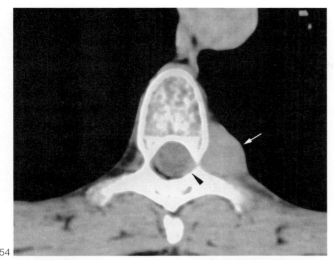

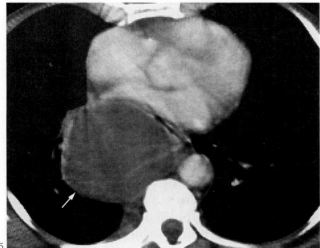

Fig. 6-54. An isolated non-Hodgkin's lymphoma (→). It displays slight contrast medium enhancement and discrete peridural spread (►).

Fig. 6-55. Neurogenic cyst. This is a hypodense retrocardial lesion with an attenuation value of 19 HU.

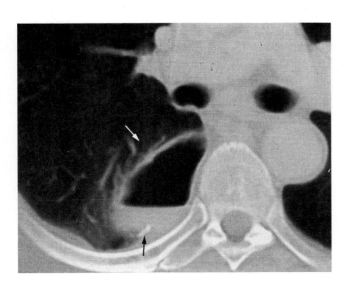

other hand, usually affect young adults. The incidence of pheochromocytomas and paragangliomas is very low. With the exception of the paraganglioma, the remaining neurogenic tumors develop exclusively in the posterior mediastinum. Calcification of these tumors is rare and primarily affects neuroblastomas and ganglioneurinomas.

• CT

In most cases, the typical paravertebral localization of these tumors can be readily demonstrated on CT scans. The masses normally have well-defined margins and attenuation values in the soft-tissue range. The CT numbers are often reduced due to liquefaction and increased lipid content. A dilated neuroforamen is a sign of neurogenic tumor origin (hourglass neoplasms). If the adjacent neuroforamen is dilated, thin sections of the tissue should be scanned. Broadening of the bony part of the vertebral canal is a sign of intraspinal origin of the tumor, which requires further investigation. Irregular bone destruction is a malignancy criterion that must be differentiated from smooth erosion of the vertebral body and ribs, which is observed in malignant as well as benign masses. Calcification occurs infrequently and predominantly in ganglioneuroblastomas.

If a hypertonic crisis occurs in conjunction with a mediastinal mass, the extremely rare *mediastinal pheochromocytoma* should be considered in the diagnosis.

Cystic Lesions

Cystic lesions in the posterior mediastinum are extremely rare. Secondary diagnostic indicators are required to distinguish these lesions.

Meningoceles are caused by unilateral or bilateral herniation of the leptomeninges through the neuroforamen. They may contain fluid and

Fig. 6-56. Upwardly displaced stomach after surgery for esophageal carcinoma. In the operation, the stomach was displaced to the mediastinum. It has a cystic appearance with fluid fluid levels in the immediate paravertebral vicinity.

be multiple. Dilatation of the neuroforamen is common; other bony defects are rare.

Histologically, *neuro-enteric cysts* are composed of pleural and enteric elements. They are normally associated with congenital defects of the thoracic spine (dysrhaphism, incomplete formation of vertebra). These smooth or lobular lesions contain a watery secretory fluid. If the gastrointestinal tract is affected, pockets of air may be present. Gastrointestinal and esophageal cysts can be differentiated only in histological tests. Neuro-enteric cysts differ from bronchogenic cysts in that their location is predominantly paravertebral which, however, is also true of cysts in the thoracic duct.

• CT

CT is normally only able to demonstrate the cystic nature of these lesions. Deformities of the spine and ribs offer additional diagnostic information. Pancreatogenic pseudocysts must be considered in the diagnosis, but usually pose no diagnostic problems when both the infradiaphragmatic findings and the patient history are clear.

Vascular Processes

Aorta

Numerous congenital deformities of the aortic arch form imposing images on conventional chest x-rays. Some examples are the *right aortic arch*, *double aortic arch*, and *coarctation*. These anomalies can be demonstrated well on CT scans.

A double aortic arch with *vascular rings* around the trachea is less common than an *aberrant left subclavian artery* with a right aortic arch. The latter causes clinical symptoms because of its course under the esophagus. In elderly patients, anomalies of the aortic arch must be differentiated from elongation and kinking. Sagittal reformatted images may facilitate the diagnosis.

Aneurysms of the Thoracic Aorta

Etiologically speaking, arteriosclerosis is the most predominant thoracic aneurysm. These aneurysms are divided into three different groups according to their location:

Type I: From the aortic valve to the exit of the brachiocephalic trunk.

Type II: From the exit of the brachiocephalic trunk to the origin of the left subclavian artery.

Type III: Directly before the point where the left subclavian artery arises to a position just above the diaphragm.

There are three different pathological and anatomical types of aortic aneurysms, namely the true aneurysm (70 to 80%), the dissecting aneurysm (ca. 25%), and the rare spurious aneurysm (peri-arterial hematoma).

Arteriosclerotic aneurysms occur more frequently than traumatic aneurysms which arise from blunt thoracic trauma. Approximately 60% of all traumatic aneurysms develop at the point of attachment of the ligamentum arteriosum, proximal to the subclavian artery, whereas 20% are found at the point of attachment of the ascending aorta and at the level of the diaphragm. Mycotic types, seen with endocarditis, are just as infrequent as aneurysms occurring with idiopathic medial necrosis. Rupture can be accompanied by pericardial tamponage, mediastinal hematomas and pleural herniation. They are the most common and most serious type of complication. Most ruptures originate in the aortic arch or the descending aorta. Their configuration is usually more fusiform than saccular.

• CT

Plain scans: Generally, one should assume that an aneurysm is present when the external aortic diameter is greater than 4 cm. A distal increase in caliber is an important distinguishing sign in borderline cases, because the physiological proportion of the antero-posterior diameters of ascending aorta and the descending aorta should be ca. 1.5. Intraluminal thrombotic deposits, especially in conjunction

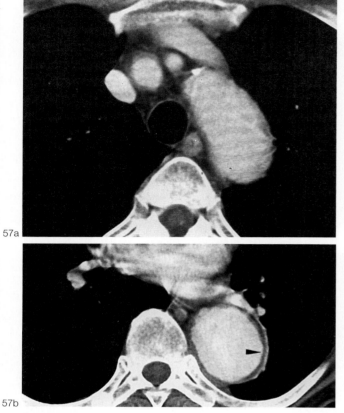

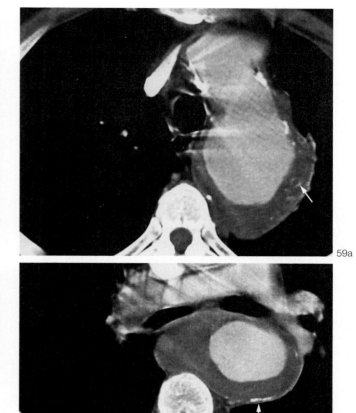

Fig. 6-57. Aortic aneurysm. In cross-sectional scans, the arch of the aorta appears wider in the dorsal region (a). In the descending segment, it is dilated to an external diameter of 5 cm. Discrete, circular thrombotic mural deposits are also visible (b).

Fig. 6-59. Extensive aneurysm of the thoracic aorta. Clear dilatation of the external and internal lumina is seen, even in the arch of the aorta. There are broad, thrombotic deposits, in some cases with ringlike intrathrombotic calcification (a→). Mural processes are also found in the descending thoracic aorta (calcification of the adventitia (b→).

Fig. 6-58. Posttraumatic aortic aneurysm. Along the lower circumference of the arch of the aorta (typically, posterior to the origin of the subclavian artery), there is spherical enlargement of the aortic lumen with wide, ringlike calcification.

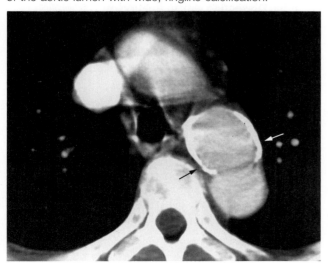

with calcific degeneration of the intima, are a further indication. Such deposits are visible even on plain scans, and they appear as hypodense zones. Sclerosis of the dilated aortic wall or of thrombotic deposits is a frequent finding. Boundaries of the aortic arch or kinking can be masked by partial volume artifacts. Thin-section scanning is then required to properly demonstrate these areas on CT scans.

Contrast-enhanced scans: After a bolus injection of contrast medium, the lumen can always be seen on axial CT scans. The lumen appears as an oval structure when the aortic tube obliquely courses through the slice plane. The scans must then be longitudinally reconstructed for exact measurement.
Rupture-related complications can be due to a mediastinal hematoma or pericardial or pleural

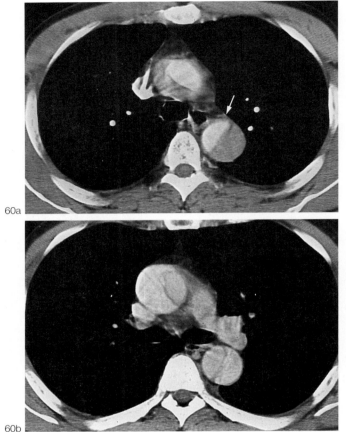

60a

60b

Fig. 6-60. Dissecting aortic aneurysm in ascending and descending sections. The true lumen is enhanced in the early phase of contrast enhancement (→), and the dissection membrane is clearly visible. Contrast enhancement is equalized in 20 seconds.

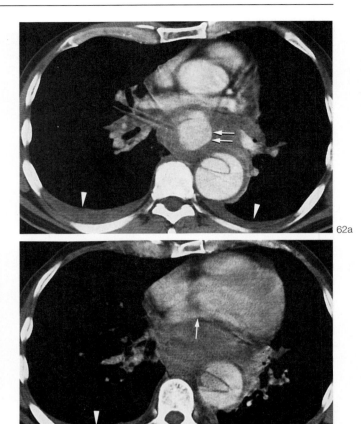

62a

62b

Fig. 6-62. Ruptured dissecting aortic aneurysm directly below the arch of the aorta. Directly superior to the aorta, there is an opaque-laden zone (⇒) corresponding to the false aneurysm. The area extending from the entire posterior mediastinum to the left atrium is enlarged by compact blood masses, thereby compressing the cardiac silhouette (→). Pleural effusions (►) are also present.

Fig. 6-61. Aortic dissection. Motion artifacts are minimized when quicker scanning times are used. However, double contour lines frequently develop (► ◄). These may complicate the evaluation and demonstration of the dissection membrane. True lumen (⇒), false lumen (→).

Fig. 6-63. Dissecting aortic aneurysm. Calcification near the dissection membrane (→) is indicative of intima calcification. This can be demonstrated on plain scans.

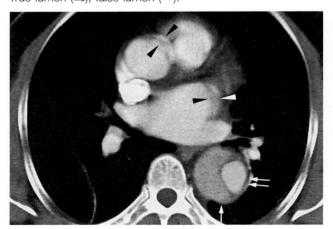

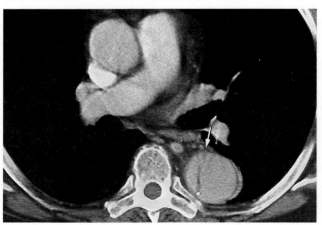

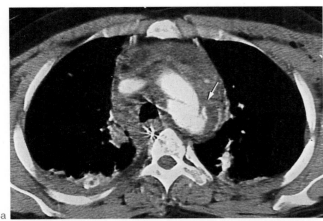

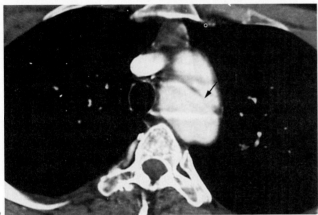

Fig. 6-64. Traumatic aortic aneurysm. After a blunt abdominal trauma, there is considerable broadening of the upper mediastinum, where the arch of the aorta can be seen as a relatively small-caliber structure with signs of a dissection membrane (a→). However, compact amounts of escaping contrast medium are not demonstrable. Six month later, a saccular aneurysm was found below the arch of the aorta (b→). The exact position of the aneurysm with respect to the left subclavian artery was determined by arteriography.

Fig. 6-65. Aortic dissection in the arch of the aorta (Type III). The dissection membrane appears broader due to the tangential angle of the section (→).

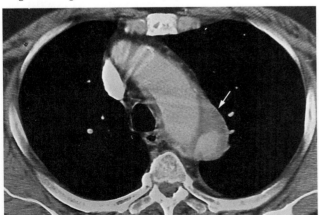

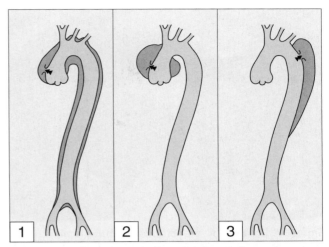

Fig. 6-66. Classification of aortic dissecting aneurysms according to de Bakey.
1 = Type I; 2 = Type II; 3 = Type III.

herniation. A traumatic aneurysm can be assumed if the aneurysm is located at the characteristic location on the distal aortic arch.

Dissecting Aneurysms

Arteriosclerosis, usually in conjunction with hypertension, is also the primary etiological factor responsible for the development of dissecting aneurysms. They only seldom arise from Marfan's syndrome, Ehlers-Danlos' syndrome and cystic medial necrosis. A dissecting aneurysm develops through a laceration in the intima wall, and the resulting intramural hematoma can spread proximally or distally. The laceration develops in the ascending aorta in ca. 80% of all cases (types I and II). The aneurysm remains restricted to this section of the vessel in ca. 10% of cases (type II), but usually extends more distally (type I). Only ca. 20% of all dissecting aneurysms arise in the upper section of the descending aorta (type III). The degree of abdominal extension is variable. A second (re-entry) laceration can develop in the periphery, thereby connecting the false and true lumina while reducing clinical symptoms. This condition is frequently accompanied by impaired flow to one kidney. Thrombosis of the intramural hematoma is rare.

According to the Stanford classification system, *Type A* dissecting aneurysms are those in

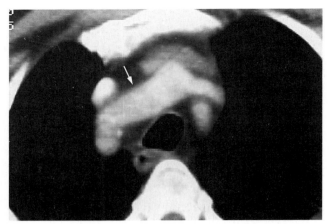

Fig. 6-67. Ectasia of the brachiocephalic trunk. There is clear dilatation of the brachiocephalic trunk (→), which branches on the left, together with the common carotid artery, from the arch of the aorta.

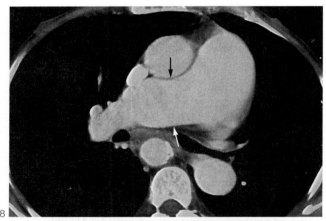

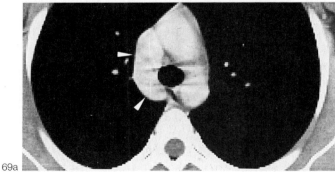

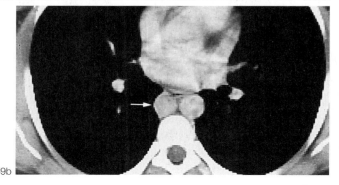

which the aneurysm affects only the ascending aorta; they require immediate surgery. *Type B* dissections are restricted to the descending aorta; there is no immediate need for surgery. Life-threatening complications include bleeding with hemopericardium, aortic valve insufficiency, acute heart failure and ruptures in conjunction with mediastinal hematoma or hemothorax.

● CT

Plain scans: Scout sections should be scanned to detect minor calcification in the (loose) dissected membrane, fresh intraluminal (hyperdense) hematoma, or possible complications (hematopericardium, mediastinal hematoma).

Contrast-enhanced scans: The classical signs of aortic dissection, namely the presence of two lumina filled with contrast medium, become visible on CT scans only after a sufficient amount of contrast medium has been administered. In some sections, images of the dissected membrane may be blurred by rapid movements and artifacts attributable to cardiac motion. Aortic dissection can be confirmed by rapid sequential scanning when there is proof of delayed filling in the false lumen at the level of the ascending aorta.

Even if no proof of an ascending aortic dissection could be found, the presence of hyperdense pericardial effusion fluid still leaves open the possibility, since the dissecting membrane could (temporarily) be masked. Enlargement of the recess of the pericardium can simulate intima loosening at the attachment of the root of the aorta, but the two conditions can be differentiated by administering more contrast medium if enhancement is insufficient.

Fig. 6-68. Ectasia of the pulmonary arteries. There is considerable dilatation of the pulmonary arteries (→). The diameter of the right pulmonary artery is 43 mm behind the ascending aorta.

Fig. 6-69. Continuity syndrome in the azygos vein. In the absence of an intrahepatic cava segment, venous drainage of the abdominal cavity occurs via the azygos vein (→). Its diameter behind the heart is similar to that of the descending aorta. It can be traced as a tubular structure extending up to the azygos arch (►).

Ectasia of the Brachiocephalic Trunk

The right side of the superior mediastinum is frequently prominent in older patients with arteriosclerosis and hypertension. This is often caused by compression of the brachiocephalic trunk or, more uncommonly, by an aneurysm in the brachiocephalic trunk. If unclear, questions regarding the etiology can be clarified by computerized tomography.

Ectasia of Pulmonary Arteries

Dilatation of the pulmonary arteries to diameters larger than 29 mm is an indication of pulmonary hypertension. Filling defects are signs of central pulmonary embolism.

Ectasia of the Azygos Vein

Dilatation of the azygos vein, which is also demonstrated on conventional chest x-rays, is normally a result of increased central venous pressure in the right atrium. If there is obstruction of the upper and lower vena cavae or occlusion of the portal vein, and abnormal disposition of the inferior vena cava, the azygos vein will become part of an extensive collateral vascular network. This results in a corresponding increase in venous caliber *(azygos vein continuity syndrome)*.

• CT

Two specific causes of the development of collateral vascular channels are frequently demonstrated by CT, especially on contrast-enhanced scans. They are 1) stenosis of the upper vena cava caused by a tumor or thrombosis and 2) the absence of an intrahepatic vena cava segment. When the azygos vein becomes part of the collateral vascular channel, a corresponding enlargement of the lumen follows.

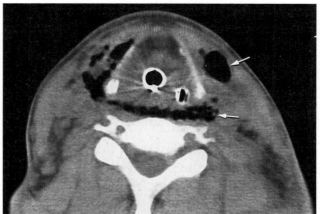

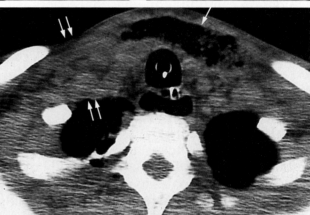

Fig. 6-70. Acute mediastinitis due to a gravitation abscess. Gas deposits (a→) are found in the cervical region near the larynx. These signalize the presence of an inflammatory process. Masking of the muscles continues caudally. Near the inlet of the thorax, gas is found to extend to the anterior mediastinum (b→). Here, also, the structure of muscles and vessels is masked due to phlegmonous permeation of fatty tissue (b ⇒).

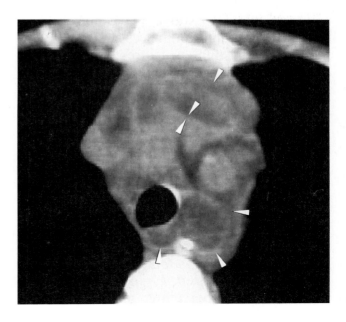

Fig. 6-71. Acute mediastinitis after phlegmonous spread of a parotic abscess. Several hypodense, ringlike structures (►) are found in the paratracheal region and anterior mediastinum; attenuation values around 15 HU. After contrast medium infusion, intensification of the ringlike structures (► ◄) indicates the presence of abscess fluid.

Mediastinal Inflammation

Acute Mediastinitis

The most frequent causes of acute mediastinitis are external traumatic injuries and perforation of a mediastinal organ (esophagus, trachea). Acute mediastinitis is more uncommonly caused by purulent processes in the fascia that spread caudal to the pharynx and neck. Direct spread of inflammation from the pleura and lungs to the mediastinum occurs relatively late. Exudation can fill the mediastinal spaces with phlegmonous material or (more uncommonly) lead to the development of abscesses, which can herniate into the hollow organs (esophagus, bronchus, pleural cavity).

• CT

Plain scans: Mediastinal phlegmons are demonstrated on CT scans as high-density areas within mediastinal fat. The distance between vessels of slender patients should be carefully analyzed, since it increases with increasing amounts of exudation. Accumulations of air may be due to a perforation or aerogenic bacteria. In patients with serious clinical complaints, local fluid collections or the development of cystoids must be considered as signs of abscess formation. Pleural effusions of varying severity accompany mediastinitis, even in the early stages.

Contrast-enhanced scans: The administration of contrast medium improves the visibility of masked mediastinal structures. Furthermore, (hypervascularized) granular tissue surrounded by abscesses can be demonstrated.

Chronic Mediastinitis

The etiology of chronic mediastinitis is heterogeneous and, in part, still unclear. It usually has an infective cause (tuberculosis, mycosis, histoplasmosis, actinomycosis, syphilis). Histologically, these disorders may also be collectively termed as *granulomatous mediastinitis*. Especially in children, lymph node enlargement due to tuberculous mediastinitis can be very extensive and may cause compression. The lymphomas may affect the airways; the clinical course is usually subacute. In adults, lymph node enlargement is normally moderate.

A diagnosis of *idiopathic fibrous mediastinitis* can be made if there is simultaneous proof of retroperitoneal fibrosis, Riedel's struma or an orbital pseudotumor. In chronic mediastinitis, the superior mediastinum is almost always affected, especially the paratracheal, carinal and hilar regions. Calcification is relatively rare.

Sclerosing fibrosis (which also indicates the terminal stages of mediastinal hematoma) has the pathological and anatomical appearance of a coarse sheet of connective tissue that encases the vessels, trachea and esophagus. Subsequent occurrence of vena cava occlusion syndrome was reported in ca. 10% of all patients with chronic mediastinitis. Sclerosing fibrosis more often occurs in connection with neoplastic lesions of the mediastinum.

• CT

Plain scans: Lymph node enlargement due to chronic mediastinitis is indistinguishable from lymph node enlargement due to other etiologies. While necrotic, hypodense, nonenhanced zones can be demonstrated in patients with extensive metastases, a specific etiology must be suspected in younger patients. The location of the affected lymph nodes should be considered in the diagnosis. Sclerosing mediastinitis appears as a soft-tissue dense zone around the vessels, trachea and esophagus, causing a variable degree of constriction. Mediastinal fat planes are also masked.

Contrast-enhanced scans: In patients with vena cava occlusion syndrome, the severity of thrombosis and collateral vascular circulation in the azygos system can be evaluated in contrast-enhanced CT scans.

Mediastinal Lesions

Pneumomediastinum
(Mediastinal Emphysema)

Air may enter the mediastinum from different routes. In spontaneous mediastinal emphysema, air enters the mediastinum through the root of the lung after an alveolar rupture has occurred along the peribronchial clefts. Lesions in the *esophagus* and *peribronchial tree* allow direct entry of air in the surrounding mediastinal connective tissue. Retroperitoneal and intraperitoneal accumulation of air and pneumothorax can lead to pneumomediastinum via different pathways.

• CT

Computed tomography can sensitively detect pockets of air, which are demonstrated without overshadowing, due to their sharply reduced (negative) density and (mixed) attenuation values. In inflammatory processes, gas-producing bacteria should be considered in the differential diagnosis.

Mediastinal Hematoma

Hemorrhage into the mediastinum is usually caused by a blunt or perforating trauma. A more uncommon cause is spontaneous rupture of an already existing aneurysm.

A blunt thoracic trauma can injure the retrosternal brachiocephalic veins and lead to a hematoma in the superior mediastinum. Ruptures of the thoracic aorta are usually caused by traffic accidents. Up to 95 % of these ruptures develop proximal to the isthmus, since the ligamentum arteriosum extends into the adventitia of the aorta beyond the point where the subclavian artery branches off. The mass of the heart combined with the force of a whiplash injury contorts the aortic arch and leads to the development of a lesion at the site of insertion of the ligament which, in turn, may give rise to a periaortic hematoma (spurious aneurysm).

Fig. 6-73. Mediastinal and soft-tissue emphysema after a bypass operation. Air deposits (→) in the chest wall and mediastinal fat, which has slightly thickened in the postoperative phase.

Fig. 6-74. Mediastinal hematoma. After a blunt abdominal trauma, the entire mediastinum is broadened (→). The blood-soaked condition of the mediastinum raises the attenuation values for mediastinal fat.

Fig. 6-72. Pneumomediastinum. After pneumothorax and drainage (Bülau method), there is a considerable amount of air in the entire mediastinum. This appears more transparent than the adjacent lung tissue (▸).

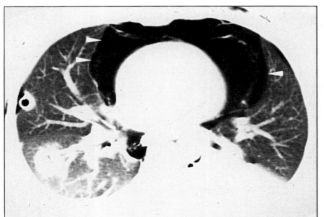

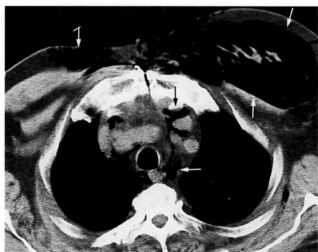

73

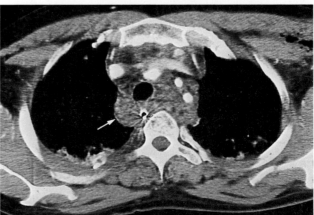

74

The lesion may extend proximally into the aortic arch, causing aortic dissection and a consequent flow deficit in the brachiocephalic artery. A chronic aneurysm is a late complication that is caused by incomplete laceration of a wall. It manifests several months after an accident.

• CT

Plain scans: On plain scans, hematomas appear as masses that variably constrict various mediastinal structures (trachea, esophagus, vessels). Layers of fatty tissue are masked by diffuse mediastinal hematoma. The attenuation value varies in accordance with the maturity of the hematoma.

Contrast-enhanced scans: In order to exclude the possibility of an aortic dissection, a bolus injection of contrast medium should be administered for better visibility of the aortic arch and the area of attachment of the ligamentum arteriosum, even in cases where the diagnosis of mediastinal hematoma could not be confirmed. In questionable cases, the origins of the brachiocephalic arteries should additionally be imaged by multidimensional angiography.

After bolus injection of contrast medium, the hematoma appears as a sharply delineated, circumscribed area. It is therefore possible to distinguish the hematoma from well vascularized neoplasms.

Chapter 7
The Heart

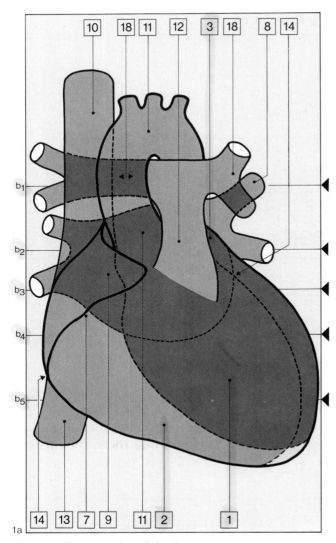

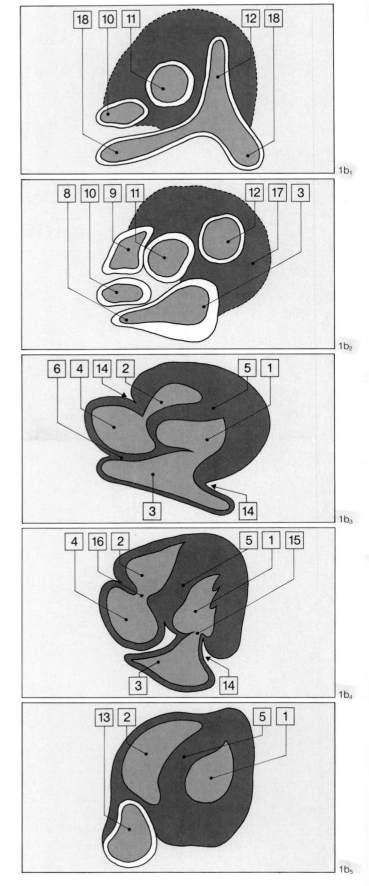

Fig. 7-1. Topography of the heart.

a) Anterior view (diagram)

b) Internal spaces and outflow tract in the transverse plane
(see a for level).

c) Analogous sectional planes for CT

Key to symbols:

 1 Left ventricle
 2 Right ventricle
 3 Left atrium
 4 Right atrium
 5 Interventricular septum
 6 Interartrial septum
 7 Coronary sulcus
 8 Pulmonary vein
 9 Right auricular apex
10 Superior vena cava
11 Ascending aorta
12 Pulmonary cone
13 Inferior vena cava
14 Atrioventricular plane
15 Mitral valve
16 Tricuspid valve
17 Transverse pericardial sinus
18 Pulmonary artery

The Heart

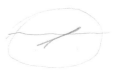

Anatomy and Imaging

The long axis of the heart runs diagonal to the horizontal CT plane. After the patient has been given a sufficient amount of *contrast medium* (CM), the individual chambers of the heart can be demonstrated on CT scans which, according to the level of the slice, will show the varying relationship of size and position of different chambers to one another. The right ventricle is scanned at its broadest point in caudal sections of the heart. The conically arched left ventricle is scanned more cranially at its point of greatest diameter. The thick left ventricular wall and the interventricular septum are readily demonstrated on CT scans. Papillary muscles are often well demarcated. Because of its thin wall, the myocardium of the right ventricle is only subtly outlined. Visualization of the *atria*, including the right cardiac auricle, is unequivocal. The maximum anteroposterior diameter of the left atrium is 4 to 5 cm in healthy individuals. Calcification of segments of the *coronal arteries* proximal to the aorta can be demonstrated on plain scans. In dynamic CT, visualization of these segments can also be enhanced by intravenous contrast medium. *Valvular calcification* can also be readily demonstrated on CT scans.

Normal scan times of 4 to 8 seconds yield satisfactory images of moving organ structures when they are produced by averaging and reformatting multiple scans. Cardiac phase-controlled scanning (ECG-gating) improves the quality of the images, thus improving the radiologist's ability to measure the actual thickness of myocardial walls in different cardiac phases. It is now possible to evaluate the systolic and end-diastolic volumes as well as the ejection fraction by means of computed tomography. In more recent developments, the imaging quality of moving cardiac structures has been improved by ultra-fast Cine-CT techniques (scan times of ca. 50 ms).

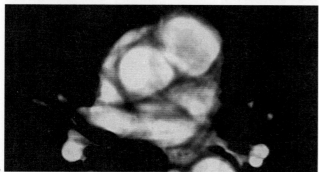

1c₁

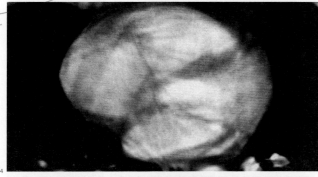

1c₂

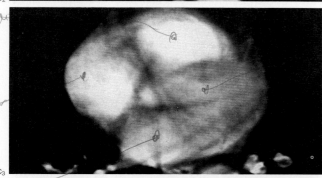

1c₃

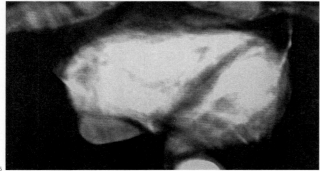

1c₄

1c₅

Current cardiologic applications of computed tomography include evaluation or confirmation of:
1. the size and shape of the heart;
2. the positional relationship of the cardiac chambers and large vessels exiting the heart;
3. the presence of intracavitary masses;
4. the patency of aortocoronary bypasses.

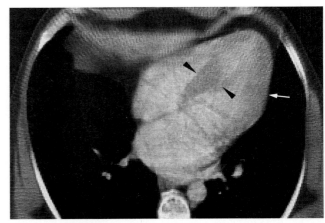

Fig. 7-2. Pressure stress. Focal thickening of the interventricular septum is found in a patient with idiopathic hypertrophic subvalvular aortic stenosis (► ◄). Hypertrophy of the remaining wall segments of the left ventricle causes moderate mural thickening (→).

Functional Conditions of the Heart

Volume Stress

Volume stress in the left ventricle is caused by pendular blood flow resulting from valvular insufficiency or a shunt. This condition first manifests as end-diastolic enlargement of a ventricle which, in patients with poor contraction, is also seen during systole. Right-sided volume stress normally occurs in conjunction with a left-to-right shunt; the condition can cause considerable ventricular enlargement.

Fig. 7-3. Cardiomyopathy (dilatative). The left ventricle shows considerable enlargement with rounding of the apex of the heart and right lateral protrusion (→) of the interventricular septum.

Fig. 7-4. Coronary sclerosis. Despite heart action, CT still sensitively detects calcification of the coronary vessels (►).

• CT

According to the severity of the condition, minor to substantial enlargement of the ventricle can be seen on CT scans. The interventricular septum rotates towards the right in patients with left-sided cardiac stress, and towards the left in those with right-sided cardiac stress. The apex of the ventricle is normally rounded, and thickening of the ventricular walls is not usually found.

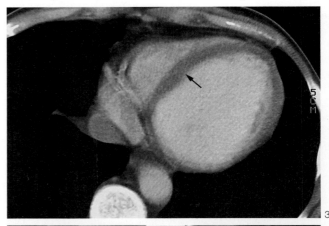

Pressure Stress

Pressure stress in the left ventricle, which is caused by hypertension or other cardiac problems, will lead to concentric hypertrophy. Idiopathic hypertrophic subvalvular aortic stenosis is a specific type in which an asymmetrical septal hypertrophy also occurs. Right-sided stress is caused by pulmonary hypertension (cor pulmonale, mitral stenosis) or aortic valve stenosis.

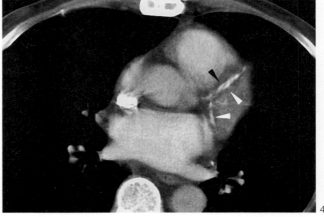

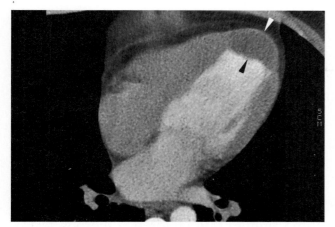

Fig. 7-5. Aneurysm of the heart wall. In the apex of the heart, there is a hypodense, sharply marginated structure that corresponds with the appearance of thrombotic deposits (► ◄).

● CT

Significant thickening of the ventricle wall and a more pronounced appearance of the trabecula is seen on CT scans of patients with a hypertrophic left ventricle. The interventricular septum may be rotated slightly to the right and have a conical configuration. Broad muscle bulging in the middle section of the interventricular septum is seen in patients with idiopathic hypertrophic subvalvular aortic stenosis. Muscular hypertrophy of the right ventricle frequently cannot be confirmed because of partial-volume artifacts and cardiac motion. Enlargement of the pulmonary trunk is an indicator of severe pulmonary hypertension.

Cardiomyopathy

Metabolic and regressive abnormalities frequently lead to ventricular enlargement and thickening of the myocardium. Contractility, which cannot be evaluated on single CT images, is usually affected in both cases. Dilatation of the affected ventricles and corresponding wall-thickening can, however, be well demonstrated.

Coronary Heart Disease

Recent myocardial infarctions can be distinguished from normal myocardium by means of ECG-gated CT with localized uptake of contrast medium. Cardiac phase-controlled scans are also necessary to confirm physiological systolic wall thickening and paradoxical reduction in diastole. This very time-consuming techni-

Fig. 7-6. Aortocoronary bypass. The implanted vein (a ► ◄) contrasts after contrast medium administration, thereby indicating its patency. With high-dose contrast medium administration, ECG triggering, and rapid, successive scanning, the venous bypasses (b, c →) can be demonstrated very graphically in various projections. The internal cardiac and intravascular spaces are shown, but not the myocardium. Bypass anastomosis along the aorta (⇒).

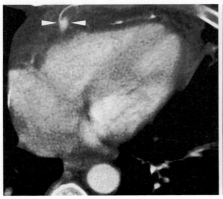

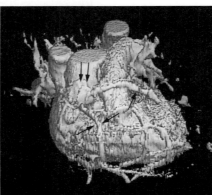

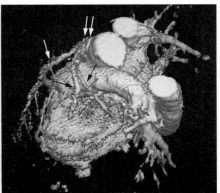

6a

6c

que has not gained wide acceptance in conventional CT, since only part of the boundary surfaces of the left ventricle are adequately demonstrated. Furthermore, new perspectives have resulted from the introduction of ultra-fast Cine-CT. The effects of infarction are frequently visible, even on CT scans with slower scan times. Scarring is demonstrated as a localized recess, the aneurysm as a protrusion which is frequently accompanied by a parietal thrombus.

The patency of *aortocoronary bypasses* can also be determined by CT. The lumen of the transplant should show punctiform enhancement, which is an indication of blood flow, after a bolus injection of contrast medium. It is not possible, however, to measure the flow rate or to diagnose stenosis. Severe stenosis may simulate an occlusion on these contrast-enhanced scans. In multiple bypasses, it may be impossible to diagnose an occlusion due to the complex morphology of the condition. Dynamic scanning is therefore recommended for postoperative follow-up examinations in asymptomatic patients.

Very rare incidences of widespread aneurysms of the coronary arteries can be demonstrated on CT scans.

Valvular Defects

A number of congenital and acquired cardiac defects can be diagnosed by analyzing the ventricles and vessels of the heart. Mitral stenosis, for example, is indicated by the following findings: small left ventricle, enlargement of the left atrium with significant dorsal impairment of the right side, valvular calcification, and concentric hypertrophy. Even though the need for cardiac pressure measurement and cardiography remains, computed tomography can be used to support equivocal echocardiograms and to check cardiac problems that are being treated.

Intracavitary Masses

The most frequent tumor is the *myxoma*, which is almost always found in the atria (75% in the fossa ovalis of the left atrium). This tumor occurs predominantly in patients in the 3rd to 6th decade of life. The cystic components within the tumor are well recognized. *Rhabdomyomas* can develop in all sections of the heart as single or multiple lesions. Rhabdomyomas which protrude into the lumen of the heart are rarely pediculated. They are diagnosed primarily in children (tuberous sclerosis).

Sarcomas of various tissue type belong to the group of primary *malignant tumors*. Their rate of occurrence is much more infrequent than that of secondary neoplasms (metastases from carcinoma of the bronchus, melanomas, malignant lymphomas).

• CT

On CT scans, these tumors are demonstrated as an intraluminal filling defect. Their CT density is not distinguishable from that of a thrombus.

Fig. 7-7. Atrial thrombus accompanying mitral valve stenosis. The left atrium is clearly dilated. Right dorsolateral, in addition to mural calcification, there is a filling defect indicative of a thrombus.

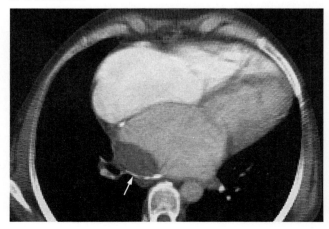

Pericardium

Anatomy and Imaging

Epicardial fat is depicted on CT scans as a hypodense space between the pericardium and the myocardium. Since the intricate structures of the myocardium are surrounded by epicardial fat, the thickness of the pad of fat is variable. It is especially prominent near the pathways of venous inflow and arterial out-

Fig. 7-8. Topography of the pericardium from a left paravertebral, sagittal view. The variable amount of subepicardial fat rounds out the contours of the heart. In some places, the parietal pericardial membrane is fused with the pleura (pleuropericardial membrane); in other areas there are additional fat-filled spaces.

Key to symbols:
 1 Parietal pericardial membrane
 2 Visceral pericardial membrane (epicardium)
 3 Subepicardial fat
 4 Adipose body
 5 Pleuropericardial membrane
 6 Left ventricle
 7 Pulmonary outflow tract
 8 Left pulmonary artery
 9 Left pulmonary vein
10 Aorta
11 Pleura

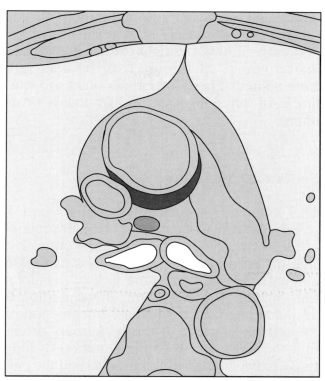

Fig. 7-9. Retroaortic pericardial pocket. Physiologically, it appears as a sickle-shaped, discretely hypodense structure dorsal to the root of the aorta. This configuration distinguishes it from an enlarged lymph node.

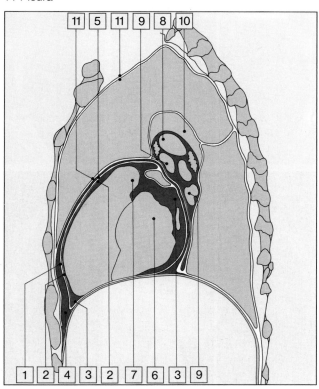

flow, but the amount of paracardiac fat and fat near the apex of the heart can vary greatly. Since the common membrane of the pericardium and the mediastinal pleura is only partial, additional spaces that are also filled with mediastinal fat can develop (e.g. epiphrenic or precardiac pads of fat). Due to the physiology of the pericardium, approximately 25 ml of fluid is found in the clefts of the pericardial space, which has a small recess in its folds.

The region of hypodense epicardial fat should be scanned tangentially in the region of maximum circumference of the heart to obtain the best CT images. In obese patients, both membranes of the pericardium can be identified as a linear densification in the vicinity of the apex of the heart. In patients with small amounts of epicardial fat and strong heart action they may occasionally be seen in a dorsolateral position around the left ventricle. Physiological pericardial fluid is usually found in the retroaortic pericardial recess, but seldom in the preaortic (aorticopulmonic) sinuses. A small area of hypodensity around the right cardiac auricle and in the vicinity of the apex of the heart are further sites of predilection for slight accumulation of physiological fluid in the pericardium.

Pericardial Anomalies

The absence of a pericardial contour on CT scans is indicative of partial or complete aplasia of the pericardium. Absence of the entire left side of the pericardium is the most common anomaly. In addition to the lack of demarcation of the left pericardium, this condition is also characterized by increased protrusion of the left main trunk of the pulmonary artery into the lungs and by an indentation of lung tissue between the ascending aorta and the pulmonary artery. Congenital pericardial cysts and pericardial diverticula are demonstrated as localized formations along the pericardium with CT numbers in the water range. Cystic teratomas must be excluded from the diagnosis.

Pericardial Fluid Collection

Acute, non-specific pericarditis, which is believed to have a viral etiology, is of clinical significance. Other forms normally accompany inflammatory processes. Bacterial pericarditis, for example, occurs preferentially in conjunction with pulmonary lesions, while the non-infectious form associated with cardiac infarction and heart surgery also accompanies rheumatoid arthritis, uremia, neoplasms, and collagenoses. Acute fluid accumulations of over 250 ml can lead to a cardiac tamponade; this may be due to perforating trauma, neoplastic aortic dissection in conjunction with hematopericardium, and bacterial, neoplastic and rheumatic pericarditis. Pericarditis occurs with serous, fibrinoserous, fibrinous, fibrinopurulent and/or purulent exudates, which can only sometimes be definitively attributed to a particular etiology.

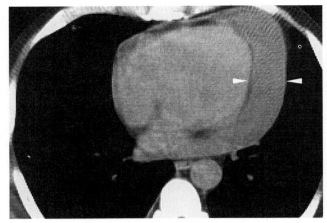

Fig. 7-10. Acute, nonspecific pericarditis. This effusion (► ◄) with an attenuation value of ca. 22 HU is located predominantly on the left side. It therefore shows a tendency for encapsulation.

Fig. 7-11. Pericardial effusion after radiotherapy. An extensive effusion is located on both sides of the heart. It extends upwards to the pulmonary outflow tract (a), has a CT number of ca. 25 HU and a delicate pericardial wall.

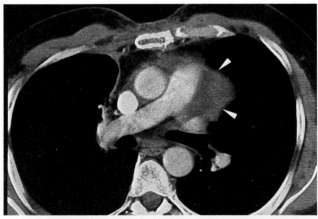

11a

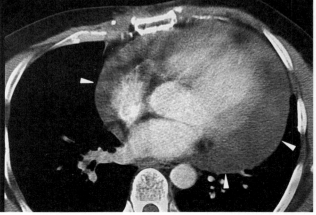

11b

Table 7-1. Causes of pericardial effusion.

- Acute idiopathic, nonspecific pericarditis
- Infectious pericarditis
  (viral, pyogenic, tuberculous, mycotic,
  parasitic, syphilitic, etc.)
- Acute myocardial infarction
  Dressler's disease
  Post-thoracotomy syndrome
  Trauma, blunt or puncture
  Aortic aneurysm
  (with pericardial involvement)
- Collagenosis
- Tumors, primary or metastasizing
  (including lymphoma and leukemia)
- Irradiation
- Uremia
- Medications
  (e.g. procainamide, hydralazine)

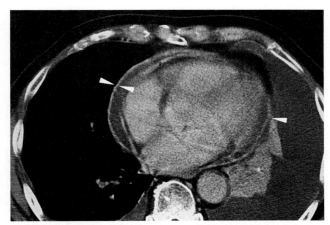

Fig. 7-12. Tuberculous pericarditis. The floridity of the process is evident in the clear contrast medium uptake in the parietal (▶ ◀) and visceral pericardial membranes. Evidence of accompanying pleural effusion.

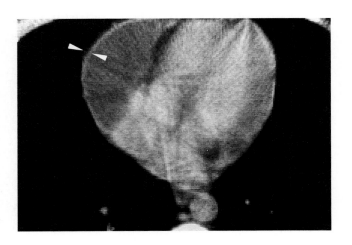

Pericardial effusions can normally be diagnosed by sonographic techniques. CT can detect dorsally situated (encapsulated) exudates and evaluate complex diagnostic situations which directly affect the pericardium and its immediate environment.

• CT

Plain scans: Fluid collections appear on CT scans as rounded, hypodense zones (as compared with the myocardium) which are located along the contour of the heart. These zones lie directly adjacent to the epicardial fatty tissue, which is intensified to varying degrees. The zone can vary in width in the different sections of the heart according to the size of the pericardial spaces. When the patient is in a supine position, recent effusions are normally found in more dorsal positions. If the epicardium and pericardium have been thickened by a fibrin coating, they are frequently demarcated from the hypodense fluid zones that lie between them. If, after a long-term observation period, the thickening of the pericardial membranes does not regress, a transformation to connective tissue may have occurred. Encapsulation of the pericardial effusion will lead to asymmetrical accumulations of fluid, which do not alter in appearance when the position of the patient is changed.

The *radiodensity* of collected pericardial fluid is slightly higher than that of water. In accordance with the protein (fibrin) content and the amount of blood mixed in, the value can rise to 10–40 HU or higher in recent hematopericardium (50 HU).

Contrast-enhanced scans: In the presence of protein-rich exudates and blood in the pericardium, it is difficult to distinguish the pericardium from the myocardium when the lamella of the epicardial fat is too thin. In such cases, the structures can be demarcated by a bolus

Fig. 7-13. Tuberculous pericarditis. Encapsulated right lateral pericardial effusion with slight thickening of the parietal membrane (▶ ◀). However, there is no clear contrast enhancement (which suggests that fibrosis has already occurred).

injection of contrast medium. It additionally opacifies parts of the pericardium that have been altered or made resorptive by inflammation, which makes it easier to identify fluid accumulations. In neighboring tumors (of the mediastinum, pleura or lungs) whose degree of spread can be evaluated on CT scans, demonstration of infiltration into the parietal membrane and possible (hypodense) pericardial exudation can normally be improved after intravenous administration of contrast medium.

Chronic Constrictive Pericarditis

As a rule, all purulent (specific and non-specific) and serofibrinous types of pericarditis as well as hematopericardium can transform into chronic constrictive pericarditis (CCP). Viral CCP has meanwhile become more common than tuberculous CCP, but the etiology usually remains unclear. Even tumor-related pericarditis can overlap with the clinical abnormality of constrictive pericarditis. Approximately half of all areas of calcification can be demonstrated on conventional x-ray pictures. Clinical differentiation of a restrictive cardiomyopathy and constrictive pericarditis can be problematic, so proof of pericardial fibrosis can be diagnostically significant. Not every pericardial thickening transforms into constrictive pericarditis after irradiation therapy, trauma or uremia.

• CT

Plain scans: Localized or circumferential pericardial thickening of inconstant width (0.5 to 2 cm) is seen on most CT scans. With only slight amounts of fluid, it may be difficult to distinguish CCP from acute pericarditis, since the attenuation values for the exudate can become as high as those of connective tissue, due to the inclusion of fibrin and blood. When calcification is also found in pericardial membranes, connective tissue development has probably occurred.

These morphological anomalies are not necessarily unequivocal signs of cardiac restriction. Signs with hemodynamic relevance are substantial broadening of the inferior and superior vena cava, hepatomegaly and ascites. Angulation of the interventricular septum with localized myocardial retraction is diagnostically indicative.

Contrast-enhanced scans: A bolus injection of contrast medium opacifies the pericardium to allow an evaluation of the inflammatory nature of the pericarditis, while demarcating the myocardial structures.

Tumors

Primary tumors – mesotheliomas and fibrosarcomas – are extremely rare. Pericardial tumors are, almost without exception, secondary occurrences from primary tumors of the mediastinum, pleura or lungs.

• CT

The purpose of the CT examination is to evaluate the pericardial involvement of secondary tumors. Clear delineation of these pericardial tumors from the myocardium is frequently possible only after a targeted bolus injection of CM has been administered. Then, deformity of heart cavities and pericardial effusion can also be demonstrated.

Chapter 8
The Lungs

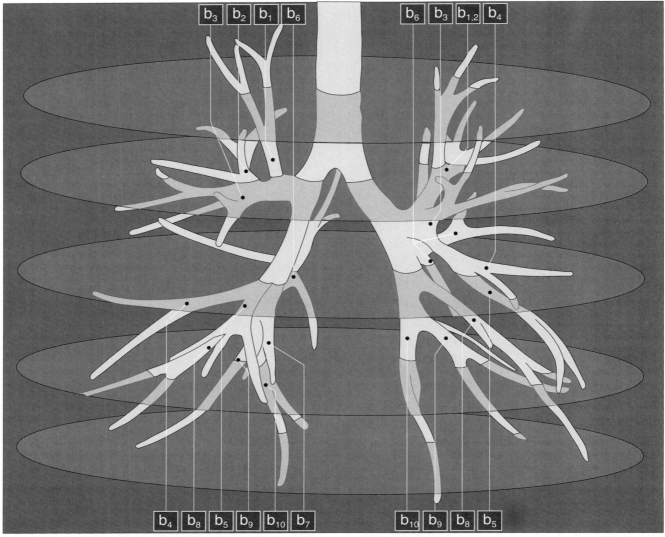

1a

Fig. 8-1. The bronchial tree. a) Spatial orientation of the bronchial structures. **b, c)** The central bronchial tree in transverse sections from cranial (b$_1$) to caudal (b$_5$) in the pulmonary window. Penumbra formation causes the bronchial structures to appear more vividly in the wide pleural window (c$_1$, c$_2$).

Key to symbols:

B$_L$	Left primary bronchus
B$_R$	Right primary bronchus
B$_{ol}$	Upper lobar bronchus
B$_{ul}$	Lower lobar bronchus
b$_{1-10}$	Segmental bronchus 1–10

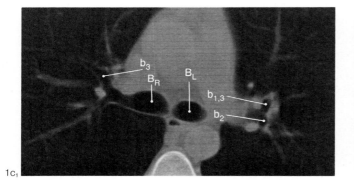

1c$_1$

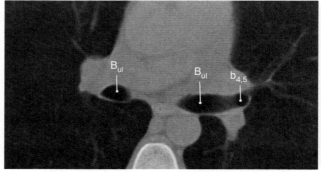

1c$_2$

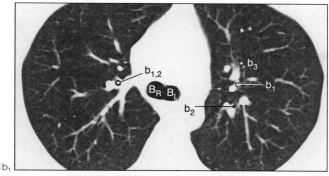

1b₁

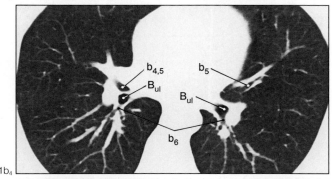

1b₂

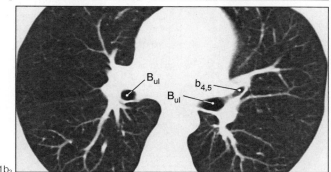

1b₃

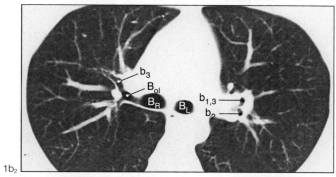

1b₄

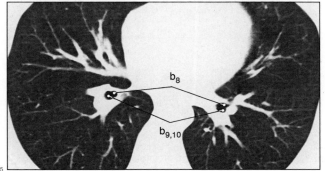

1b₅

The Lungs

Anatomy and Imaging

Computed tomography can now provide high-quality, artefact-free images of lung structures, which makes CT scans superior to plain radiographs and conventional tomography. By adjusting the window setting, transitions from lung tissue to soft tissue to bone can be demonstrated in detail. When complex pulmonary lesions display patchy areas of shadow, computed tomography is often required for further diagnosis.

Bronchial Tree

CT analysis of the lungs begins with the bronchial tree. The anatomy of bronchial structures is best analyzed at normal slice thicknesses of 8 to 10 mm. Longer stretches of the horizontal passages can then be viewed in one slice, while the oblique bronchial passages appear more vividly, due to penumbra formation caused by partial-volume effects. Images of all passages of the main and segmental bronchi, including the carina, can be obtained by sequential scanning. Thin-slice CT makes it possible to demonstrate secondary and tertiary branches of the bronchi in the periphery and evaluate unclear or distorted passages, even those of the central bronchial tree.

Septa

The septa of the lungs are contiguous visceral pleural membranes which enclose each lung. The primary septa lie oblique to the axial CT plane, while the secondary septum runs parallel. At slice thicknesses of 10 mm, the septa can be identified only by indirect reference to the lung structure, which becomes more finely structured (subpleural) and transparent near the septa. Virtually unstructured lung layers are therefore seen above and below the secondary septum. In thin-section tomography, the primary septa, which appear as discrete lines, can be directly demonstrated.

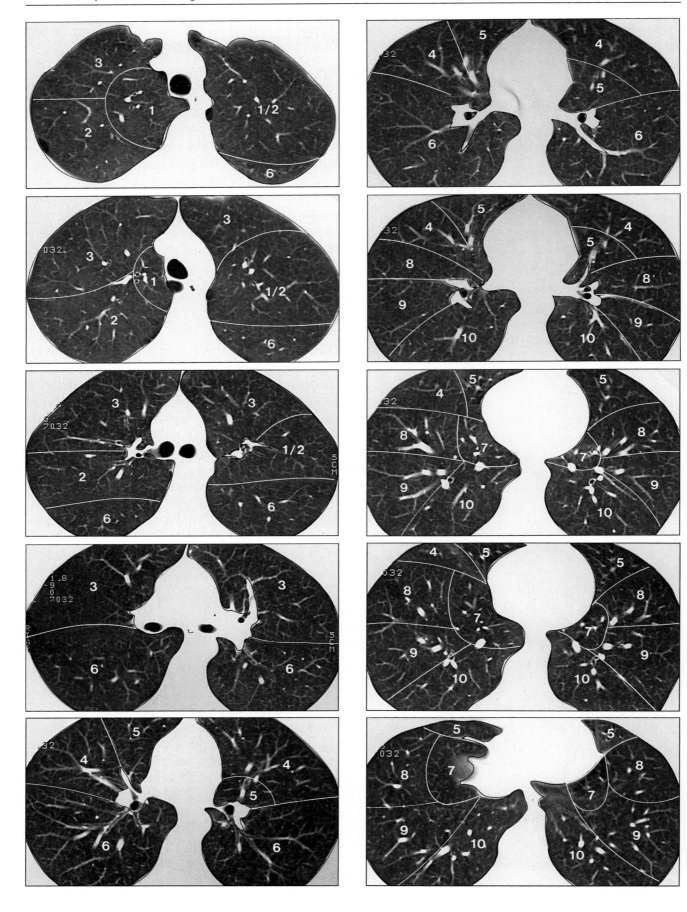

A small, cuneiform pleural extension near the chest wall and mediastinum proximal to the lungs often serves as an additional reference to the position of the primary septum. Pulmonary ligaments comprise pleural folds below the hilum of the lung which may extend all the way down to the diaphragm, thus mediastinally attaching the lower lobes.

Bronchovascular Structures – Hilum of the Lung

Once the bronchi and the central course of the pulmonary arteries have been identified, evaluation of complex hilar structures is facilitated in that each bronchus is escorted by its corresponding artery. At the level of the segmental bronchi, the artery appears as a dense structure (especially near the lower lobes) which is interrupted by clearly outlined bronchial lumina. In contrast to the pulmonary arteries, the pulmonary veins of the lower lobe run relatively horizontal to the atrium. They therefore have an elongated appearance on CT scans. The main veins of the upper lobe, on the other hand, run a steep caudal course in front of the primary bronchi, which makes them clearly distinguishable.

The right lobar bronchus branches from the right primary bronchus directly below the level of the carina. In contrast, the left lobar bronchus and the lingual segmental bronchus branch somewhat deeper. Therefore, the bronchovascular structures in the left upper lobe appear less bunched than those on the opposite side. The veins in the lower lobe, which are displayed as horizontal, thick strands, are easy to find. Their venous branches mark segmental borders. The course of the main pulmonary arteries ventrolateral to the right bronchi and dorsolateral to the left bronchi is readily demonstrated, even on plain

Fig. 8-2. Bronchopulmonary segments in CT scan. The lobe borders in the upper and lower lobes can be readily located once the primary septum has been located. Approximate segmental boundaries can be determined with the help of vascular landmarks. Here, note that the pulmonary veins run between segments and lobes.

scans, so it normally is not difficult to identify enlarged lymph nodes.

In equivocal cases, a bolus injection of contrast medium may be necessary to clearly identify lymph nodes.

Bronchopulmonary Segments

The primary and secondary septa are the only clearly distinguishable lobe borders. Segmen-

Fig. 8-3. Segment boundaries on the surface of the right (a) and left (b) lungs.

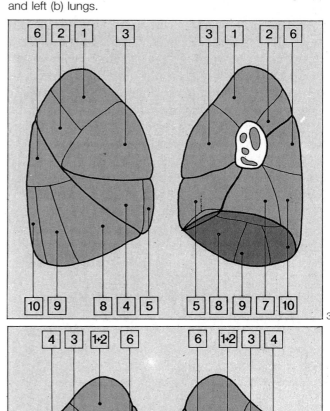

3a

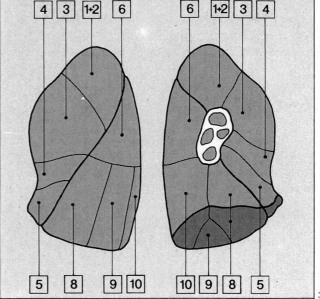

3b

tal borders cannot be identified in normal, evenly aerated lungs. The central course of the bronchi and the intersegmental arrangement of drainage veins mark the boundaries of bronchopulmonary segments, each of which extends as a wedge-shaped structure toward the hilum. Individual segments differ considerably in shape and size.

Lobules of the Lung (Secondary Lobules)

A secondary lobule (hereafter called lobule) is comprised of 30 to 50 primary lobules, which are the smallest functional units of the lung distal to the respiratory bronchioles. The structure of a lobule is equivalent to that of a bronchopulmonary segment: it is wrapped in connective tissue septa and contains veins and lymphatic vessels and receives its central air and blood supply from a secondary bronchus and accompanying artery. The size of lobules varies from 1 to 2.5 cm; the acini subelements measure ca. 7 to 8 mm. On CT scans lobules are best demonstrated in the peripheral lung, where they appear as polygonal, normally 5-cornered, broad-based structures on the visceral pleura. In healthy individuals, normal septal borders are demonstrated only indirectly or not at all on high-resolution CT scans. The nucleus of the lobule, including the artery and the bronchiolus, is demonstrated on axial CT scans as a punctiform figure approx. 1 cm away from the pleural border. On non-axial scans, the artery of the lobule appears as a finely branched figure which, unlike the septa, does not reach the pleural border.

Pulmonary Nodules

Computer tomographic sensitivity in detecting pulmonary nodules is dependent on the location of the nodules. Oblique vessels can mimic a pulmonary nodule. In subpleural regions, pulmonary nodules 1 to 2 mm in diameter and larger can be identified after careful examination. In the vicinity of the hilum, it becomes difficult to identify very small nodular structures contiguous with larger vessels. Only with thin- section scanning and detailed image ana-

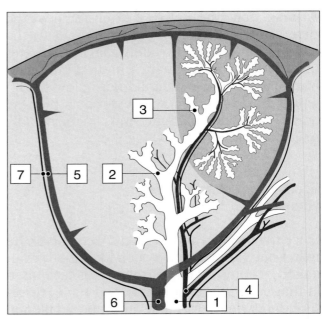

Fig. 8-4. Secondary pulmonary lobule. In the central region, the bronchiolar lobule (1) merges with the lobule and branches via the terminal bronchiole (2) into the alveolar duct (3). The lobular artery (4) follows the branches of the bronchiolus. Peripheral veins drain the lobule; the veins run along the interlobular septum (5), converging to form the interlobular vein (6). Lymph drainage is both interlobular (7) and central along the arteries.

Fig. 8-5. The secondary lobule in CT scan. In cross section the interlobular arteries appear as punctiform structures approx. 1 cm from the pleural boundary. Some branching structures are also discretely visible. In a healthy lung, neither the bronchiolar lobule nor the interlobular septa are distinguishable. The lobule has a polygonal shape in cross section.

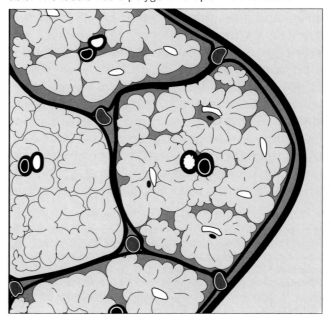

lysis can nodules measuring 3 to 4 mm in diameter be detected.

The outer margins of larger pulmonary nodules must be observed closely since even the smallest ramifications extending to contiguous interlobular and lobular structures must be properly assessed, as is also the case with calcification and air inclusions. The evaluation of small pulmonary nodules by thin-section tomography is complicated, since it is difficult to reproduce the same inspirational conditions in different scans. Rapid scanning within a single inspirational phase (spiral CT) can facilitate the diagnosis.

Because the *CT density* of pulmonary nodules varies greatly from the density of the surrounding lung tissue, the attenuation values must be interpreted carefully. Partial-volume artifacts can be excluded by adjusting the slice thickness. The diameter of the investigated nodules should be at least twice the thickness of the slice. Furthermore, the accuracy of different scanners will vary, so phantom tests should be performed beforehand. CT techniques have a high sensitivity for detecting ringlike calcification and, in particular, diffuse calcification.

Lung Density

The CT density of the lung is greatly dependent upon the degree of inspiration (among other factors). The ventrodorsal CT density gradient, which is influenced by fluctuations in perfusion, is low during full inspiration (ca. 20 HU/10 cm stretch of lung). The gradient rises with increasing expiration as a result of regional variation in ventilation. Such density increases occur symmetrically in the respective lung segments and, if the lung structure is otherwise normal, they are readily distinguishable from infiltrations.

Fig. 8-7. Pulmonary histogram. When the attenuation values of the pulmonary surfaces are plotted according to frequency, the result is a typical lung density curve with a maximum at -850 HU. With successive expiration, the histogram widens and the peak of the distribution curve shifts toward higher attenuation values, indicating the decreasing air content and nonuniform regional ventilation.

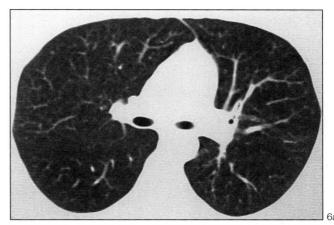

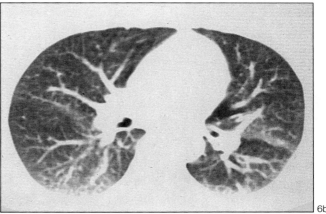

6a

6b

Fig. 8-6. The lung density is greatly dependent on the degree of inspiration. At maximum inspiration (a), even the respective dorsal sections of the lung are virtually transparent. Physiologically, there is a slightly increasing ventrodorsal CT density gradient of about 30 HU. At expiration (b), the attenuation values in the respective sections of the lung increase significantly and can simulate dorsal infiltration.

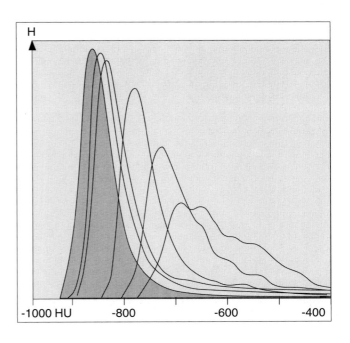

H

-1000 HU   -800   -600   -400

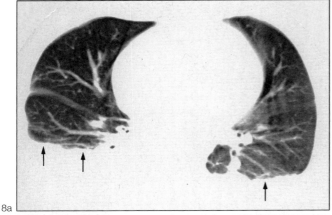

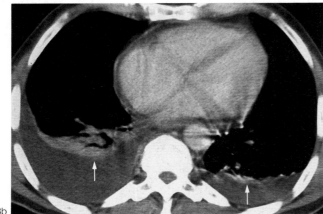

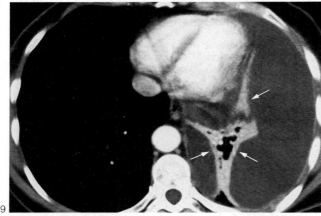

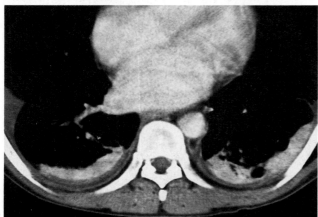

Respiration Defects of the Lungs

Partial Loss of Volume

Healthy alveolar spaces may become under-aerated when the respiratory function of a lung segment decreases or when a supplying airway is constricted. This condition is usually found in bedridden patients with reduced motility of the diaphragm. Pneumothorax, compression of lung tissue (e.g. via development of pleural effusions), or scar contraction in shrivelling lung tissue can lead to a partial lung collapse with regionally reduced perfusion. Narrowing or obstruction of bronchi can lead to (sub)segmental reduction in pulmonary ventilation.

• CT

Radiologic signs of underventilation can be demonstrated on CT scans as well as on conventional chest radiographs. Radiologic signs include shrinkage of the affected hemithorax or mediastinal displacement, distortion of the septa or bronchovascular structures, compensatory over-ventilation in adjacent portions of lung and elevation of the diaphragm. Early signs of reduced or increased ventilation, respectively, can be identified on CT scans as areas of increased or decreased density of lung tissue (with lateral view for comparison). Computed tomography displays a high degree of sensitivity in detecting striated under-aerated zones that run parallel to the borders of motion (squamous cell atelectasis) as well as the frequently accompanying alveolar infiltrates.

Fig. 8-8. Partial loss of volume (dystelectasis). Lungs with loss of volume and lobar collapse of different degrees of severity are accompanied by pleural effusion. The compressed lung tissue appears soft-tissue dense with pockets of air. The adjoining vascular lung framework is distorted (a→). Atelectatic, noninflammatory lung tissue contrasts clearly and homogeneously (b→).

Fig. 8-9. Partial loss of volume (dystelectasis). This shows a strong homogeneous enhancement.

Fig. 8-10. Compression atelectasis. The entire left lower lobe is compressed by adherent pleural effusions. The central sections of the lung still contain air.

Atelectasis

Long-term underventilation can give rise to lung collapse. The alveolar spaces then become void of air.

• CT

In the absence of ventilation in a bronchopulmonary segment or lobe due to occlusion of the supplying bronchus, the borders of that segment of lobe are sharply demarcated on CT scans. Depending on the degree of volume loss, mediastinal displacement and elevation of the diaphragm may result. Airless lung areas are demonstrated on CT scans as structures of soft-tissue density which, after the administration of contrast medium, become clearly enhanced in the presence of compressed vessels. These signs can be absent, however, when the bronchial system is filled with retained secretions (exudation). In that case, depending on the efficacy of the remaining supply vessels, the collapsed lung may display a marble-like appearance.

Various patterns of atelectasis can be differentiated on CT scans.

In atelectasis of the *left upper lobe*, the border facing the main septum migrates ventrally to form a bordering wedge along the anterior mediastinal contour. The tip of the wedge points towards the hilum, while the left pulmonary artery is distorted superiorly and anteriorly. Clear mediastinal distortion to the left, hyperdistension of the left lower lobe, and herniation of the right lung above the anterior mediastinal contour comprises the total clinical picture of atelectasis of the upper lobe.

Atelectasis of the *right upper lobe* appears on cross-sectional images as a triangular structure. The anterior border represents the raised secondary septum, the frequently concave or convex structure of the posterior contours represents the main septum. The primary bronchus migrates more sharply caudad, and the right hilum is clearly raised.

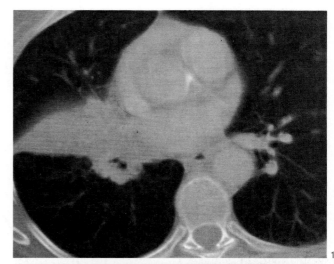

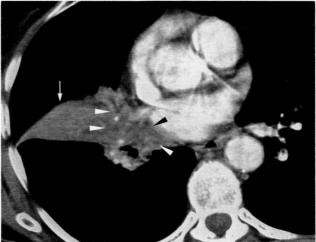

Fig. 8-11. Middle lobe atelectasis with typical wing-shaped appearance (b→). The segment bronchi are blocked by a tumor, which can only be indistinctly discerned against the poorly contrasting collapsed lung (b ►).

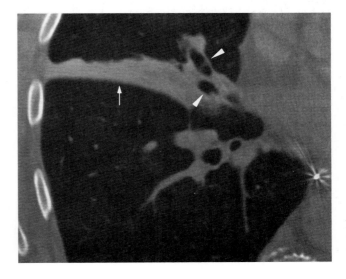

Fig. 8-12. Partial atelectasis of the middle lobe. The segment bronchi (►) remain open in the center. The dorsal boundary of the shadow is the main septum (→).

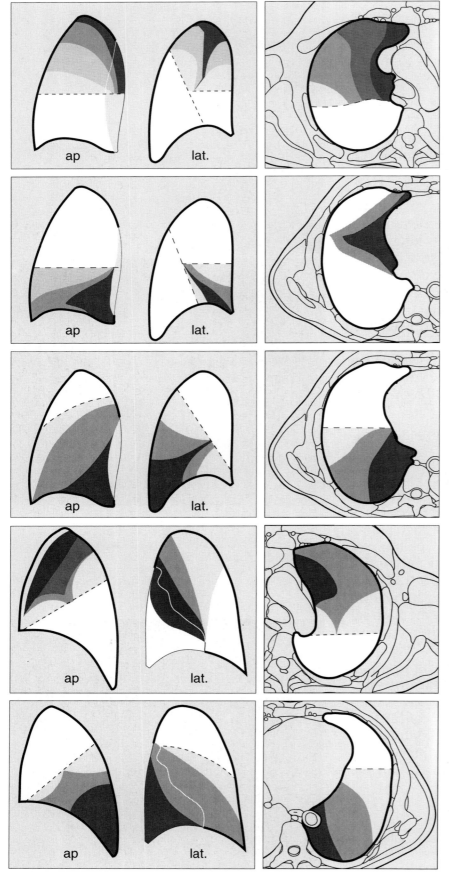

Fig. 8-13a. Right upper lobe atelectasis. As ventilation decreases, the boundary of the main septum migrates ventrally and medially until, finally, a small secondary shadow touches the mediastinum.

Fig. 8-13b. Middle lobe atelectasis. As ventilation decreases, the anterior segment of the upper lobe migrates in front of the boundary of the middle lobe so that the secondary septum forms a border. The main septum migrates ventromedially. In the transverse section, a prominent triangular opaque structure on the mediastinum becomes apparent. This structure varies in size depending on the degree of ventilation.

Fig. 8-13c. Right lower lobe atelectasis. As ventilation decreases, the main septum migrates dorsomedially, until it appears as a paravertebral soft-tissue structure and the lower pole of the hilum is rotated dorsally on the right.

Fig. 8-13d. Left upper lobe atelectasis. At the onset of the ventilation disorder, the overinflated apical segment of the lower lobe displaces the medial portion of the main septum ventrally, first forming a V-shaped dorsal boundary. The upper lobe ultimately joins the mediastinum as a lateroconvex or lateroconcave structure.

Fig. 8-13e. Left lower lobe atelectasis. As on the opposite side, the lower lobe in the posterior mediastinum appears on the aorta, distorting the hilum vessels to the dorsal side.

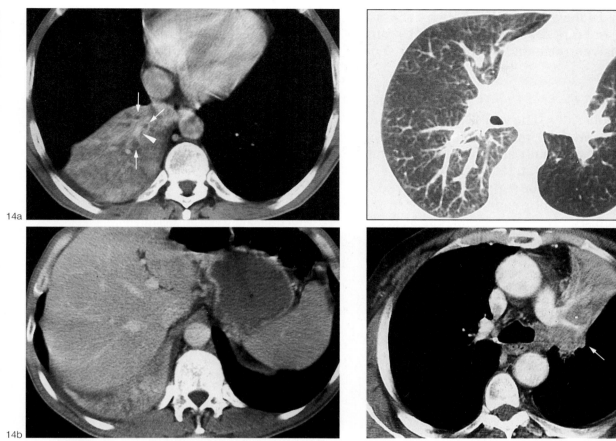

Fig. 8-14. Right lower lobe atelectasis. After a bolus injection of contrast medium, the secretion-filled bronchi inside the collapsed area appear hypodense (a→), and the contrasting vessels (a►) in the diaphragm (b) can be traced into the periphery.

Fig. 8-15. Upper lobe atelectasis with a central bronchial carcinoma. The tumor (→) cannot be clearly distinguished from collapsed tissue after a bolus injection of contrast medium, but the larger vessels branching into the collapsed area can. Distinct left lateral displacement of the mediastinum is apparent in the pulmonary window (a), and the hyperinflated left lower lobe exhibits reduced attenuation values.

Fig. 8-16. Rounded atelectasis. The pulmonary window setting (a) shows pleural thickening (scarring following tuberculous pleurisy) on a round shadow. The bronchovascular bundle can be seen streaking like the tail of a comet into it. In the soft-tissue window (b), the round figure exhibits strong, homogeneous enhancement.

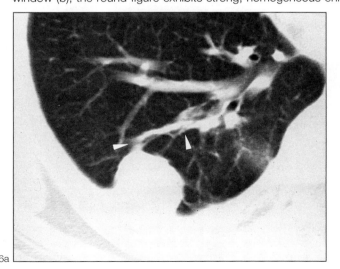

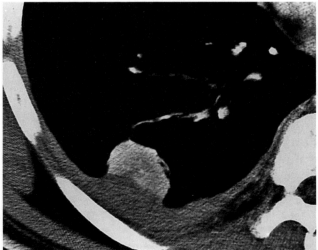

Atelectasis of the *middle lobe* also appears as a triangular or trapezoid structure on CT scans which runs ventrocaudad to the anterior thoracic wall.

Atelectasis of the lower lobes forms a similar image on both sides. The lobes lie flat along the dorsal paravertebral mediastinum; the main septum rotates medially and caudad and forms the lateral border of atelectasis.
Central occlusion of the supplying lobar or segmental bronchus is normally found in obstructive atelectasis. In *compression atelectasis*, however, reduced ventilation occurs in the peripheral region, so the central bronchial structures of the atelectatic region normally appear to be still aerated. The cause of lung compression (usually effusion) can also be clarified by computed tomography. Since the adhesive strength of the pleural membranes is eliminated, the airless lobes of lung contract evenly in the direction of the hilum, but portions of the lower lobes are basally fixed to the pulmonary ligaments.

Round Atelectasis

Compressive atelectasis subsequent to an effusion can also become persistent (e.g. after scar formation) if the effusion recedes and the lung unfolds. The visceral pleura then invaginates, spiralling into the lung. On the CT scan, bronchovascular structures streak like the tail of a comet throughout the soft-tissue dense atelectic areas of the pleura.

Parenchymal Lung Abnormalities

Infiltrations

Here the diagnostic criteria of plain chest radiography can again be applied to computed tomography. Infiltrations are demonstrated as homogeneous areas of density enhancement. Patchy shadows around air bronchograms provide definitive proof of alveolar infiltration (airspace pattern). Evidence of an interstitial process is given when images of the subpleural

space that are free of artefacts demonstrate structural changes at lung window settings. These changes can be demonstrated at normal slice thicknesses. Thinner slices improve the chances of making this diagnosis at the lobular

Fig. 8-17. Broncho-alveolar infiltration. This creates map-like shadows on CT scans. Where there is diffuse permeation of the airspace, one can see areas of reduced transparency similar to milk glass.

Fig. 8-18. Broncho-alveolar infiltration. In pathological and anatomical terms, this corresponds to nonuniform or diffuse permeation of the acini with exudation.

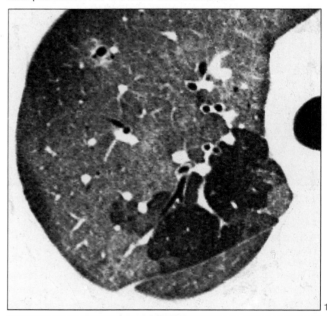
17

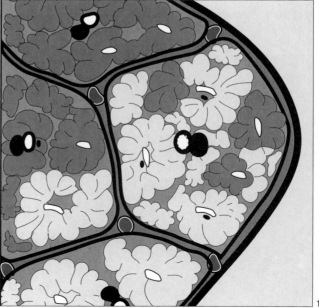
18

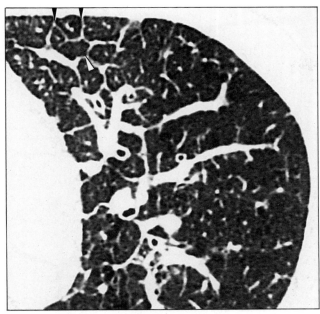

Fig. 8-19. Interstitial infiltration. Depending on the cause, it primarily affects the intralobular lung framework or the interlobular septa. These structures therefore become readily detectable on CT scans (►). In tumor-related infiltration, fine nodules are often found.

Fig. 8-20. Interstitial edema. In acute to chronic disorders, hemodynamic, inflammatory and neoplastic infiltration of varying severity can be found throughout the lung framework. Interstitial reactions will therefore produce a variety of structural patterns on CT scans. Interstitial edema is characterized by uniform (and reversible) thickening of all septa.

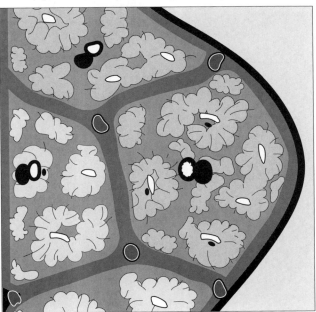

level. *Broncho-alveolar infiltrations* primarily affect the air space, i.e. the bronchiolus, its ramifications and the connecting alveoli. Correspondingly, infiltrations can thicken the alveolar space or the walls of the bronchiolus, thus making them detectable on CT scans. Depending on the type of process inducing the inflammation, groups of acini, whole lobuli or larger, connected air spaces may be filled with the exudate.

Thin-section CT scans demonstrate various patterns:
– poorly defined *circular* lesions (of up to 1 cm in diameter) which form isolated or confluent structures in the lobule,
– *subtle areas* of ground-glass appearance or cloudy opacification which affect the entire lung or individual lobuli,
– *air bronchograms* which become more clearly visible with increased opacification,
– *map-like* distribution patterns which respect individual (sub)segmental borders, but permeate the air space of the core and periphery of the lung unevenly.

Perivascular (usually inflammatory) *infiltration* arising from the vessels primarily affects the interstitial space, which is thereby broadened while the air space remains unaffected. Depending on the degree of infiltration, interstitial structures (especially the intralobular septa) are thickened, and a honeycombed pattern is observed.

Lymphatic dissemination occurs along interstitial lymph vessels which primarily drain to the interlobular septa, but also occurs in peribronchial regions. Tumor-related infiltrations broaden the interstitial tissues, thus making them readily detectable on CT scans. If signs of inflammation are absent, the aerated alveolar space is relatively sharply delineated from plump interstitial structures. The interlobular septum is also involved in this process. Localized tumor accumulations and granulomas are demonstrated as micronodular distensions. They may be distributed in peripheral (also intraseptal) or centrilobular (peribronchial) areas.

Interstitial edema is caused by hemodynamic processes or obstruction of the lymph tracts.

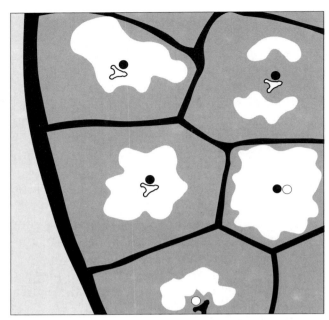

Fig. 8-21. Centrilobular emphysema. The emphysema originates in the core of a lobule and spreads unevenly throughout the lung.

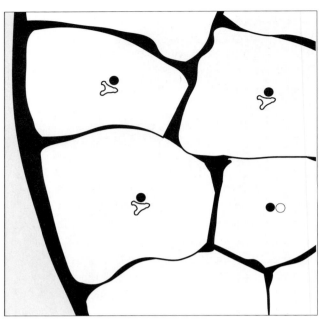

Fig. 8-22. Panlobular emphysema. All lobules are pathologically and anatomically affected by the emphysema development. The septa are deformed due to the resulting hyperinflation.

Fig. 8-23. Panlobular emphysema. Segmental distribution of emphysema development.

Fig. 8-24. Centrilobular emphysema. Following the pathological and anatomical pattern of involvement, the hypodense emphysematous regions are spread unevenly throughout the lung.

Fig. 8-25. Panlobular emphysema. Structural changes in the entire lung with a coarse reticular pattern between the overinflated airspaces.

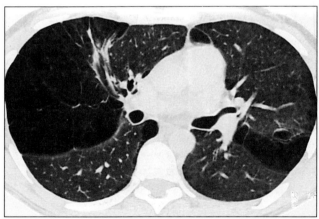

23

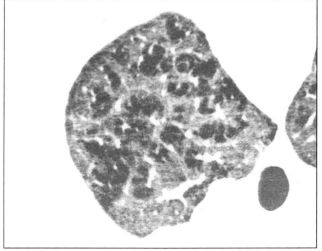

24

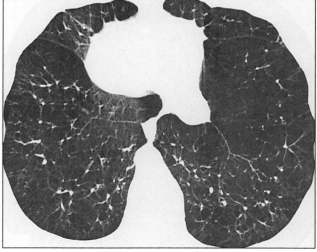

25

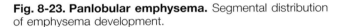

An interstitial edema is demonstrated on CT scans as a uniform thickening of septal structures which, in part, are accompanied by a hazy reduction in transparency of the alveolar space. The Kerley B lines seen on (plain) survey radiographs are a summation of the thickened and layered interlobular septa.

Images of nodular, reticulonodular and reticular patterns, also obtainable on plain chest radiographs, are improved by thin-section CT techniques. One can thus diagnose the development of a nodular structure through a localized, centrilobular (peribronchial, perivascular) infiltration of the alveolar space or through filling of individual subsegments (acini). Purely reticular patterns at the level of the lobule are related to the interstitial tissues (interlobular septum, intralobular connective tissue structure). Due to improved imaging by CT, abnormalities of these structures can be detected earlier.

Emphysema

Emphysema is characterized by enlargement of peripheral air spaces distal to the terminal bronchioli accompanied by an irreversible loss in substance of the lung. Pathological and anatomical distinctions are made between panlobular, centrilobular, periseptal and cicatricial emphysema. Although small blisters and bullae are often found in conjunction with emphysema, they can also be found in normal lung tissue.

Centrilobular emphysema predominantly affects the upper lobe and originates at the center of a lobule of the lung. These pathological changes spread unevenly throughout the normal lung with tiny localized to large confluent foci which can lead to distortion of the vascular system.

Panlobular emphysema is found predominantly in the lower lobe of the lung. The condition can lead to uniform rarefaction of tissue of the lobule of the lung.

Periseptal emphysema is characterized by involvement of air spaces of the lobuli along the

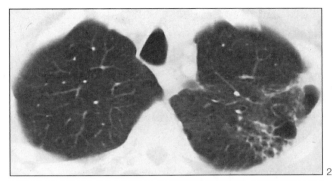
26

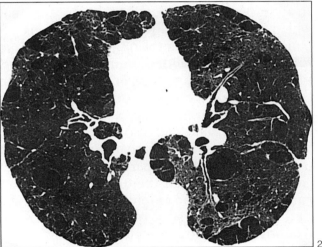
27

Fig. 8-26. Bullous emphysema in the tip of the left lung. Subpleural and periseptal emphysema blisters can be sensitively detected and, in applicable cases, identified as the cause of pneumothorax.

Fig. 8-27. Bullous emphysema which has spread uniformly throughout the lung. Structural changes can be seen in great detail at high resolution.

Fig. 8-28. Destructive emphysema with a significant degree of bullous structural changes.

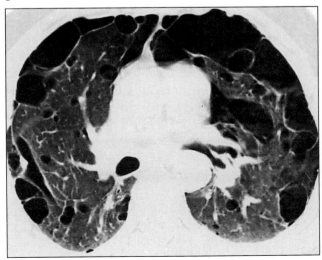

septa and pleura. These can transform into 0.5 to 2 cm large bullae which often can be traced as beaded structures along the septa.

In *cicatricial emphysema*, corresponding air spaces are found along scar contractions, especially in cirrhotic forms of tuberculosis and silicosis.

• CT

In addition to the classical signs of emphysema, which is characterized by emphysematous expansion of the peripheral lung, dilatation of the retrosternal space with thinning of the mediastinal folds between the lungs, dilatation of the central pulmonary vessels due to arterial pulmonary hypertension, an increase in diagnostic peribronchial signs can also be demonstrated. When thin sections are scanned, destructive transformation of lung parenchyma in the region of the lobuli can therefore be diagnosed early. Centrilobular emphysema is characterized by the dispersion of variably sized, increasingly transparent portions of lung (especially in the upper lobe). Areas of increased lucency are indicative of panlobular emphysema, which is most intensely expressed in a symmetrical pattern in the lower lobe of patients with alpha$_1$-antitrypsin deficiency. Computed tomography displays sensitivity in detecting subpleural blisters formed by bullous emphysema and increased lucency related to localized cicatricial emphysema in the vicinity of scars and contractions. The large number of peribronchial signs that can be demonstrated on plain radiographs can be better traced to their initial sites on CT scans, and the images are more prominent. As on plain chest radiographs, emphysema in conjunction with invasive pulmonary inflammation is demonstrated on CT scans as an area of increased reticular shadows (honeycombed in some places), which occurs due to the changes in lung structure.

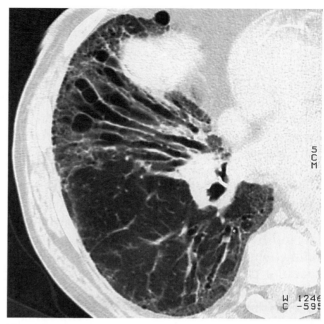

Fig. 8-29. Varicose bronchiectasis. The greatly dilated bronchi, some of them bundled, extend in irregular caliber into the periphery of the lung, which has been changed by fibrous sheaths and sustains the spread of bronchiectasis with traction.

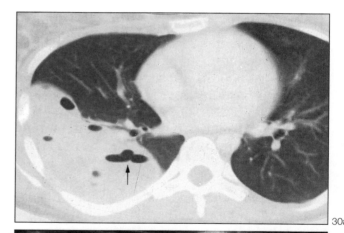

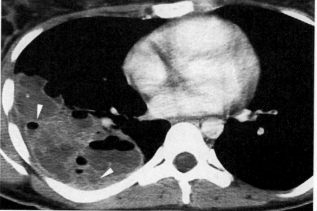

Fig. 8-30. Pulmonary sequestration. Segmental densification in the lower right segment with small air fluid levels (a→) inside individual honeycombed spaces. This altered pulmonary structure becomes apparent after injection of contrast medium (b►). Aortic arterial supply of the sequestrum cannot be readily demonstrated in the CT scan.

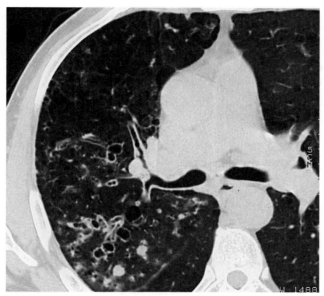

Fig. 8-31. Cystic bronchiectasis. Relatively spherical, thick-walled dilatation of the bronchi in the periphery of the lung, some of which are filled with secretion and are recognizable as round shadows.

Fig. 8-32. Cystic bronchiectasis. Chronically inflamed lung tissue changes are often detected in the vicinity of the bronchiectasis, here with fibrotic lung tissue changes (b→) with accompanying subpleural emphysema.

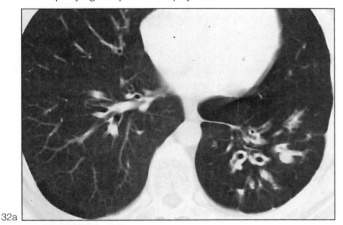

32a

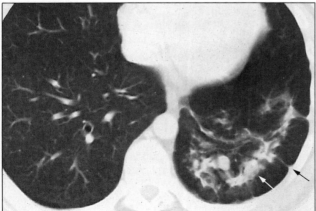

32b

Bronchopulmonary Anomalies

Pulmonary Sequestration

In pulmonary sequestration, the tissue formed during lung development does not communicate with the bronchial system. Pulmonary sequestration is found predominantly in the left, basal epiphrenic region and more infrequently in subdiaphragmatic regions. In *intralobular* types, the blood supply normally comes from the thoracic aorta in up to 75% of cases, and from the abdominal aorta in the rest; drainage is to the pulmonary veins. Clinically, pulmonary sequestration is found in adults after recurring infections, hemoptysis, secondary communication with the bronchial system and cystic transformation. *Extralobular* types have their own envelope of pleura and have venous drainage to systemic veins. Clinical complaints are infrequent.

• CT

Plain scans: Pulmonary sequestration is demonstrated as a subsegmental, epiphrenic zone of soft-tissue density found especially in the left basal paravertebral region. Sequestration frequently has the appearance of atypically structured atelectasis. The major CT findings are a honeycombed pattern or cystically transformed basal pulmonary regions with or without air fluid levels. Calcification may occur. Accompanying infiltrations often mask the morphological etiology of sequestration, making it difficult to make the diagnosis on the basis of plain scans.

Contrast-enhanced scans: A bolus injection of contrast medium will normally enhance the image, especially when atelectatic types are investigated. Systemic arterial supply is then readily demonstrable, and the diagnosis can be made.

Bronchiectasis

Bronchiectasis is found predominantly in basal bronchopulmonary segments. It can cause re-

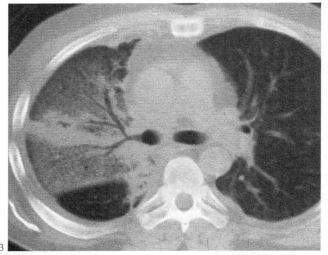

33

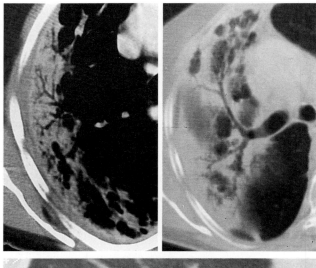

35

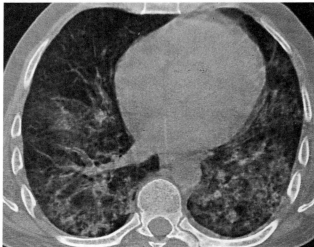

34

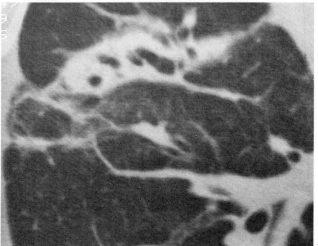

36

Fig. 8-33. Bronchopneumonic infiltration. Typical segment-oriented infiltration pattern with demonstrable air bronchogram.

Fig. 8-34. Pneumonia. Chronic pneumonia caused by fungus superinfection exhibits both alveolar and interstitial patterns of enhancement with reticular thickening following the bronchial structures.

Fig. 8-35. Organizing pneumonia. Located near the shrivelled right hemithorax is a dense, primarily subpleural shadow of the reduced lung in which the bronchogram structures can be seen. The non-infiltrated areas of the lung are overinflated.

Fig. 8-36. Post-pneumonic fibrosis. Cases of chronic pneumonia lead to the development of cordlike structures and distortion of the lung framework, including bronchiectasis.

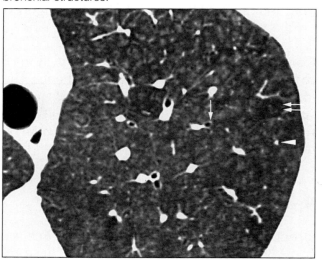

Fig. 8-37. Extrinsic allergic alveolitis. Extremely fine, indistinct and discrete flocculent points of reduced transparency are uniformly distributed throughout the entire lung without evidence of septal thickening. Lobular artery (►). Due to the overall reduced transparency in the lung, even the lumina of smaller bronchi contrast clearly as hypodense structures (→). Noninfiltrated lobule (⇒).

curring bronchopneumonia, which frequently aggravates the primary condition.

Bronchiectasis is an irreversible dilatation of medial and small bronchi. It is divided into three different morphological and anatomical types on the basis of appearance:

- *cylindrical* bronchiectasis creates tubular structures that extend to the peripheral lung without causing a reduction in caliber;
- *varicose* bronchiectasis causes irregular dilatation and therefore has a wave-like surface contour.
- in *saccular* bronchiectasis, the medial bronchi terminate in cystic (subpleural) spaces.

• CT

Thickening or dilatation of the bronchi that extends to the pleural surface is the most frequent sign of bronchiectasis. Computed tomography can more sensitively detect this disorder when bronchial structures lie on the axial scanning plane. The segmental bronchi are most frequently affected. The deformed bronchi are crowded together and distort the structure of the lung. CT can differentiate this disorder of the bronchi from localized alveolar expansion, since the bronchi and their accompanying arteries exhibit a thick-walled appearance. Saccular projections may be filled with mucus. Thin-section tomography is recommended for demonstration of cylindrical bronchiectasis, which is not as clearly demonstrated by normal scanning techniques. Computed tomography can clearly demonstrate the different configurations displayed by varicose and cylindrical bronchiectasis when the bronchi lie on a horizontal plane.

Pulmonary Inflammation

Pneumonia

Pneumonia is divided into three basic types which are identified according to their pattern of dissemination and mode of infiltration.

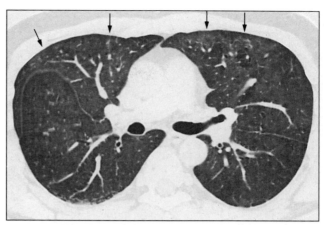

Fig. 8-38. Pneumocystis carinii pneumonia. In the ventral sections of the lung there are extremely fine reticular and foggy points of reduced transparency (→) representing both interstitial and alveolar infiltration (alveolitis).

Fig. 8-39. Pneumocystis carinii pneumonia. The areas of reduced transparency are primarily in alveolar areas, which are affected in varying degrees and thus exhibit a maplike density pattern.

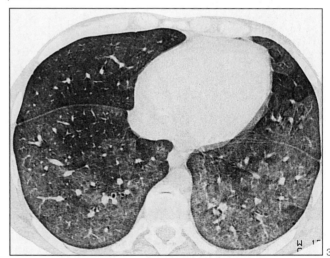

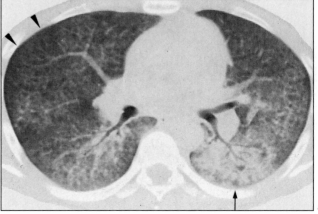

Fig. 8-40. Pneumocystis carinii pneumonia. Alveolar infiltration pattern with dense infiltrates, particularly in the left dorsal area with positive bronchogram structures (→). A slight interstitial component can be detected in the ventral sections (▸).

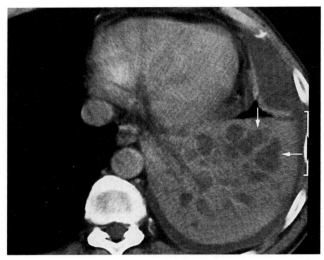

Fig. 8-41. Poststenotic suppurative pneumonia. After injection of contrast medium, the suppurations in the left lower lobe contrast against the lung tissue that is well supplied with blood as a hypodense area with a marginal enhancement.

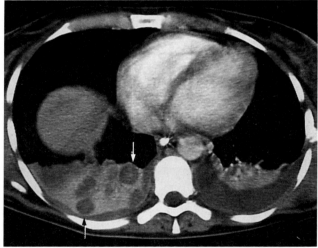

42

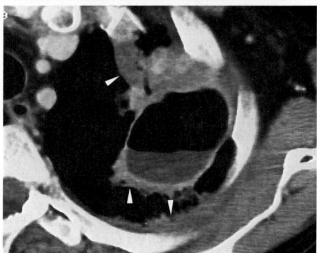

43

Lobar pneumonia is rare and is usually caused by pneumococcal infection, which uniformly infiltrates patches of the affected lobe.

In *bronchopneumonia*, the air spaces of the secondary lobules display multilocular infiltration. Aerated and non-aerated tissue zones are in juxtaposition.

Interstitial pneumonia is primarily caused by viral, mycoplasmic, and rickettsial infections. It disseminates interstitially and via the interlobular septa. Peribronchial alveoli demonstrate mixed degrees of exudation.

• CT

In patients with *lobar pneumonia*, the alveolar space of several lung segments or of one complete lobe of the lung displays a homogeneous shadow. Air bronchograms are usually present in hilar areas.

In patients with *bronchopneumonia*, segmentally oriented shadows are frequently distributed inhomogeneously throughout the lungs.

Characteristic signs of *interstitial pneumonia* are lobar and interlobular septal thickening with finely stippled, predominantly central opacification expressing perivascular and lymphatic infiltration. Mixed clinical pictures with increasingly interstitial (reticular) characteristics of the bronchopneumonial infiltrates are observed in patients with chronic disease.

Pulmonary Abscess

Abscesses are usually postpneumonic occurrences (staphylococcus, klebsiella) which develop through demarcation of necrotic lung

Fig. 8-42. Suppurative pneumonia. After injection of contrast medium, round hypodense structures indicative of foci of liquefaction can be distinguished on the right inside the partially collapsed areas of the lung.

Fig. 8-43. Pulmonary abscess. Large thin-walled abscess cavity with air fluid levels representing the connection to the bronchial system. The wall of the abscess is thin, but it shows a clear enhancement due to an inflammation-related increase vascularization. Lung infiltration (►).

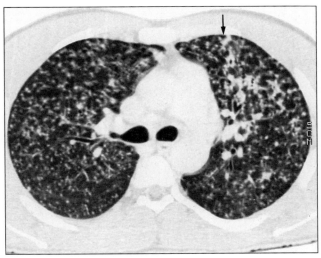

Fig. 8-44. Miliary tuberculosis. Extremely small nodules measuring approx. 1 mm are distributed throughout the entire lung and exhibit a slight confluence in the left upper lobe (→).

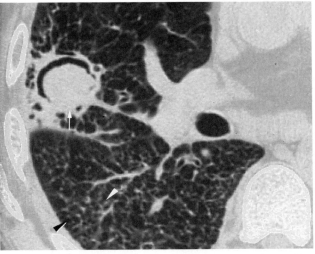

Fig. 8-45. Aspergilloma. Typical aspects of an Aspergillus mycetoma inside the pulmonary cavity (→). Finely structured pulmonary fibrosis can be seen in the lower lobe (►).

segments. Additional pathogenic causes of pulmonary abscess development are pulmonary infarction, septic pulmonary embolism, aspiration and bronchiectasis.

In the further course of disease, the abscess usually develops a smooth membrane which, when it communicates with the bronchial system, can be identified as a hollow space (cavity) having a demonstrable fluid level. The development of empyema after the abscess herniates into the pleural cavity is a serious complication. After the symptoms of inflammation have subsided, the cavity collapses and retracts, forming a scar. In children an abscess can lead to the development of valvular stenosis and, ultimately, a pneumatocele.

• CT

Plain scans: In the stage of demarcation, air fluid levels and air inclusions that do not stay within the bounds of the alveolar borders are the first indications of a pulmonary abscess.

Fig. 8-46. Tuberculous cavity. In the posterior segment of the right upper lobe, a ringlike figure is detected with peg-shaped induration of the cavity wall (a ►). In the surrounding area, a slight pulmonary infiltration (→) and cordlike structures in the upper right area (⇒) are apparent. There is a significant enhancement of the cavity wall after injection of contrast medium (b ►).

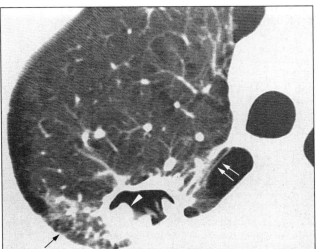

46a

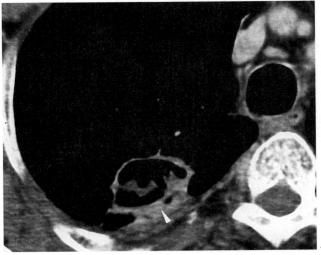

46b

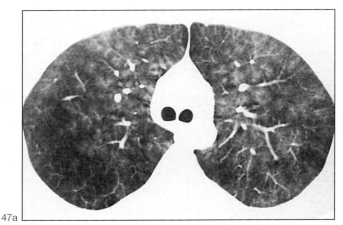

47a

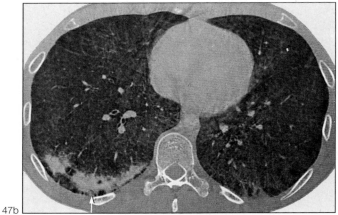

47b

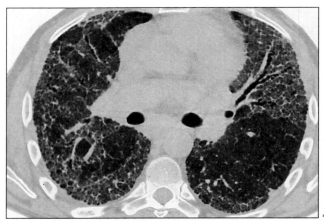

49

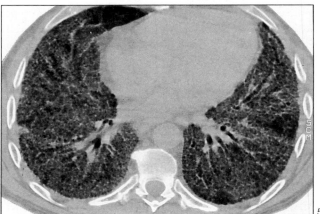

50

Fig. 8-47. Desquamative alveolitis in the upper areas with existing fibrosis in the respective parts. Here, more compact fibrotic infiltrates (→) are found.

Fig. 8-48. Idiopathic pulmonary fibrosis. Typical distribution of the fibrotic zone in the pleural space in a honeycombed pattern. This scan shows cystic tissue transformations of varying size with development of emphysema. The form of the accompanying subpleural emphysema varies as a result of traction.

Fig. 8-49. Idiopathic pulmonary fibrosis with generalized pattern of involvement.

Fig. 8-50. Idiopathic pulmonary fibrosis with a generalized, very fine, reticular pattern. Here, accompanying chronically inflammatory processes increase the density of the lung as a whole.

Fig. 8-51. Idiopathic pulmonary fibrosis. Generalized pattern of involvement. The fibrosis enhances the polygonal shape of the interlobular septa. In this case the overinflated alveolar space appears transparent without any signs of inflammation.

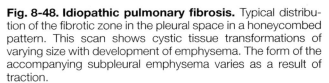

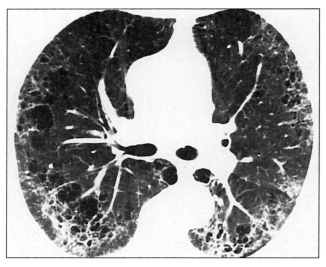

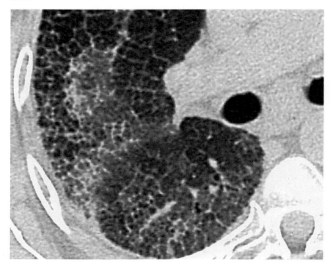

Contrast-enhanced scans: If the abscess is inside a thick pneumonic infiltrate, evidence to confirm the diagnosis can usually be obtained after the administration of contrast medium. The abscess tissue is then demarcated as a hypodense tissue zone with a hyperdense ring structure (abscess membrane), which makes it distinguishable from hyperperfused lung tissue. Possible involvement of the pleural cavity of the bronchial system can be safely diagnosed and quantitatively assessed. There is usually no peripheral enhancement in patients with pulmonary liquefaction in conjunction with necrotizing pneumonitis or gangrenous pneumonia.

Differential diagnosis: If the enhanced abscess membrane is relatively smooth, the evidence is usually sufficient to differentiate between an abscess and a necrotic tumor.

Interstitial Lung Diseases

Interstitial lung diseases have neither a neoplastic nor an infective cause. They affect the septa of the alveolar space, run a chronic course and transform into fibrosis of varying severity.

Idiopathic Pulmonary Fibrosis

In middle-aged women, this disease frequently begins insidiously as an interstitial, proliferating pneumoid disease (usual interstitial pneumonia, UIP) or as acute, desquamative alveolitis (DIP). Interstitial infiltration causes a broadening of the alveolar septa. If the cells of the alveolar wall respond with a severe inflammation, the clinical picture of alveolitis may also be observed.

• CT

Involvement of the alveolar space in acute alveolitis is seen on CT scans as a dense, normally symmetrical shadow in the air space which becomes unevenly confluent with the lobuli. As the ventilation of the alveolar space increases, the interstitial process involving

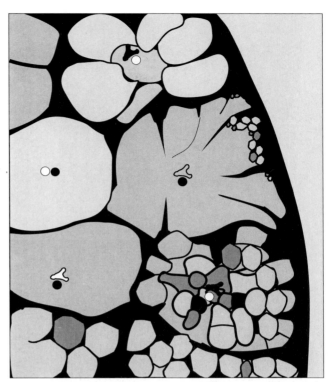

Fig. 8-52. Pulmonary fibrosis. The structural patterns are varied and can only be roughly correlated with individual clinical pictures. The severity and course of the disorder can be established readily in CT scans on the basis of the loss of parenchyma and emphysema development.

broadening of the septal structures becomes more readily visible. Evidence of incipient fibrosis can be found in increased numbers of non-septal, arciform subpleural lines, thickening and distortion of the lobule septa, and expansion of the adjacent alveolar space. The subpleural cavity characteristically shows a larger emphysematous tissue area with cystic air inclusions of 2 to 4 mm diameter. As the disease progresses, the transformation spreads in the same manner to the central lung tissue. In the final stage, a honeycomb pattern (severity may vary) has developed in the lung framework.

Differential diagnosis: The morphological picture of *rheumatoid arthritis*, *scleroderma*, and other *collagen diseases* are very similar.

Sarcoidosis

The formation of epitheloid cell granulomas is characteristic of sarcoidosis. First the granulo-

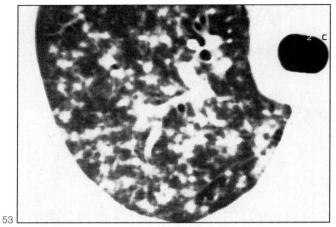

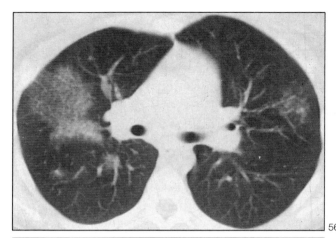

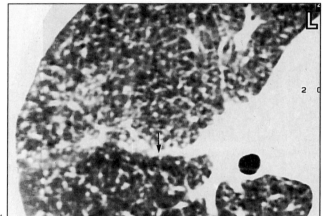

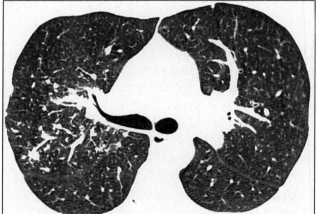

Fig. 8-53. Disseminated sarcoidosis. The individual granulomas are located both in the subpleural space and in the vicinity of the bronchovascular bundle.

Fig. 8-54. Fine nodular disseminated sarcoidosis. The subpleural space is frequently afflicted so that the main septum is demarcated (→). A discretely reticulo-nodular structure is already apparent in the ventral sections of the lung.

Fig. 8-55. Fine nodular sarcoidosis. A slight confluence of the granulomas can be seen in the periphery. A clear bronchovascular form of dissemination is apparent. These structures appear prominent and exhibit mantle-like thickening.

Fig. 8-56. Sarcoidosis. Detection of dense localized infiltrates affecting both the interstitial tissues and the alveolar space in lymphadenopathy.

Fig. 8-57. Sarcoidosis. Detection of a primarily bronchovascular spread on the right involving the right hilum. In addition to this, individual central and subpleural granulomas can be distinguished in the lung.

Fig. 8-58. Sarcoidosis. Fine-nodular, disseminated pattern of involvement. The subpleural space forms a prominent recess with slight thickening of the interlobular septa as an initial indication of the onset of interstitial fibrosis.

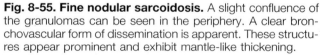

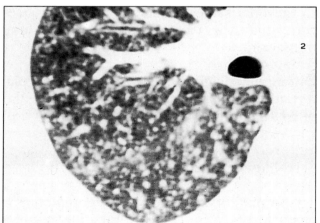

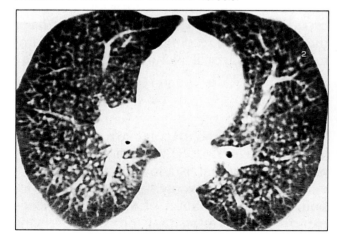

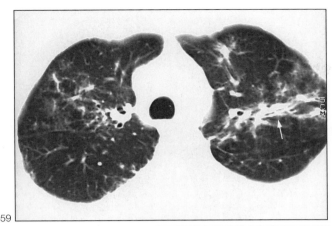

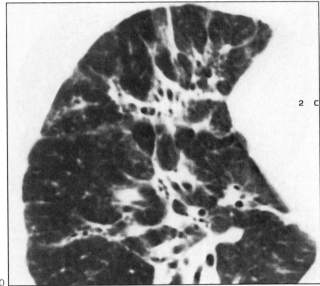

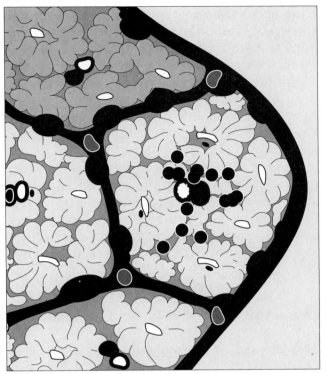

Fig. 8-61. The spread of sarcoidosis in interstitial tissues of the lung may be primarily perivasal, peribronchial or intraseptal.

Fig. 8-59. Phase III sarcoidosis. Prominent, primarily peribronchial enhancement of the lung framework with distortion of the bronchial system and development of bronchiectasis. Cords extend into the periphery of the lung with attendant hyperinflation of the adjacent airspaces.

Fig. 8-60. Phase III sarcoidosis. Prominent fibrotic cords of the bronchovascular bundle extending to the pleura as a band-shaped structure. Significant distortion of the entire lung framework with focal emphysema development and bronchiectasis.

mas permeate (usually symmetrically) the lymph nodes of the hilum of the lung and disseminate to the pulmonary interstitial tissues along the peribronchial, perivascular, intraseptal and subpleural lymph tracts. These very small granuloma can merge together, forming stippled shadows of different sizes. Fine nodules typically appear on chest radiographs. Pleural effusion can occur. The progression of the interstitial anomalies can lead to pulmonary fibrosis (severity may vary).

• CT

Areas of densification filled with fine nodules as well as hilar (and mediastinal) lymph node enlargement are typical signs of sarcoidosis. A predilection for the midzones of the lung and the subpleural regions is observed. Pathological changes occur predominantly in the interstitial tissues, which means that the interlobular septa and centrilobular, perivascular regions will appear as a finely nodulated structure in high-resolution CT (according to the pattern of distribution). Confluent nodules can form even more dense conglomerates, which form prominent round shadows on plain radiographs. They sometimes merge to form loose, localized infiltrates with visible air bronchograms. Predominantly peribronchial dissemination is frequent when various infiltration types are combined. The latter is characterized by a broadening of the bronchovascular bundle that extends into the lung periphery; the structure of the bronchus is prominent and distortion of the surrounding lung tissue is observed.

Rare alveolo-acinar types can also be demonstrated by computed tomography. These types are characterized by an intralobular shadow filled with very tiny dots; their is no visible septal involvement.

Incipient *fibrosis*, on the other hand, is demonstrated by thickening of the septa of the lobule, including localized expansion of the adjacent air spaces. An increasingly reticular structure results, possibly with a honeycombed appearance. More prominent zones of fibrosis can furthermore be limited to regions of a single lobe. Cirrhotic transformation zones affect the severity of bronchiectasis and cicatricial emphysema.

Histiocytosis X (Eosinophilic Granuloma)

This disease of unclear etiology begins as an exudative alveolar process with atypical pulmonary symptoms. Pneumothorax occurs in up to approx. 25% of cases. Granulomas arising from eosinophilic granulocytes develop in the peribronchial, paravascular, and interlobular tissues. They primarily affect the midzone and upper zone. The disease begins in an exudative alveolar phase; it seldom transforms into coarse reticular fibrosis. Hilar lymph node enlargement may occur.

• CT

In the proliferating stage, fine nodules are located throughout the entire lung. Small, thick-walled cystic spaces which may also be found in the periphery are typical. Some may become confluent with nodular structures. Larger, thin-walled cysts are occasionally seen. A reticular pattern shows the transition to fibrosis, which can be very extensive and further characterized by a honeycomb pattern and cicatricial emphysema.

Pulmonary Lymphangiomyomatosis

Pulmonary lymphangiomyomatosis almost exclusively affects young women. It is characterized by proliferation in the unstriated muscles in the alveolar septa, vessel walls and lymph

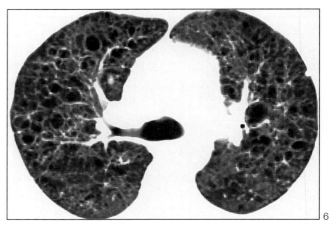

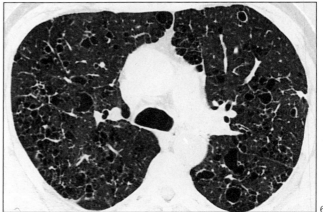

Fig. 8-62. Histiocytosis X. CT revealed reticular enhancement of the entire lung framework, throughout which cystic spaces of various sizes are distributed.

Fig. 8-63. Histiocytosis X. Irregularly shaped cysts with recognizable walls, some of them confluent, are distributed within the lung framework with only discrete reticular enhancement of the lung tissue.

Fig. 8-64. Lymphangiomyomatosis. Numerous thin-walled cysts of various sizes are distributed throughout the entire lung.

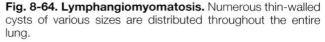

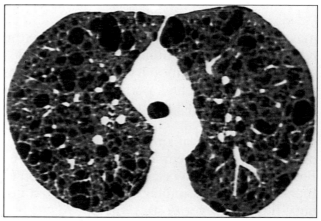

tracts. Due to the narrowing of the smaller bronchioles, emphysematous blisters and cysts develop in the lungs, which can lead to pneumothorax. Even the musculature near the mediastinal and retroperitoneal lymph nodes can become involved, thus leading to lymph node enlargement and chylous effusions.

• CT

Cystic changes measuring between a few millimeters and centimeters uniformly permeate the lung parenchyma without predilection for the periphery of the lung. The cyst walls are smooth and accentuated; (fibrotic) reticular components are normally absent.

Asbestosis

Asbestos fibers are inhaled into the alveolar space, where they are phagocytosed. After several years of exposure, the tissues react with peribronchiolar fibrosis, which spreads to the alveolar septa and later reaches the interlobular septa. These changes are more extensive in the lung bases than in apical sections, and are normally accompanied by pleural changes. Nodular granulomas are not found.

• CT

Fibrosis begins in the periphery, demonstrating various structural patterns. Fine reticular lines are found in the intralobular region, in addition to thickened septa (ca. 1 to 2 cm long) extending towards the pleura. Additionally, curvilinear lines of densification can be found, especially in the affected lung sections. These lines run at an interval of less than 1 cm parallel to the pleura. In order to exclude respiratory defects, these areas should be inspected with the patient lying prone, at constant maximum inspiration. Advanced asbestosis is characterized by fibrotic bands, honeycombing and confluent zones of fibrosis in conjunction with

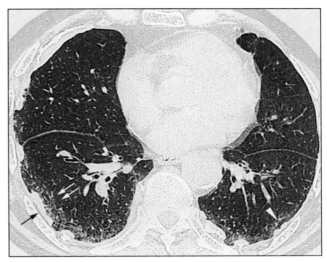

Fig. 8-65. Asbestosis. Above the sharply defined pleural plaques (→) there is an increased fine reticular pattern (⇉) with a discrete, curvilinear dense line running parallel to the pleural borders (►) on the left.

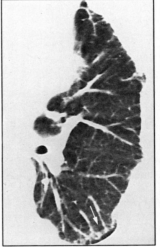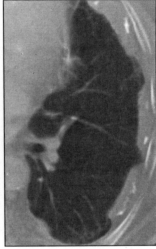

Fig. 8-66. Asbestosis. Next to the 1 cm long septal enhancements running vertical to the pleura, distortion and elongation of the blood vessels can be detected. The pleural border is relatively angular due to plaque formation (curved secondary shadow →).

Fig. 8-67. Silicosis. Fine punctiform enhancement can be seen in almost all areas of the lung. The interlobular septa are thickened (►); the secondary septum on the right has been intercepted tangentially and thus appears as an oval ring figure (⇉). The subpleural space exhibits very fine septal enhancement indicative of a slight fibrotic component.

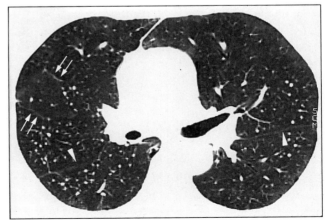

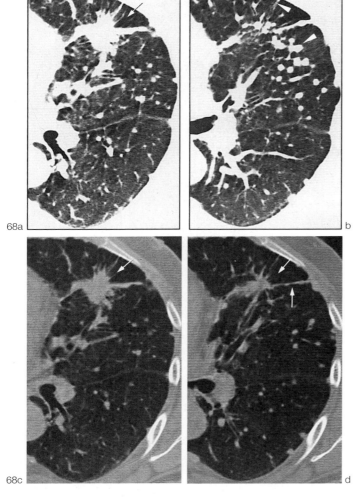

68a

b

68c

d

Fig. 8-68. Silicosis. In addition to fine nodular, well delineated structures with a retracting tendency (b ►), cord structures and a distortion of the lung framework are also detected. Approx. 1 cm caudal, a star-shaped enhancement with fine radial ramifications involving the pleura can be discerned (a→, c→). It extends caudally (d→) so that this stellate figure similar to a bronchial carcinoma corresponds to a silicotic fibrotic zone.

cicatricial emphysema and bronchiectasis. The latter and the more frequently occurring circular atelectasis or plaque formation in the main septa are characterized by lenticulated or wedge-shaped configurations. Their appearance is distinguishable from that of the more round or star-shaped bronchial carcinomas which frequently occur in patients with asbestosis.

Silicosis

Inhaled quartz dust is absorbed by alveolar macrophages. In the interstice, the dust causes fibroblast reactions that lead to the formation of nodules from collagen fibers. These proliferating lesions first affect the finer septal structures and produce a nodulo-reticular pattern on radiographs. With time, up to 20% of these intrapulmonary nodules calcify. Broad confluent lesions (conglomerates) form in the final stage. The draining hilar lymph nodes become reactively enlarged and may display typical "eggshell" calcification.

• CT

Pulmonary changes occurring in patients with silicosis can be detected much earlier in high-resolution CT than in conventional chest radiography. A reticular pattern of thickening in the intralobular and interlobular septa is a sign of increased fibrosis, which uniformly affects the core and periphery of the lung. This pattern can change to form a honeycomb pattern. These sharply delineated nodular densifications which are normally only a few millimeters large have a predilection for the upper zones of the lung. They are uniformly distributed throughout the lung parenchyma. Calcification can be better demonstrated by thin-section techniques. Punctiform densification structures located directly on top of the pleura are indicative of fibrosis of the very fine bron-

Fig. 8-69. Carcinomatous lymphangitis. Detection of thickening of the septum with club-shaped distension (→) in addition to extremely fine palisade-like and arc-shaped subpleural lines (►) and nodules (⇒).

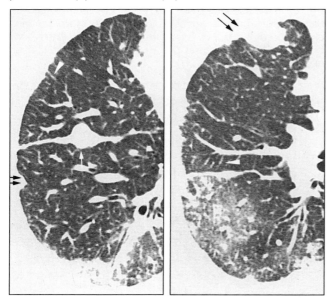

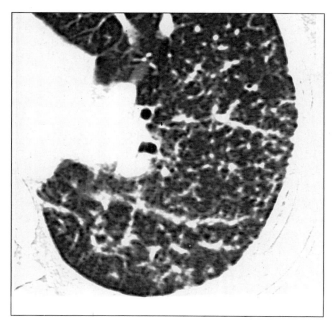

Fig. 8-70. Carcinomatous lymphangitis. Generally increased reticulo-nodular structure in which the septal structures are thickened like strings of pearls. The visceral pleura also contains very small nodules.

chioles in conjunction with involvement of the adjacent alveolar space. CT scans can provide detailed information on the size and shape of the lesions, accompanying cicatricial emphysema, and cavitation of the fibrotic zones.

Fig. 8-71. Carcinomatous lymphangitis. Thickening of the interlobular septa, the frontal ones in particular, making the polygonal structure of the lobules (►) readily visible. In addition to this, nodular structures in the core of the lobule are detected.

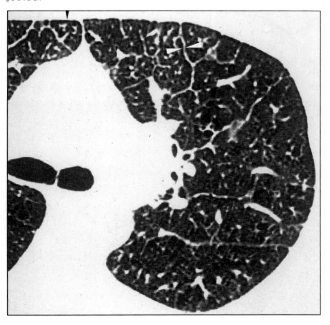

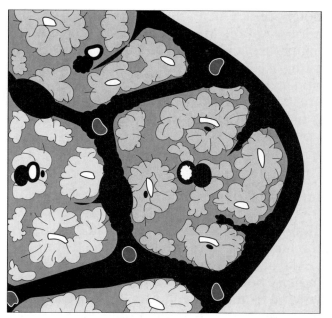

Fig. 8-72. Dissemination pattern of carcinomatous lymphangitis. Dissemination along the lymph vessels causes defined distensions of the interlobular septa that appear beadlike. In addition to this, the interlobular septa are thickened. They are represented as arc-shaped structures on the pleural border.

Carcinomatous Lymphangitis

Carcinomatous lymphangitis is frequently found in conjunction with carcinoma of the breast, stomach, pancreas and prostate. The tumor spreads via the lymph vessels to the root of the lung or the visceral pleura to the pulmonary interstice. Reticulated and striated shadows, including Kerley B lines, are often difficult to differentiate from infiltrates.

• CT

When the lymph vessels become filled with tumor cells, lymphostasis and generalized expansion of the affected interlobular septa occur. The septal pattern is extended, which means that the polygonal structure of the lobuli is also evident near the hilum. Localized proliferation of small tumor foci will cause nodular thickening of the interlobular septa and parts of the alveolar septa. Peribronchial distension of the center of the lobule is also frequently observed. Some of the subpleural lobules form cuneiform shadows, while some of the septa form arciform shapes on top of the pleura. In advanced stages, the nodular nature of tumor dissemination becomes increasingly prominent. The upper lobe of the lung is affected by the infiltrating process only later. In accordance with the path of dissemination, either the lung periphery or the bronchovascular (axial) paths are more prominently affected. Bronchiectasis is only rarely found within the infiltrated portions of lung.

Interstitial Tumor Infiltration

Tumors can infiltrate the interstitial tissues of the lungs by routes other than the lymph vessels. Especially in patients with an intrapulmonary tumor focus, infiltration occurs via the visceral pleura or the lung base. In such cases, the tumor tissue grows adjacent to areas of connective tissue. The septal structures become thickened and some have a triangular appearance.

Pulmonary Embolism and Infarction

Thrombembolic occlusion of the pulmonary arteries will only cause pulmonary infarction if ischemia develops due to secondary left cardiac insufficiency. Due to perfusion, the peripheral and (sub)segmental portions of lung are first affected. They form a cuneiform or coniform structure with their base situated towards the pleura. Infection (infarction pneumonia), an abscess, or communication with the bronchial system (infarction cavity) may develop in the infarcted lung area.

• CT

Plain scans: A perfusion deficit itself normally cannot be detected by computed tomography. Compensatory hyperperfusion of the non-affected lung segments, which is seen on CT scans as lightly dotted areas of reduced transparency, are detectable on CT scans only if a massive embolism has occurred. The appearance of a broad soft-tissue structure adjacent to the pleura which protrudes convexly against the lungs, has a wedge-shaped, blunt tip that points towards the hilum with hiloradial bands

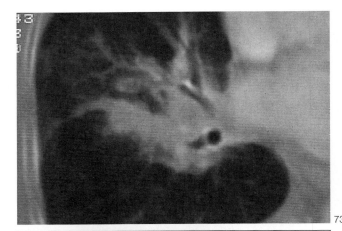
73a

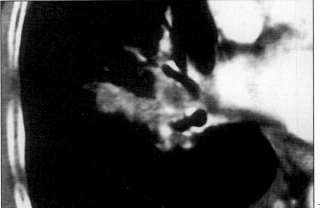
73b

Fig. 8-73. Interstitial tumor infiltration. The tumor located in the hilum is spreading primarily along the bronchovascular bundle.

Fig. 8-74. Central pulmonary embolism. Detection of a filling defect in the vicinity of the greatly enlarged pulmonary artery on the right, indicating a large central thrombus (→).

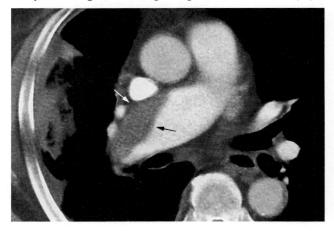

is indicative of hemorrhagic infarction or infarction pneumonia.

Contrast-enhanced scans: After a bolus injection of contrast medium and after careful scanning, central embolisms can be identified on CT scans as a filling defect within the central pulmonary artery. Peripheral, cuneiform shadows on the pleura, enhancement of central hypodensity and peripheral enhancement indicate that an infarction has occurred.

Differential diagnosis: The presence of a peripheral wedge- shaped structure is not a specific sign of infarction, since such lesions also are observed in patients with hemorrhage, pneumonia, focal edema and a focal tumor. If a blood vessel lies within the cuneiform densification structure (vascular sign; also observed in septic infarction embolisms), infarction is probably the cause.

Lung Injuries

External trauma can cause small localized injuries in the lung parenchyma and hemorrhaging into the alveolar space (lung contusion). If the trauma has made a larger laceration in the lung tissue, a cavity develops after retraction of the elastic lung tissue. This traumatic pulmonary cyst can fill with blood, thus becoming a pulmonary hematoma. After resorption has occurred, the hematoma can be demonstrated on CT scans as an area of shadow (globular

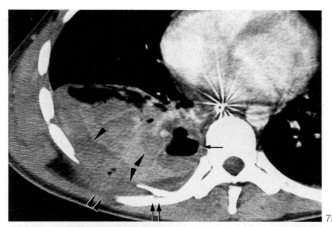

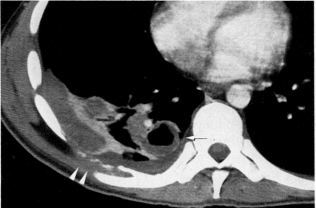

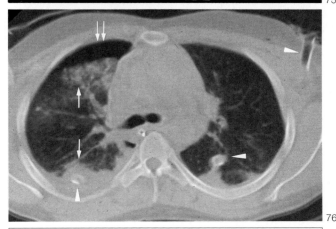

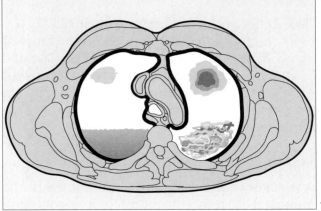

Fig. 8-75. Extensive pulmonary contusion. After a bolus injection of contrast medium, the injured regions (a ►) appear hypodense and are thus delineated from viable, collapsed lung tissue. On plain scans, these areas had exhibited hyperdensity due to hemorrhage. Twelve days later (b), the areas of contusion were smaller. They appear more hypodense than the atelectatic lung tissue. A persistent air cavity within a hypodense zone represents a traumatic pulmonary cyst (→). Additional findings: fractured rib (a⇉) with epipleural hematoma (a, b ►).

Fig. 8-76. Pulmonary contusion with pneumothorax. After insertion of a drainage tube (►), residual pneumothorax remains (⇉). The infiltrated areas (→) correspond to foci of contusion.

Fig. 8-77. Pulmonary contusion. Depending on their severity, pulmonary contusions exhibit different patterns of infiltration, which may vary from loose to compact shadows that, additionally, may be veiled by aspirated blood.

bleeding). Aspirations and foci of contusion become absorbed within days, but because of its size, a pulmonary hematoma takes weeks to become absorbed.

Traumatic pneumothorax develops through a laceration in the visceral pleura.

The possibility of a bronchial injury must always be excluded when there is a large segmental shadow and volume reduction in the corresponding hemithorax.

• CT

Plain scans: In trauma patients, poorly defined infiltrations of the alveolar space are frequently found in the affected areas; these are primarily indicative of aspiration. Compact, airless portions of lung are probable signs of contusion.

Contrast-enhanced scans: Healthy lung tissue can be differentiated from a hematoma or pleural effusion after a bolus injection of contrast medium.

Pulmonary Neoplasms

Benign Tumors

A *lipoma* can be readily identified due to its characteristic tissue density. *Chondromas* are characterized by calcification, while *osteomas* are marked by osseous components of greatly varying intensities. Because of their distinct central areas of fusiform or "popcorn-shaped" calcification, *hemartomas* can usually be identified on conventional chest radiographs.

The status and specificity of most benign tumors cannot be reliably judged on the basis of their CT appearance, however. When located in endobronchial locations, they cause cough, hemoptysis and poststenotic pneumonia. In peripheral, parenchymal sites, however, they normally produce no symptoms.

• CT

Atelectasis and narrowing of the lumen of the bronchial system (the latter in patients with

centralized tumors) can be demonstrated on CT scans. Peripheral benign tumors appear as sharply demarcated, sometimes lobular shadows which seldom exceed 4 cm in size. With the exception of a lipoma, the CT density offers no reliable clue as to the type of neoplasia. The popcorn type of calcification is characteristic of hamartomas, while osseous structures are indicative of an osteoma.

Bronchial Adenoma

Bronchial adenomas are classified as semi-malignant, since they metastasize predominantly

Fig. 8-78. Hamartoma. Smoothly marginated circular neoplasm containing central calcification, the structural aspects of which cannot be further evaluated due to movement artifacts caused by the aorta. However, a conventional tomographic image revealed typical, dumbbell-shaped calcification.

Fig. 8-79. Broncho-adenoma. A very small intraluminal tumor fills most of the bronchus of the right lower lobe (→). Spread beyond the dorsal boundaries of the wall of the bronchus was not detected.

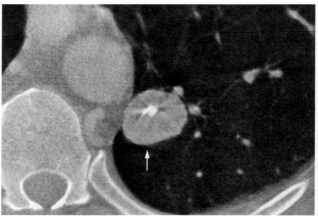

78

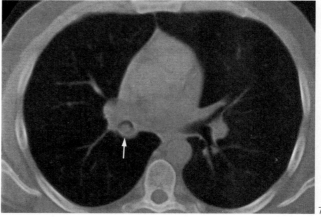

79

in the regional lymph nodes and only seldom in the extrathoracic lymph node chains. This is especially true of the *cylindroma*. The largest group comprises the *carcinoid tumors*. Up to 80% of all bronchial adenomas arise from the central bronchial system. They can obstruct the bronchial system so severely that poststenotic pneumonia and atelectasis can develop.

After the site, size and spreading of the tumor have been determined by CT, the histological diagnosis is normally secured by bronchoscopy.

• **CT**

Plain scans: These normally centrally located tumors appear as intraluminal soft-tissue structures, especially in patients with accompanying poststenotic pneumonia or atelectasis. They are normally identified as a characteristically broad-based structure on the bronchial wall. However, they can exceed these limits and be-

come large, central masses which then can no longer be distinguished from malignant tumors. Even smoothly marginated or lobulated peripheral masses can grow to a considerable diameter. The CT densities for these structures lies within the range of 80 to 180 Hu. They are frequently demonstrated as stippled areas of calcification.

Contrast-enhanced scans: Because of the high degree of vascularization of carcinoid tumors, there is significant enhancement after the administration of contrast medium.

Bronchial Carcinoma

In industrialized nations, bronchial carcinoma is the most frequent type of malignant growth

Table 8-1. Staging of bronchial carcinoma via computed tomography.

Tumor Stage		CT Staging
T1	Carcinoma < 3 cm	◗
T2	Carcinoma > 3 cm	◗
T2	Carcinoma > 3 cm (no atelectasis)	●
T2	Carcinoma > 3 cm (with collapse)	◒
T2	Involvement of primary bronchus, 2 cm or further distal	◗
T2	Infiltration of visceral pleura	◒
T3	Infiltration of mediastinal pleura	◗
T3	Infiltration of chest wall	◗
T3	Infiltration of diaphragm, mediastinal pleura and parietal pericardium	◒
	Infiltration of the primary bronchus within 2 cm of the carina	◗
	Total atelectasis of the entire lung	●
T4	Infiltration of mediastinum	◗
	Infiltration of heart and large vessels	◗
T4	Infiltration of trachea	◗
T4	Infiltration of esophagus	◒
T4	Infiltration of body of vertebra	●
T4	Infiltration of carina	◗
T4	Malignancy of pleural effusions	○

∅ = not possible; ○ = seldom possible; ◒ = not reliable; ◗ = usually accurate;

● = accurate

Fig. 8-80. The typical CT appearance of a **bronchial carcinoma** is that of a peripheral circular focus with radial, corona-like ramifications. Scar-forming pulmonary processes must be considered in the differential diagnosis, especially when there is known focal emphysema.

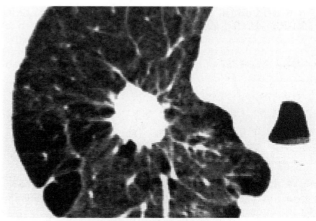

80a

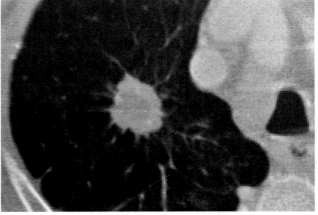

80b

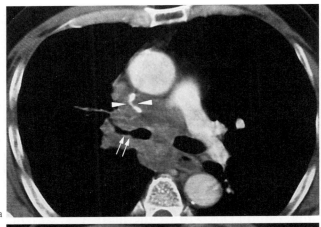

81a

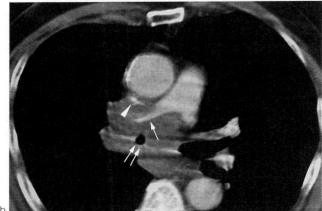

81b

Fig. 8-81. Central bronchial carcinoma. Small-cell bronchial carcinoma encasing the lower lobar bronchus (a, b ⇉) and right pulmonary artery (→). In cranial sections (a), the tumor extends into the mediastinum and surrounds the superior vena cava (►). Individual lymph node metastases cannot be distinguished from the tumor.

Fig. 8-82. Central bronchial carcinoma. This small-cell tumor extends a cone-shaped projection into the mediastinum (►) and surrounds the pulmonary artery (→).

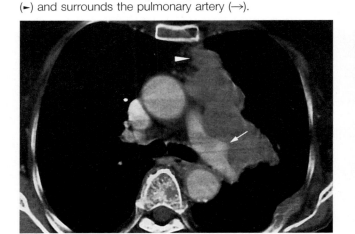

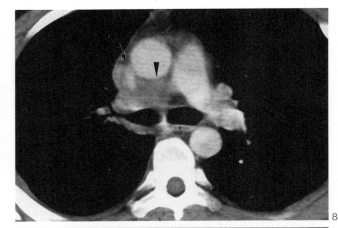

83a

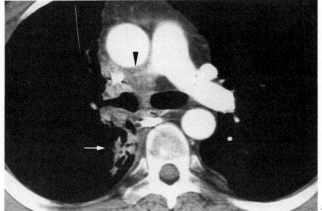

83b

Fig. 8-83. Central bronchial carcinoma under radiotherapy. Since the regression of this small-cell carcinoma (a ►) was still incomplete, chemotherapy was continued. The carcinoma surrounds the superior vena cava (a →). After radiotherapy was completed (50 Gy), the size of the soft-tissue mass was reduced (b ►). However, residual tumor tissue cannot reliably be differentiated from fibrotic tissue. Paramediastinal pulmonary fibrosis (b →).

Fig. 8-84. Paramediastinal pulmonary fibrosis after radiotherapy. After radiogenic pneumonitis had subsided, CT revealed a shrunken right hemithorax with an area of lung thickening corresponding to the radiation field. This exhibited clear absorption of contrast medium and contained air bronchograms.

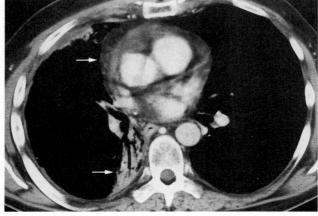

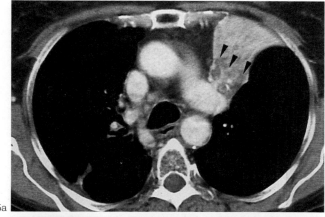

85a

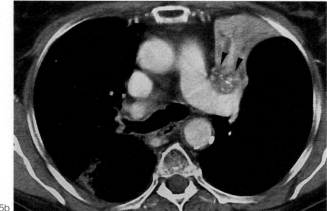

85b

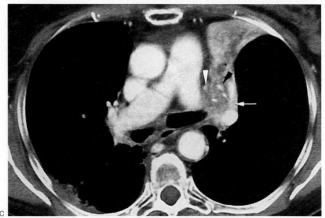

85c

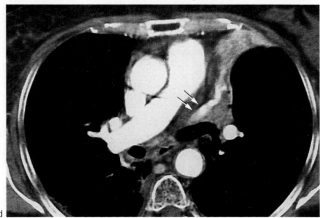

85d

with a lethal outcome. While its incidence is still higher in males, its rate of occurrence is rising in females, partly because more and more women smoke. The number of patients with squamous cell carcinoma is greater than the number with small-cell (oat cell) carcinoma, adenocarcinoma and large-cell carcinoma. Within in the group of adenocarcinomas, one distinguishes the bronchiolar adenocarcinoma, which can have a solitary focus or can occur as a multicentric or pneumonic type. The primary treatment for small-cell carcinoma is chemotherapy. Types which are not small-cell are surgically treated (resection). Staging of non-small-cell bronchial carcinomas should therefore be rigorously performed (TNM system) in order to determine precisely the resectability of the tumor.

It is sufficient to classify small-cell carcinomas into limited disease groups (tumor limited to one hemithorax, including the lymph nodes, but with no pleural effusion) and extensive disease groups (malignancy has spread beyond these regions). On the whole, the lymph node status is a better long-term indicator of the patient's prognosis than the primary tumor size.

Besides determining the severity of known bronchial carcinomas, CT is frequently a decisive factor in the diagnosis and differentiation of inflammatory and neoplastic lesions. It has now replaced conventional hilum tomography in this respect.

• CT

On the basis of their symptomatology, bronchial carcinomas are classified as either central or peripheral.

The *central bronchial carcinoma* is defined as a carcinoma located in the central bronchial tree,

Fig. 8-85. Central bronchial carcinoma. The tumor obstructs the left upper lobe and lingular bronchus 3 cm distal to the carina. This can be distinguished from upper lobe collapse by virtue of its rounded configuration (►) and its discreetly hypodense appearance as compared with the clearly enhanced collapsed tissue. The supplying artery (→) and draining vein (⇒) of the latter are also visible.

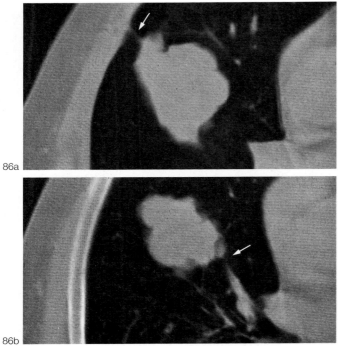

86a

86b

Fig. 8-86. Peripheral bronchial carcinoma. The tumor appears as a lobulated structure. There is pleural (a→) and hilar involvement (b→) with corresponding distortion of the pulmonary vessels.

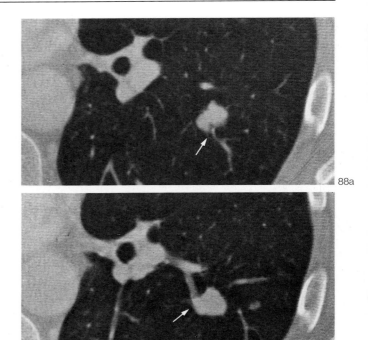

88a

88b

Fig. 8-88. Peripheral bronchial carcinoma. Slightly lobulated, relatively centrally located tumor. The pulmonary vessels are drawn toward the tumor (→).

Fig. 8-87. Peripheral bronchial carcinoma. A peripheral, round tumor nodule with ramifications and calcification can be seen on the pleura.

Fig. 8-89. Peripheral bronchial carcinoma in the apical segment of the lower lobe characterized by fine extensions. Pleural involvement and slight thickening of pleural structures (►) can be seen as well as clear traction of vascular and bronchial structures (in the direction of the tumor).

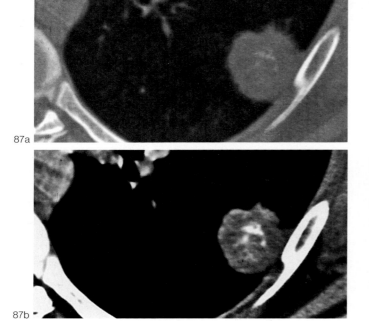

87a

87b

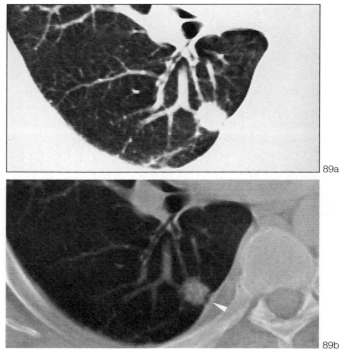

89a

89b

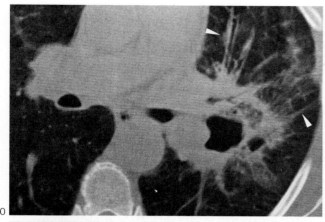

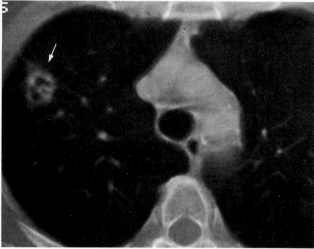

Fig. 8-90. Bronchial carcinoma. Large cavity of necrosis with irregular, thickened walls. Additionally, several tumor extensions project into the periphery (►).

Fig. 8-91. Peripheral bronchial carcinoma (necrotic squamous cell carcinoma). The relatively small tumor with a diameter of 2 cm already exhibits necrosis and extends fine ramifications toward the pleura (→).

Fig. 8-92. Necrotic bronchial carcinoma. The wall of the cavity is broad and of nonuniform density (→).

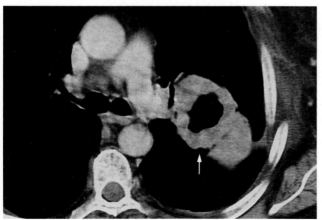

including its branches in the bronchopulmonary segments. The most frequent CT indicator is a *soft-tissue dense mass in the presence of bronchial distortion*.

Bronchial stenosis leads to reduced ventilation with segmentally oriented loss of volume and poststenotic infiltration. Poststenotic distension of bronchopulmonary segments is rarely found. In the initial search for the tumor, it is particularly important to carefully look for circumferential bronchial wall thickening in the absence of any considerable constriction of the lumen.

Finally, the development of *bronchial occlusion* gives rise to *atelectasis*, which appears at the typical site and is demonstrated as a soft-tissue dense formation. According to the extent of spreading, a shadow in the core of the tumor can appear as a round, cuneiform protrusion of the central borders of atelectasis that converges at the hilum.

If the tumor is surrounded by the lung or pleura, the tumor diameter and also the *tumor stage* (T1 to T4) can normally be reliably diagnosed. If endobronchial spreading is present, the distance between the tumor and the carina must be carefully evaluated. The thickness of the posterior wall of the primary bronchi can be adequately assessed by comparison with the surrounding lung.

Tumor invasion into the mediastinum, heart, larger vessels, trachea, esophagus and vertebrae can be assumed only if the contours of these organs are interrupted. The only criterion for reliable diagnosis of mediastinal invasion is obliteration of mediastinal fat by tumor extension. The demonstration of pleural or pericardial effusion is an unreliable indicator of pleural infiltration. An intact mediastinal contour along the tumor borders is not sufficient for exclusion of incipient infiltration.

The tumor is normally still resectable when the surface contact of the tumor does not exceed 3 cm on CT scans. For preoperative determination of the size of surface contact, one should therefore utilize thin-section techniques when border surfaces cannot be imaged tangentially (curved or horizontal).

Contrast-enhanced scans: After administration of contrast medium, recently collapsed lung becomes clearly visible as an area of homogeneous enhancement, which allows differentiation of the hypodense tumor as it is seen against the background of the collapsed parenchyma. If infiltration has led to congestion of secretions, enhancement can be absent, and an inhomogeneous pattern of opacification is observed. The shadow at the core of the tumor is no longer distinguishable.

If a filling defect of the vessel lumen exists, tumor herniation into a large vessel can be demonstrated on CT scans after a bolus injection of contrast medium.

A *peripheral bronchial carcinoma* normally appears as a rounded opacity inside lung tissue. Since the CT appearance of bronchial carcinomas is that of a variably demarcated, soft-tissue dense focus, a carcinoma cannot be differentiated from benign solitary neoplasms on CT scans per se, without confirmation of secondary signs of malignancy as regards the definition of the tumor borders, determination of the relationship of the tumor to the pleura, and mediastinal invasion.

In 85 to 95 % of these cases, however, the carcinoma will have a diffuse focus. A *radiating corona* is a typical sign of peripheral bronchial carcinoma whereby fine 2 to 8 mm ramifications radiate from the periphery of the circular focus into the lung, thus giving the structure a corona-like appearance. These interstitial structural densifications can be more sensitively detected on thin-section CT scans than on conventional sections. Interstitial ramifications near the pleura can become thickened due to interstitial reactions (connective tissue reactions), and they appear as cord-like *pleural fingers* or *flaps* extending to the visceral pleura. A unilateral, eccentric indentation in the external surface *(Rigler's umbilical sign)* signifies the site of entrance of the vessels and is seen predominantly in malignant tumors. Smaller vessels can also be drawn into the vicinity of the circular focus, and they serve as further proof of malignancy. Infiltrating growth is seen more frequently in connection with adenocarcinoma

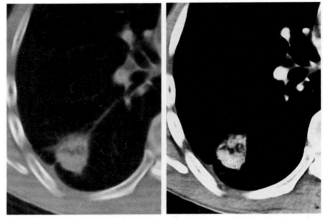

Fig. 8-93. Bronchio-alveolar carcinoma. Peripheral tumor with fine, strandlike projections and small pockets of air representing air bronchograms.

Fig. 8-94. Bronchiolar adenocarcinoma. Multicentric spread with numerous round tumor foci (some compact and confluent) with small cavities of necrosis (→).

Fig. 8-95. Bronchiolar adenocarcinoma. Pneumonic type. Relatively broad, subsegmental shadow with discrete bronchogram structures.

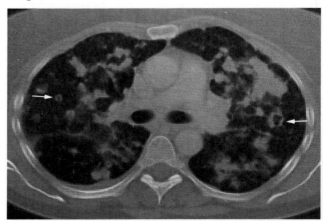

94

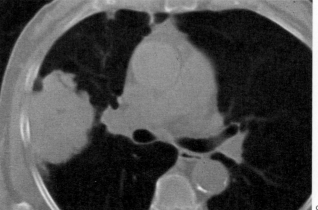

95

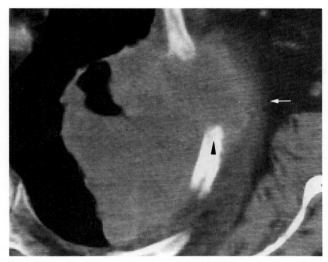

Fig. 8-96. Peripheral bronchial carcinoma with involvement of the chest wall. The large tumor makes broad surface contact with the visceral pleura, has also transmigrated the intercostal space, and infiltrated thoracic muscles (→). The cortex of adjacent ribs exhibits erosion (►).

Fig. 8-97. Sensitivity in demonstrating lymph node metastases as related to the transverse diameter of the nodes in non-small cell bronchial carcinoma. When lymph nodes of a transverse diameter of 10 mm or more are considered pathological, a 70% level of specificity can be achieved with 95% sensitivity. When the pathological transverse diameter is set at 15 mm, the level of specificity is raised to 95%, whereas sensitivity drops to 80% (Glazer 271).

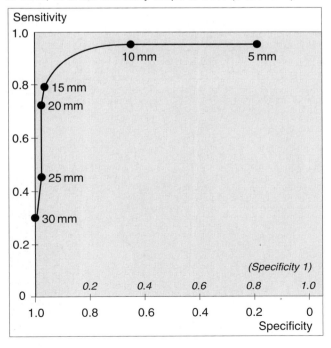

and squamous cell carcinoma than with small-cell and large-cell types.

The *attenuation* of malignant growth is normally in the soft-tissue range which, however, can also be true of benign forms of abnormal growth. Attenuation values exceeding 165 to 200 HU indicate fine areas of calcification and are a sign of benign growth. This is an insufficient criterion for excluding malignant growth, however, as intrafocal, localized, punctiform or amorphous areas of calcification are found in up to approx. 6% of malignant tumors diagnosed by thin-section tomography. These calcifications are eccentric-peripherally localised and take up less than 10% of the transverse tumor area. Central areas of "dumbbell-shaped" calcification, on the other hand, are almost always found in benign lesions (tuberculomas, hamartomas).

Tumor necrosis is predominantly associated with squamous cell carcinoma. The irregular borders of the necrotic cavity normally lie eccentrically and wall thickness is therefore irregular. Since signs such as a drainage bronchus altered by inflammation or accompanying inflammation are normally absent, these tumor cavities are normally readily distinguishable from abscesses and tuberculous cavities. Most of the associated findings are caused by secondary inflammation. However, inflammatory changes can also occur in connection with infected tumor cavities. As a rule, the area of necrosis must be differentiated from *air inclusions* (pseudocavities) which lie in the intact bronchoalveolar space. The latter are especially frequent occurrences in solitary bronchiolo-alveolar carcinoma, and they lead to heterogeneous CT densities.

Bronchial carcinomas can also appear as *pulmonary infiltrates*, but these are observed much more infrequently than solitary pulmonary nodules. The appearance of highly localized areas of infiltration can correspond with that of *bronchio-alveolar carcinoma*, which frequently displays centralized air bronchograms, while retraction phenomena, radial extension, and a pleural flap create an irregular, star-shaped figure. Larger (lobar) areas of infiltration of the alveolar carcinoma may also be observed. In that case, the central bronchial tree may be ventilated while the periphery demonstrates compact shadowed areas. The carcinoma, which remains in the matrix and fills the air space, displays somewhat reduced attenuation values (ca. 30 HU) in comparison to the usual forms of atelectasis. After the *administration of contrast medium*, the vessels of the lungs are clearly enhanced as compared with the homogeneously hypodense parenchyma (angiogram sign). The profusion of mucus produced by the tumor may cause bulging in the affected bronchopulmonary segment.

The diagnosis of *thoracic wall infiltration* can be made only if there is evidence that the infiltration has clearly infiltrated the tissue borders. Radiologic masking of extrapleural fat is a very sensitive indicator of carcinomatous infiltration. For this purpose, it is very important to obtain a tangential image of the tissue interface. When the tumor/pleura interface exceeds a diameter of 3 cm and a blunt angle of infiltration toward the pleural boundary is observed, the probability of pleural invasion is increased. In the inlet of the thorax, nerve infiltration occurring with Pancoast's tumor will lead to Horner's syndrome.

Contrast-enhanced scans: The administration of contrast medium only brings about minor, nonspecific enhancement of the peripheral tumor. These images are, however, of diagnostic value. In patients with bronchiolo-alveolar carcinoma, the pulmonary vessels contrast sufficiently against the homogeneous, hypodense, infiltrated parenchyma (angiogram sign).

Differential diagnosis: Varices, arterio-venous anomalies and granulomas enhance more strongly than the peripheral bronchial carcinoma.

• *Lymphatic Spread*

Lymph node enlargement is well demonstrated on CT scans. Metastatic and inflammatory abnormal lymph nodes, however, cannot be dis-

tinguished from one another exclusively on the basis of their CT densities and size, although the probability of metastatic invasion rises in proportion with the degree of enlargement of the lymph node. Numerous authors consider lymph nodes with a transverse diameter of over 10 mm to be infiltrated with tumor. One should keep in mind that lymph nodes that drain the tumor area are preferentially affected (which, however, is also the case with accompanying, extensive poststenotic pneumonias). In small-cell bronchial carcinoma, certain lymph node regions are skipped over. Very extensive metastases, which can also become calcified during therapy, may calcify.

Fig. 8-98. Multiple pulmonary metastases from a chondrosarcoma. Sharply marginated, round shadows are diffusely spread throughout the lung. In the periphery of the lung, a very small round focus of 1–2 mm diameter was also detected.

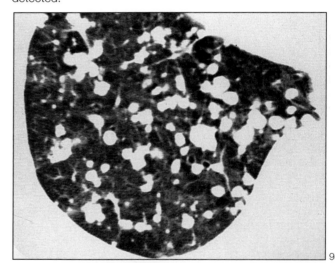

98

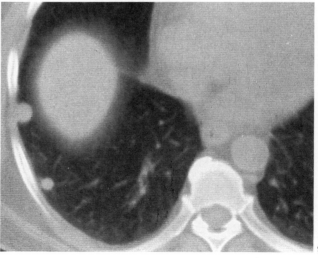

Fig. 8-99. CT sensitively detected **pulmonary metastases** in the phrenicocostal sinus.

99

In many cases, CT is used to diagnose and find the exact location of enlarged lymph nodes before mediastinoscopy and surgery. Thin-section tomography and, when necessary, a bolus injection of contrast medium should be used, at least when scanning critical regions such as the aorto-pulmonary window. When the mediastinal structures are clearly demonstrated and there is no evidence of abnormal lymph node structure, mediastinoscopy can be dispensed with.

• *Distant Metastases*

Bronchial carcinomas metastasize preferentially in the adrenal gland, and therefore it should be included in staging. Additionally, metastases are frequently found in the liver, skeleton and cerebral parenchyma.

Pulmonary Metastases

Pulmonary metastases larger than ca. 6 mm can be demonstrated on conventional chest radiographs. However, computed tomography is much more sensitive in detecting them and is also clearly superior to conventional tomography. Computed tomography has therefore become the more widely accepted method in diagnosing occult pulmonary nodules, especially prior to performing invasive treatments.

• **CT**

In patients with a known tumor, multiple, soft-tissue dense pulmonary nodules are indicative of pulmonary metastases. Subpleural metastases can be demonstrated when they are larger than 2 mm, while those in the core of the lung must have a diameter of over 4 mm. On 8 mm scan slices, solitary nodules are clearly marginated, and the surrounding lung structure is only slightly altered. In thin-section tomography, one can frequently observe radial extensions with very fine, nodular thickening of the neighboring septa which can change to form a lymphangitic pattern (carcinoma of the breast or colon).

Fig. 8-100. Dignity of a solitary round tumor nodule depends on the degree and pattern of calcification and the shape and sharpness of contour of the nodule.

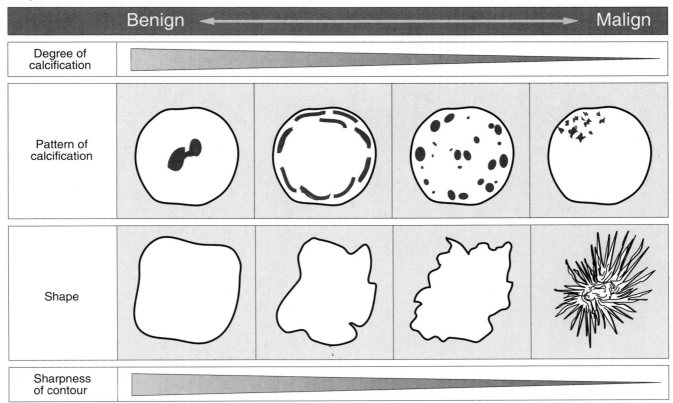

Tumor necrosis is diagnosed in approximately 5% of pulmonary metastases. Calcification, which regularly occurs in connection with metastases from osteosarcomas and chondrosarcomas, is also very rarely observed in metastases from mucogenic carcinomas (carcinoma of the colon or breast).

Differential diagnosis: Calcified pulmonary nodules with cicatricial surrounding lung tissue are typical signs of chronic inflammatory granulomatous lesions, especially in long-standing tuberculosis.

Solitary Nodules

Dense, solitary soft-tissue nodules may be due to bronchial carcinoma, benign pulmonary neoplasms and granulomas. The diagnosis of a pulmonary nodule can frequently be supported by the evidence of additional, similar circular foci found on conventional chest radiographs. At the same time, CT demonstration of non-calcified granulomas which cannot be distinguished from metastases leads to an increased rate of false-positive diagnoses with respect to metastases, which must be taken into consideration. The presence of multiple soft-tissue dense nodules reduces the probability of a peripheral bronchial carcinoma being responsible.

For qualitative evaluation of a solitary nodule, one must take the following factors into consideration:
1. The *sharpness of the margins*; in benign tumors, the external contours demonstrated by high-resolution CT are smooth on all sides.
2. The *configuration* of the nodule can be lobulated, serrated, or stellate.
3. *Proof of calcification*, which is best demonstrated by thin- section techniques. The probability that the nodule will be benign rises proportionally with the degree of calcification. The cross-sectional area of malignant tumors normally contains less than 10% calcification.
4. Evaluation of *calcareous structures*. Central areas of calcification (especially popcorn or dumbbell-shaped calcification and ringlike peripheral calcification) indicate benign growth. So do finely plaqued, stippled areas of calcification that are distributed evenly throughout the nodule. Eccentric, fine calcification that is found predominantly along the periphery is a sign of malignancy, especially when found in nodules that are larger than 3 cm.

Chapter 9
The Pleura

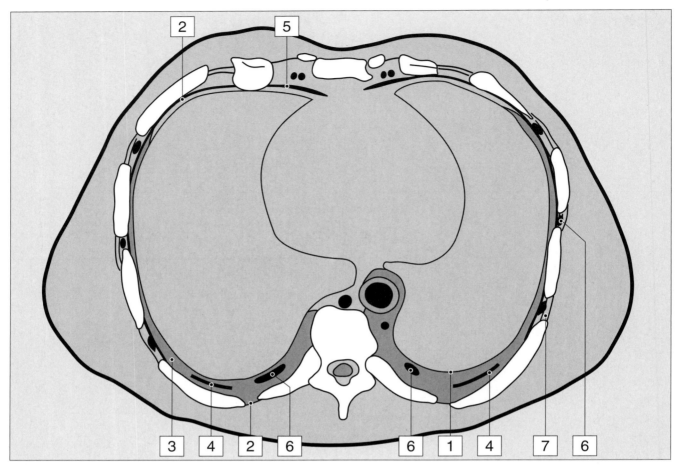

Fig. 9-1. Extrapleural tissue layers. In the transverse plane, diagonally coursing muscles and vessels in extrapleural fat appear as linear structures. Unlike pleural plaques, they cause no pleural protrusion. The endothoracic fascia forms a common tissue layer with the innermost layer of the intercostal muscles.

Key to symbols:

1 Parietal pleura
2 Endothoracic fascia
3 Extrapleural fat

4 Subcostal muscle
5 Transverse thoracic m.
6 Intercostal vein
7 Intercostal muscles

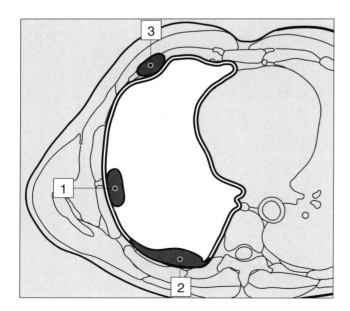

Fig. 9-2. Differentiation of pleural processes. Identification of the pleural borders and the configuration's angle with the lung (acute or flat) makes it possible to determine whether masses belong to the lung (1), pleura (2) or chest wall (3).

The Pleura

Anatomy and Imaging

The visceral membrane of the pleura encloses the lobe of each lung and, thereby, the double layers form the various septa (fissures) of the lung. The fissures divide the lung into the characteristic compartments seen on CT scans. Together with the parietal membrane which lines the pleural cavity, a fine, soft-tissue dense interface is found which, in healthy individuals, is recognizable as a subtle structure in costoparietal and mediastinal regions. Thin-section tomography is improved by selecting a wide window setting. Further outward, a delicate layer of fat (extrapleural and subpleural fat) is located between the costoparietal pleura and the endothoracic fascia. This layer of fat can be several millimeters thick in obese patients and can then be demonstrated on CT scans. The intercostal veins and the innermost layer of the subcostal and intercostal muscles lie directly adjacent to and outside the fascia. The outer margins of these soft-tissue structures, which normally traverse obliquely through the CT layer, are clearly demarcated by intercostal fatty tissue of varying thickness. This must not be confused with pleural thickening. On the retrosternal side, the transverse thorax musculature also forms a prominent boundary surface. The apices of the pleura, diaphragmatic pleura, and the secondary septum cannot be seen in healthy individuals. When free or encapsulated fluid collections are present in the pleural space, horizontal and semi-axial border surfaces can also be demonstrated.

Pleural Effusion

The accumulation of fluid inside the pleural cavity is a nonspecific sign that may arise from a number of different disorders. In order of frequency, transudation arising from cardiac insufficiency and serous or purulent effusions caused by pneumonia are the most frequent

Tabelle 9-1. Causes of pleural effusion (according to the Fraser-Paré model, ref. 3453).

● frequent ◒ occasional ○ rare

Cause	Transudate	Serous	Purulent	Serofibrinous	Serosanguinous	Other thoracic diseases	Extrathoracic diseases
Infectious							
Bacteria							
Klebsiella, Enterobacter, Serratia genera			●			●	
Pseudomonas, Salmonella			●			●	
E. coli, Actinobacter			●			●	
Hemophilus, M. mallei			●			●	
Anaerobes, C. perfringens		●				●	
Str. pneumoniae, Fr. tularensis		●				●	
Staphylococcus aureus		◒	●		◒	●	
Streptococcus pyogenes		●	●			●	
M. tubercolosis		●	●			◒	
Pancreatitis, subphr. abscess		●					●
Mycotic							
Actinomyces, Nocardia			●			●	
Blastomyces, Cryptococcus		●				●	
Histoplasma, Aspergillus		●				●	
Viral (incl. mycoplasma)		●				◒	
Parasitic							
Entamoeba histolytica				○	●	●	
Echinococcus granulosus					●	●	
Immunologic							
Syst. lupus erythmatodes		●				◒	
Rheumoid disease		●				◒	
Wegener's granulomatosis		●				●	
Neoplastic							
Bronchial carcinoma		●			◒	●	
Alveolar cell carcinoma		●			●	●	
Malignant lymphoma					●	◒	●
Metastases		●			●	◒	●
Mesothelioma					●	●	
Multiple myeloma					●	●	
Thrombembolic					●	◒	
Cardiovascular							
Cardiac insufficiency	●					●	
Constrictive pericarditis	●					●	
Venous occlusion (SVC, azygos vein)	●					●	
Traumatic							
Blunt chest trauma					●	●	
Abdominal surgery		●					●
Other causes (rare)							
Asbestosis			●		○	◒	
Sarcoidosis			●			●	
Nephr. syndrome, cirrhosis	●					●	
Myxedema, hydronephrosis			●			●	
Familiar polyserositis					●	●	
Uremic pleurisy			●		○	●	

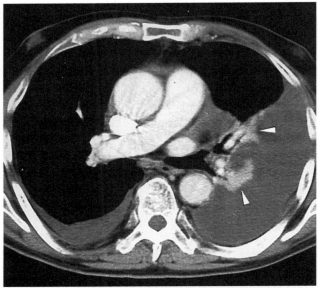

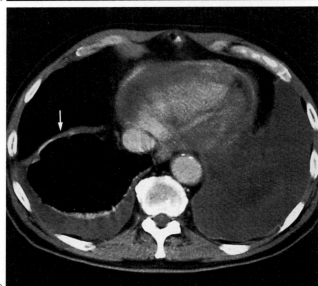

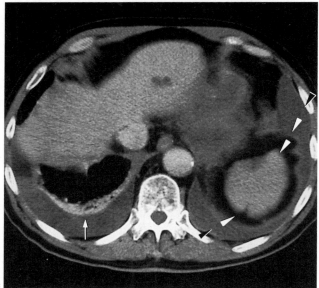

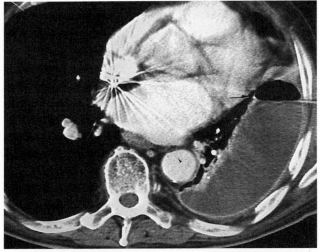

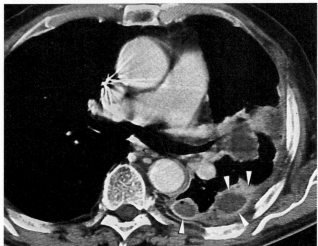

Fig. 9-4. Loculated pleural empyema. The basal empyemal cavity extends ventral to dorsal (a). Encapsulated fluid is found in the cranial region. There is a clear loss of volume in the entire left lung, together with signs of compressive lung collapse. Partial loss of volume and accompanying lung infiltration can be seen in upper areas (b ►). Air in the empyemal cavity entered due to puncture biopsy (a→).

Fig. 9-3. Pleural effusion. The structure on the right has the typical sickle-shaped configuration of a leaking pleural effusion; CT numbers are in the water range. The effusion on the left extends higher and compresses the lung (compression collapse). The lingula and lower lobe (a ►) therefore appear as small soft-tissue zones. In the left basal region (b), the pleural cavity is entirely filled with effusion fluid; on the right, part of the fluid is seeping into the main septum (b→). Effusion fluid surrounds the dome of the diaphragm in the diaphragmatic sinus; therefore, the spleen and surrounding fat form imposing structures in the scan (c ►). Partial loss of volume (c→).

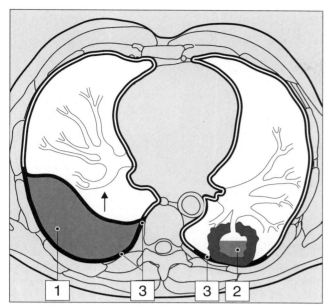

Fig. 9-5a. In order to differentiate an empyema (1) from a secondary pulmonary abscess involving the pleura (2), it is important to evaluate the configuration (empyema is usually convexoconcave) and primary location of the disease. Expanding pleural processes displace the bronchial tree (→). Thickened, partially adhesive pleural membrane (3).

causes. The latter can lead to empyema, as can serosanguilent effusions associated with tumors and embolism.

• CT

Florid dry pleuritis usually cannot be detected by computed tomography. CT diagnosis is pos-

Fig. 9-5b. Infected emphysemic bulla. This can be distinguished from an empyema due to the primary intrapulmonic location of the fluid, identifiable on the basis of the acute angle of its external contours with the pleura (→).

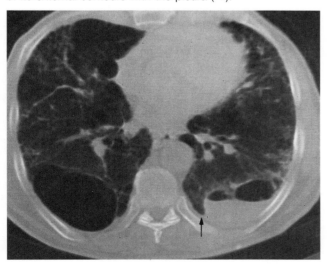

sible only when free fluid is present in amounts of 15 to 50 ml or more. The fluid should accumulate posteriorly when the patient is placed in the supine position.

Fibrinous deposits are characterized by thickening of the visceral and parietal pleural membranes. They can become encapsulated and eventually reorganize. Enhancement of the pleura after the administration of contrast medium is indicative of an inflammatory disorder (empyema).

The *attenuation* of effusion fluid clearly increases when the fluid contains large amounts of blood. It is therefore possible to distinguish between hemothorax and other pleural abnormalities. A minor rise in the attenuation value (ca. 30 HU) is a nonspecific sign. It is indicative of an increase in protein content, which may be caused by serofibrinous, serosanguilent and purulent effusion. The low lipid content of a chylous effusion does not specifically cause density reduction. Furthermore, motion and induration artifacts often falsify CT numbers.

Empyema

Pleural empyema is usually caused by extension of pneumonic infection or super-added infection following pulmonary infarction. It is infrequently caused by spread of inflammation from the thoracic wall. In exudative stages, the exudate is found to have clearly increased leucocyte levels. In the subsequent fibropurulent stage, the pleural membranes become thickened with accumulation of fibrin. Granulation tissue spreads inward, and an abscess cavity finally develops. In the stage of reorganization, which starts approximately two to three weeks after successful treatment, fibrosis of the granulation tissue occurs. Fistulae projected toward the bronchial system develop, and are usually seen together with obliteration of the empyema cavity (pleural lesion). Empyema is normally accompanied by bronchopneumonic infiltration, which is why CT is increasingly preferred over conventional chest radiography for diagnosis of complex cases.

• CT

Plain scans: Analogous to pleural effusion, empyema has a convexoconcave, sickle-shaped CT appearance. As the disease progresses, increased adhesion of pleural membranes is observed, and the amount of exudate increases, distorting the configuration to a biconvex or even rounded shape which leads to increased displacement of the lungs. Thickening of the normally delicate pleural membranes increases over the course of disease, but seldom exceeds 5 mm. Especially in chronic empyema, the volume of extrapleural fat increases slightly, and a uniform increase in attenuation is observed. The parietal pleura maintains its smooth, outer contours.

When the CT number is around 30 HU, the *attenuation* of empyema fluid lies in the abscess range. However, the attenuation of empyema fluid is subject to fluctuations and is, therefore, of only minor diagnostic significance. *Air* contained in the vesicles is a sign of viscous secretion and occurs predominantly in conjunction with gas-forming bacterial diseases. Fluid fluid levels indicate the presence of bronchopleural fistulae.

Invasion of a pulmonary abscess into the pleural cavity is probable when a primary intrapulmonary disorder exists. Empyema seldom occurs after thoracic wall infection, and the spread of an empyema through the chest wall is also rare.

Contrast-enhanced scans: After the administration of contrast medium, the pleural membranes display homogeneous enhancement which heightens towards the pleural cavity. Because the visceral pleura and lung tissue have different attenuation values, empyemic fluid can be distinguished from the surrounding lung

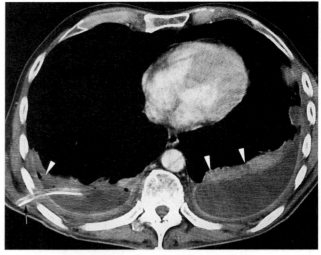
Fig. 9-6. Bilateral pleural empyema (right; Bülau drainage method→). The pleural membranes are clearly thickened. Peripheral enhancement seen vis-a-vis the pleural cavity is an expression of an inflammatory reaction. There is partial loss of lung volume (►).

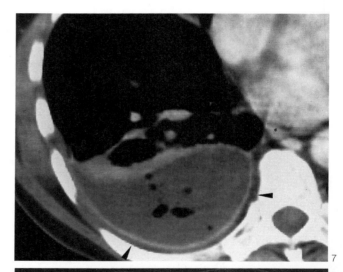

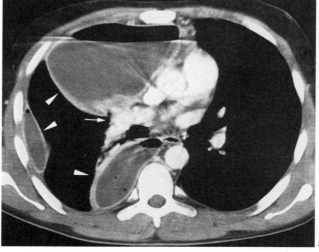

Fig. 9-7. Pleural empyema. Typical configuration with thickened, contrasted pleural membranes. The presence of gas is indicative of infection, whereas the increased CT number of extrapleural fat (►) signifies that the process is long-standing.

Fig. 9-8. Pleural empyema. Multiloculated fluid accumulation (►) with partial loss of lung volume (→).

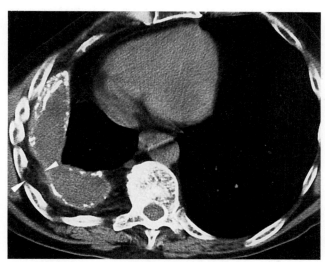

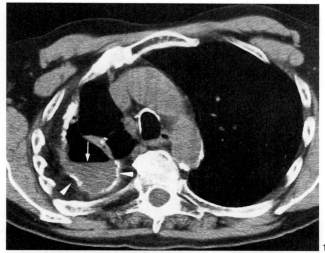

10a

Fig. 9-9. Broad zone of pleural callosity due to tuberculosis. Both the visceral and parietal membranes are calcified. The attenuation value of the pleural cavity is 50–65 HU, and is probably fibrotized. There is reactive proliferation of epipleural fat (▶ ◀).

tissue, which is mostly altered by bronchopneumonic lesions. This also makes it possible to identify collections of pus within the lung.

Pleural drainage, which is frequently difficult to demonstrate on conventional chest radiographs, can usually be reliably demonstrated on CT scans, which helps determine the origin of the underlying problem.

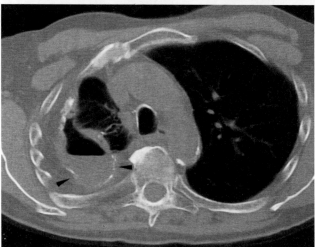

10b

Fig. 9-10. An **empyema** (a→) within an area of tuberculous pleural callosity (▶). A pulmonary infection spread to the tuberculous, broad, calcified area of pleural thickening. Even after fibrosis and calcification have occurred, the contents of the indurated pleural cavity may remain liquid for years. Infection may easily develop via the usual portals of entry.

Pleural Thickening

Pleural thickening frequently occurs when previous inflammatory processes heal, thereby causing fibrosis. The basal region near the costophrenic recess is the usual site of occurrence. Apical pleural thickening is more likely to be due to nonspecific causes than underlying tuberculosis. Broad, circular thickening (fibrothorax) normally arises from connective tissue reorganization in conjunction with hemothorax or pyothorax (empyema). Later, plaque-like or broad areas of calcification develop on the fibrotic pleural membranes. *Pneumonectomy* is a special case: The empty pleural cavity

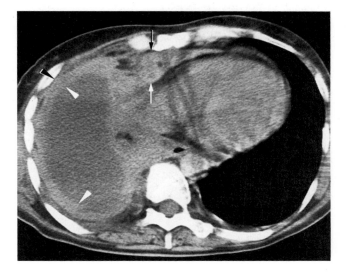

Fig. 9-11. After **pneumonectomy**, pleural thickening (▶) and nodular structures have developed in the cardiodiaphragmatic angle (→), thereby signalizing a recurrence.

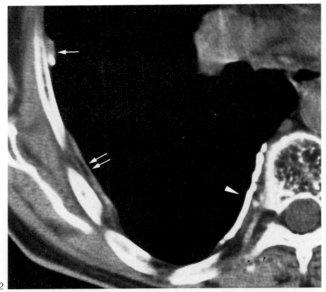

12

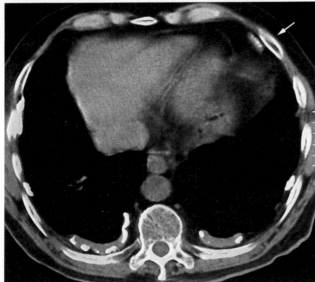

13a

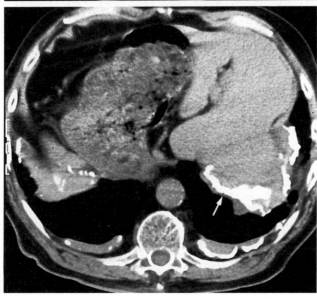

13b

fills with fibrous exudate and later displays parietal reorganization. Normally after only incomplete resorption of fluid, the mediastinum rotates in the direction of the fluid-filled pleural cavity.

● CT

On CT scans a circular, predominantly smoothly marginated soft-tissue zone with an incomplete ring of calcification extends along the margins of the pleural cavity. There is no significant amount of contrast enhancement.

A cavity following pneumonectomy is characterized by a sickle-shaped pleural cavity that is reduced in size and has a soft-tissue dense coating. In the center of this structure, a hypodense zone which indicates the presence of residual fluid is found.

Asbestosis

After exposure to asbestos dust, changes in the pleura normally become visible after a latent period of two decades. The disorder is characterized by localized, parietal pleural thickening (plaques) made of fibrotic hyalinized, largely calcified tissue. Adhesion to the visceral pleural membranes is rare. The location of plaques is costoparietal (6th to 9th rib), paraspinal, mediastinal and diaphragmatic. They are only rarely located in the interlobar septa or the angles of the diaphragm. Changes in lung structure, the basic characteristic of asbestosis, are present in up to 10% of cases without any accompanying changes in pleural structure. In asbestosis, diffuse pleural thickening affecting both pleural membranes is just as infrequent as serous pleural effusion.

Fig. 9-12. Asbestosis. Pleural plaques usually appear dense and sharp-edged. They may be fully (►) or partially (→) calcified or noncalcified.

Fig. 9-13. Asbestosis. Sharply marginated and edged areas of pleural thickening (plaque- and ringlike) have developed in the parietal pleura. The extent of plaque-like calcification is variable. Calcified structures usually are located behind the ribs (a→) and on the diaphragmatic pleura (b→).

• CT

The rather sharply marginated pleural densifications, including their frequent lamellar or punctiform areas of calcification, are best detected at a pulmonary window setting. Calcified and noncalcified plaques frequently coexist. They can be as broad as 10 mm and, if they contain soft-tissue components, a mesothelioma must be suspected. Effusion, which is rarely associated with asbestos-related pleural disease, can lead to diffuse, uncharacteristic pleural thickening. Reticular anomalies of the lung parenchyma can normally be demonstrated on high-resolution CT scans.

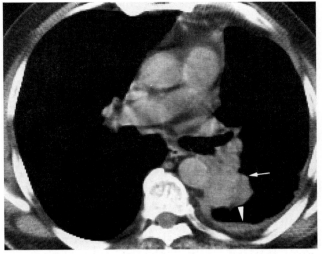

Fig. 9-14. Mesothelioma. A polycyclic, demarcated soft-tissue structure lies directly contiguous with the aorta (→). Dorsally, there is a broad area of pleural thickening (►).

Primary Neoplasms of the Pleura

Benign Neoplasms

The *localized benign mesothelioma* is the most common benign pleural tumor, and it is most frequently found in patients over forty. It is pedunculated in 30 to 50% of cases, originates in the visceral pleural membrane, and has a smooth surface. Localized mesotheliomas are usually found in the inferior hemithorax, but are sometimes located in the interlobar space. Localized mesotheliomas are frequently accompanied by hypertrophic osteo- arthropathy. Tumor calcification is very rare.

In pleural *hyaloserositis*, multiple nodulated, hyaline pleural thickening occurs in the parietal membrane (iced pleura). Typical round, ringlike calcification is a frequent finding. Lipomas occur more frequently than the rare, usually 3 to 4 cm large *fibrin bodies* and *multiple fibroma* (which have a round to oval configuration and can spontaneously degenerate). *Lipomas* originate from subpleural parietal fat and can lead to costal erosion.

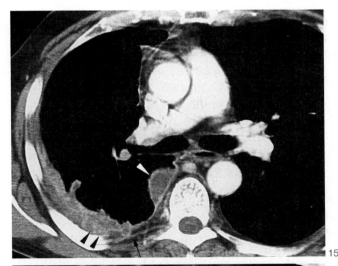

15a

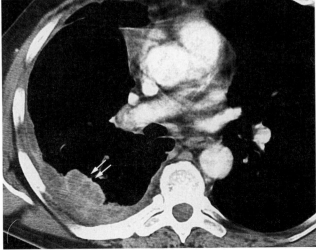

15b

Fig. 9-15. Mesothelioma. Vascularized tumor tissue (⇒) is demarcated via contrast medium administration. This extends paravertebrally inside the pleural cavity, and small pockets of fluid are seen (►). One tumor nodule encroaches the pleural border (→), another rests against a rib. Beginning bone erosion therefore cannot be excluded (⊫).

• CT

Plain scans: The good demonstrability of the pleura usually makes it possible to demonstrate the pleural origin of a mass. A *lipoma* can be distinguished from other lesions simply by comparing CT numbers. Fibrin bodies and fibromas usually appear as multiple occurrences, while *benign mesotheliomas* are solitary. Because of its intrapleural locations, the latter cannot be directly demonstrated.

Contrast-enhanced scans: Because of the relatively high degree of vascularization of benign mesotheliomas, they display homogeneous enhancement after the administration of contrast medium.

Malignant Mesothelioma

The diffuse mesothelioma is a highly aggressive malignant tumor. It affects men five times more frequently than women. The patient will often have a history of asbestos exposure. According to the stage of disease, this neoplasm may display pathological and anatomical signs of tuberous and plaque-shaped components. It permeates the entire pleural cavity, totally or partly encloses the lung, and may invade the interlobar fissure. Flat, usually multiple tumors that are frequently accompanied by a sanguinolent effusion may also be found. When the malignant mesothelioma causes a fulminant and therefore unfavorable course of disease, the thoracic wall and the pericardium are breached and destroyed. Histological differentiation between mesotheliomas and fibrothorax or metastasizing adenoid carcinomas is often difficult.

• CT

Plain scans: The preferentially unilateral attack and circular, lamellar or tuberous pleural thickening of over 1 cm are characteristic signs that distinguish malignant mesotheliomas from fibrothorax, which tends to demonstrate a more uniform and more minor degree of pleural thickening. Malignant mesotheliomas will usually lead to significant volume reduction on the affected side. They penetrate pleural fis-

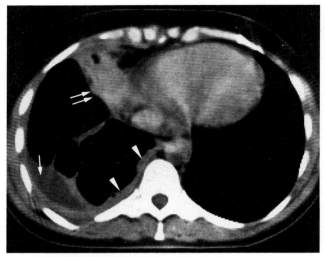

Fig. 9-16. Mesothelioma. The right dorsolateral pleural membranes are thickened and surrounded by encapsulated effusion fluid (→). Plaque-like pleural thickening extends paravertebral (►). In the right ventral region, there is a broad soft-tissue zone (⇒) with strand-like structures projecting into the lung. These soft-tissue structures correspond to tumor tissue. They become moderately enhanced after contrast medium administration, which facilitates the identification of effusion fluid.

sures and, in the final stages, frequently spread to the contralateral pleural cavity. Localized linear areas of calcification, especially those found on the contralateral side, are indications of asbestos-related pleural disease which, how-

Fig. 9-17. Mesothelioma. Reduction of the left hemithorax. There is bulbous thickening in the visceral pleura and anterior pleural fold (→) as well as clear enhancement after contrast medium administration. There is no evidence of osseous destruction. The visceral pleura displays tumorous thickening (►).

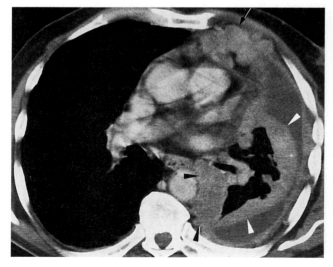

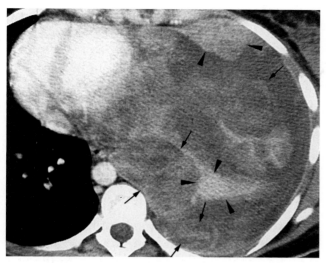

Fig. 9-18. Metastasizing synovioma. Hemorrhagic and some necrotic metastases were found in the pleura and lungs. CT examination revealed broad, vascularized soft-tissue formations in the pleural cavity and hypodense formations (→) inside the collapsed lung (►). The attenuation value of the effusion fluid was raised due to hemorrhage.

ever, may also occur within the tumor. Infiltration of subpleural lung tissue occurs infrequently, because of effusion-related lung compression and the frequent occurrence of accompanying pulmonary fibrosis. Advanced malignant mesothelioma is characterized by thoracic wall invasion accompanied by costal destruction, mediastinal, retrosternal and/or diaphragmatic lymph node enlargement and spreading of the tumor outside of the affected hemithorax.

Contrast-enhanced scans: After the *administration of contrast medium*, the tumor tissue becomes clearly and sometimes inhomogeneously enhanced. Circumscribed effusions are thereby demarcated. Since the invasion into the thoracic wall, diaphragm or pericardium is often underestimated, a bolus injection of contrast medium is recommended for improved diagnosis.

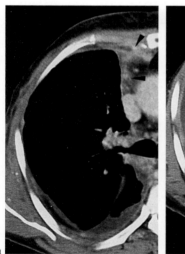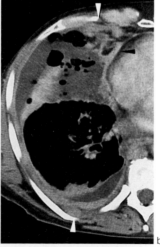

19a

b

Fig. 9-19. Pleural carcinosis in a metastasizing carcinoma of the breast. After contrast medium administration, there is clear, in some places nodular, thickening of the enhanced parietal pleura (a, b►). Micronodular structures are scattered throughout the mediastinal pleura, where they coalesce to form small nodules (c►). This is an important indicator of pleural carcinosis.

Fig. 9-20. Pleural carcinosis in a muciferous carcinoma. CT revealed broad pleural thickening with bulbous structures (→); the internal contours (►) are strikingly smooth and absorb contrast medium.

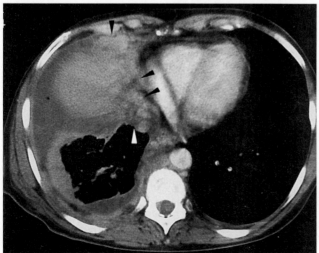

19c

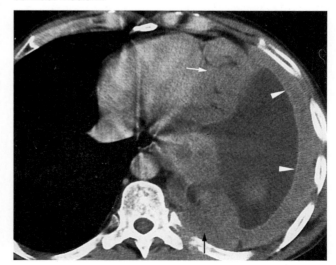

Pleural Metastases

40 to 50% of all pleural metastases arise from bronchial carcinoma; they are followed in frequency by carcinomas of the breast, malignant lymphoma, carcinoma of the ovary and tumors of the gastrointestinal tract. Pleural metastases are frequently accompanied by pleural effusions, which regularly appear as the disease progresses. Pleural exudates (frequently hemorrhagic) have a high protein content. Usually, a lymphoma involves the pleura during the late stages of systemic disease.

• CT

Plain scans: Pleural metastases or pleural carcinomatosis can be demonstrated only after solid components have been located in the pleural membranes. Pleural metastases can usually be differentiated from accompanying effusions after contrast medium has been administered. If multiple nodular components are found, it is highly probable that the condition is malignant. Unstriated, medium-grade pleural thickening with accompanying pleural effusion is a nonspecific sign. When thickening is greater than 1 cm, a tumor is strongly suspected. In the pleuropericardial angle in particular, extrapleural fat may swell due to accompanying lymphatic distension, carcinomatosis or small lymph nodes, which are further signs of malignancy. Additional evidence of bone destruction or carcinomatous lymphangiosis provides strong proof of a malignant pleural disorder.

In patients with malignant lymphomas, (chylous) pleural effusion can make evaluation even more difficult. A considerable number of intrapleural and extrapleural soft-tissue masses may be found.

Contrast-enhanced scans: A bolus injection of contrast medium demarcates solid components and pleural membranes from effusion, which is especially important when absorption of contrast medium is inhomogeneous in soft-tissue masses.

Chapter 10
The Chest Wall

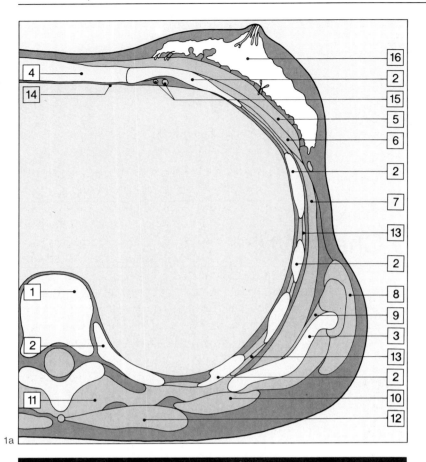

1a

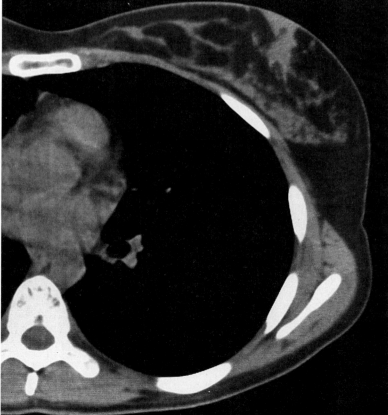

1b

Fig. 10-1. Topography of the chest wall.
a) Transverse section.
b) CT scan

Key to symbols:

 1 3rd thoracic vertebra
 2 Rib, sternum
 3 Scapula
 4 Sternum
 5 Pectoralis major muscle
 6 Pectoralis minor muscle
 7 Sup. serratus anterior muscle
 8 Teres major muscle
 9 Subcapularis muscle
10 Rhomboid major muscle
11 Erector spinae muscle
12 Trapezius muscle
13 Intercostal muscles
14 Endothoracic membrane
15 Internal thoracic vein/artery
16 Breast

The Chest Wall

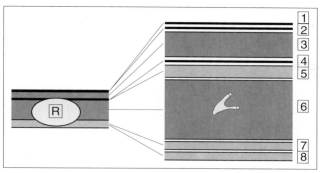

Fig. 10-2. Tissue layers in the chest wall (according to Im, ref. 720). 1 = visceral pleura; 2 = parietal pleura; 3 = extrapleural fat; 4 = endothoracic fascia; 5 = innermost intercostal muscle (intercostales intima muscle); 6 = intercostal fat and vessels; 7 and 8 = internal and external intercostal muscles.

Fig. 10-3a, b. Thoracic surgery. After rib resection, there is clear asymmetry of the bony thorax and widespread pleural calcification (►). The lower angle of the scapula (b→) protrudes deep into the thoracic cavity together with the surrounding soft-tissues when the arm is raised.

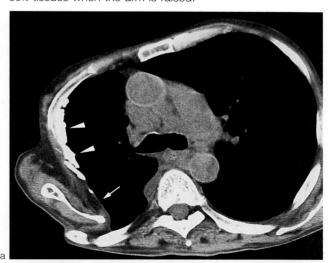

3a

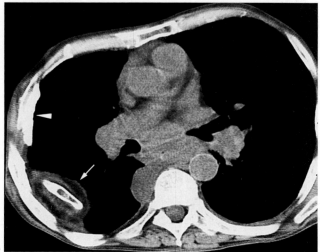

3b

Anatomy and Imaging

The chest wall, with its cylindrical configuration, is a good object for computer tomographic scanning. Its inner surface, lined with costoparietal pleura, the anterior and posterior borders of the sternum, and the sternoclavicular joints can be demonstrated clearly and in detail. The streak-like, cortical layer and seemingly open medullary spaces of the ribs, which lie diagonal to the scanning plane, are not clearly demonstrated on CT scans. Slice phenomena may simulate rib destruction.

The thoracic musculature can be evaluated in detail when there is a sufficient amount of delineating fat. The individual muscle fibers can be demonstrated, which makes it possible to identify infiltrative processes. In the upper section of the chest wall, the soft-tissues of the thoracic girdle can clearly be demonstrated on CT scans, even in locations which were previously poorly demonstrated by conventional radiography (subcapsular space, axilla).

Tumors

Primary chest wall neoplasms are rare and usually arise from the ribs. Chondrogenic tumors like *(osteo)chondromas, chondrosarcomas* and *enchondromas* are the most common (ca. 40% of all cases). Osteogenic *osteoblastomas, endostomas* and *osteogenic sarcomas,* on the other hand, are rare in comparison.

Next in order of frequency are malignant neoplasms of the hemopoietic and reticulo-endothelial systems, such as *myelomas, Hodgkin's lymphoma, Ewing's sarcoma* and *reticulum cell sarcoma.* The more rare benign entities are, in order of decreasing frequency, *fibrous dysplasia, Paget's disease, hemangioma, eosinophilic granuloma* and *aneurysmal bone cyst.*

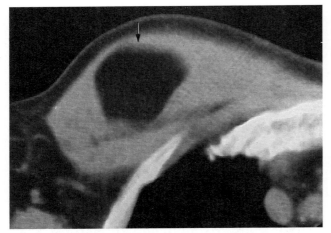

Fig. 10-4. This **lipoma** in the pectoralis major muscle has homogeneous attenuation values in the fat range.

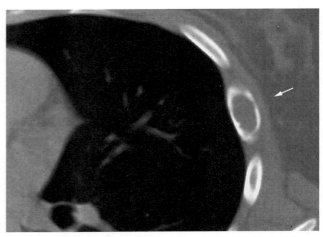

Fig. 10-6. Enchondroma. The affected rib is slightly dilated. Typical chondrogenous calcification is absent here.

Fig. 10-7. Plasmocytoma of the clavicle. The affected end of the clavicle is dilated; the cortex is still free and absent of soft-tissue structures.

Fig. 10-5a, b. Aneurysmal bone cyst. The affected rib is dilated and honeycombed in appearance. After contrast medium administration, the soft-tissue clearly enhances, thereby demarcating variably sized, cystoid chambers indicative of hemorrhage.

Fig. 10-8. Eosinophil granuloma of the rib. Evidence of osteolysis with subpleural soft-tissue structures. The tumor demonstrates homogeneous tissue structure after administration of contrast medium.

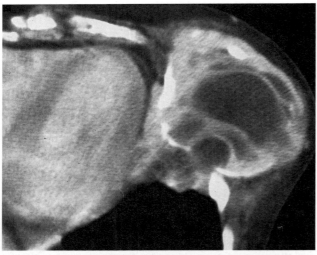

5a

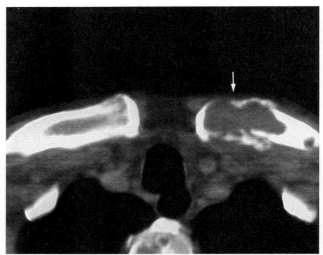

7

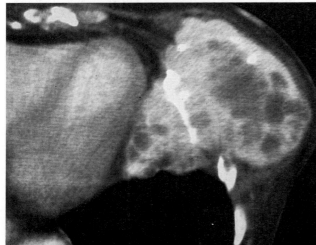

5b

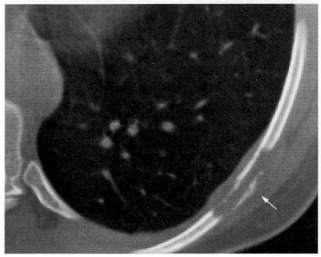

8

Primary soft-tissue tumors, such as *lipomas, liposarcomas* and *fibrosarcomas,* are even more uncommon.

Secondary intra-osseous neoplasms are more common. They arise from primary tumors of the breast, lungs, prostate, kidney, thyroid, and stomach and are preferentially located in the ribs and sternum.

It is not unusual to observe relatively early invasion of the chest wall in conjunction with peripheral pulmonary tumors and malignant mesotheliomas. Late infiltration, however, is usually seen in malignant tumors of the mediastinum and in breast cancer.

• CT

Plain scans: Since the majority of primary and secondary chest wall neoplasms originate from tissue of the cartilage, bone and medullary space, the indications for computer tomographic examination are similar to those indications applicable in other skeletal areas. Bone deformity and destruction can clearly be demonstrated with high-resolution CT scans, which are performed when conventional radiographs were questionable. Important diagnostic indicators such as cartilage destruction and (extra-osseous) soft-tissue components can be reliably evaluated by computed tomography. Proof of the absence of soft-tissue components, as in Tietze's syndrome, can even be of diagnostic significance.

Tumor invasion appears on CT scans as masking of the individual muscle layers which are separated by fat. Since extrapleural fat can also be masked by hemorrhage and accompanying fibrosis, it is more difficult to differentiate incipient infiltrations from pulmonary and pleural tumors. The diagnosis of recurrent breast carcinoma is complicated by the presence of scar tissue, post-radiotherapeutic fibrosis, and the absence of delineating fat.

The most reliable indicator of all invasive malignant processes is bone destruction.

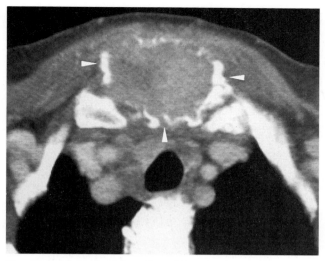

Fig. 10-9. Metastasizing thyroid carcinoma. After bolus contrast medium administration, CT revealed clearly enhanced tumor tissue and a dilated sternum (►).

Fig. 10-10a, b. Metastasizing pheochromocytoma with rib destruction. This hypervascularized tumor tissue clearly absorbs contrast medium (b).

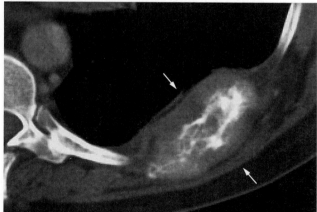

10a

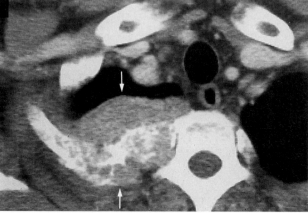

10b

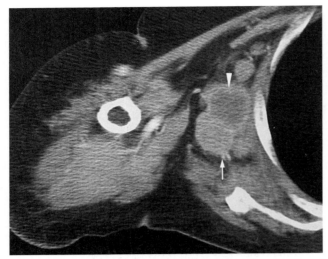

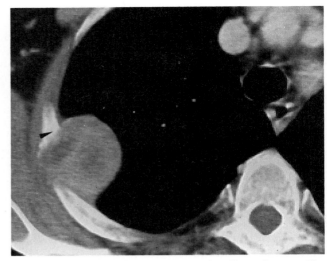

Fig. 10-11. Non-Hodgkin's lymphoma on the chest wall (→); regressive changes (►).

Fig. 10-12. Metastasizing carcinoma of the breast. Contrast medium absorbing tumor tissue (→) infiltrates the axilla; hypodense areas (regressive changes) are also visible (►).

Fig. 10-13. Metastases in the chest wall from recurrent breast cancer (→). Fine projections from the tumor connect the recurrent carcinoma to an enlarged lymph node (►) and the thickened pleura (⇒).

Fig. 10-14. Metastases from a renal cell carcinoma. The hypervascularized tumor tissue shows clear enhancement after bolus contrast medium administration. There are signs of bone erosion (►).

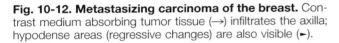

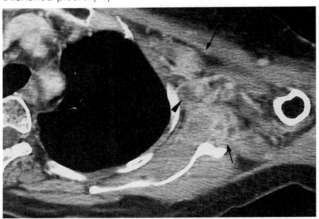

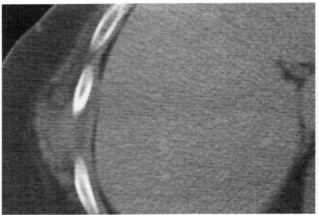

12

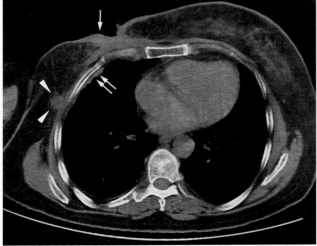

13

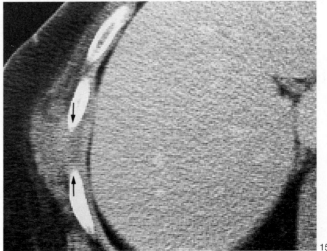

15a

15b

Contrast-enhanced scans: The individual fascial structures often become clearly visible after intravenous contrast administration. This makes its easier to distinguish distension and deformity of soft-tissue structures. In extensive intrathoracic tumor processes, chest wall infiltration can be demonstrated rather accurately on contrast-enhanced CT scans, because the demarcation of tumor tissue is thereby improved. Computer tomography's increased sensitivity for detecting slight enlargement of parasternal lymph nodes can be an essential factor in the diagnosis of tumor recurrence.

Inflammations

Infection rarely originates within the chest wall itself. Inflammation of the lungs or pleura, usually in association with *tuberculosis* or *fungal infections*, often affects the chest wall. This is manifested as osteomyelitis, phlegmons, and suppuration. Primary (hematogenous) *osteomyelitis* of the ribs or sternum (rare) can also spread to contiguous soft-tissues.

Inflammatory changes in soft-tissue are, frequently, only nonspecific signs that must always be differentiated from neoplastic processes of the chest wall. If there are no apparent signs of infection and the skeleton is intact, the possibility of malignant infiltration must always be considered in the diagnosis.

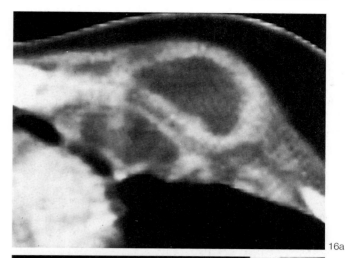

16a

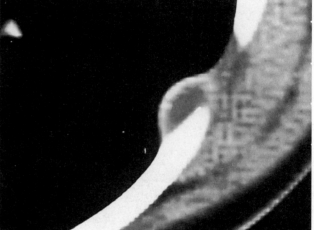

16b

Fig. 10-16a, b. Tuberculous abscess in the chest wall. Within the dilated wall, there are hypodense areas (ca. 25 HU) that are sharply demarcated by broad peripheral zones of granulation tissue (a). There is an additional epipleural focus (b).

Fig. 10-15a, b. Soft-tissue metastases from a primary carcinoma in the body of the uterus (after an extended postoperative period). The borders of the dilated intercostal space with the endothoracic fascia are smooth; there is moderate displacement of the serratus anterior muscle. A striated structure appears in the intercostal space after contrast medium administration. Since osseous destruction was absent and bone scintigraphic findings were positive, an inflammatory process was initially suspected.

◄─────────

Fig. 10-17. Phlegmon in the chest wall after a chest operation. Even after bolus contrast medium administration, the muscles remain nonuniformly hypodense (→) and masked; fatty tissue shows strandlike densification. Air (►).

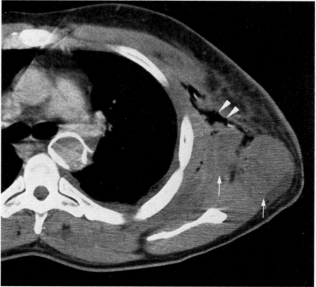

17

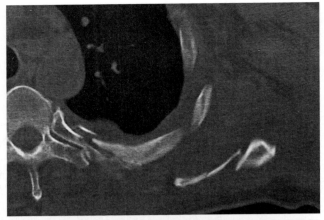

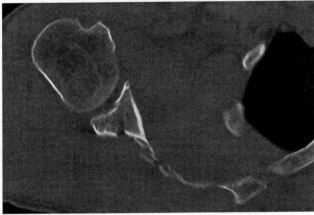

Fig. 10-18. Chest trauma. CT sensitively revealed fractures, especially in the scapula and its socket, avulsion in the head of the humerus, and complex paravertebral fractures as well as a fractured sternum.

Fig. 10-19. Massive chest trauma. In addition to locating fractures (→), CT can be used to reveal masked fatty tissue corresponding to blood-soaked soft-tissue (►), air (▻), and raised CT numbers indicating hemorrhages in muscle tissue.

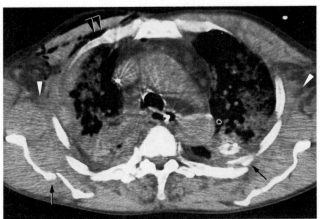

• CT

Plain scans: Structural (osteomyelitic) changes in the ribs can be demonstrated with thin-section, high-resolution CT bone scanning techniques. Spongy sclerosis must be differentiated from normally reaction-free, malignant destruction. Inflammatory soft-tissue invasion is manifested on CT scans as masking of the muscle layers that are separated by fat and regional distension of the chest wall.

Soft tissue processes associated with actinomycosis are less circumscribed and more widespread.

Contrast-enhanced scans: The inflamed tissue becomes enhanced after the administration of contrast medium. Hyperdense demarcation of the margins, as seen in an abscess, can be demonstrated.

Trauma

External injuries to the chest primarily affect the thoracic wall. Most rib fractures, local hematomas and soft-tissue emphysema can be demonstrated on conventional radiographs.

However, when there is a complicated thoracic trauma, computed tomography is the least invasive and most comprehensive diagnostic method. With CT, it is possible to assess all injuries to the spinal column, mediastinum, lungs and pleura in a single examination.

• CT

Hematomas usually appear on CT scans as homogeneous, soft-tissue structures, but they may also be slightly hyperdense. They mask muscle structures and lead to dilatation of the chest wall. *Fractures* of the ribs and sternum can be identified only in association with dislocation. *Sternoclavicular dislocation* can also be diagnosed reliably.

Furthermore, injuries to the spinal column, mediastinum, lungs, and pleura can also be assessed in the same examination.

Chapter 11
The Liver

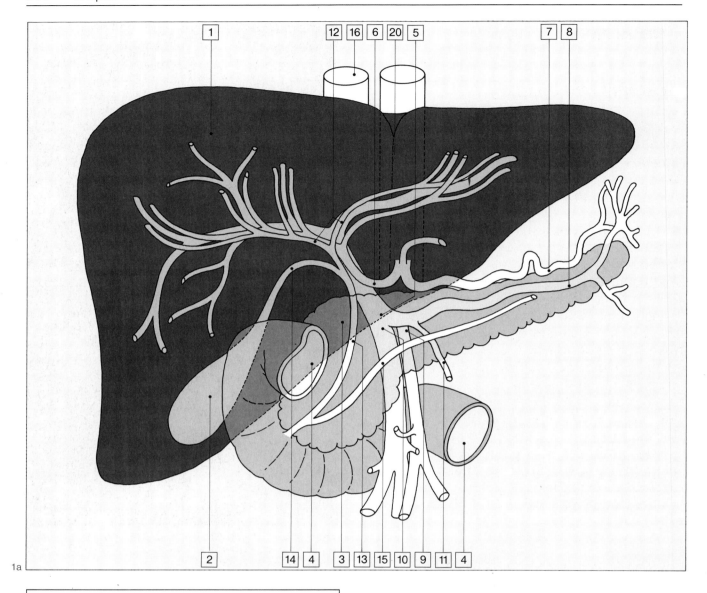

1a

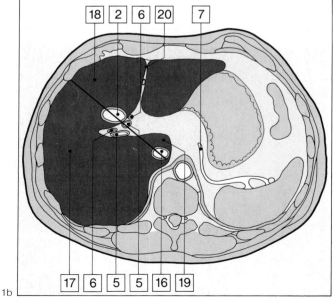

1b

Fig. 11-1a. Topography of the porta hepatis.

Fig. 11-1b. The border between the right and left lobes of the liver is defined by an imaginary line running from the inferior vena cava to the gallbladder.

Key to symbols:

1 Liver	12 Hepatic duct
2 Gallbladder	13 Common bile duct
3 Pancreas	14 Cystic duct
4 Duodenum	15 Pancreatic duct
5 Portal vein	16 Inferior vena cava
6 Hepatic artery	17 Right lobe
7 Splenic vein	18 Quadrate lobe
8 Splenic artery	19 Caudate lobe
9 Superior mesenteric artery	20 Falciform ligament
10 Superior mesenteric vein	(longitudinal fissure)
11 Inferior mesenteric vein	

The Liver

Anatomy and Imaging

The liver occupies the greater part of the upper abdomen, weighing 1350 to 1500 g in adults. It appears on CT scans as an extensive soft-tissue zone. Since the shape and size of its left lobe are variable, the CT configuration of the liver can be extremely variable. *Fissures* converging at the *porta hepatis* divide the organ into segments that are visible even on plain scans. The longitudinal fissure extends right paramedian and contains the *ligamentum rotundum* of the liver, which frequently can be identified as a punctiform soft-tissue structure, provided there is an adequate amount of surrounding fat. The extension of the ligamentum rotundum, namely the *falciform ligament*, extends through the liver and along its upper surface. The actual border between the right and left lobes of the liver often cannot be seen, but its location can be inferred from an incomplete recess on the lower edge of the liver. For topographic orientation, an imaginary line can be drawn between the inferior vena cava and the gallbladder. The continuation of the ligamen-

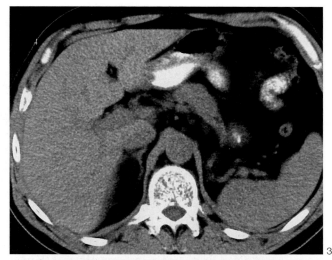

3a

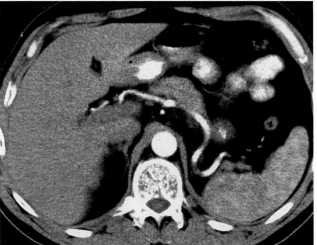

3b

Fig. 11-3a-c. Portal structures appear hypodense on plain scans (a). After the hepatic arteries are briefly contrasted (b), the portal veins are contrasted (c).

Fig. 11-2. Contrast enhancement of hepatic structures after a bolus injection of contrast medium. The aorta (1) and branches of the hepatic artery (2) become enhanced, as do the portal veins (3), within approximately 40 to 60 seconds. The enhancement of liver tissue corresponds to the surface curve (modified according to 3357).

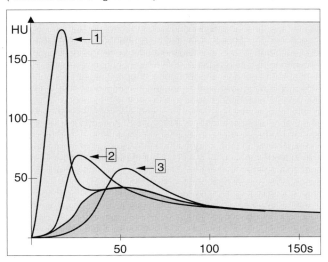

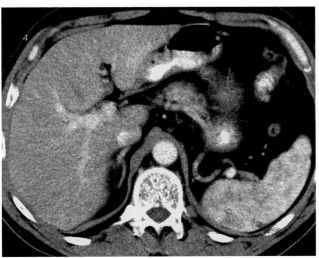

3c

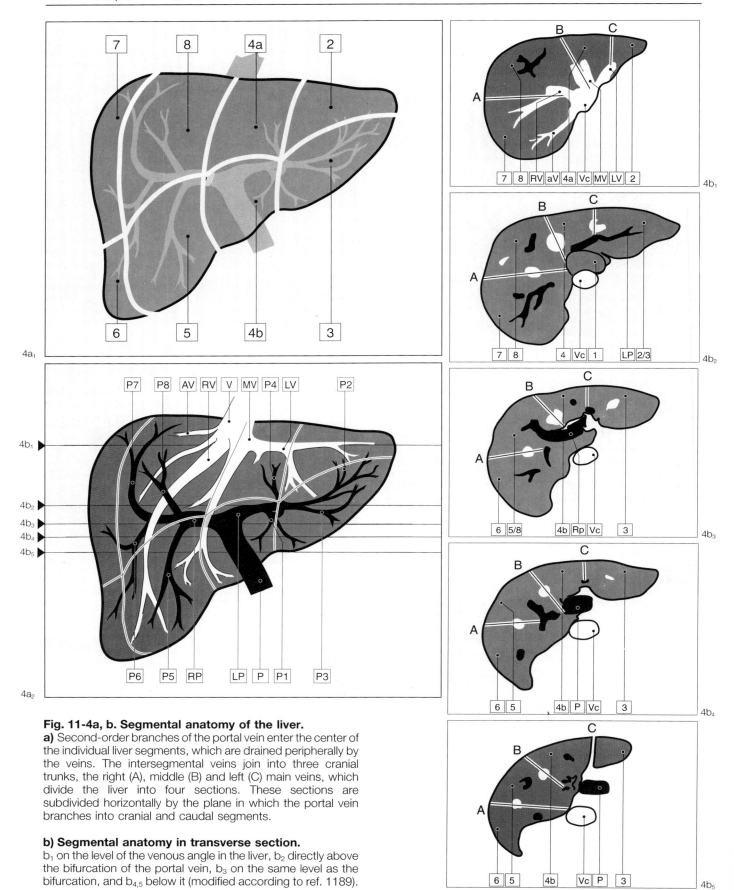

Fig. 11-4a, b. Segmental anatomy of the liver.

a) Second-order branches of the portal vein enter the center of the individual liver segments, which are drained peripherally by the veins. The intersegmental veins join into three cranial trunks, the right (A), middle (B) and left (C) main veins, which divide the liver into four sections. These sections are subdivided horizontally by the plane in which the portal vein branches into cranial and caudal segments.

b) Segmental anatomy in transverse section.

b₁ on the level of the venous angle in the liver, b₂ directly above the bifurcation of the portal vein, b₃ on the same level as the bifurcation, and b₄,₅ below it (modified according to ref. 1189).

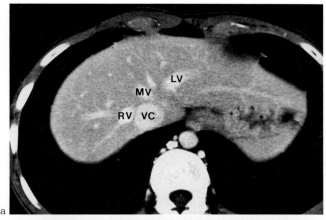

5a

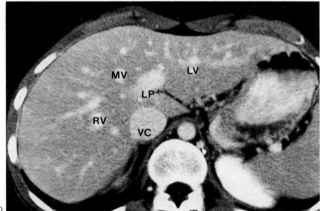

5b

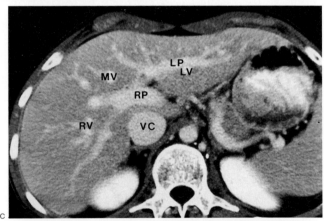

5c

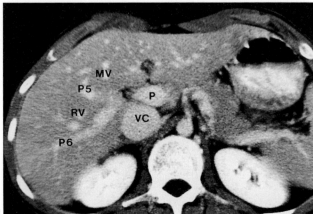

5d

tum rotundum on the lower edge of the liver, i.e. the ligamentum venosum, forms the outer border between the quadrate lobe and the caudate lobe. This structure appears on a cross-sectional view as a frontally coursing fissure and is the most prominent structure of the porta hepatis.

The left *lobe of the liver* usually extends on the left to the medioclavicular line, but does not reach the anterior pole of the spleen. The right lobe occupies the entire right subphrenic space. More caudal, it has a lateroconvex recess which provides room for the kidney. The gallbladder lies below the porta and against the medial contour of the right lobe of the liver; it may extend as far as the abdominal wall.

The larger *blood vessels* can be seen in normodense, noncontrasted hepatic tissue as hypodense structures with a typical configuration. They may be invisible on CT scans when parenchymal density is even slightly reduced (fatty infiltration, etc.). However, they appear hyperdense as fatty infiltration increases. Bolus administration of contrast medium ensures reliable demonstration of even small vascular rami. The variable shape of the porta hepatis is extensively filled out by the vascular band of the *portal vein*, which is accompanied on the left side by the *hepatic artery* and on the right side by the *bile ducts*. This triad relationship is also seen in further branches located in the liver periphery. The supply areas of tertiary rami correspond to the eight *hepatic segments*, which can be localized via computed tomography when one has a good knowledge of venous topography. Similar to the lungs, each segment

Fig. 11-5. Hepatic segments in CT.

Key to symbols:
(11-4 and 11-5)

P   = Portal vein
LP   = Left main branch of the portal vein
RP   = Right main branch of the portal vein
P1-8 = 1st–8th segmental branch of the portal vein
V   = Hepatic vein(s)
RV   = Right main vein of the liver (= sector boundary A)
MV   = Middle main vein of the liver (= sector boundary B)
LV   = Left main vein of the liver (= sector boundary C)
AV   = Accessory liver veins
VC   = Inferior vena cava

is drained via intersegmental veins. Normally, the three main branches of the hepatic veins drain below the diaphragm (stellate pattern) into the inferior vena cava. Therefore, left, middle and right main hepatic veins can usually be demonstrated on one section. They divide the liver into four sectors. The *left main hepatic vein* extends partly in the longitudinal fissure and thus marks off the caudate lobe (segment 4) from the left lateral segments 2 and 3. The *middle main hepatic vein* forms a border between the left and right lobes and marks off a vertical plane that ends caudally at the bed of the gallbladder. The *right main hepatic vein* divides the right lobe of the liver on the one side into anterior segments 5 and 8 as well as into dorsally located posterior segments 6 and 7. Segments 7 and 8 form the dome of the liver. The caudate lobe comprises the first liver segment, which drains via smaller veins directly into the *inferior vena cava* (IVC). Here, the IVC courses axially through the hepatic tissue and can be identified as a sharply marginated, hypodense oval structure.

The *attenuation value* of normal hepatic tissue (65 ± 5 HU) is higher than that of all other organs and muscles in the epigastrium. Structures containing blood or bile therefore appear hypodense.

Adjacent structures are usually easily identifiable. When thicker slices are scanned, narrow horizontal and curved fissures on the upper and lower surfaces of the liver are hard to visualize and are poorly defined, especially in the region of the porta hepatis. Cautious interpretations must be made in such cases, and thin-section CT should be performed in questionable cases. A nondistended subphrenic space can be evaluated only along the lateral circumference of the liver.

Contrast Enhancement of Hepatic Structures

Maximum contrast of the aorta is seen 12 to 17 seconds after bolus administration of 50 to 70 ml of contrast medium, and brief, isolated demonstration of the hepatic arteries occurs. Via the mesenteric vessels, the vena porta is con-

trasted after a further 15 to 20 seconds, and the larger vessels ca. 40 to 60 seconds later. After protracted bolus contrast administration, mixed images of the arterial and portovenous phases appear due to simultaneous enhancement of the hepatic arteries and the portal vein. The hepatic parenchyma reaches maximum enhancement 40 to 60 seconds after contrast enhancement and drops to about 50% of maximum in approximately 5 minutes.

A high level of contrast enhancement that extends as far as the liver periphery is achieved after selective injection of contrast medium in the hepatic arteries. In proportion with the administered dose, contrast enhancement of the hepatic parenchyma can be considerably increased by means of selective injection of contrast medium in the superior mesenteric artery or splenic artery (*CT portography, computer tomographic arterial portography (CTAP)*). However, (laminar) circulatory phenomena in the portal vein can lead to non-uniform enhancement of the parenchyma, so it may be advisable to simultaneously inject contrast medium in the superior mesenteric and splenic arteries. In *delayed scans* after administration of high doses of contrast medium (more than 60 g iodine), the density of the hepatic parenchyma is just sufficiently enhanced for diagnostic purposes (ca. 20 to 25 HU).

Fig. 11-6. Cystic liver. Numerous sharply marginated hypodense structures of water density of various sizes are distributed throughout the liver. The simultaneous appearance of renal cysts is indicative of a hamartosis.

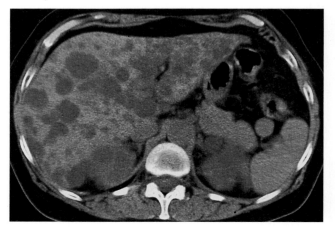

Cystic Liver Diseases

Dysontogenetic Cysts

Dysontogenetic cysts are part of a hamartosis, which frequently occurs in combination with multiple pancreatic and renal cysts. The liver is permeated with numerous, variably sized (epithelialized) cysts containing a clear liquid. Complications such as superinfections or hemorrhages are rare.

• CT

Plain scans: CT scans show delicate, smooth or thin-walled hypodense zones organized in rosette-shaped or tufted configurations of water density. Partial volume artifacts may falsify the attenuation value.

Contrast-enhanced scans: There is no enhancement of hypodense zones or contiguous sections of the liver after contrast administration.

Solitary Hepatic Cysts

Solitary hepatic cysts most frequently occur in women in the 4th to 5th decade. The cysts may reach a diameter of up to 20 cm. An epithelial layer, a firm fibrous capsule, and a well vascularized tissue layer can be seen vis-a-vis the hepatic parenchyma. These cysts have serous contents. Developmental anomalies and retention are considered to be the main etiologies of the solitary hepatic cyst.

• CT

On CT scans, these cysts demonstrate the usual CT appearance of cystic lesions.

Differential diagnosis: The following must be considered in the diagnosis: *choledochal cysts; bile accumulation due to leakage; abscesses; necrotic metastases; echinococcus cysts.*

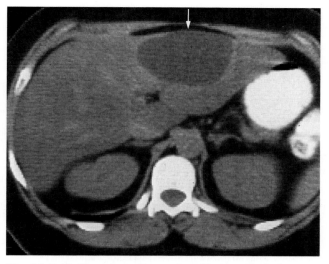

Fig. 11-7. Solitary hepatic cysts with smooth, but accentuated walls.

Table 11-1. Vascularity of hepatic tumors (angiographic criteria).

Primary Hepatic Tumors		Metastatic Hepatic Tumors
Hepatocellular carcinoma (in adults)	hypervascularized	Renal cell carcinoma
Focal nodular hyperplasia		Carcinoid
		Islet cell tumor
Adenoma		Carcinoma of the thyroid
Hemangioma		Transitional cell carcinoma
Hemangio-endothelioma		Papillary carcinoma (pancreas)
Hemangio-endothelial sarcoma		Leiomyosarcoma (colon)
		Carcinoma of the adrenal glands
		Adenocarcinoma of the breast
		Seminoma (carcinoma of the testis)
Adenocarcinoma of the biliary tract	hypovascularized	Adenocarcinoma – pancreas – gallbladder
Hepatocellular carcinoma (in children)		Carcinoma – colon – esophagus – lung
		Malignant melanoma
		Wilm's tumor

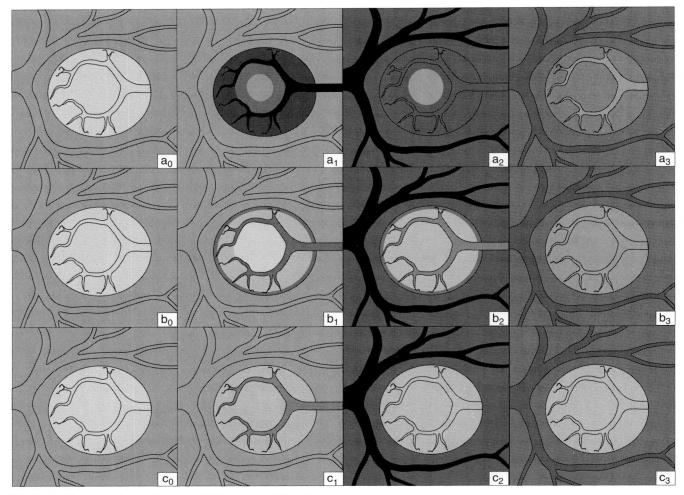

Fig. 11-8. Contrast behavior of solid tumors of the liver.
Supplied by the branches of the hepatic artery, the tumor contrasts positively in the arterial phase. During portovenous contrast medium uptake, contrast enhancement is limited to the surrounding liver parenchyma. Tumor recognition depends on the time expired after contrast medium injection and the vascularity of the tumor.

a) *Hypervascularized tumors:*
a_1: Plain scan
a_2: In the arterial contrast medium phase, the liver parenchyma becomes slightly enhanced, while the hypervascularized tumor is greatly contrasted and, thus, more clearly visible.
a_3: In the portovenous phase, the increased opacification of the hepatic parenchyma leads to a partial masking of the tumor, which often remains detectable only in the center (reduced in size) as a hypodense structure.
a_4: In the portovenous phase, the tumor is often isodense unless avascular necrotic areas counteract the loss of contrast.

b) *Isovascular tumors:*
b_1: Plain scan
b_2: During the arterial contrast medium phase, Isovascular tumors generally exhibit only minimal peripheral enhancement and scarcely differ from the slightly contrasted hepatic parenchyma.
b_3: The greatest contrast to the tumor is achieved in the portovenous phase.
b_4: In the late phase, the contrast diminishes due to reduced opacification of the hepatic parenchyma and reduced uptake of contrast medium by the tumor.

c) *Hypovascularized tumors:*
c_1: Plain scan
c_2: There is no recognizable opacification of the tumor during the arterial contrast medium phase.
c_3: Maximum contrast of the tumor to the parenchyma is achieved in the portovenous phase.
c_4: Contrast diminishes in direct proportion to the venous opacification of the parenchyma.

Solid Tumors of the Liver

CT confirmation of hepatic tumors is determined by the difference in density of the tumor and surrounding hepatic tissue. As can be seen on plain scans, a reduction in protein concentration, increased water content, mucoid or fatty degeneration and necrosis lead to reduced density of the tumor as compared with the protein-rich healthy hepatic tissue, even in cases with increased tumor vascularization. The attenuation value increases after intravenous contrast medium administration, thus representing the intravascular space in the first arteriovenous contrast medium passage. The particular nature of the liver's vascular supply, however, creates a time-shifted enhancement pattern. Arterial contrast medium flooding occurs via the hepatic artery 12 to 15 seconds after injection and is joined by portal enhancement, which occurs via the portal vein 40 to 60 seconds after injection. Approximately 25% of the blood volume of the liver is supplied by the hepatic artery, and ca. 75% by the portal vein.

Contrast enhancement correspondingly occurs via these two vascular systems. Of diagnostic importance is the fact that tumors of the liver are almost always supplied by the branches of the hepatic artery. Angiography classifies the tumors according to their degree of vascularization as compared with the non-altered branches of the hepatic artery. The tumors are thus defined as hyper-, iso- and hypovascularized.

Hypervascularized regions reach maximum enhancement in the arterial phase before a relatively intense enhancement, usually occurring in the portovenous phase, also develops in the surrounding tissue (contra-timed enhancement, Fig. 11–8a_1-a_3). When there is a high degree of vascularization and a large cavity of blood (poling), the positive enhancement sometimes, but rarely, persists even during the portovenous contrast phase.

Isovascularized regions are dependent on portovenous enhancement; they show no enhancement during the arterial phase (portovenous enhancement; Fig. 11–8b_1-b_3).

Hypovascularized regions become hypodense during the arterial phase, which is further emphasized by contrast enhancement of the surrounding hepatic tissue during the portovenous phase (same type of maximum enhancement; Fig. 11–8c_1-c_3).

The arterial and portovenous phases can sometimes be demonstrated separately by means of short injection times and rapid scanning sequences. Analogous to selective angiographic scans, this usually makes it possible to demonstrate hypervascularized regions as hyperdense hepatic lesions during the arterial phase. Time-shifted waves of contrast medium flooding overlap when the injection time is extended. Enhancement is then dependent on the stronger portovenous blood flow. Hypo- and isovascularized regions become more clearly demarcated from the enhanced hepatic parenchyma, while the additional arterial enhancement of hypervascularized lesions diminishes or dispenses with the contrast difference of the surrounding tissue. A targeted bolus injection is especially suitable for isolated demonstration of hypervascularized hepatic processes during the brief arterial phase.

CT portography or computed tomographic arterial portography (CTAP) is currently the most reliable means of demonstrating hepatic tumors and the best method for defining tumor borders. This technique is performed as a supplement to presurgical arteriography of the liver. Optimum images are obtained when enhancement of the liver is uniform. This can be achieved via simultaneous injection of contrast medium in the superior mesenteric and splenic arteries. Perifocal, inferiorly contrasted, sharply marginated regions of the hepatic parenchyma may be due to compression of the portal vein and should not be interpreted as infiltration. *Intra-arterial scanning*, in which contrast medium is injected into the hepatic artery, can be an unsatisfactory diagnostic method in problematic regions containing peripheral vessels. Therefore, the method is hardly ever used today.

In contrast, *delayed scans* taken 6 hours after contrast medium injection are reported to yield

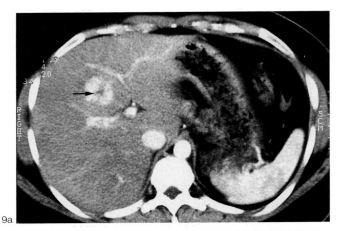

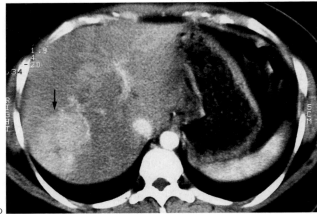

Fig. 11-9a, b. Focal nodular hyperplasia. Discretely hypodense, sharply defined regions were revealed on plain scans. After bolus injection of contrast medium, they demonstrate sharp, brief contrast enhancement (→). One of the two lesions exhibits a typical central scar (a→).

Fig. 11-10. Focal nodular hyperplasia. The pediculate tumor (a→) at the lower edge of the liver (a►) contains a hypodense central structure, as can be seen on this plain scan (a). It becomes more clearly demarcated after bolus injection of contrast medium. In the early arterial contrast medium phase (b), the peripheral vessels (b, c►) and a pluricentric fascicular contrast structure (b→) can be seen. Compared to the liver tissue, the mass enhances most strongly during the early arterial contrast medium phase. It becomes isodense within ca. 70 to 100 seconds.

results comparable to those of bolus contrast administration. However, ca. 60 g of iodine (= 200 ml 30% CM) must be administered in order to achieve enhancement of healthy hepatic parenchyma (20 to 25 HU). Small hepatic lesions as well as hemangiomas can be difficult to diagnose.

Not only does computed tomography make it possible to identify tumors, but it can be used to classify and grade them as well. Additionally, the resectability of malignant tumors can be determined when the segmental anatomy is taken into consideration. The true extent of the tumor along the virtual segmental borders is, however, often underestimated.

Adenomas and Focal Nodular Hyperplasia (FNH)

Adenomas of the liver are rare neoplasms that arise either from liver cells (hepatic adenoma) or the bile ducts *(biliary adenoma)*. The extremely rare biliary adenoma is of differential diagnostic interest, because it may contain cystic components *(cystadenoma* of the liver).

The *hepatic adenoma*, which consists of solid tissue, is most common in young women and more infrequently in children and men. Single or multiple adenomas are found with increased frequency in women who have taken oral contraceptives containing the drug mestranol for more than 5 years. They can lead to necrosis, infarction, and spontaneous hemorrhage.

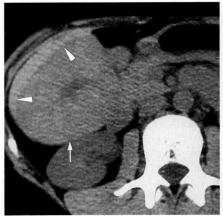

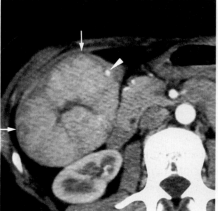

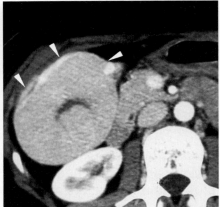

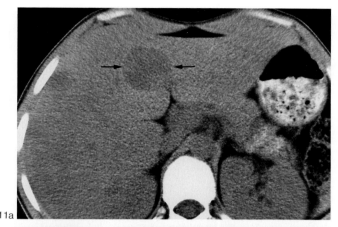

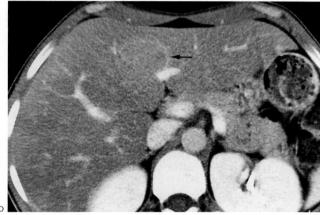

Fig. 11-11a, b. Hepatic adenoma. The sharply demarcated hypodense structure that was also recognizable on the plain scan (a) exhibits discrete, harmonious contrast enhancement after bolus injection of contrast medium. The surrounding blood vessels have been displaced in a circular pattern due to tumor expansion (a→).

Avascular regions are then found in these normally hypervascularized tumors. Resection is recommended in view of the risk of hemorrhage and malignant transformation.

Like the hepatic adenoma, *focal nodular hyperplasia (FNH)* can be single or multiple. This also occurs preferentially in women in the 3rd to 6th decade. These masses can reach a diameter of up to 8 cm; they differ histologically from adenomas in that bile ducts are absent. Malignant degeneration of FNH has not yet been reported.

Adenomatous hyperplasia develops from postnecrotic cirrhosis or hepatic dystrophy. These lesions differ from hepatic adenomas in that they have vascular supply lines that extend from the periphery to the center of the lesion.

The extent of this usually nodular hyperplasia is determined by tissue loss due to necrosis.

Differential diagnosis: Since bile ducts are absent and stellate Kupffer cells only rarely develop in hepatic adenoma, the possibility of FNH can be excluded by performing sulfur colloid scans and functional scintigraphy of the bile ducts.

• CT

Focal Nodular Hyperplasia (FNH)

Plain Scans: Isodensity of FNH is rare. It normally appears as a hypodense area that is relatively sharply demarcated from surrounding tissue. Pedunculated forms are known to occur.

Contrast-enhanced scans: Strong but brief homogeneous tumor enhancement that significantly diminishes one minute after contrast medium administration is a typical finding in FNH. In around half of all cases, a stellate hypodensity pattern is found in the central tumor region, corresponding with the vascular pedicle of the adenoma. A centrifugal enhancement pattern can sometimes be demonstrated when a dynamic CT sequence is performed.

Fig. 11-12. Hepatic lipoma. A mass near the posterior lobe of the liver (→) with density values in the fatty range accompanied by a sharply defined hypodense structure in the water density range (cyst ►).

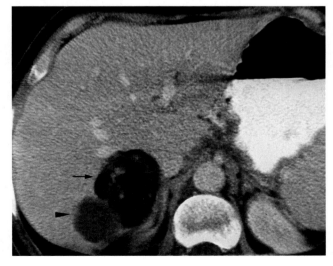

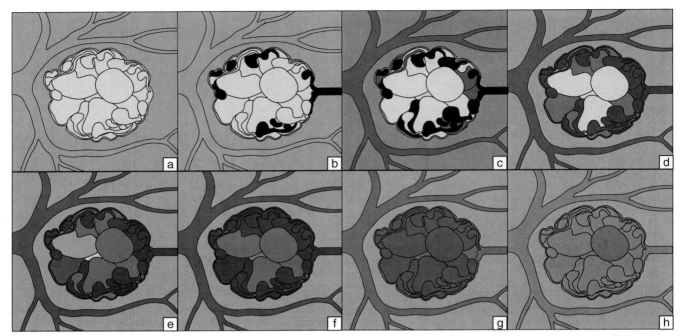

Fig. 11-13. Contrast behavior of a hemangioma. The hemangioma generally appears hypodense and sharply delineated from healthy liver tissue on plain scans. In the arterial contrast medium phase, the periphery of the hemangioma is partially enhanced with sharply contrasted, enlarged blood spaces (b). During the portovenous contrast medium phase (c) the peripheral enhancement of the hemangioma intensifies, but the overall contrast difference is less. The central blood spaces gradually become filled with contrast medium in accordance with their size and anatomy. This creates a hyperdense zone that contrasts more sharply against the less opacified liver (g). As time progresses, the contrasted blood pool is diluted with less highly contrasted blood and the CT numbers fall to the density of the hepatic parenchyma (resulting in isodensity).

In individual phases, a hemangioma can simulate a malignant tumor because of its ring-shaped contrast pattern. In the early contrast medium phase, with good demarcation of individual blood spaces, distinct delineation of the tumor from the hepatic parenchyma and overall favorable contrast medium kinetics, a reliable diagnosis can normally be made. Isodensity, even of hypervascularized tumors, may be observed.

Hepatic Adenoma

Plain scans: The identification of areas of necrosis or fresh hemorrhage, which appear as hyperdense areas, frequently makes it possible to distinguish *hepatic adenomas* from focal nodular hyperplasia.

Contrast-enhanced scans: Vital adenoma tissue is usually hypervascularized. It therefore becomes temporarily hyperdense after bolus contrast administration.

Differential diagnosis: It may be necessary to perform additional scintigraphic examinations for a definitive diagnosis of the adenoma.

Hepatic Lipoma

The hepatic lipoma is the only type of extremely rare mesodermal tumor described to date. It can be diagnosed on the basis of its attenuation value (in the fat range) and its smoothly marginated appearance.

Hemangioma

The *hemangioma* is the most common benign tumor of the liver. Its size ranges from a few millimeters to a considerable mass. Cystic degeneration sometimes, but rarely, occurs as they mature. The most common type is the cavernous hemangioma, which has a tendency for thrombosis, hyalinization, and occasional calcification. With frequent multiple findings, the possibility of liver metastases must often be considered, especially when ultrasound examinations fail to reveal the typical hemangioma structures or when the patient has a history of tumor malignancy. *Hemangio-endotheliomas* most commonly occur in children, and involvement of other organs is frequent. These tumors

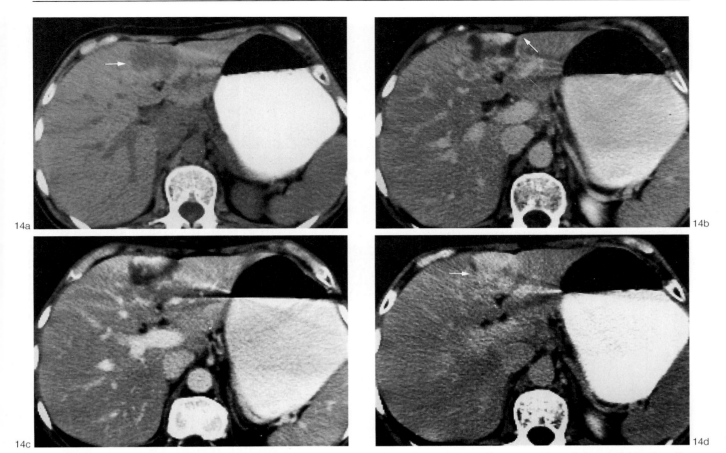

Fig. 11-14a-d. Hemangioma on the longitudinal fissure of the liver. Two minutes after contrast medium administration, the sharply demarcated hypodense structure (a→) exhibits peripheral hyperdensity that slowly spreads. (c) Four minutes after injection. The lesion first shows complete contrast medium filling 15 minutes after injection (d→).

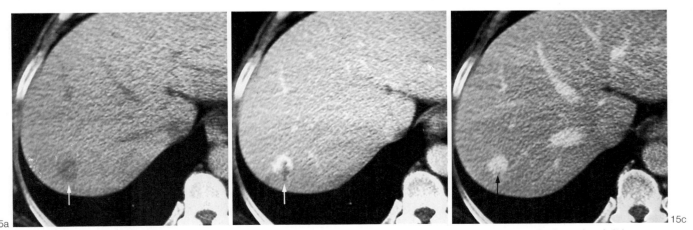

Fig. 11-15a-c. Hepatic hemangioma. Plain scans revealed a sharply demarcated hypodense area of 1.2 cm (a→). It becomes strongly enhanced after contrast medium administration, and a small filling defect is revealed (b→). In the late film, the defect is filled with contrast medium and forms a homogeneous hyperdense structure (c→).

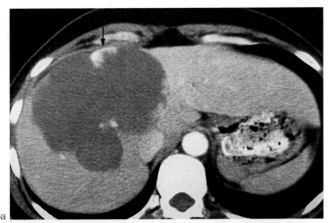

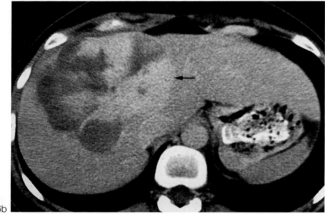

Fig. 11-16a, b. Large hepatic cavernoma. After administration of a contrast medium (a), the lobulated, sharply marginated hypodense mass gradually fills with contrast medium. It contains lacunar hyperdense structures, which become confluent within 20 minutes. They occupy the greater part of the loculated mass (b).

are characterized by amorphous calcification, wide nutritive arteries with arteriovenous shunting and a multicentric configuration.

• CT

Plain scans: A sharply marginated *hypodense area* of uniform tissue density is usually demonstrable on plain scans. Any inhomogeneity within the lesion is sharply demarcated and appears "structured". Rarely demonstrable, circumscribed areas of hyperdensity, the density of which may even equal that of calcium, are an indication of regressive tissue change.

Contrast-enhanced scans: With regards to hemangiomas, it is essential that the (bolus) dose of contrast medium be large enough to secure a reliable diagnosis. Round, sometimes belt-like

areas of enhancement that are sharply demarcated from the liver are initially seen in the periphery of the lesion. Concentric interflow patterns in the periphery (iris phenomenon) later lead to the formation of an isodense zone ca. 3 (to 30) minutes after injection. This type of contrast behavior is associated with bolus contrast administration; longer lasting *hyperdensity* is achieved only occasionally.

This kinetic behavior pattern can be attributed to the accumulation of contrast medium in cavernous spaces and the slow mixation of contrast medium with the pools of blood contained in those spaces. Large hemangiomas therefore require an extended contrast medium administration period (up to 15 min.) related to the size of their blood spaces and structure if homogeneous hyperdense enhancement as compared with the surrounding hepatic tissue is to be obtained. Therefore, hyperdensity usually occurs more quickly in small hemangiomas than in large ones.

The hemangiomas appear *isodense* when the dose of contrast medium is insufficient or during the wash-out phase. This may make it difficult to distinguish hemangiomas from other solid lesions. A hemangioma can be unequivocally diagnosed when a non-temporary and extensively homogeneous hyperdensity pattern is observed. This corresponds with the radiodensity of the (portovenous) blood pool.

Mesenchymal Hamartoma

The mesenchymal hamartoma is an anomaly of hepatic connective tissue that incorporates myxomatic and cystic components. In childhood years, they tend to form avascular cystic spaces and display rapid growth.

Hepatocellular Carcinoma (HCC)

Hepatocellular carcinomas (HCC) are found in ca. 1% of all autopsy examinations. They usually arise from cirrhosis, and the incidence of HCC was observed to rise as the incidence of cirrhosis increases. Hepatocellular carcinomas

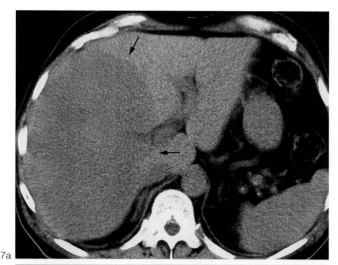

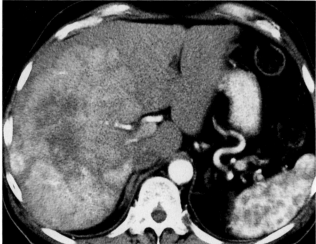

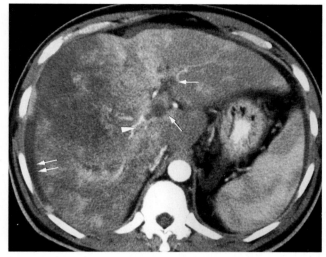

Fig. 11-18. Hepatocellular carcinoma. A large mass occupies the entire right lobe of the liver, which appears distended. During the early portovenous contrast medium phase, irregular blood vessel structures (►) were detected within the tumorous hypodense structure, indicating the development of an arteriovenous shunt. The portal venous thrombosis is apparent in the sharply marginated hypodense structures (→). Perihepatic ascites is detected (⇒).

Fig. 11-17a-c. Hepatocellular carcinoma. The plain scan demonstrates a large hypodense, sharply marginated mass in the right lobe of the liver (a→). In the arterial contrast medium phase (b), it exhibits somewhat lobulated structural hyperdensity. During portovenous contrast medium distribution, peripheral enhancement and capsular structures appear accenting the capsular structures (c→). Regressive changes appear as hypodense areas in the late film.

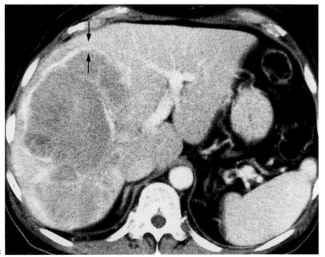

most frequently manifest in patients in the 5th to 7th decade; they occur three times more often in men than in women. The association of cirrhosis with hepatocellular carcinoma is clearly lower in the U.S.A. but is significantly higher in Japan.

Hepatocellular carcinomas can be divided into three categories:
1. Multicentric; intrahepatic metastases due to venous invasion.
2. Solitary large masses (20 to 40% of all cases).
3. Diffuse involvement of the liver (relatively rare). Large tumor formations may be surrounded by a capsule and/or show necrotic destructions. Fatty degeneration of tumor areas has been reported; calcification is occasionally observed.

Spreading of the tumor is initially lymphogenous, extending via the porta hepatis and the hepatoduodenal ligament into the bed of the pancreas and mesenteric root. Larger tumors directly attack adjacent organs like the diaphragm, abdominal wall and pancreas. Blood-borne metastases are mainly seen in the lungs, bone and spleen.

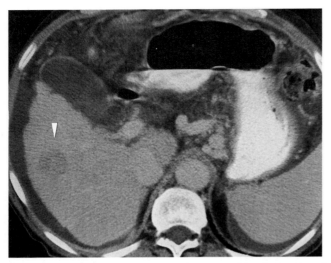

Fig. 11-19. Hepatocellular carcinoma with cirrhosis of the liver. A hypodense structure measuring 3 cm is detected in hepatic tissue exhibiting nodular transformation.

• CT

Plain scans: With pre-existing cirrhosis of the liver, one usually finds larger, slightly hypodense or isodense lesions that distend one lobe of the liver causing clear contour deformation; the lesion is usually sharply demarcated from the remaining hepatic tissue. When the patient has cirrhosis of the liver with the corresponding deformation of liver contour, the tumor tissue

Fig. 11-20. Hepatocellular carcinoma. The liver shows signs of cirrhosis, i. e., distortion of the left lobe. The mass in the right lobe of the liver appears irregularly hypodense in a plain scan and does not sharply contrast against the liver, even after bolus injection of a contrast medium. Satellite tumor expansion (→) is detected. The arrangement of blood vessels near the porta hepatis appears irregular, indicating cirrhotic transformation of liver tissue.

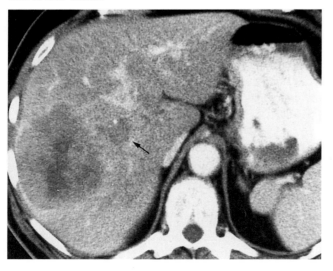

is often only discretely visible or not at all distinguishable from surrounding tissue on plain scans. Areas of necrosis and fatty degeneration can lead to marked hypodensity.

Contrast-enhanced scans: Ca. 1 minute after bolus contrast administration, a general or ring-like pattern of enhancement with capsule-like margins is observed. The lesion sometimes appears hypodense against the background of enhanced hepatic tissue. Additionally, satellite nodules are also demarcated along the borders of the lesion. In one third of all patients, the tumor invades the portal veins, thus leading to thrombosis. This is seen as a hypodense, sometimes ringlike structure oriented towards the portal veins, and it leads to a segmental, portovenous reduction in contrast enhancement of the hepatic parenchyma. (Wedge-shaped) areas of the liver that are not affected by the tumor can be more strongly contrasted by opening arterioportal shunts. When the patient has cirrhosis of the liver, however, even bolus contrast administration does not always lead to clear demarcation of the hepatocellular carcinoma.

Differential diagnosis: In patients with multicentric spreading, the possibility of liver metastases or regenerating nodules must be taken into consideration. Regional portovenous thrombosis and, especially, proof of regional lymph node enlargement are indications that a hepatocellular carcinoma is the primary tumor.

Cholangiocarcinoma

The cholangiocarcinoma is much rarer than the hepatocellular carcinoma, and it affects women twice as often as men, usually in the 5th to 7th decade of life. There is usually a poorly vascularized adenocarcinoma with strongly emphasized fibrous components. The disease is predominant in patients with gallstones, biliary carcinoma and sclerosing cholangitis. The cholangiocarcinoma is usually found in the region of the hepatic bifurcation and, from there, it can lead to biliary obstruction (Klatskin's tumor, see bile tract).

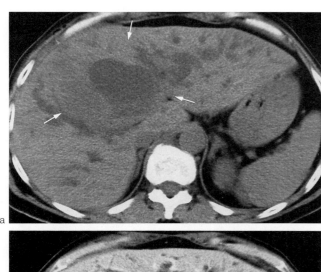

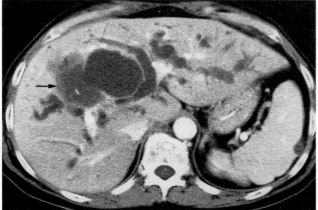

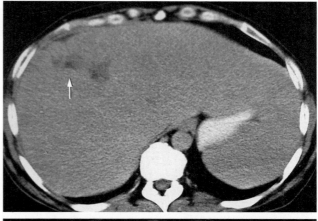

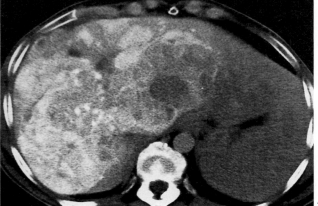

Fig. 11-21a, b. Cholangiocarcinoma. The plain scan reveals a broad mass between the lobes of the liver. This is interrupted in the center by a sharply marginated hypodense structure corresponding to cystic expansion of the biliary system. All intrahepatic bile ducts display dilatation and contortion. After administration of contrast medium, the tumor is not clearly demarcated. A more prominent hypodense structure can be seen in the center (→).

Fig. 11-23a, b. Fibrolamellar hepatocellular carcinoma. A large tumor has infiltrated both lobes of the liver. The tumor exhibits hypodense regressive changes that are visible, even in the plain scan (a→). After bolus injection of a contrast medium, it is distinctly demarcated from the liver as a hyperdense structure with an extremely nonuniform parenchyma structure (b).

Fig. 11-22. Cholangiocarcinoma. The sclerosing cholangitis detected with ERPC appears in the form of slightly expanded bile duct structures. After administration of contrast medium, a discrete hypodense structure corresponding to a central cholangiocarcinoma is detected in the center of the liver (→). Cystic dilatation of a central bile duct (⇒).

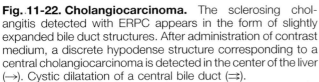

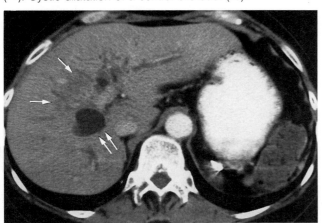

• CT

Plain scans: When the tumor is located centrally in the hepatic bifurcation, cholangiectasis is the leading diagnostic sign. This usually small tumor can frequently be demonstrated only by means of targeted, thin-section scanning in the region of the porta hepatis, where it appears as a moderately hypodense structure.

Contrast-enhanced scans: When the tumor location is peripheral, it usually becomes more clearly defined as a hypodense zone after contrast medium administration. In patients with strictured bile ducts, localized, dilated ducts are sometimes identifiable within the tumor.

Fibrolamellar Hepatocellular Carcinoma

This rare, malignant tumor affects young patients without hepatic cirrhosis who are in the 2nd and 3rd decade of life. It contains eosinophilic hepatocytes and collagen structures and is calcified in ca. 30% of all cases. These tumors often have a good prognosis after resection.

• CT

Plain scans: The lesion usually appears as a hypodense mass that is sharply demarcated from hepatic tissue. Amorphous calcification is located centrally.

Contrast-enhanced scans: Variably intense enhancement develops. Centrally located,

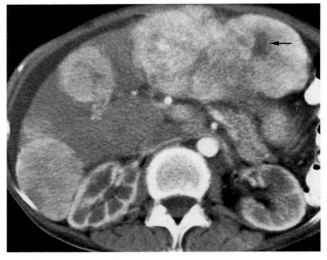

Fig. 11-25. Hepatic metastases from a carcinoid. In the early arterial contrast medium phase, a sharply marginated hypervascularized mass is visible in both lobes of the liver. Only slight, centrally located regressive changes (→) can be detected as focal areas of hypodensity.

Fig. 11-24. Metastases from a carcinoma of the colon. A clearly demarcated hypodense structure exhibiting peripheral hyperdensity (→) was detected during the early portovenous contrast medium phase. A central concentration of contrast medium is observed in the late portovenous phase, thus making the tumor appear smaller.

Fig. 11-26. Metastases from a malignant schwannoma. Sharply marginated hypodense structures are detected below the diaphragm. A round hyperdense structure with only slight central enhancement becomes visible after contrast medium administration. The larger of the two lesions exhibits regressive changes that are not affected by the contrast medium (→). (See also, hemangioma).

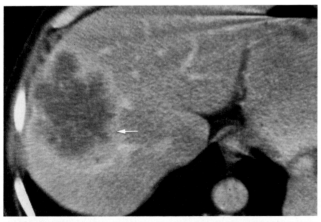

24a

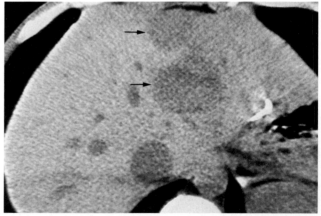

26a

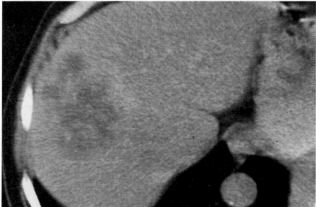

24b

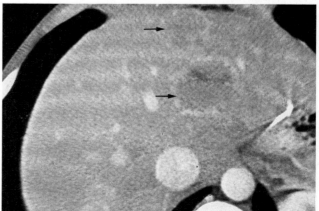

26b

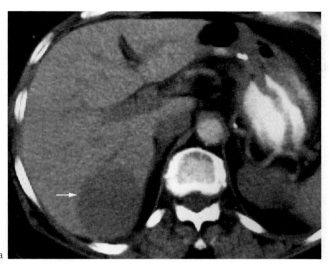

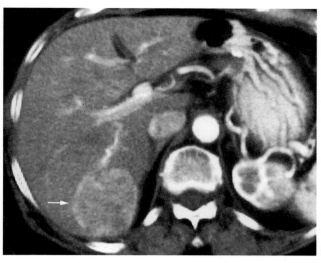

Fig. 11-27a, b. Metastases from a gastrinoma. The sharply marginated homogeneous hypodense structure in the right dorsal lobe of the liver exhibits a homogeneous hyperdense structure indicative of hypervascularization during the early arterial phase (see also, focal nodular hyperplasia).

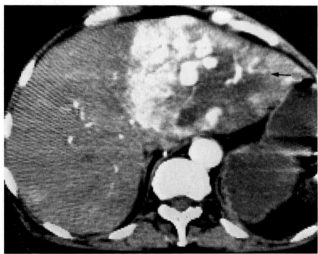

Fig. 11-28. Metastases from a hypernephroma. Indications of increased vascularization and widened arterial vessels within the mass of the left lobe of the liver (a→) become visible in the arterial contrast medium phase. In the early portovenous phase, a hyperdense structure briefly appears in the right lobe of the liver (b→). This structure is no longer detectable in the late portovenous phase (c). Due to the pronounced hypervascularization and the shunts within the tumor, the hyperdense structure persists throughout the portovenous phase, excluding necrotic regions that appear as hypodense zones (c→).

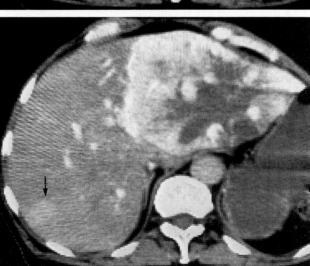

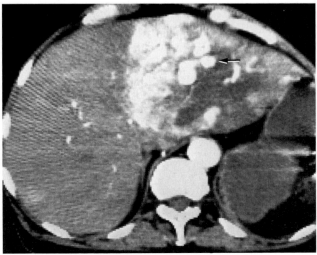

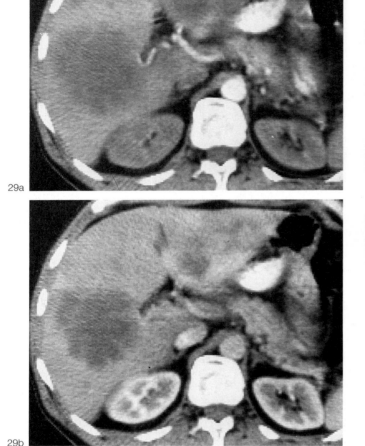

29a

29b

Fig. 11-29a, b. Metastases from a carcinoma of the co-lon. The metastases appear as hypodense regions in the early arterial contrast medium phase (a). Within 30 seconds, they appear more clearly demarcated but smaller (b). Septa and tumor borders are more accentuated because of peripheral enhancement in the later portovenous phase.

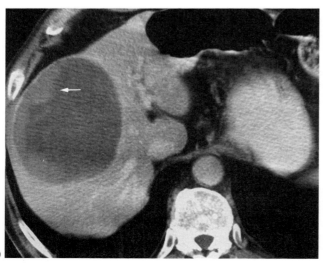

30

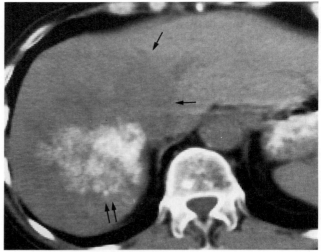

31

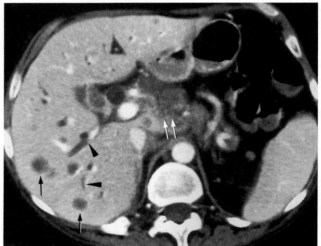

32

Fig. 11-31. Calcified hepatic metastases from a colonic carcinoma. The broad hypodense structure (→) contains amorphous calcification indicative of necrobiotic metaplastic processes (⇒).

Fig. 11-32. Metastases from a tonsillar carcinoma (→). Multiple round hypodense structures are detected in the liver during the early portovenous contrast medium phase. The congested bile ducts appear as sharply marginated, hypo-dense cordlike structures (►). This is attributable to lymph node metastases in the porta hepatis (⇒).

Fig. 11-30. Regressive changes due to metastases. Ne-crosis can cause a homogeneous reduction in attenuation value, resulting in a cystic appearance. In this case (bronchial carcinoma), viable tumor tissue exhibits peripheral enhance-ment (→).

strand-like structures are demarcated and appear either hyper- or hypodense. Therefore, they may simulate the CT appearance of focal nodular hyperplasia with central scar formation.

Secondary Tumors of the Liver (Metastases)

Tumors of the gastrointestinal tract (in this case, mainly colonic cancer), breast cancer, bronchial and renal carcinomas as well as uterine tumors metastasize preferentially in the

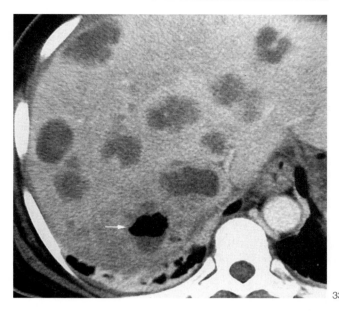

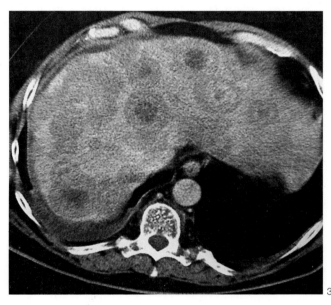

Fig. 11-33. Infected metastases from a colonic carcinoma. Hypodense structures in the anterior sections of the right lobe of the liver appear in the early portovenous phase with typical peripheral enhancement and central hypodense structures. In the dorsal lobe of the liver there are additional air pockets representing anaerobic superinfection of the metastases (→).

Fig. 11-34. Metastases from small-cell bronchial carcinoma. Diffuse distribution of metastases throughout the hepatic parenchyma. Administration of contrast medium reveals a round structure.

Fig. 11-35a, b. Detection of metastases after CT portography and on a delayed film.
a) After CT portography (computed tomographic arterial portography), the metastases from a carcinoma of the colon is demarcated as a markedly hypodense region (→) within the uniformly contrasted hepatic parenchyma. The angular configuration is caused by a portovenous perfusion disorder resulting from a tumor; this disorder can also appear more prominently.
b) On delayed scans made six hours after intravenous injection of contrast medium, the metastases (→) appear as discrete, sharply marginated hypodense structures against the slightly contrasting hepatic parenchyma.

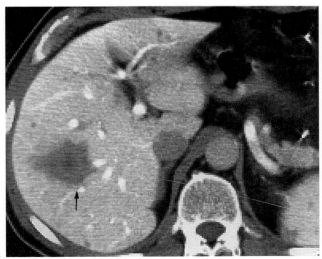

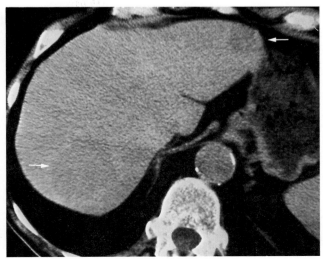

liver. When multiple hepatic lesions occur in tumor patients, they indicate metastatic disease. They may be highly circumscribed, but may also be evenly distributed as small nodules throughout the liver (e.g. carcinoma of the breast). The pathological and anatomical structure of the metastatic tissue resembles that of the primary tumor (e.g. mucinous permeation of metastases in colon and stomach cancer). Vascularization usually corresponds to that of the primary tumor, so when searching for metastases of a primary tumor, one can also expect to see the known vascular pattern reflected in the hepatic lesions.

• CT

Plain scans: On plain scans taken at a narrow window setting, mostly multiple changes should be demarcated as round, sometimes confluent, frequently indistinctly demarcated areas of variable hypodensity. Metastases of mucinous carcinomas tend to calcify. In slowly growing tumors, large zones of calcification may result.

Contrast-enhanced scans: Because of possible isodensity, a *bolus dose of contrast medium* is generally necessary for localization of metastases. The first areas scanned are those that looked suspicious on plain scans. The majority of all metastases have better circulation in their periphery, so the hypodense center becomes more prominent after contrast medium administration. The size of the lesion may therefore be underestimated. The uptake of contrast medium is delayed in the highly fibrous center of metastases of adenocarcinomas. Therefore, a slight central zone of hyperdensity with a hypodense margin appears after ca. 10 minutes. Zones of necrosis do not enhance in metastases with liquefaction, which means that ringlike images (similar to those of abscesses) can appear. *Hypervascularized* metastases (e.g. in renal cell carcinoma, gastrinoma) temporarily appear hyperdense in the early (arterial) bolus phase, and then become isodense within 1 to 2 minutes.

In questionable cases, the bolus series can be followed by a delayed scan performed 4 to 6 hours later. The latter, however, requires a high dose of contrast medium.

When there is fatty degeneration of the liver, primarily hypodense metastases may become isodense due to a drop in radiodensity of the surrounding tissue. Then, contrast medium administration is the only means of demonstrating the metastases.

Lymphoma Manifestation in the Liver

Primary malignant lymphomas of the liver are very rare, but secondary lymphoma involve-

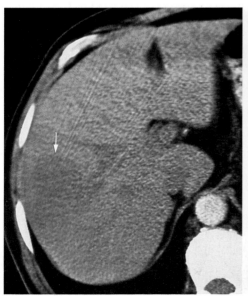
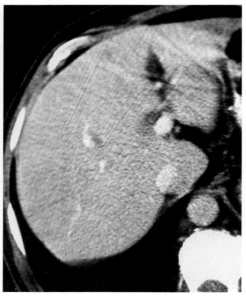

36a,b

Fig. 11-36a, b. Hepatic manifestations of Hodgkin's disease. In the plain scan the infiltrated region appears discretely hypodense (a→), becoming isodense after administration of contrast medium.

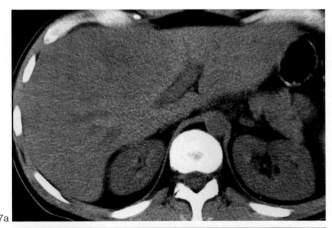

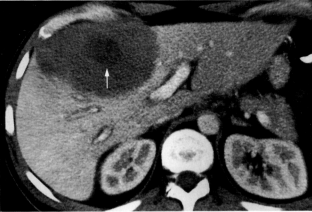

Fig. 11-37a, b. Manifestation of a non-Hodgkin's lymphoma in the liver. Discrete hypodense structures of varying density appearing in the plain scan become clearly demarcated after injection of contrast medium with a persisting central hypodense structure indicating necrobiotic metaplastic processes (b→).

ment in the late stages of disease is found in 50 to 80% of all patients. One third of all lymphoma patients have hepatomegaly, but liver involvement can be demonstrated histologically in only ca. 60%. Enlargement of the liver alone is therefore not sufficient to support a diagnosis of diffuse lymphoma manifestation in the organ.

• CT

Plain scans: As in the diagnosis of carcinomatous metastases, it is difficult to demonstrate the finely nodular, diffuse involvement due to primary disease on CT scans. Even circumscribed, larger hepatic foci are frequently isodense, but may be seen on plain scans as hypodense areas of rather variable intensity with or without organ deformation.

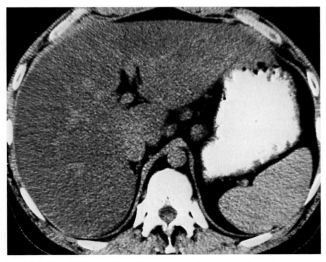

Fig. 11-38. Fatty infiltration of the liver. On the plain scan the liver exhibits overall enlargement. It appears hypodense with the portal structures contrasting as hyperdense regions. The density of the hepatic parenchyma has been greatly reduced in comparison to the spleen.

Contrast-enhanced scans: After bolus contrast administration, the tumor areas are frequently demarcated as round, sharply marginated zones of hypodensity the vascular architecture of which often remains intact. Even broad hyperdense regions may be found. Non-Hodgkin's lymphomas are frequently hypervascularized. They may have nodular protrusions, thereby resembling hepatocellular carcinomas.

Fig. 11-39. Focal fatty degeneration of the liver. A hypodense structure is detected in the vicinity of the enlarged caudal lobe (⇒). An additional circular hypodense structure is visible in the right lobe of the liver (→). The round formation can be differentiated from the other focal liver changes by taking the kinetics of contrast medium into account.

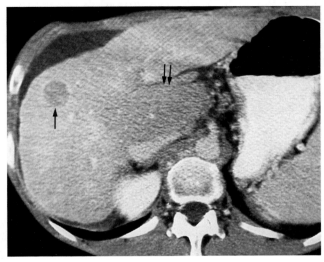

Differential diagnosis: Metastases, hepatocellular carcinoma, and focal steatosis (which is seldom problematic when the primary disease is known) must be considered in the diagnosis.

Inflammatory Regressive Changes in the Liver

Fatty Infiltration of the Liver

The deposition of fat in hepatocytes occurs in patients with general obesity, Cushing's disease, diabetes mellitus, hyperalimentation, malnutrition, chronic infection, and chemotherapy. This is usually associated with an increase in organ size.

• CT

Plain scans: A *diffuse* reduction in CT density of hepatic tissue is usually seen. Fatty degeneration of the liver can be diagnosed via plain scans when the radiodensity of the liver is lower than that of the spleen. Measurement of the density of the hepatic parenchyma allows a sufficient evaluation of the degree of fatty infiltration. The vessels frequently have a higher CT number than the parenchyma (contrast inversion). Neoplasms (metastases, FNH, hemangiomas, etc.) do not become involved in fatty infiltration, and these areas can be seen as hyperdense zones on plain scans. On the other hand, fatty infiltration of the liver can mask metastases on plain scans.

Focal fatty infiltration (steatosis areata) is variably pronounced and either localized or wide areas may be affected. Due to the accumulation of fat, these areas may resemble a mass lesion, but they generally maintain their vascular architecture.

Contrast-enhanced scans: The density difference between normal and fatty tissue remains constant after contrast administration.

Differential diagnosis: Reduction in density of hepatic tissue also occurs in amyloidosis and glycogen storage diseases.

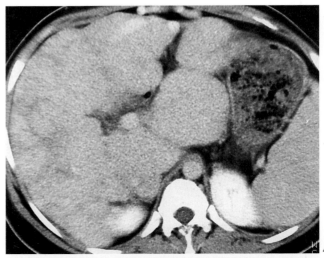

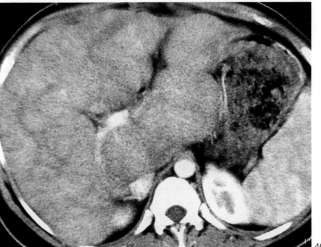

40a

40b

Fig. 11-40. Cirrhosis of the liver. Typical metaplastic processes of (postnecrotic) cirrhosis of the liver with numerous regeneration nodules, enlargement of the caudal lobe and deformation of the porta hepatis. After injection of contrast medium, the nodular structure of the liver appears more distinct, and the regeneration nodules are more clearly distinguished from the surrounding scar tissue than in the plain scan.

Hepatitis

Neither purulent nor non-purulent hepatitis is a primary indication for CT examination. Segmental inflammation due to radiation therapy appears as a sharply marginated, hypodense area that corresponds to the irradiation field; no increase in enhancement occurs after contrast medium administration. Calcification due to a granulomatous inflammation (tuberculosis, brucellosis, sarcoidosis) can be more sensitively detected by CT than by conventional radiography of the abdomen. Purulent bacte-

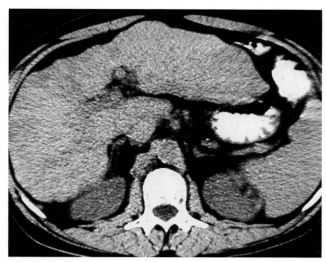

Fig. 11-41. Typical deformation that accompanies cirrhosis of the liver showing a significant enlargement of the quadrate lobe as well and a relative reduction in the size of the right lobe of the liver.

rial hepatitis should be diagnosed by CT only if abscess formation has occurred.

Cirrhosis

Cirrhosis of the liver is found in ca. 8% of all patients during autopsy examination. The septal form is the most common (57%), followed by the cholangitic (biliary) type (20%), and the

postnecrotic (postdystrophic) type. Septal cirrhosis develops due to fatty infiltration of the liver, which constantly decreases in size due to the incorporation of fibrous tissue. Biliary cirrhosis, however, leads to enlargement of the liver. Depending on the degree of tissue loss, variably large, bulbous regenerating nodules are found with the postnecrotic type. The increase in intrahepatic resistance determines the extent of portal hypertension with splenomegaly, collateral circulation, and ascites.

● CT

Plain scans: Although the shape and size of the liver can be evaluated on CT scans, the extent of structural tissue change cannot, since the CT number of the regenerating nodules seldom differs from that of cirrhotically changed liver tissue. The porta hepatis appears to be constricted by the typical enlargement of the lateral segment of the left lobe of the liver and the caudate lobe, occurring together with shrinkage of the remaining segments of the liver. This change in the relationship of the hepatic segments can be quantitatively defined via a quotient. Deformity of the left lobe can lead to considerable displacement of adjacent organs and the gall bladder. As a result of vas-

Fig. 11-42. Ratio of the caudal lobe to the right lobe (according to ref. 1236). The ratio of distances A (caudate lobe) to X (right lobe) in healthy individuals is 0.37 ± 0.16 and in cirrhosis patients 0.88 ± 0.20. Reference lines: 1 directly lateral to the main trunk of the porta hepatis, 2 tangential to the medial border of the caudal lobe, 3 vertical to both parallels in the center between the portal vein and the vena cava (white).

Fig. 11-43. Hemochromatosis. Clear increase in density of the hepatic parenchyma > 90 HU strongly accentuating the portal structures. The enlargement of the caudal lobe and the slight deformation of the arrangement of the blood vessels indicate cirrhotic metaplastic processes.

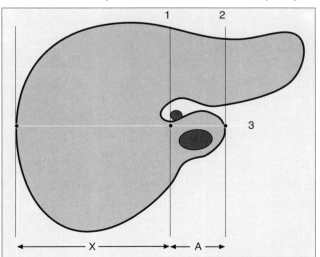

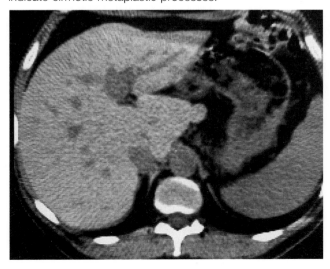

cular contortion due to structural tissue change, the portal structures become more difficult to visualize. The CT diagnosis becomes more evident with the appearance of ascites, splenic enlargement, prominent splenic vessels, and collateral circulation channels (reopened umbilical vein). Esophageal varices are usually visible only in extensive cases. When hepatomegaly is found, any possible malignant growth must also be identified.

Contrast-enhanced scans: Further non-equivocal sings of cirrhosis are generalized, inhomogeneous and reduced parenchymal enhancement after bolus contrast medium administration. Only in the healing phase of acute (or subacute) hepatitis are tissue areas with inflammatory changes demarcated from regenerating nodules.

Hemochromatosis

Idiopathic hemochromatosis is characterized by increased, pathogenetically inexplicable intestinal absorption of iron, which is stored in parenchymatous organs (liver, pancreas, myocardium). In 100 g of tissue, the hepatocytes contain 1 to 10 mg of iron, i.e., 5 to 50 times the normal value. The reaction of the parenchymatous organs to these deposits is cirrhotic metaplasia. In secondary *hemosiderosis*, this increased absorption of iron is caused by chronic anemia (thalassemia), congenital atransferrinemia, and (rarely) because of (alcohol-related) cirrhosis. When organ function is impaired, the condition is diagnosed as secondary hemochromatosis, in which iron accumulation is much less severe than in the primary form.

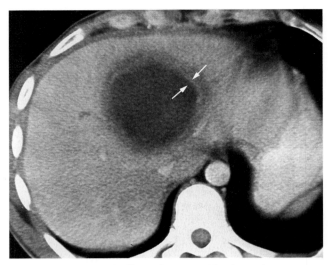

Fig. 11-44. Pyogenic liver abscess. The hypodense structure is contrasted by a sharply delineated peripheral enhancement (abscess membrane →). The structure is demarcated against the liver tissue by a broad hypodense border corresponding to the granulation tissue. The density values of the contents of the abscess are approx. 25 HU.

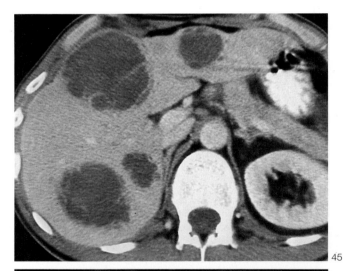

45

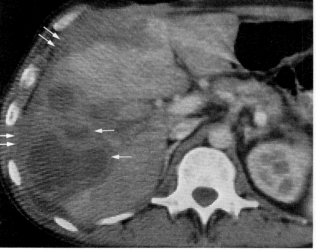

46

Fig. 11-45. Multiple liver abscesses. The hypodense structures are sharply demarcated against the hepatic parenchyma. Hyperdense septal structures corresponding to the abscess membranes are also detectable inside the formations. The granulation tissue is less prominent against the liver as compared to Figure 11-43.

Fig. 11-46. Liver abscess with perihepatic extension. The individual chambers of the abscess appear as irregular hypodense regions with fine peripheral enhancements (→). Granulation tissue surrounds these structures and the liver (⇒).

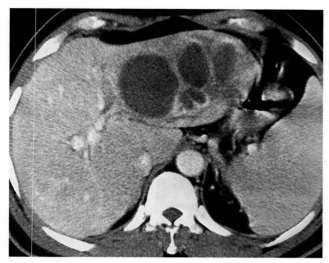

Fig. 11-47. Amebic abscess. Subphrenic multiloculated abscess with slight peripheral enhancement. The granulation tissue is less sharply contrasted against the distended left lobe of the liver. Loculation is rare in amebic abscesses.

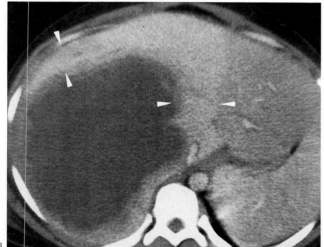

48

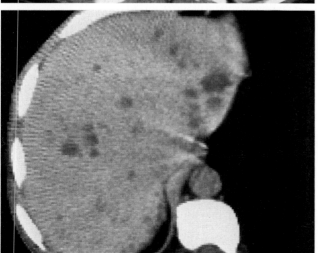

49

• CT

Plain scans: The increase in the iron content causes a significant increase in the CT number of hepatic tissue. With values of 100 to 140 HU, the figure is frequently twice that of the normal value. Density wise, the portal structures become more prominent, and not infrequently, there are also signs of portal hypertension and cirrhosis.

Differential diagnosis: When the CT number of the liver is increased, other storage diseases must be considered in the diagnosis: *gold storage* within the reticulo-endothelial system (RES) after treatment of rheumatoid arthritis, *glycogen storage disease*, effects of *hemodialysis* or chronic *arsenic poisoning*.

Abscesses

A *pyogenic abscess* may be due to various factors: abscess-forming infections in the course of obstruction of the biliary tract, hematogenous dissemination in systemic, septic infections (endocarditis, pneumonia), or purulent inflammations in the drainage area of the portal vein (appendicitis, diverticulitis, colitis, Crohn's disease). Rare findings include bacterial inflammations that spread from the immediate vicinity of the liver (e.g. the gallbladder) and direct infections due to an injury. The etiology remains unclear in around 50% of all cases (*cryptogenic abscess*). E. coli is the most common pathogen, and anaerobes are frequently involved. Pyogenic abscesses can be uni- or multilocular. They are most often found in elderly patients with diabetes mellitus, cardiac insufficiency, or cirrhosis of the liver.

Fig. 11-48. Amebic abscess. The hypodense mass occupies the greater portion of the right lobe of the liver with density values around 29 HU. After injection of contrast medium, a broad hyperdense border zone (► ◄), corresponding to prominent granulation tissue, is detected.

Fig. 11-49. Fungal microabscesses. Detection of numerous, sharply marginated hypodense structures distributed throughout the liver. Neither a hypodense border nor granulation tissue is detected on plain or contrast enhanced scans.

Amebic abscesses occur in patients predominantly from South and Central America, the Near East, and parts of Africa. The pathogen gains access to the liver via portal vein circulation. Once in the liver, it causes necrosis made of thick consistent medium that ultimately liquefies (anchovy sauce). The clinical picture may be complicated by thrombophlebitis in individual branches of the liver vessels. A superinfection caused by pyogenic pathogens occurs in ca. 20% of all cases.

Fungal microabscesses are found mainly in immunocompromised patients. They are caused by Candida albicans, Aspergillus, and Cryptococcus. Numerous small foci of inflammation are distributed evenly throughout the liver; this can also be seen in the spleen.

• CT

Abscess formation begins with fresh *inflammatory infiltration*. This is seen as a discrete, hypodense zone on plain scans which, after contrast administration, may demonstrate slight, widespread enhancement. The degree of hypodensity increases after the onset of inflammatory necrosis and the area becomes more clearly demarcated from surrounding tissue. In perifocal regions, as an expression of the inflammatory reaction, a ringlike, indistinctly demarcated zone of enhancement appears.

Final *demarcation* of the abscess is due to the formation of a pyogenic wall. It is seen, on the one side, as a zone that is hypodense as compared with the contiguous liver tissue and, on the other side, as a sharply demarcated, hyperdense rim around the cavity of the abscess. An inflammatory co-reaction, the severity of which corresponds with the stage of inflammation, occurs in the surrounding hepatic tissue.

The abscess cavity itself does not become enhanced. The attenuation value depends on the age of the abscess. Fresh abscesses are only moderately hypodense. The CT number decreases as colliquation of the necrotic areas increases and as a result of absorbent pro-

cesses. *Gas*, which is a sign of the presence and growth of anaerobic bacteria, is a pathognomonic indicator of abscesses.

This results in:

Plain scans: Slight hypodensity in the early phase. This increases in later phases and can ultimately reach water density values. These zones become more sharply demarcated from the liver and can assume the CT appearance of a cyst if absorption does not occur.

Contrast-enhanced scans: There is an area of discrete enhancement in the early phase, then increasing hypodensity in the center of the lesion. A hyperdense, sharply marginated inner ring with an indistinct hypodense outer rim is seen (abscess wall, double target sign). This cyst wall, which absorbs only a slight amount of contrast medium, again becomes smooth after the inflammation subsides (postinflammatory cysts).

Differential diagnosis: In *pyogenic* abscesses, uni- and multilocular formations are seen with relatively thin pyogenic walls, occasional gas bubbles, and CT numbers of ca. 20 to 30 HU.

Amebic cysts are usually unilocular, the CT number ranges from 0 to 20 HU, there is a broad abscess membrane or granulation tissue layer; the location is frequently subphrenic.

Fungal microabscesses are usually small, disseminated, and have only discretely visible abscess walls. The CT number is around 30 HU.

Necrotizing metastases can mimic the appearance of an abscess, especially in view of the fact that they too can display septic superinfection. In such a case, the patient's clinical picture will frequently be the decisive factor in making the diagnosis. Cholangitic abscesses are found in the biliary system.

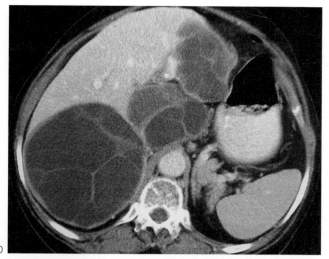

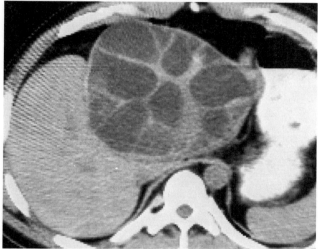

Echinococcosis (Hydatid Disease)

Echinococcosis develops from the larvae of the Echinococcus alveolaris (multilocularis) and E. granulosus (cysticus unilocularis). Variable morphological symptoms arise that primarily affect the liver. Other organs of involvement are, in order of frequency, the lungs, brain, spleen, and other parenchymatous organs.

● *Echinococcus granulosus (cysticus unilocularis)*

This infection is endemic to the Mediterranean region, the Soviet Union and Australia. Echinococcus granulosus leads to the formation of large cysts which can be recognized by their typical three-layered structure (germinal layer; endocyst of hyalin and ectocyst, which is highly vascularized as an expression of their floridity; and granulation tissue).

Secondary daughter cysts develop within the primary cyst as well as in adjacent cysts via protuberances in the germinal layer. Ringlike, polycyclic calcification usually results from calcification of the cyst walls and is seldom caused

Fig. 11-50. Echinococcosis granulosus. Several cystic structures are detected in the liver. A capsule is sharply demarcated from liver tissue. Typical cordlike septa can be seen.

Fig. 11-51. An echinococcus cyst involves the entire left lobe of the liver. The septa are broader and more prominent.

Fig. 11-52. Echinococcus cyst with mural calcification (→). The secondary cysts appear as small, round hypodense areas that form a wreathlike structure below the capsule (⇒).

Fig. 11-53. Echinococcus alveolaris. Broad calcified structures that are sharply demarcated from the hepatic parenchyma are detected in the right lobe of the liver. In the center of calcification, irregular map-like hypodense structures corresponding to necrosis are found.

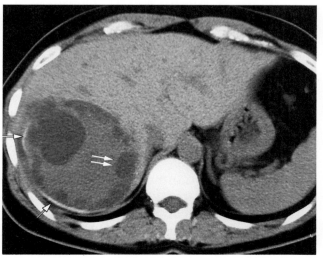

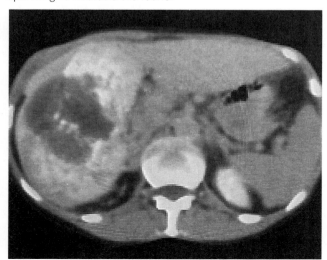

by amorphous calcareous deposits produced by thickening of the cyst contents.

• CT

Plain scans: The typical structure of loculated cysts is seen on plain CT scans. Secondary cysts usually have a round or ellipsoid configuration and are delineated by variably thick septa. The cyst wall, which sometimes appears thicker than the surrounding hepatic parenchyma, is sharply demarcated from the parenchyma. Characteristically partial or total wall calcification may be absent, which makes it difficult to differentiate these cysts from other types. CT numbers lie in the water range or slightly higher (10 to 45 HU).

Contrast-enhanced scans: A sign of floridity that is occasionally seen after contrast administration is a ringlike enhancement pattern in the region of the external cyst wall.

• *Echinococcus alveolaris*

Infection with E. alveolaris (endemic to central and southern Europe, South America, Australia, and Southeast Asia) occurs in childhood years and is localized preferentially in the right lobe of the liver. Most of the infected hepatic tissue becomes necrotic. Its macroscopic appearance is that of spongy tissue permeated by small cysts. The tissue is often yellowish in color due to xanthomatous perifocal inflammation.

• CT

Plain scans: Diseased tissue appears on CT scans as an indistinctly delineated, irregular zone of hypodensity (20 to 40 HU) that usually has small, nodular to extensive, perifocal, amorphous calcification. In up to 40% of the cases, more strongly hypodense zones of necrosis (0 to 10 HU) can be distinguished. Cholangiectasis is found in around 50% of these patients.

Contrast-enhanced scans: The accompanying inflammation is often marked by perifocal enhancement that clearly demarcates it from the mass, which absorbs hardly any contrast medium.

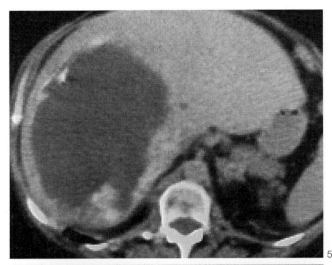

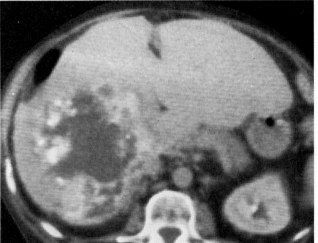

Fig. 11-54. Calcified structures surround a central area of hypodensity in the right lobe of the liver. This area expands to form a larger cystic structure inferior to the diaphragm. Calcification is detected in the surrounding capsule region.

Differential diagnosis: When calcification and necrosis are absent, it is hardly possible to differentiate infected areas from a malignant tumor. The clinical findings, especially the patient's serology, determine which steps must be taken next.

Trauma

Blunt abdominal trauma after traffic accidents is the most common cause of liver injury. Rupture of the parenchyma with an accompanying or later occurring capsule rupture can lead to a life-threatening hemorrhage in the abdominal

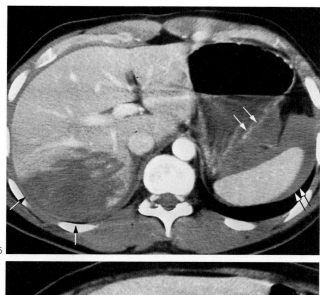

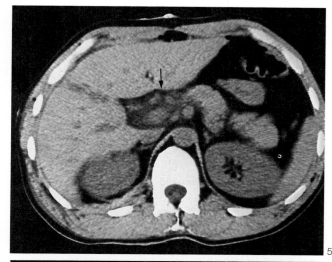

55

57a

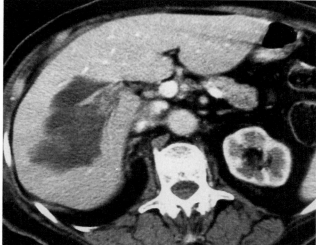

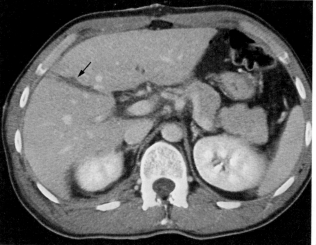

56

57b

Fig. 11-55. Blunt hepatic trauma after a traffic accident. Plain scans revealed a slightly hyperdense hematoma. After bolus contrast medium injection, this appears as an irregularly marginated hypodense region (→). It is thereby demarcated from the vital hepatic parenchyma, which is partially lacerated. Evidence of fluid (blood) in the abdominal cavity (⇒).

Fig. 11-56. Ruptured solitary hepatic cyst. Hypodense structure with irregular margins and increased attenuation values (around 35 HU). It is demarcated as an avascular space after injection of contrast medium.

Fig. 11-57a, b. Hepatic trauma following a stab wound. Plain scans revealed a hypodense structure between the lobes of the liver. The structure is demarcated more sharply after injection of contrast medium (b→). In the plain scan, the hematoma is seen masking the structures of the porta hepatis (a→).

cavity. A piercing gunshot, knife or lance wound or surgery can lead to separation of the capsule of the liver from the abdominal wall, thereby opening the peritoneal cavity.

The capsule of the liver usually remains intact in less severe blunt traumas. Small parenchymal lacerations in the periphery of the liver lead to the development of localized, frequently subcapsular, *hematomas*. A *central-*

ized parenchymal rupture may develop in more severe abdominal trauma with a localized trauma zone, but the organ capsule usually remains intact. Lacerations occur mainly in the cranial segment of the right lobe of the liver, and they may be accompanied by injuries to the inferior vena cava and the central hepatic vein. Aerobilia as well as clinically demonstrable hemobilia, both of which can be demonstrated well on CT scans, show the lacerations of even larger bile ducts. The liver may *rupture* or *fragment*, accompanied by rupture of the capsule and hemorrhaging in the abdominal cavity, in piercing injuries as well as very severe blunt abdominal trauma. Injuries of the hilum of the liver, usually caused by piercing trauma, can also lead to considerable bleeding. Chronic cases with bile leakage and oozing hemorrhages usually result from surgical intervention.

• CT

Plain scans: Fresh hematomas cannot always be diagnosed on the basis of their CT density when the radiodensity of the liver is normal. Hematomas can often be seen as hypodense zones on plain scans. Extensive hematomas

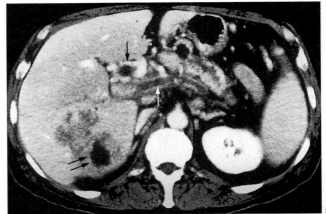

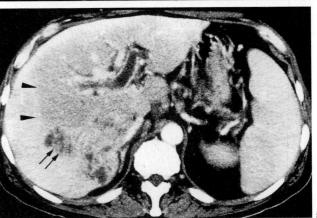

Fig. 11-58a, b. Cavernous transformation after a portal venous thrombosis in a young child. In the bolus contrast medium phase, irregular maplike enhancement of the liver results from altered arterial perfusion (a). In the late portovenous phase, collateral vessels of the portal veins appear as broadened hyperdense structures of the porta hepatis with finger-shaped ramifications. Hypodense bile duct structures are detected inside these ramifications (b→).

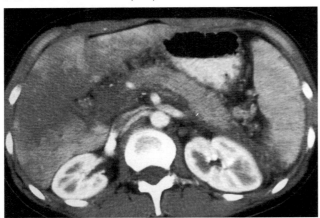

58a

Fig. 11-59a, b. Fresh portal venous thrombosis in a patient with a metastasizing carcinoma of the pancreas. The splenic and portal veins contain a cordlike hypodense structure within the lumina. This is surrounded by a delicate hypodense border (→) on contrast enhanced scans. Hepatic perfusion is irregular in the portovenous contrast medium phase (►). Metastases from the pancreatic carcinoma (⇉).

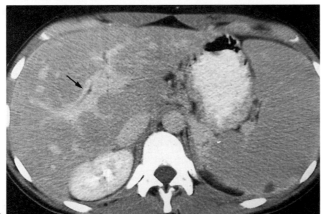

58b

(e.g. in central parenchymal rupture) are inhomogeneously hyperdense and sometimes have a linear configuration. Subcapsular hematomas have a typical, lenticulate configuration. Larger hematomas can become posttraumatic cysts. The peritoneal cavity should be investigated for (hyperdense) fluid accumulations. *Gas* within the bile ducts is indicative of a biliary lesion. Biliary pseudocysts (biliomas) are frequently subcapsular or perihepatic. In the postoperative phase, they appear as thin-walled fluid collections with a CT number of around 10 HU.

Contrast-enhanced scans: It is generally necessary to administer contrast medium in order to demarcate the hepatic parenchyma from he-

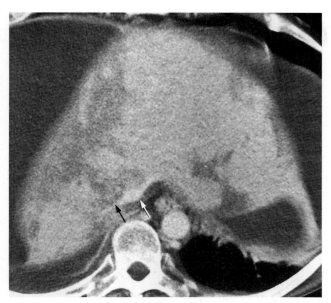

Fig. 11-60. Budd-Chiari syndrome. In this case, a tumor causes occlusion of the hepatic veins. Therefore, at the angle of the hepatic veins, the parenchyma becomes inhomogeneously hypodense after contrast medium administration. Due to impression, the inferior vena cava appears as a slit-like structure (→). Evidence of considerable amounts of ascitic fluid.

matomas. When there is a central laceration of the liver, one should watch for uniform parenchymal enhancement, lacerations that may extend to larger vessels, and intact confluence of hepatic veins.

Vascular Processes

Portal Venous Thrombosis

In adult patients, hematologic diseases and infections now and then lead to thrombotic occlusion of the portal vein, which is also caused by direct tumor compression and invasion.

• CT

Plain scans: Plain scans are not usually helpful.

Contrast-enhanced scans: Portal venous thrombosis can be clearly demonstrated after targeted bolus contrast administration and, if necessary, thin-section scanning. Depending on the age of the thrombosis, the portal vein as well as its branches show no contrast enhancement; a central hypodense area may be seen. Occlusion of the portal vein usually develops slowly and, when periportal collateral channels have developed (cavernous transformation), they become visible as hyperdense strands on CT scans.

Budd-Chiari Syndrome

Various diseases accompanied by stenosis or obstruction of the hepatic veins with a concomitant increase in coagulability can lead to vascular thrombosis. Some of these diseases are: congenital membranous stenosis of the inferior vena cava (IVC), absence of the transhepatic segment of the IVC, obstruction of the suprahepatic segment of the IVC, right ventricular failure, constrictive pericarditis, allergic vasculitis, polycythemia, leukemia, and tumors at the site of entry of hepatic veins.

• CT

Plain scans: Enlargement of the liver with accompanying ascites is visible on plain scans.

Contrast-enhanced scans: Absence of enhancement in the hepatic veins after bolus administration of contrast medium is indicative of occlusion. In the late portovenous phase, a maculated pattern of parenchymal enhancement, especially in the periphery, appears in the liver.

Differential diagnosis: Right ventricular failure must be differentiated from macular changes in the liver which, however, is extensively visible in the lumina of the hepatic veins.

Chapter 12
The Biliary System

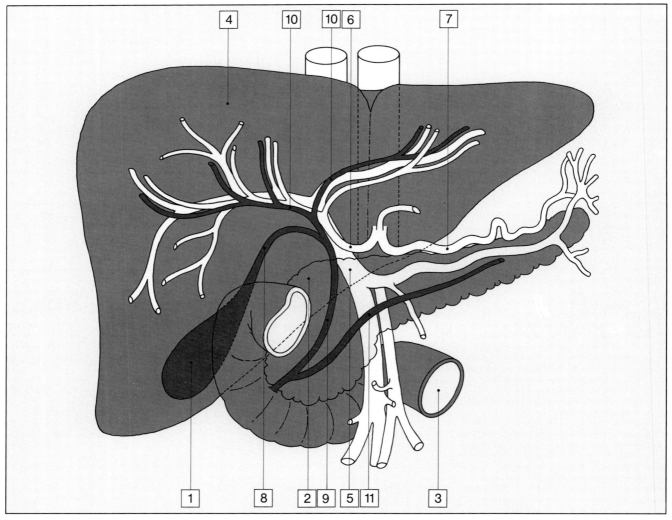

Fig. 12-1. Topography of the biliary system.
a) Anterior view of situs.
b) Transverse sections (for level, see a).

Key to symbols:

1 Gallbladder	4 Liver	8 Cystic duct
2 Pancreas	5 Portal vein	9 Bile duct
3 Duodenum	6 Hepatic artery	10 Hepatic duct
	7 Splenic artery	11 Pancreatic duct

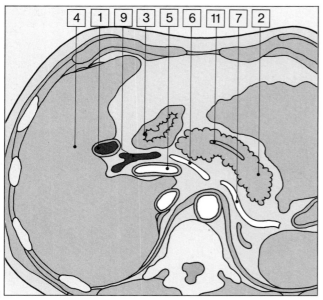

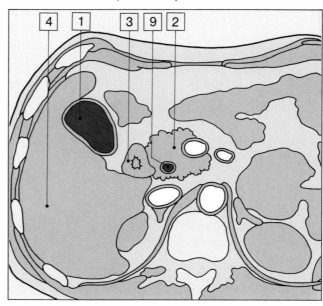

The Biliary System

Anatomy and Imaging

The shape and position of the *gallbladder* vary in relation to its degree of function. On CT scans, the gallbladder is located on the medial contour of the right hepatic lobe caudal to the porta hepatis. The CT density of the lumen is normally slightly above that of water (0 HU), but attenuation values may rise to ca. 25 HU as the viscosity of bile increases. Surrounding fatty tissue is usually absent, so the wall of a normal gallbladder is seldom visible on CT scans. The gallbladder then has a cystic appearance on CT scans.

The *common bile duct* traverses the duodenum in the hepatoduodenal ligament and runs an almost vertical caudad course through the head of the pancreas. The inclination of this section of the bile duct determines how well it can be scanned. The common bile duct can be demonstrated on CT scans when its course is virtually axial, its diameter is 3 mm or larger, and pancreatic tissue has been opacified. Image quality is reduced due to partial volume artifacts when the diameter of the tubular lumen is small and the common bile duct deviates from the CT axis by ca. 30° or more. At calibers of 8 mm or wider, CT demonstration of the common bile duct is no longer course-dependent. Prepapillary sections of the common bile duct are readily demonstrable on thin-section CT scans after enhancement of the parenchyma of pancreatic tissue.

The (hypodense) intrahepatic ducts lie in front of the ramifications of the portal veins. After intravenous administration of urographic contrast medium (CM), intrahepatic ducts with a caliber of 2 mm or larger can be demonstrated on thin-section slices (3 to 5 mm). They then appear as delicate hypodense structures lying in front of the opacified vessels. In some healthy individuals, ducts in the periphery of the liver may also be as large in caliber.

Gallbladder Enlargement

The size of the gallbladder is function-dependent and is not a specific diagnostic criterion. After long periods of fasting or in patients with diabetes mellitus or acromegaly, the gallbladder is frequently enlarged and often reacts significantly to gastric stimulants. After a negative cholecystogram, other causes of gallbladder enlargement must be taken into consideration (e.g. cystic duct occlusion). If no gallstones are found, hydrops and acute cholecystitis are primary diseases for consideration in the diagnosis.

• CT

The gallbladder is considered to be enlarged when its horizontal diameter exceeds 5 cm on CT scans. When hydrops is suspected, longitudinal distension should also be assessed. Functional enlargement of the gallbladder usually does not cause wall thickening.

Inflammatory Changes of the Gallbladder

Cholecystitis

Cholelithiasis is the most frequent cause of cholecystitis with cholestasis. Cholecystitis is characterized by considerable thickening (up to 10 mm) of the gallbladder wall. The lumen, too, is usually enlarged. If the acute inflammatory phase persists for a long period of time, increased exudation of leukocytes may lead to *empyema*. The leukocytes may also invade neighboring organs. In cases of (very rare) *emphysematous* cholecystitis arising from anaerobic bacteria, gas is found not only in the lumen, but also in discrete amounts in the gallbladder wall, itself. *Chronic* cholecystitis is almost always accompanied by gallstones; the gallbladder wall adheres to surrounding tissue and becomes permeated with fibrous tissue. Calcification of the gallbladder wall and limy bile are frequent findings in patients with chronic gallbladder inflammation. The final stage consists of sclero- atrophic cholecystitis.

• CT

Plain scans: The primary sign of acute chole-cystitis is thickening of the gallbladder wall. This is usually 3 to 5 mm thick, but may even exceed 10 mm in thickness. Enlargement of the lumen, gas and hypodense fluid in the direct vicinity of the gallbladder are frequent accompaniments. Chronic inflammatory wall processes lead to contraction of the gallbladder and striation of pericystic fatty tissue. Small deposits of calcium and peripheral encrustations (which can lead to porcelain gallbladder) can be diagnosed early, but must be differentiated from calculi. However, when a contracted gallbladder is very small, its demonstration may be impossible. Emphysematous cholecystitis is characterized by intramural inclusions of gas.

The *attenuation* of bile is usually raised to values greater than 25 HU, and may reach values of up to 80 HU.

Contrast-enhanced scans: A bolus of contrast medium usually gives rise to clear enhancement of a thickened gallbladder wall. A well contrasted inner layer can normally be distinguished from the hypodense outer layer, the appearance of which corresponds to serous edema.

In patients with empyema, strong contrast enhancement and distended, irregular, partially stratified walls are seen.

Perforation and pericholecystic abscesses in the vicinity of the gallbladder appear on CT scans as hypodense, encapsulated zones with enhanced margins. In non-acute stages, chronic indurative processes involving the gallbladder wall are only slightly enhanced. In some cases, a hypodense seam (halo) is seen.

Differential diagnosis: *Thickening of the gallbladder wall* in absence of signs of acute in-

Fig. 12-4. Chronic cholecystitis. An irregularly thickened gallbladder wall is seen after contrast medium administration. The border with the liver is indistinct. It was concluded that a gallbladder carcinoma had arisen from the chronic cholecystitis. In surgery, however, only chronic, scarred changes in the bed of the gallbladder were found.

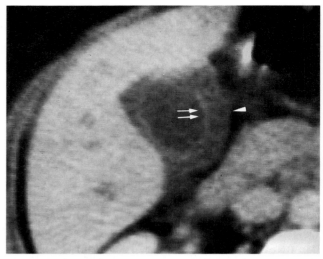

Fig. 12-2. Cholecystitis. After contrast medium administration, an enhanced, 1–2 mm thick hypodense rim (►) is seen along the inner wall of the gallbladder (⇒).

Fig. 12-3. Empyema of the gallbladder with an abscess of the abdominal wall. After CM administration, a thickened, irregularly layered gallbladder wall (► ◄) can be seen. The dilated muscles of the abdominal wall are enhanced (→).

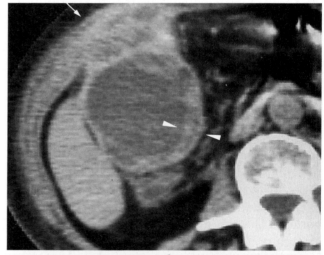

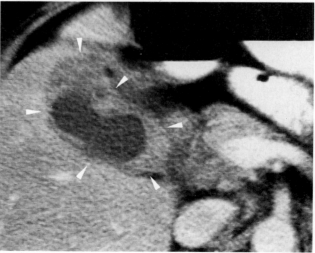

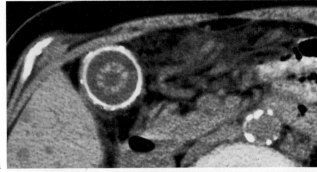

5a

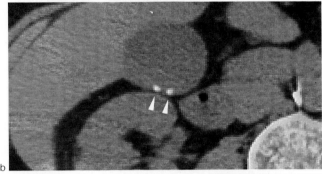

5b

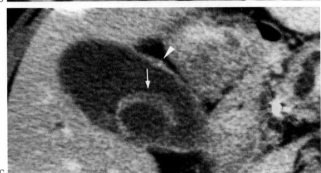

5c

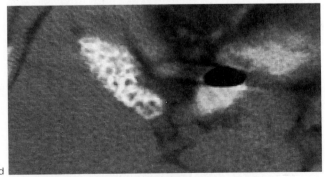

5d

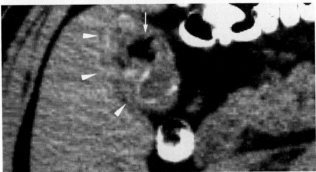

5e

flammation may also be seen in patients with hepatitis, pancreatitis, hypoproteinemia, and adenomyomatosis.

Cholelithiasis

Most gallstones contain cholesterol or bilirubin (pigment calculi) and show amorphous calcification. Pure cholesterol stones, on the other hand, display ringlike or central deposits of calcium. Most gallstones can be diagnosed by ultrasound. The global accuracy of computed tomography in diagnosing gallstones is 80 to 90%.

• CT

The typical radiological patterns of calcification in gallstones can also be demonstrated in larger concrements via computed tomography. The radiodensity of bile, which is dependent on its degree of viscosity, fluctuates between 0 HU and a maximum of 80 HU. The degree of contrast difference between bile and gallstones is, therefore, inconsistent. Sometimes, gallstones even appear isodense. The radiodensity of cholesterol calculi usually ranges from ca. -60 to 140 HU, but may be significantly higher when the calculi contain larger amounts of calcium. Vacuum phenomena can reduce attenuation to -370 HU. This negative attenuation of calcium-free gallstones sometimes renders them demonstrable in non-enhanced bile.

Intraductal calculi are more sensitively detected by thin-section computed tomography.

Differential diagnosis: When the attenuation of bile is raised (> 50 HU), limy bile, biliary sludge, post-angiographic conditions, and hemobilia (65 to 90 HU) must be considered in the diagnosis.

Fig. 12-5a-e. Cholecystolithiasis. a) Multiple ringlike calcification of a solitary gallstone. **b)** Two punctiform, calcified gallstones (►). **c)** Large gallstone with ringlike calcification (→); the attenuation value in the center is equal to that of bile. **d)** Multiple gallstones. **e)** "Vacuum" phenomena within gallstones (→). Thickening of the gallbladder wall due to chronic cholecystitis (c, e ►).

Gallbladder Tumors

Next to gallstones, cholesterosis *(cholesterol papillomas)* is the second most common filling defect diagnosed on cholecystograms. These usually multiple lesions are normally 3 to 5 mm large, but can reach a maximum size of 10 mm. *Adenomyomatosis* consists of focal or generalized hyperplasia of the gallbladder wall. True *papillomas* and *adenomas* (can be as large as 4 cm) are rare as compared with *cholesterol papillomas* (cholesterosis). *Gallbladder carcinomas*, ca. 95% of which are adenocarcinomas, frequently develop due to underlying chronic cystitis. Gallstones are therefore found in up to around 75% of these cases. Women over sixty are frequently affected. The tumor spreads in the bed of the gallbladder even before any clinical symptoms become apparent, thereby infiltrating the hepatoduodenal ligament, liver, and regional lymph nodes. The prognosis of these tumors is, therefore, generally unfavorable. *Sarcomas* of all the various tissue types are extremely rare. Metastatic spread into the gallbladder is normally attributable to a melanoma.

• CT

Plain scans: *Adenomyomatosis* appears on CT scans as generalized or focal thickening of the gallbladder wall. In rare cases, it can also lead to soft-tissue dense intraluminal thickening. The outer contours of the gallbladder wall, however, remain smooth. Because of their small diameters, cholesterosis *polyps* and *papillomas* can be demonstrated in non-enhanced gallbladders without biliary contrast medium only when their diameter is larger than 5 mm.
Gallbladder carcinomas frequently appear on CT scans as a more or less inhomogeneous soft-tissue structure in the bed of the gallbladder that is weakly distinguishable from the surrounding hepatic parenchyma. An (irregularly) thickened gallbladder wall and intraluminal lesions are two further signs of gallbladder carcinoma. Dilatation of intrahepatic ducts is relatively common and suggestive of biliary tract obstruction due to a lymphoma or tumor invasion into the porta hepatis.

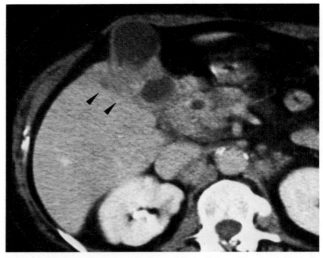

Fig. 12-6. Carcinoma of the gallbladder. Intravesical soft-tissue mass compromising the gallbladder. The border with the liver is indistinct (►), which is indicative of infiltrative growth into the liver.

Fig. 12-7. Carcinoma of the gallbladder. The lumen of the gallbladder displays an irregular configuration. The thickened wall extends towards and into the liver as an indistinct, hypodense zone – a sign of infiltrative growth.

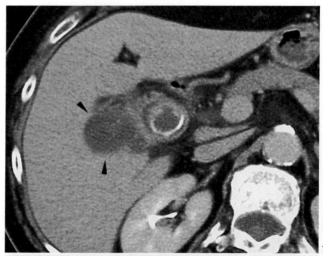

7a

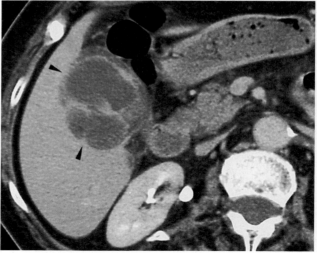

7b

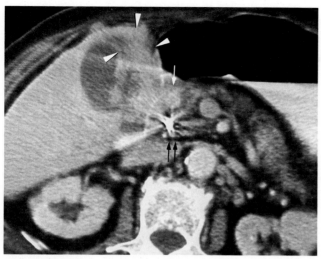

Fig. 12-8. Carcinoma of the gallbladder. The tumor (►) has spread to the porta hepatis (→), making it necessary to insert a bile duct replacement.

Fig.12-9. Carcinoma of the gallbladder. The gallbladder walls are thickened and indistinctly delineated (b→). The tumor has spread to the liver and displays slightly hyperdense peripheral enhancement (a►).

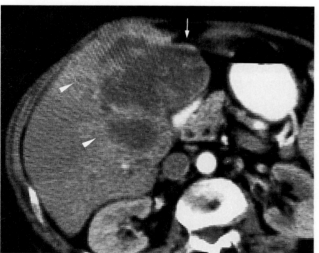

9a

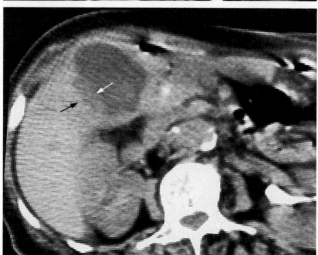

9b

The possibility of infiltration in the direction of the pancreas or duodenum can be evaluated only after sufficient intestinal opacification via oral contrast medium has been achieved. Because of the complex anatomical position of these structures, portal and hepatoduodenal lymph node enlargement can be evaluated only when there is sufficient delineating fat and when the lymph nodes are 1 cm and larger. If infiltration of the liver is extensive, the primary site of the neoplasm can no longer be determined by means of computed tomography (infiltrating gallbladder carcinoma or malignant tumor spreading to the porta hepatis). When the gallbladder wall facing away from the liver is involved, local peritoneal carcinomatosis develops early.

Contrast-enhanced scans: A bolus of contrast medium is needed to better differentiate structures of the porta hepatis, contours of the gallbladder, and intrahepatic metastases. Contrast enhancement of the tumor tissue, itself, is extremely variable.

Differential diagnosis: When the gallbladder wall is thickened or the gallbladder bed shows abnormality, a wide range of diseases must be considered in the diagnosis. They include: gallbladder carcinoma, chronic cholecystitis, and colonic cancer in the right flexura. Less common diseases are adenomyomatosis and xanthogranulomatosis cholecystitis.

Biliary Obstruction

Obstruction of the biliary tract is rarely caused by anomalies such as gallbladder septa or choledochal cysts. Biliary obstruction is more commonly caused by calculi, strictures, stenosis, and primary or secondary tumors in the porta hepatis and pancreas. The most common sign seen in diagnostic imaging is dilatation of the bile ducts which, however, may be absent in patients with a clear clinical picture of obstruction. A morphologically detailed evaluation by means of endoscopic retrograde cholangiopancreatography (ERCP) or functional radionuclide imaging of the gallbladder may be required to clarify the diagnosis.

• CT

Extensive dilatation of the bile ducts can be unequivocally diagnosed on plain scans. Minor intrahepatic dilatation, however, can be diagnosed only after a sufficient dose of *contrast medium* has been administered. Then, even peripheral bile ducts become apparent as punctiform hypodense structures. In contrast to local thrombosis of the portal vein, obstructed bile ducts are slightly distorted and sharply demarcated from the liver parenchyma. Consideration of the spatial relationship of enhanced, adjacent branches of the portal vein permits an analysis, even of unclear regions of the porta hepatis. Small, soft-tissue dense lesions can then be diagnosed from sizes of ca. 10 mm and larger.

A choledochal width of 7 to 8 mm is classified as borderline, and widths exceeding 9 mm are considered pathological, both before and after cholecystectomy. If bile ducts can be seen in the periphery of the liver after contrast medium administration, intrahepatic biliary dilatation must be concluded.

When dilatation (diffuse or focal) of the biliary tract is found, one must always investigate the possibility of obstruction due to calculi (intra or extrahepatic). As was the case in the gallbladder, gallstones of the biliary tract can be clearly identified only when calcified. Since the common bile duct passes axially through the CT section, computed tomography can sensitively detect concretions in prepapillary choledochal areas. These calculi often have a rosette-shaped configuration. In patients with Mirizzi's syndrome, the porta hepatis and neck of the gallbladder should be carefully scanned via thin-section CT, if necessary, on a lateral view. It is thereby possible to reveal the gallstone and its position with respect to the hepatocholedochal duct.

Biliary Tract Infections

Obstructions caused by calculi, strictures, ascariasis, and tumors provide favorable conditions for the development of pyogenic biliary

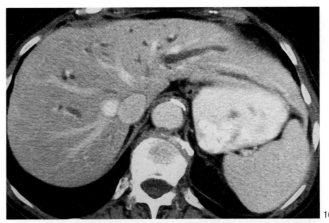
10a

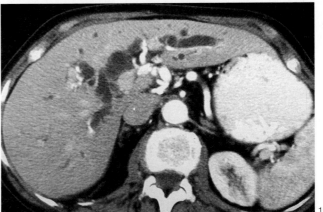
10b

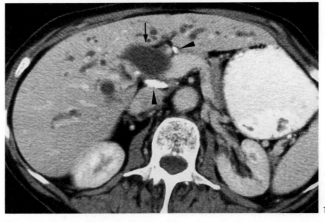
10c

Fig. 12-10a-c. Biliary obstruction. A stenotic process in the head of the pancreas is causing considerable intrahepatic dilatation of the bile ducts; they appear contorted. Their position with respect to portal vessel structures is essentially maintained. Hepatic artery (►), hepatocholedochal duct (→).

tract infections. Periductal abscesses, especially in hepatic regions, are serious complications of cholangitis. In chronic cases or with frequent recurrences, strictures can develop in the peripheral bile ducts, leading to secondary sclerosing cholangitis. Stenosing papillitis, which is seen as an accompaniment of adjacent

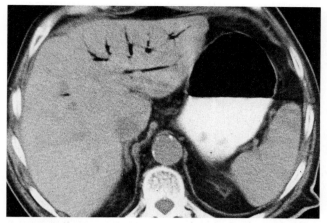

Fig. 12-11. Aerobilia. Air in the bile ducts, especially due to papillotomy, can be very sensitively detected by CT.

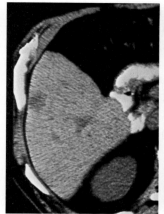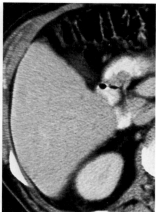

Fig. 12-13. Pericholangitis. CT reveals very fine, punctiform hypodense areas inside the right lobe of the liver (a), which become masked after contrast medium administration (b). The typical clinical symptoms of cholangitis receded after antibiotic treatment, and the hypodensity found in CT disappeared.

Fig. 12-12. Pericholangitic abscess. In the early bolus phase, hypodense zones around the bile ducts (→) are delineated by zones of increased perifocal contrast enhancement (a►), which becomes less visible in the portovenous phase (b). When bile ducts are scanned orthograde, a discrete, crestlike structure can be seen.

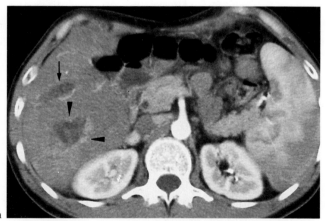
12a

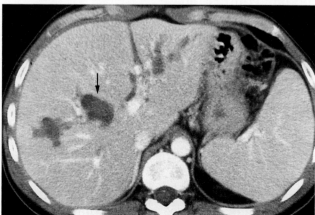
12b

inflammatory processes, leads to dilatation of the common bile duct. *Primary obliterative cholangitis* is commonly observed with ulcerative colitis, retroperitoneal fibrosis, and Riedel's struma. Cirrhosis with portal hypertension develops as the disease progresses.

• CT

Extrahepatic: An acute infection of the *common bile duct* is readily demonstrable in intrapancreatic areas. Clear enhancement of wall thickening is usually clearly visible on thin-section CT scans taken after the *administration of contrast medium.*

Intrahepatic: Acute intrahepatic pericholangitic infections can be demonstrated on CT scans if abscess formation has begun. In recurrent cholangitis, primary and secondary bile ducts are frequently found. A spotty parenchymal pattern develops in contiguous hepatic tissue. CT scans are usually able to demonstrate intrahepatic gallstones and areas of gas formation that cannot be seen on plain radiographs. The symptoms they cause include focal atrophy and focal fatty degeneration of the liver. *Obliterative cholangitis* is characterized by focal dilatation, which appears on CT scans as wormlike or fusiform areas of diffuse of focal hypodensity in the liver parenchyma. Reactions are often absent in surrounding tissue, and the degree of enhancement of duct walls will vary in proportion to the severity of the process.

Contrast-enhanced scans: Enhancement of ductal walls or widespread or focal opacification of the liver parenchyma (surrounding reaction) is seldom successful in providing unequivocal proof of inflammatory biliary abnormalities.

Differential diagnosis: A tumor should be suspected when wall thickening is eccentric and caliber reduction abrupt, even if no soft-tissue components are found.

Tumors of the Biliary Tract

Biliary tract tumors are 2 to 3 times rarer than gallbladder tumors and 8 times less frequently than pancreatic carcinomas. Benign neoplasms are rarities. These tumors are usually adenocarcinomas (cholangiocarcinomas) displaying cirrhotic infiltrating, circular stenosing (exopythic), or polypoid growth forms. In order of frequency, the distal common bile duct, ampulla of Vater, proximal hepatic duct near the bifurcation, cystic duct and, finally, the hepatic duct are most commonly involved. In ca. 30% of these cases, regional metastases are found at the time of surgery.

• CT

Plain scans: Depending on the tumor location, there is either generalized, lobar, or focal obstruction of intra and extrahepatic bile ducts. Lobar hepatic atrophy may also be observed. The lesions themselves can be demonstrated on CT scans from sizes of 1 cm and larger. Infiltrating tumors normally appear isodense to hyperdense, whereas expansile tumors are hypodense. Regional lymph nodes in the porta hepatis, lesser omentum and hepatoduodenal ligament are often affected.

Contrast-enhanced scans: Small polypoid tumors do not enhance clearly. Ringlike hyperdensity comes from the surrounding, dilated bile duct. In more extensive processes, en-

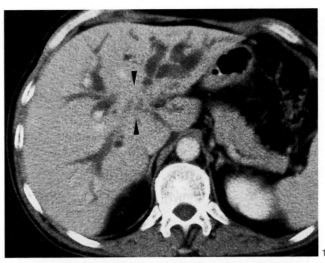
14a

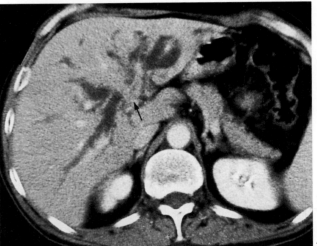
14b

Fig. 12-14a, b. Klatskin's tumor. At the level of the hepatic bifurcation, a circumscribed lesion is seen (→). It diffusely extends cranially through the left lobe of the liver (►), thereby leading to constriction and regional dilatation of the bile ducts. The attenuation value is more or less equal to that of the enhanced liver.

hancement is seen in the center of the tumor in the late contrast phase.

Differential diagnosis: In extensive processes, these lesions are no longer distinguishable from metastatic lymphomas of the porta hepatis, malignant lymphomas, or carcinomas of the pancreatic head.

Choledochal Cysts

Like choledochal diverticula and choledochoceles, the choledochal cyst is a congenital ano-

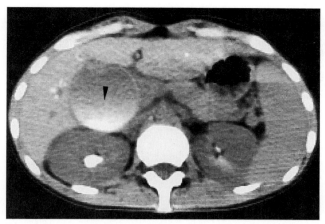

Fig. 12-15. Choledochal cyst. This cystic, thick-walled mass in the region of the porta hepatitis enhances after administration of biliary contrast medium. Stratification and sedimentation phenomena are detected (▸).

Fig. 12-16a, b. Caroli's disease. Generalized dilatation of the bile ducts extends into the periphery of the liver (→) in a young adult male with no signs of biliary obstruction. Near the porta hepatis, slightly saccular areas of dilatation are seen (▸). Pericholangitic abscess formation is a typical complication (▹).

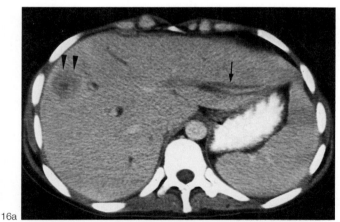

16a

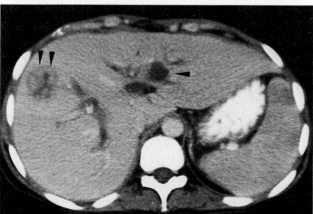

16b

maly that causes focal dilatation of the common bile duct. The location of these cysts is usually supraduodenal, and walls show fibrous thickening. Since they cause compression and displacement, choledochal cysts are usually discovered in childhood and adolescent years.

• CT

The CT findings are those of a thick-walled cyst that enhances after intravenous administration of biliary contrast medium. Choledochal cysts can become as large as 10 cm.

Caroli's Disease

Caroli's disease is a congenital abnormality of the biliary tract that usually presents with cystic renal transformation (medullary sponge kidney). This disease is a type of communicating cavernous ectasis of the biliary tract. It causes saccular dilatations which often lead to the development of intrahepatic calculi or cholangitis. Another type that presents with cirrhosis and portal hypertension causes proliferation of dilated terminal bile ducts. Central biliary tract dilatation, cholelithiasis and cholangitis, on the other hand, do not occur. Clinical symptoms usually manifest in childhood or adolescence.

• CT

Multiple saccular dilatations of bile ducts can usually be demonstrated as (normally focal) sharply marginated, polycyclic or fusiform areas of hypodensity. They are often bunched together. These hypodense ductal dilatations form a cuff around normal-caliber branches of the portal vein. This is a typical sign that can be seen when vascular contrast enhancement occurs after a bolus of contrast medium. Gallstones can be seen only if they are calcified. In doubtful cases, biliary contrast media can clarify whether the calculi belong to the biliary system by contrasting the hypodense zones. When cystic renal changes are detected in children or adolescent patients with cirrhosis and portal hypertension, the possibility of Caroli's disease should be considered.

Chapter 13
The Pancreas

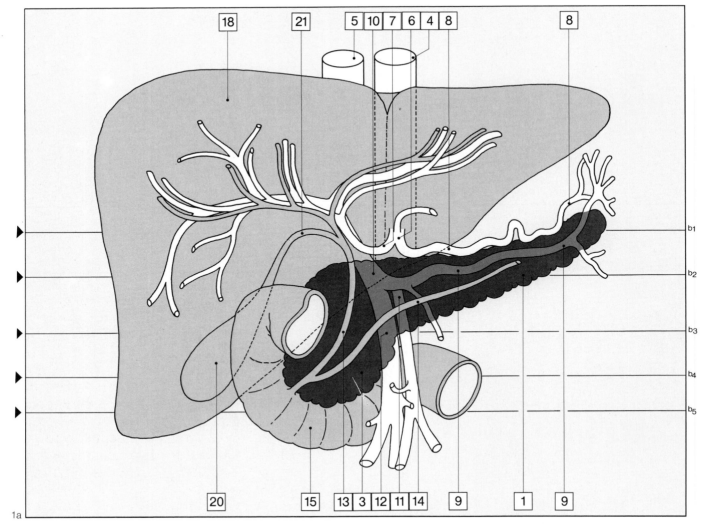

1a

Key to symbols:

1 Tail of pancreas
2 Body of pancreas
3 Head of pancreas (uncinate process)
4 Abdominal aorta
5 Inferior vena cava
6 Celiac trunk
7 Hepatic artery
8 Splenic artery
9 Splenic vein
10 Portal vein
11 Sup. mesenteric artery
12 Sup. mesenteric vein
13 Bile duct
14 Pancreatic duct
15 Duodenum
16 Stomach
17 Spleen
18 Liver
19 Small and large intestine
20 Gallbladder
21 Cystic duct
22 Kidney
23 Renal artery
24 Renal vein
25 Parathyroid gland

Fig. 13-1. Topography of the pancreas.
a) Anterior view of situs.
b) Transverse sections; for level see a).

c) Pancreatic parenchyma after contrast medium administration. Homogeneous enhancement after bolus contrast medium injection.

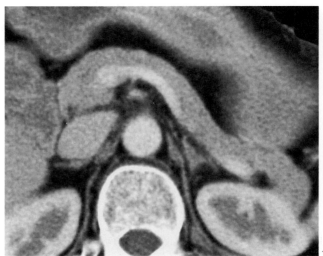

1c

1b₁

1b₂

1b₃

1b₄

1b₅

The Pancreas

Anatomy and Imaging

The weight and length of the adult pancreas range from 60 to 100 g and 12 to 15 cm, respectively. On CT scans, the pancreas slopes slightly upward from the splenic hilum, crossing the abdominal aorta and vena cava, extending to the right. Therefore, the pancreas can be demonstrated on CT scans only in horizontal sections.

A pad of surrounding fat clearly defines the *margins of the pancreas*, which are smooth in adolescents, but become lobulated with increasing age or obesity as more fat accumulates. The surrounding fat is absent in thin or emaciated patients and children, and intravenous contrast medium (CM) must then be administered to demarcate the pancreatic borders. The internal structure of pancreatic tissue is also affected by the patient's constitution and age. The texture of pancreatic parenchyma in older or obese patients is uniformly inhomogeneous as compared with adolescent patients. The *configuration* of the pancreas is quite variable, though the diameter generally decreases from the pancreatic head to the tail. Minimal fluctuations in caliber are normal and may simulate abnormalities on different sectional planes of a curved organ. Clear physiological narrowing of the pancreas (the neck) is found anterior to the superior mesenteric vein and artery. Embedded in the lower curve of the duodenum, the *uncinate process* forms the lower prolongation of the pancreatic head, which appears as a beaklike structure on cross-sectional scans. The uncinate process lies behind the superior mesenteric vein, which molds the contours of the process. The borders of the superior mesenteric vein are not clearly demarcated by fat. Depending on the parenchymal density, the borders of the vein may therefore be masked on plain scans. In contrast, a layer of fat normally clearly demarcates the dorsal contour of the head of the pancreas from the inferior vena cava.

The *main pancreatic duct* (duct of Wirsung) extends along the center of the tail and body of the pancreas. In the pancreatic head, the configuration of the main pancreatic duct and accessory duct (duct of Santorini) is variable. The main pancreatic duct, the diameter of which ranges from 1 to 3 mm, unites with the common bile duct in the prepyloric region. The pancreatic duct, which also must be imaged in sections, is seldom or just barely visible on thin-section plain scans (3 to 5 mm sections). An intravenous bolus of contrast medium is necessary and close examination required to identify the pancreatic duct on CT scans. A dilated pancreatic duct exceeding 5 mm in diameter can sometimes be visualized on plain scans as linear streaks of hypodensity. The layer of fat between the splenic vein and parenchymal border often runs a parallel course, thus simulating dilatation of the pancreatic duct (false duct). A good knowledge of vascular anatomy can therefore prevent this interpretive error.

Proper evaluation of *neighboring structures* is an essential prerequisite for correct image analysis. Even in the thinnest patients, the superior mesenteric artery is an easily identifiable landmark for locating the body of the pancreas, which lies in front of the vessel. The splenic vein normally passes along the posterior border of the pancreas, extending to the splenic hilum, but it can sometimes be encased in pancreatic tissue. Dorsal displacement of the splenic vein may indicate an intrapancreatic process, while ventral displacement is an indicator of retropancreatic lesions (adrenal, renal, para-aortic). The splenic artery, on the other hand, usually curves along the upper surface of the pancreas and therefore can be demonstrated only in several portions. Neither the superior mesenteric vein nor the portal vein is demarcated from the pancreatic parenchyma by fatty tissue, so their visibility on plain scans will vary in accordance with parenchymal structure. They become distinctly visible, however, when fatty deposits build up (pancreatic lipomatosis). Changes in wall structure, caliber, and branches of vessels (duodenojejunal artery) can be demonstrated after bolus injection of contrast medium. The left renal vein extends along the upper contours of the infe-

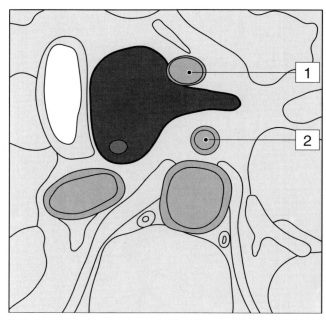

Fig. 13-2. Uncinate process. Beaklike configuration; that of the dorsal contour is ventroconvex. The superior mesenteric artery (2) is surrounded by fatty tissue, but not the superior mesenteric vein (1).

Fig. 13-3a, b. Physiological fatty infiltration of the pancreas. Interlobar fatty infiltration occurs with increasing age. This leads to increased lobulation and inhomogeneity of pancreatic tissue.

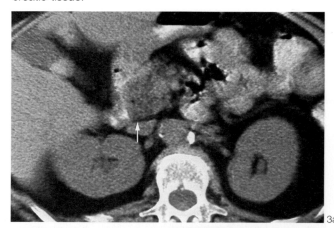

3a

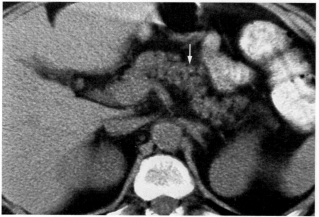

3b

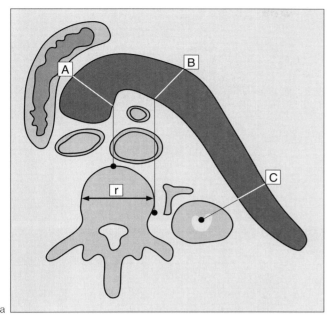

4a

Fig. 13-4a, b. Dimensions of the pancreas. As a rule, the transverse diameter of the pancreas, from head to tail, decreases in each individual. Individual variation can be evaluated by comparison with a reference structure, i.e., vertebral body (r). The pancreatic dimensions have been shown to be greatly age- dependent (compiled from data by von Heuck et al., ref. 1403).

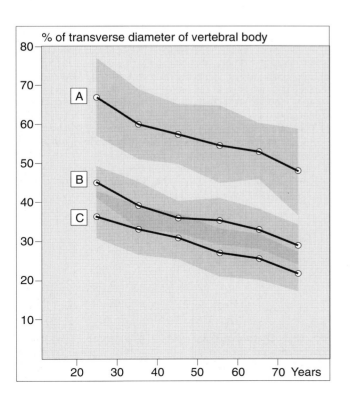

rior part of the duodenum and unites with the inferior vena cava behind the head of the pancreas. The duodenum itself, which molds the lateral and caudal contours of the head of the pancreas, must be completely opacified with oral contrast medium. Only then can the caudal boundary of the uncinate process be distinguished from the inferior part of the duodenum, which extends behind both the superior mesenteric artery and vein. Especially in very thin patients, the tail of the pancreas cannot be clearly distinguished from the proximal jejunum convolution without oral contrast medium. These structures may mimic a mass lesion.

In the arterial phase after *intravenous bolus injection of contrast medium*, there is homogeneous enhancement of pancreatic parenchyma, which demonstrates, on the whole, a homogeneous granular pattern of internal structure. Since the embedded or surrounding larger vessels are opacified as compared with unenhanced fluid within the pancreatic duct, the general conspicuity of the pancreas is improved. A rapid scanning sequence (e.g. spiral CT) must be used to fully demonstrate the entire organ during maximum enhancement.

The *dimensions* of the pancreas are measured vertical to its axes. The orientational values for the antero-posterior diameter of the head and tail of the pancreas are 2.5 and 1.5 cm, respectively. Pancreatic size is clearly age-related. Individual variation can be reduced by comparing pancreatic size with the transverse diameter of the vertebrae. The pancreas can be easily displaced towards the retroperitoneum, which means that pancreatic configuration and size may changes when the patient is placed in a right lateral position. The body and tail of the pancreas are thus extended, providing a better overview of the organ. Thus, the relative amount of displacement of the pancreatic borders towards adjacent organs can also be used as a diagnostic aid.

A *divided pancreas* (pancreaticum divisum) occurs in ca. 5 to 10% of the population when the dorsal and ventral buds of the pancreas do not fuse. Generally, the pancreatic head ap-

pears swollen. Sometimes a thin, almost coronal recession or interface is seen. Regressive
abnormalities on both sides of the pancreas can
cause further demarcation.

Cystic Pancreatic Diseases

Dysontogenetic Cyst

The dysontogenetic cyst is a type of hamartoma that frequently occurs with multiple renal
and kidney cysts and occasionally is associated
with cerebellar angioma and encephalocele.

• CT

Several large, delicately walled, water-filled
spaces of various sizes are found on CT scans;
they have the CT appearance of benign
cysts.

Retention Cysts and Pseudocysts

Around 20 to 25% of patients with inflammatory pancreatic disease, especially chronic pancreatitis, develop retention cysts and/or pseudocysts.

A *retention cyst* arises from stenosis or obstruction of the pancreatic duct; its initial location is
thus intrapancreatic.

Pseudocysts develop after necrosis of pancreatic parenchyma, which first becomes demarcated by granulation tissue. Fibrosis of

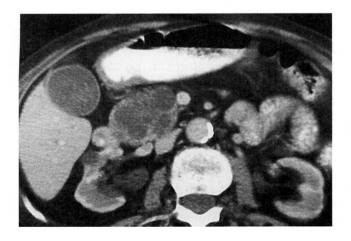

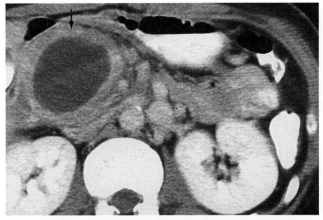

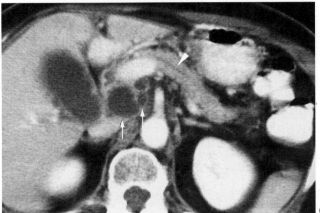

Fig. 13-6a-f. Pancreatic pseudocysts.
a) Large, sharply marginated pseudocyst (→) in the head of the
pancreas; the inner walls become slightly enhanced. Its homogeneous attenuation value is slightly above that of water.
b) Small pseudocysts (→) which also have attenuation values
in the water range. The cyst walls become clearly enhanced.
Pancreatic duct (►).
c) False cysts with considerable wall calcification (►) and
slightly raised, homogeneous attenuation values.
d) Large pseudocyst in the superior recess (→) of the omental
bursa. The walls are discretely enhanced and, therefore,
sharply demarcated from the homogeneous, water-dense
contents.
e) This pseudocyst is atypically located in the porta hepatis
(→), which is therefore dilated. The configuration of the cyst is
predetermined by the shape of the space.
f) Hemorrhage in a pancreatic pseudocyst. Vascular erosion
led to the development of the hematoma-like lesion that can be
identified on the basis of its increased attenuation value.

Fig. 13-5. Dysontogenic cysts. These cysts found in the
head of the pancreas have a mulberry-like configuration, are
hypodense and have delicate walls. Their CT number is slightly
above that of water.

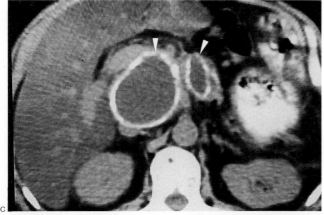

6c

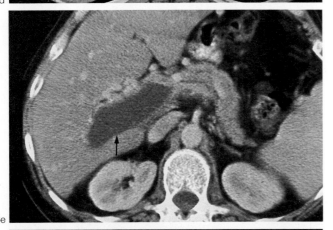

6d

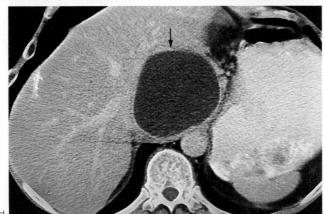

6e

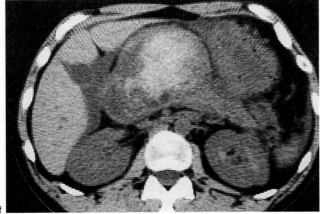

6f

older lesions occurs, thereby coarsening the walls, which then adhere to surrounding tissue. The contents of the cyst may have a liquid or gelatinous consistency; if blood has entered, the contents may be colored brown. Cysts sometimes develop due to exudation of fluid from the peritoneum into the omental bursa. These fluid collections are not pseudocysts in the true sense, because they occupy a pre-existing (encapsulated) space.

Pseudocysts more often develop in the pancreatic head than tail and, as their size increases, tend to involve the omental bursa. Spreading to the porta hepatis, perirenal space, or mediastinum is less common. In acute pancreatitis, pseudocysts may develop in the zone of exudation (necrotic route). Pseudocysts are sometimes found in intramural locations of the intestinal wall. Superinfection of a pseudocyst gives rise to abscess, and erosion of intracystic vessels may give rise to an arterial pseudoaneurysm.

• CT

Retention cysts and pseudocysts display the CT appearance of hypodense, relatively smoothly demarcated cyst-like masses, the walls of which are usually thickened (maximum of several centimeters). These cysts are of water *attenuation*. CT numbers rise significantly when recent necrosis and hemorrhage exists, making it hard to distinguish the zone of liquefaction from the pancreatic parenchyma. A bolus contrast medium injection will then be necessary to demarcate the necrotic zone (which does not take up any contrast medium) from pancreatic tissue or granulation tissue. *Partial or ringlike calcification* is frequently seen on CT scans. Spots of hyperdensity within the cyst are indicative of hemorrhage.

A *traumatic* pseudocyst arises from intrapancreatic hematoma, which is often accompanied by pancreatitis. In the early stage of disease, it appears on CT scans as a slightly hyperdense or isodense mass. Within the first few weeks after development, the attenuation of these cysts will decrease.

Differential diagnosis: Due to the varied morphology of pseudocysts, the entire spectrum of other cystic masses that may occur in or near the pancreas must be considered in the differential diagnosis.

Pancreatic Tumors

Microcystic Adenoma

This benign neoplasm, which was formerly classified as serous cystadenoma, develops preferentially in men and women over the age of sixty. When discovered, microcystic adenomas are normally around 5 cm in size, but can become much larger. A microcystic adenoma is composed of very small cysts with hypervascularized septa. A macroscopically solid appearance can result. Malignancy of these neoplasms has not been reported.

• CT

Plain scans: According to the tissue composition of the microcystic adenoma, the conglomerate of small cysts may display a honeycomb appearance or may have a more solid appearance if the cysts are beyond the limits of resolution. Radial calcification with a central area of cicatrization is frequently observed.

Contrast-enhanced scans: Rich enhancement occurs after a bolus injection of contrast medium, especially in the areas of septation.

Differential diagnosis: Islet cell tumors must be excluded from the differential diagnosis.

Macrocystic Adenoma

This benign tumor was previously known as mucinous cystic tumor and occurs primarily in women between the ages of 40 and 60. Macrocystic adenomas are located almost exclusively in the pancreatic tail or body and have usually already become large masses when they are discovered. In contrast to the microcystic adenoma, these tumors may transform into a malignant one and should be surgically removed.

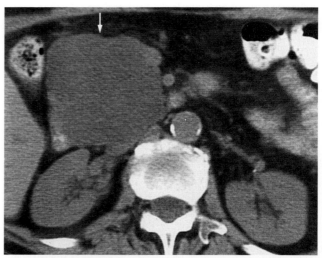

7a

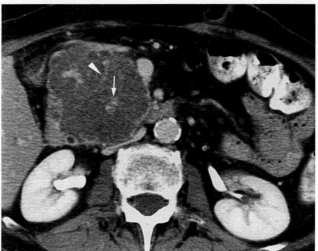

7b

Fig. 13-7. Microcystic adenoma. This large mass measures 6 x 7 cm. It appears hypodense in plain scans, but clear septal structures (b►) with highly vascularized centers (b→) can be seen after contrast medium administration.

Fig. 13-8. Microcystic adenoma. Typical configuration with multiple cysts; these have central areas of calcification.

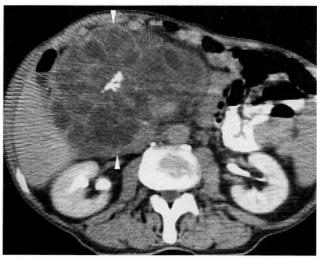

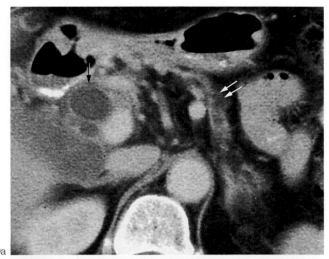

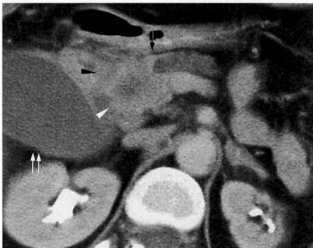

Fig. 13-9. Carcinoma in head of the pancreas. The slightly enlarged head of the pancreas (b, c ►) becomes increasingly indistinct in cranial regions; it encases the superior mesenteric vein (c→). The pancreatic duct breaks off abruptly (b→), and the proceeding pancreatic organs are atrophied (a ⇉). The supraduodenal choledochus is considerably dilated (a→) and the gallbladder is enlarged (b ⇉). Clear enlargement of regional lymph nodes could not be demonstrated.

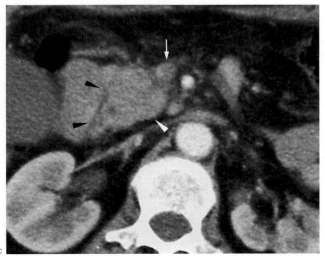

• CT

Plain scans: Macrocystic adenoma appears on plain scans as a large, multilocular cyst or a conglomerate of cysts that is significantly larger than 2 cm. The septa of macrocystic adenoma may be calcified and are normally thicker than the septa of microcystic adenoma. If these septal signs are absent, the macrocystic adenoma may mimic a pseudocyst.

Contrast-enhanced scans: After administration of contrast medium, macrocystic adenomas are characterized by their distinct, hypervascularized septa.

Pancreatic Carcinoma

The incidence of pancreatic carcinoma is rising, and it currently accounts for ca. 5% of all carcinomas in humans. Since the majority of pancreatic carcinomas (60%) are found in the pancreatic head, clinical abnormalities arise from obstruction of the bile duct. Of the 20% of pancreatic tumors located in the body-tail region, most are discovered too late for curative treatment. The remaining 20% affect the entire pancreas. The most frequent histological finding is a variably differentiated, hypovascularized adenocarcinoma; anaplastic forms are rare. Regional dissemination occurs early, following the routes of the perineural and peripancreatic lymph tracts into the periaortic, gastric and portal lymph nodes and, later, the mediastinal lymph nodes. Hematogenous dissemination of the tumor first affects the liver and lungs, then the bone and adrenal glands. Direct invasion of adjacent organs (stomach, colon, spleen and liver) occurs in advanced stages of the disease.

In order to diagnose pancreatic carcinoma at a resectable stage, a painstaking clinical examination and good ultrasound images are needed in addition to a detailed CT examination. When results are even slightly questionable, an additional endoscopic retrograde cholangiopancreatography (ERCP) must be performed.

• CT

A circumscribed *mass* is the primary sign, but not an early sign, of pancreatic carcinoma. Normal pancreatic dimensions described here are only a rough orientational guideline, so all aspects of the organ must be evaluated. An increase in caliber and inharmonious organ configuration are unreliable indicators of pancreatic carcinoma that may be evident on plain scans; an intravenous bolus of contrast medium is needed for further diagnosis. If the margins of the pancreas remain indistinct after *intravenous contrast administration*, the patient should be placed in a lateral position or, if necessary, given a dose of oral contrast medium. In particular, any round enlargement of the uncinate process must be carefully evaluated.

On unenhanced scans, the *attenuation* of the tumor tissue is generally equal to that of healthy parenchyma. In the presence of interlobular fatty infiltration, especially pancreatic lipomatosis, masses with nondeformed contours can be identified on the basis of their relative hyperdensity. After a bolus of contrast medium, hypodense tumor tissue can be distinguished from the opacified pancreatic parenchyma in the early bolus phase. Any additional contour deformity deepens the suspicion of carcinoma. Since 10% of all patients with carcinoma have accompanying pancreatitis (possibly with pseudocysts), any structural inhomogeneity including pseudocysts should be critically evaluated, even if only one section of the pancreas is affected.

Intrapancreatic infiltration often has to be deduced from dilatation of the *pancreatic duct* or

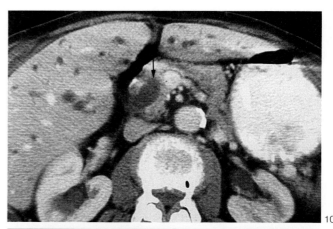

10a

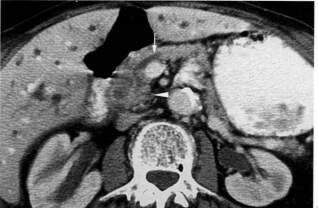

10b

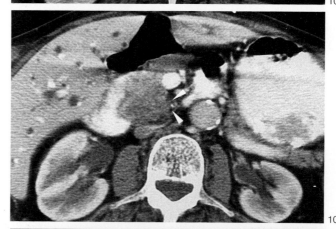

10c

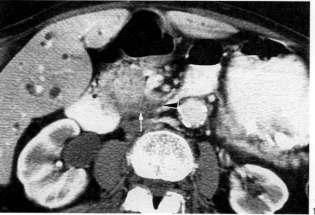

10d

Fig. 13-10. Carcinoma in head of the pancreas. The head of the pancreas is enlarged with a slightly hypodense central area (c) as well as slight unsharpness of its dorsal borders (d→). Tiny, archlike mural contours in the mediodorsal region of the dilated uncinate process (b,c,d ►). Very slight enlargement of peripancreatic lymph nodes is suspected. Dilatation of the pancreatic duct (b→) and considerable enlargement of the supraduodenal portion of the bile duct (a→) are signs of prepapillary encasement of the biliary system, which later was clearly documented by ERCP.

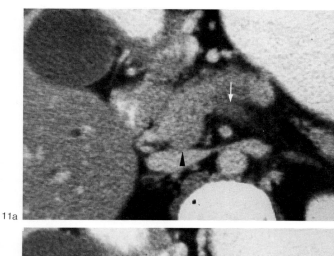

11a

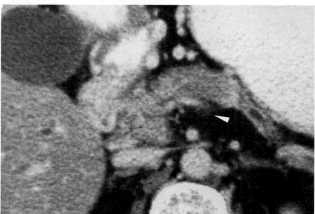

11b

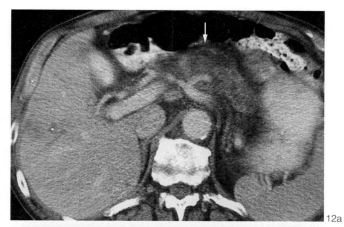

12a

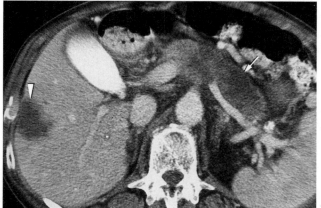

12b

Fig. 13-11. Carcinoma in head of the pancreas. The pancreatic head is altogether enlarged (c). Medially, a slightly indistinct projection surrounds the superior mesenteric vein (→), which does not become enhanced. Besides having two ramifications, very discrete nodular structures can be seen along the margins of the head (►). Angiography confirmed that this tumor was not resectable.

Fig. 13-12. Carcinoma in body of the pancreas. After contrast medium administration, the tumor is demarcated as a hypodense zone in the pancreatic head/tail region (b→). In cranial sections, there is encasement of the celiac trunk (a→). Metastases are demonstrated in the lymph nodes (c→) and liver (b►).

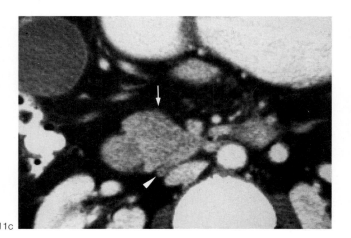

11c

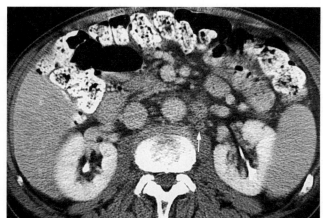

12c

common bile duct. An abrupt increase in caliber in one or both ductal systems is critically indicative of malignancy. A smooth or bead-like CT appearance of duct walls is indicative of tumor. Irregular, distorted ductal contours must be critically evaluated when further signs of chronic pancreatitis are absent. After *intravenous contrast enhancement*, dilatation of the biliary tract becomes clearly visible and the contours of the pancreatic duct can be better evaluated.

Peripancreatic infiltration initially causes localized strands of poor definition along the borders of the mass, which makes it difficult to diagnose minor degrees of infiltration in thin patients. Masking of the cuff of fat around the superior mesenteric artery is an important sign. A targeted bolus injection is then required to demonstrate the mantle-like zones of *encasement* associated with constriction of the lumen – an indication that the tumor is no longer resectable. Masking in the regions of the superior mesenteric vein, portal vein, inferior vena cava and abdominal aorta has the same diagnostic significance. In individual cases, it may help to place the patient in a lateral position to better diagnose infiltration into adjacent organs on the basis of relative pancreatic displacement with respect to those structures.

Secondary signs like regional metastases, hepatic metastases, or (malignant) ascites consolidate the diagnosis of malignancy. In most cases, these signs indicate inoperability of the tumor.

The tumor is considered *resectable* when peripancreatic infiltration, vascular encasement, and all secondary signs are absent. The bed of the uncinate process should be carefully examined after *pancreatectomy*, since new growths, i.e. lymph node metastases, preferentially occur there.

Differential diagnosis: The *solid epithelial neoplasm* (very rare, and occurring almost exclusively in women under 30) is a hypovascularized, expansively spreading tumor of low malignancy. It normally displays cystic degeneration arising from hemorrhagic necrosis.

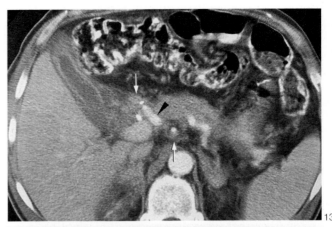

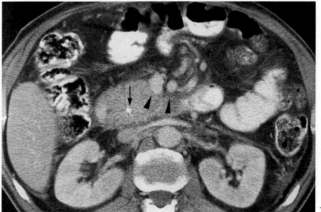

Fig. 13-13. Carcinoma in head of the pancreas. In the enlarged head, the endoprosthesis can be seen as a central punctiform, hyperdense structure (b→). From the medial aspect, the mass is indistinctly demarcated and causes involvement of mesenteric vessels (b►). Encasement of the hepatic and mesenteric arteries (a►) and lymph nodes in the region of the hepatoduodenal ligament (a→) was demonstrated. The wall of the gallbladder is thickened as in chronic cholecystitis.

Fig. 13-14. Carcinoma in body of the pancreas. CT revealed compact lymph node conglomerates (→) along the celiac trunk (►), an indication of non-resectability.

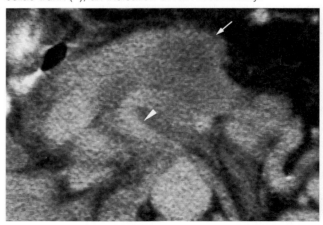

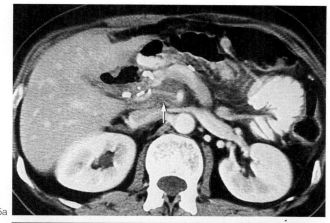

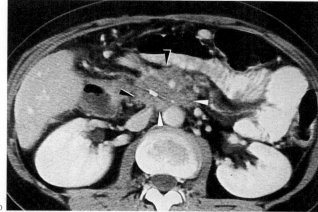

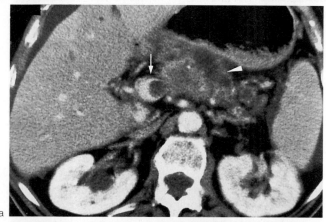

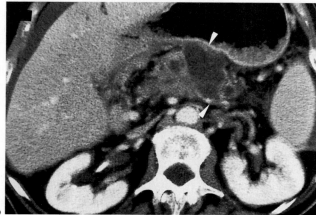

This neoplasm can be diagnostically differentiated from other solid and cystic pancreatic masses when the tumor has a large volume but no metastases, a low degree of contrast enhancement and irregular cysts showing no septation.

In patients with localized pancreatic (head) dilatation with regional lymph node enlargement, the possibility of *metastatic spread* from other tumors (e.g. seminomas) or *malignant and benign lymphomas* (including plasmocytomas, Castleman's disease) must be excluded. The lymphoma conglomerate may align with the pancreatic head in such a way that simulates a mass lesion. Malignant lymphomas displace the pancreas in such a way that, after contrast administration, the pancreas is deformed, but the pancreatic dimensions remain normal.

Cystadenocarcinoma

The rare cystadenocarcinoma occurs preferentially in the tail of the pancreas. Upon macroscopic examination, its appearance resembles that of its benign variant, the macrocystic adenoma. The malignancy of the cystadenocarcinoma manifests via the formation of metastases and infiltration of surrounding tissue.

• CT

Plain scans: More solid components with poor vascularization are found on CT scans in addition to the usual signs of macrocystic adenoma. Regional lymph node enlargement must be found to confirm the diagnosis of malignancy.

Fig. 13-15. Recurrence of a carcinoma in the head of the pancreas. Only 6 months after pancreatectomy, a soft-tissue formation was found in the former site of the head of the pancreas (b ►). This extends with the vessels into the porta hepatis (a→). Metal clips make it more difficult to evaluate the situation.

Fig. 13-16. Cystadenocarcinoma of the pancreas. After contrast medium administration, hypodense zones are marked off inside the tumor (►), which polycyclically protrudes into retroperitoneal tissue and has also infiltrated the portal vein (a→). In surrounding areas, small, nodular structures corresponding to enlarged lymph nodes can be seen.

Contrast-enhanced scans: Contrast medium must be administered to demonstrate hypervascularized septa and, more commonly, hypovascularized tumor sections, and to evaluate surrounding structures.

Islet Cell Tumors

Insulin-secreting (B cell) insulomas account for up to 80% of all pancreatic islet cell tumors; they are localized in the body-tail region of the pancreas in up to 60% of cases. The remaining islet cell neoplasms are found in the head-body region and may secrete glucagon (A cells), gastrin (Zollinger-Ellison syndrome) or serotonin (Verner-Morrison syndrome). Around three-quarters of all islet cell tumors are hormonally active (secretory). Multiple growths are found in 10 to 15% of cases, and the tumors generally have a size of 1 to 2 cm. The condition normally manifests in the 3rd to 6th decade of life.

Ca. 10% of all insulomas transform, while the rate of malignant transformation of gastrinomas is significantly higher (ca. 60%). *Malignant* types tend to be hormonally nonfunctional and are diagnosed late. They therefore may reach a size of up to 25 cm and metastasize in regional lymph nodes and the liver before they are discovered. As regards malignancy, the histology of the tumor is of less significance than tumor infiltration. With very few exceptions, almost all islet cell tumors are highly vascularized, regardless of their hormonal activity and malignancy.

• CT

Plain scans: These normally large *malignant tumors* cause a corresponding deformation of the pancreas. Calcification is seen in ca. 20% of all islet cell tumors. Vascular structures are rarely encased in tumor tissue.

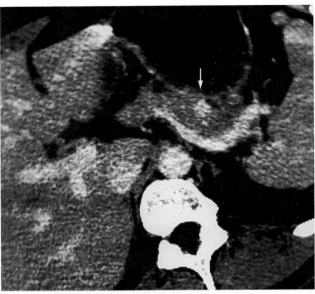

Fig. 13-17. Insulinoma. This tumor, measuring just 1 cm, can be demonstrated only in a certain, short period of the arterial bolus phase. It is then visible as a hyperdense region (→).

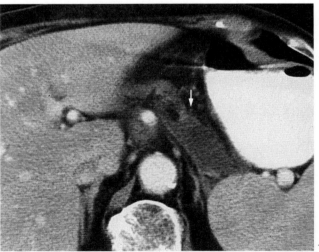

18a

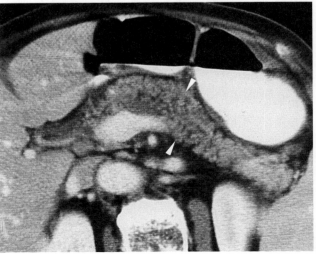

18b

Fig. 13-18. Edematous pancreatitis. Lobulation of pancreatic structures is the earliest detectable sign, since fatty tissue is masked (▸). In this case, there is additional accumulation of fluids in the region of the omental bursa (a→).

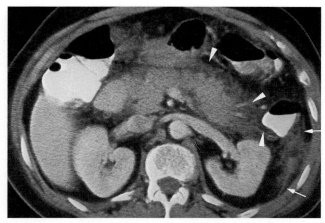

Fig. 13-19. Edematous pancreatitis. Overall dilatation of the organ with unsharpness of contour of direct peripancreatic fat (►) and fascial thickening (→).

Fig. 13-20. Edematous pancreatitis. Small peripancreatic edemas can be identified due to the unsharpness of pancreatic contour and slight thickening of the retroperitoneal fasciae and mesenteric structures (►). In many cases, these thickened structures are the only identifiable remnant of past pancreatitis.

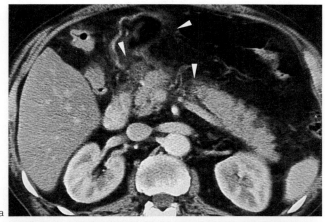

20a

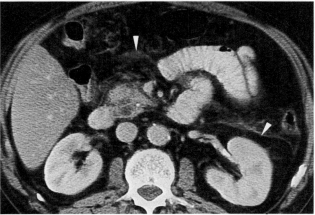

20b

Contrast-enhanced scans: Because of their isodensity, *small, hormonally active islet cell tumors* are rarely demonstrable on plain scans. When clinical abnormalities have been diagnosed, multiple targeted scans, each after a bolus of contrast medium, must be obtained before all portions of pancreatic parenchyma can be evaluated in thin sections. When this technique is used, islet cell tumors are demonstrated in the early bolus phase as circumscribed, irregular hyperdense zones. Because of their high degree of vascularization, centralized necrosis is relatively infrequent in the larger mass lesions. Lymph node and liver metastases are indicative of malignancy. These hypervascularized lesions appear as hyperdense areas on bolus contrast medium scans.

Secondary Tumors

Distant metastases are occasionally diagnosed in the pancreas. They may arise from primary tumors of the lung, breast, thyroid, liver, ovary and testis or malignant melanomas. The pancreas is normally affected by advanced tumors in adjacent organs (stomach, colon, kidney). Malignant lymphomas may infiltrate the pancreas, but rarely occur as isolated mass lesions.

• CT

Plain scans: When they occur as isolated mass lesions, secondary tumors cannot be differentiated from primary pancreatic neoplasms.

Contrast-enhanced scans: Since they are poorly vascularized, metastases can be differentiated from enhanced parenchymal tissue after a targeted bolus injection of contrast medium.

Differential diagnosis: A probable diagnosis can often be made when there is evidence of other metastases, when the pattern of spread and, in some cases, the type of primary tumor is known.

Pancreatitis

Acute Pancreatitis

While the cause of acute pancreatitis remains unknown in about one quarter of all cases, the presence of gallstones shows the most frequent association with acute pancreatitis, followed by alcohol-related problems. A clinical distinction is made between acute and acute relapsing types. During healing, both types cause a medium-term decrease in pancreatic function, but rarely lead to pancreatic atrophy. These types do not evolve into chronic pancreatitis.

Pathological and anatomical distinctions are made between edematous (interstitial) pancreatitis and hemorrhagic (necrotizing) pancreatitis. The severity of the clinical picture is determined by the extent of necrosis, which can cover the greatly enlarged organ or entire parts of an organ like a mantle. Both forms are accompanied by various amounts of exudative fluid, which can permeate into the retroperitoneal space and become encapsulated there.

Infection from necrosis or exudate (suppuration) leads to complications. The amount of serous or hemorrhagic ascites varies. Since CT is able to demonstrate the majority of these lesions, it is possible to make a prognosis on the basis of CT findings.

• CT

Plain scans: One of the leading CT signs of acute pancreatitis is excessive swelling of the

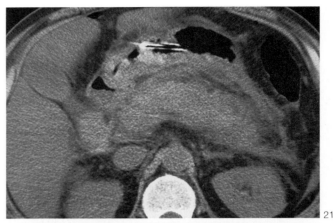

21a

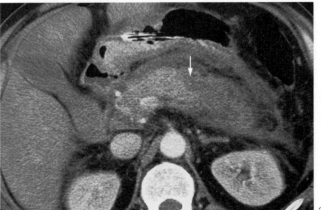

21b

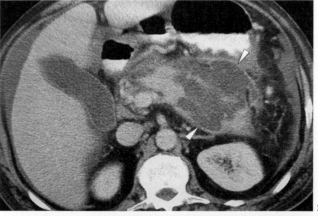

21c

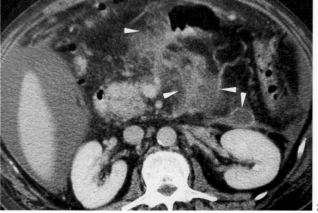

21d

Fig. 13-21. Hemorrhagic, necrotic pancreatitis. When the condition is acute, the pancreas displays an inhomogeneous increase in attenuation value, with CT numbers slightly higher than those of the kidney. It is, at the same time, dilated and indistinctly delineated from the surroundings (a). After contrast medium administration, an attenuation defect can be seen in the region of the body-to-tail junction; this corresponds to a local reduction in blood flow or beginning necrosis (b→). 14 days later, one can see parenchymal loss in conjunction with organ dilatation (c ►). Viable pancreatic tissue now displays better circulation and is therefore more clearly demarcated. An additional finding is encapsulated exudation (d ►) in the following regions: anterior pararenal space, mesenteric root, and anterior renal fascia. Considerable amount of ascitic fluid.

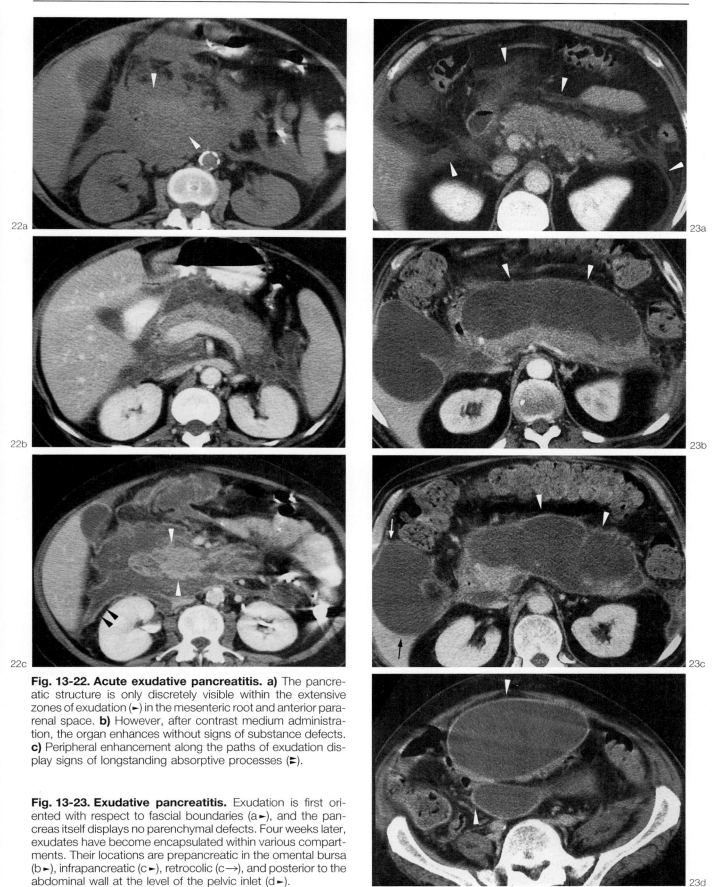

Fig. 13-22. Acute exudative pancreatitis. a) The pancreatic structure is only discretely visible within the extensive zones of exudation (▸) in the mesenteric root and anterior pararenal space. **b)** However, after contrast medium administration, the organ enhances without signs of substance defects. **c)** Peripheral enhancement along the paths of exudation display signs of longstanding absorptive processes (▸).

Fig. 13-23. Exudative pancreatitis. Exudation is first oriented with respect to fascial boundaries (a ▸), and the pancreas itself displays no parenchymal defects. Four weeks later, exudates have become encapsulated within various compartments. Their locations are prepancreatic in the omental bursa (b ▸), infrapancreatic (c ▸), retrocolic (c →), and posterior to the abdominal wall at the level of the pelvic inlet (d ▸).

pancreas. In acute pancreatitis, the pancreas is usually surrounded by isodense or slightly hypodense exudative zones. The extent to which these zones spread out in the anterior and posterior pararenal space is extremely variable. When acute pancreatitis is accompanied by ascites (even in small amounts), a narrow halo can be found around the lower pole of the lobe of the liver, even in early stages.

Edematous and Serous Exudative Forms

Plain scans: *Edematous* pancreatitis has a favorable prognosis and is characterized by localized or generalized organ enlargement. The organ contours remain identifiable and are often surrounded by a delicate, exudative halo of low density. The density of pancreatic tissue is either slightly reduced or not reduced. Since interlobular fat structures are masked, the organ has a plump appearance. Perirenal fasciae are visible and thickened. Encapsulation, as seen with pseudocysts, does not develop. The edematous form has a tendency for quick regression and may evolve into the *serous-exudative* form. The latter is characterized by great enlargement of the pancreas and collections of hypodense exudate, the regression of which take considerably longer.

Contrast-enhanced scans: A bolus of contrast medium homogeneously enhances the pancreatic parenchyma. There is no evidence of a localized perfusion deficit.

Hemorrhagic Necrotizing Forms

Plain scans: Hemorrhagic necrotizing acute pancreatitis leads to considerable swelling of the pancreas, and the margins of the gland overlap with surrounding exudative or necrotic masses. Since purely hemorrhagic, macroscopically non-necrotizing forms exist, the homogeneity of tissue density must be carefully evaluated. Hemorrhage may cause a local or general increase in the attenuation of the pancreas; however, parenchymal attenuation may be normal, due to density averaging of edemas and hemorrhages. When inhomogeneity exists, necrosis should be suspected. Since the attenuation of exudate is somewhat higher (over 10 – 20 HU), the margins of the pancreas

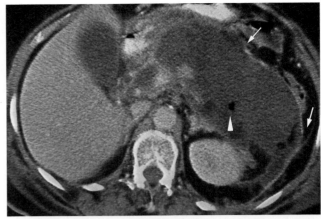

24a

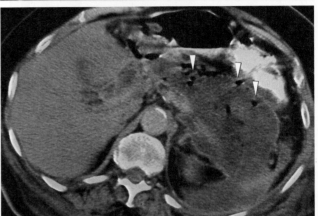

24b

Fig. 13-24. Abscess formation in acute exudative pancreatitis. a) Pancreatitis of several weeks' duration has led to the accumulation of large amounts of encapsulated fluid within the anterior pararenal space. The contrast-enhanced border membranes are still very delicate (→), so the configuration still has not assumed the appearance of a false cyst. A small amount of gas was also found (a ►). **b)** 14 days later, the formation contains numerous small pockets of gas (►), a definite sign of abscess formation.

Fig. 13-25. Past acute pancreatitis. In some places, the pancreas is still masked by exudates and fibrin. Thickening of the absorptive border surfaces (►) is indicative of a long-standing absorptive process.

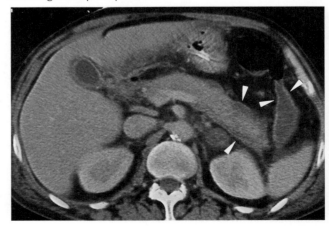

will be less distinct than is the case with serous-exudative types.

Contrast-enhanced scans: In patients with hemorrhagic necrotizing pancreatitis, a bolus of contrast medium facilitates the further diagnosis, since vital, enhanced pancreatic tissue can be clearly differentiated from zones of necrosis and ischemia. Border surfaces of exudative zones (e.g. fasciae and peritoneum) are delicately enhanced in initial stages, but as the disease progresses, these zones become broader and absorb more contrast medium as a result of their increased absorbent activity. After a long course of disease, when increased inhomogeneity is observed within the zones of exudation or especially in the direct vicinity of the pancreas, fibrin sequestration must be suspected.

Spread of Exudation and Complications

In both forms of acute pancreatitis, extrapancreatic *exudative or necrotic spread* occurs in basically the same manner, both of which can exactly demonstrated on CT scans. Exudates normally respect the fascial borders of the anterior pararenal space, the perirenal space and the posterior pararenal space. The initial degree of abnormality in the anterior pararenal space is variable; exudates also occur along the mesenteric root, the paracolic gutter, and the gastrohepatic, gastrosplenic, and gastrocolic ligaments. Involvement of the posterior pararenal space is caused by caudal migration of the renal fascial infundibulum. Because it is shielded by the renal fascia, the perirenal space is usually not affected. However, if the ferment activity of the exudate is strong, the fasciae or peritoneal membranes can become perforated, and the perirenal spaces, the omental bursa and even the mediastinum may become filled with exudate. Absorption of exudate can take several weeks. Fluid inclusions that are not absorbed assume the CT appearance of *pseudocysts* when a wall clearly encloses the absorption tissue. When this encapsulated fluid accumulates in intramural locations in the duodenum, stomach or colon, it may lead to obstruction of the gastrointestinal tract. *Hemorrhage* into the cyst, caused by vascular erosion and pseudoaneurysm, must be suspected when hyperdense areas are found.

Abscess formation is a serious complication (suppurative pancreatitis). Abscesses develop because of superinfection of exudates which become increasingly encapsulated and cystic in appearance. Since it is not possible to distinguish an absorptive border surface from an abscess membrane, only the presence of gas accumulations can provide a clear diagnostic indication of abscess. Communication of the abscess with the gastrointestinal tract must be suspected when extensive fluid fluid levels are observed in cystic formations.

Chronic Pancreatitis

In an etiological sense, chronic pancreatitis is more often caused by alcoholism than biliary disease. 30 to 50% of all cases of chronic pancreatitis calcify (chronic calcifying pancreatitis). A distinction is made between chronic relapsing pancreatitis and progressive (insidious) pancreatitis. Both forms lead to insufficiency of exocrine and endocrine functions. Pathological and anatomical findings indicate a multifocal inflammation which may not necessarily alter the external appearance of the pancreas, even when clinical symptoms are clear. When the disease has a progressive character, fibrous tissue reorganization will cause predominantly perilobular fibrosis. Generalized

Fig. 13-26. Severe ductal dilatation (►) in chronic pancreatitis. Contortion of the duct leads to the development of a honeycomb-like structure.

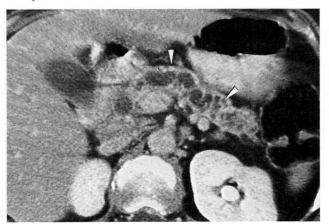

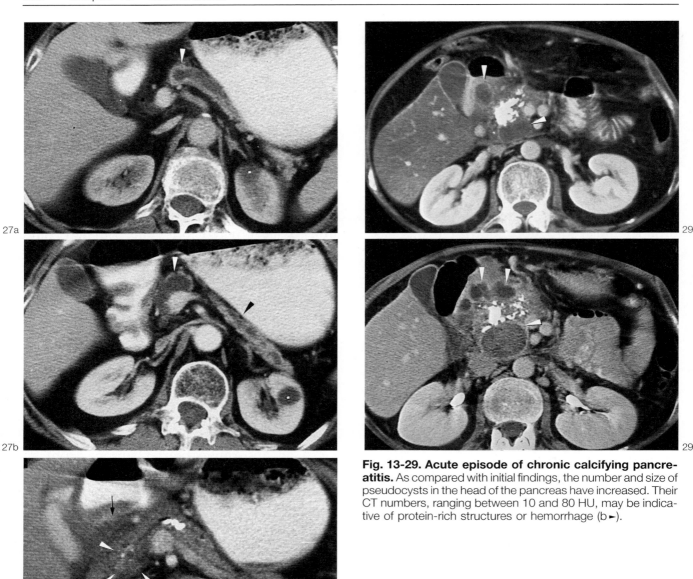

Fig. 13-29. Acute episode of chronic calcifying pancreatitis. As compared with initial findings, the number and size of pseudocysts in the head of the pancreas have increased. Their CT numbers, ranging between 10 and 80 HU, may be indicative of protein-rich structures or hemorrhage (b ►).

Fig. 13-27. Chronic pancreatitis. Almost complete loss of pancreatic tissue, which surrounds the altogether dilated pancreatic duct in a tubelike manner. Calcification was not found.

Fig. 13-28. Chronic pancreatitis. The diameter of the body and tail of the pancreas is only moderately reduced. The slightly dilated main pancreatic duct is just barely visible (►). Findings include fine and course calcification throughout the entire organ. The head of the pancreas appears slightly plump and contains small nodules (►). Its borders with the duodenal wall, which is thickened by inflammation (→), cannot be reliably demarcated.

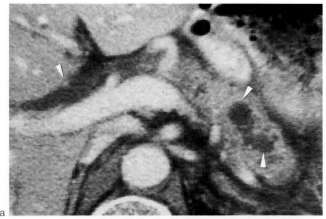

30a

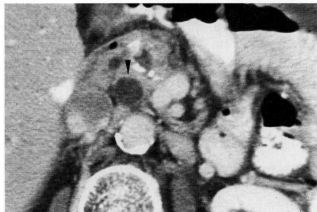

30b

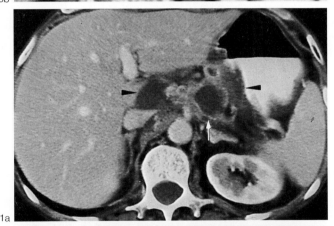

31a

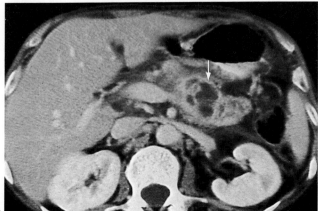

31b

or localized swelling of the pancreas due to underlying sclerolipomatosis and/or dilatation of the pancreatic duct may occur in the further course of disease. Pancreatic atrophy is often observed in the advanced stage of disease.

Dilatation may be caused by stenosis of the pancreatic duct or by traction from the scarred and shrivelled pancreatic parenchyma. Calcification localized mainly in the ductal system occurs more frequently in alcohol-related chronic relapsing pancreatitis (ca. 40%) than in biliary forms (ca. 22%). In the literature, some authors have made a distinction between calcification and true lithiasis. In the latter case, individual, larger calculi are found within the main pancreatic duct. Statistical and clinical observations indicate that chronic pancreatitis is a pathogenic factor for the development of pancreatic carcinoma, which occurs in ca. 2 to 3% of patients with chronic calcifying pancreatitis.

• CT

Plain scans: *Calcification* is the primary diagnostic sign of chronic pancreatitis. Areas of calcification frequently have a linear configuration corresponding with the course of the pancreatic duct.

Pancreatic *atrophy*, the terminal stage of chronic pancreatitis, manifests on CT scans as reduction of the entire organ with sharply demarcated, normally smooth borders. Interestingly, in surgically confirmed cases, enlargement of the pancreas is more commonly found than atrophy. Sometimes the pancreas appears as only a fibrous sheath around the pancreatic duct. Partial atrophy of the tail and body is a frequent result of duct displacement, indicating an underlying malignant process in the head of the pancreas. Obstruction-related

Fig. 13-30. Chronic pancreatitis. The organ is relatively plump with irregular dilatation of the pancreatic duct and common bile duct (▸); calcification can be seen in the head of the pancreas.

Fig. 13-31. Recurrence of chronic pancreatitis. In addition to a conglomerate of pseudocysts, peripancreatic exudation was also found (▸). The organ itself is deformed and, in some places, destroyed due to pseudocyst formations (→).

atrophy of the pancreas can be caused by the replacement of fatty tissue in the pancreatic lobule by interlobular connective tissue (sclerolipomatosis). The transition to pancreatic lipomatosis is smooth.

The diagnosis of chronic pancreatitis can be reliably made when there is evidence of general pancreatic atrophy, which also involves the head of the pancreas, as well as extensive parenchymatous calcification and dilatation of the pancreatic duct.

Pancreatic *swelling* due to a chronic proliferating inflammation normally affects the entire gland, which then has a slightly plump appearance. An isolated mass is occasionally found in the pancreatic head. If the normally sharply demarcated pancreatic margins become ill-defined, an acute inflammation must be suspected (pancreatitis of the pancreatic head).

Lymph node enlargement is observed only in isolated cases.

Contrast-enhanced scans: *Dilatation of the pancreatic duct* can be better demonstrated after administration of contrast medium. Dilatation occurring during chronic pancreatitis may be caused by atrophy or obstruction of the pancreas (calcified and noncalcified calculi, strictures). Because of scarred distortion, the contours of the pancreatic duct are more irregular than in tumor-related obstruction. Dilatation of the suprapancreatic portion of the common bile duct, showing fusiform intrapancreatic constriction, is not an unusual finding associated with the proliferating form of pancreatitis. ERCP is then needed for a detailed evaluation.

Pseudocysts accompany more than 30% of all cases of chronic pancreatitis. Especially after administration of contrast medium, they appear as small, sharply marginated low density zones within the pancreatic tissue. Pseudocysts can reach sizes as large as 15 cm or more. It is not unusual to find them in other epigastric regions, even those distant from the pancreas.

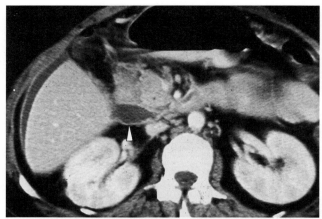

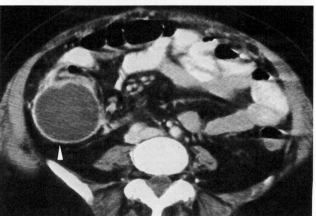

Fig. 13-32. Pseudocysts in chronic pancreatitis. Pseudocysts are often the only visible remnant of a past chronic pancreatitis. Their location is usually peripancreatic, but they can be found in all sections of the abdomen and peritoneum. In this case, a retroduodenal pseudocyst (a ►) was found; it extends caudally and retrocolically (b ►).

Differential diagnosis: In patients with chronic pancreatitis, isolated areas of organ dilatation should be further diagnosed by ERCP.

Pancreatic Abscess

Pancreatic abscess normally occurs due to infection of a pseudocyst (during acute or chronic pancreatitis) and is only seldom caused by an infection infiltrating from an adjacent organ (kidney, colon).

• CT

Plain scans: Neither the configuration nor the attenuation of an infected pseudocyst makes it distinguishable from a noninfected pseudocyst.

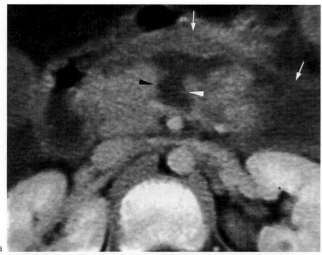

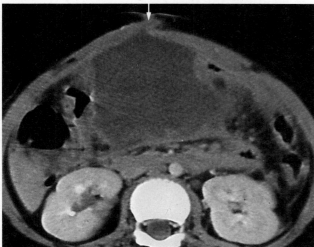

Fig. 13-33. Blunt abdominal trauma. After contrast medium administration, findings include pancreatic rupture and hypodensity in the body of the pancreas (a ►). Additional findings include peripancreatic exudation, i.e., hemorrhage (a→). A pseudocyst has developed 7 days later; it fills the entire upper abdominal space (b→). Six months after implantation of the body of the pancreas into the stomach (c ►), normal structure has returned to the head and body of the pancreas.

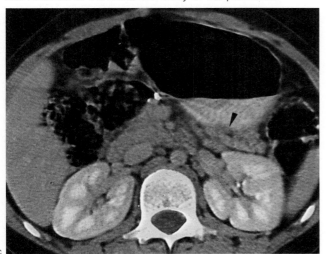

Both appear as an isolated, moderately hypodense mass within and in the vicinity of the pancreas. Gas accumulation is the only pathognomonic distinguishing factor.

Contrast-enhanced scans: The walls of an abscess display border enhancement, but this sign may also be observed in active absorptive processes without infection and is thus not conclusive.

Pancreatic Trauma

The effects of abdominal trauma, especially blunt trauma, manifest primarily in the pancreatic tail, normally in combination with other internal injuries. Distinction is made between contusions, incomplete pancreatic rupture (capsule not ruptured) and complete pancreatic rupture (parenchyma and capsule ruptured, with or without rupture of pancreatic duct).

A traumatic pseudocyst often develops in patients with incomplete pancreatic rupture. Complete ruptures can lead to tail sequestration, pseudocysts, and a fistula with the omental bursa. Depending on how extensive the effects of contusion are, pancreatitis may develop.

• CT

Plain scans: A hematoma which develops after trauma injury can normally be demonstrated on plain scans as an isodense to hyperdense zone which later develops into a hypodense mass. The degree of extension and spreading of the hematoma into the retroperitoneal space can be evaluated by CT. However, this type of traumatic pseudocyst is not distinguishable from inflammatory forms. Edematous pancreatitis with minor amounts of exudate is a common accompaniment.

Contrast-enhanced scans: Contrast medium enhances vital pancreatic tissue, thereby accentuating traumatic parenchymal defects. Furthermore, contrast medium can demarcate pseudocysts and other fluid collections.

Lipomatosis and Atrophy

Lipomatosis is usually an accompanying symptom of generalized adiposity. A further cause of lipomatosis is occlusion of the pancreatic duct. Sections of the pancreatic parenchyma located in the area of occlusion become atrophied and the individual lobules of the gland are replaced by fat. Lipomatous glandular permeation also occurs in the final stage of chronic pancreatitis and is termed sclerolipomatosis because fibrosis accompanies the condition. Late stages of cystic pancreatic fibrosis may also evolve into lipomatosis. *Lipomatous pancreatic atrophy*, which is thought to be of viral etiology, is a rare pancreatic disease occurring in children.

• CT

Plain scans: A lobular parenchymal structure is normally found in the pancreas of obese patients. The individual lobules of the gland are pushed apart by fatty tissue accumulating between them. During the stage of lipomatous atrophy, there is a loose connective tissue matrix, but the original contours of the organ are still distinguishable.

Contrast-enhanced scans: Although lipomatous structures can be easily recognized as areas of low enhancement after the administration of contrast medium, enhancement is not required for diagnosis.

Chapter 14
The Gastrointestinal Tract

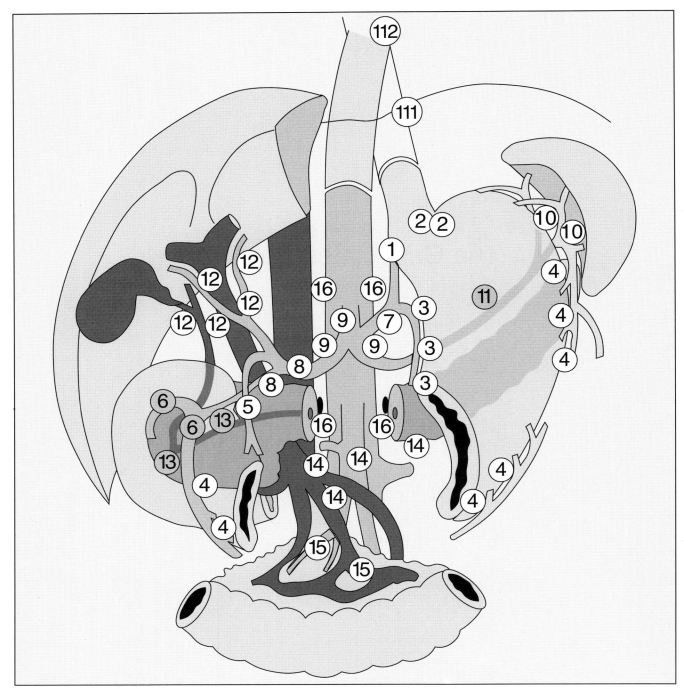

Fig. 14-1. Lymph node stations affected by stomach cancer. (Numeration in accordance with the recommendations of the Japanese Research Society for Gastric Cancer).

Key to symbols:

1 Right cardiac lymph node
2 Left cardiac lymph node
3 Lymph nodes of the lesser curvature
4 Lymph nodes of the greater curvature
5 Suprapyloric lymph nodes
6 Subpyloric lymph nodes
7 Lymph nodes of the left gastric artery
8 Lymph nodes of the common hepatic artery
9 Lymph nodes of the celiac trunk

10 Lymph nodes of the splenic hilum
11 Lymph nodes of the splenic artery
12 Lymph nodes of the hepatoduodenal ligament
13 Retropancreatic lymph nodes
14 Mesenteric lymph nodes
15 Lymph nodes of the middle colic artery
16 Paraaortic lymph nodes
111 Diaphragmatic lymph nodes
112 Lymph nodes of the posterior mediastinum

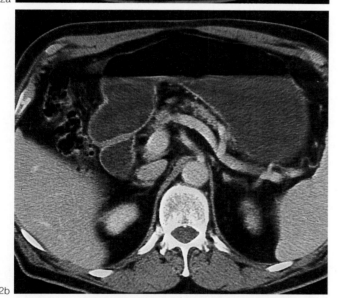

2a

2b

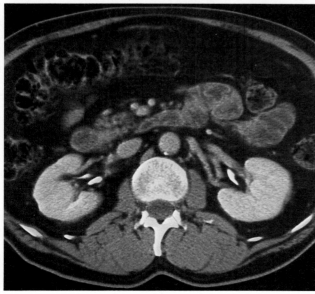

2c

The Gastrointestinal Tract

Anatomy and Imaging

The upper *esophagus* is directly adjacent to the membranous part of the trachea. The outer margins of the esophagus are often not clearly demarcated from surrounding structures in the cervical region, because very little fat is positioned between them. In difficult cases, contrast medium may be administered to better demarcate the esophagus from the thyroid gland and adjacent muscles and vessels. Below the level of tracheal bifurcation, the esophagus lies in juxtaposition to the left atrium, which means that demarcation of esophageal walls will be complicated by motion artifacts. Proceeding downward, the esophagus passes through the hiatus of the diaphragm and enters the abdominal cavity. The site where the phrenico-esophageal ligament attaches the esophagus to the diaphragm normally cannot be visualized on CT scans. Below the level of the diaphragm, the esophagus is attached by the gastrohepatic ligament, which passes in front of the caudate lobe into the porta hepatis. When the esophagus is filled with air and slightly dilated, wall thickness should not be greater than 3 mm.

The shape and configuration of the *stomach* is extremely variable. When the stomach is full, the dorsal gastric fundus distends greatly, so it comes in contact with the diaphragm and is molded by the contours of the spleen. The body of the stomach extends to the ventral abdominal wall. The number of sections required to scan the stomach will vary in accordance with the position of its main axis. The pylorus and duodenal bulb are contiguous with the head of the pancreas.

When the patient is placed in a right lateral position, the gastric antrum is more evenly spread, and tangential demonstration of the

Fig. 14-2. After the stomach was filled with water, and an antiperistaltic agent and contrast medium were administered, the gastric wall was scanned tangentially. It appeared as a homogeneously enhanced, sharply marginated structure and could, therefore, be easily differentiated from the lumen and surroundings. (c) Folds of the small intestine become visible after a bolus injection of contrast medium.

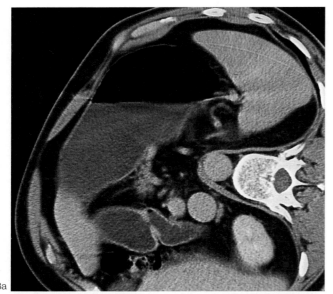

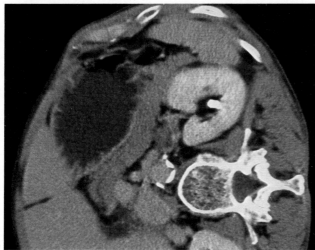

Fig. 14-3. With the patient in the lateral position, other sections of the gastric wall can also be demonstrated tangentially. In particular, this makes it easier to distinguish it from the pancreas (b).

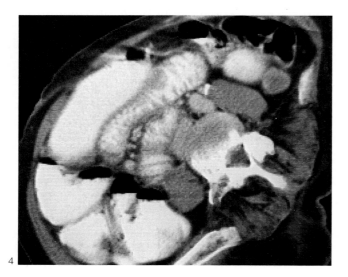

relationship of the gastric antrum to the pancreas is improved. Conversely, pathological abnormalities of the esophagogastric junction can be better demonstrated in a left lateral position when supine imaging yields inadequate results.

As a rule, the stomach must be fully distended before gastric wall lesions can be assessed. After antiperistaltic agents have been administered and sufficient filling has been achieved, the normal *gastric wall* should not be thicker than 4 mm. The walls of a collapsed stomach can be as thick as 10 mm or more. Detailed images of the gastric wall are best obtained when the stomach is filled with water, distended, and enhanced by intravenous contrast medium. Gastric walls enhance homogeneously, and the folds of the mucous membrane can be easily distinguished from the hypodense gastric lumen. When the intestine is opacified with oral contrast medium, familiar radiologic signs can be observed throughout the entire tract, from the *duodenum* to the *rectum*. Kerckring's folds, haustra, and the appendix can be demonstrated in relatively good detail, although the high resolution quality of conventional gastrointestinal examinations cannot be achieved. However, the extraluminal sections of the intestine and the peritoneal cavity are also demonstrated on CT scans.

The *thickness of the intestinal* wall is determined by the degree to which the corresponding intestinal segment is distended. The walls are approx. 3 mm thick in the normally distended intestine, but can be reduced to a thickness of 1 to 2 mm when there is more marked distension, especially in the colon or rectum. Like the stomach, the rectum can also be filled with water to obtain more detailed images of lesions and to better distinguish them from the lumen and surrounding structures; intravenous contrast medium also helps. Insufflation of air into the rectum or colon results in poorly reproducible images, even when antiperistaltic agents have been used.

Fig. 14-4. The administration of Gastrografin® and a bolus injection of contrast medium reduces the level of contrast, i.e. the richness of detail, of the image.

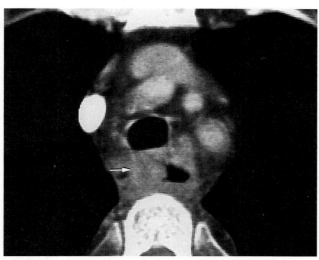

5a

Fig. 14-5. Carcinoma of the esophagus. Eccentric lumen with irregular external contours (a, b→). This is attributable to periesophageal lymph node enlargement. The aorto-pulmonary window exhibits reticular thickening with strandlike, lymphangiotic structures (c►). The membranous part of the trachea is protruded (b►). In this case, beginning infiltration cannot be excluded.

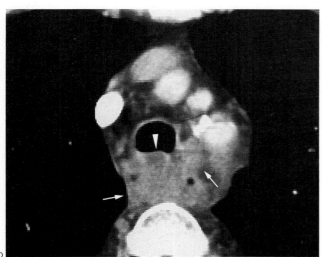

5b

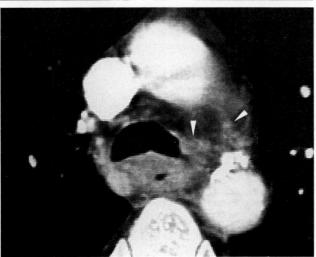

5c

The Esophagus

Esophageal Tumors

The most common esophageal tumor is the (squamous cell) carcinoma, which occurs primarily in older male patients. It develops preferentially at the three physiological constrictions of the esophagus. Sarcomas, on the other hand, are rarely found in the esophagus. The most common type is the leiomyosarcoma. Benign growths are also rare, and when they do occur, their location is either intraluminal (polyps, adenomas, papillomas) or intramural (myomas, neurinomas, lipomas, hamartomas).

Lymphatic spread of esophageal carcinomas first occurs in the submucous membrane, then proceeds from peri-esophageal regions into the mediastinum or soft tissues of the neck. Cervical and supraclavicular lymph nodes are therefore classified as regional lymph nodes (N1) of the cervical esophagus. The regional lymph nodes for the intrathoracic esophagus include the mediastinal and perigastric lymph nodes, but not the celiac lymph nodes. A tumor with its focus in the upper third of the esophagus will frequently affect the infradiaphragmatic lymph node chains. Lymph-borne and blood-borne distant metastases (M1) are primarily found in the lungs, liver, kidneys, and bone.

Tumor resection is no longer indicated after the tumor has clearly invaded the tracheobronchial system or adjacent vascular structures (e.g. aorta, vena cava, pericardium, pulmonary artery), or after extensive metastases has occurred.

• CT

Plain scans: Wall thickening and passage obstruction associated with prestenotic dilatation are the primary signs of esophageal carcinoma. Eccentric wall distension greater than 3 to 5 mm is a primary indication of a tumor process. Ill-defined or localized infiltration into the surrounding structures (T3) is readily recognizable on CT scans when the cuff of surrounding fat is sufficient. Infiltration of the adventitia of the descending aorta is very probable when more than 90° of the circumference of the aorta is surrounded by tumor tissue, but improbable when less than 45° is surrounded. Broken contour lines or intraluminal contour abnormalities are signs that the tumor has invaded the tracheobronchial tree or vascular system. Evidence of broad surface contact between the tumor and these structures can only tentatively support the diagnosis of wall infiltration. Diagnosis of tumor infiltration is difficult and unreliable in patients lacking mediastinal fat.

Contrast-enhanced scans: Border surfaces can often be better demonstrated after a bolus dose of contrast medium has been administered, since vital tumor tissue becomes clearly enhanced. Structural irregularities become more evident, and tumor borders can be more clearly distinguished from adjacent lymph node structures and vascularized border surfaces.

Submucous *lymphatic tumor spread* cannot be demonstrated on CT scans. Peri-esophageal (peritumoral) lymph nodes larger than 10 mm indicate metastatic involvement. Netlike nodulo-reticular densifications in the direct vicinity of the tumor are indicative of lymphatic spread. The infradiaphragmatic lymph nodes (perigastric, celiac trunk, hepatoduodenal ligament) should always be examined when the tumor focus is in the upper esophagus. Metastatic involvement is proven when these lymph nodes have a transverse diameter of 8 mm or more.

The lung and the liver should always be examined for metastases, since they are the organs primarily affected by *hematogenous* spreading.

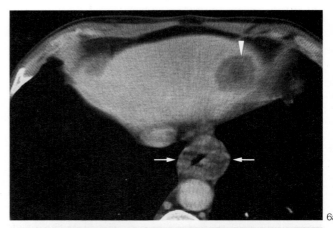

6a

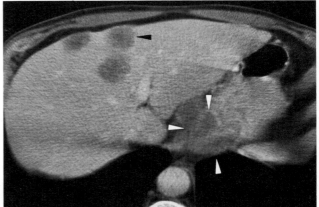

6b

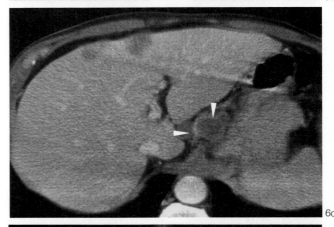

6c

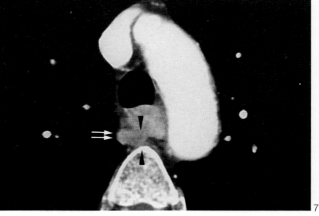

7

Fig. 14-6. Distal esophageal carcinoma. The sharply marginated, circular tumor (a→) has walls of 1.5 cm thickness. It has infiltrated the cardiac orifice (b► ◄). Evidence of metastatic spread to retrogastric lymph nodes (c►) and the liver.

Fig. 14-7. Esophageal carcinoma. After contrast medium administration, there is discrete, hypodense enhancement of a periesophageal lymph node (► ◄). Azygos vein (⇒).

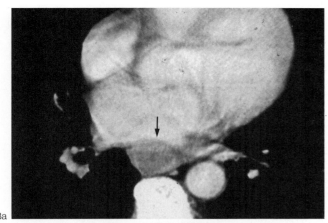

8a

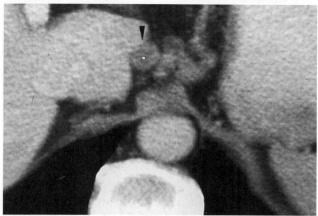

8b

Fig. 14-8. Distal esophageal carcinoma. The esophagus is sharply marginated (a→), and its walls are only slightly thickened. However, lymph node metastases is detected in the celiac trunk (b ►).

Fig. 14-9. Esophagitis due to an alkaliburn. A bolus injection of contrast medium reveals a dilated, thin-walled esophagus (►). Slight obliteration of periesophageal fat and discrete amounts of pleural effusion fluid (bilateral) (→) are detected. This suggests mediastinal and pleural involvement.

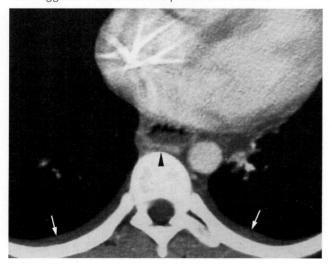

Differential diagnosis: A *benign esophageal lesion* is demonstrated on CT scans as a smoothly marginated area of focal wall thickening. Enhancement is slight yet homogeneous in *leiomyomas*, but is more strongly pronounced in *hemangiomas* and *fibroepitheliomas*. The presence of an esophageal *duplication cyst* can be deduced only if oral contrast enhancement has excluded a diverticulum from the diagnosis. It normally is difficult to distinguish a uniformly circular, sharply marginated malignant tumor from an area of *inflammatory wall thickening*.

Inflammatory Esophageal Abnormalities

Reflux esophagitis arises from increased gastroesophageal reflux or a hiatus hernia. The disease primarily affects the lower third of the esophagus. Chronic reflux esophagitis can lead to ulcers, esophageal stricture, and wall thickening. *Candidial esophagitis* affects the entire esophagus, and accompanying wall edemas and infiltration lead to thickening of the entire esophageal wall. Other mycoses can cause a similar clinical picture. *Tuberculosis* and syphilis, which may cause secondary esophageal involvement, can lead to segmental thickening of the esophageal wall due to intramural granulomas.

● CT

Uniform, circular wall thickening can be demonstrated during the florid stages of disease which, in more *localized* cases, cannot be distinguished from a spherical carcinoma restricted to the esophageal wall (T2 stage). When esophageal stricture develops as a result of chemical burns, Crohn's disease or ulcer, the esophageal walls do not become thickened during the stage of cicatrization, so the external diameter of the esophagus is normally reduced.

Generalized esophageal wall thickening is observed in patients with candidial esophagitis. This condition must be differentiated from rare intramural pseudodiverticulosis, which is characterized by the occurrence of numerous intramural pseudodiverticula that are 1 to 3 mm in size. Both can be demonstrated on CT scans. Idiopathic muscular hypertrophy of the esophagus is rare.

Esophageal Varices

The submucosal esophageal veins form collateral vascular channels in patients with portal hypertension. They drain via the peri-esophageal veins into the azygos vein system. "Downhill" varices are rare occurrences observed after obstruction of the superior vena cava. They are part of the venous drainage channels for the inlet of the thorax. The caliber of esophageal varices can become rather large and cause thickening the esophageal wall. Esophageal varices are usually sclerosized endoscopically.

• CT

Plain scans: Wall thickening is frequently found in the distal esophagus and in the esophagogastric junction. The outer margins may have a nodular appearance on plain scans.
Contrast-enhanced scans: When there is sufficient enhancement after a protracted intravenous dose of contrast medium, the intramural veins and the dilated peri-esophageal veins can be demonstrated at the level of the diaphragm. These veins can usually be traced as dilated venous convolutions passing along the stomach (gastro-esophageal, retrogastric), pancreas, and splenic pedicle (perisplenic, mesenteric, retroperitoneal).
Inflammatory reactions often develop in the treated esophageal segment after *sclerosis* has occurred. The effects of such a reaction may range from localized thickening of the esopha-

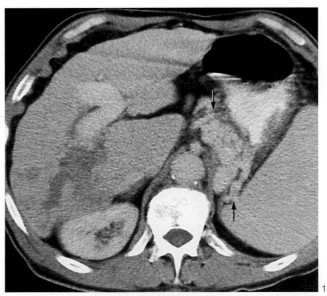

10a

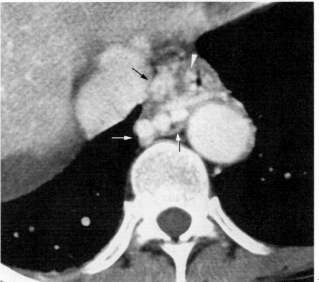

10b

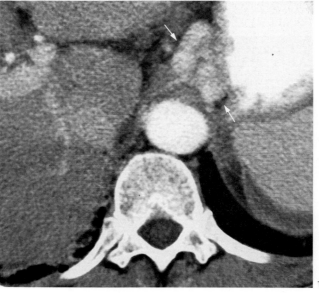

10c

Fig. 14-10. Varices of the esophagus and fundus.
a) In a patient with cirrhosis of the liver, a filling defect is found in the fundus of the stomach. After protracted contrast medium administration, contrast medium filling is observed in broad venous convolutions. This corresponds to varices of the fundus (→).
b, c) Periesophageal and submucous esophageal varices. Medial to the cardiac orifice, venous convolutions become opaque-laden after protracted administration of contrast medium (c→). They extend cranially into the periesophageal region (b→). Submucous veins are also visible inside the esophagus (b ►).

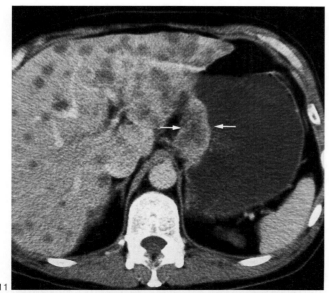

11

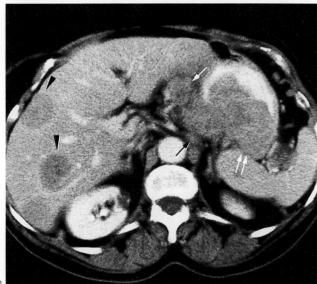

12

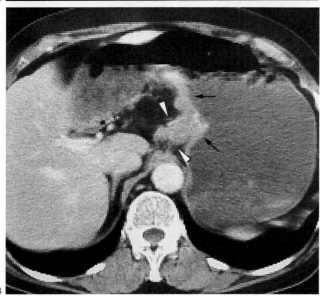

13

geal wall to exudation in the surrounding mediastinum, obliteration of adjacent fat, or pleural reactions with pleural effusion. These processes are usually better demonstrated on contrast-enhanced CT scans (with consideration for potentially infradiaphragmatic spread).

The Stomach

Tumors of the Stomach

Gastric Carcinoma

Gastric carcinoma is the third most common tumor of the gastrointestinal tract. On the whole, the incidence of this tumor has receded in the last decade. However, the number of carcinomas at the cardia is increasing as compared with antral carcinomas. Because many endoscopic examinations are now performed, gastric carcinomas are more often detected in early stages. In most cases, however, gastric carcinomas have already reached an advanced stage with infiltration of the muscles of the stomach wall by the time of diagnosis.

Relatively early *lymphatic* spread occurs in the submucous and serous membranes. It first affects regional lymph nodes of the gastric wall (N1 stage), then perigastric chains along the vessels (common hepatic artery, left gastric artery, splenic artery; N2 stage). Invasion of the hepatoduodenal ligament, the mesenteric root, para-aortic lymph nodes, or diaphragmatic lymph nodes is classified as distant metastases (M1). *Hematogenous* distant metastases are found most frequently in the liver and lung, but may also be found in the bone and kidney. The purpose of computer tomography is not merely to confirm the presence of the tumor, but to define the extent of spread.

Fig. 14-11. Cardiac carcinoma. The tumor spreads to the side of the lesser curvature. It has already given rise to multiple hepatic metastases.

Fig. 14-12. Large cardiac carcinoma (⇒) with large retrogastric lymph node metastases (→) and hepatic metastases (▸).

Fig. 14-13. Cardiac carcinoma (→) with lymph node metastases that surround the celiac trunk (▸).

• CT

Plain scans: The stomach must be fully distended before good diagnostic images of the gastric wall can be obtained. The average thickness of the normal stomach wall is then 4 mm. (It is advisable to place patients with cardia carcinoma in a left lateral position to provide a better overview of the gastro-esophageal junction.) When the stomach is fully distended, the majority of T1 tumors will be demonstrated as localized areas of wall thickening. Large tumors appear as lumpy or smooth soft-tissue formations. The attenuation of mucinous carcinomas is low. The serous membrane has probably been breached when the wall is distended by more than 2 cm. Infiltrative tumors (Bormann IV), which are difficult to diagnose endoscopically, appear on CT scans as areas of segmental or complete gastric wall thickening. Tumor infiltration into the *serous membrane* itself usually cannot be reliably demonstrated. When the outer margins of the stomach are knobby and fine, or radial extensions are seen, infiltration of the serous membrane must be assumed. Evidence of peritoneal (circumscribed) ascites is an indirect sign of serosa infiltration, especially when the peritoneal membrane is thickened.

Direct *dissemination* of the tumor beyond the gastric wall occurs at the surfaces of contact with the liver, transverse colon and, most frequently, the pancreas. When the dividing layer of fat is free of cordlike structural thickening, infiltration into surrounding structures is unlikely. It is therefore difficult to assess whether the tumor has invaded adjacent organs of cachetic patients. Infiltration is also unlikely when mobility of the gastric wall with respect to adjacent structures is free. This can be demonstrated by turning the patient. Adhesion due to inflammation is not an uncommon finding. It is difficult to demonstrate the *lymph nodes* of the gastric wall (N1) on CT scans, but they are not diagnostically relevant, since they, too, will probably be removed during surgery. Large lymph nodes near the hepatoduodenal ligament (e.g. mesenteric and para-aortic lymph nodes) are classified as distant metastases (M1), and should therefore be carefully investigated. Conglomerates of lymph nodes enlarged to 8 to 10 mm in diameter also indicate metastatic involvement.

Local recurrence of gastric carcinoma may be found at the anastomosis, regardless of whether partial resection or gastrectomy has been performed. An irregularly marginated soft-tissue dense mass is demonstrated on CT scans. However, metastases with lymph node conglomerates, hepatic metastases and peritoneal carcinomatosis with ascites are more frequently observed.

Contrast-enhanced scans: Tumor areas can be demarcated from the healthy gastric wall after

Fig. 14-14. Cirrhous carcinoma of the stomach with circular mural infiltration in the antrum and body of the stomach. With the patient in the right lateral position, a good image was obtained. There was no evidence of spread beyond the gastric wall (b ►). With the patient in the dorsal position, retrogastric lymph nodes surrounding the celiac trunk were demonstrated. They became slightly opaque-laden (a→).

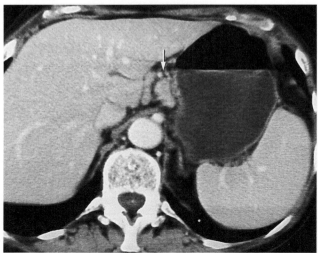

14a

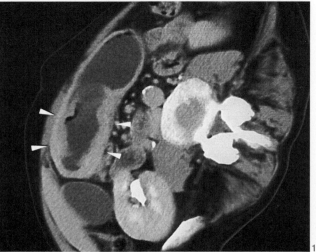

14b

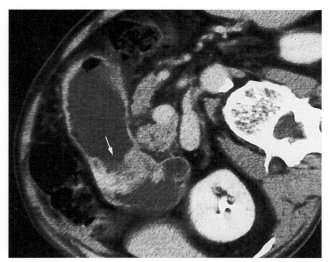

Fig. 14-15. Carcinoma of the antrum exhibits circular extension without evidence of spreading beyond gastric wall.

Fig. 14-16. Prepyloric carcinomas of the antrum. The circular mass of the tumors obstructs contrast medium passage into the stomach. In neither case was there evidence of tumor spread beyond the gastric walls or of regional lymph node enlargement.

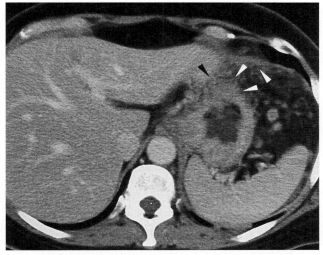

Fig. 14-17. Cardiac carcinoma with evidence of extensive lymphangiosis extending to the lobes of the liver.

Fig. 14-18. Local recurrence of stomach cancer after B-II operation. In the vicinity of the anastomosis (►), a soft-tissue mass is detected. Part of it extends into the pancreas (→). The retroperitoneal space is masked by infiltration. Lymph node metastases (a⇒).

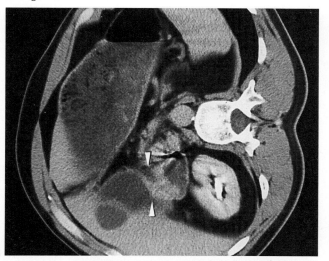

16a

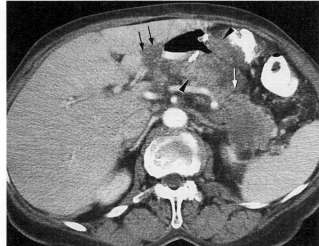

18a

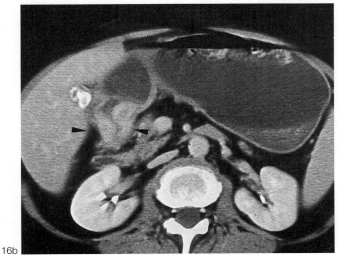

16b

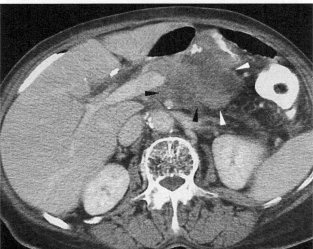

18b

administration of contrast medium, especially when the stomach is filled with water. With the exception of mucinous carcinomas, the tumor exhibits slightly increased, inhomogeneous absorption of contrast medium, which is especially pronounced in diffuse, cirrhotic types. A bolus of contrast medium also helps differentiate lymphatic from vascular structures. Furthermore, inflammation-related lymph node enlargement should demonstrate less enhancement than metastatic lesions.

Gastric Sarcomas

Approximately 3% of all malignant gastric tumors are sarcomas. The stomach is the most frequent gastrointestinal site of manifestation of *malignant lymphomas*, which normally include histocystic or lymphocytic non-Hodgkin's lymphomas or Hodgkin's disease. Macroscopic distinctions are made between infiltrating, ulcerating and polypoid types. Isolated or generalized involvement of the stomach may be observed. Lymphadenopathy is a common accompaniment.

Around 25% of all gastric sarcomas are *leiomyosarcomas*. Their location is usually submucous, but can also be subserous, submucous and subserous, and intramural. Direct tumor invasion into adjacent organs is observed with larger tumors. Regional metastases often arise as a result of peritoneal implants (more often hematogenous than lymphatic). This is first seen in the liver and later in the lungs.

● CT

Plain scans: Gastric *lymphoma* is characterized by pronounced segmental or generalized gastric wall thickening to an average of 5 cm (range = 2.5 to 8 cm). Circumscribed or polypoid forms of malignant lymphoma are occasionally found. The outer margins of the tumor are usually sharply demarcated from the surroundings. Most of the surfaces toward the lumen have a wavy or undulating appearance. Deep ulcerations frequently occur in polypoid lesions. Fistulae and perforation of the abdominal cavity are not seen as often as in small bowel involvement.

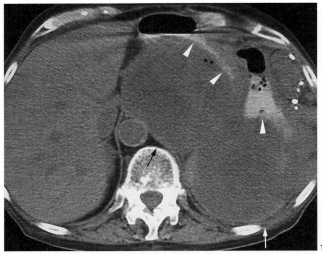

19a

Fig. 14-19. Leiomyosarcoma of the stomach. The plain scan reveals a large, bullous structure that deforms the stomach (►) and contains ulcers. After bolus contrast medium injection, the tumor displays considerable peripheral enhancement (→), which demarcates large, hypodense zones of necrosis.

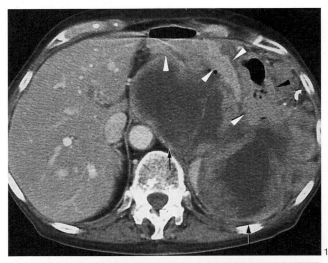

19b

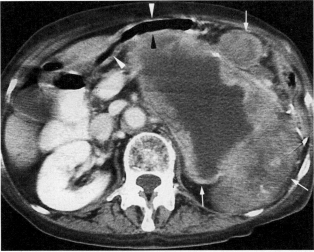

19c

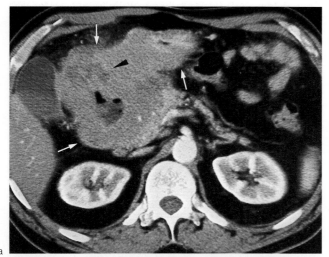

20a

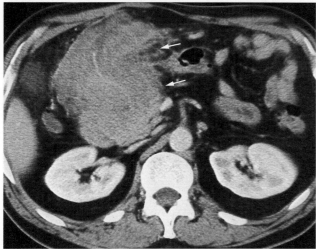

20b

Fig. 14-20. Malignant lymphoma of the stomach (lymphoblastic lymphoma). The gastric wall in the antrum is over 2 cm thick (a→). After contrast medium administration, it exhibits only slight, macculated enhancement (a►). The lymphoma extends to the duodenum (b→). Regional enlargement of lymph nodes was not detected.

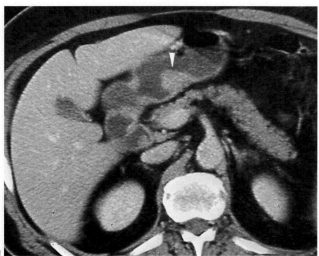

21

Leiomyosarcomas can involve large sections of the gastric wall and are characterized by their pedunculated appearance. Expansion has been described to be as large as 5 to 18 cm. Leiomyosarcomas create an irregular density pattern on plain scans. When communication exists with the gastric lumen, low density areas in the water range containing air or liquid may give the mass a cystic appearance. Calcification is occasionally observed.

Contrast-enhanced scans: Intravenous administration of contrast medium leads to only low-grade enhancement of *malignant lymphomas* (10 to 20 HU). Their frequently recognizable central zone of hypodensity is poorly demarcated, since it contains lymphomatous tissue instead of necrotic tissue. Vital tissue from a *leiomyosarcoma* becomes strongly enhanced, thus clearly demarcating hypodense zones of necrosis, cystic degeneration and/or hyalinization.

Differential diagnosis: When gastric wall thickening is severe, *malignant lymphomas* can be distinguished from *leiomyosarcomas* because of the absence of necrotic zones and calcification, a low degree of parenchymal enhancement, and evidence of regional lymph node enlargement. The CT appearance of lymphoma infiltration differs from that of infiltrative cirrhous *adenocarcinoma* in that the external margins are sharply demarcated (usually no perigastric infiltration), there is considerable wall thickening, pronounced enlargement of affected lymph nodes, and a minor degree of contrast enhancement.

Benign tumors cannot be differentiated when there is a focal lesion on the gastric wall with absence of metastases.

Benign Gastric Tumors

The most common benign gastric tumors are, in order of frequency, leiomyomas, neurogenic

Fig. 14-21. Leiomyoma of the stomach. Demonstration of a 1.5 cm mass on the gastric wall. It displays homogeneous enhancement, and there is no evidence of tumor spread beyond the gastric wall.

tumors (schwannomas, neurofibromas), fibromas, lipomas, hemangiomas and other vascular tumors.

• CT

Gastric *leiomyomas* are usually discovered when they reach a size of 5 cm, but they can become much larger. The leiomyoma first manifests as an endoluminal mass which, in contrast to the leiomyosarcoma, seldom develops with necrosis. Ulceration of this submucous tumor is a more common finding. Homogeneous enhancement is seen after administration of contrast medium.

The rare *lipoma* can be positively identified, due to its characteristically hypodense tissue density.

When enhancement of an area of the gastric wall is unusually strong, a *vascular tumor* of the stomach must be suspected. Their characteristic location makes them distinguishable from extragastric varices.

Fibromas and *neurinomas* are normally not distinguishable from common gastric *polyps* and *adenomas*.

Gastric Inflammation

Gastric wall thickening only rarely occurs in systemic *granulomatous* diseases like tuberculosis, sarcoidosis, and Crohn's disease. Localized wall thickening is demonstrable, especially on contrast enhanced CT scans, even in patients with gastric ulcers. Extensive wall thickening may occur in exudative *pancreatitis*, and the individual layers of the stomach can be visualized after contrast medium has been administered. These rare causes may be of importance when considering a differential diagnosis.

Small Intestine and Colon

Cysts

Duplication cysts are rare anomalies of the small bowel. They lie contralateral to the me-

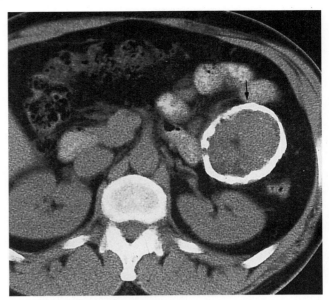

Fig. 14-22. Mesenteric cyst. Mesenteric cyst measuring 6 cm is found in the left epigastric region. It exhibits ringlike calcification and inhomogeneous CT numbers of ca. 40 HU.

senteric attachment and have walls that are usually smooth and a few millimeters in thickness. CT numbers for these cysts normally fall within the water range.

Mesenteric cysts may be single or multiple occurrences. They develop with virtually equal frequency in the jejunum and ileum. These

Fig. 14-23. Paraganglioma of the duodenum. In the second part of the duodenum, findings after bolus injection of contrast medium include dorsal wall thickening (→), smooth boundaries and a low-density center (▶).

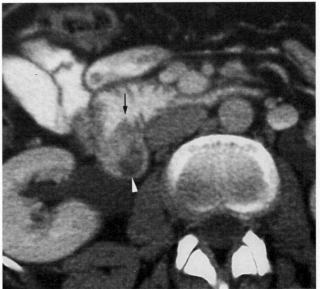

cysts arise from diverse tissue types and therefore may contain serous, chylous or mucinous fluid, so density values may either fall in the water range or higher (0 to 40 HU).

Solid Tumors

Benign Tumors

The range of benign tumors in the small and large bowel overlaps with those of the stomach. Adenomas and lipomas are therefore the most common types.

• CT

See: benign gastric tumors

Malignant Tumors

Small bowel tumors are rare and make up about 5% of all gastrointestinal neoplasms. The most common is the *carcinoid tumor*, a lesion with a low degree of malignancy. It is followed in frequency by the malignant lymphoma and leiomyosarcoma. *Carcinoma of the colon*, on the other hand, is one of the most common forms of cancer (second most frequent cause of cancer in women, and third in men, although men are more often affected than women).

The number of *malignant lymphomas* and *myosarcomas* is much smaller, as is the number of benign mesenchymal tumors.

Malignant Lymphomas and Myosarcomas

The morphology and differential diagnosis of sarcomas of the colon and small bowel is identical to that of those in the stomach. Fistulae occur more frequently in malignant lymphomas with extensive invasion of the small bowel, giving rise to a tumor conglomerate that encases intestinal loops. The tumor normally does not penetrate into the free abdominal cavity.

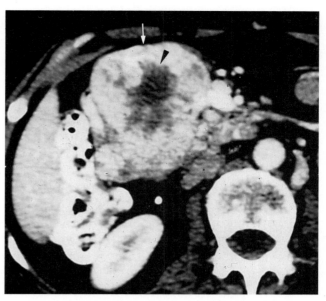

Fig. 14-24. Duodenal carcinoid. Rare location. The tumor exhibits brief, but strong, peripheral contrast enhancement (→). The center of the tumor remains hypodense, an indication of regressive change (►). Enlargement of regional lymph nodes was not found.

Small Intestine Carcinoids

Small bowel carcinoids arise from neuroendocrine cells of the submucous membrane, normally in the region of the terminal ileum. They can reach a size of 5 cm or more, but most are relatively well circumscribed. Lymphatic spread into the mesentery gives rise to large areas of regional lymph node invasion in the mesenteric, para-aortic and paracaval regions. The tumor becomes clinically manifest after metastases into the liver has occurred, with a corresponding rise in serotonin levels.

• CT

Regional lymph node enlargement within the mesenteric root, its para-aortic or paracaval regions are CT characteristics that help to identify the carcinoid tumor. Typical computer tomographic signs are stellate retraction phenomena near regional lymph node enlargements, which create a wheel-spoke effect inside mesenteric fatty tissue. The intestinal tumor itself appears as an area of localized or circular wall thickening in the affected intestinal loop. Because they are highly vascularized, intrahepatic metastases normally appear as hyperdense areas on contrast-mediated CT scans (bolus injection).

Colorectal Carcinoma

Colorectal carcinomas arise due to malignant transformation of polyps and are located primarily in the rectum and sigmoid colon. Almost all colorectal carcinomas are adenocarcinomas. Metastases develop primarily in regional lymph nodes. Distant metastases occurs relatively late in the liver and lungs. As is the case with stomach diagnosis, the primary role of CT is not to confirm the presence of the tumor, but to determine how far the metastases has spread. Colorectal tumors are often an incidental finding.

• CT

Plain scans: The loops of the colon, with variably distended haustra and flexures, are generally poor scanning objects, even with good homogeneous filling of contrast medium. Only the rectal ampules can be reproducibly opacified in such a manner that the intestinal wall can be demonstrated tangentially when distended. Under those conditions, minor wall thickening (5 mm or more) can be demonstrated on *high-resolution scans*. Unreliable results are often obtained when an attempt is made to distinguish early infiltration of fat *(T4)* from a tumor restricted to the wall *(T3)*. This is because minor changes in perirectal fat can also arise from inflammation. In other sections of the colon, colorectal tumors that are 2 cm and larger can be identified as filling defects after homogeneous intestinal opacification has been achieved. Depending on its location, localized and spherical wall thickening can be demonstrated from thicknesses of 0.5 to 1.5 cm.

Surrounding structures have been infiltrated when the border surfaces between the tumor and contiguous fat appear ill-defined, lobulated or straggly. Gas accumulation inside larger tumors is a sign of putrefaction and must be differentiated from abscess-forming diverticulitis.

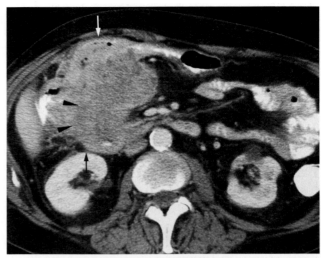

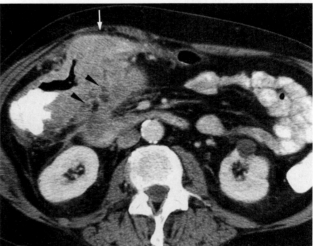

Fig. 14-25. Carcinoma of the transverse colon in the right flexura, with infiltration of the gastrocolic ligament and duodenum (→). Regressive Changes (▸) in the center of the tumor.

Fig. 14-26. Tumor recurrence after sigmoidectomy. Superior to the site of anastomosis, there is eccentric wall thickening without tumor spread beyond the physiological walls.

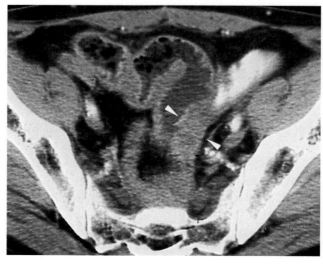

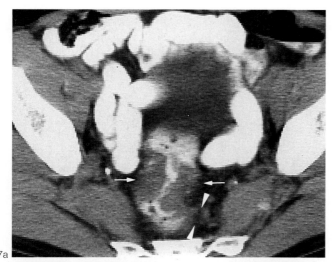

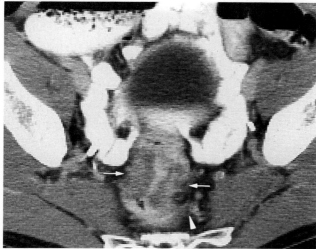

27a

27b

Fig. 14-27. Circular sigmoid carcinoma (→). The tumor becomes slightly enhanced (b), with the exception of small ramifications (►); this corresponds to infiltration. No clear enlargement of regional lymph nodes.

Fig. 14-28. Anal carcinoma. The tumor distends the sphincter (►). Further evidence of a lymph node metastases in the left inguinal region (→).

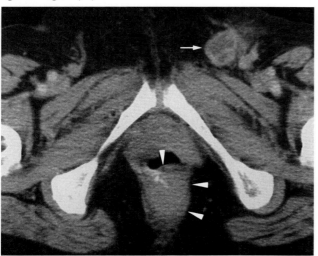

Infiltration of the levator ani muscle or ischiorectal fossa is a factor that determines the resectability of a deeply seated rectal carcinoma, so the status of these muscles must be assessed prior to surgical resection. In order to diagnose *infiltration into adjacent organs*, unequivocal proof of parenchymal invasion, cortical defects in bone, or disruption of the contours of the bladder must be found. A *bolus of contrast medium* is often necessary to improve demarcation of the organ borders. When *lymph nodes* are larger than 1 cm, or when several smaller lymph nodes are clustered in the drainage area of the tumor, a diagnosis of metastases can be made. Metastatic spread is often underestimated. Furthermore, accompanying inflammation complicates the diagnosis. A sufficiently high and protracted *dose of contrast medium* must be administered to distinguish between peritumoral inflammation (characterized by increased vascular supply) and fibrous tissue or lymphatic structures. The presence of the latter must be assumed when additional (non-vascular) nodular structures permeate the neighborhood of the tumor. Cranially located mesenteric lymph nodes (N3) are easier to diagnose because there is a sufficient amount of demarcating fat.

The liver should always be examined during staging, since it is the likely site of *blood-borne* metastases.

Careful examination techniques must be employed in order to obtain proof of local *tumor recurrence*. Good contrast enhancement and filling of the region of anastomosis must be maintained in colon resection, because local recurrences often lie in extraluminal locations. Any asymmetrical soft-tissue formation that was not caused by surgical anastomosis warrants suspicion of tumor recurrence.

Differential diagnosis: The benign *villous adenoma* is seen on CT scans as an intraluminal, polycyclic tumor resting broadly against the intestinal wall. Attenuation values for this tumor are uniformly reduced to levels below 10 HU.

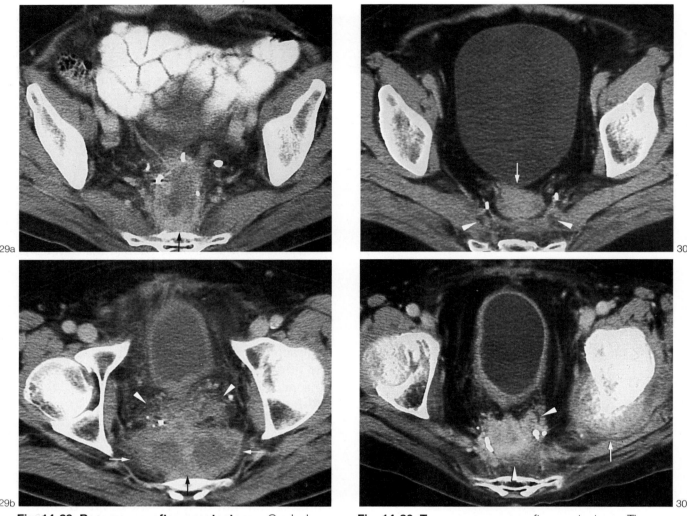

29a

29b

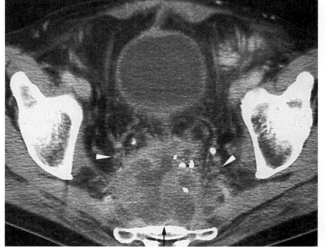

29c

Fig. 14-29. Recurrence after proctectomy. Gradual enlargement of the soft-tissue structure in front of the sacrum. Six months later (b→) it appears more nodular and, except for the tumor center, it absorbs more contrast medium than the adjacent muscle tissue. One year later (c), there is an increase in the tumor's soft-tissue constituents, hypodense zones (colliquation) and fatty infiltration (►).

30a

30b

Fig. 14-30. Tumor recurrence after proctectomy. The presacral space appears normal, with the exception of small scar tissue zones (a ►). The uterus is dorsally displaced (a→). 1 1/2 years later, signs of infiltration in the region of the uterus (b ►) and osseous destruction of the acetabulum (b→) are found.

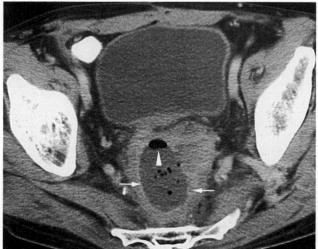

31

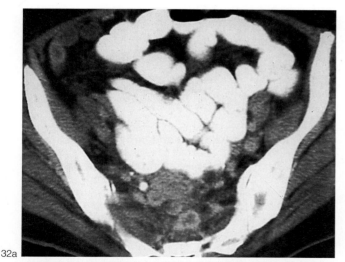

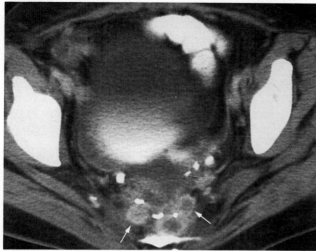

Fig. 14-32. In a proctectomized patient, a tumor recurrence with multiple small soft-tissue structures was found. They had central areas of necrosis and exhibited peripheral contrast medium enhancement.

Tumor Recurrence after Proctectomy

Computer tomography is an especially suitable method for demonstrating local recurrences following proctectomy. During postoperative healing, especially in response to abscess formation, considerable, sometimes expansive, scar tissue formation can develop. Late abscesses and fistulae are not unusual occurrences. This is why it is advisable to make an

◄
Fig. 14-31. Infected recurrence. After proctectomy, findings include evidence of a gas-containing cavity (►) and peripheral enhancement (→), which are signs of an abscess. During surgery, the broad, irregular wall of the cavity was found to be tumorous. Regional lymph node enlargement was not detected.

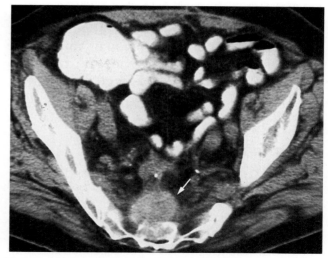

Fig. 14-33. Presacral metastases in a proctectomized patient (→).

initial base examination at the earliest two months after surgery, but preferably four to six months after proctectomy, when it can be safely concluded that the healing process has ended.

• CT

When no scar tissue is present, tumor recurrence can be safely excluded. Various amounts of scar tissue are usually found, however, but are divided from the sacrum by a narrow layer of fat. The uterus and prostate gland can normally be readily differentiated from this strand-like or smoothly demarcated soft-tissue structure.

A tumor recurrence is demonstrated on CT scans as an expansive, homogeneous, spherical soft-tissue structure. Any irregular, asymmetrical or eccentric borders substantiate suspicion of tumor recurrence. This is especially applicable if inhomogeneous enhancement of these structures exceeds muscle tissue attenuation on contrast-enhanced scans. Air inclusions normally correspond to abscesses, but their presence may be attributable to a tumor recurrence, especially when the patient is undergoing radiation therapy (necrotic gas). When it is difficult to distinguish tumor recurrence from fibrosis, the postoperative base examination may provide a helpful comparison.
Unequivocal signs of tumor recurrence include bone destruction in the sacrum, infiltration of

adjacent organs (bladder, piriformis muscle, obturator internus muscle, gluteal muscles), or indisputable evidence of regional lymph node enlargement. Late occurrence of hydronephrosis must also be considered as a sign of recurrence.

Inflammatory Diseases

Acute inflammatory processes of the small bowel and colon do not require computer tomography, since they lead to only temporary, reversible, minor swelling of the intestinal mucosa. Chronic granulomatous diseases can lead to thickening of the intestinal wall. In these cases, CT scans can provide additional information after enteroclysis of the small bowel.

Crohn's Disease

This disease most frequently affects the terminal ileum, but can affect all other sections of the intestine as well. In the course of the disease, the development of intestinal follicles first leads to nodular swelling of the submucosa. This, in turn, leads to corresponding changes in the surface of the mucous membrane. In its further relapsing course, Crohn's disease progresses to a *deep stage*, which is characterized by fissures, wall fibrosis, and narrowing of the lumen. Fistulae and adhesion of intestinal loops are typical signs of the disease, and the development of abscesses in intestinal convolutions is a typical complication. The lymph nodes on the mesenteric attachment are enlarged by either granulomatous or inflamed lesions. Chronically inflamed lesions can also develop into the mesenteric root, thereby causing dilatation and sclerosis of lymph vessels.

• CT

Plain scans: The primary sign of Crohn's disease is segmental *intestinal wall thickening*, which is seldom greater than 1.5 cm. In an acute episode the outer margins of the intestinal wall are often not easily distinguishable from mesenteric fat, which is densified by edema and strand formation. During the inflammatory phase, the intestinal wall becomes

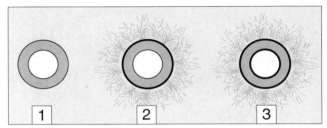

Fig. 14-34. Double halo sign and targetlike appearance. The appearance of an affected intestinal wall, as seen in CT sections after bolus administration of contrast medium, is variable. It may become homogeneously enhanced (1), have a low-density center and a hyperdense external rim (2 = **double halo**), or exhibit internal and external rings of hyperdensity (3 = **double-ring**, **targetlike**, or **target board signs**).

Fig. 14-35. Crohn's disease. Clear wall thickening in the terminal ileum at Bauhin's (iliocecal) valve (a→). Caudally (b), the lumen is intersected transversely (→). The contiguous fatty tissue shows an increasingly fine, reticulonodular structure (►).

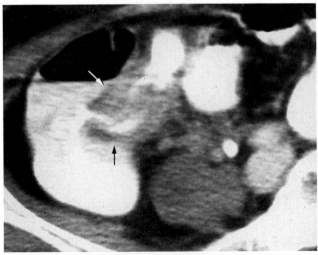

35a

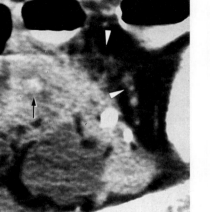

35b

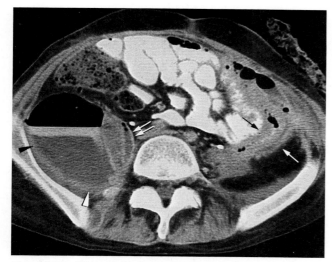

Fig. 14-36. Abscess in Crohn's disease. Clear thickening of the wall of the small intestine with homogeneous contrast enhancement (→). In the right pelvic inlet, a retrocolic abscess with a large cavity (►) and loculation (⇒) are found.

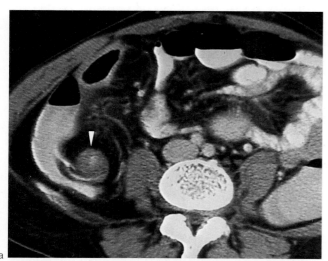

37a

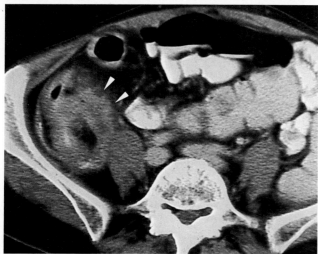

37b

more sharply demarcated, and fine, fibrotic projections may be seen. Approximately one third of all regional (mesenteric and retroperitoneal) lymph nodes are moderately enlarged to sizes of up to 2 cm. *Fibrolipomatous proliferation* is a frequent sign that can be demonstrated as local hypertrophy of surrounding mesenteric fat. The *fistulae* characteristic of Crohn's disease are easily distinguishable as cordlike structures, since they contain either air or contrast medium. They can lead to the development of sizable zones of necrosis, especially in perirectal regions. The abdominal wall, muscles of the back, ischiorectal fossa, and presacral space should then be thoroughly examined. Good bowel opacification is required in order to demonstrate the resulting *abscesses*.

Contrast-enhanced scans: After a bolus of contrast medium has been administered, the ring-like intestinal tube is seen on cross- sectional scans as a double halo with a hypodense inner ring (representing an edema in the submucous membrane) and a hyperdense outer ring (inflamed, hypervascularized muscle). This stratification vanishes during chronic stages. The administration of contrast medium additionally facilitates identification of abscesses by demarcating the zones of liquefaction.

Differential diagnosis: *Ulcerative colitis* must be excluded from the diagnosis (see page 334).

Yersiniosis causes lymphonodular hyperplasia without ulceration of the mucosa. Segmental wall thickening is normally seen, but is absent when there is an inflammation-related change in surrounding mesenteric fat. As compared with Crohn's disease, yersiniosis more frequently causes moderate enlargement of lymph nodes near the mesenteric attachment and root. Enlarged lymph nodes are hypodense in *Whipple's disease*, which causes only

Fig. 14-37. Crohn's disease. The terminal ileum exhibits a greatly reduced lumen, wall thickening, and an increased amount of surrounding fat (a►). The mesenteric root is displaced. The constricted segment of the ileum continues caudally in an arch- shaped configuration. There are strandlike projections on the surface of the mesenteric attachment (b►). Contrast medium is uniformly absorbed in the intestinal wall.

minor thickening of the intestinal wall. *Intra-mural hematomas*, which may arise after trauma, anticoagulant therapy, or hemorrhagic diathesis, are normally located in the proximal small bowel and lead to the development of a cuff of homogeneous thickening in the affected bowel segment. Intramural hematoma is usually accompanied by (hemorrhagic) ascites, and regression normally begins 1 to 2 weeks after the onset of disease.

Ulcerative Colitis

Ulcerative colitis continuously affects the colon all the way from the rectum proximally and leads to the development of infiltrative inflammation and erosion of the intestinal wall. Intermittent ulceration or areas of ulceration develop in the further course of disease and can lead to localized or extensive fibrosis of the intestinal wall. The course of ulcerative colitis is usually chronic (intermittent or continuous) and is seldom acute or fulminant. Ulcerative colitis is classified as a precancerous lesion.

• CT

Plain scans: In acute ulcerative colitis, circumferential areas of wall thickening that are sharply demarcated from the surroundings are

Fig. 14-38. Ulcerous colitis. The entire intestinal wall is clearly thickened. Scans in the transverse plane reveal a discrete, double-ring structure (► ◄), the internal and external contours of which are hyperdense. There is an increase in surrounding fat, which contains numerous vessels. Regional lymph node enlargement is not detected.

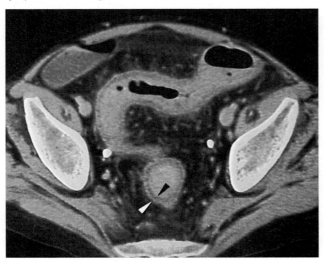

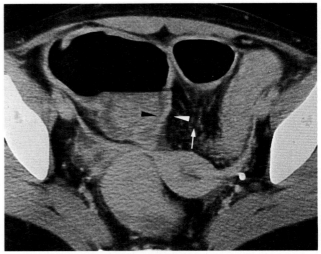

Fig. 14-39. Colitis with shigellosis and amebiasis. The sigma and rectum are dilated. The intestinal wall is thickened and becomes enhanced after contrast medium administration (►). Due to the contrast enhancement of the intestinal lumen, the double-ring sign is not visible. Clearly increased intravascular injection at the mesenteric attachment (→).

typically seen. Depressions caused by ulceration and raised areas indicating mucosal swelling or pseudopolyps can be identified on CT scans when the intestine is well enhanced by contrast medium. Smooth external and internal wall borders are found in subacute and inflammation-free phases of the disease. Wall thickening is more pronounced than in Crohn's disease and is normally less than 1 cm. A ring-like area of density reduction due to fatty infiltration may be seen on plain scans, resulting in the appearance of a rosette-shaped struc-

Fig. 14-40. Colitis. Endoscopy revealed nonspecific colitis as an accompaniment of infiltrative spread of a liposarcoma of the mesocolon. Here, too, is a typical "targetlike" sign (►).

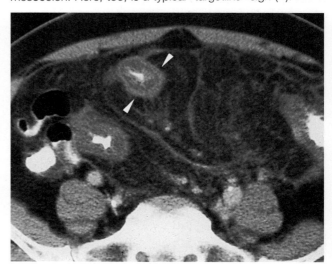

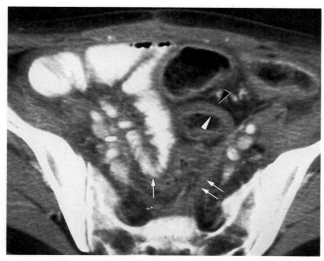

Fig. 14-41. Radiation colitis. In addition to narrowing of the intestinal lumen (→) and fibrotic broadening of the fasciae (⇒), areas of frank wall thickening (► ◄) were also found. The boundary layer proximal to the lumen exhibits delicate contrast enhancement after bolus contrast medium injection.

ture with hyperdense internal and external borders. Moderate regional lymph node enlargement is less frequently observed.

Contrast-enhanced scans: A relatively typical sign in the acute phase of disease is stratified wall enhancement with ringlike enhancement of the outer margins. This can be observed after intravenous administration of contrast medium.

Differential diagnosis: Differentiation of *Crohn's disease (granulomatous colitis)* must be based on the analysis of essential CT signs. The "halo" sign, smooth walls, continuous involvement (rectum) and only minor wall thickening (ca. 8 mm) indicate ulcerative colitis, whereas discontinuous segmental involvement, homogeneous enhancement of the intestinal wall, more severe wall thickening (ca. 13 mm), fistulae, abscess formation, and moderate lymph node enlargement substantiate a diagnosis of Crohn's disease.

Ischemic colitis leads to the development of polypoids or homogeneous segmental wall thickening in the colon. Patient history and proof of vascular disease (sclerosis, aneurysm) can facilitate the evaluation of these nonspecific findings.

Appendicitis

Appendicitis is a disease afflicting younger patients. The appendix is obstructed by a fecal concretion in 50 to 80% of all cases. The position of the appendix is retrocecal or retroperitoneal in ca. 30% of cases, and intraperitoneal in 70% of cases.

In retroperitoneal appendicitis, the inflammation invades retroperitoneal fat and can permeate fasciae and fatty tissue by means of inflammation, which eventually leads to abscess formation. In intraperitoneal appendicitis, the inflammation causes localized adhesion of peritoneal membranes and intraperitoneal abscess.

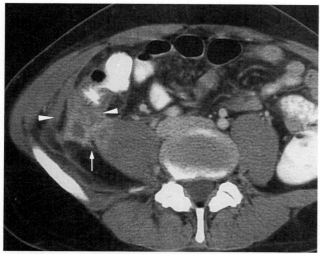

42a

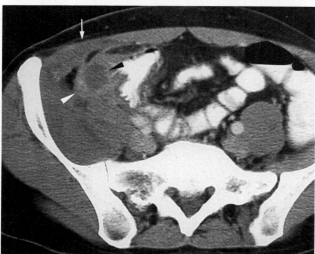

42b

Fig. 14-42. Postoperative (**appendectomy**) occurrence of a perityphlitic, multiloculated abscess (►). Involvement of the psoas muscle (a→) as well as the abdominal wall (b→).

• CT

Plain scans: In infiltrative phases, the normally readily demonstrable retrocecal fatty tissue is seen on CT scans as a streaky, reticulated area which becomes more demarcated when abscesses are present. A retrocecal appendix can sometimes be identified as a finger-shaped soft-tissue structure. Calcific densification corresponding to fecal concretion may be seen in the central region. Intraperitoneal abscesses are fluid collections that are demonstrated as sharply marginated, hypodense areas. While the masking of surrounding fat is initially less pronounced, the amount of masking can increase as the disease progresses. Protracted processes can cause wall thickening in the pole of the cecum.

Contrast-enhanced scans: After the administration of contrast medium, an abscess membrane or inflamed peritoneal tissue appears on CT scans as a hyperdense membrane. Gas accumulations are a reliable sign of abscess formation. Thickened walls of the affected section of the intestine are clearly demarcated due to the absorption of contrast medium.

Diverticulitis

Diverticulitis develops from underlying diverticulosis, a disease predominantly occurring in elderly inhabitants of industrialized nations. Inflammation normally spreads from the diverticulum to surrounding tissue (peridiverticulitis) and can eventually attack more distant segments of the intestine (pericolitis). Typical complications associated with the disease are perforations in the free abdominal cavity, sealed perforation with fistulae and abscess, and vascular erosion with hemorrhage. Diverticulosis and diverticulitis are focused mainly in the sigmoid colon. The frequency of occurrence decreases as proximity to the cecum increases.

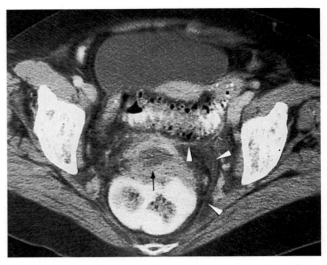

Fig. 14-43. Diverticulosis. The sigma exhibits multiple diverticulation and only moderate wall thickening. Thickening of surrounding fasciae (►) represents multiple development and healing of inflammation. Now, there are signs of abscess development at the rectosigmoid junction (→).

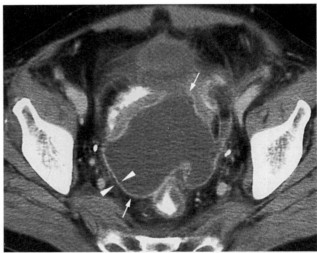

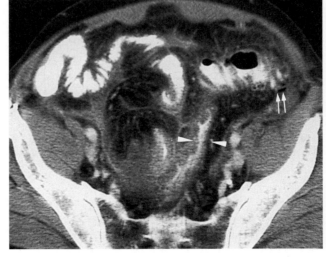

Fig. 14-44. Diverticulitis and peridiverticulitic abscess. The inflamed segment of the intestine is narrowed with thickened walls (b ►). The ventral section of the pelvic colon still exhibits isolated diverticula (⇉). Further cranial, an irregular, partially lobulated fluid accumulation with a contrasting membrane is seen. This corresponds to a large abscess (a→).

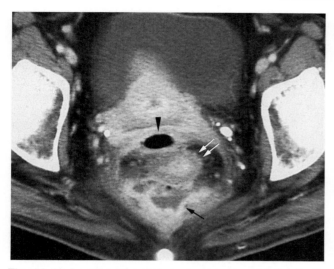

Fig. 14-45. Large perirectal abscess in sigmoid diverticulitis. Perirectal fat is permeated and exhibits multiple loculations from the abscess (→). It contains granulation tissue and air, which are typical signs of perforation (►). Overall inflammatory thickening of the rectal wall (⇉).

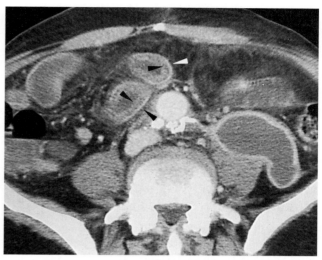

Fig. 14-47. Small intestinal ischemia after aortic aneurysmorrhaphy. All loops of the small intestine are dilated and contain fluid. One loop exhibits wall thickening and the typical double-ring sign (►). This is an expression of mucosal swelling in the course of mechanically stimulated vascular congestion.

• CT

Plain scans: Diverticulosis can often be demonstrated without further contrast medium when individual diverticula are found after the colon (sigma) has been filled with air or contrast medium. The inflammation normally causes moderate wall thickening (0.5 to 1.5 cm) with diffuse or straggly masking of surrounding fat structures and thickening of bordering fasciae. Thin-section scanning techniques should be

Fig. 14-46. Ileus of the small intestine with clearly dilated intestinal loops and evidence of fluid. Wall thickening was not detected.

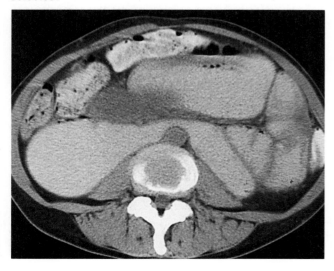

used to provide better evidence of the diverticulum and more accurate images of wall contours in poorly visible areas (of the pelvis). Inflamed vesicocolic fistulae can be readily demonstrated because of intravesicular gas.

Contrast-enhanced scans: A diffusely marginated mass can usually be identified as part of the intestine after intravenous contrast medium administration. These masses frequently contain small, intramural rows of gas, which is characteristic of diverticula.

Fusion of the inflamed diverticulum or liquefaction of inflamed pericolic tissue can lead to the development of *large abscesses*. Intravenously administered contrast medium can demonstrate these multiloculated, colliquated spaces by demarcating the abscess membrane. Accompanying fluid is usually found in the adjacent peritoneal cavity during this stage and is a sign of local peritonitis.

Differential diagnosis: Compact, circumferential wall thickening without air inclusions but with minor signs of surrounding inflammation are generally suspicious, especially when the wall thickness is greater than 2 cm (colon carcinoma). Additional examinations must be performed for clarification.

Functional Diseases of Intestine

Computer tomographic signs of obstruction in the small bowel are generally the same as those from conventional abdominal radiography. However, the cause of obstruction is usually also identifiable on CT scans.

Herniation through the abdominal wall (femoral or inguinal hernia) and internal hernias are identified by displacement of sections of the intestine, especially when the vessels of the mesenteric root are distended.

Mesenteric Ischemia

Mesenteric ischemia arises less frequently from arterial embolism (cardiac abnormalities, endocarditis, cardiac infarction) than from mesenteric vein occlusion (thrombosis due to tumor compression, inflammation, trauma or thrombosis). In patients with mesenteric vein thrombosis, it leads to hemorrhagic infarction in the affected intestinal segment with migratory edema, intramural hemorrhage, intestinal ileus, and bloody ascites.

• CT

Plain scans: Dilated, fluid-filled intestinal loops with circular, homogeneously thickened walls are sometimes surrounded by weakly hyperdense ascitic fluid. These are classical, yet nonspecific, radiologic signs of mesenteric ischemia. The more uncommon finding of gas in the intestinal walls is much more sensitive to CT detection. The degree of masking of mesenteric fat due to accompanying edema is variable.

Contrast-enhanced scans: As is the case in granulomatous intestinal inflammations, a bolus of contrast medium will lead to a ringlike or rosette-shaped enhancement pattern which, depending on the degree of wall hemorrhage, will be variably pronounced. Direct proof of mesenteric vein thrombosis, especially of the superior mesenteric vein or portal vein, can often be obtained.

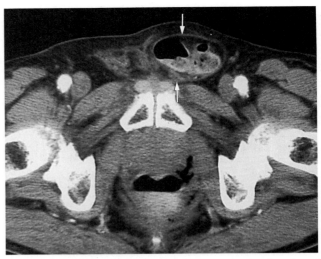

Fig. 14-48. Inguinal hernia. Due to considerable dilatation of the inguinal canal (→), the large intestine has dislocated caudally up to the scrotal attachment.

Differential diagnosis: *Intestinal pneumatosis* is also observed with ileus, enteritis, colitis, chronic obstructive lung disease, and subsequent to gastrointestinal endoscopy. The disease must therefore be diagnosed in a clinical context. Simultaneous proof of gas in the intestinal walls and veins of the mesentery are pathognomonic signs of intestinal infarction.

Fig. 14-49. Abdominal hernia. A loop of the bowel (→) protrudes through a broad gap in the muscles (▸).

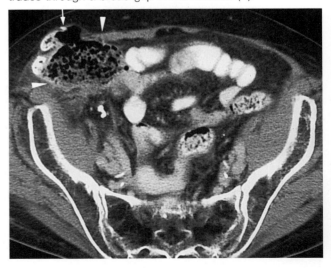

Chapter 15
The Peritoneal Cavity

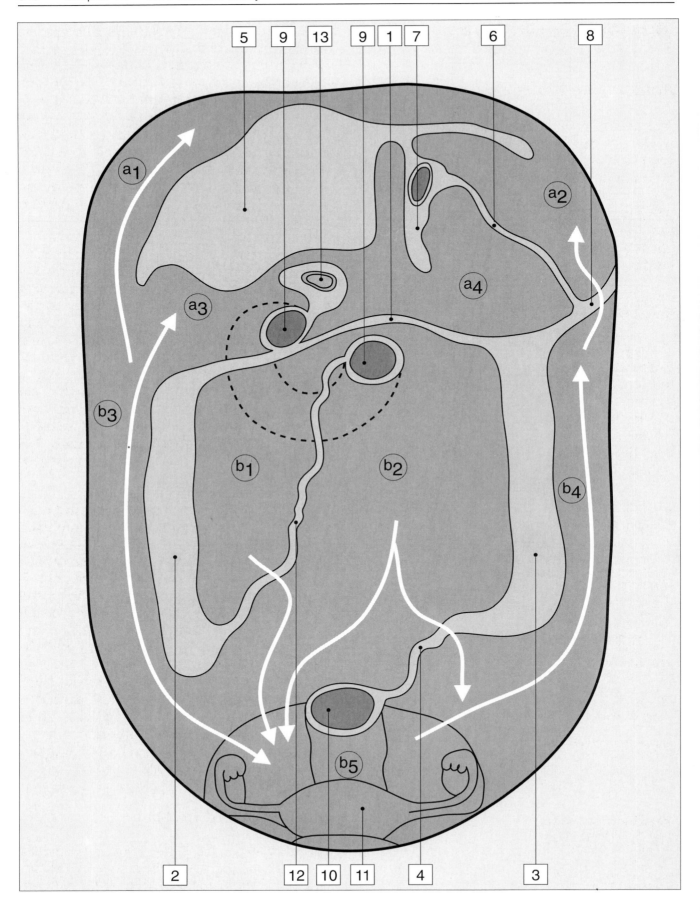

The Peritoneal Cavity

Anatomy and Imaging

The abdominal cavity is a complex object for scanning. It is difficult to demonstrate on transverse sections, because peritoneal folds are normally curved through the plane. Peritoneal compartments can be visualized, however, when they contain a sufficient amount of effusion fluid. The peritoneal cavity is divided by the transverse colon into two main compartments.

Supramesocolic Compartment

The right dorsal surface of the liver is attached to the diaphragm by the coronary ligament, thus creating subphrenic and *subhepatic compartments* that communicate ventrally. The falciform ligament forms an incomplete medial barrier separating the *right subphrenic space* from the left, so communication still exists. Intrahepatic fluid may collect in the anterior and

◄ ─────────────────────────────

Fig. 15-1. Topography of the posterior abdominal wall.

Key to symbols:
1 Transverse mesocolon
2 Attachment of ascending mesocolon
3 Attachment of descending mesocolon
4 Sigmoid mesocolon
5 Attachment area of the liver with diaphragma
6 Gastroplenic ligament
7 Gastropancreatic fold (with esophagus)
8 Phrenicocolic fold
9 Duodenum
10 Rectum
11 Uterus and adnexa
12 Root of the mesentery
13 Hepatoduodenal ligament (with portal vein)

Supramesocolic Compartment
a_1 Right subphrenic compartment
a_2 Left subphrenic compartment
a_3 Subhepatic compartment
a_4 Omental bursa

Inframesocolic Compartment
b_1 Right infracolic space
b_2 Left infracolic space
b_3 Right paracolic gutter
b_4 Left paracolic gutter
b_5 Pouch of Douglas

posterior subphrenic and subhepatic spaces. From the left cranial aspect, the upper surface of the liver is separated by the very narrow coronary ligament, which extends towards the diaphragm. The *lesser omentum (gastrohepatic ligament)* connects the posterior surface of the liver, including the porta hepatis, to the lesser curvature of the stomach and contains the left gastric artery, the hepatic artery, and the portal vein. The lesser omentum lies in front of the lesser sac *(omental bursa)* of the peritoneum.

The lesser sac is limited dorsally by the pancreas, laterally by the gastrosplenic and splenorenal ligaments, caudally by the mesocolon and gastrocolic ligament, and ventrally by the posterior stomach wall, lesser omentum, and caudate lobe of the liver. A prominent fold around the left gastric artery divides the lesser sac into upper and lower compartments. The lesser omentum attaches the intraperitoneal section of the esophagus. From the epiploic foramen, the lesser omentum extends to the hepatoduodenal ligament and contains the portal vein, hepatic artery, and common bile duct.

On CT scans, the lesser omentum can be located by identifying the vessels contained within it. The lesser omentum itself is only occasionally recognizable as a delicate, streaklike structure. The hepatoduodenal ligament is clearly identified by the course of the portal vein. The *left subphrenic space* contains the lateral and cranial convexities of the spleen and extends to the surface of the left lobe of the liver, where it is medially limited by the falciform ligament. From its dorsomedial aspect, the spleen is attached to the diaphragm by a fold of the phrenicosplenic ligament. More caudally, the phrenicocolic ligament incompletely separates the left subphrenic space from the left paracolic gutter.

Inframesocolic Compartment

The inframesocolic compartment is divided into right and left infracolic spaces by the mesentery of the small intestine. The compartment lies below and behind the mesocolon, and the ascending and descending colon are located on either side. Infracolic fluid flows caudad across the sigmoid mesocolon into the *pouch of Douglas*. From there, it may rise laterally from the ascending and descending colon to the diaphragm via the *paracolic gutters*, the preferred route being on the right. In bedridden patients, fluids readily accumulate in the lower recesses (pouch of Douglas and

posterior subhepatic space). As more and more effusion fluid accumulates, the ventro-lateral circumference of the liver and spleen and the paracolic gutter will also become filled.

Mesentery

The mesentery of the small intestine is a broad, fan-shaped peritoneal fold that contains vessels, nerves and lymph nodes. It attaches the loops of the small intestine to the posterior abdominal wall. The root of the mesentery begins to the left of midline and extends from the flexures of the duodenum and jejunum to the right sacro-iliac joint.

Fig. 15-2a–d. Topography of the upper abdominal cavities.
a) Right paravertebral section.
b) Median section.
c) Transverse section at level of porta hepatis.
d) Transverse section above the renal hili
(5 cm caudal from c).

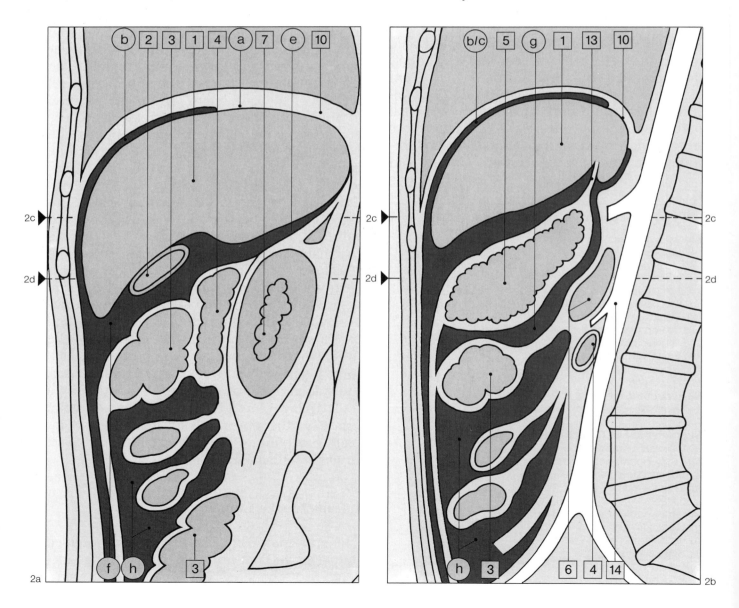

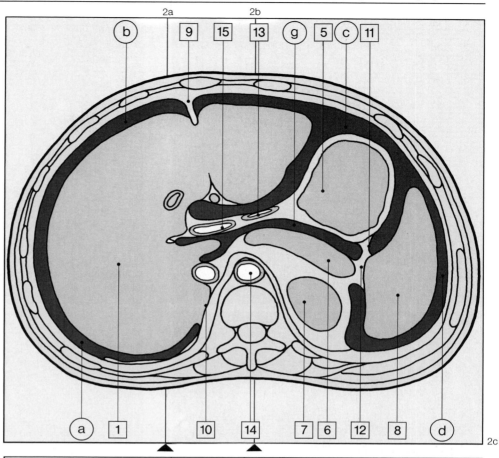

2c

Key to symbols:
1 Liver
2 Gallbladder
3 Colon
4 Duodenum
5 Stomach
6 Pancreas
7 Kidney
8 Spleen
9 Falciform ligament
10 Coronary ligament
11 Gastrosplenic ligament
12 Lienorenal ligament
13 Lesser omentum
14 Abdominal aorta
15 Portal vein

Subphrenic Compartment
a) Right dorsal
b) Right ventral
c) Left ventral
d) Left lateral

Subhepatic Space
e) Right dorsal (Morison's pouch)
f) Right ventral
g) Omental bursa
h) Inframesocolic compartment

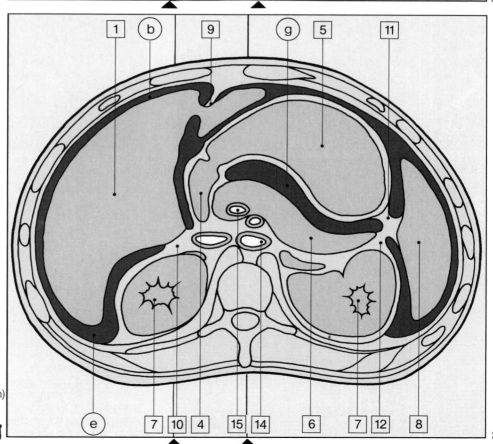

2d

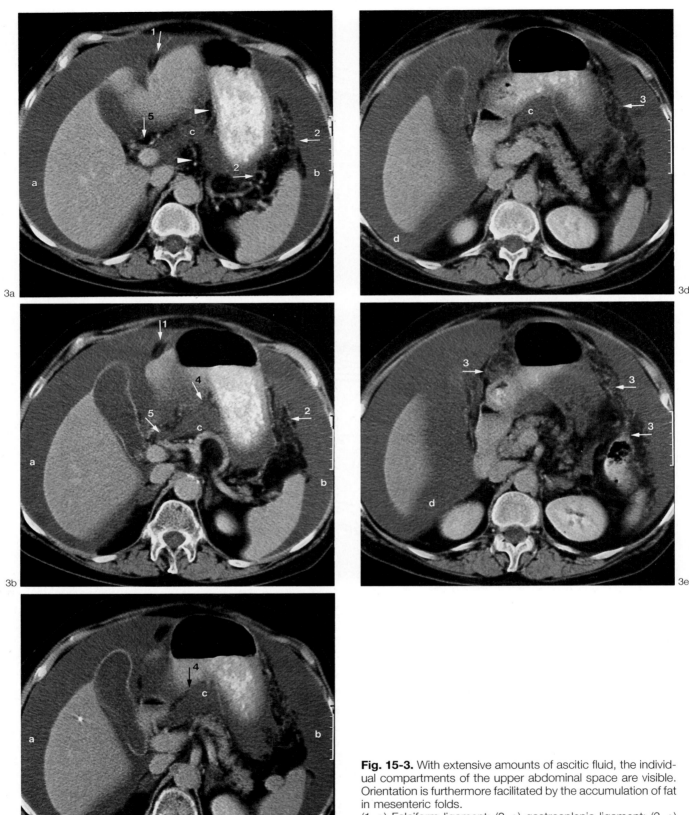

Fig. 15-3. With extensive amounts of ascitic fluid, the individual compartments of the upper abdominal space are visible. Orientation is furthermore facilitated by the accumulation of fat in mesenteric folds.

(1→) Falciform ligament; (2→) gastrosplenic ligament; (3→) gastrocolic ligament; (4→) lesser omentum; (5→) hepatoduodenal ligament; (a) right subphrenic space; (b) left subphrenic space; (c) omental bursa; (d) subhepatic space. (►) Left gastric artery (omental fold).

• CT

The position of peritoneal folds must be deduced on the basis of organs and vessels contained within them. The transverse mesocolon horizontally traverses the second part of the duodenum and can frequently be identified with reference to the transverse colic artery, which courses in front of the pancreas.

Intraperitoneal *fluid* can be demonstrated in amounts of 50 ml or more. The spaces of the peritoneal cavity can then be visualized, and peritoneal folds are indirectly demonstrated as compartment borders. Folds in the subphrenic space and dorsal subhepatic recess can be visualized as a seam of hypodensity with a width of 0.5 cm. Small amounts of fluid in other compartments of the peritoneal cavity can be reliably demonstrated only when the intestinal lumen becomes clearly distinguishable after administration of oral contrast medium. This is especially important in the infracolic space, which is difficult to visualize because of the folds of the mesenteric root. Intestinal loops and fat-containing mesenteric membranes are pushed apart when large amounts of effusion fluid collect. The lesser sac is less severely distended in patients with free ascites. When the fluid is confined (e.g. in pancreatitis, peritoneal carcinomatosis), the lesser sac has a bulging, cyst-like appearance.

Inflammation can lead to adhesions in each of the above compartments, and infection may lead to the development of an abscess. The location of encapsulated fluid is determined by the site of the primary lesion (perforation, inflammation), the corresponding intraperitoneal compartment, gravitational forces, and the position of the body. Infected fluid therefore usually accumulates in the pelvis, right subhepatic space, and right subphrenic space. In peritoneal carcinomatosis, however, it is found primarily in the pouch of Douglas, near

Fig. 15-4. Inframesocolic compartment. The paracolic gutters (a,b) are found superior to the ascending and descending colon (→). The inframesocolic compartment commences below the mesenteric root. (a) Right paracolic gutter, (b) left paracolic gutter, (c) inframesocolic compartment, frame of the colon (→), sigmoid mesocolon (▸).

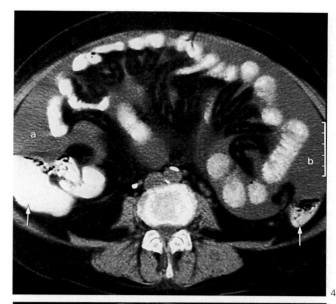

4a

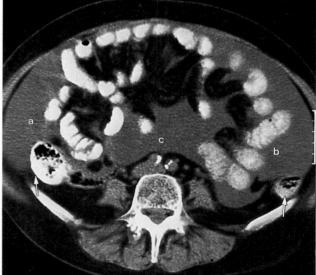

4b

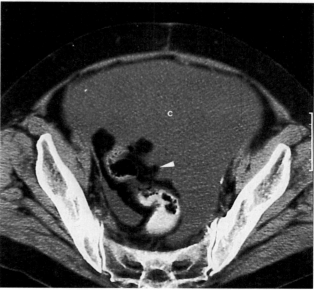

4c

the ileocecal junction, the sigmoid mesocolon, and the right paracolic gutter.

Solid infiltrating processes also spread along the above-mentioned folds, which are then rendered visible.

Ascites

Ascites is a common accompaniment of numerous diseases. Low- protein transudates develop due to an increase in venous blood pressure or reduced colloid osmotic pressure. The exudate, which accumulates as a result of peritoneal inflammation, has a protein content of more than 30 g/l. Neoplastic metastases lead to the development of ascites by causing direct peritoneal irritation or by blocking lymph drainage.

• CT

Ascites appears on CT scans as a hypodense rim around intraperitoneal organs. The degree to which the physiological compartment becomes filled with fluid depends on how much fluid has accumulated. As pressure increases, the intestine becomes eccentrically and laterally displaced, and is thereby compressed. Loculated ascites develops as a result of postoperative inflammatory or neoplastic adhesions. This leads to the development of cystic formations that cause corresponding displacement of bowel loops and compression of parenchymatous organs. The lesser sac is normally only moderately filled with ascitic fluid. When pancreatic and gastric findings are normal, carcinomatosis is probable when the amount of ascitic fluid in the lesser sac is much larger than that in the infracolic spaces. In patients with peritoneal carcinomatosis, solid components can be sensitively detected on the smooth surfaces of parenchymatous organs from a diameter of ca. 0.5 cm and larger. This size is indicative of malignancy.

Fig. 15-5. Ascites in peritoneal carcinomatosis. Peritoneal adherence leads to non-uniform distribution of ascites. Falciform ligament (►), stomach (► ◄), greater omentum (⇒), mesenteric root (→).

Table 15-1. Diseases accompanied by ascites.

Cardiovascular diseases (incl. hypoproteinemia)
• Right heart failure • Occlusion of inferior vena cava • Portal vein occlusion • Budd-Chiari's syndrome • Constrictive pericarditis • Hypoalbuminemia • Cirrhosis of the liver • Myxedema
Inflammatory Diseases
• Peritonitis • Familial paroxymal peritonitis • Abdominal vasculitis • Eosinophil gastroenteritis • Tuberculosis • Pancreatitis • Intestinal perforation • Whipple's disease • Glomerulonephritis
Neoplastic Diseases
• Peritoneal carcinomatosis (malignant growths in the stomach, colon, ovaries, pancreas) • Blockage of lymph flow (incl. malignant lymphomas) • Pseudomyxoma peritonei • Mesothelioma • Meigs' syndrome

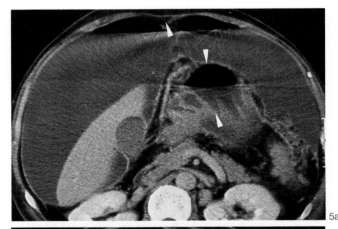
5a

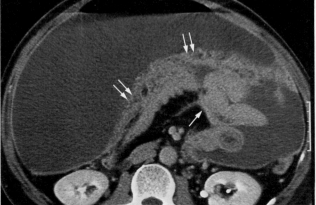
5b

The *attenuation value* of ascitic fluid fluctuates in accordance with variability of the protein content, with values normally ranging from 0 to 30 HU. Very dense ascites can be detected in patients with tuberculosis and intraperitoneal hemorrhage (bloody ascites) or in patients with ureteroperitoneal fistulae after the administration of contrast medium.

Peritonitis – Intraperitoneal Abscess

Peritonitis usually arises from an infection of the abdominal cavity after injury or bacterial infiltration of the peritoneum. Acute peritonitis can cause severe inflammatory reaction with fibrino-purulent exudates in the entire mesentery and peritoneum.

An intraperitoneal *abscess* is basically infected local peritonitis that develops after perforation of the gastrointestinal wall (ulcer, diverticulum), adjacent inflammation (pancreatitis, tubovarian, pericholecystitis), or surgery. The abscess develops in the vicinity of the affected organ, becomes encapsulated, and may spread in the corresponding peritoneal compartment. Abscesses in the lesser sac result from ulcer perforation of the posterior gastric wall or pancreatitis. Abscesses are found in the left subphrenic space after ulcer perforation of the anterior gastric wall, anastomotic insufficiency, or colon perforation. Depending on the drainage paths of intraperitoneal fluid, abscesses may be found in the *subphrenic* or *subhepatic* spaces when there is inframesocolic or supramesocolic involvement. The right space is affected two to three times more frequently than the left. The (posterior) subhepatic space (Morrison's pouch) is the deepest point of the abdominal cavity and is preferentially affected in bedridden patients. *Douglas'* abscess arises not only from inflammation of

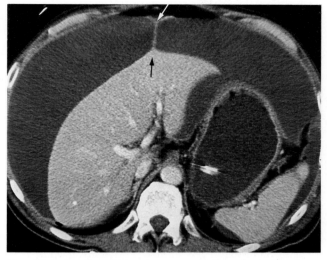

Fig. 15-6. Ascites. Extensive accumulation of subphrenic ascites, divided by the falciform ligament (→). Insignificant amount of ascitic fluid within the omental bursa.

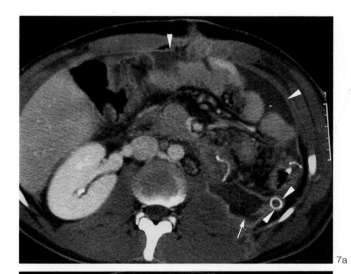

7a

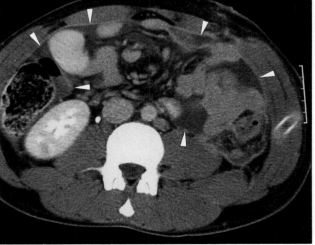

7b

Fig. 15-7. Peritonitis after gunshot injury. After nephrectomy and surgery, fluid with a slightly raised attenuation value (17–25 HU) is found in the abdominal cavity. The peritoneal membrane shows clear enhancement after contrast medium administration, thereby signalling inflammation (►). The bed of the kidney has a hypodense zone corresponding to an old hematoma (a→). The drainage tube (► ◄) lies next to this accumulation of fluid.

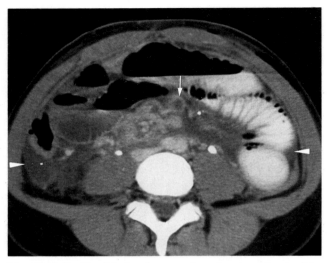

Fig. 15-8. Peritonitis in abscess-forming lymphadenitis. After contrast medium administration, there is only discrete enhancement of the peritoneum (▻). The peritoneal fluid has an attenuation value of 15 HU. Abscess fluid can be found in the region of the mesenteric root (→).

Fig. 15-9. Peritoneal abscess. On the left, behind the abdominal wall, there is a lenticulate area of hypodensity, the margins of which clearly absorb contrast medium (▻ ◅). The attenuation value is ca. 25 HU.

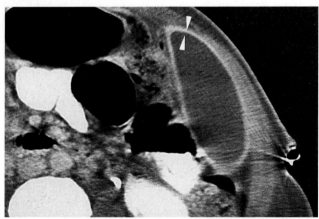

9

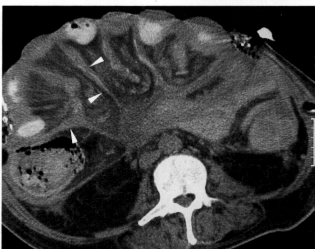

10

pelvic organs, but also as a result of inframesocolic exudation.

• CT

Acute *peritonitis* is characterized by a generalized collection of intraperitoneal fluid. After the administration of contrast medium, this severe inflammation is marked by dilatation of the mesenteric vessels, indistinctness of mesenteric fat, and opacification of peritoneal membranes. Chronic peritonitis can lead to extensive thickening of the peritoneum.

A *developing* intraperitoneal abscess behaves like loculated ascitic fluid, so it is initially difficult to differentiate between the two. Preferential locations for abscess formation are the right subphrenic and right subhepatic spaces and the pouch of Douglas. When clinical symptoms are obvious, any localized, isolated fluid collection in the peritoneal cavity is suspicious. To be able to tell whether an *intestinal loop* contains free fluid or an *abscess*, optimal contrast preparation of the intestine is necessary. *Gas bubbles* within an extraluminal hypodense mass is pathognomonic of an infectious lesions. Elongated gas shadows inside a circumscribed mass can, however, be due to underlying fistulization in the intestinal lumen. The surrounding peritoneal membrane broadens when *abscesses* become chronic. Contrast administration opacifies the membrane, and the typical rim enhancement of abscesses can be seen on the CT scan.

The *attenuation value of abscesses* normally ranges between 20 and 40 HU, but can be much lower, especially when the patient is receiving treatment. It may therefore be difficult to differentiate pseudocysts, liquefying hematoma, biloma, and loculated ascites radiographically. Fine-needle aspiration or radionuclide imaging can be performed as an additional diagnostic measure as required.

When abscess formation spreads to solid organs or the retroperitoneal space (perityphlic

Fig. 15-10. Peritonitis with fanlike fibrinous inflammation. The peritoneal membrane, thickened by fibrinous deposits, displays a fanlike configuration in the mesenteric root (▻).

abscess), masking of fatty tissue and the formation of a clearly visible abscess membrane make it much easier to diagnose abscess formation.

Differential diagnosis: Cystic intraperitoneal masses due to abscesses, hematomas, peritoneal carcinomatosis, pancreatic pseudocysts, mesenteric cysts, lymphoceles (e.g. after kidney transplant), retroperitoneal lymphadenectomy and urinomas (after rupture of the bladder) must be considered in the diagnosis.

Hemorrhage in the Abdominal Cavity

Hemorrhages in the abdominal cavity may arise from blunt abdominal trauma (liver, spleen), intestinal perforation with vascular erosion, spontaneous rupture of a vascularized tumor, extrauterine pregnancy or excessive anticoagulant therapy.

• CT

Intraperitoneal blood collects at the previously mentioned sites (see anatomy section) and can be demonstrated especially well in the subhepatic recess. The *attenuation values* of blood from a fresh hemorrhage, like that of flowing blood, are much higher than the attenuation values of *ascites*. A true hematoma with blood aggregation is rare, and attenuation values may be as high as 70 or 80 HU (e.g. encapsulated blood). Inhomogeneous attenuation values can be observed within intraperitoneal fluid after incomplete coagulation, but the attenuation drops sharply within days (provided no secondary hemorrhage occurs). The attenuation value usually drops to a level of 0 to 20 HU after a week or two. The position of circumscribed hyperdensity areas within accumulated fluid gives clues as to location (organ) of the initial hemorrhage. In encapsulated areas of the peritoneal cavity, sedimentation phenom-

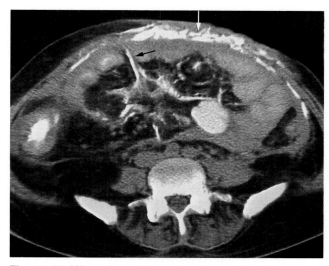

Fig. 15-11. When there is longstanding fanlike, fibrinous inflammation, **calcification** of the peritoneal membrane frequently occurs (→).

Fig. 15-12. Mesenteric hematoma after blunt abdominal trauma. The attenuation value of 75 HU and the masking of mesenteric fat are the primary diagnostic signs of mesenteric hematoma.

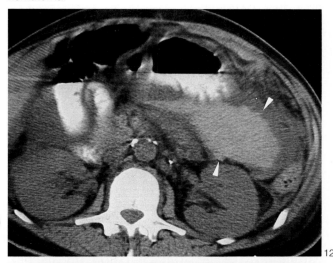

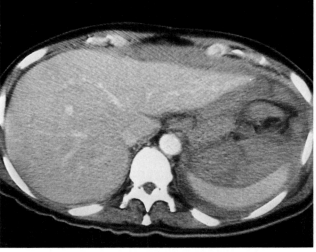

Fig. 15-13. Hemoperitoneum. The abdominal cavity is filled with hyperdense fluid with an attenuation value of 50 HU. The parenchymatous organs are clearly demarcated after contrast medium administration.

ena sometimes occur which are similar to those observed with hematomas.

Biliary Ascites

Leakage of bile into the peritoneal cavity is usually due to iatrogenic causes, but this may also arise due to trauma or spontaneous rupture of a bile passage. The leaked bile produces a local inflammatory response that quickly leads to encapsulation of the fluid. Therefore, intraperitoneal bile is usually found as localized effusion fluid located near the porta hepatis or in the epigastric region (biloma).

• CT

Biliary ascites usually appears on CT scans as a simple unilocular (seldom multilocular), low density area near the liver. The CT number is around 20 HU.

Pseudomyxoma Peritonei

Pseudomyxoma peritonei is an intraperitoneal accumulation of gelatinous, mucinous material. The mucin-producing cells that cause this disorder usually originate from an adenocarcinoma. The most common cause is the spread of a mucinous cystadenocarcinoma of the ovary to the peritoneal cavity, but malignant degeneration of an appendicular mucocele occasionally can also be seen. Peritoneal pseudomyxomas rarely originate from other mucinous carcinomas (of the stomach, colon, uterus, bile ducts, or pancreas). An abscess may develop within a pseudomyxoma.

• CT

Plain scans: The peritoneum is usually filled with hypodense formations, and surrounding organs show local displacement. Lenticular indentations due to encapsulation of fluid can develop on the surface of the liver. Irregular septation of hypodense areas is a characteristic sign, but is frequently not clearly visible.

The attenuation value of the intraperitoneal mass ranges from 15 to 30 HU, i.e., slightly

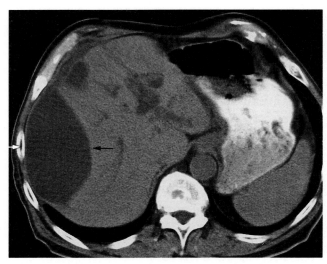

Fig. 15-14. Biloma. CT after liver transplantation. Patient has the clinical picture of cholestasis. A primarily subcapsular accumulation of bile is found (→).

Fig. 15-15. Pseudomyxoma peritonei. There is a considerable amount of nodular thickening in the greater omentum (a ►) and peritoneum in the region of the pelvis (b ►).

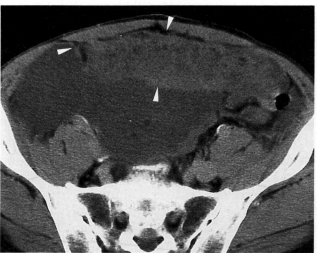

15a

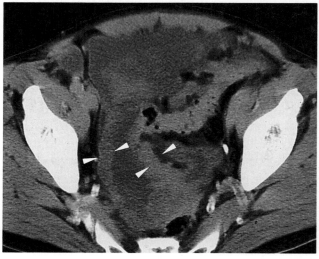

15b

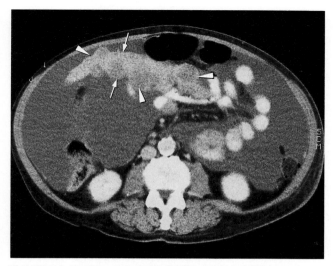

Fig. 15-16. Peritoneal mesothelioma. In addition to extensive ascites, there is knobby thickening of the greater omentum (→). The tumor tissue clearly absorbs contrast medium, and bulbous tumor components can be seen (►). The remaining sections of the peritoneal membrane are not clearly thickened.

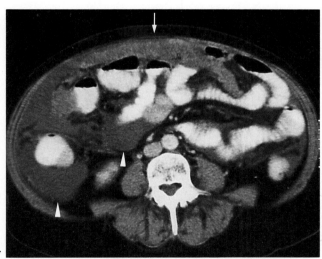

17

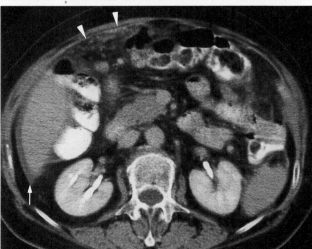

18

above that of water. Calcification may be observed in chronic disease, especially in the vicinity of the greater omentum.

Contrast-enhanced scans: Septation is seen. The solid components are slightly enhanced and therefore distinguishable from mucinous deposits. The masses, themselves, remain unenhanced. The most common underlying cause of pseudomyxoma peritonei, namely ovarian cancer, can frequently be identified in the pelvis after contrast administration.

Differential diagnosis: Peritonitis and cystic intraperitoneal masses must be excluded from the diagnosis.

Primary and Metastatic Peritoneal Neoplasms

Although primary peritoneal mesothelioma is very rare, other tumors frequently metastasize in the peritoneum. The primary site of a metastatic peritoneal carcinoma is usually the ovary. Other primary locations include gastrointestinal organs (colon, stomach, pancreas and liver). Sarcomas are most commonly associated with non-Hodgkin's lymphoma, followed by leukemia, Hodgkin's lymphoma and leiomyosarcoma. Spread is initially subperitoneal, then intraperitoneal after the peritoneum has become involved. Solid tumor components vary from finely granular to coarsely nodular types and may be disseminated or localized. An effusion of variable severity is a frequent accompaniment.

● CT

Plain scans: Evidence of solid components within ascitic fluid usually means that there is a

Fig. 15-17. Peritoneal carcinomatosis in ovarian carcinoma. The major omentum shows flat, pancake-like thickening (→). Ascites is also found (►). Visible sections of the peritoneal membrane are accentuated, but lack clear evidence of nodular formations.

Fig. 15-18. Peritoneal carcinomatosis in ovarian carcinoma. The only major findings were veillike, dense structures in the gastrocolic ligament and greater omentum (►). Only slight amount of ascitic fluid (→).

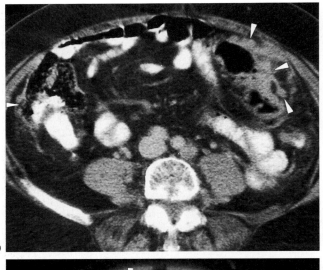

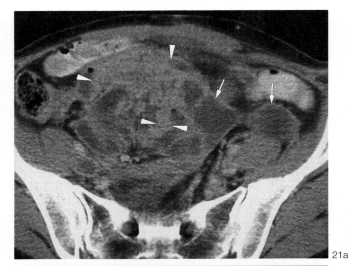

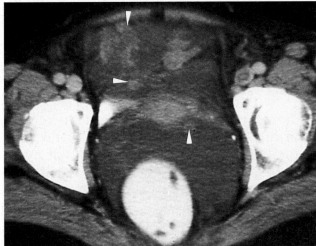

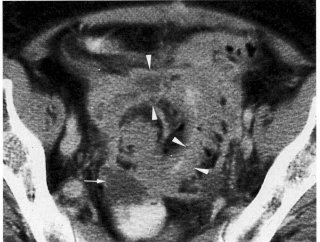

Fig. 15-19. Peritoneal carcinomatosis without ascites. Small, nodular dense structures can be seen near the colon (►).

Fig. 15-20. Peritoneal carcinomatosis in ovarian carcinoma. Ascitic fluid with disseminated tumor nodules (►) is visible in the true pelvis.

Fig. 15-21. Peritoneal carcinomatosis in ovarian carcinoma of the true pelvis. In both patients, the walls of the intestine are thickened due to deposits that have accumulated during peritoneal carcinomatosis (►). They surround loculated accumulations of ascitic fluid (→).

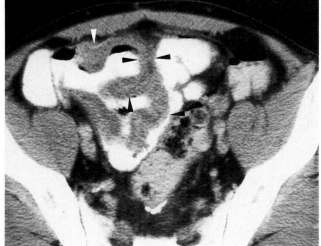

Fig. 15-22. Peritoneal carcinomatosis after colon carcinoma. In absence of hypodense ascitic fluid, cufflike, contrast medium absorbing soft-tissue structures are found between loops of the intestine.

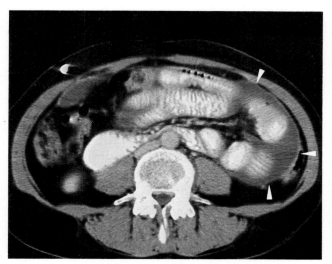

Fig. 15-23. Peritoneal carcinomatosis. Focal, encapsulated fluid collections with small, discrete nodular densification in the parietal membrane (►).

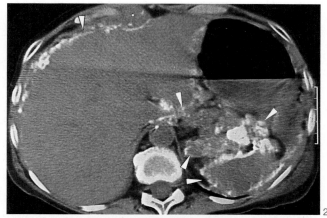

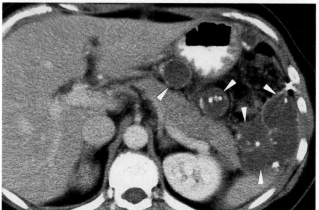

peritoneal neoplasm. Discrete solid components inside ascitic fluid are best demonstrated on smooth surfaces of organs like the liver, where they can be demonstrated when of a diameter of 0.5 cm and larger. Nodular soft-tissue structures located between intestinal loops are not as sensitive to detection. They can be demonstrated from a diameter of 1.5 cm only after optimum homogeneous opacification of the bowel. Sensitive proof of ascites must be critically evaluated in patients with corresponding tumor diseases, since peritoneal metastases measuring only a few millimeters in size can be overlooked. Calcification of peritoneal metastases is occasionally observed in cancer of the ovary.

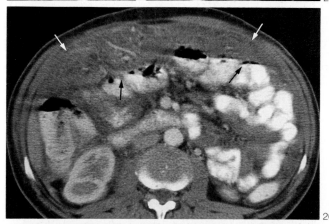

Fig. 15-24. Calcified peritoneal metastases. Within ascitic fluid, there are calcified structures on peritoneal and hepatic tissues (►); these occur preferentially in ovarian carcinoma.

Fig. 15-25. Peritoneal carcinomatosis in conjunction with a muciferous carcinoma of the ovary; this is located within encapsulated pockets of ascites (►).

Fig. 15-26. Peritoneal and mesenteric manifestations of lymphoma after HIV infection. Strandlike tumor structures that absorb contrast medium are disseminated throughout the entire abdominal cavity, where they cause thickening of the major omentum (a→), and throughout the mesenteric root, where bulbous growth of lymph nodes is seen on the mesenteric attachment (b→).

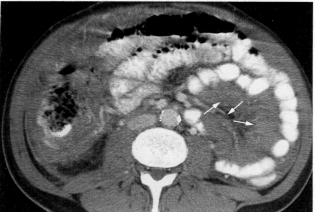

Involvement of subperitoneal *mesenteric fat* can lead to four different clinical pictures: Finely reticular, streaklike opacification (1) is an expression of interstitial spread. These areas are variably permeated by (2) fine or coarse nodules. These structures can merge to form (3) inhomogeneous soft-tissue zones. The large surface area of the greater omentum presents a broad, boardlike (pancake) appearance on tangential scans. (4) A stellate configuration may be seen at the mesenteric root due to stretching and swelling of vessels. This occurs more commonly in association with carcinomas, whereas rounded, nodular densifications predominate in lymphomas.

Contrast-enhanced scans: In addition to demonstrating the primary tumor, bolus administration of contrast medium also facilitates the diagnosis by enhancing soft-tissue elements and peritoneal border surfaces. It also makes it easier to identify slightly enlarged lymph nodes in the mesenteric root.

Chapter 16
The Spleen

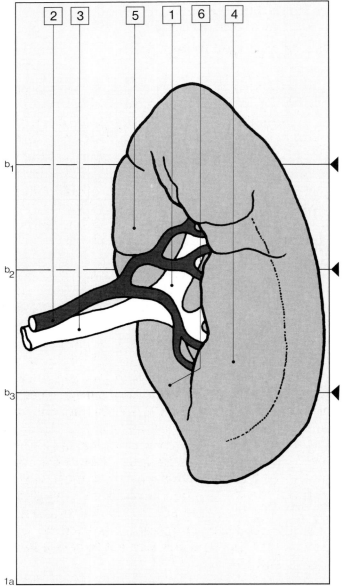

1a

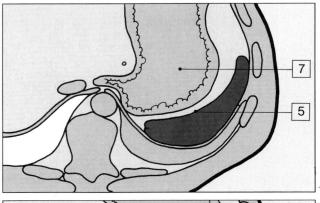

1b₁

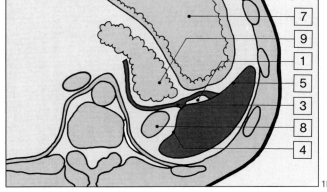

1b₂

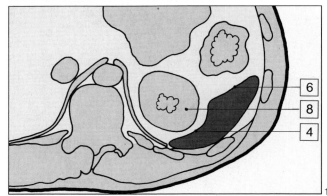

1b₃

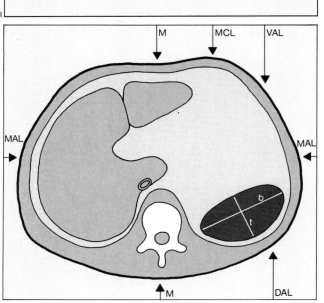

1c

Fig. 16-1. The normal spleen.
a) Ventral view.
b) Configuration in transverse section (for level, see 1a).

c) Normal dimensions of
the spleen
w = 7–10 cm
d = 4–6 cm
l = 11–15 cm

d) Splenic index
w × d × l = ca. 300
range = 160–440
(according to Lackner)

Key to symbols:
1 Hilum
2 Splenic artery
3 Splenic vein
4 Renal fascia
5 Gastric fascia
6 Colic fascia
7 Stomach
8 Kidney
9 Pancreas

w = width (x-axis of the ellipsoid
splenic diameter)
t = depth (y-axis of the ellipsoid
splenic diameter)
l = longitudinal length
(= scan route)

M   = Median line
MCL= Medioclavicular line
AAL = Anterior axillary line
MAL = Middle axillary line
DAL = Dorsal axillary line

The Spleen

Anatomy and Imaging

The normal adult spleen does not weigh more than 200 g. Its shape conforms to the contours of the organs adjacent to it, e.g. the stomach, kidney, diaphragm and splenic flexure of the colon. The outer capsule of the spleen is covered by the peritoneum. The supplying vessels reach the spleen via the splenorenal ligament and fan out in the hilar region. The vessels extend with the gastrosplenic ligament to the greater curvature of the stomach.

Since the size of the spleen is variable, it is a difficult to assign *standard values for normal size*. The transverse oval spleen is normally less than 10 cm in length and 6 cm in breadth. As a rule, however, the craniocaudad length of the normal spleen should not exceed 15 cm, as can be adequately demonstrated by normal scanning techniques. Splenomegaly can be diagnosed when the size of the spleen exceeds at least two of these standard values. The splenic index (Fig. 16–1) has proven its practical value. However, its numbers do not represent the actual weight of the spleen, but a linearly proportional value. The normal-sized spleen usually does not extend beyond the mid-axillary line, and only in splenomegaly or hepatomegaly is there surface contact between the spleen and the liver.

The splenic parenchyma has a homogeneous appearance on plain scans. The *attenuation value* of the spleen is a mean 45 ± 5 Hounsfield Units (HU). Immediately after the *administration of contrast medium*, the spleen shows a mottled or inhomogeneous enhancement pattern, which corresponds to the red pulp and trabecula of the spleen. 90 to 120 seconds later, the initial enhancement pattern fades to a more homogeneous one.

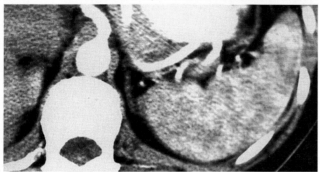
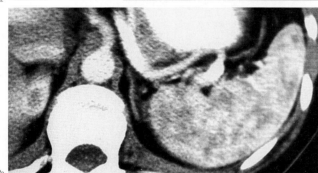
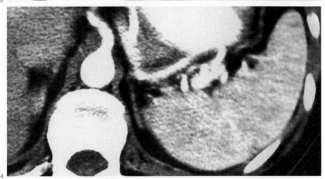
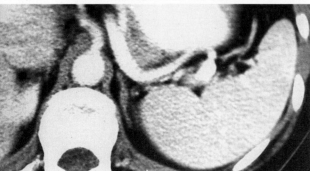

$1e_1$
$1e_2$
$1e_3$
$1e_4$
$1e_5$

Fig. 16-1e. Contrast enhancement of the splenic parenchyma after a bolus injection of contrast medium. Brief demonstration of "partitioning", which corresponds to trabecular and pulpar parenchymal structures. (e_2 = 10 s; e_3 = 20 s; e_4 = 30 s, e_5 = 60 s).

Table 16-1. Causes of splenomegaly, based on model by Harrison.

Splenomegaly due to inflammations	**Acute (subacute) infection** Septicemia, bacterial endocarditis, abscess, mononucleosis, etc.) **Chronic infection** Tuberculosis, syphilis, histoplasmosis, brucellosis, malaria, leishmaniosis, etc.) **Other causes** Lupus erythematosus, rheumatoid arthritis, sarcoidosis, histiocytosis, etc.
Splenomegaly due to intrasplenic obstruction	Cirrhosis of the liver, thrombosis, stenosis of the portal vein, splenic vein, right heart insufficiency
Splenomegaly due to increased storage	Nieman-Pick's disease, Gaucher's disease, amyloidosis, hemosiderosis, hemochromatosis
Splenomegaly due to disturbed hematopoiesis and blood decomposition	Hemolytic anemia, thalassemia, myelofibrosis, polycythaemia vera, thrombocytopenic purpura
Splenomegaly due to neoplasms	Cysts (neoplastic pseudocysts), benign solid tumors (hemangiomas, etc.), reticulum cell sarcoma, malignant lymphoma, leukemia, myeloma

Table 16-2. Diseases from which **splenic calcification** can arise.

Infections	Echinococcus cysticus Abscess Granulomas (multiple) in – Tuberculosis – Brucellosis – Histoplasmosis
Tumors	Lymphangioma Hemangioma Nonparasitic cysts
Vascular diseases	Arteriosclerosis Aneurysm (splenic artery) Hematoma Pseudocyst Infarction Phleboliths
Other diseases	Sickle-cell anemia Hemosiderosis Capsular calcification

Fig. 16-4. Echinococcus cyst. This calcified echinococcus cyst has shrivelled. Spicula-like projections therefore extend from the chitin membrane.

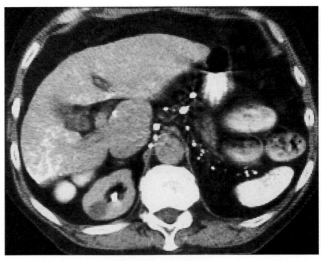

Fig. 16-2. Thorotrast spleen. Small spleen with a diffuse increase in attenuation value (250 HU). The splenic lobe as well as the right lobe of the liver are opaque-laden. Compensatory hypertrophy of the caudate lobe can be seen.

Fig. 16-3. Calcified splenic cysts, probably of parasitic origin.

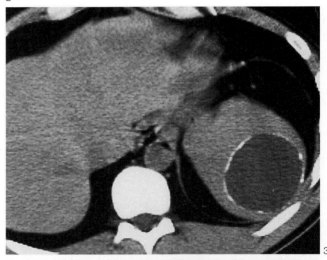

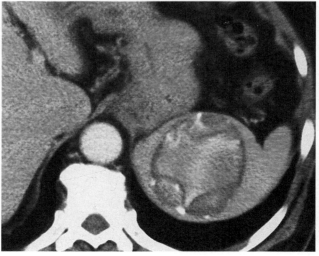

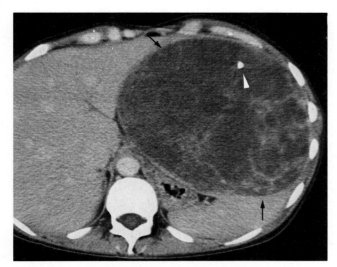

Fig. 16-5. Lymphangiomatosis of the spleen. Large mass of 12 cm diameter (→), with capsule, is located on top of the spleen. Several fine septations, which become visible after contrast medium administration, are detected. A single, small, isomorphic area of calcification was found (►).

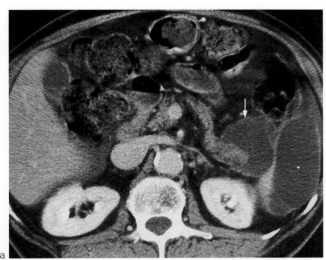

6a

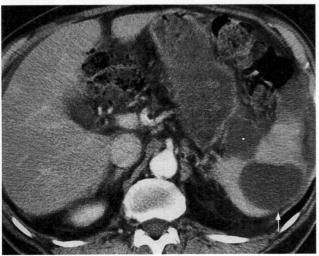

6b

Cystic Splenic Diseases

Splenic cysts are rare and are sometimes parasitic in nature (e.g. echinococcus cysts). Benign congenital splenic cysts are epidermoid cysts that have an epithelial lining (true cysts). They occur more often in women than in men. False cysts lack an epithelial lining and may develop as a result of trauma or infarct. Some benign splenic neoplasms such as lymphangiomas and hemangiomas also have cystic elements.

• CT

Cysts of the spleen display the usual CT characteristics of benign cysts. In very large cysts, the splenic parenchyma is flattened and claws develop along the edges. Ringlike calcification occurs occasionally in epidermoid cysts and pseudocysts, but preferentially in parasitic cysts, which have the same CT appearance as those found in the liver. Depending on the longevity of the preceding hematoma, the attenuation value of posttraumatic pseudocysts may be slightly higher than that of water.

Solid Tumors of the Spleen

Although malignant lymphomas and plasmocytomas can develop in the splenic parenchyma, primary splenic tumors are extremely rare. The frequency of hemangiomas is greater than that of lymphangiomas. Hemartomas, fibromas, myxomas, chondromas, osteomas, malignant hemangio-endotheliomas, and fibrosarcomas, on the other hand, are rarities.

When splenic metastases occurs, the underlying primary tumor is usually in the late stages of development. Splenic metastases is usually characterized by multiple lesions that are disseminated hematogenously. Lymphatic spread occurs only in isolated cases. Splenic metas-

Fig. 16-6. Splenic metastases from a carcinoma in the tail of the pancreas. Liquid and necrotic areas near the tail of the pancreas (a→) and inside the spleen (b→) in a patient with peritoneal carcinomatosis.

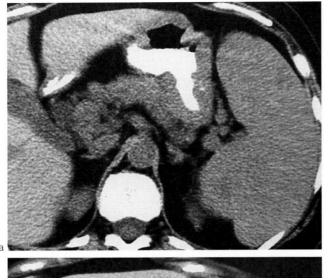

7a

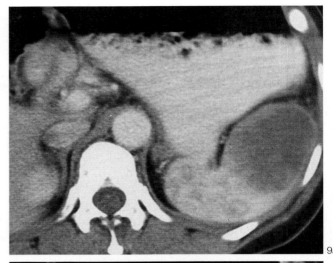

9a

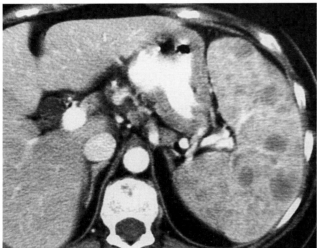

7b

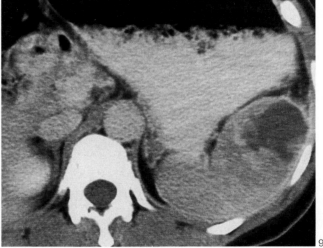

9b

Fig. 16-7. Non-Hodgkin's lymphoma. Splenic enlargement with multiple lesions which become delineated as hypodense zones after bolus contrast medium administration.

Fig. 16-8. Splenic involvement in Hodgkin's disease. Slight hypodensity after contrast medium administration and slight deformity of contour.

Fig. 16-9. Non-Hodgkin's lymphoma. A hypodense, delineated mass shows stronger peripheral enhancement (b) in the late bolus contrast medium phase.

Fig. 16-10. Non-Hodgkin's lymphoma. The lower pole of the spleen is enlarged and becomes clearly demarcated (hypodense) after contrast medium administration. Enlarged lymph nodes were also found along the splenic vessels.

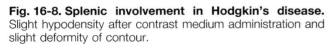

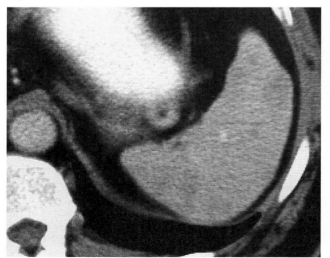

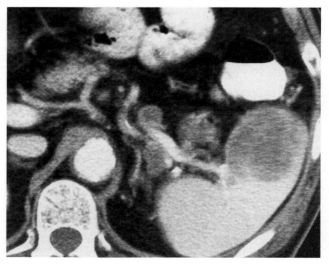

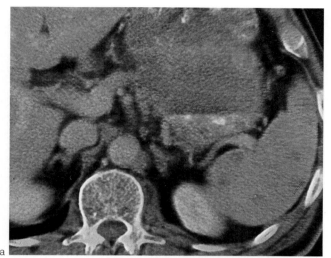

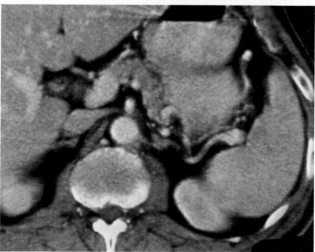

Fig. 16-11. Non-Hodgkin's lymphoma. Very fine hypodense structures could be seen after contrast medium administration. They were no longer demonstrable after chemotherapy (b).

Fig. 16-12. Metastases from a melanoma. A large, hypodense mass displays inhomogeneous enhancement after bolus contrast medium administration.

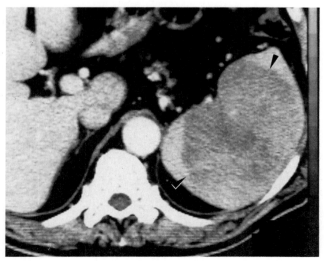

tases often arise from primary tumors of the skin (malignant melanoma), lungs and breast. They more infrequently arise from primary tumors of the ovaries, testes, prostate, colon and rectum.

Splenic metastases can lead to considerable enlargement of the spleen, although almost one third of them are so small that they must be detected microscopically.

• CT

Malignant Lymphomas

Plain scans: Most non-Hodgkin's lymphomas (NHL) cause splenomegaly, whereas only ca. 65 % of Hodgkin's lymphomas cause an abnormal increase in splenic size. The external splenic contours may remain unchanged, or a ball-shaped nodule may develop. In the majority of cases, the CT density of the splenic parenchyma is homogeneous, which correlates with diffuse organ permeation. Nodular implants, which more frequently develop in NHL than in Hodgkin's disease, appear as focal low-density zones.

Contrast-enhanced scans: A bolus of contrast medium demarcates tumor lesions as circumscribed low-density zones. During the scan sequence, it is possible to verify diffuse organ involvement when trabeculation is not found during the arterial phase and when a fine, nodular pattern is observed during the parenchymal phase.

Rare splenic *angiosarcomas* and *hemangiotheliomas* are demonstrated on plain scans as hypodense, variably extensive masses. Hypervascularization in these tumors can be demonstrated by injecting a bolus of contrast medium. When Thorotrast accumulation is present, there is probably a concomitant angiosarcoma.

Hemangiomas frequently form multiple masses that appear on CT scans as sharply demarcated, variably configured hypodense areas. Only slight enhancement occurs after a protracted bolus of contrast medium is administered. Round areas of calcification and phleboliths have been reported in isolated cases.

Multiple, localized *metastases* are found in most cases. The degree of hypodensity and post-constrast enhancement of the lesions is determined by the type of underlying primary tumor as well as the degree of vascularity and/or necrosis of the lesions.

Inflammatory Splenic Diseases

In acute and chronic infections, hyperplasia occurs in various cell elements and leads to variably severe splenomegaly. Granulomatous infection causes only moderate splenic enlargement.

Disseminated micronodular calcification frequently develops, especially in the healing stages of diseases such as *tuberculosis*, *histoplasmosis* and *brucellosis* (possibly concentric stratification in brucellosis). A *splenic abscess* often develops in the course of generalized infection (e.g. septicemia), especially in immunosuppressed patients. Abscesses rarely develop in necrotic splenic tissue (infarct, pseudocyst, hematoma).

• CT

Granulomatous infiltrates lead to an abnormal enlargement of splenic size and may occasionally be observed as disseminated low-density areas after bolus administration of contrast medium. In many cases, dense, round areas of calcification are the only signs of a past infection.

Splenic abscesses are demonstrated on CT scans as circumscribed hypodense zones that do not enhance after the administration of contrast medium. Depending on the stage of their development, they may be clearly demarcated from surrounding tissue and have a characteristic abscess wall. The attenuation value, which changes as the abscess ages, ranges from 20 to 40 HU. Proof of infection is obtained when gas is found in pockets of liquefaction.

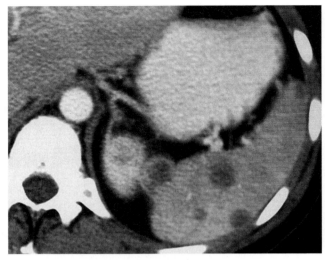

Fig. 16-13. Epithelioid cell granulomatosis of the spleen **(sarcoidosis).** After bolus contrast medium administration, round, hypodense structures which were only discretely visible on plain scans become sharply demarcated.

Fig. 16-14. Splenic abscess. Hypodense subcapsular regions contain small amounts of gas (►), a sign of abscess formation.

Fig. 16-15. Splenic abscess. Subcapsular hypodense structure with subtle amounts of gas (►).

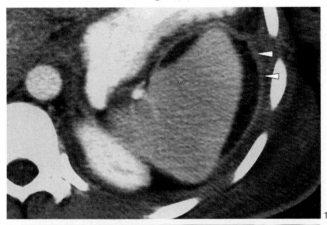

14

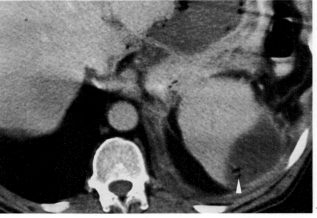

15

After bolus administration of contrast medium, micro-abscesses arising in fungal infections are demonstrated on CT scans as multiple, small, sharply delineated hypodense zones that lack a well-defined abscess wall. These abscesses may be as large as 2 cm. Micro-abscesses often occur simultaneously in the spleen and liver.

Differential diagnosis: It may be difficult to distinguish abscesses from long-standing hematomas or pseudocysts when pathognomonic signs of gas accumulation are not found. The clinical findings must then be used to substantiate the diagnosis.

Trauma

The majority of splenic lacerations are caused by blunt abdominal trauma. Lacerations are usually incurred in traffic accidents, but occasionally arise from stab or goring wounds. When the spleen is enlarged due to inflammation (e.g. in mononucleosis), a splenic rupture may spontaneously occur without significant trauma. When the vessel pedicle is damaged, large vessels may rupture or thrombosis may develop. Depending on the severity of these effects, infarction or the development of collateral vascular circulation may occur. In splenic injuries resulting from contusion, subtle tears in a vessel may be seen, but are of little clinical significance. Evidence of a splenic hematoma, on the other hand, is a very serious clinical sign, since a ruptured splenic capsule can lead to a life-threatening hemorrhage into the abdominal cavity.

Splenic Hematoma

Plain scans: Although fresh splenic hematomas may appear hyperdense, they are more often isodense as compared with the normal spleen. Long-standing hematomas are demonstrated as hypodense areas that usually are well distinguishable.

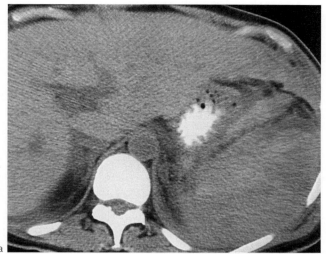

16a

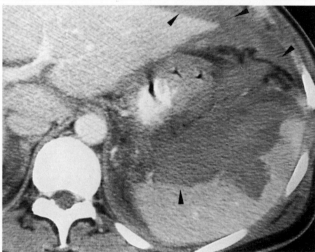

16b

Fig. 16-16. Acute splenic rupture. The irregular contours of the spleen within slightly hyperdense subphrenic fluid can be seen even on plain scans. After bolus contrast medium administration, viable splenic tissue is demarcated from surrounding blood (►).

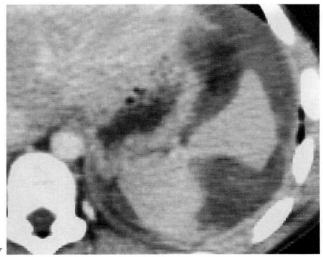

17

Fig. 16-17. Splenic rupture. Parenchymal laceration is made evident by the convexity of the spleen. The surrounding fluids, with attenuation values exceeding 50 HU, indicate the presence of blood in the abdominal cavity.

Compression and deformation of the splenic parenchyma is usually observed with a *subcapsular* hematoma. The capsule of the spleen usually appears on CT scans as a demarcated, circular structure that gives the hematoma a sickle-shaped appearance. *Intraparenchymal* hematomas have irregular margins and a sometimes wedge-shaped appearance. If a parenchymal rupture is not discovered and the capsule of the spleen does not rupture, the hematoma may transform into a (false) cyst. Intraperitoneal collection of fluid is an important indicator of *splenic rupture*. When there is a fresh secondary rupture, the CT number of hyperdense intraperitoneal blood will be higher than that of the intrasplenic or perisplenic hematoma. As a rule, the status of adjacent structures (liver, kidney, pancreas, bone) must be evaluated for further damage.

Contrast-enhanced scans: A bolus of contrast medium must be administered to demarcate masked parenchymal lacerations (isodense) caused by a recent traumatic injury.

Vascular Processes

Splenic Infarction

Splenic infarctions result from thrombo-embolic occlusion of the splenic artery or its branches. The embolism normally originates from within the heart (defect of the mitral valve, myocardial infarction) or from an aortic lesion. Thrombosis may arise from arteriosclerosis, subendothelial infiltration in patients with myeloid leukemia, inflammatory or neoplastic pancreatic disease, or trauma and hemagglutination in patients with sickle-cell anemia. Areas of infarction may liquefy, develop into pseudocysts and (infrequently) calcify.

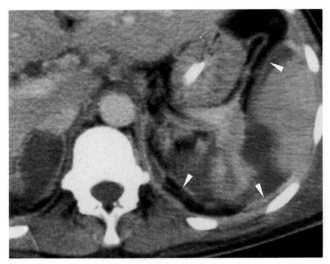

Fig. 16-18. Splenic hematoma. An intrasplenic hematoma becomes demarcated after bolus administration. However, the location of the bloody fluid is still subcapsular (▶).

Fig. 16-19. Splenic infarction. After bolus administration, a sharply marginated, segmented area of hypodensity can be seen in the enlarged spleen, as well as a slight recess in the splenic capsule.

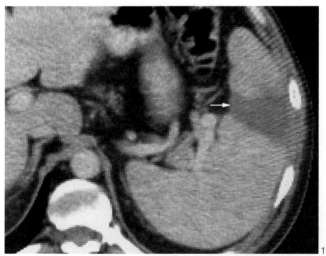

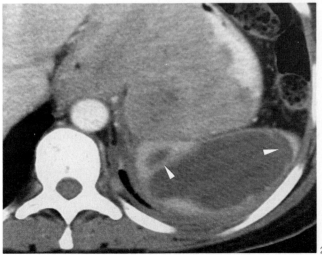

Fig. 16-20. Extensive splenic infarction. A complete infarction of the spleen has occurred as a result of encasement of an extensive gastric carcinoma. Only the peripheral areas of the parenchyma are supplied by capsular vessels (▶).

19

20

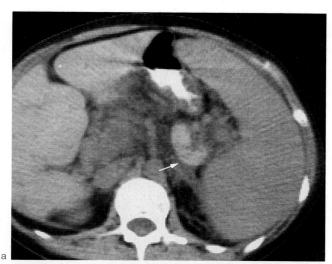

21a

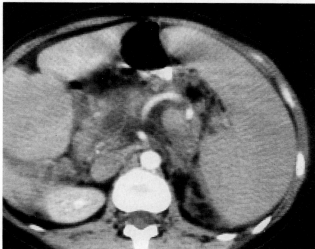

21b

Fig. 16-21. Fresh splenic vein thrombosis. Considerable enlargement of the spleen. In conjunction with chronic pancreatitis, the splenic vein appears dilated and hyperdense, thereby corresponding to fresh thrombosis (→). After bolus contrast medium administration (b), delayed contrast enhancement of the spleen was recorded. The dilated splenic vein shows no enhancement.

• CT

Plain scans: Areas of infarction may have a wedge-shaped, round, or linear appearance on CT scans. Disseminated distribution occurs preferentially in myeloproliferative disease. Areas of fresh infarction are usually hypodense, but may temporarily display a speckled hyperdensity pattern as the result of a hemorrhage. During later cellular reorganization, the tissue density rises as the volume decreases. This process is identifiable as an indentation in the capsule located above the area of infarction. Amorphous calcification can also be observed in the advanced stages of infarction.

Contrast-enhanced scans: Fresh (segmental) perfusion deficits appear as hypodense zones after the administration of contrast medium. Later scans will demonstrate a lightly speckled enhancement pattern in the infarction area and more intense enhancement along the margins and capsule of the spleen (rim sign).

Splenic Vein Thrombosis

Splenic vein thrombosis may arise from an inflammatory or neoplastic pancreatic process that infiltrates the splenic vein. Two further causes are peritonitis and trauma. The condition may lead to the development of collateral vascular channels (including the varices of the esophagus) and severe splenomegaly.

• CT

Plain scans: Fresh splenic vein thrombosis is characterized by abnormal enlargement of the spleen, hyperdensity, and distension of the splenic vein.

Contrast-enhanced scans: The patency of the splenic vein can be evaluated after the administration of contrast medium. Collateral vascu-

Fig. 16-22. Accessory spleen. Small, round structure along the splenic border has the same pattern of contrast enhancement as the primary spleen.

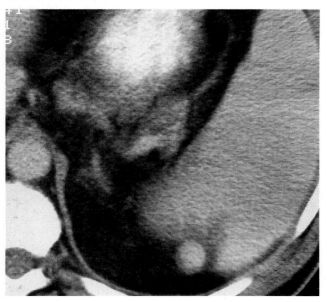

lar channels, which develop primarily in the fundic, gastro-epiploic and gastro-esophageal veins are also enhanced.

Splenic Anomalies

Asplenia is a very rare disorder that is usually accompanied by various cardiovascular and abdominal anomalies. In *polysplenia*, the spleen is separated into 2 to 10 individual parenchymal lobes. *Accessory spleens* are more frequently found. They consist of nodules of functional splenic parenchyma that can range from a few millimeters to 10 cm in diameter. 75% of all accessory spleens are localized in the hilar region, and 20% are found in the tail of the pancreas. Marked compensatory hypertrophy may occur when the nodules are isolated from the spleen or when the spleen is removed.

Splenosis occurs when splenic tissue is disseminated and implanted in the peritoneal cavity after trauma or surgery.

• CT

Plain scans: An *accessory spleen* appears as a homogeneous, smoothly marginated soft-tissue structure with a CT number equal to that of the parenchyma of the primary spleen. An accessory spleen is a diagnostically significant finding that must be distinguished from mass lesions of the pancreas, kidney, and adrenal gland.

Contrast-enhanced scans: After bolus administration of contrast medium, these anomalies can usually be demonstrated well on CT scans, since enhancement of the accessory spleens is synchronous and equal to the enhancement of the primary spleen. The surrounding vessels, renal parenchyma and contours of the pan-

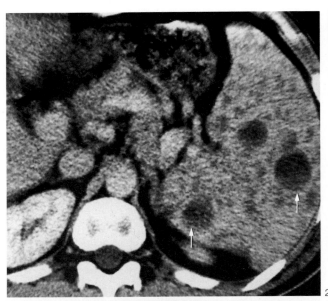

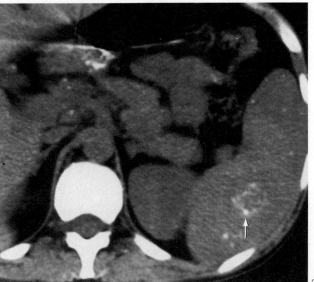

Fig. 16-23. Pneumocystosis of the spleen after pneumocystis carinii infection in an AIDS patient. Splenomegaly with areas of hypodensity (a→). Disseminated calcification is found after treatment (b→).

creas can be positively identified. Questionable cases can be clarified by radionuclide imaging of the spleen.

Chapter 17
The Kidney

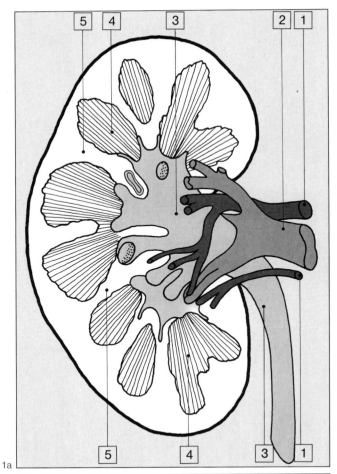

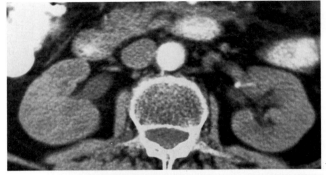

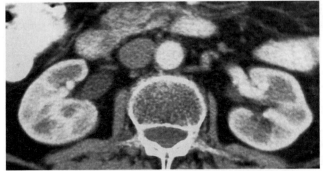

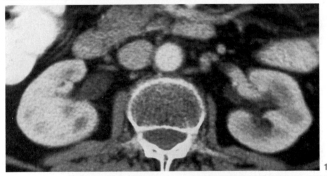

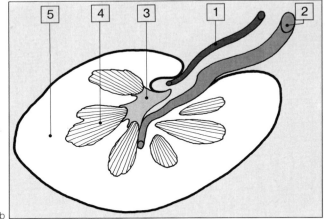

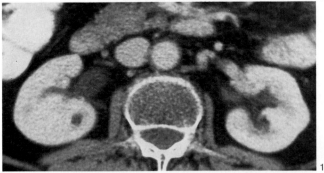

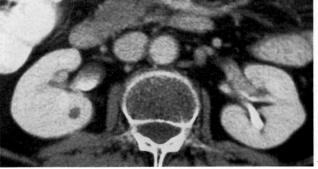

Fig. 17-1. Topography of the renal hilum.
a) Longitudinal section.
b) Transverse section.

Key to symbols:

1 Renal artery	3 Renal pelvis and ureter
2 Renal vein	4 Renal (medullary) pyramids
	5 Renal cortex

c) Contrast enhancement of the renal parenchyma after bolus contrast medium injection. The well supplied renal cortex exhibits maximum enhancement after 25 seconds. The renal medulla enhances 60 to 80 seconds p.i., and is predominantly isodense as compared with the renal cortex. ($c_1 = 15$ s, $c_2 = 25$ s, $c_3 = 50$ s, $c_4 = 75$ s, $c_5 = 125$ s after injection).

The Kidney

Anatomy and Imaging

An average adult kidney weighs about 150 g. The renal parenchyma is organized in segments around the renal sinus and it contains up to 18 renal (medullary) pyramids which, in turn, accommodate the system of renal collecting tubules. The tubules fuse to form 6 to 12 renal papillae in the region of the renal sinus. The renal cortex is well vascularized and envelops the renal pyramids. It also contains the system of renal vessels, glomeruli and tubules. The pelvi-calyceal system extends throughout the renal sinus and unites within the kidney to form the renal pelvis. The main renal arteries lie dorsal to the renal veins. They separate near the hilum into ventral and dorsal branches. The vessels run between the papillae in front of and behind the renal collecting system to the points where they enter the parenchyma as interlobar vessels.

• CT

Plain scans: On transverse scans, the kidneys appear oval near the renal poles and sickle-shaped in the hilar region. When viewed tangentially, the external boundaries of the kidney are smooth. The craniocaudad length of the kidney ranges from 10 to 12 cm, the average width of the renal parenchyma is ca. 1.5 cm in healthy adults. The normal diameters at the level of the hilum are 5 to 6 cm (transverse) and ca. 4 cm (anteroposterior).

Contrast-enhanced scans: The renal parenchyma appears homogeneous on plain scans. Depending on the degree of hydration, the attenuation of the renal parenchyma on contrast-enhanced scans is an average 30 ± 10 HU. After enhancement, the observations are similar to those at arteriography. After a bolus injection of contrast medium (CM), the cortical region becomes enhanced ca. 10 seconds after the aortic peak in the early arterial phase. The renal (medullary) pyramids initially appear hypodense, but are approximately equal to the attenuation of the cortical parenchyma

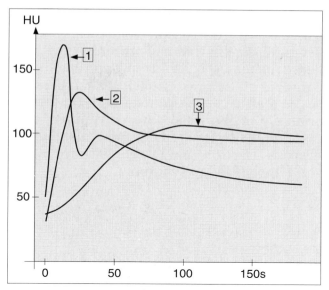

Fig. 17-2. Time-density curve for the normal renal parenchyma. After a bolus injection (8 ml/s), the first maximum density peak (1) is seen in the aortic lumen within 15 seconds. Maximum density of the renal cortex occurs later (2), then the attenuation values gradually decrease. The renal medulla takes longer to reach maximum enhancement (3) but, 120 seconds after injection, its density slightly exceeds that of cortical tissues.

after approx. 60 seconds. Only at the level of the hilum of the kidney are the renal pyramids demonstrated in full length as triangular structures from their base to the apex. Near the poles of the kidneys, they are intersected at different levels along their longitudinal axis. The configuration of the surrounding, contrast-enhanced renal cortex therefore varies from oval to ringlike. The fibrous capsule does not become enhanced with contrast medium and cannot be demonstrated on CT scans.

Cystic Renal Diseases

Renal Cysts

Renal cysts are benign, non-neoplastic renal lesions. Simple renal cysts are rare in children, but are more commonly acquired as the age of the patient increases. Renal cysts are found in over 50% of all adults over 50, usually as an incidental finding. They can form multiple lesions that are randomly distributed throughout the entire renal parenchyma, or they can accumulate in subcapsular or peripelvic locations.

The frequency of *multiple renal cysts* rises in patients with renal insufficiency who are undergoing dialysis therapy. whereby the incidence increases in direct proportion to the duration of therapy. Renal cysts are rarely larger than 2 cm in diameter and are located primarily in the renal cortex. Multiple renal cysts frequently occur in patients with tuberous sclerosis (Bourneville-Pringle syndrome) or von Hippel-Lindau syndrome.

• CT

Simple renal cysts have the following CT characteristics:
1. They have smooth, thin walls that are not always clearly defined (either before or after CM administration).
2. They have water-dense cystic contents (15 HU max.).
3. Internal or peripheral calcification is absent. 4. The attenuation value does not rise after intravenous administration of contrast medium.

Note: Especially when the lesions are small, partial volume averaging and overshadowing of artifacts can falsify the attenuation value.

Table 17-1. Differential diagnosis of renal cysts.

Thickened or irregular margins or septa	Renal cell carcinoma, Cystadenoma, Complicated renal cysts (after hemorrhage or infection), Abscess, Echinococcus cyst
Raised attenuation value	Post-inflammatory or infected cyst, Cyst associated with hemorrhage Lime milk cysts (some with sedimentation), Echinococcus cyst, Tuberculosis
Calcification	Post-inflammatory or infected cysts, Cysts developing after hemorrhage, Colliquated hematoma, Multicystic kidney, Polycystic kidney, Renal cell carcinoma, Echinococcus cyst, Tuberculosis

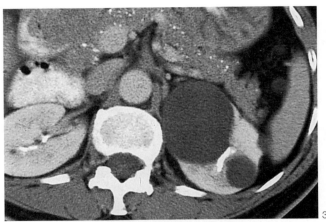

3a

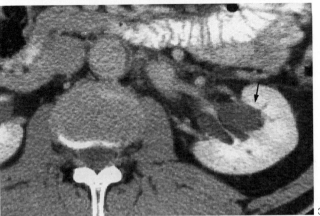

3b

Fig. 17-3a, b. Renal cysts. 1. On plain scans, cysts (a) can be recognized as masses that appear hypodense as compared with the renal parenchyma. 2. After administering a sufficient amount of contrast medium, they become sharply demarcated from the renal parenchyma, still exhibiting water density. When measuring their density via CT, minor artifact formation must be taken into account. 3. Frequently, parapelvic cysts (b) can be detected only after appropriate contrast medium administration. They usually cause deformity and impression of the renal collecting structures.

Fig. 17-4a. Complex cyst (lime milk cyst). In this patient, renal tuberculosis had occurred and was treated in the distant past. Now, a cyst with shell-like calcification and sedimented contents (→) can be seen.

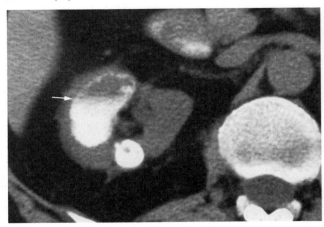

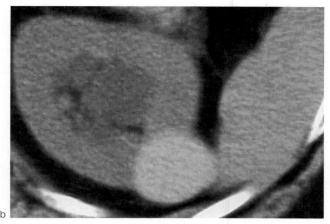

4b

Fig. 17-4b. Complex cyst. On plain scans, the complex cyst appears hyperdense, but sharply marginated from the contiguous renal parenchyma. No increase in density is registered after contrast medium administration.

Fig. 17-5. Cystic kidney. Both kidneys are enlarged (a→), and the renal cortex is deformed by cystic masses. Plain scans (a) reveal calcification and spotty areas of hyperdensity corresponding to post-hemorrhagic complex cysts (a ►). After contrast medium administration (b), hypodense cysts of various sizes are sharply demarcated from the renal parenchyma.

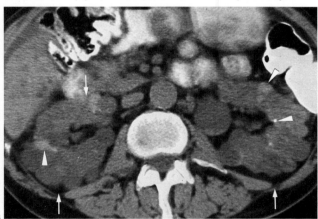

5a

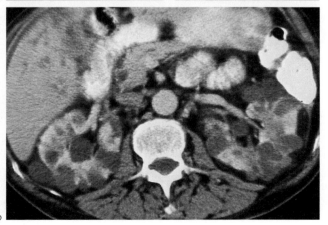

5b

Differential Diagnosis: If only one of the above CT characteristics is missing, a wide range of other lesions must be considered in the diagnosis (Table 17–1).

Anomalies that have a cystic appearance and pathological processes of the efferent urinary passages such as calyceal cysts, calyceal diverticula, hydronephrosis, or pyonephrosis are often first detected on plain scans. They usually become unequivocally visible after administration of contrast medium.

Polycystic Renal Disease in Children (Cystic Kidney)

Childhood polycystic renal disease is genetically acquired (autosomally recessive) and has a non-uniform clinical picture. It is accompanied by variably severe liver disease with proliferation of portobiliary connective tissues and choledochectasia. Neonatal types are characterized mainly by polycystic renal degeneration which, after only a few months, leads to death as a result of uremia.

• CT

Plain scans: CT scans show clear, bilateral enlargement of the kidneys and a moderately reduced attenuation value in the renal parenchyma. However, the 1 to 2 mm cysts, themselves, cannot usually be identified on CT scans.

Contrast-enhanced scans: A fine, radial structure appears on cross-sectional images after the administration of contrast medium. Depending on the stage of disease, the medulla and cortex may not be easily differentiated.

Polycystic Renal Disease in Adults (Cystic Kidney)

This autosomally dominant disease is usually bilateral, and clear asymmetry of renal volume is frequently observed in the early stages. The number and size of the cysts increases as the disease progresses. The kidney can increase to several times its normal weight. Accompanying cysts are found in the liver and biliary tract of 30 to 60% of all patients, and in the pancreas in 10% of all patients. Cerebral and abdominal aneurysms and cerebral arteriovenous anomalies frequently occur. In the later stages of disease, terminal renal insufficiency develops in the 5th to 6th decade.

• CT

Plain scans: The enlarged kidneys have a mottled enhancement pattern. Since cystic formations merge to form hypodense areas, individual cysts can be identified only along the margins. Cystic hemorrhages with consecutive infections are a common complication. The affected cysts have a characteristic, hyperdense appearance. Thickened cyst walls, usually a result of this complication, can be distinguished from calyceal calculi because calcification of the former is usually ringlike.

Contrast-enhanced scans: The renal parenchyma becomes clearly enhanced after a bolus injection of contrast medium. Depending on the severity of cystic degeneration, the parenchyma may appear as a hyperdense residual structure or display a reticular pattern. The larger the kidneys, i.e. the more extensive the cystic change, the smaller the amount of demarcated parenchyma. The individual, linear, distorted calyces are markers that help to identify the collecting structures. When focal enhancement of a rounded figure is seen within hypodense areas of a cystic kidney, an accompanying tumor must be suspected, especially when the lymph nodes near the hilum of the kidney are enlarged.

Differential diagnosis: Multiple renal cysts must be considered in the diagnosis.

Multicystic Renal Dysplasia

(Bulbous kidney, blastemic cysts)

Multicystic renal dysplasia is not genetic in origin. It develops unilaterally and is urographically and arteriographically silent. These cysts

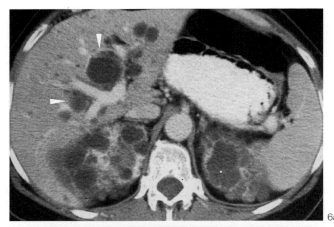

6a

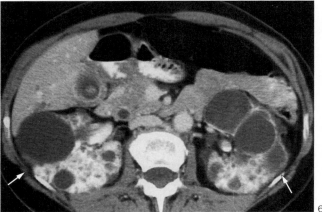

6b

Fig. 17-6. Cystic kidney. Cysts of various sizes are distributed throughout the kidneys (→). Very small cysts become visible after contrast enhancement of the renal parenchyma. Additional finding: hepatic cysts (►).

Fig. 17-7. Cystic kidney with generalized hamartosis. Cysts are distributed through most of the kidneys (→) as well as the liver. Therefore, only small remnants of the parenchyma (►) can be found. There is renal and hepatic insufficiency with ascites.

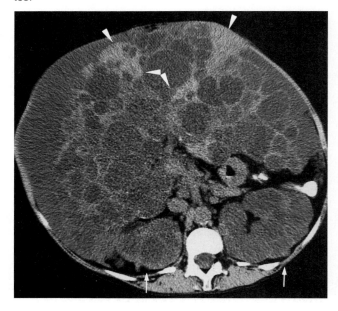

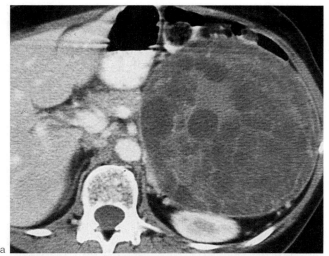

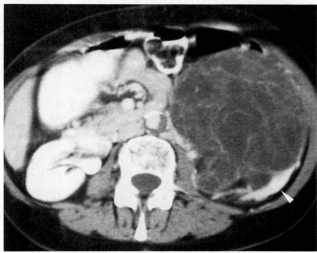

8a

8b

Fig. 17-8. Multiloculated cystic nephroma. 8 x 10 cm, sharply marginated mass contains numerous round, hypodense zones representing cysts. They are delineated from the contrasted, trabecular stroma (kidney ►).

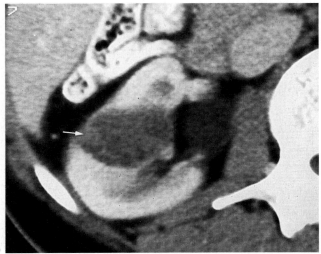

9

form racemose structures and typically show ringlike calcification. The efferent urinary passages are either atretic or blind.

• CT

Plain scans: Multiple, large, unilateral cysts, usually with peripheral calcification, display racemose organization.

Contrast-enhanced scans: Enhancement of the parenchyma cannot be demonstrated.

Multilocular Cystic Nephroma

(Multilocular renal cyst, cystic adenoma, cystadenoma, segmental polycystic kidney)

The multilocular cystic nephroma develops predominantly in young boys and in women between the ages of 40 and 60. The clinical symptoms of this cystic tumor include hematuria, infection, and rapid growth. Sarcomatous degeneration has been reported in rare cases. The affected kidney has only focal cystic changes. The septa and capsule of the mass are hypervascularized and surround the spaces filled with myxomatous material. Angiographic differentiation of malignant masses is not possible. Multilocular cystic nephromas are often discovered only after they have reached a size of ca. 10 cm in diameter. They can, however, become much larger.

• CT

Plain scans: Most of the cystic cavities are relatively large and contain variably broad, soft-tissue dense septa. The mass is sharply demarcated from the surrounding renal tissue and the perirenal cavity. It frequently distends into the renal sinus. The septa are several millimeters thick, reticulated, smooth in appearance, and have no nodular components.

Fig. 17-9. Recurrence of cystic nephroma. Three years after tumor resection, a hypodense, discretely honeycombed structure was found on CT scans. It exhibits the same structural texture as the primary tumor and corresponds to a tumor recurrence.

Contrast-enhanced scans: The septa become moderately enhanced, thereby demarcating the adjacent cystic cavities.

Differential diagnosis: In some cases, the cysts may be small and contain mostly solid components. It is then impossible to distinguish them from malignant neoplasms in the absence of secondary malignancy criteria.

Solid Tumors

Renal Cell Carcinoma

(Hypernephroma, hypernephroid renal carcinoma, adenocarcinoma, renal carcinoma, Grawitz's tumor)

The majority of all solid tumors that develop in the renal parenchyma are malignant. Approximately 90% of all malignant renal tumors are renal cell carcinomas. They are found primarily in men between the ages of 50 and 70, and they very rarely occur in children and adolescents. Since about half of all patients have no signs of macrohematuria at the time of diagnosis, renal cell carcinoma is frequently discovered incidentally. Approximately 35 % of all patients with von Hippel-Lindau syndrome develop renal cell carcinoma in the course of the disease. The prognosis depends on how extensive the tumor is. A prognosis can be made according to Robsen's staging system (Table 17–2).

Metastases is initially lymphatic and regional. Then spread extends successively to the me-

Table 17-2. Staging of renal cell carcinomas according to Robsen.

I	Tumor within the fibrous capsule
II	Perforation of the fibrous capsule, Infiltration of the ipsilateral adrenal gland
III	Infiltration of the renal vein, Metastatic spread to regional lymph nodes
IV	Perforation of Gerota's fascia, Involvement of surrounding muscles and/or Distant metastases

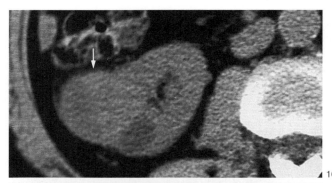
10a

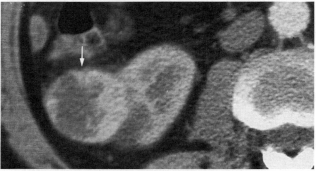
10b

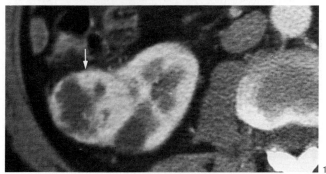
10c

Fig. 17-10. Renal cell carcinoma.
a) A tumor with a diameter of 3 cm protrudes beyond the lateral renal contours and communicates with the renal fascia. It appears slightly hyperdense as compared to the healthy renal parenchyma.
b) At the same time as the renal parenchyma (25 s p.i.), the tumor exhibits hyperdense peripheral enhancement.
c) Even after 60 seconds, the peripheral enhancement of the tumor resembles that of the renal cortex.
d) Only 300 seconds after injection the tumor becomes hypodense as compared with the renal parenchyma.

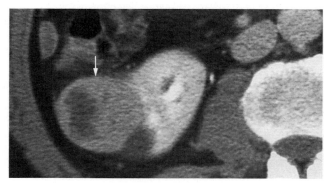
10d

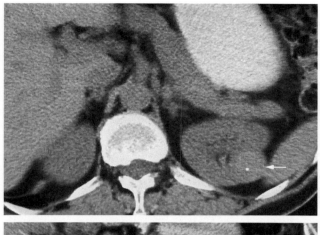

11a

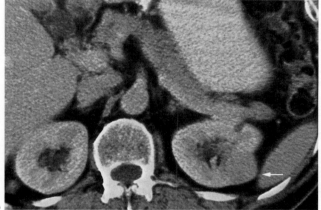

11b

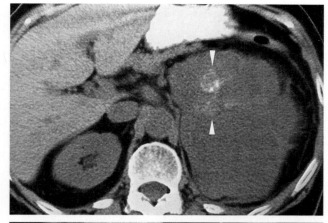

13a

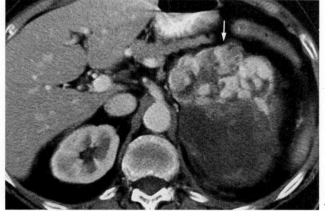

13b

Fig. 17-11. Renal cell carcinoma. The plain scan (a) reveals a sharply marginated, slightly hyperdense (50 HU) mass (→), the appearance of which corresponds to a renal cyst. After contrast medium administration, the attenuation value increased by 35 HU (b).

Fig. 17-13. Large renal cell carcinoma.
a) Plain scans reveal calcification corresponding to regressive changes (►).
b) After bolus contrast medium injection, a hypervascularized tumor was found (→). It extends caudally as a smoothly marginated mass with considerable zones of necrosis. The center has an attenuation value of ca. 25 HU.
c) The possibility of local capsular perforation and infiltration of the psoas muscle cannot be excluded (►). However, the borders of the renal fascia are intact. Enlargement of lymph nodes was not found.

Fig. 17-12. Renal cell carcinoma. Rather hypovascularized, bulbous tumor. The tumor absorbs only moderate amounts of contrast medium (20–30 HU), which confirms the diagnosis of hypovascularization. The renal collecting system is infiltrated (→).

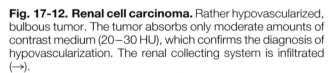

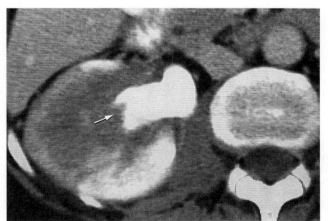

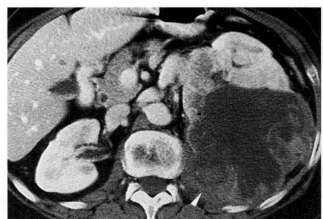

13c

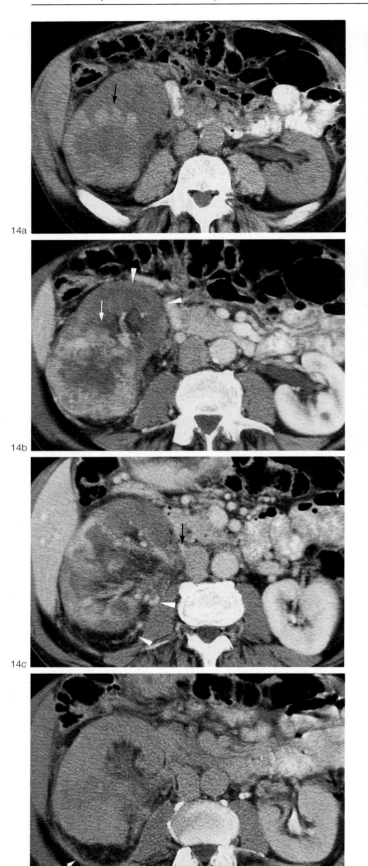

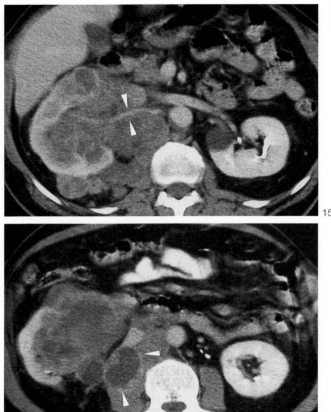

Fig. 17-15. Renal cell carcinoma with multiple regional metastases that extend into the psoas muscle (b ►). They also surround and ventrally displace the vena cava and the renal artery (a ► ◄). The individual lymph node metastases exhibit clear peripheral enhancement.

diastinum, affecting regions up to the hilum of the lungs and the supraclavicular fossa. In the terminal stages of renal cell carcinoma, there are primarily hematogenous metastases in the lung (over 50%), liver and bones (30%), adrenals (20%), contralateral kidney (10%), and brain (5 %).

Fig. 17-14. Renal cell carcinoma. A 5 cm large, slightly hyperdense mass is found on plain scans (a→). It exhibits strong, rim enhancement (b→), whereas the renal parenchyma only slowly enhances (►). A compact mass causing slight compression of the inferior vena cava (c→) surrounds the entire vascular pedicle. This gives rise to occlusion of the renal artery. The tumor and kidney are supplied by collateral (►) and capsular vessels. Only in delayed scans made 15 minutes after contrast medium injection (d) a slight, uniform enhancement of the renal parenchyma is observed. The renal fascia is clearly thickened (→), but there is no tumor spread beyond its boundaries.

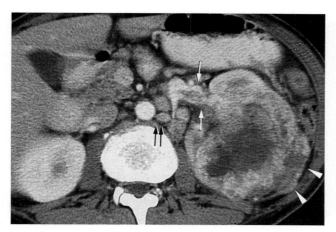

Fig. 17-16. Renal cell carcinoma. The renal fascia shows clear laterodorsal protrusion (►), but appears to be intact. Invasion of the renal vein (→) and proof of regional lymph node enlargement (⇉).

Fig. 17-17. Renal cell carcinoma. A hypervascularized, relatively sharply demarcated, hyperdense mass is located in the upper pole of the kidney (→). The renal tissue surrounding it appears hypodense and indistinct on the side facing the liver (►). This suggests the presence of inflammatory processes. Intraoperative findings revealed a gelatinous, hemorrhagic tumor reaction. (a) Bolus contrast medium phase; (b) parenchymal phase.

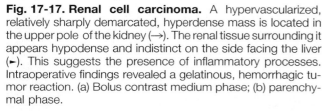

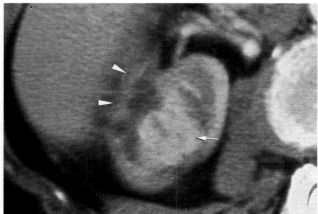

17a

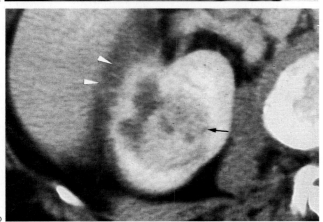

17b

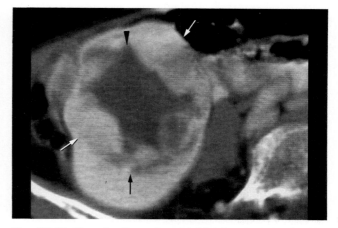

Fig. 17-18. Renal cell carcinoma. Highly vascularized tumor tissue marginates the periphery (→). This contrasts sharply against the hypodense, necrotic tumor center (►).

• CT

Plain scans: Renal cell carcinoma can be identified when their is clear deformation of the renal cortex due to protrusion of the tumor into the perirenal space or renal sinus. Due to the increased vascularization of the tumor, the tumor tissue usually appears more dense than the renal parenchyma. Large renal cell carcinomas tend to create several (hypodense) necrotic zones, which can undergo cystic transformation. Regressive changes lead to the development of calcification, which may be amorphous at the tumor center or ringlike around the periphery. Hemorrhage into the tumor parenchyma leads to an inhomogeneous increase in attenuation value. Hemorrhage can additionally lead to the development of a subcapsular hematoma and masking of the tumor.

Contrast-enhanced scans: A bolus injection of contrast medium makes it possible to differentiate renal cell carcinomas. When expansile, these tumors are relatively sharply demarcated from the renal parenchyma. However, the tumor borders are sometimes ill-defined. Depending on its degree of vascularity, the tumor may temporarily appear hyperdense as compared with the surrounding renal parenchyma, however, it is usually hypodense. Zones of necrosis appear more sharply hypodense after a bolus injection. The tumor walls can be better evaluated when a cystic configuration has developed. The walls are usually irregularly vascularized.

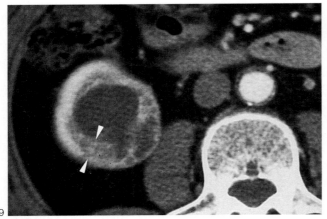

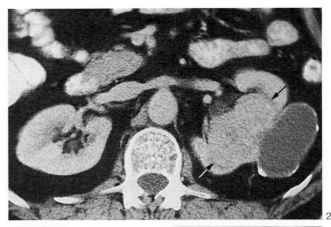

19

22

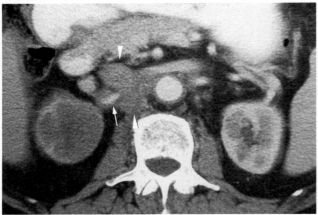

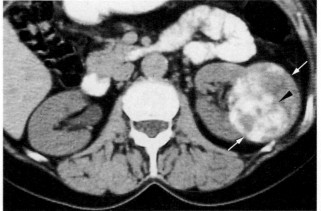

20

23

Fig. 17-19. Cystic renal cell carcinoma. The lower pole of the right kidney exhibits several round, low-density areas (around 18 HU) with no significant increase in density after CM administration. Solid tumor components found in the peripheral region exhibit moderate contrast medium uptake (►).

Fig. 17-20. Renal cell carcinoma. The upper pole of the kidney shows generalized enlargement. After CM administration, this region exhibits only moderate enhancement (ca. 40 HU) as compared with the kidney. The right renal artery is surrounded (→), and the inferior vena cava is compromised. However, sonographic findings revealed that the latter was not infiltrated. Lymph node metastases were detected (►).

Fig. 17-21. Contralateral metastases after nephrectomy of the right kidney. The small mass (→) has the appearance of a small renal cell carcinoma.

Fig. 17-22. Renal cell carcinoma with hematoma. In the late contrast medium phase, the tumor (→) appears slightly hypodense as compared with the renal parenchyma. The adjacent, hypodense structure with peripheral calcification does not enhance. This corresponds to a longstanding hematoma.

Fig. 17-23. Calcified renal carcinoma. Within the smoothly marginated tumor (→), dense, maplike calcification was detected on plain scans (►) (rare finding).

Fig. 17-24. Post-nephrectomy metastases. Inferior to the bed of the kidney, there is a 2 to 4 cm large soft-tissue structure located on an adhesive loop of the bowel. This absorbs only slight amounts of contrast medium (→).

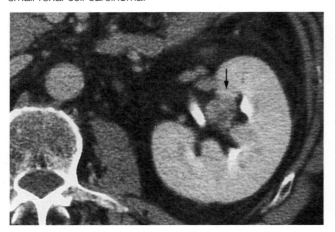

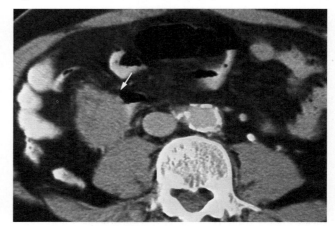

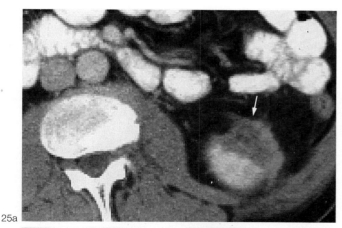

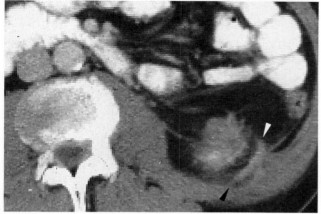

Fig. 17-25. Post-operative phase of renal cell carcinoma. Three months after resection of the lower pole of the kidney, a hoodshaped soft-tissue structure that exhibits peripheral enhancement is found in the renal parenchyma (a→). This corresponds to scar tissue. Also the moderate, strandlike structures in the surroundings (►) are suggestive of a cicatricial process. Further follow-up examinations show increasing retraction of scar tissue.

Fig. 17-26. Renal adenoma. Soft-tissue dense mass is 1.3 cm large (→). It exhibits slight enhancement (30 HU).

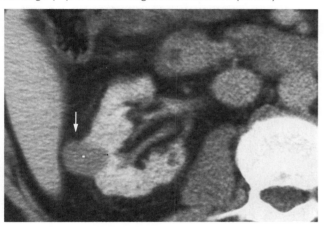

Evaluation of tumor extent: After administration of contrast medium, the patency of the *renal vein* must always be checked in order to determine whether the renal venous system has been infiltrated. Contrast enhancement of perirenal vessels usually makes it possible to differentiate collateral vascular channels from tumor-related or inflammatory *cord* formation in the renal capsule. Direct invasion or *infiltration* of the tumor into adjacent organs in unequivocally demonstrated when the internal structure of muscles or bone displays abnormalities. Since *lymph node metastases* of a hypernephroma can be well vascularized, lymph node enlargement must also be considered in areas of contrasted soft-tissue. Sufficient preparation of the bowel is essential for unequivocal diagnosis of pathological lymph node changes.

Differential diagnosis: Because of its polymorphic variability, the tumor may simulate benign diseases of the kidney (e.g. complex renal cysts, hematomas, inflammations). When diagnosing renal cell carcinoma, the following lesions must be considered in the differential diagnosis: *carcinoma of the renal pelvis, oncocytoma, renal lymphoma, renal metastases, complex renal cysts, renal abscess, multilocular cystic nephroma, adrenal adenoma and mesenchymal tumor.*

Nephradenoma

Nephradenoma is a frequent autopsy finding (7–23% of all autopsies); multiple occurrence is not rare. Nephradenomas often occur in conjunction with benign nephrosclerosis or pyelonephritis, and they frequently develop in dialysis patients. Nephradenomas are usually microscopic in size, but can become as large as several centimeters. These lesions are considered to be potentially malignant when their diameter is 3 cm or larger. Histological differentiation is made between papillary, tubular and alveolar nephradenomas, and it is often difficult to distinguish them from carcinomas.

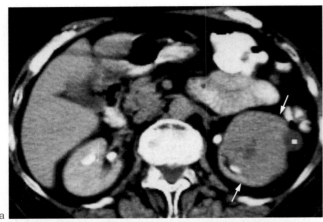

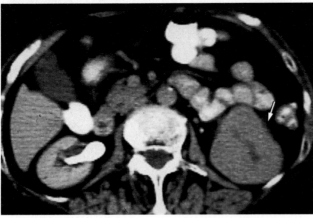

Fig. 17-27. Oncocytoma. A mass is located in the left kidney. After contrast medium administration, it exhibits moderate, homogeneous enhancement with a sharply marginated, linear central low-density zone. This corresponds to central scar formation, which is characteristic of oncocytomas.

Fig. 17-28. Angiomyolipoma. A mass is located in the upper pole of the right kidney. It is sharply delineated from the kidney and is slightly lobulated. The attenuation values lie mainly in the fat range (→), but are somewhat increased by fine, reticular structures. A small, peripheral soft-tissue zone was also detected (►). Is this due to hemorrhage?

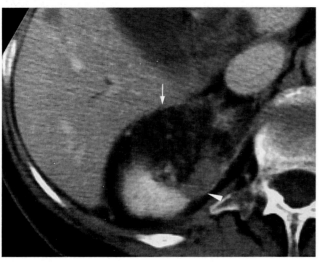

• CT

Adenomas appear on CT scans as soft-tissue dense masses which absorb variable amounts of contrast medium. Low density areas correlate with central areas of necrosis. Calcification is a rare finding in these tumors. Differential diagnostic characteristics that unequivocally distinguish these tumors from renal cell carcinomas have yet to be found.

Oncocytoma

The oncocytoma is a relatively large epithelial cell that has an eosinophilic, granular cytoplasm and originates from the proximal tubular epithelium. In the strictest histological sense, renal oncocytomas must be classified as benign lesions. They range from 1 cm in diameter to considerable sizes. The oncocytoma affects men more frequently than women. The peak occurrence is in the 6th and 7th decade, which is similar to that of the renal cell carcinoma.

• CT

Oncocytomas appear on CT scans as marginated, variably large renal masses. Centralized, stellate scar tissue is frequently found on CT scans, but cannot be considered as diagnostic of oncocytoma, because it cannot always be reliably distinguished from an area of central necrosis. Administration of contrast medium sometimes helps to delineate the cicatricial structure. A spoke wheel configuration may also be seen on contrast-enhanced scans.

Mesenchymal Tumors

• Angiomyolipoma

The angiomyolipoma is classified as a hamartoma. This mixed tumor contains fatty tissue as well as arteries with wall anomalies (aneurysmal degeneration) and atypically well-differentiated muscle fibers. They are found in 50 to 80% of all patients with tuberous sclerosis (Bourneville-Pringle syndrome) and are usually either bilateral or multifocal. Otherwise, their growth is unilateral.

The possibility of malignant sarcomatous transformation has been discussed. This is generally rejected, however, even when angiomyolipomatous tissue can be demonstrated in adjacent lymph nodes.

● CT

The primary diagnostic sign of angiomyolipoma is the presence of fatty components, which are present in variable proportions, depending on the overall composition of the tumor. In accordance with their degree of vascularity, soft-tissue structures of the tumor become variably enhanced after bolus administration of contrast medium. This usually sharply demarcates the fatty components of the tumor from the surrounding soft-tissue. In some cases, aneurysmal deformation of the vessels can also be seen on the CT image.

One frequent complication is rupture of the aneurysmal vessels, which leads to hemorrhage into the tumor and perirenal cavity. This can be demonstrated on CT scans.

● Other Mesenchymal Tumors

The fibroma, lipoma, leiomyoma and hemangioma are small, benign tumors which usually do not become larger than 1 cm in diameter. On the whole, they are very rare and clinically insignificant. The lipoma is the only one of these tumors that can be reliably diagnosed by CT, since it consists entirely of low attenuation tissue and has no other tissue components. When evaluating a lipoma, an angiomyolipoma should also be considered in the diagnosis.

Tumors of the Renal Pelvis

Papillary tumors of the renal pelvis, like those of the urinary bladder, have a tendency to undergo malignant transformation. Carcinomas of the renal pelvis constitute 8 to 10% of all malignant renal tumors. Around 80% of them are transitional cell carcinomas. Squamous cell carcinomas are more infrequent and tend to cause early infiltration of the renal parenchyma. Approximately 25 to 40% of all carcino-

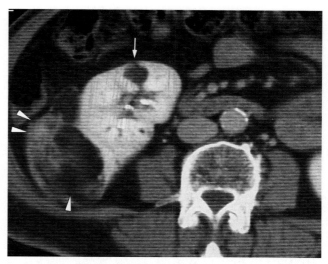

Fig. 17-29. Angiomyolipoma. The mass, which displaces the kidney, is sharply marginated and has a maplike tissue texture. Hypodense areas correspond to fat, and soft-tissue structures (▷) probably contain fibrous constituents as a result of hemorrhage. Prominent vascular structures are found in the periphery (▶). A second low-density area within the kidney is also fat-dense. This corresponds to an additional angiomyolipoma (→).

Fig. 17-30. Lipopenic angiomyolipoma (→). The primary tumor constituent may be angiomatous or myomatous. This tumor, therefore, can be diagnosed only on the basis of very small fat deposits (▶).

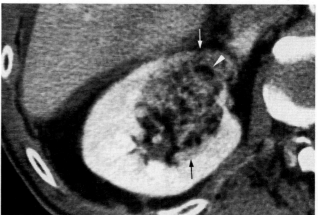

30a

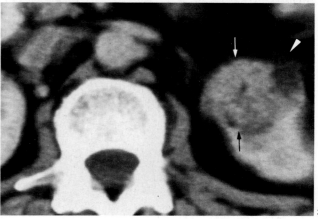

30b

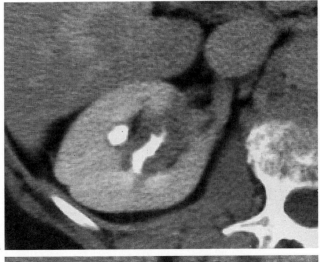

31a

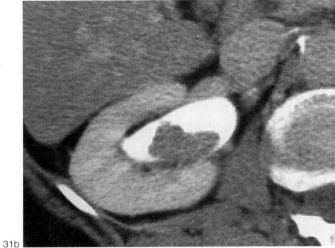

31b

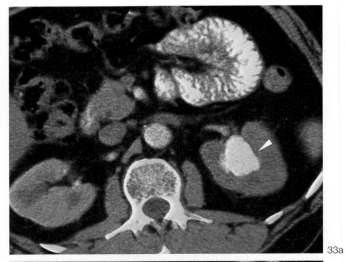

33a

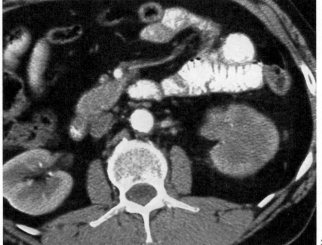

33b

Fig. 17-31. Carcinoma of the renal pelvis. The tumor extends like a cuff around the middle calyceal group (a). It creates
a filling defect in the renal pelvis (b).

Fig. 17-32. Carcinoma of the renal pelvis. In the hilum of
the kidney, there is a sharply marginated, soft-tissue dense
mass that is 2 cm in size. It causes displacement of the collecting structures. No regional lymph node enlargement.

Fig. 17-33. Carcinoma of the renal pelvis. The tumor has
caused diffuse infiltration of the lower pole of the kidney. This is
manifested by the obliteration of cortical structures that is observed after bolus injection of contrast medium (b). Retention of
urine in the renal pelvis (a ►).

Fig. 17-34. Carcinoma of the renal pelvis. The tumor extends into the renal parenchyma (►).

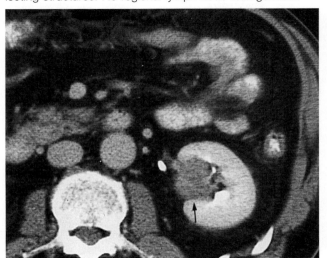

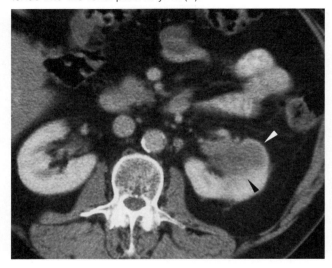

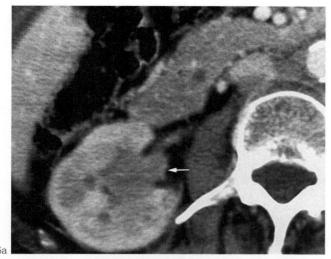

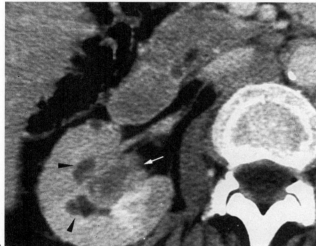

Fig. 17-35. Urothelial carcinoma. The invasive tumor (a, b→) is indistinctly demarcated from the renal parenchyma. On late scans (b), some calyces (►) remain unenhanced, since they are surrounded by tumor tissue. Evidence of retrocaval lymph node metastases (c ►).

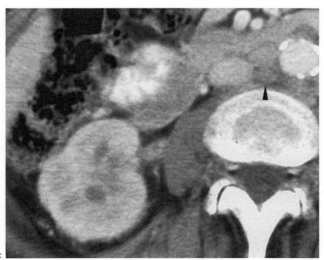

mas of the renal pelvis are multiple. They are frequently accompanied by carcinomas of the ureter. Regional (para-aortic) lymph nodes are usually infiltrated, even by very small tumors. Hematogenous metastases occur preferentially in the lungs and bone.

These tumors affect men more frequently than women and occur preferentially in the 5th to 8th decade. Children and juveniles are very rarely affected.

Macrohematuria is the most common clinical symptom. The diagnosis of pelvic tumor is suggested when a filling defect is found on a urogram. However, the urogram is accurate in only one out of two patients.

• CT

Plain scans: Deformity of the renal calyces or dilatation of the renal pelvis accompanied by a slight rise in attenuation as compared with urine is characteristic of renal pelvic tumors. In some cases, the attenuation of these tumors will be increased as compared with that of the noncontrasted renal parenchyma (30 HU). Normally, pericalyceal fat is either discretely visible and flattened or cannot be demonstrated on the CT scans. Stippled calcification has been reported in isolated cases. Extensive hyperdense areas inside the tumor signify a hemorrhage.

If the tumor continues to spread, the muscle layer of the renal pelvis will be infiltrated (stage T3) and the renal parenchyma or the renal sinus will become involved. In large tumors of the renal pelvis, one can only guess the primary site of the tumor, i.e. the center of growth. It then is impossible to distinguish large renal pelvic carcinomas from renal cell carcinomas.

Contrast-enhanced scans: Tumors of the renal pelvis are usually hypovascularized, so contrast enhancement is only moderate. In a few cases, however, attenuation values of around 50 HU have been reported. After the administration of contrast medium, renal pelvic neoplasms usually appear as a parietal filling defect (possibly lobulated) within the opacified renal collecting tubules. Because of the extensive, wallpaper-like growth of the tumor, there is often an area of circumscribed or circular wall thickening which can lead to constriction of a group of calyces. In that case, one calyx or an entire group becomes obstructed. The segmental blockage of drainage in the kidney is characterized by delayed parenchymal enhancement and accumulation of contrast medium.

Thin-section scanning is generally required for densitometry of an intrapelvic tumor, but measurements are still imprecise because of beam hardening artifacts due to high concentrations of contrast medium in surrounding tissue.

Renal Lymphoma

Primary lymphomas of the kidney are rare, because the renal parenchyma contains no lymphoid tissue. Secondary renal lymphomas frequently arise from non-Hodgkin's lymphomas, especially in the later stages of disease, and are predominantly bilateral.

• CT

Plain scans: Renal lymphomas have several different CT manifestations, which are as follows:
- In approx. 50% there are multiple, nodular masses. The renal parenchyma is dilated and deformed by the nodular protrusions.
- Next in order of frequency (25%) are renal lymphoma that develop from implants of a lymphoma from adjacent lymph nodes. The kidney is usually displaced. The non-affected kidney retains its normal structure and excretory function.
- In around 10% of all cases, diffuse infiltration leads to generalized enlargement of the kidney and reduced excretory function.
- Additional manifestations include diffuse infiltration of the perirenal space, isolated infiltration of the renal sinus and encasement of the proximal ureter, and a unilateral parenchymal lesion.

Contrast-enhanced scans: The attenuation values of a renal lymphoma is frequently moderately reduced as compared with healthy renal

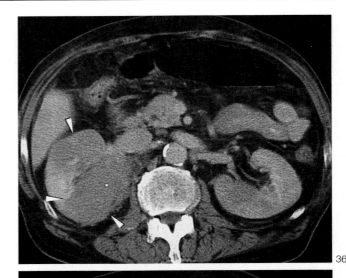
36a

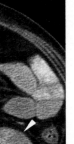
36b

Fig. 17-36. Renal lymphoma. Multinodular invasion with bilateral dilatation of the renal cortex, more so on the right than on the left. This is caused by sharply marginated, low-density zones which correspond to lymphomatous infiltration.

Fig. 17-37. Renal lymphoma. This film shows infiltration into the kidney with extensive retroperitoneal tumor manifestation.

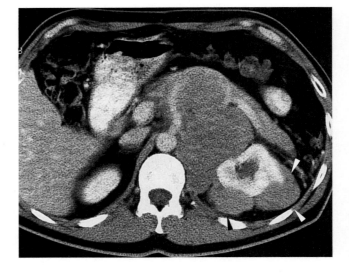

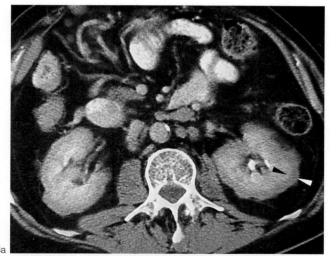

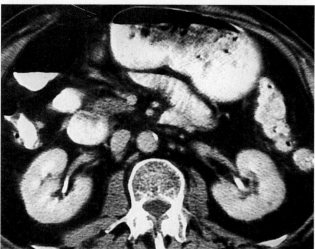

Fig. 17-38. Renal lymphoma. Diffuse infiltration. After CM administration, there is cortex-like additional broad zone in the renal parenchyma. This becomes slightly hypodense as compared with the parenchyma (a ►). Complete regression after completion of chemotherapy (b).

Fig. 17-39. Renal lymphoma. Diffuse infiltration in conjunction with generalized non-Hodgkin's lymphoma.

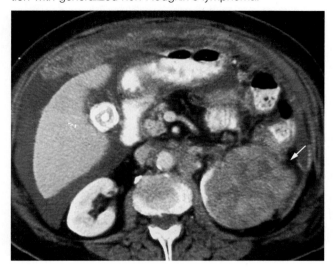

parenchyma as seen on plain CT scans. After the administration of contrast medium, the lymphoma becomes indistinctly demarcated from the opaque-laden renal parenchyma and demonstrates a lightly speckled or inhomogeneous enhancement pattern with an attenuation value of 10 to 30 HU.

Differential diagnosis: Since renal lymphomas are usually secondary manifestations (metastases), the involvement of other organs is usually generally known from clinical findings. Therefore, despite having several clinical manifestations, renal lymphomas are usually not difficult to diagnose.

Renal Metastases

Renal metastases are three times more common than primary tumors at post mortem examinations. They generally occur in connection with generalized carcinomatosis. Their size at the time of autopsy is usually only a few millimeters. Bilateral involvement of the kidneys is demonstrated in ca. 50% of all cases. Bronchial carcinomas are the most frequently metastasing followed in order of frequency by metastases from carcinomas of the breast, contralateral kidney, colon, stomach, cervix, ovaries, pancreas, and prostate.

● CT

Plain scans: Focal and sometimes considerable deformation of the contours of the renal parenchyma may be demonstrated, but this is a nonspecific sign.

Contrast-enhanced scans: These mostly focal lesions can best be demonstrated after administration of contrast medium. They show slight, homogeneous enhancement and are therefore hypodense as compared with the surrounding renal parenchyma. The normal structure of the kidney becomes increasingly destroyed in proportion with the degree of infiltration. This results in a reduced and uneven pattern of enhancement in the slightly enlarged kidney.

Differential diagnosis: It is easier to make the diagnosis when there is bilateral growth, proof of additional metastases, and knowledge of a primary tumor. A solitary hypodense metastases in the renal cortex cannot be reliably distinguished from a hypovascularized renal cell carcinoma.

Nephroblastoma

The nephroblastoma, or Wilms' tumor, is the most common abdominal tumor in children. Both kidneys are affected in approx. 7% of all cases, and most nephroblastomas have reached a size of over 5 cm by the time they are discovered. Nephroblastoma are histologically classified as mixed tumors, and they contain variably differentiated tissue components. The tumors often show areas of hemorrhage, necrosis, and cystic degeneration, but are seldom calcified. Nephroblastomas invade the venous system in early stages, and regional lymph node involvement tends to occur. Metastases develop primarily in the lungs.

• CT

Plain scans: Nephroblastomas are usually demonstrated as extensive tumors that completely fill the bed of the kidney, thereby displacing adjacent organs. Because children normally have only slight amounts of delineating fat, it is often difficult to diagnose the tumors on plain scans. Sufficient bowel opacification is required. The attenuation value of the nephroblastoma usually ranges from 30 to 40 HU, and therefore correlates with that of muscle tissue. Their density usually is not homogeneous and is either reduced by necrosis and cystic degeneration or is slightly raised due to hemorrhage. In very extensive tumors, the boundary between adjacent organs and the upper pole of the tumor may be masked by partial volume artifacts. Thin sections should be scanned to prevent this.

Contrast-enhanced scans: Because of the extremely variable tissue composition of nephroblastomas, their appearance on CT scans is rather variable. Areas of severe cystic degeneration or necrosis are clearly demarcated. Frequently, the margins of the normal kidney

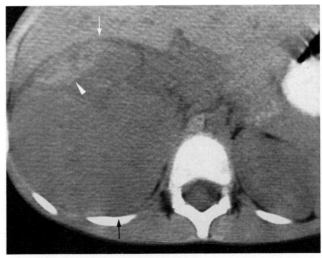

40a

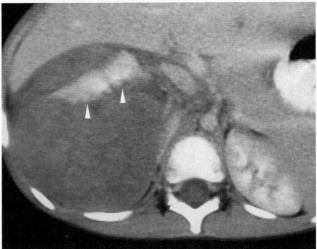

40b

Fig. 17-40. Wilm's tumor. Large mass (→) in the right kidney bed. Plain scans (a) reveal a narrow high-density zone (►) that is suggestive of hemorrhage. The bolus injection of contrast medium (b) leads to enhancement of still functional, noninvaded sections of the renal parenchyma (b ►).

can be identified only after the administration of contrast medium. A diagnostically and prognostically important factor is invasion of the venous system. This manifests as dilatation of the veins and as a filling defect, which can be seen after administration of contrast medium.

→

Fig. 17-42. Renal abscess. A mass (►) with low-density spots is located in the lower pole of the left kidney. Thickening of Gerota's fascia (→) and slight, streaky densification of the perirenal space are also observed. In the region of inflammation, less contrast medium is absorbed than in the normal parenchyma.

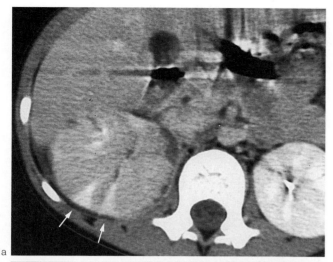

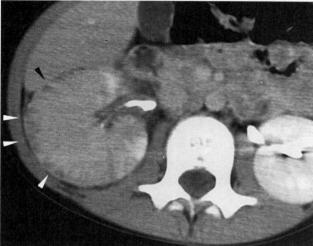

Fig. 17-41. Focal bacterial nephritis. Considerable enlargement of the right kidney. Mostly reduced contrast after contrast medium administration, but contrast medium accumulates in the typical radial or wedge-shaped areas of the parenchyma (a→). Low-density spots are located directly inferior to the fibrous capsule (b►). They are suggestive of incipient abscess formation. The perirenal space is not yet masked.

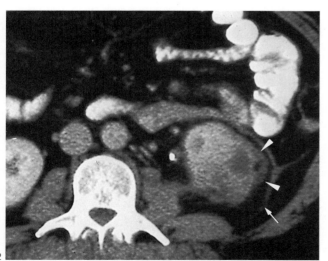

For unequivocal demonstration of lymph node enlargement, good bowel preparation is required in addition to adequate intravascular contrast enhancement.

Inflammatory Renal Diseases

When acute renal infections such as glomerulonephritis, abacterial interstitial nephritis, and pyelonephritis cause no clinical complications, there is usually no need for CT examination.

Acute Pyelonephritis – Local Bacterial Nephritis

These acute infections arise due to ascension of bacteria from the collecting tubules to the renal cortex. Interstitial infiltrates first compromise the tubules, causing tubular stasis in the affected sections of the parenchyma. As the disease progresses, liquefaction leads to the development of microabscesses which ultimately merge to form visibly abnormal areas (abscesses, abscess-forming pyelonephritis). By initiating effective antibiotic therapy, leukocytic infiltration can be quickly reversible, but abscesses require a longer period of healing.

● CT

Plain scans: In the early stages of these normally unilateral infections, the renal parenchyma is diffusely or focally dilated, depending on the degree of involvement of the renal parenchyma. The renal capsule is poorly defined, and a strand enhancement pattern is seen within perirenal fatty tissue. Gerota's fascia may also be thickened. These are additional and unreliable signs of acute infection.

Contrast-enhanced scans: After administration of contrast medium, a speckled or sometimes striated area of hypodensity can be seen. It obliterates the structure of the renal medulla and cortex can be seen in the areas of inflammation. Follow-up scans a few hours later show a reversal of enhancement: Because of tubular stasis, the attenuation in the infected regions is slightly hyperdense as compared with no lon-

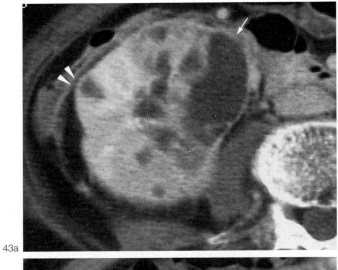

43a

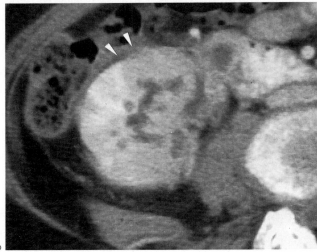

43b

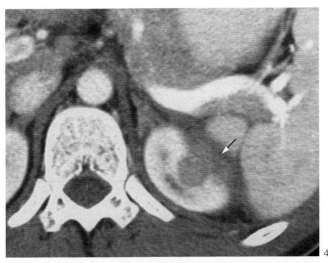

45a

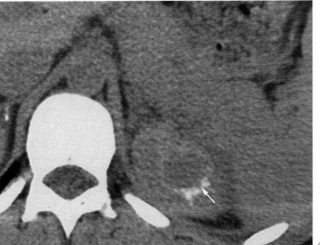

45b

Fig. 17-43. Multiple renal abscesses. Demonstration of numerous, sharply marginated low-density areas. Some of them are located beneath the capsule (a→). Enhancement of the inflamed areas of the kidney is slightly less than that of the normally functioning renal tissue, which appears hyperdense. Perirenal fat is only slightly masked by fine, dense radial structures. Gerota's fascia is also slightly thickened (a►). After 14 days of antibiotic treatment, the condition is clearly improved (b).

Fig. 17-45. Renal abscess. In patient undergoing treatment, a hypodense, sharply marginated, 1–2 cm large zone was found in the upper pole of the left kidney. Obliteration of the adjacent perirenal fat was also observed. On late scans, tubular stasis was also found in the vicinity (b→).

Fig. 17-44. Abscessed nephritis and perinephritis. There is only slight contrast enhancement with slight excretory insufficiency. The kidney lies within a fluid zone (→) corresponding to a purulent cavity. This is demarcated by a broad zone of granulation tissue (►). Gerota's fascia is thickened (►). Additional finding: abdominal abscess (⇒).

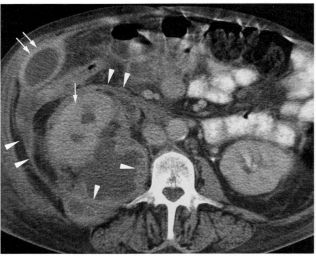

44

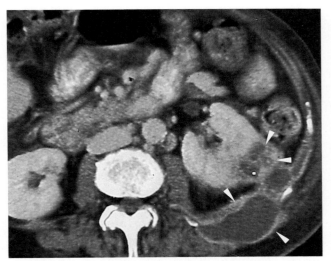

Fig. 17-46. Renal abscess with abdominal abscess. Distension of the renal contours was found in the dorsal region of the left kidney. Hypodense zones and abscess walls (►) were demarcated. This process communicates with the dorsolateral abdominal wall, thereby leading to zones of hypodensity inside the abdominal wall. These are also demarcated via granulation tissue (► ◄).

ger enhanced, properly functioning renal parenchyma. When there is diffuse infection of the entire kidney, the medullary and cortical contrast enhancement is already neutralized in the bolus phase. The pathologically abnormal enhancement pattern can still persist for weeks after the clinical symptoms have subsided.

Renal Abscess

If acute pyelonephritis or focal bacterial nephritis is allowed to progress, the leukocytic infiltrates develop into microabscesses, which ultimately fuse to form larger abscesses. In the further course of disease, abscesses may spread to the renal collecting system or to the perirenal space. When successfully treated, they transform into fibrous tissue.

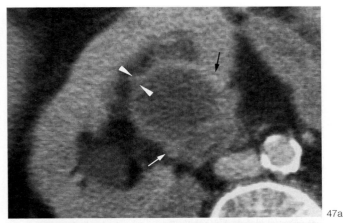

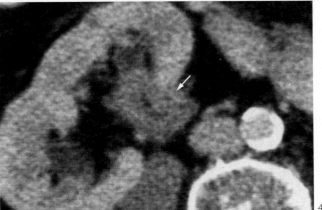

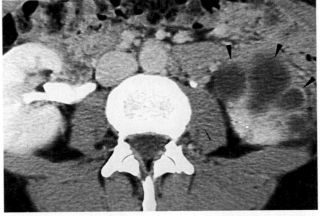

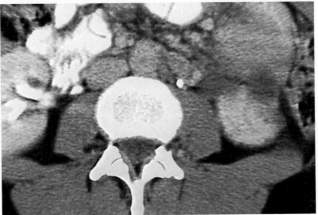

Fig. 17-47. Healing renal abscess. This already thick-walled process (a ► ◄) exhibits clear retraction and reduction (b→) after protracted antibiotic treatment.

Fig. 17-48. Superinfected renal cysts. The cysts exhibit a "cloverleaf" configuration and are located in the lower pole of the left kidney (a ►). They exhibit peripheral enhancement. After a long period of antibiotic treatment, significant reduction is seen three months later (b). There has been no change in size of the other thin-walled renal cysts.

A superinfection associated with cysts or hematomas can directly lead to abscess formation without causing focal bacterial nephritis. Renal carbuncles, which develop hematogenously, are characterized by dry necrosis and large amounts of granular tissue.

Spontaneous healing may occur after the renal collecting system has been infiltrated. Pyonephrosis frequently develops when the drainage of fluid is obstructed by necrotic material or pus.

• CT

Plain scans: On CT scans, the abscess zones appear hypodense as compared with the surrounding renal parenchyma. Depending on the extent of the lesion, a renal mass and/or perirenal changes may be seen. Gas formation within the lesion is a reliable sign of abscess. The attenuation value of renal abscesses ranges from 20 to 30 HU.

Contrast-enhanced scans: After a bolus injection of contrast medium, hypodense abscesses are demarcated from the enhanced renal parenchyma. After a short time (5 to 8 days), the abscess membrane appears on CT scans as a ringlike, sharply marginated structure. Masking of contiguous perirenal fat is due to infectious infiltration of surrounding tissues. It may also indicate invasion of the perirenal space.

Differential diagnosis: When very small lesions are found, local bacterial nephritis should be considered in the diagnosis. In questionable cases, late contrast-enhanced scans may help secure the diagnosis when tubular stasis or filling of contrast medium is not demonstrable within the abscess.

Emphysematous Pyelonephritis

Emphysematous pyelonephritis frequently occurs in diabetic patients and leads to severe clinical symptoms with sometimes even lethal outcome. Obstruction of the efferent urinary passages by papillary necrosis, strictures, or calculi are favorable conditions for bacterial spreading in association with fermentative anaerobic decomposition. Gas accumulates near renal pyramids and spreads to the perirenal space, resulting in a radial, streaky configuration.

• CT

Plain scans: Intrarenal gas, which can also be detected on conventional radiographs, is more sensitively detected by computed tomography. Direct proof of the cause of obstruction (calculi, fungal mycelia, retroperitoneal mass) can more often be obtained.

Contrast-enhanced scans: The (usually) enlarged kidney shows reduced contrast enhancement and an obstruction-related delay in excretion.

Differential diagnosis: Gas may accumulate after urological surgery, but this should be limited to the collecting system. Intraparenchymal (aseptic) gas may also develop after tumor embolization or extensive renal infarction.

Xanthogranulomatous Pyelonephritis

Xanthogranulomatous pyelonephritis is a disease of unclear etiologic origin and is characterized by chronic urinary disorder and an accompanying infection that originates in the renal pelvis. The inflamed renal parenchyma is replaced by a yellowish tissue containing lipids and macrophages (xanthoma cells). Parenchymal tissue is replaced by fibrous tissue. This rare disease predominantly affects women from the 3rd to 6th decades. Diffuse, unilateral kidney involvement is usually reported. Focal xanthogranulomatous pyelonephritis is usually seen in women and children. It is not uncommon for the inflammatory process to spread to the perirenal space. In patients with long-standing disease, the perirenal borders to the pararenal space, diaphragm and intestine are frequently infiltrated. Fistulae have also been reported.

• CT

Plain scans: The affected kidney is usually only moderately enlarged, but extensive enlargement has been reported in isolated cases. The kidney may also be deformed. Approximately 80% of these patients have a renal pelvic stone (with or without calyceal calculi). In the renal parenchyma, there is sometimes a central, cloverleaf-shaped hypodense area (with attenuation values ranging from -15 to +25 HU) which can resemble hydronephrosis. In focal xanthogranulomatous pyelonephritis, the process is limited to renal segments or one pole of the kidney.

The infiltrating infection masks the perirenal fatty tissue. A complex mass may develop in extensive processes where there is thickening of Gerota's fascia, infiltration of the psoas muscles and spread of infection to involve loops of the bowel.

Contrast-enhanced scans: After administration of contrast medium, the hypodense regions can be distinguished from the more dense cortical areas and from the usually dilated and slightly enhanced or nonenhanced structures of the renal collecting system.

Chronic Pyelonephritis

Chronic pyelonephritis is diagnosed primarily by clinical and urographic examination. The CT diagnosis is based on the usual radiologic features, such as:
- Loss of parenchyma (ranging from narrowing of the parenchymal cortex to organ atrophy).
- Scarred indentation above the deformed calyces, extending to the fibrous capsule.
- Nodules of regeneration product (acquired pseudotumors).
- Reduced excretory function.

Although calyceal deformity can be demonstrated on CT scans, this diagnosis remains the domain of urography.

Renal Tuberculosis

Postprimary renal tuberculosis manifests in the kidney 5 to 20 years after initial hematogenous

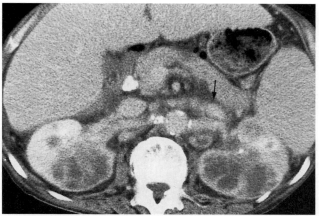

49a

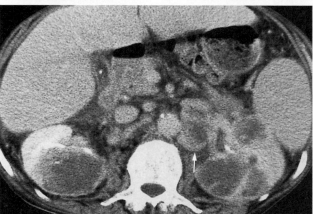

49b

Fig. 17-49. Florid renal tuberculosis. In contrast-enhanced scans, there is bilateral dilatation of the renal parenchyma with low- density areas in the region of the renal pyramids. These contain discrete septa and displace the collecting structures. On the left side, enlarged lymph nodes (→) with central low-density areas are observed. This is indicative of caseation.

Fig. 17-50. Ulcero-cavernous renal tuberculosis. Inflamed sections of the kidney appear hypodense, thereby demarcating a tuberculous abscess (→). The renal pelvis exhibits delicate parietal enhancement as an expression of an accompanying inflammation (▸).

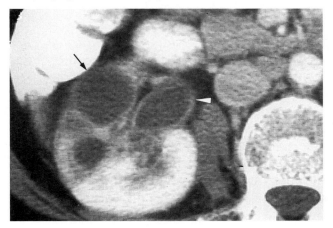

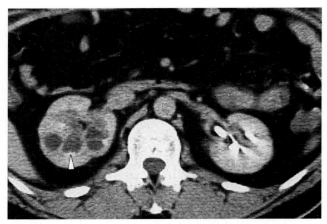

Fig. 17-51. Remnants of past ulcerocavernous renal tuberculosis. The right kidney exhibits sharply marginated areas of hypodensity characterized by their "cloverleaf" configuration. These become enhanced after contrast medium administration (►), which suggests communication of the tuberculous cavities with the renal collecting system. Caseous lymph nodes, a sign of floridity, are not found. Discrete calcific deposits are detected in the renal parenchyma on plain scans.

dissemination. Productive renal tuberculosis is characterized by tubercles (usually miliary) which diffusely permeate the renal parenchyma, whereas parenchymal loss is the main feature of liquefying, caseogenous renal tuberculosis. Calyceal destruction detected in a urogram is normally due to extensive parenchymal changes in the affected renal segment. Typical accompaniments of tuberculosis include productive processes or strictures, which can lead to distortion of the renal collecting system and encapsulation of groups of calyces. In more advanced stages, the disease ultimately leads to tuberculous pyonephrosis (caseous pyonephrosis after inspissation of necrotic material).

• CT

Plain scans: The late stages of *productive renal tuberculosis* are usually characterized by bilateral renal atrophy. Punctiform areas of calcification may develop after a granulomatous inflammation has run its course.

The *ulcerative cavernous form* of the disease gives rise to a varied clinical picture. Within the parenchyma of the usually normal-sized kidneys, low-density areas located along the renal pyramids give the structures a mulberry-

shaped or clover-leaf appearance. The cause is usually hydrocalices that develop as a result of calyceal stricture. Attenuation values greater than 40 HU and especially prominent peripheral calcification are signs suggestive of closed cavities. Depending on the extent of calcification of the caseous necrotic material, widespread or ringlike opaque structures may be seen. As was the case in pyonephrosis, obstruction of the renal pelvis results in an irregular, distended pelvicalyceal system. The appearance of the kidney can vary greatly when masses of detritus become calcified (tuberculous infarction kidney, caseous pyonephrosis).

Contrast-enhanced scans: In advanced renal tuberculosis, administration of contrast medium improves the demonstration of the renal parenchyma and, thereby, gives a more detailed image of tissue transformation processes and deformation of the renal collecting system.

Renal Transplants

Doppler ultrasound, renal radionuclide imaging, and renal biopsy are the methods of choice for evaluation of renal transplants. They may be supplemented by additional angiographic and computer tomographic examinations.

Fig. 17-52. Transplanted kidney. Homogeneous enhancement is observed after contrast medium administration. This indicates normal excretory function of the kidney. The appearance of the bed of the kidney is normal.

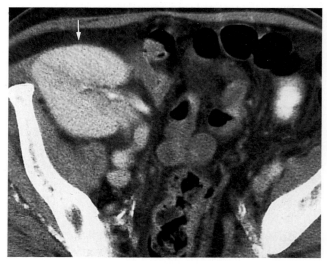

Acute and chronic organ rejection is the most important complication to watch for after renal transplantation. Direct postoperative complications include collections of fluid near the transplant (hematoma, urinoma, lymphocele, or abscess). In principle, all of these complications can be detected by sonography.

• CT

Plain scans: A renal transplant may still be normal-sized in acute rejection. A rapid growth in size increases the likelihood of organ rejection. Chronic rejection is characterized by gradual organ shrinkage, which may be accompanied by calcification.

Direct postoperative complications may include hematoma, abscess and lymphocele. The raised attenuation value of hematomas, the development of abscess walls, and the configuration of fluid collections usually facilitate the diagnosis. Gas collections suggestive of an abscess must be differentiated from surgically related air inclusions.

Contrast-enhanced scans: In sequential computed tomography, a quantitative analysis of contrast medium passage in the kidney is performed in five minutes. Rejection of the renal transplant is evaluated by assessing changes in renal function.

Fibrolipomatosis

Fibrolipomatosis is characterized by proliferation of fatty tissue or connective tissue in the renal sinus. When the renal parenchyma is atrophied, fatty tissue fills the renal sinus. An additional fibrous tissue element may develop due to obstruction-related, repeated extravasation of urine in the peripelvic space or pericalyceal space. This theory is supported by the high coincidence of fibrolipomatosis with prostatic adenoma, chronic pyelonephritis and nephrolithiasis.

• CT

CT scans show clear dilatation of the renal sinus, usually demonstrating splaying of the

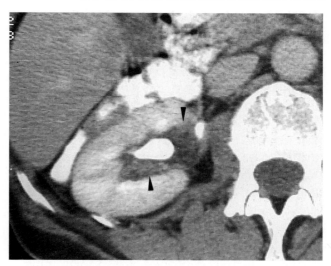

Fig. 17-53. Fibrolipomatosis. The renal collecting structures are surrounded by hypodense tissue, some of which absorbs contrast medium (►). Signs of displacement, as seen in the case of peripelvic cysts, are not found.

(contrasted) renal collecting system within. These changes are usually equally developed in both kidneys. In contrast to peripelvic cysts, there are no clear signs of displacement. Fibrolipomatous tissue develops like a cuff around the calyces and renal pelvis. Depending on the percentage of fat and fibrosis tissue, the CT numbers may vary from -100 to +20 HU. It can therefore sometimes be difficult to distinguish fibrilopomatosis from peripelvic cysts.

Renal Trauma

Trauma (usually blunt) can lead to a *contusion* or *rupture* of the renal parenchyma. A more rare complication is *transection* of the arterial or venous renal pedicle. Isolated lacerations in the renal collecting system or ureter are rare; they are usually found in connection with other injuries. Vascular injury is usually accompanied by *hematomas* of variable extent and can lead to local thrombosis. Lacerations in renal collecting structures lead to extravasation of urine, especially when an obstruction has also developed.

Renal Contusion

Pathological and anatomical examinations show a focal parenchymal laceration with minor hemorrhage and urine accumulation. The distribution may be local or diffuse, depending on the site affected by trauma. More severe parenchymal lacerations can lead to intrarenal and subcapsular hematomas. Postcontusional parenchymal injuries often manifest only weeks after the initial contusion.

• CT

Plain scans: CT scans usually show a kidney whose external contours are poorly margined (and deformed when there is a perirenal hematoma). With minor hemorrhage, the attenuation value is not always raised; there is considerable variation here.

Contrast-enhanced scans: The renal parenchyma shows inhomogeneous opacification after the administration of contrast medium. This enhancement pattern is a result of perfusion disturbances, i.e. local extravasation of contrast medium. This is confirmed when hyperdense areas appear on late contrast-enhanced scans taken a few hours later. Low-density zones, especially those that are segmental, are suggestive of perfusion disturbances in the segmental arteries. They are due either to a vascular constriction or vessel laceration with infarction.

Renal Pedicle Injuries

The renal pedicle is injured in 5% of all renal traumas. A laceration that damages the intima of arteries frequently leads to thrombotic occlusion. Arterial lacerations usually lead to contraction and, therefore, abrupt cessation of the artery. It is not unusual for a laceration in larger veins to cause an extensive retroperitoneal hematoma.

• CT

Plain scans: The most common sign of pedicle injuries is a perirenal or retroperitoneal hematoma that masks the renal sinus.

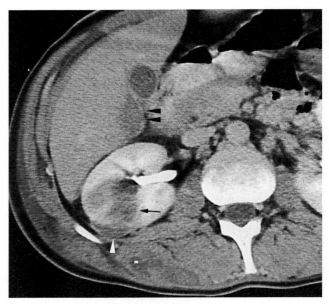

Fig. 17-54. Contusion of the kidney. Segmental hypodensity is observed after contrast medium administration. This corresponds to the focus of contusion (→). Further findings include discrete, subcapsular hematomas in the kidney (►) as well as the liver (⊫). A focus of contusion is also found in the region of the right erector spinae.

Contrast-enhanced scans: The extent of renal vascular injuries can be assessed when there is a coincidental segmental perfusion deficit. Collateral circulation channels in the capsular arteries have developed when peripheral cortical contrast enhancement is demonstrated.

Renal Hematoma

Nephritis, neoplasms, aneurysms of the renal artery, arteriosclerosis, hydronephrosis, polyarteritis nodosa, tuberculosis, renal cysts, and coagulopathies can lead to nontraumatic hematomas in the bed of the kidney. Approximately 20 % of these hematomas are subcapsular. Besides the more common abdominal traumas, penetrating wounds and iatrogenic punctures are additional causes of traumatic hematomas. The renal capsule (fibrous capsule) may remain intact after a parenchymal rupture, thus leading to the development of a subcapsular hematoma. An initially subcapsular hematoma can always cause secondary complications by invading the perirenal space. Frequently, the only clinical sign of subcapsular or perirenal hematomas are symptoms of

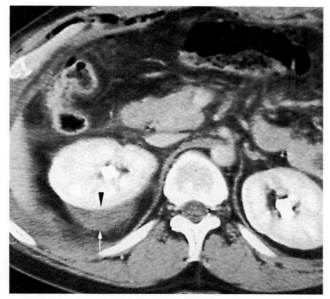

Fig. 17-55. Subcapsular renal hematoma after blunt abdominal trauma. On plain scans, the protrusion appears discretely hyperdense (→). On contrast-enhanced scans, it exhibits the typical lenticulate configuration and is hypodense (►) as compared with the opaque-laden renal parenchyma.

hypertension resulting from compression (page kidney), especially in the case of spontaneous hemorrhage.

• CT

Plain scans: Intrarenal hematomas are only rarely demonstrable on plain scans, where they appear as hyperdense zones which can later display sedimentation phenomena. Because the renal capsule is so rigid, hematomas usually

Fig. 17-56. Laceration of the kidney. As a result of abdominal trauma, not only the hepatic parenchyma, but also the renal parenchyma, was lacerated. There is a pronounced perirenal hematoma which also masks the renal pedicle (→).

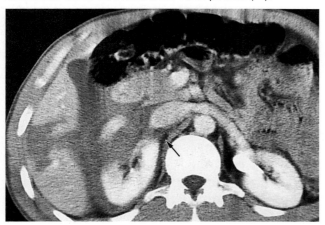

develop in subcapsular areas. The hematoma develops below the capsule, thereby displacing and flattening the renal parenchyma. This results in the typical, sickle-shaped configuration.

The attenuation of a hematoma depends on its age and type (compact hematoma, diffuse hemorrhage). As compared with healthy muscle and renal tissue, fresh, compact hematomas appear hyperdense for several days. As more and more time passes, the hematomas become increasingly hypodense and may liquefy (density reduction, capsule formation), calcify, and become absorbed or reorganized.

Contrast-enhanced scans: Since they are avascular lesions, hematomas do not enhance after administration of contrast medium. Fresh hematomas are displayed as poorly marginated zones of hypodensity.

Obstructive Uropathies

Hydronephrosis

The most common causes of urinary obstruction are various mechanical causes such as obstruction of the lumen (lithiasis, tumor, trauma), intramural processes (congenital, inflammatory, radiation strictures, atresia), or compression of the efferent urinary passages (retroperitoneal tumor, lymphoma, retroperitoneal fibrosis, pelvic tumor, hematoma, trauma, atypical ureteral course). Purely functional causes of hydronephrosis (neurogenic, ureterovesical reflux) are rare and occur preferentially in younger patients.

Depending on the location of the obstruction, individual calyces, the renal pelvis, a ureter, or the bladder may be affected. Increased intraluminal pressure leads, initially, to atrophy of the papillae with consecutive excavation and flattening of the renal pyramids. Ultimately, only the renal columns remain as parenchymal bridges.

Chronic, insidious hydronephrosis causes variable enlargement of the kidneys. When renal

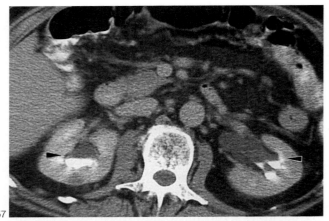

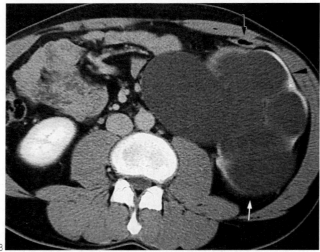

Fig. 17-57. Slight urinary obstruction. After contrast medium administration, contrast medium stratification phenomena are observed bilaterally in the slightly dilated renal collecting structures (►). The excretory function is not affected.

Fig. 17-58. Hydronephrosis. Considerable dilatation of the renal collecting system (→) has led to flattening of the renal parenchyma. The latter, however, still absorbs contrast medium (►).

function is reduced, they are frequently smaller than normal. Compensating hypertrophy of the contralateral kidney occurs. The concept of purely inflammation-related renal atrophy in hydronephrosis is still controversial. The onset and duration of obstruction and the age of the patient seem to be important pathogenetic factors.

• CT

Plain scans: CT scans show the dilated collecting system as a central zone of hypodensity (approximately water-dense) oriented along the calyces. The duration and the extent of (chronic) obstruction are factors which determine the degree of deformation of collecting structures, which ultimately fuse to form a lobulated configuration. The recesses correspond to atrophied renal pyramids. In the final stages, the collecting system has a fluid-filled, fibrous, saccular appearance.

Minor dilatation of collecting structures cannot always be demonstrated on CT scans because of their unsuitable scanning geometry. In relatively early stages, the renal pelvis protrudes extrarenally and medially. When the obstruction is low, the dilated ureter can be traced caudally, provided that its course is axial and the lumen is greater than 0.3 to 0.5 cm in width.

Contrast-enhanced scans: Dilatation of renal collecting structures may be absent when the renal collecting system and the ureter are surrounded. In these cases, obstruction can be identified on the basis of layering phenomena (caused by the specific gravity of contrast medium) in the renal collecting system. In patients with reduced renal function, persistent, long-lasting enhancement of the parenchyma (obstructive nephrogram) is characteristic of obstruction.

Pyonephrosis

Pyonephrosis occurs when there are simultaneous effects of obstruction and inflammation, e.g. with inflammatory changes in the parenchyma (pyelonephritis, tuberculosis, abscess), after secondary obstructions caused by necrotic material or strictures, and from secondary infections arising with hydronephrosis. In pyonephrosis, the collecting system is filled with pus, and has a variably saccular appearance, which is determined by the degree of obstruction and parenchymal obliteration. Inflammatory changes are often seen in the perirenal and pararenal spaces. Cirrhosis of the kidney may develop in chronic cases, and amorphous or ringlike areas of calcification can be seen on conventional radiographs.

• CT

Plain scans: As was the case with hydronephrosis, pyonephrosis is characterized by variable dilatation of renal collecting structures. The inflammation-related reduction or obliteration of the renal parenchyma can also be assessed. In cases of hydronephrosis, the attenuation value of the collecting system is approximately equal to that of water. It rises, however, in pyonephrosis, and can reach values of 20 to 70 HU, depending on the degree of inspissation of necrotic material. Sedimentation is indicative of variable particle size and a raised protein content in impacted fluid.

Differential diagnosis: Tuberculous and nonspecific pyonephrosis cannot be differentiated by computed tomography, even though more severe calcification is seen in the healing stages or renal tuberculosis. Although invasion of the perirenal space and pararenal space can be demonstrated in early stages, this only rarely occurs in renal tuberculosis. Hypertrophy of perirenal fat in response to chronic inflammation has been described.

Urolithiasis

Approximately 90% of all renal calculi are composed of calciferous carbonates, phosphates, oxalates, and magnesium ammonium phosphate. The remaining 10% contain uric acid or urate. Only ca. 1% of all renal calculi are cystine stones.

• CT

Plain scans: When the scanned sections are thin enough, all renal calculi can be demonstrated on plain CT scans. They appear as hyperdense structures with attenuation values greater than 200 HU. Uric acid calculi and xanthine calculi have attenuation values less than 500 HU and can therefore be differentiated from cystine stones (450 to 650 HU) and other calciferous stones.

There is still no definite method of making a pretherapeutic assessment for extracorporal

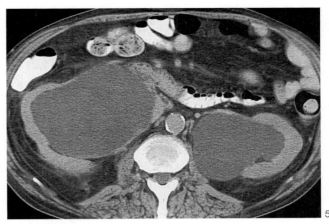

Fig. 17-59. Considerable bilateral hydronephrosis.

Fig. 17-60. Pyonephrosis with perirenal hematoma. The hydronephrotic, shrunken kidney still exhibits a small seam of parenchyma. Fluid contained in the dilated collecting system has a CT number of 25 HU. The dilated perirenal space (→) has similar, somewhat maculate, but higher (▸) CT numbers that are suggestive of hematoma, but could also be due to abscess.

Fig. 17-61. Calyceal concrements. Very small concrements were sensitively detected on plain scans.

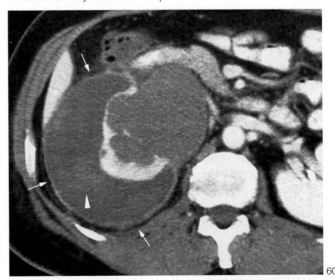

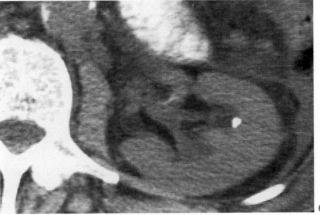

shock wave lithotripsy as to the likely fragility and outcome.

Differential diagnosis: In general, calculi should be differentiated from other types of calcification. Vascular stenosis in the renal sinus can be identified on the basis of its linear configuration. The appearance and configuration of papillary calcification and calcifications of medullary sponge kidney may sometimes cause diagnostic difficulties.

Vascular Processes

Arteriosclerosis

Vascular sclerosis can be demonstrated by CT while still at an early stage. This also holds true for the renal artery, provided thin sections are used. In the final stages of the disease, atrophic kidneys with generalized reduced parenchyma and an increased amount of fat in the renal sinus are observed.

Renal Artery Stenosis

• CT

Contrast-enhanced scans: A perfusion difference with the contralateral kidney is visible on CT scans only after hemodynamic effects of renal artery stenosis have become apparent. The late and reduced filling of contrast medium leads to a delay and reduction of enhancement on the affected side of the cortical compartment as well as the medullary compartment. Depending on the extent of stenosis, the parenchymal enhancement of the affected kidney is variably extended as compared with that in the contralateral, healthy kidney.

Renal Infarction

Thrombo-embolic occlusion of the renal artery or its branches causes renal infarction. Embolisms usually originate from the cavity of the heart (mitral valvular insufficiency, myocardial infarction, atrial myxoma) or from an aortic

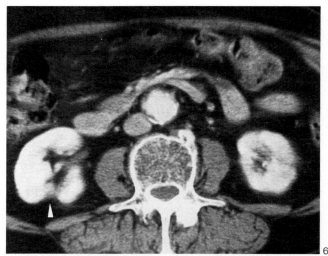

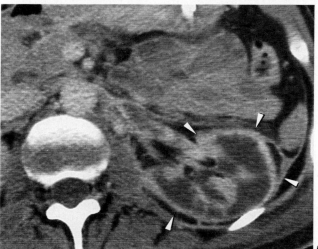

Fig. 17-62. Parenchymal scars (►) were detected **after renal infarction**.

Fig. 17-63. Renal infarction. Total infarction of the left kidney due to embolism. After contrast medium administration, it becomes evident that the periphery of the renal parenchyma is still supplied. This is indicated by peripheral enhancement (►).

aneurysm. Thrombotic occlusions are found in conjunction with arteriosclerosis, trauma, and iatrogenic intimal lesions and embolization.

• CT

Plain scans: In the early stages, the contours of the kidney are only rarely deformed. Slight hyperdensity, especially in subcapsular regions, may point to an underlying hemorrhage.

Contrast-enhanced scans: After the administration of contrast medium, the affected areas of the parenchyma become relatively sharply

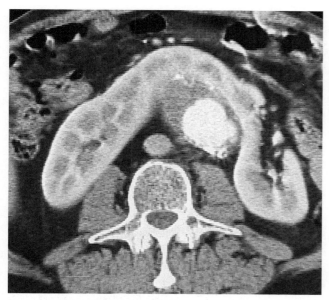

Fig. 17-64. Horseshoe kidney. Broad parenchymal bridge in front of the aorta, which exhibits aneurysmatic change. Characteristic of the disease, the renal collection system is opened ventrally.

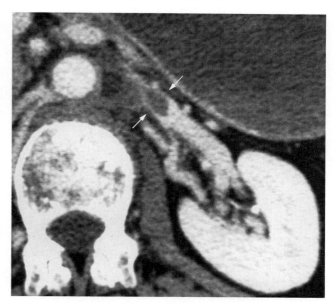

Fig. 17-65. Renal vein thrombosis in carcinoma of the pancreas. With careful scanning, it is usually possible to demonstrate the intravascular thrombus.

demarcated from healthy renal parenchyma. In minor infarctions, these areas often have a wedge-shaped appearance and correspond to the supply area of the segmental arteries of the renal pyramids. The perfusion deficit does not, however, extend all the way to the renal capsule, because the capsular vessels are able to supply a narrow, subcapsular area of the cortex (cortical rim sign). In later stages, infarcted regions of the parenchyma become atrophied and scar tissue develops. Superinfection of the infarcted areas, which may be accompanied by intrarenal abscesses, is a possibility to be considered when diagnosing a septic embolism.

Renal Vein Thrombosis

Renal vein thrombosis can develop in conditions causing increased blood coagulation, e.g. plasmacytoma, renal and retroperitoneal tumor, inflammation, nephrotic syndrome, and amyloidosis. In chronic disease, extensive collateral circulation channels develop in capsular and gonadal veins.

• CT

Plain scans: The complete clinical picture of renal vein thrombosis develops only after com-

plete obstruction of the renal vein and appears as a broad cord of soft-tissue that is usually larger than 2 cm. The kidney is enlarged and inhomogeneously dense. The perirenal space frequently contains strandlike opacities.

Contrast-enhanced scans: Several collateral and gonadal vessels become visible after the administration of contrast medium. The renal vein itself, however, does not become enhanced, but the thrombus becomes visible in the contrasted inferior vena cava. Edematous tissue in the enlarged kidney displays variable enhancement: The cortical regions show more intense parenchymal enhancement than the central sections of the kidney.

When occlusion of the renal vein (which usually maintains its normal caliber) is incomplete, it usually is possible to diagnose renal vein thrombosis with careful scanning.

Congenital Variations, Anomalies

Congenital anomalies of the kidney include *agenesis*, or absence of the kidney, and *aplasia*, which occurs when the kidney fails to develop. *Lobar dysmorphism* occurs when there is hy-

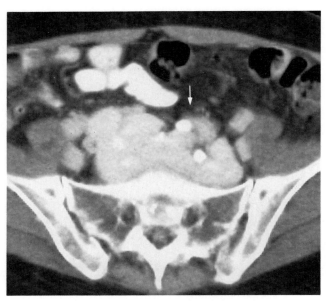

Fig. 17-66. Pelvic kidney. The irregularly contorted organ exhibits a ventrally oriented, branched collecting system (→).

pertrophy or doubling of a renal segment (renal pyramid and surrounding cortex).

Malposition (ectopia) of the kidney can be congenital or acquired (ptosis). Crossed *dystopia* occurs when one kidney is displaced to the contralateral side; malrotation and an abnormal shape may also be observed. In *"horseshoe" kidneys*, the lower poles of the kidneys are fused together, and the collecting system has a typical, ventral orientation. The vascular supply is extremely variable.

• CT

With a unilaterally silent kidney, it is normally possible to distinguish between a simple non-functioning kidney and *agenesis* or *aplasia*, because the renal bed can be demonstrated on CT scans. The presence of a small, soft-tissue dense structure with aortic vascular supply across from the exit of the renal artery is suggestive of aplasia. However, it is rarely possible to differentiate between aplasia and agenesis. The adrenal gland appears enlarged in over 90% of all cases.

A *hypoplastic kidney* appears basically as a smaller version of a normal kidney. Abnormal changes in the parenchyma may be used as a criterion to distinguish a hypoplastic kidney from a pyelonephrotic atrophic kidney.

The diagnosis of *horseshoe kidney* is secured with evidence of bridge formation across the lower poles of the kidneys and renal malrotation, which can be demonstrated on plain CT scans. Parenchymal and fibrous bridging can be distinguished after a bolus injection of contrast medium has been administered. Preoperative angiography is necessary, because the vascular supply from the aorta is extremely variable.

Lobar dysmorphism of a kidney, which can cause the appearance of a tumor-like mass in the renal parenchyma, behaves like normal renal tissue. Medullary and cortical structures can be distinguished after a targeted bolus injection of contrast medium, and the nature of the anomaly is more clearly visible. The diagnosis of fetal lobulation can also be secured by similar contrast enhancement.

Chapter 18
The Adrenal Glands

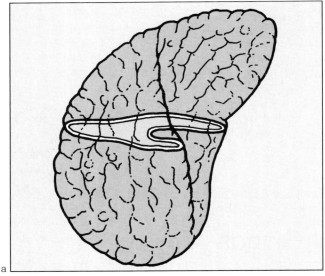

1a

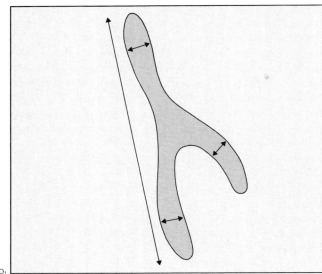

1b₁

Limb length	Left (mm) ± SD	Right (mm ± SD
Karstaedt	21.5 ± 4.6	22.8 ± 6.3
Montagne	21.5 ± 3.2	22,1 ± 4.6
Heuck	24.3 ± 7.9	26.8 ± 6.4

Limb lenght	Left (mm) ± SD	Right (mm ± SD
Karstaedt	6.7 ± 1.7	5.1 ± 1.1
Montagne	~ 10	~ 10
Heuck	5.7 ± 1.2	5.5 ± 1.0

1b₂

Fig. 18-1a-c. Normal adrenal glands.

a) Ventral view of left adrenal gland.
b) Measurement of limb length and thickness in the transverse plane.
c) Configuration of normal-sized adrenals according to data by various researchers.

Right:

Triangular (3 %)

Linear (9 %)

Linear (36–87 %)

V-shaped (9–52 %)

Left:

V-shaped (50–60 %)

Deltaic (32 %)

Triangular (9–40 %)

1c

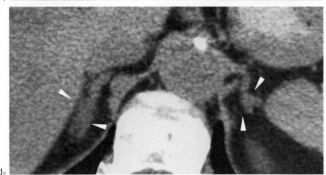
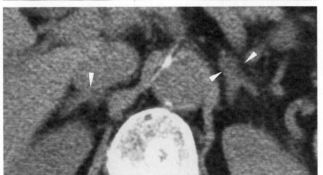
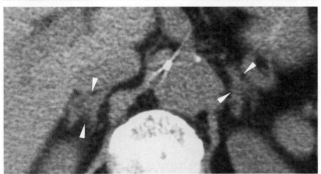
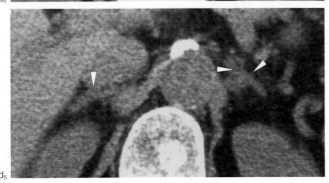

1d₁

1d₂

1d₃

1d₄

1d₅

The Adrenal Glands

Anatomy and Imaging

Normal adrenal glands weigh 12 to 16 g in adults. They are almost always identifiable on thin CT sections. Imaging difficulties arise only in cachectic patients with severely reduced amounts of retroperitoneal fat or when artifacts degrade the scan. The CT appearance of the adrenals is variable, the basic forms being linear, V-shaped, deltoid and triangular. Due to the complicated infolding of the adrenal gland surface, cross-sectional configurations of the same organ will vary, depending on the level of the section. The left adrenal is located ca. 0.5 cm away from its ipsilateral kidney, and it extends somewhat lower than the right adrenal. The right adrenal is situated directly opposite, and it appears as a streak-like, contralateral structure situated between the diaphragm and Glisson's capsule. Adjacent splenic vessels may simulate enlargement of the left adrenal (contrast medium administration may be required). The location of the adrenals remains unchanged, even in cases of renal ectopia.

Due to the variety of CT configurations of the adrenal glands, the length of the left and right limbs is greatly variable. The craniocaudad length ranges from 20 to 40 mm. The thickness of each respective gland is homogeneous (5 to 8 mm). A thickness of more than 10 mm is indicative of abnormal pathology.

False tumors: A protruded, non-opacified, and atypically shaped fundus of the stomach, a gastric diverticulum, increased lobulation of the spleen, portosystemic collateral vessels or an atypically located loop of the colon can simulate a mass (false tumor) in the adrenal bed.

Fig. 18-1d. Demonstration of adrenal glands in CT scan, proceeding cranial (d₁) to caudal (d₅). On plain scans, the adrenal glands appear as linear structures inside perirenal fat.

Hyperplasia and Tumors of the Adrenal·Cortex

Hyperplasia of the adrenal glands is normally a result of increased hormone production. All primary cortical tumors may be endocrinologically active or silent. A histological section cannot demonstrate whether a neoplasm produces hormones. In order to judge the hormonal activity of an adrenal neoplasm, certain indirect signs, like accompanying hypoplasia or atrophy of other adrenal tissue, must be evaluated. A clinical examination (suppression test) is normally required to distinguish nodular hyperplasia from multiple adrenal adenoma. Histological differentiation of malignant and benign adrenal tumors can also be difficult if unequivocal evidence of metastatic spread is absent.

Cushing's syndrome arises from an ACTH-producing pituitary adenoma in up to 75% of cases and is characterized by diffuse or nodular hyperplasia. About 20% of all adrenocortical adenomas and 5 to 10 % of all adrenocortical carcinomas are associated with increased glucocorticoid levels.

The most frequent causes of primary *hyperaldosteronism* (PHA) are adenomas (classical Conn's syndrome), micronodular and macronodular hyperplasia. Carcinoma is a very rare cause. In adult patients with PHA, adenomas are diagnosed three to four times more frequently than hyperplasia. Extra-adrenal, aldosterone-producing adenomas are rare. Bilateral nodular hyperplasia is more frequently responsible for Conn's syndrome in pediatric patients with PHA than adenoma.

Adrenogenital syndrome (AGS) is caused either by congenital hyperplasia (enzyme defect) or by a cortical tumor. When AGS occurs in children, it is normally tumor-related (carcinomas more frequent than adenomas). Adrenal feminization usually arises from carcinoma of the adrenal cortex.

Adrenocortical Hyperplasia

Occurrence: Prevalent in Cushing's syndrome, adrenogenital syndrome, and Conn's syndrome; more infrequent in thyrotoxicosis, acromegaly, diabetes mellitus, and malignant disease.

• CT

Generalized enlargement of an adrenal gland must be evaluated under consideration of its horizontal and vertical dimensions. The length and width of the limbs of the organ are the proper parameters of measurement. However, the majority of clinically diagnosed bilateral adrenocortical hyperplasias do not show any clear signs of enlargement on CT scans. Macroscopic adrenal gland enlargement occurs more frequently in Cushing's syndrome than in Conn's syndrome.

Due to the variety of configurations of the adrenal glands, only unequivocal, bilateral enlargement of the adrenals should be interpreted as hyperplasia.

Adrenocortical Adenoma

Patients with Cushing's syndrome, adrenogenital syndrome, and Conn's syndrome display a clinical picture of hyperadrenalism.

Benign adrenocortical neoplasms are normally discovered at a size of 2 to 5 cm, however, they can become much larger. Larger neoplasms frequently display necrosis and cystic degeneration. Cushing's adenomas are normally larger than Conn's adenomas, which are rarely larger than 2 cm in diameter. Bilateral adenomas have been diagnosed in isolated cases (ca. 1 to 2%). Calcification occurs very infrequently in Conn's adenoma.

• CT

Plain scans: Under favorable scanning conditions (sufficient periglandular fat, peripheral location), adrenocortical adenomas can be detected when they are as small as 10 mm, but must be at least 15 mm in diameter before they

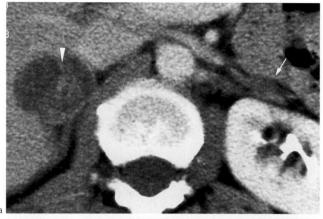

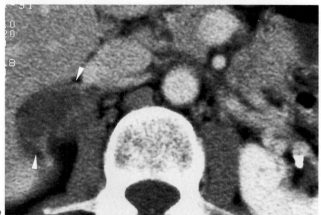

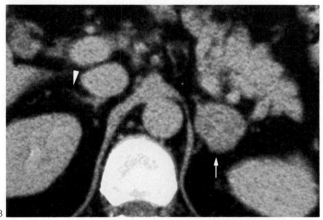

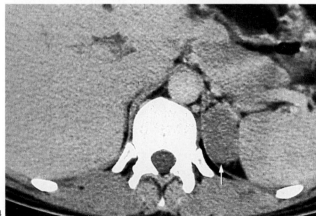

can be reliably diagnosed. Adrenocortical adenomas are round, smoothly marginated masses that are homogeneous in thickness.

Since adrenocortical adenomas are especially rich in lipoids, there is a lipoid-related reduction in tissue density ranging from 50 HU in adenomas with low lipoid levels to ca. -20 HU in those with high lipoid levels. These adenomas are sometimes water-dense.

Contrast-enhanced scans: When the CT numbers of adrenocortical adenomas drop to the water range, contrast medium must be used to differentiate fatty tumors from avascular cysts. Because of their good vascularization, Cushing's adenomas usually become intensely enhanced by contrast medium. The enhancement of Conn's adenomas is approx. 30 HU lower. The whole length of the adrenal glands should be thoroughly scanned to avoid overlooking any adenomas possibly located at the ends of the limbs.

Adrenocortical Carcinoma

Clinical picture in hyperfunction: Cushing's syndrome, adrenogenital syndrome (AGS) frequently mixed pictures.

More highly differentiated, hormonally active carcinomas are predominant in pediatric patients. Clinical abnormalities associated with hormonally active malignancies are frequently absent in adult patients. Adult adrenocortical

Fig. 18-2. Nodular hyperplasia in a patient with clinically diagnosed Cushing's syndrome. A large adenoma has developed on the right (a). The more highly vascularized organ matrix within the adenoma becomes discretely visible after contrast medium administration (a, b►). Only smaller dilated nodules have developed on the left (a→).

Fig. 18-3. Cushing's adenoma. A sharply marginated, slightly hypodense adenoma (→) is easily identifiable within increased amounts of fatty tissue. Compensatory hypoplasia has occurred on the opposite side (►).

Fig. 18-4. Conn's adenoma. A sharply marginated, hypodense and homogeneous mass in the left adrenal gland shows slight contrast enhancement (→).

carcinomas are therefore often discovered in inoperable stages with metastatic spread. Extensive necrosis, hemorrhage, and calcification are more frequently associated with carcinomas than adenomas. These carcinomas are often diagnosed late, which contributes to the overall unfavorable prognosis.

• CT

Plain scans: Small carcinomas are normally indistinguishable from small adenomas based on their CT appearance. Infiltration of neighboring organs and the para-aortic space, spread into veins and regional nodes are reliable, but late, signs of malignancy. Lipids may accumulate within the tumor, causing a corresponding reduction in tissue density. Hypodense areas signify zones of necrosis. Amorphous calcification is present in ca. 35% of all cases.

Contrast-enhanced scans: Viable tumor tissue displays only slight enhancement. Necrotic zones remain unenhanced and become sharply demarcated, in contrast to areas of low attenuation associated with lipid accumulation.

Nonfunctioning Adenoma

Hormonally inactive adrenocortical adenomas are termed nonfunctioning adenomas. They are discovered as an incidental finding in 2 to 8% of all autopsies. These adenomas are found most often in older, obese diabetic patients, elderly women, and hypertensive patients.

• CT

Nonfunctioning adenomas are usually small (less than 3 cm), but they can become as large as 6 cm in diameter. They are sharply marginated, have a CT number of ca. 20 HU (range = 10 to 40 HU), and become moderately enhanced after the administration of contrast medium (20 to 30 HU). The development of nonfunctioning adenomas is usually unilateral, and they frequently contain calcium. On the whole, nonfunctioning adenomas do not have a characteristic CT appearance that makes them distinguishable from endocrinologically active adenomas.

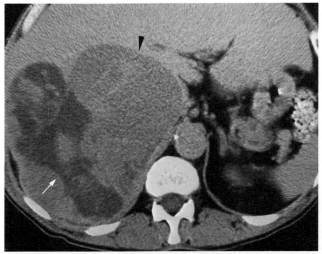
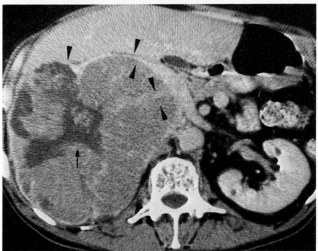

Fig. 18-5. Adrenocortical carcinoma. This large tumor displaces the liver. After bolus contrast medium administration (b), subcapsular structures (►) and hypodense zones (→) corresponding to necrosis become visible on the CT scans.

Differential diagnosis: Nonfunctioning adenomas that are smaller than 5 cm in diameter with smooth, well defined borders and homogeneous parenchymal density are not likely to be malignant. A six-month follow-up to confirm the absence of progression is normally sufficient. However, patients with a known history of a tumor should undergo a percutaneous biopsy when proof of adrenal metastatic spread might have therapeutic consequences.

Adrenal Medullary Tumors

Myelolipoma

Myelolipomas are rare, benign tumors that can be classified as a mesenchymal metaplasm with myeloid and erythroid elements. Myelolipomas usually evoke no clinical symptoms unless they have become extremely massive (they can become as large as 12 cm in diameter). Endocrinologic disturbances are rare. Hemorrhage, calcification and ossification can develop in the predominantly fatty components of myelolipomas.

• CT

Plain scans: A myelolipoma appears on CT scans as a fatty mass enclosed in a smooth capsule. The attenuation value of its fatty tissue components is equal to or slightly above that of the retroperitoneal space (-50 to -80 HU). Calcification, which is rare, is usually ringlike or punctiform. Hemorrhagic areas may be reorganized or calcified and are sharply demarcated from fatty tissue components.

Contrast-enhanced scans: Soft-tissue components (myeloid tissue) show clear enhancement.

Differential diagnosis: Renal angiomyolipoma, retroperitoneal lipoma and liposarcoma must be considered in the diagnosis.

Pheochromocytoma

These chromaffin tumors are located within the adrenal glands in 90% of cases and extra-adrenally in 10% of all cases. Around 10 % of all pheochromocytomas develop bilaterally. In contrast, ca. 30% of all pheochromocytomas in children are extra-adrenal, and 30 to 70% develop bilaterally.

Pheochromocytomas are frequently associated with autosomally dominant, inherited multiple endocrinologic neoplasms (Werner's syndrome, Sipple's syndrome) or occur in combination with neoplasms of other endocrinologic organs. These lesions are frequently bilateral, and extra-adrenal location is rare. Non-hereditary pheochromocytomas frequently manifest in the 5th decade of life. Pheochromocytomas are highly vascularized, and even small lesions tend to become necrotic or display cystic degeneration. Fibrosis, hemorrhage and peripheral calcification (often ringlike) are not uncommon findings.

Fig. 18-6. Myelolipoma. Mass in the bed of the right adrenal gland; it has predominantly homogeneous, fat-dense attenuation values; cordlike structures (→) can also be seen. A small area of calcification is seen in the adrenal gland (►).

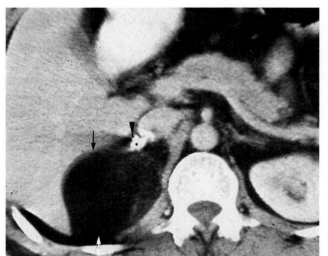

Fig. 18-7. Pheochromocytoma. After bolus contrast medium administration, there is intense contrast enhancement in the periphery of the tumor (→). Hypodensity is an indication of necrosis or hemorrhage.

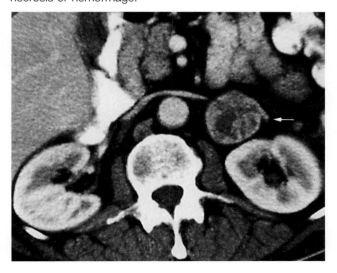

• CT

Plain scans: These masses, which are normally larger than 2 cm, have smooth margins. Plain scans reveal variable reduction in CT numbers due to necrosis and/or cystic degeneration. Punctiform or coarse peripheral calcification is found in ca. 35% of all patients. Most pheochromocytomas are larger than adrenocortical adenomas.

Contrast-enhanced scans: A bolus of contrast medium usually leads to strong enhancement

Fig. 18-8. Malignant pheochromocytoma (pheochromoblastoma). A large mass was found in the left epigastric region. The periphery of the tumor is highly vascularized, and there are large, hypodense zones of necrosis (a ►). In caudal areas, peritumora veins (b ►) drain the hypervascularized tumor. Invasion of the adrenal vein, which was demonstrated angiographically, could not be confirmed. a) Plain scan; b) bolus contrast medium administration.

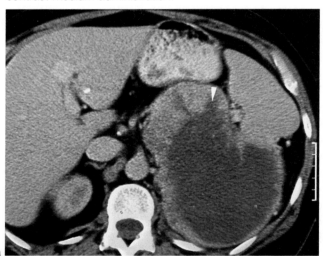

8a

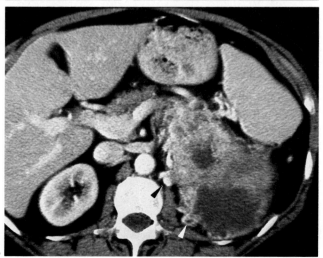

8b

which may, however, be limited to viable areas. Areas of cystic degeneration and necrosis are sharply demarcated.

Differential diagnosis: Symptoms (hypertensive crisis) and laboratory tests (catecholamines, vanillic acid-mandelic acid) considerably narrow the number of other adrenal tumors that must be considered in the diagnosis. Multiple endocrinologic neoplasms may, however, lack clear diagnostic signs.

If a pheochromocytoma is suspected but no mass can be found, possible extra-adrenal locations, especially the para-aortic region and the region of the aortic bifurcation, should be investigated.

Pheochromoblastoma (Malignant Pheochromocytoma)

The pheochromoblastoma is the malignant version of the pheochromocytoma. This tumor is characterized by early metastatic spread and is usually hormonally active. Approximately 40% of all extra-adrenal pheochromocytomas are found to be malignant.

• CT

Computer tomographic evidence of metastatic spread, infiltrative growth, and extension into the vascular system must be found to substantiate the diagnosis of a malignant pheochromocytoma.

Neuroblastoma

The neuroblastoma is the second most common abdominal tumor in children. It originates in immature cells of the sympathetic system. Around 50% percent of all neuroblastomas localize (usually unilaterally) in the adrenal glands, while 25% localize in extra-adrenal, intra-abdominal areas of distribution of the sympathetic system. Large neuroblastomas tend to develop hemorrhage, necrosis, cystic degeneration, and calcification. Early metastatic spread occurs in the liver, skin, and

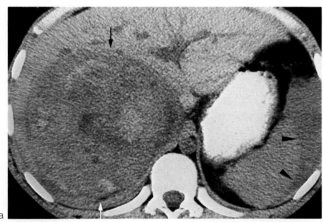

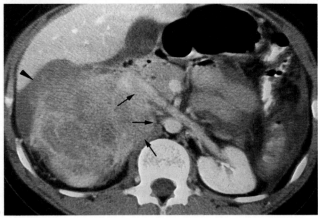

Fig. 18-9. Primitive neuroectodermal tumor (PNET). Plain scans revealed hyperdensity (hemorrhage) within the tumor (a→) and fluid in the abdominal cavity (blood a, b ►). After bolus contrast medium administration, a greatly hypervascularized tumor was found to invade surrounding tissues (b→).

The tumor usually spreads along vessels into the portal fissure and across the midline to the contralateral side. Herniation into the spinal canal causes enlargement of the intervertebral foramen. Enlarged lymph nodes are frequently included in the tumor conglomerate, and the intestine must be sufficiently opacified before a diagnosis can be made. The stage of the tumor is essentially determined by the degree of regional metastases in lymph nodes and the presence or absence of distant metastases. Tumors which do not surround larger vessels are more often resectable than those which have crossed the median line.

Contrast-enhanced scans: Inhomogeneous enhancement is observed after the administration of contrast medium. Localized areas of hypodensity signify necrosis or cystic degeneration.

Differential diagnosis: Wilm's tumors must considered in the diagnosis.

Metastases into the Adrenals

Adrenal lesions frequently are attributable to metastases. Metastases into the adrenals most arise from primary carcinomas of the bronchial system, followed by those of the breasts and contiguous organs (kidney, pancreas, stomach), and from lymphomas and melanomas. Metastases into the adrenals develop due to hematogenous spread, which is why they are bilateral in over 50% of all cases. Metastases into the adrenals normally produce no clinical symptoms, but extensive lesions can lead to adrenal insufficiency.

• CT

Plain scans: The configuration of metastatic masses can vary greatly from localized dilatation of a limb of an adrenal gland to the development of round to ovoid soft-tissue structures which are usually small, but can reach a size of 10 cm. These frequently bilateral lesions usually have smooth margins. When the lesions are small, the masses appear homogeneous. They become more inhomogeneous

bones, particularly in the skull and orbits. A tentative clinical diagnosis is often made on the basis of catecholamine metabolites in urine. The stage of the tumor determines whether resection or chemotherapy should be performed.

• CT

Plain scans: Neuroblastomas are frequently diagnosed when they have become large masses that severely displace the kidney. Coarse and, in some cases, ringlike calcification is found in 80% of cases. The tumor attenuation is normally reduced as compared with muscle tissue.

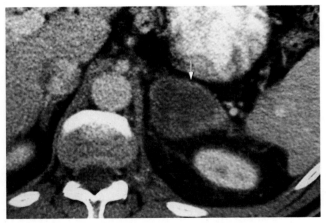

Fig. 18-10. Metastases in the adrenal arising from a primary bronchial carcinoma. The adrenal gland is enlarged and shows only discrete peripheral enhancement after contrast medium administration.

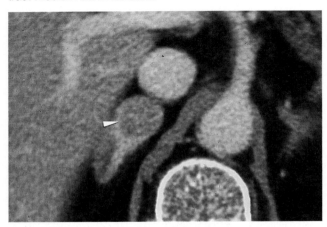

Fig. 18-11. Metastases in the adrenal. This mass is clearly vascularized, yet appears hypodense as compared with the more strongly enhanced adrenal gland (►). Its appearance corresponds to that of contralateral metastases after renal cell carcinoma.

as their size increases (due to necrosis). Hemorrhage can cause a temporary increase in the attenuation value. Calcification is very rare.

Contrast-enhanced scans: Moderate, inhomogeneous, mostly marginal enhancement which occurs after the administration of a bolus dose of contrast medium is a criterion (although ambiguous) for distinguishing metastases into the adrenals from adenomas. Zones of necrosis are clearly demarcated.

Differential diagnosis: Evidence of bilateral lesions, a history of a primary tumor and proof of metastatic spread in other organs often helps to

differentiate metastases into the adrenals from primary adrenal carcinomas and nonfunctioning adenomas. When lymphomas invade the adrenals, extensive enlargement with absence of necrosis are frequent findings. When a primary source is known, the diagnosis of metastases into the adrenals normally is not problematic.

Adrenal Cysts

Cystic lesions are very rare in the adrenal glands. They are usually 3 to 4 cm in size, but can become much larger. Ringlike calcification develops in ca. 15% of all adrenal cysts (i.e. more frequently than in renal cysts). Only a small portion of adrenal cysts are epithelial in origin. Endothelial cysts (lymphangiomatous, angiomatous) and pseudocysts (after traumatic hemorrhage, tumor necrosis) are more common, whereas parasitic cysts (echinococcus) are more infrequent.

• CT

Plain scans: Adrenal cysts have the usual CT appearance of benign cysts. Thin-walled cysts are usually indistinguishable. A thick-walled appearance is indicative of a pseudocyst. Concentric areas of septation and calcification indicate that the cyst is of parasitic origin.

Contrast-enhanced scans: When the mass has a thick-walled appearance, the possibility of a necrotic tumor (pheochromocytoma) must be considered in the diagnosis. The vascularized (or hypervascularized) marginal tissue of necrotic tumors can be identified after a bolus of contrast medium has been injected.

Differential diagnosis: Pheochromocytomas must be excluded from the diagnosis.

Hemorrhage

Blunt trauma, coagulopathy, anticoagulant therapy, malignant hypertension, septic abortion, toxicemia, and organ transplantation are

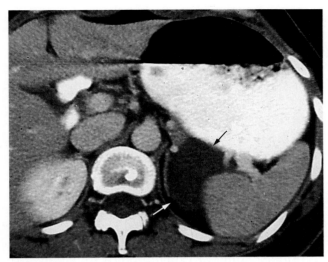

Fig. 18-12. Adrenal cyst. Sharply marginated, homogeneous hypodense area between the limbs of the adrenal gland. The cystic mass is compressed by the medial pole of the spleen.

Fig. 18-13. Hemorrhage into the adrenal gland. After blunt abdominal trauma, CT revealed contusion of the spleen (►) and a hypodense, dilated right adrenal gland (→). The limbs of the adrenal glands are thereby pushed apart, which was clearly demonstrated after contrast medium administration.

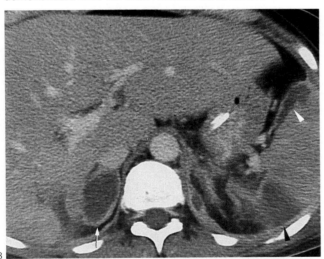

13

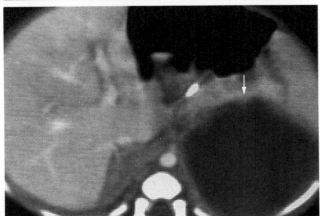

14

amongst the primary causes of adrenal hemorrhage. When bilateral, these hemorrhages can lead to adrenal insufficiency. In patients with Waterhouse-Friderichsen syndrome (classical meningococcal septicemia) and forms of septicemia arising from other pathogens, massive bilateral hemorrhage will eventually lead to complete destruction of the adrenal glands.

• CT

Plain scans: Fresh hemorrhage appears on CT scans as homogeneous or streaky, hyperdense, swollen areas of an adrenal gland. The organ boundaries may be intact or be diffusely demarcated from surrounding fat. As the hemorrhage progresses, its CT density drops and can no longer serve as a computer tomographic criterion for differentiating hemorrhages from other adrenal masses. A hemorrhage may either be absorbed or transform into a hypodense hematoma with CT numbers in the water range (pseudocysts).

Contrast-enhanced scans: After a bolus of contrast medium has been injected, the hypodensity of a hematoma makes it distinguishable from the adrenal parenchyma.

Differential diagnosis: Hemorrhagic metastases that absorb contrast medium must be considered in the diagnosis.

Inflammations

Exudative inflammation does not develop in the adrenal glands, because of the high levels of adrenal corticosteroid. The course of granulomatous infections is protracted, and focal necrosis tends to occur. In order of frequency, tuberculosis, infantile toxoplasmosis, leprosy, histoplasmosis, blastomycosis and coccidioido-

Fig. 18-14. Hemorrhage. CT of an infant revealed a large hypodense area located above the left kidney. It fills the left epigastric region, has an attenuation value of ca. 30 HU and capsule-like borders. The spleen and kidney are displaced. The cystlike adrenal hemorrhage was a result of birth trauma.

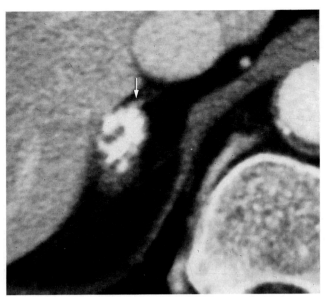

Fig. 18-15. Calcification. Calcification can be seen throughout most of the adrenal gland. This was caused by a past (granulomatous) inflammation (e.g. tuberculosis).

mycosis are the primary causes of inflammatory adrenal enlargement. Fibrosis, partial calcification, and atrophy may develop as the enlarged adrenals heal. Idiopathic atrophy, which is more often demonstrated by CT, should be regarded as a result of lymphocytic infiltration in the course of an autoimmune disease.

• CT

Plain scans: In the florid stages of inflammation, general enlargement of the adrenals is seen. A rounded hypodense or isodense mass is frequently seen in patients with mycosis. A healed granulomatous infection develops areas of calcification that may cause shrinkage (atrophy) of the adrenal gland.

Contrast-enhanced scans: Florid inflammation usually appears on CT as areas of faint homogeneous enhancement; inhomogeneous enhancement sometimes occurs.

Hypoplastic Atrophy

Hypoplasia may be congenital or may develop during childhood (idiopathic Addison's disease). Atrophy often arises as a result of chronic infection, auto-immune disease or hemorrhage. The normal weight of the adrenal gland can drop by ca. 1.5 g. Anterior pituitary insufficiency can lead to secondary adrenal atrophy (Sheehan's syndrome). When pituitary function is normal, a hormonally active adrenal adenoma can lead to atrophy of non-autonomous adrenal tissue.

• CT

When thin sections are scanned and the diameter of the scanning field is reduced, even atrophied adrenal glands can be demonstrated computer tomographically. Tissue attenuation may be raised in patients with secondary hemochromatosis.

Chapter 19
The Urinary Bladder

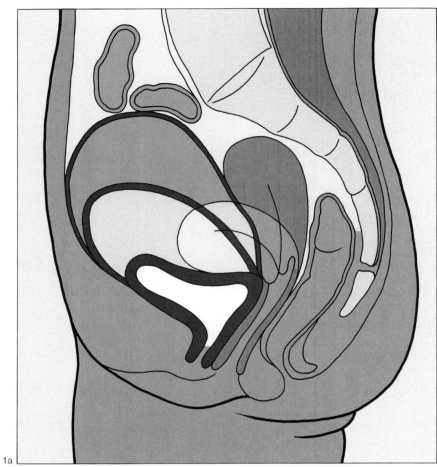

1a

Fig. 19-1a, b. Normal urinary bladder. When more fully distended, a larger area of the bladder wall is more axially oriented and can therefore be better demonstrated on CT scans. With similar alignment, the vesico-uterine region and the circumference of the uterus (b ►) can be more precisely evaluated.

Fig. 19-1c. Trabeculated bladder. A prostatic adenoma (c_1→) has caused considerable thickening of the bladder wall (► ◄).

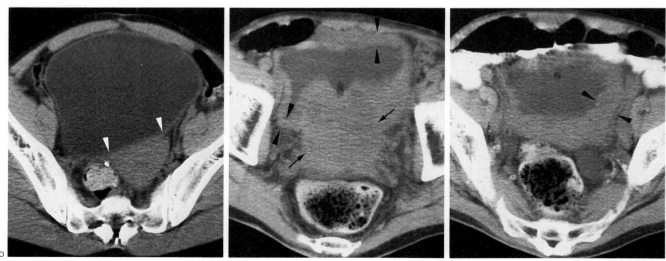

1b

$1c_1$, $1c$

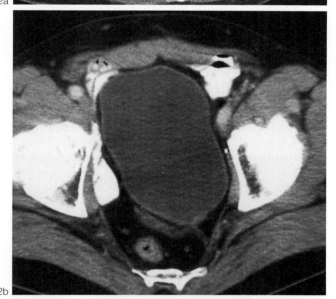

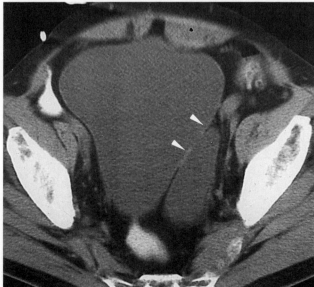

The Urinary Bladder

Anatomy and Imaging

The configuration of the urinary bladder is dependent on the degree of filling. When the bladder is empty, the fundus sinks and it lies virtually horizontal (transverse). If scanned when empty, only a small portion of the bladder wall would be visible on tangential CT scans. When fully distended, however, most of the bladder wall extends axially through the sectional plane, and the imaging conditions are greatly improved. Only a small area of the fundus and base of the bladder are ill-defined due to partial volume artifacts. A fully distended bladder wall is normally 1 to 3 mm thick. The outer contours are delineated by perivesical fat. Assessment of the bladder is complicated by effects of compression from the loops of the bowel, especially when the bladder is not fully distended. After filling the lumen with diluted contrast medium to an opacity of 150 to 200 HU, the internal contours of the bladder wall can be clearly visualized. When water is instilled prior to bolus contrast medium administration, the contrasted wall structures can be clearly distinguished from the lumen and surrounding structures.

Displacement

Displacement of the bladder can also be diagnosed by urography and ultrasound. This is caused by various lesions in adjacent organs, including tumors in the female genitalia, prostatic lesions, tumors and abnormal masses in the intestines (especially the sigmoid colon and rectum), aneurysms in pelvic vessels, primary and secondary tumors of the bony pelvis, pelvic lipomatosis, and neurofibromatosis.

Fig. 19-2a, b. Ileal bladder duplication. The duplication has a nonuniform, non-centered lumen (a→). In this case, the bladder duplication has a virtually normal physiological configuration (b).

Fig. 19-3. Large bladder diverticulum. The neck of the diverticulum is located along the fold of the bladder wall (►).

Anomalies

A *persistent urachus* can be found along the midline between the navel and top of the bladder, where it appears, either as a cystic formation, or as a diverticulum arising from the fundus of the bladder. A persistent urachus is usually diagnosed incidentally. *Bladder diverticula* may be congenital or acquired. They appear as sacculations of the (lateral) bladder wall which frequently become carcinomatous.

Infections

A clinical diagnosis of bladder infection usually can be made on the basis of the patient's complaints of dysuria. Thus, there normally is no need for CT. Most bladder infections are bacterial. They are only rarely caused by parasites, chemical substances or irradiation. The various acute types (necrotising, hemorrhagic, purulent) can all become chronic (proliferating) and lead to wall thickening and contraction. *Bilharziosis* leads to the formation of scar tissue and polypoid filling defects of the bladder lumen. In *cystitis cystica*, one usually finds thin-walled, water-dense cysts with diameters of 1 mm to a maximum of 10 mm. *Calcification* of the bladder wall is sometimes seen, especially after bilharziosis or tuberculosis, but rarely after irradiation, amyloidosis, echinococcus infection, cytotoxic cystitis, or malacoplakia.

• CT

Plain scans: The thickness of the bladder wall is dependent on the degree of filling. Therefore, only retrograde cystography can provide comparable examination conditions. When fully distended, the normal bladder wall is a several millimeters thick. Thicknesses exceeding 0.5 cm must be considered pathological.

In *acute* infections, the filling capacity of the bladder is usually not restricted, and the wall thickness is borderline. Focal swelling of the mucous membrane can develop when tumors penetrate the bladder from the outside (bul-

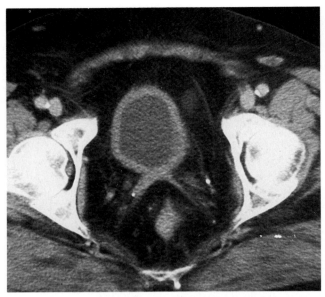

Fig. 19-4. Inflamed contracted bladder. After extirpation and irradiation due to a uterine neoplasm, the urinary bladder has thickened walls and is clearly contracted.

Fig. 19-5. Colovesical fistula. This scan documents peridiverticular abscess formation (a→). Inflammation has spread to the wall of the bladder and fistula are evident. CT revealed focal wall thickening (b ►) and tiny intravesical deposits of air (b→).

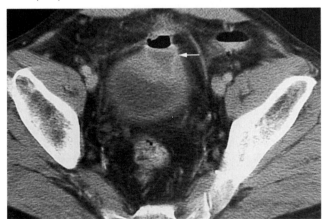

5a

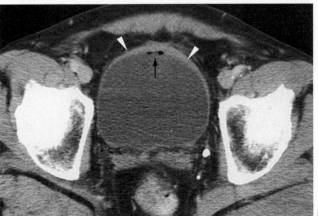

5b

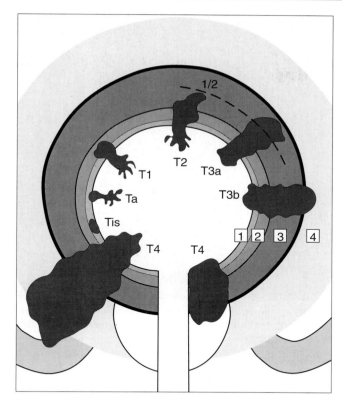

Fig. 19-6. Tumor classification. ·

1 Mucosa, submucosa
2 Inner muscle layer
3 Outer muscle layer
4 Perivesical fat

Tumor spread beyond the outer limits of the wall of the bladder can be demonstrated via CT (modified according to the TNM system).

Table 19-1. Staging of bladder cancer via computed tomography.

Tumor Stage		CT Staging
T_{is}	Carcinoma in situ	Ø
Ta	Papillary, noninvasive	O
T1	Subepithelial tumor invasion	◓
T2	Infiltration of deep muscles	◓
T3A	Infiltration of superficial muscles	◓
T3B	Infiltration of perivesical fat	●
T4	Infiltration of prostate gland, vagina Infiltration of uterus, pelvis and abdominal wall	◕
		●
N1	Solitary lymph node metastases, >2 cm	●
N2	Solitary metastases larger than 2–5 cm; multiple metastases <5 cm	●
N3	Metastases >5 cm	●

Ø = not possible; O = seldom possible; ◓ = not reliable; ◕ = usually accurate;

● = always accurate

lous edema). The bladder wall can then become as much as 1 cm thick.

Lumen reduction and wall thickening are primary signs of *chronic* infection. These changes are uniform in radiation-related cystitis, mainly on the anterior wall in bilharziosis, and irregular in tuberculosis.

Contrast-enhanced scans: When the bladder is full, a small hyperdense rim is seen on the interior side of the bladder wall in patients with acute infection (CM bolus). This corresponds to hypervascularization of the mucosa.

Differential diagnosis: *Focal wall thickening* may be observed in patients with granuloma related tuberculosis, candidial cystitis due to fungal infection, and cystitis cystica. They must be differentiated from tumors of the urinary bladder. *Calcification* is frequently found in conjunction with bilharziosis and tuberculosis, but seldom with radiation-related cystitis. Calcification is more severe in alkaline, encrusted cystitis.

Enterocolic fistulae can be diagnosed when there is gas in the bladder lumen. They are a relatively common complication of inflammatory conglomerate tumors occurring in Crohn's disease or sigmoid diverticulitis.

Tumors of the Urinary Bladder

Papillomas, Carcinomas

Over 90% of these tumors, ca. 80% of which are papillary carcinomas of the epithelium of the urinary tract, arise from the mucous membrane. They occur primarily in older patients, and their overall frequency is increasing. Twenty-five percent of these tumors are multifocal. The lateral bladder wall is involved in 45 to 50% of all cases, the trigone and the neck of the bladder in ca. 25%, and the fundus of the bladder in 5 to 10%. Metastases are initially lymph-borne and involve the parametrial, iliac, and para-aortic lymph nodes. The extent and degree of tumor metastasis do not correlate. Histological malignancy criteria are used to grade the tumor, but tumor staging, which is performed via computed tomography, is also essential for successful treatment.

• CT

Plain scans: Extensive tumors can be demonstrated on plain scans, where they appear slightly hyperdense as compared to urine.

Contrast-enhanced scans: Highly detailed images of the bladder wall can be achieved after a bolus injection of contrast medium. The wall structures are enhanced compared with the distended, unenhanced (hypodense) lumen. In most cases, the tumor has already been diagnosed by cystoscopy. It appears as a soft-tissue structure, the internal and external structures of which absorb contrast medium. It is therefore well delineated.

Stage T1 polypoid tumors do not change the overall configuration of the urinary bladder. When wall infiltration has occurred *(stages T2 and T3)*, the fully distended bladder is inharmoniously protruded or depressed (plateau phenomena).

Incipient wall invasion *(T3 a/b)* can be diagnosed when the soft- tissue tumor mass clearly exceeds the external margin of the non-affected, adjacent bladder wall. If fine, reticular opacification is found within the perivesical fat along the exterior tumor borders, this must be taken as an clear indication of early lymphatic spread.

More severe tumor extension into perivesical fat is normally readily demonstrable by CT. *Stage T3b* tumors can be easily diagnosed, and those which infiltrate the stomach and pelvic walls *(T4b)* are especially easy to identify. As a rule, the base and fundus of the urinary bladder can be only poorly demonstrated on the axial CT scanning plane, so tumor staging is, in some cases *(T4a)*, restricted. Full distension of the urinary bladder improves the image definition in these areas, and clearer diagnostic images can be obtained when thin sections are scanned. It may also be necessary to place the patient in a lateral position.

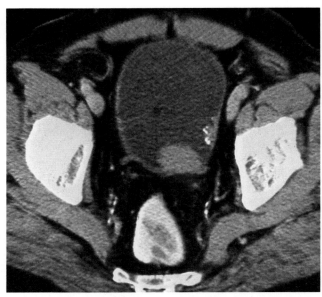

Fig. 19-7. Papilloma of the urinary bladder with calcific incrustations. Histologic stage T1, no evidence of regional lymph node enlargement.

Fig. 19-8. Large papilloma of the right wall of the bladder. The papillary nature of the growth is made evident by its configuration. No abnormality was detected outside the bladder wall (histologic stage T2).

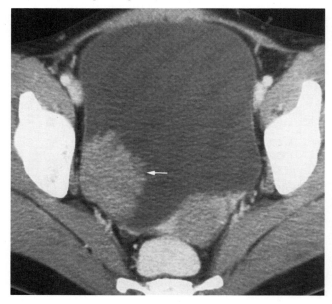

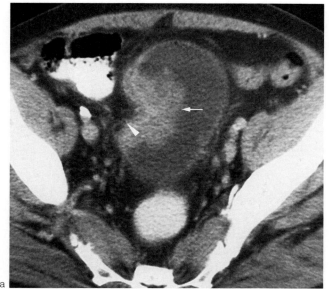

9a

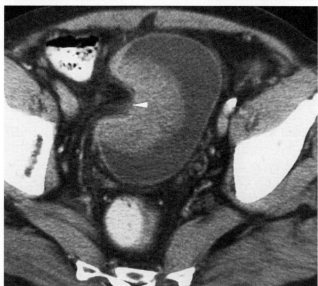

9b

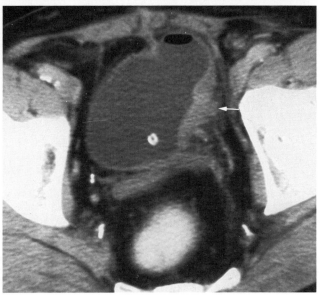

10

Differentiation of stage *T3a* tumors from *T3b* tumors is correct in ca. 80% of all diagnoses. Tumor extension is usually underestimated in higher grade tumors. It is difficult to distinguish tumor invasion of adjacent organs when only minimal perivesical fat is present. It may be necessary to scan the patient in additional positions to make the correct diagnosis. Obliteration of fatty tissue between the seminal vesicles and posterior bladder wall is a sign of tumor infiltration in the seminal vesicles.

When enough intravenous *contrast medium* is administered, *enlarged lymph nodes* 1 cm and larger can be reliably distinguished from vessels. Even if unequivocal signs metastatic lymph node involvement are absent, lymphatic metastasis should be suspected when there are numerous slightly enlarged lymph nodes in the drainage area of the tumor. Lymph nodes larger than 1.5 cm should be considered to be metastatic changed, because simple reactive change (e.g. inflammation) in lymph nodes becomes less likely as their size increases. Lymph nodes near the ipsilateral obturator muscles and the middle external iliac vessels are first affected by lymph-borne metastasis, which then spreads pronally to the lymph nodes around the internal and common iliac vessels and presacral regions.

After *cystectomy*, all sections of the intestine in the minor pelvis must be completely opacified so that blind loops will not be mistaken for recurrent tumor. Any asymmetry in muscle and lymph node structures must be critically evaluated.

Differential diagnosis: *Focal wall thickening* (inflammation), *mesenchymal tumors*, and

Fig. 19-9. Carcinoma of the bladder. A large, broad-based tumor can be seen on the right bladder wall (→); this has led to retraction of the bladder wall. Fine projections (►) indicative of regional carcinomatous lymphangiosis (stage T3b) can be seen.

Fig. 19-10. Carcinoma of the urinary bladder (T3b). The tumor has attacked the left side of the bladder wall, and micronodular growths are visible in perivesical fat (→). The fat also exhibits increased vascularization and reticulation.

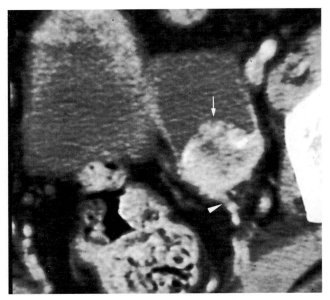

Fig. 19-11. Diverticular carcinoma. A tumor located within the diverticulum (→) has irregular outer contours. A vessel touches the tumor (►), so beginning tumor infiltration can be assumed (stage T3b).

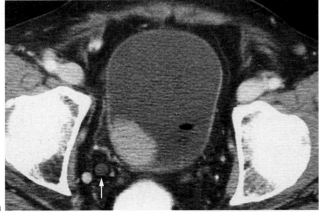

12a

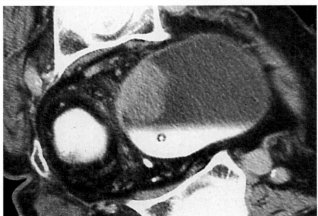

12b

urachal carcinomas (fundus of the bladder) must be considered in the diagnosis. The latter are usually extravesical, and lie along the midline between the umbilicus and the urinary bladder. They may be solid or cystic lesions and frequently display calcification of the mucin secreting epithelium. Infiltration into the small intestine and bladder and regional lymph nodes confirms malignancy.

Mesenchymal Tumors

Mesenchymal tumors are rare lesions that originate in muscle tissue. Benign types, such as the *leiomyoma* and the *rhabdomyoma*, are smoothly marginated and sometimes pediculate. They are clinically relevant only if there are accompanying signs of obstruction. Malignant types, such as the *leiomyosarcoma* and the *rhabdomyosarcoma*, display rapid, tuberous, sometimes ulcerating growth. Their overall prognosis is poor.

The above tumors usually manifest in the 4th decade of life, but there is also an early childhood type, called the embryonal rhabdomyosarcoma. This tumor is characterized by especially aggressive infiltration of adjacent organs. *Pheochromocytomas* and *primary malignant lymphomas* of the urinary bladder are rarities.

Fibromas, neurofibromas, lipomas, and hemangiomas are occasional incidental findings. Except for the (extremely) rare *lipoma* of the urinary bladder, a specific differential diagnosis usually is not possible. The tumor size, extent, and possible malignancy can be diagnosed by CT after metastatic spread has occurred.

Fig. 19-12. Carcinoma of the bladder (stage T3a). A tumor of 2 cm diameter is located in the trigone of the bladder and does not spread beyond the bladder wall. CT revealed ureteral obstruction (→). Slight perivesicular striation exhibits equal bilateral distribution and, therefore, is not indicative of carcinomatous lymphangiosis. Even when the patient is in a lateral position (b), there is no evidence of a change in configuration or infiltration beyond wall boundaries.

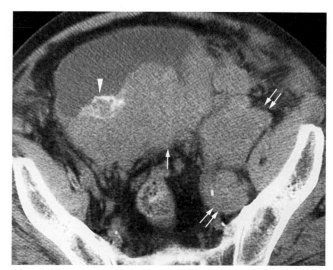

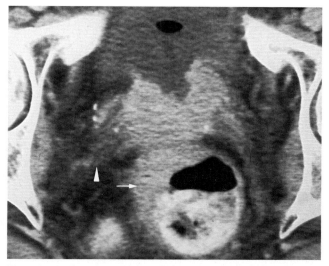

Fig. 19-13. Very large carcinoma of the bladder. A tuberous tumor can be seen protruding into the lumen of the bladder (→). It exhibits calcific incrustation (►) and large, regional lymph node metastases (⇒).

Fig. 19-14. Carcinoma of the bladder (stage T3a). The tumor causes slight left lateral protrusion of the bladder wall (b→). In upper areas, however, it leads to retraction of the bladder wall, an expression of tumor infiltration (a→). Tumor spread beyond the limits of the bladder wall was not detected. An increased number of fine nodules (►) were detected in perivesical fat, so the possibility of carcinomatous lymphangiosis cannot be excluded.

Fig. 19-15. Carcinoma of the bladder (stage T4). This tumor is located in the dorso-basal region. The increased number of strandlike structures seen in the surrounding fat (►) is an indication of tumor infiltration. The tumor infiltrates the right lateral wall of the rectum (→).

Fig. 19-16. Postoperative scan (cystectomy). After a bolus injection of contrast medium, soft-tissue zones exhibiting circular enhancement can be seen in the bed of the urinary bladder (→). This is an indication of tumor recurrence. There are additional, large soft-tissue structures in the region of the internal and external iliac lymph nodes that correspond to the appearance of lymph node conglomerates (►).

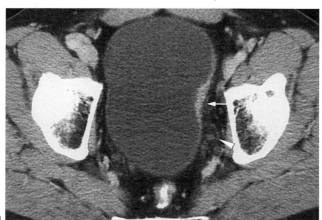

14a

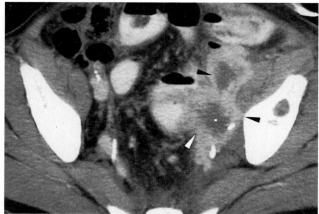

16a

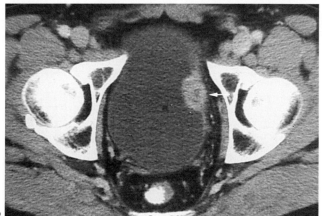

14b

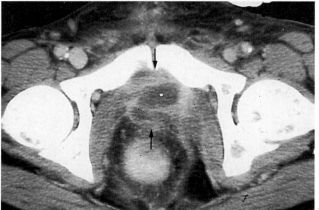

16b

Chapter 20
The Prostate and Seminal Vesicles

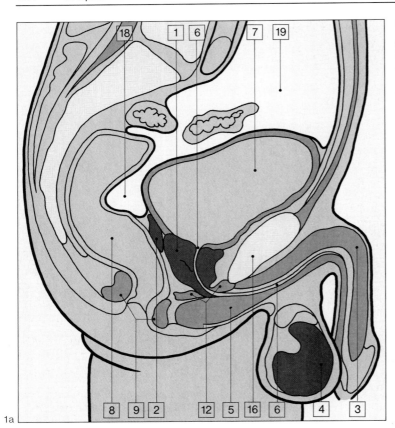

1a

Fig. 20-1. Topography of the male pelvis.

a) Lateral view.
b) Frontal view. b_1 is situated 3 cm above b_2.
c) Transverse CT sections.

Key to symbols:

 1 Prostate
 2 Seminal vesicle
 3 Corpus cavernosum of the penis
 4 Testes
 5 Corpus spongiosum of the penis
 6 Urethra
 7 Urinary bladder
 8 Rectum
 9 Sphincter ani muscle
10 Obturator internus muscle
11 Levator ani muscle
12 Deep transverse perinei muscle
13 Ischiocavernosus muscle
14 Pudendal artery and vein
15 Ischiorectal fossa
16 Pubic bone
17 Prostatic plexus
18 Rectovesical space
19 Abdominal cavity
20 Deferent canal
21 Hip bone
22 Obturator vein and artery
23 Dorsal artery of the penis
24 Ischial tuberosity

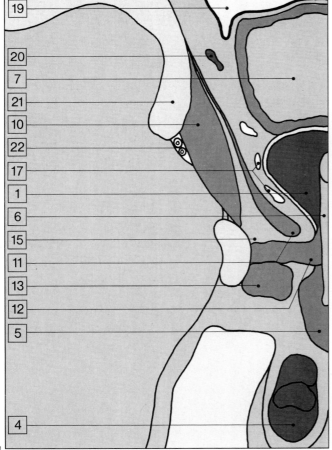

$1b_1$

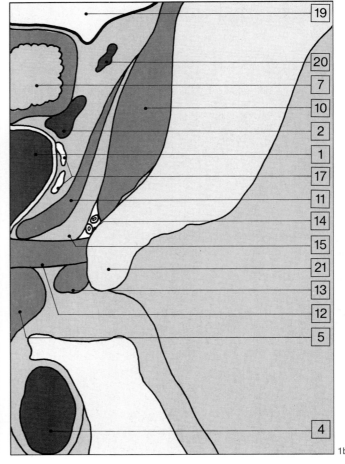

$1b_2$

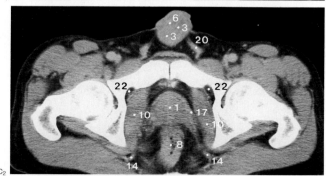

1c₁

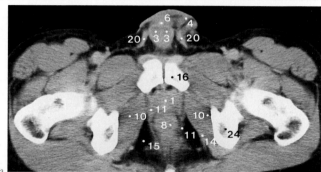

1c₂

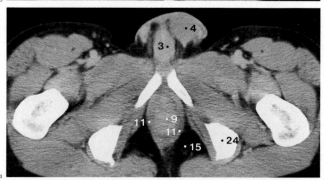

1c₃

1c₄

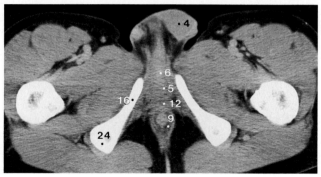

1c₅

The Prostate and Seminal Vesicles

Anatomy and Imaging

The prostate appears on CT scans as a homogeneous, smoothly marginated, oval, infravesical soft-tissue structure. The size of the organ increases with age. The anteroposterior diameter increases from 2.5 to 3 cm, and the lateral, craniocaudal diameter increases from 3 to 5 cm. The lateral contours of the prostate are usually masked by the contiguous ligament of the levator ani muscle, but can sometimes be demarcated when thin sections are scanned. The border oriented towards the urinary bladder is either virtually horizontal or it rises slightly cranial from the supine aspect. Partial volume artifacts arising from these structures can mask slight irregularities on the bladder wall or contours of the prostate. The parenchymal density is ca. 40 to 65 HU. Peripheral calcifications on the capsule of the prostate usually correspond to phleboliths within the periprostatic plexus.

The seminal vesicles lie directly above the prostate dorsal to the urinary bladder. These ca. 5 to 6 cm long glandular lobes are separated from the posterior wall of the bladder by a thin layer of fat. When the patient is placed in a supine position, this layer of fat becomes wedge-shaped and extended, thus forming the "angle" of the urinary bladder and seminal vesicles through which the ureters extend to the trigone of the bladder. The high degree of mobility of the seminal vesicles often gives them a slightly asymmetrical appearance, which is a normal finding. The deferent canals extend to the prostate from the midline of the seminal vesicles. They can be visualized only if they are calcified.

Prostatic Cysts

Prostatic cysts may be congenital or acquired. Only rarely do congenital anomalies cause dilatation of the prostatic utricle (mega-utriculus). When constriction occurs, a cystic structure develops which is known as a utriculocele. Müllerian cysts, which arise from the Müllerian ducts, lie in the midline posterior to the prostate. They may become larger than 5 cm in diameter and thereby compromise the urinary bladder and rectum.

Prostatic Adenoma
(Benign Prostatic Hyperplasia)

The prostatic adenoma a type of benign, adenomatous hyperplasia that involves the central sections of the prostate, the tuberous structures of which compress the base of the bladder. This is the most common cause of infravesical obstruction, and it can lead to significant enlargement of the prostate. The compromised prostatic tissue remains within the capsule after enucleation.

• CT

Plain scans: The only visible sign of prostatic adenoma is enlargement of the prostate, the borders of which are sharply delineated from surrounding fat and the ligaments of the levator ani muscle. Asymmetry and curved protru-

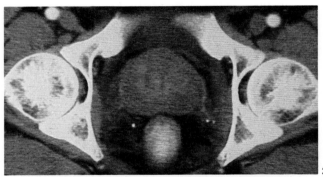

3a

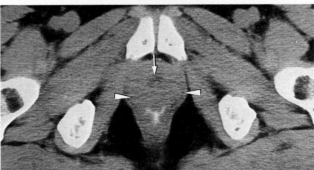

3b

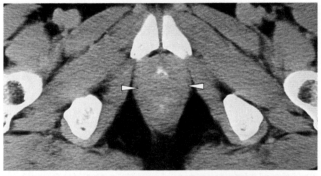

4a

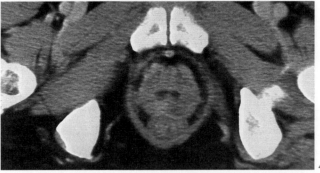

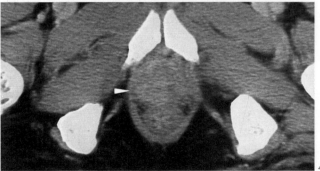

4b

Fig. 20-2. Hyperplasia of the prostate. Symmetrically enlarged, smoothly marginated prostate. After contrast medium administration, a central, stippled, yet symmetrical pattern of enhancement is observed.

Fig. 20-3. Carcinoma of the prostate (stage T1). Normal-sized, smoothly marginated prostate with homogeneous CT values (►). The prostate enhances homogeneously after contrast medium administration. The central area of hypodensity (a→) is due to transurethral resection.

Fig. 20-4. Carcinoma of the prostate (stage T2). In the upper image (a), the prostate appears sharply marginated and symmetrical. In the lower image taken after contrast medium administration, the tissue exhibits inhomogeneous enhancement, and the right lobe of the prostate appears somewhat more prominent (►). Histological findings: carcinoma in the region of the right lobe of the prostate; hyperplasia of left lobe; chronic prostatitis.

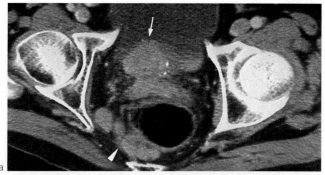

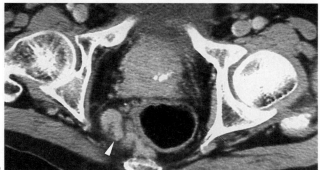

Fig. 20-5. Carcinoma of the prostate (stage T3). The cranial pole of the prostate (b) is already enlarged. The soft-tissue figure converges with the seminal vesicles, which are not clearly enlarged in the upper scan. Histological findings: infiltration of the seminal vesicles. The part of the tumor protruding into the urinary bladder (a→) has infiltrated, but not yet perforated the wall. The calcification corresponds to multiple prostatic concrements. In this patient with known cirrhosis of the liver and portal hypertension, the soft-tissue structure in the right perirectal region (b►) corresponds to convolution of the perirectal veins.

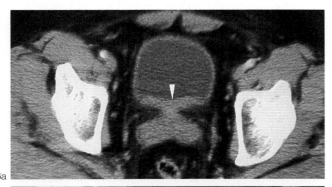

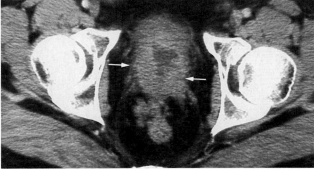

sions in the base of the urinary bladder are sometimes found.

Contrast-enhanced scans: A bolus of contrast medium creates homogeneous enhancement and allows for reliable differentiation between adenomas and peripheral, compromised prostatic tissue.

Prostatic Tumors

The *prostatic carcinoma* is the second most common malignant tumor in men. Like prostatic hyperplasia, it most often occurs very late in life. Prostatic carcinomas develop in peripheral parenchymal areas. When their size increases, they breach the capsule of the prostate and, according to their location, invade either periprostatic fat, the seminal vesicles, the neck of the bladder, or the floor of the pelvis. Eventually, the regional lymph nodes near the obturator internus muscles and, subsequently, the internal, presacral, and external iliac muscles become metastatically involved. Blood-borne metastases initially affect the skeletal system, then the lungs and liver in later stages. *Sarcomas* are much rarer than carcinomas, and they usually affect younger men. Rhabdomyosarcomas develop in children, whereas leiomyosarcomas usually present in middle-aged patients. In addition to aggressive growth, they are further characterized by hematogenous metastases in the lungs, liver, and skeleton.

● **CT**

Plain scans: In addition to enlargement of the organ, an eccentric, fine nodular protrusion on the contours of the prostate is also an important, but nonspecific, sign of these tumors. These findings are suggestive of stage T2 tumors, but may be difficult to differentiate from incipient periprostatic infiltration of stage T3 tumors. Clear organ invasion can be recog-

Fig. 20-6. Carcinoma of the prostate (stage T3). A nodular tumor (b→) has infiltrated the wall of the bladder (a►) and seminal vesicles. The latter appear symmetrical, but are clearly thickened and compact.

nized as irregular, sometimes streaklike, masking of periprostatic or perirectal fat. Asymmetrical dilatation of the seminal vesicle is suggestive of tumor invasion, especially when there is visible obliteration of the angle of the urinary bladder and seminal vesicles. Only in tumors which extend cranially and grow rapidly the border facing the urinary bladder can be reliably assessed for a possible early diagnosis of bladder wall infiltration. Proper filling of the urinary bladder is, therefore, important for good results. Infiltration (T4) of the rectum, pelvic wall, and ureter can usually be diagnosed with confidence.

Contrast-enhanced scans: Since a bolus of contrast medium enhances tumor tissue to the same extent as normal prostatic tissue, intracapsular tumors (T1, T2) will not be identifiable. In extensive tumors (T3, T4), the bladder wall or walls of other hollow organs are enhanced, which makes it possible to determine the extent of infiltration. When necrotic regions are delineated, tumor regression and lymph node enlargement can be better distinguished from ectatic vessels.

The criteria pertaining to the evaluation of possible *lymph node involvement* are similar to those of other pelvic tumors. Metastases can be concluded only if the lymph nodes have reached a size ca. 1.5 cm or larger (specificity: 70 to 90%). Multiple smaller lymph nodes and

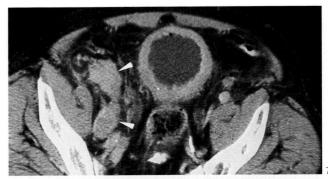
7a

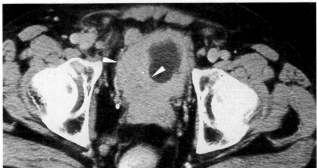
7b

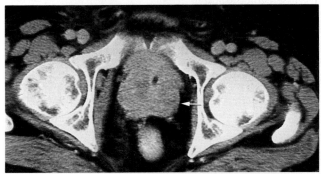
7c

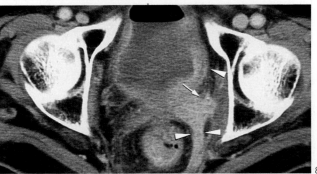
8a

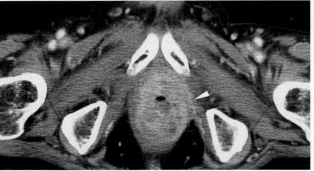
8b

Fig. 20-7. Carcinoma of the prostate (stage T3) with extensive lymph node metastasis. CT revealed nodular enlargement of the prostate (c→) without involvement of periprostatic tissue. The tumor infiltrates the seminal vesicle and, primarily, the right wall of the urinary bladder (b►). In higher sections, a trabeculated bladder with clearly thickened walls was seen, and the mucosa exhibited seamlike enhancement, a sign of an accompanying inflammation. The right external iliac lymph nodes were considerably enlarged and the surrounding lymphatic vessels are enlarged too (a►).

Fig. 20-8. Recurrent prostatic carcinoma. The tumor infiltrates the pelvic floor, especially the left levator ani muscle (b►). The tumor appears as a hyperdense hypervascularized structure that is demarcated from surrounding muscle tissue. In cranial sections, cordlike infiltration of perirectal fasciae (a ► ◄), the dorsal bladder wall (a►), and the lateral pelvic wall (a→) were detected on the left. There is a spread of the tumor along the lymphatic vessels in the right perirectal section. Trabeculated bladder.

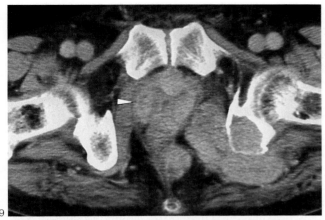

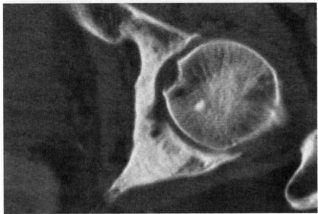

Fig. 20-9. Recurrent prostatic carcinoma with extensive tumor growth and osseous destruction in the left hip joint.

Fig. 20-10. Osteoplastic metastases of a prostatic carcinoma with irregular densification of the joint cavity.

Fig. 20-11. Chronic prostatitis. CT revealed multiple, coarse, ringlike calcification inside the normal-sized prostate, which is sharply marginated. The prostate clearly absorbs contrast medium as an expression of current prostatitis.

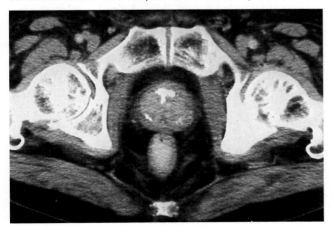

localized streaks in fatty tissue may also raise the suspicion of malignant infiltration.

Sarcomas are usually diagnosed after they have already become rather extensive. Assessment of their extent is similar to that of carcinomas. Since they usually show early blood-borne metastases, the liver, lungs, and skeleton should be included in the staging examination.

Prostatic Infections

Intracanalicular, blood and lymph-borne infection of the prostate leads to diffuse inflammation. Depending on the pathogen, phlegmons or abscesses may develop. The most common complications of chronic prostatic infection include the formation of fibrous tissue and scar tissue and, ultimately, atrophy of the prostate.

Genital tuberculosis is frequently accompanied by prostatitis. The ulcerous, cavernous type of this disease can lead to fistulization of the urethra, rectum, and perineum. Calcification of tuberculous necrosis is sometimes also found. Because of their compact, amorphous nature, these secondary prostatic calculi can usually be differentiated well from primary prostatic calculi (products of prostatic secretion).

• CT

Plain scans: In the acute stages of prostatitis, there is uniform enlargement of the prostate that does not displace the urethra. Prostatic adenomas cannot be diagnosed on the basis of attenuation differences. Inflammatory liquefaction leads to the appearance of areas of hypodensity. When these areas increase in size, the contours of the organ may protrude and the capsule may, ultimately, be breached. Periprostatic infection results in temporary, ill-defined masking of surrounding fat.

Contrast-enhanced scans: After the administration of contrast medium, these zones are demarcated as hypodense, often loculated zones which display the type of rim enhancement typical of abscesses.

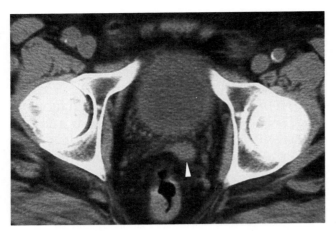

Fig. 20-12. Aplasia of the right seminal vesicle. The right seminal vesicle is not established, and there is agenesis of the right kidney.

Seminal Vesicles

Agenesis of the seminal vesicles is a congenital anomaly that is frequently combined with other types of agenesis of the origins of the mesonephric duct (agenesis of the ureter or kidney, deferent canal, or epididymis). *Cysts of the seminal vesicles* are usually congenital retention cysts. They often occur in association with ipsilateral agenesis or dysplasia. They become clinically relevant only in middle-aged patients with accompanying infection of the seminal vesicle, prostate, or epididymis. *Abscesses of the seminal vesicles* are very rare. Malignant *tumors* (adenocarcinomas and leiomyosarcomas) are further rarities.

Chapter 21
The Female Genital Organs

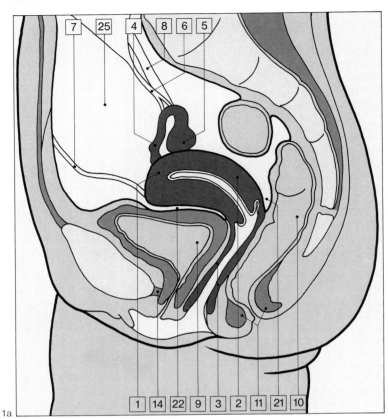

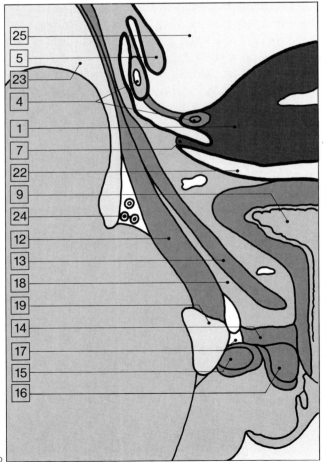

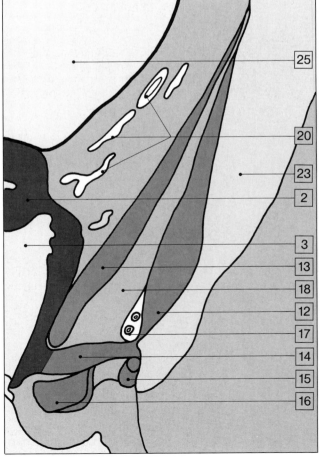

Fig. 21-1a-d. Topography of the female pelvis.

a) Median section.
b) Frontal section.
c) Frontal section 5 cm behind b).
d) Transverse CT sections.

Key to symbols:

1 Uterine corpus
2 Uterine cervix
3 Vagina
4 Uterine (Fallopian) tube
5 Ovary
6 Suspensory ligament of the ovary
7 Round ligament of the uterus
8 Ureter
9 Urinary bladder
10 Rectum
11 Sphincter ani muscle
12 Obturator internus muscle
13 Levator ani muscle

14 Deep transverse perinei muscle (urogenital diaphragm)
15 Ischiocavernosus muscle
16 Bulbocavernosus muscle
17 Pudendal artery and vein
18 Ischiorectal fossa
19 Pubic bone
20 Uterovaginal plexus
21 Recto-uterine pouch
22 Uterovesical pouch
23 Hip bone
24 Obturator artery and vein
25 Abdominal cavity
26 Sacrouterine ligament

1a

1b

1c

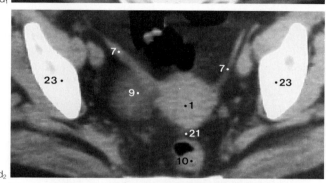

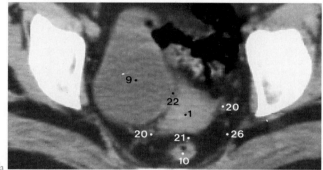

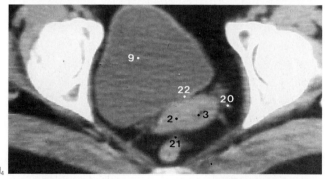

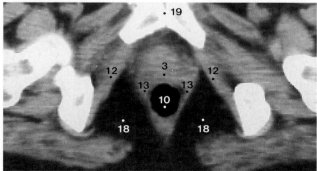

The Female Genital Organs

Anatomy and Imaging

The *vagina*, urethra and rectum are bounded laterally by ligaments of the levator ani muscle. Because there is only a slight amount of delineating fat, the transverse oval structure of the vagina is variably distinguishable from these adjacent structures. The lumen can be demarcated by inserting a tampon (which contains air). The tampon often will not lie in the center, especially when the position of the fornix is high, because it is displaced by the neck of the uterus. Clinical assessment of the thickness of the vaginal wall or evaluation of the vaginocervical junction should, therefore, performed with care.

The *uterine cervix*, which is located more cranially, has a longitudinal length of ca. 2 cm. In transverse sections, it appears as a transverse oval soft-tissue structure, the diameter of which usually does not exceed 3 cm. After bolus contrast medium administration, the uterine cervix shows homogeneous enhancement and is sharply demarcated from surrounding fat. The cervical canal can sometimes be identified on the basis of the air within it.

Demonstration of the *corpus of the uterus* depends greatly on the degree of filling of the urinary bladder. When the bladder is fully distended, the axis of the uterus tilts upward and the circumference of the uterus can be scanned tangentially. From this position, the cross-sectional diameter of the uterus of healthy women of reproductive age should not be larger than 5 cm. When the bladder is empty, the axis of the uterus can extend into the transverse plane, thereby making measurement of the uterus unreliable. After a bolus of contrast medium, the *cavity of the uterus* also becomes visible as a discrete, T-shaped structure. The borders with the urinary bladder (vesico-uterine recess) and with the rectum (recto-uterine recess) cannot be evaluated in this horizontal position.

The fibrous tissue layer that lies between the sheaths of the *broad ligament* is called the *parametrium*. It extends from the sides of the uterus to the extraperitoneal fasciae of the pelvic wall. The parametrium is bounded cranially by the peritoneal fold around the uterine (Fallopian) tube, and caudally by the cardinal ligament (lateral cervical ligament). The *round ligament of the uterus* is located in the ventral aspect of the parametrium. It extends laterally from the fundus of the uterus to the pelvic wall and the inguinal canal. The ligament of the ovary, which is also located in the parametrium, extends from the angle of the uterus to the ovary. The fatty fibrous tissue and peritoneal layer of the broad ligament are not visible on CT scans, but the ligamentous elements are, probably due to their course. The round ligament of the uterus can, therefore, be traced as far as the inguinal canal when there is sufficient fat. The broad ligament sometimes appears as a broad hyperdense zone within the para-uterine fat that extends, in a triangular configuration, to the pelvic wall. At the level of the cervix, this configuration corresponds to the cardinal ligament. Additionally, the broad ligament contains numerous vessels of the uterus and ovaries (uterovaginal plexus), lymph vessels and lymph nodes of the first drainage areas. These structures appear on CT scans as areas of subtly increased attenuation. They can usually be identified as vessels after bolus administration of contrast medium. Areas of structural thickening of more than 3 to 4 mm which absorb no contrast medium must be considered pathological.

The support apparatus of the uterus also includes the *uterosacral ligaments*, which are attached postero-lateral to the cervix at the level

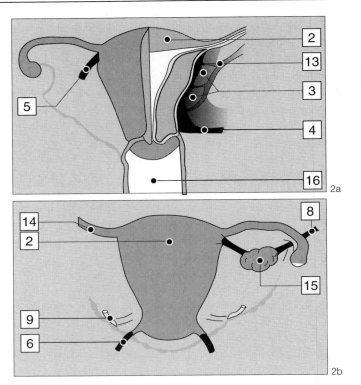

2a

2b

Key to symbols:
1 Uterine cervix	7 Uterovesical ligament	12 Rectum
2 Uterine corpus	8 Suspensory ligament of the ovary	13 Parametrial vessels
3 Broad ligament		14 Uterine (Fallopian) tube
4 Cardinal ligament	9 Ureter	15 Ovary
5 Round ligament of the uterus	10 Umbilicovesical fascia	16 Vagina
6 Sacrouterine ligament	11 Urinary bladder	

Fig. 21-2a, b. Position of the ligamentous apparatus with respect to the uterus. a) Ventral view; **b)** dorsal view.

Fig. 21-3. The supporting apparatus of the uterus in a transverse section. This is marked only by fasciae and vessels in CT. The parametrial enforcement at the level of the cervix corresponds to the cardinal ligament. The ureters enter the urinary bladder in front of the uterus. They are surrounded by a fine layer of fat, which can be demonstrated in thin-section CT scans.

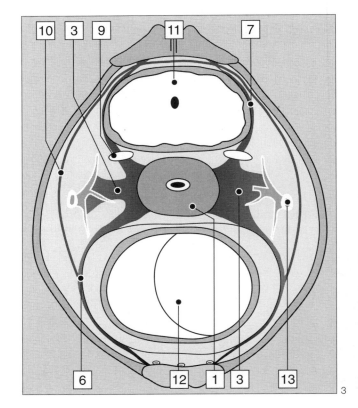

3

of the fornix of the vagina. Some of these ligaments intermesh with fibers of the cardinal ligament, and all extend together with the perirectal fascia to the sacrum. In healthy individuals, these ligaments and fasciae appear as thin opaque structures within fatty tissue.

The *adnexae* can be analyzed when one has good knowledge of the anatomy of the parametrium and the above ligaments. By locating the trapezoid configuration of the fundus of the uterus, one frequently is able to identify the origin of the Fallopian tube or the ovarian ligament. Normal-sized, flatly ellipsoid ovaries measuring ca. 3 x 1.5 cm are soft-tissue structures which frequently cannot be clearly distinguished from the surrounding intestine. They usually lie posterolateral to the uterine angle in the *ovarian fossa*, a peritoneal niche located between the internal and external iliac arteries. The position of the ovaries, like that of the uterus, depends on the degree of filling of the urinary bladder. Since the ureter lies directly behind the ovaries, the ovaries can be more easily identified when it is opaque. The *pelvic ureter* traverses the iliac vessels, passes medial to the internal iliac vessels, extends medially alongside the uterosacral ligament, then passes 1 to 2 cm lateral to the cervix before it finally reaches the trigone of the bladder in front of the uterus. The prevesical part of the ureter is surrounded by a delicate layer of fat that delineates it from the ventral margins of the cervix.

Contrast enhancement of the small and large intestine is an essential precondition for clear identification of uterine and ovarian abnormalities. The only place where intestinal contrast is not required for diagnosis is the subperitoneal cavity, including the ischiorectal fossa. When involvement of the urinary bladder is suspected, the lumen should be fully distended before starting the CT examination. This ensures not only good tangential scanning of the bladder wall, but also provides better scanning conditions for demonstrating the uterus, parametrium, and adnexes.

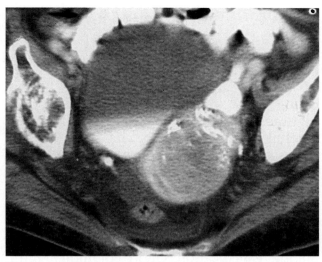

Fig. 21-4. Uterine myoma. The fundus of the uterus appears slightly hypodense and exhibits peripheral calcification after bolus injection of contrast medium.

Fig. 21-5. Uterine myoma. In the region of the uterine fundus are slightly arched, isodense protrusions (►), some of which are calcified.

Fig. 21-6. Uterine myoma. After contrast medium administration, muscle tissue in the center of the uterus becomes enhanced. Variable vascularization of uterine myoma is observed; they may exhibit hypervascularization.

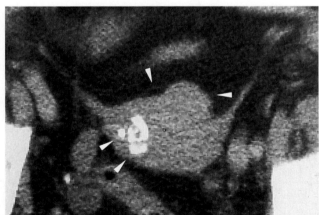

5

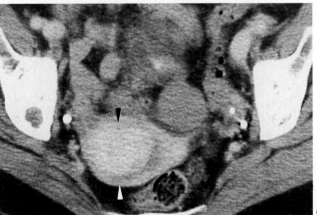

6

Uterine Tumors

Myomas (Uterine Leiomyoma)

Myomas are found in ca. 20% of all women over 30. 95% of these lesions are subserous or intramural. The size of myomas ranges from a few millimeters to over 20 cm. Pediculate varieties are found in submucous and subserous locations. They are sometimes found in the broad ligament or the cervix.

Approximately one third of all myomas display benign changes, e.g. hyaline or fatty degeneration, necrosis, or hemangiomatous transformation. Calcification is more common in intramural and subserous types. Calcification is, at first, punctiform and disseminated, but as degeneration increases, larger areas of plaque-like or ringlike calcification will develop. An infection causing the formation of abscesses or putrefaction of degenerated (submucous) myoma tissue will cause serious clinical symptoms. Poorly or well vascularized myomas can be distinguished from uterine tissue. Sarcomatous degeneration is rare (ca. 0.5%).

• CT

Plain scans: Depending on its size, a myoma may deform and displace the uterus. Tuberous protrusions that are isodense as compared with uterine tissue can be unequivocally diagnosed as fibromyomatas only after evidence of calci-

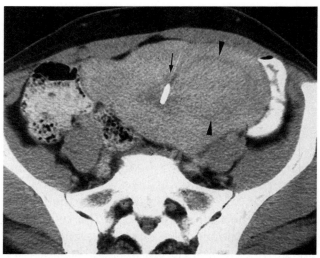

Fig. 21-7. Uterus myomatosus. Inside the polycyclic uterus, a myoma nodule becomes slightly hyperdense after a bolus injection of contrast medium (►). Intrauterine pessary (→).

fication has been found (occurs rarely in solid malignant tumors). The absence of regional lymphadenopathy and absence of symptoms supports the diagnosis of fibromyoma.

Regressive changes (hyaline or cystic degeneration) or centrally located edema lead to the appearance of hypodense zones. These can be sharply demarcated, which gives the lesion a cystic appearance. The presence of gas inside the lesion is usually an important indication of infection or gangrene. However, small amounts of gas can be attributed to necrosis within large myomas.

Fig. 21-8. Cervical carcinoma (stage Ib). The cervix exhibits general enlargement and smooth margins. Adnexal structures are normal in appearance (►).

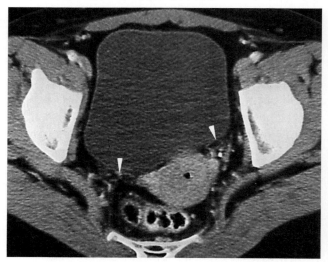

Table 21-1. Staging cervical carcinoma via computed tomography.

Tumor Stage		CT Staging
T1	Carcinoma limited to the uterus	○
T2 a	Infiltration of upper two-thirds of the vagina	○
T2 b	Infiltration of parametrium	◑
T3 a	Tumor extends into lower third of the vagina	◒
T3 b	Carcinoma extends from parametrium to pelvic wall	●
T4	Carcinoma extends into bladder/ rectum or beyond the pelvic boundaries	●
N1	Regional lymph node metastases	◑
M1	Distant metastases	◑

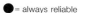 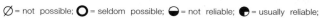

∅ = not possible; ○ = seldom possible; ◒ = not reliable; ◑ = usually reliable;
● = always reliable

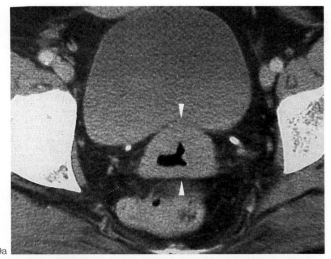

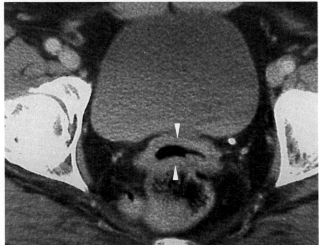

Fig. 21-9. Cervical carcinoma (stage IIa). Compact, smoothly marginated cervix with irregular, fissured lumen (a ►). The adjacent, cufflike vagina exhibits generalized thickening (b ►).

Fig. 21-10. Cervical carcinoma (stage IIa). Dilated cervix. The discrete projection (►) represents the attachment of the cardinal ligament, not infiltration.

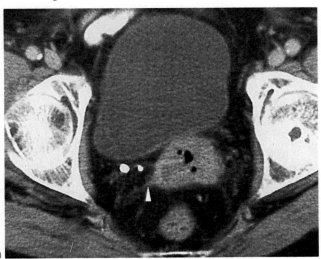

Contrast enhanced scans: Even in hypervascularized myomas, the tumor borders become only discretely visible after bolus contrast medium administration. Regressive changes are more strongly contrasted, but this does not provide any specific information for the differential diagnosis.

Differential diagnosis: It usually is not possible to clearly distinguish a submucous fibromyoma from a lesion caused by *adenomyomatosis*. Multiplicity and a young age of the patient would exclude a *corpus adenoma* and substantiate the diagnosis of myoma. Rapidly expansive tumor growth, especially in post-menopausal patients, is suggestive of a *uterine sarcoma*. Regional lymph node enlargement is a further sign of a malignant tumor. Although rare, ascites has been described in association with fibromyomas.

Cervical Carcinoma

Carcinoma of the cervix, the most common form being squamous cell carcinoma, most frequently affects women between the ages of 45 and 55. These tumors usually spread locally from the lateral wall in the direction of the vagina. They are considered to be resectable as long as they have not breached the lateral borders of the organ (stage II A). Radiotherapy is usually indicated when infiltration of parametrial and paravaginal tissue (stages II B, III B) has taken place.

Metastases in the regional lymphatics can occur as early as stage II A. Firstly, the hypogastric and obturator lymph nodes, then the iliac and para-aortic lymph node regions become involved. The para-uterine lymph nodes often remain unaffected by regional metastases. Distant metastases, especially those in the liver, lungs, brain, and skeleton, develop only in advanced stages.

• CT

A good overview of the cervical region can be obtained when the urinary bladder is adequately distended. Inserting a vaginal tampon also makes it easier to identify *stage II A* tumors. Eccentric dilatation of the normally ring-shaped cervix is usually the first evidence of a lesion, which has probably already been diagnosed clinically. One may assume that the tumor is restricted to the cervix only if the contours of the organ are unquestionably smooth and sharply delineated. An large bolus of contrast medium usually delineates the tumor as a slightly hypodense formation within healthy cervical tissue. A dilated (hypodense) uterine cavity is indicative of (tumor-related) obstruction of the cervical canal.

Protrusion of the organ contours into the *parametrium (stage II B)* usually excludes the possibility of surgical resection. This is characterized by ill-defined organ contours in early stages, and by the appearance of dense soft-tissue strands in the parametrium or paravaginal soft-tissue in later stages with more pronounced infiltration. Solid, strand-like lesions in the parametrium that are larger than 4 mm and nodular malformation of the external contours of the cervix should be interpreted as tumor infiltration. However, these criteria are applicable only if there has been no previous inflammation (with scar tissue formation) and no previous pelvic surgery or radiotherapy.

When the tumor spreads to the pelvic wall *(stage III B)*, it appears as an extensive soft-tissue dense mass accompanied by obliteration of parametrial fat, which can become so extensive that the muscle borders of the obturator internus or piriformis muscles can be masked. Stage III B tumors are soft-tissue dense parametrial lesions that are still separated from the wall of the bony pelvis by a thin layer of fat. When obstruction of the *ureter* extends through the infiltrated parametrium, the tumor must also be classified as stage III B.

When making an evaluation of parametrial infiltration, the previous medical history of the patient must be taken into consideration, since

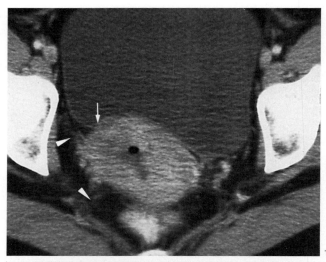

11a

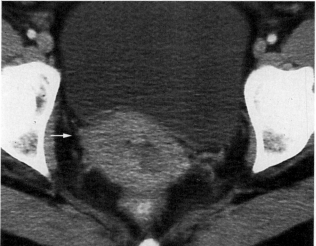

11b

Fig. 21-11. Cervical carcinoma (stage IIb). Eccentrically enlarged cervix with hypodense, demarcated tumor tissue (→). In the right parametrial region, there are clearly more striated structures, with ramifications extending along the sacrouterine (►) and broad ligaments (►).

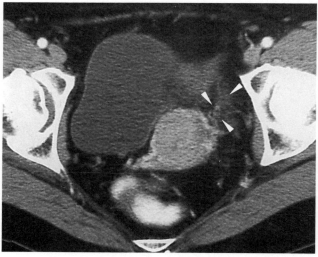

12

Fig. 21-12. Cervical carcinoma (stage IIb). Dilated cervix. Incipient infiltration of the parametrium exhibiting reticular ramifications projecting from parametric connective tissue (►).

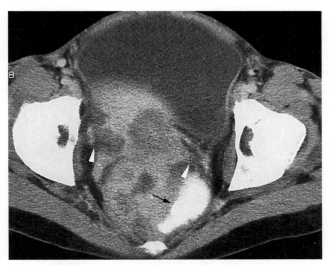

Fig. 21-13. Extensive cervical carcinoma (T4) with para-metrial (▶) and rectal involvement (→).

Table 21-2. Staging of carcinoma of the uterus via computed tomography.

Tumor Stage		CT Staging
T1	Carcinoma limited to uterine corpus	
T1 a	Cavum < 8 cm	◑
T1 b	Cavum > 8 cm	●
T2	Carcinoma extends into the cervix	○
T3	Carcinoma spreads beyond the uterus into the Vagina	◑
	Parametrial tissues	
	Adnexae	◑
T4	Carcinoma extends into bladder/ rectum or beyond the pelvic boundaries	●
N1	Regional lymph node metastases	◐
M1	Involvement of distant organs	◐

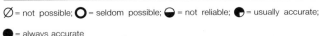

Ø = not possible; ○ = seldom possible; ◑ = not reliable; ◐ = usually accurate;

● = always accurate

the *effects of irradiation and infection* can also lead to blurring of organ contours and to structural changes in contiguous fatty tissue. Homogeneous thickening of the ligaments, especially the uterosacral ligament, is often found as a result of irradiation, but also occurs in association with invasive tumor growth or lymphatic metastases. Additional nodular structures along the fascia and ligaments must always be recognized as tumor indications.

A vaginal tampon must be inserted to better demonstrate the uterovaginal junction for a

precise evaluation of tumor extension into the vagina. Then, tumor-related wall thickening can be reproducibly demonstrated. Clear demonstration, however, is possible only in advanced tumor stages (II B, III B).

Computed tomography can also demonstrate invasion of adjacent organs like the bladder and rectum *(stage IV A)*. In early tumor stages, tangential scanning of border surfaces is necessary to be able to clearly distinguish tumor invasion from the effects of compression.

Regional, *lymph-borne tumor spread* must be assumed when the *transverse diameter* of a lymph node in the primary areas is larger than 1 cm, or when the para-iliac lymph nodes are larger than 1.5 cm. When asymmetry is found, lateral comparison scans can make it possible to diagnose even slight lymph node enlargement. Computed tomography shows sensitivity in demonstrating lymph node enlargement of lymph nodes proximal to the obturator muscles, presacral regions and, in later stages, in the paralumbar region. Nodular structures in the ligaments are frequently attributable to regional lymphogenous metastases.

Contrast-enhanced scans: In stage II B, a bolus of contrast medium makes it possible to differentiate between vessels and malignancy related structural densification. Contrast enhancement of the pericervical ureter is required for identification of peri-uterine fat. When this is masked (false thickening of the ureter), tumor infiltration is indicated. A protracted intravenous injection of contrast medium (or late bolus phase) will make it easier to distinguish convolutions of the iliac vessels from enlarged lymph nodes in all tumor stages.

Carcinoma of the Body of the Uterus

Carcinomas of the body of the uterus are three times rarer than carcinomas of the cervix. They remain restricted to the cavity of the uterus for a relatively long time, then spread ultimately to the cervix. The abdominal cavity is rarely penetrated. Lymph node metastases usually occur subsequent to infiltration of the external third of the uterus wall. Metastases, like those of ovarian cancer, are found predominantly in the para-aortic and lumbar regions, but seldom in the regional external iliac chain. Simultaneous tubal carcinomas or ovarian carcinoma are found in 13 % of all patients with carcinoma of the uterine body. Pyometra may arise as a complication (infection of necrotic tumor tissue).

• CT

Plain scans: These tumors usually have already been diagnosed at the time of CT examination. Depending on the tumor size, the effects of the tumor are seen on CT scans as deformation and dilatation of the uterus. This somewhat nonspecific sign does not distinguish these tumors from uterine myomas.

Contrast-enhanced scans: After intravenous *contrast medium administration*, the tumor frequently appears as a hypodense, eccentrically spread region in the myometrium. The extent of infiltration can, therefore, be assessed. A central, non- contrasted, low-attenuation region that is thereby demarcated from the tumor and surrounding uterine tissue is often found. This corresponds to the presence of necrotic tissue components or congested secretory fluid in the dilated lumen of the uterus. *Infiltration* of adjacent tissue (parametrium, pararectal fat, bladder, rectum) can be demonstrated in advanced tumors.

Enlargement of regional lymph nodes (external and common iliac chains, presacral chains) and para-aortic *lymph node chains* is usually well demonstrated. Therefore, the clinical staging must often be reviewed after the CT examination.

Differential diagnosis: When diagnosing a carcinoma of the body of the uterus, the following lesions must be considered in the diagnosis:
– Chorionepitheliomas infiltrate the uterine wall in early tumor stages and cause moderate enlargement of the organ. Pulmonary

Fig. 21-15. Endometrial carcinoma and adenomyomatosis. Broad area of tumor invasion (3 mm). Dilatation of the cavity of the uterus was the only finding.

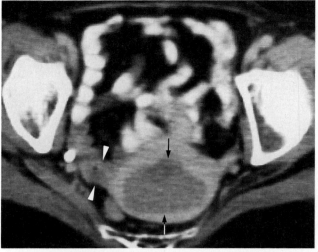

14a

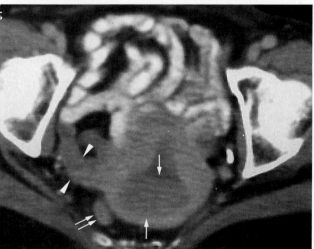

14b

Fig. 21-14. Corpus carcinoma (T3). Considerable enlargement of the fundus and uterine corpus. Carcinoma appears as eccentrically shaped zone (→), as does the cavity of the uterus. Carcinoma extends right laterally into the uterine tube (►). The rectum is clearly displaced (⇒).

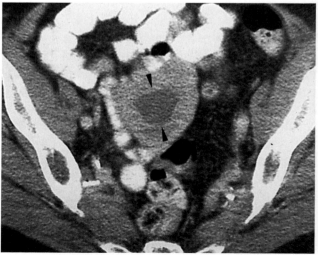

15

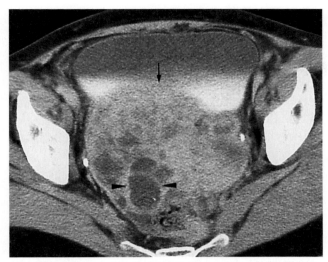

Fig. 21-16. Recurrence of a leiomyosarcoma of the uterus. After contrast medium administration, a very large mass (→) shows signs of cystic degeneration inside well vascularized tumor tissue (►).

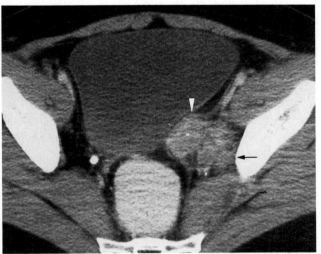

17a

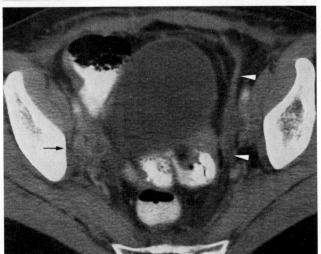

17b

metastases develop early. Previous history of abortion, birth, or vesicular mole.

– The *uterine sarcoma* (2% of all malignant tumors of the uterus) constitutes a sarcoma of the mucous membrane that leads to considerable enlargement of the uterus and early necrotic liquefaction.

– *Fibromyosarcomas* cannot be distinguished from fibromyomas (myomas) in early tumor stages. The former is distinguished by its tendency for rapid growth.

– The appearance of *uterine adenomyomatosis* can be similar to that of a carcinoma of the body. The central hypodense areas of the former are attributable to mucous membrane hyperplasia caused by endometriosis. Lymph node enlargement is absent in this benign lesion.

– *Pyometra* and *hematometra* can be found in various necrotic tumors.

Recurrent Malignant Uterine Tumors

Tumor recurrences usually develop on the vaginal stump and, less commonly, on the pelvic side-wall. Advanced tumors ultimately spread to the pelvic side-wall, infiltrate the ischiorectal fossa, urinary bladder or rectum, and metastasize via regional and para- aortic lymph node chains. Depending on the location of tumor tissue, hydronephrosis and bone destruction can develop and severely aggravate the clinical picture.

• CT

Two to three months after (radical) hysterectomy, only a narrow layer of connective tissue corresponding to the vaginal stump should be seen on CT scans. Most of the bed of the uterus is filled with fatty tissue, but sometime with strands of dense scar tissue. Recurrent tumors appear as soft-tissue dense, rounded, lobulated or irregular masses that may lie in the bed of

Fig. 21-17. Recurrence of a cervical carcinoma at the pelvic wall. a) Soft-tissue dense structure (→) on the pelvic wall. Histological diagnosis: infiltration of adjacent ovary (►). **b)** Inhomogeneous soft-tissue mass on the right (→) into which the dilated ureter terminates. Clear thickening of fasciae due to irradiation (►).

the uterus or on the pelvic side-wall. The central attenuation of larger lesions is often reduced by necrosis. When there is only slight tumor expansion, recurrence can be diagnosed only after the intestine has been well opacified by contrast medium. It may also be necessary to change the patient position. Depending on how much pelvic fat is present, recurrent tumors can be demonstrated by CT when they attain sizes of 2 to 4 cm and larger.

Differential diagnosis: *Postoperative scars* (which usually appear as dense streaks), but especially extensive *radiation fibrosis* complicate the diagnosis of tumor recurrence. The diagnosis is significantly improved when baseline (comparison) CT findings were obtained after surgery or radiotherapy. If regional lymph node enlargement is found in association with a soft-tissue mass, the lesion must be diagnosed as malignant.

Hematomas and *abscesses* usually appear as hypodense, ring-shaped structures that are organized along fascial structures. They are clearly delineated after the administration of contrast medium. When the configuration of these structures is relatively spherical and fibrous tissue develops very slowly, it may be difficult to distinguish them from recurrent tumors. Follow-up examinations are then necessary to clarify the diagnosis.

Ovarian Tumors

Cysts

• *Functional Cysts and Retention Cysts*

Retention cysts are the most common type of ovarian lesion. *Follicular*, *lutein*, and *corpus luteum cysts* are thin-walled masses that contain serous secretions. They are usually only a few centimeters in size and are seldom larger than 6 to 7 mm in diameter. *Chocolate cysts*, on the other hand, are usually bilateral and can become very large and measure up to 12 cm in diameter. They contain thickened blood secreted by ectopic endometrial aggregates *(endometriosis)*.

Bilateral polycystic ovaries *(Stein-Leventhal syndrome)* are characterized by the development of small cysts and are, therefore, only moderately (at most, two times larger than the normal diameter) and uniformly enlarged. The very small retention cysts contained within the ovaries usually do not measure more than 0.5 cm in diameter.

• *Neoplastic Cysts*

The *simple serous cystadenoma* is the most common type of cystic ovarian neoplasm and accounts for 20 to 25% of all ovarian tumors. *Cilial glandular serous cystadenomas* are less common (5 to 12%), but have a high rate of degeneration (20 to 30%). Very fine areas of calcification (psammomas) are found within the cyst wall in 12% of all serous cystadenomas. Depending on the severity, they can build up to form a fine "veil" on the image. Serous cystadenomas may be unilocular or multilocular; 20 to 50% are bilateral. *Pseudomucinous cystadenomas* are usually multilocular and have a characteristically glassy, gelatinous content. Their incidence (10 to 18%) is somewhat lower than that of the serous cystadenoma. Pseudomucinous cystadenomas are seldom bilateral (12%) and degenerate in 5 to 15% of cases. A feared complication that occurs in 7% of all pseudomucinous cystadenomas is rupture of the tumor with the development of a *peritoneal pseudomyxoma*, which can occasionally display amorphous calcification (calcified mucin).

• CT

When they are specifically sought and when there is sufficient bowel contrast, small *retention cysts* can be identified from diameters of 1 to 2 cm. The scanning section must include the fundus of the uterus as well as the ovarian fossa. These lesions present the usual CT characteristics of cysts (except for chocolate cysts).

The *cystadenoma* is usually quite large and can be reliably demonstrated by on CT scans. The walls of cystadenomas are usually just barely recognizable, whereas those of mucinous cystadenomas are often prominent or moderately and homogeneously thickened. Calcification is

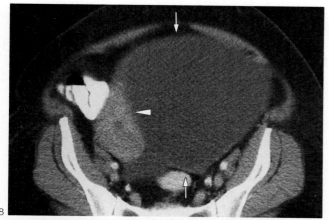

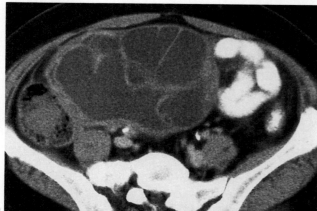

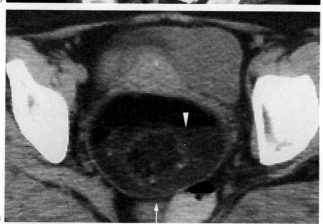

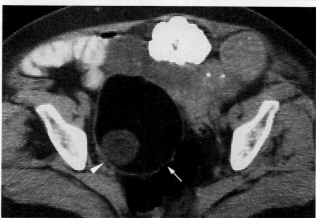

a recognized feature of serous cystadenoma; so, too, is a bilateral presentation.

Unequivocal computer tomographic differentiation between serous (ca. 15 HU) and mucinous cystadenomas solely on the basis of *attenuation* is only sometimes possible. The more solid nature of chocolate cysts can be demonstrated well on CT scans, however, because their attenuation values fall in the soft-tissue range.

Contrast-enhanced scans: The administration of contrast medium demonstrates the avascular nature of these lesions (absence of enhancement of the cyst walls and contents).

Differential diagnosis: Benign cystadenomas must be differentiated from mucinous and serous cystadenocarcinomas.

Parovarian and *paro-ophoron cysts* are remnant cysts that originate in the Wolffian (mesonephric) duct. Their attenuation values lie in the water range, and they are further characterized by their periovarian location.

• *Dermoid Cysts*

Dermoid cysts comprise 5 to 10% of all ovarian neoplasms and are, thus, relatively common tumors. Approximately 25% of these cysts are bilateral, and they are usually 12 to 15 cm in diameter at presentation. They contain organ tissue of various types. Approximately 50% of all histologically tested specimens contained lipoid and sebaceous material. Calcification is

Fig. 21-18. Serous cystadenoma (13 cm in diameter) with no evidence of loculation (→). It displaces the uterus (►).

Fig. 21-19. Mucinous cystadenoma. Multiloculated cystic mass in the pelvis. Septa are still thin, yet some appear prominent (borderline type).

Fig. 21-20. Dermoid cyst. Behind the uterus, there is a 6 x 8 cm cystic mass (→) exhibiting calcification within solid tumor components. Shadow indicative of fatty fluid level (►); fatty components lie on top.

Fig. 21-21. Dermoid cyst. On the right in the bed of the ovary, there is a lipoferous mass that is 7 cm in diameter (→). It has a soft-tissue nidus (►) and smooth, cystic walls.

just as common and appears either in a ringlike formation or is organized (30%), e.g., in teeth and bones. These cysts should be surgically removed because they may later become malignant.

• CT

Plain scans: Computed tomography is superior to conventional radiography in reliably demonstrating fatty substances (with negative CT attenuation). If ringlike (eggshell-like) calcification is also found on the cyst walls, the diagnosis is confirmed. The demonstration of ectodermal vestigia (bones, teeth) can be considered pathognomonic, as is the case with the fat-liquid level, which is only very rarely observed within the cyst.

Cystic Solid and Solid Tumors of the Ovary

• Tumors of the Germinal Epithelium

These tumors comprise ca. 68% of all ovarian tumors and are thus the largest group of primary ovarian tumors. The most common type is the *cystadenoma*, which, according to their histological type, degenerate into *cystadenocarcinomas* in 20 to 30% of all cases. The initially thin walls of these cysts are replaced by neoplastic strands. The tumor then ultimately contains both solid and cystic components.

The nature of rare endometrioid tumors is similar. These homogeneous, solid malignant tumors of the germinal epithelium account for only ca. 3% of all cases. The incidence of these tumors increases in patients over 40; they most commonly affect women over seventy. These tumors spread in the peritoneum, omentum, and mesentery. They can be found in the contralateral ovary in 50% of all cases, and in the Fallopian tubes in 45%. Lymph-borne metastatic spread to iliac and para-aortic chains occurs in only ca. 15%. One of the main purposes

Table 21-3. Staging of ovarian carcinoma via computed tomography.

Tumor Stage		CT Staging
T1	Limited to ovaries	
T1 a	Limited to one ovary, <3 cm	○
T1 a	Limited to one ovary, >5 cm	●
T1 b	Limited to both ovaries, <3 cm	○
T1 b	Limited to both ovaries, >5 cm	●
T1 c	Ascitic fluid also found	●
T2	Carcinoma extends into the pelvis	
T2 a	Uterus and tube	○
T2 b	Sigmoid colon, bladder, rectum	◑
T2 c	Ascitic fluid also found	●
T3	Carcinoma extends into the small intestine	◑
	Carcinoma extends into the omentum	◕
	Intraperitoneal metastases	◑
	Intraperitoneal metastases > 1 cm, ascitic fluid also found	◕
N1	Spread to regional lymph nodes	◕
M1	Distant metastases	◕

∅ = not possible; ○ = seldom possible; ◑ = not reliable; ◕ = usually accurate;

● = always accurate

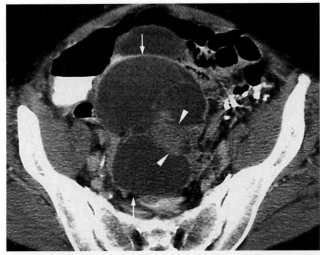
22a

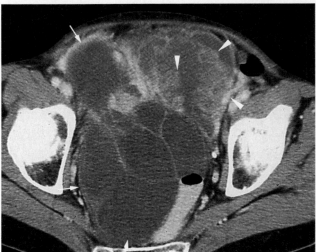
22b

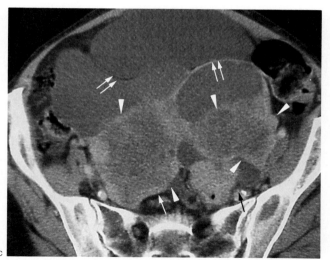

22c

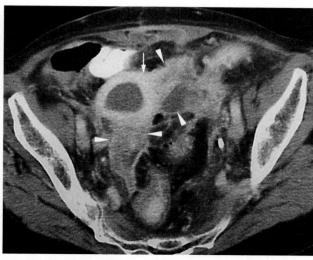

23a

Fig. 21-22a-e. Ovarian carcinoma. A large cystic mass that fills some portions of the pelvis (→) contains septa. Attenuation values in the hypodense zone range from 10 to 20 HU. A common factor for such masses seen in several patients is variably prominent solid tumor components (►) that clearly absorb contrast medium. Urinary bladder (⇒).

Fig. 21-23. Metastasizing ovarian carcinoma, post-operative film (a, b). The uterus (→) is united in a conglomerate formed by peritoneal carcinosis with small encapsulations of ascitic fluid (►). In the perirectal region, evidence of infiltration via the lymphatic vessels is seen (⇒). After termination of chemotherapy (c), all traces of intra- and extraperitoneal infiltration have disappeared.

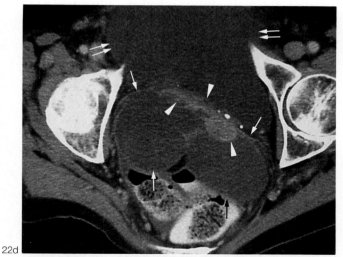

22d

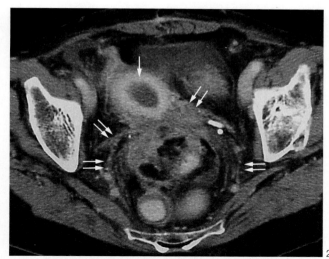

23b

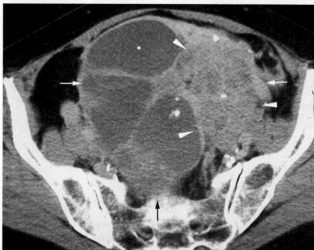

22e

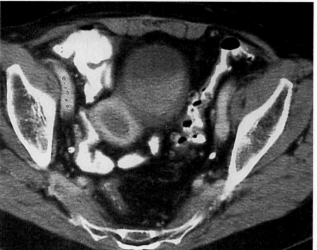

23c

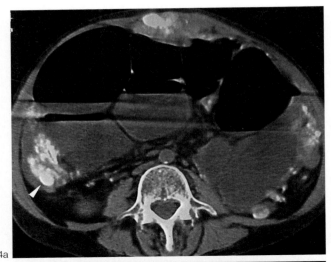

24a

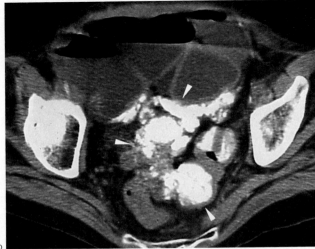

24b

Fig. 21-24. Calcified metastases in the peritoneum from an ovarian carcinoma are distributed throughout the abdominal cavity (►). Intestinal shadows represent intestinal obstruction (ileus).

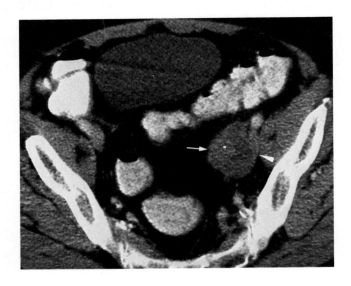

of CT, in addition to confirming the primary diagnosis and staging lymph nodes as a supplement to "second-look" operations, is to identify tumor recurrence.

● CT

Plain scans: Ovarian tumors appear as solid or cystic lesions that may be unilateral or bilateral and are located ca. 2 to 3 cm from the angle of the Fallopian tube. When their size increases, the uterus is displaced from the median plane and can sometimes no longer be seen in the vicinity of the extensive tumor. Ascites develops in the early stages of peritoneal involvement. The solid nodules formed by peritoneal seedings can be identified within ascitic fluid when their size is 0.5 cm or larger when they lie on smooth peritoneal surfaces such as the liver and the pouch of Douglas. They frequently merge to form conglomerates, especially in the vicinity of the greater omentum. They can also invade the mesentery, where they can be diagnosed on the basis of typical signs. Calcification is usually observed in serous carcinomas.

Contrast-enhanced scans: A bolus of contrast medium relatively clearly delineates solid and cystic tumor components, demonstrates focal wall thickening in cystadenomas ("borderline" tumors), and facilitates the diagnosis of lymph node enlargement.

Solid and cystic-solid tumors of the ovary with a size of 3 cm or more should always be considered malignant until proof of the opposite has been found. Lymph node enlargement confirms malignancy. All lymph nodes in the entire retroperitoneal cavity must be evaluated.
Because of the difficulty in recognizing discrete peritoneal seedings and lymphatic micrometastases, normal CT findings do not preclude the necessity of a second-look operation or laparoscopy.

Fig. 21-25. Recurrence from ovarian carcinoma. Six months after resection, chemotherapy and full remission, a cystic (►), somewhat solid, sharply marginated structure is seen in the bed of the left ovary (→).

Differential diagnosis: *Krukenberg tumors* are ovarian metastases that arise from stomach, breast, and colon carcinomas. These cystic solid tumors cannot be differentiated by computer tomography from primary ovarian tumors.

• *Tumors of the Ovarian Stroma*

Most tumors of the ovarian stroma are hormone secreting. The most common types are *granulosa cell tumors* and *thecal cell tumors* (thecomas), which may become as large as 15 cm. Approximately 25% of these tumors transform into malignant tumors, usually in the 7th decade of life. These mostly solid, usually unilateral tumors then contain cystic components due to necrosis, especially when their size is large. The clinical picture of these tumors is characterized by a raised estrogen level.

The rare *arrhenoblastoma* produces androgens and causes virilization of females, usually in the ages of 20 to 30. This lesion is usually unilateral, may have cystic components, and is only a few centimeters in size. A further rarity is the *gonadoblastoma*, which also causes masculinization. This lesion is sensitive to early radiologic detection because of its characteristic calcification (psammomas). Approximately 30% of all gonadoblastomas are unilateral, and they are generally benign.

Masculinizing *hypernephroid tumors* display a tendency for necrosis. Similar to *ovarian stroma* that causes hyperthyroidism, these tumors usually display malignant growth.

Malignant tumors arising from differentiated mesenchymal tissue grow slowly and their recurrences are more localized. Metastases usually occur only in very late stages.

• **CT**

These solid, usually lobulated tumors are located near one or both of the ovaries. Their appearance is nonspecific and they cannot be reliably differentiated from solid types of ovarian carcinoma. This is because cystic degeneration of stroma tumors can also resemble the appearance of a cystadenocarcinoma. The strong tendency for calcification of gonadoblastomas and evaluation of the patient's hormone status may provide diagnostic information.

• *Germ Cell Tumors*

Dysgerminomas are found predominantly in younger women (2nd to 3rd decade). This malignant tumor causes relatively large lymph node metastases.

The *malignant teratoma* is a solid tumor composed of all three germinal layers. It has an invasive nature and tends to metastasize early.

Fig. 21-26. Krukenberg tumors. With known stomach carcinoma, both ovaries are found to be dilated. They become discretely hypodense after contrast medium administration (▸).

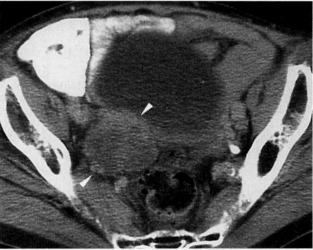

26a

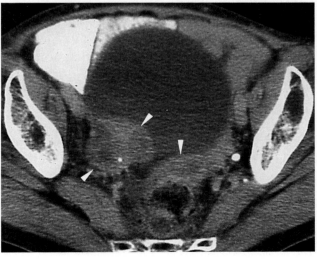

26b

• CT

Whereas dermoid cysts very rarely show degeneration, the malignant teratoma is a solid tumor that is characterized by infiltration and metastases. On the basis of their CT appearance, malignant teratomas are indistinguishable from other solid malignant tumors.

Inflammatory Processes

Uterine Inflammations

Due to obstruction of secretion in inflammatory conditions or infection of necrotic material in carcinomas of the body, tissue debris collects in the uterine cavity. This condition leads to pyometra with considerable enlargement of the uterus and acute clinical symptoms.

• CT

Plain scans: The degree of obstruction determines whether the uterus is merely enlarged or "ballooned". The dilated cavity of the uterus is hypodense.

Contrast-enhanced scans: After contrast enhancement of the myometrium, the uterine cavity is more clearly delineated and appears relatively smooth. Stronger luminal and peripheral enhancement is suggestive of the presence of empyema.

Differential diagnosis: When an area of hypodensity has irregular margins and partially permeates the myometrium, *carcinoma of the body* must be considered in the diagnosis.

Adnexal Inflammations

Ascending and hematogenous infections cause exudative thickening of the salpinx, which can become blocked as the disease progresses which, in turn, leads to intraluminal accumulation of purulent material *(pyosalpinx)*. When treated with the proper medications, the purulent material transforms to serous fluid, usually

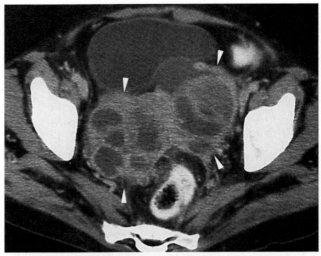
27a

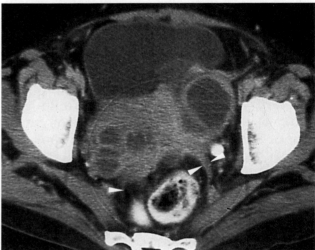
27b

Fig. 21-27. Tubo-ovarian abscess. Both adnexae are greatly dilated and exhibit rounded areas of hypodensity, the wall of which show clear peripheral enhancement (a ►). The adjacent uterus also shows contrast medium uptake indicative of inflammatory involvement. The uterosacral ligaments are thickened (b ►). Ascites was not found. Acute clinical signs often facilitate the differential diagnosis of ovarian carcinoma, in which the solid tumor components absorb greater amounts of contrast medium than the cyst walls.

with simultaneous thinning of the walls *(hydrosalpinx)*. Adhesions may develop near the focus of infection *(perisalpingitis, peri-oophoritis)*, or liquefaction can spread *(tubo-ovarian cysts, Douglas abscesses)*. Inflamed conglomerate masses that involve sections of the bowel are a sign of involvement of distant surrounding structures *(pelvic peritonitis)*. Natural abscess drainage can occur spontaneously into the vault of the vagina or rectum.

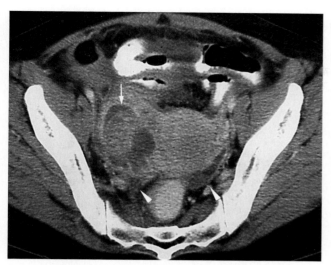

Fig. 21-28. Abscessed adnexitis. Appendicitis has spread to the adnexae, leading to abscess formation, i.e., local peritonitis. Abscess membrane (→) with accompanying ascites in the pouch of Douglas (►).

Parametrial Inflammations

The portals of entry for these infections are wounds and lacerations of the cervix and vagina after childbirth or surgery. Only seldom do intestinal and bladder infections spread to the parametrium. Exudation can be spread via many pathways: into the lateral sections of the parametrium (*lateral parametritis*), the dorsal parametrium (*posterior parametritis*), in the fat of the neck of the bladder (*anterior parametritis*), and into perirectal fat (*paraproctitis*). In long-term processes with expansive growth, the exudate may ultimately infiltrate the psoas muscle, or ascend to the retroperitoneal space (as opposed to the path of descending processes) as well as the pararenal, perirenal, and properitoneal spaces. After liquefaction and encapsulation, the abscess can spontaneously drain into hollow organs (rectum, bladder, uterus) or permeate the anterior or posterior abdominal wall.

• CT

Plain scans: When the bowel is properly filled with contrast medium, hydrosalpinx and pyosalpinx can be demonstrated from a size of 2 to 3 cm when CT scans are carefully obtained. They appear as variably hypodense cystic lesions in the angle of the uterus. The attenuation value of lesions with serous contents falls within the water range (5 to 20 HU), and is somewhat higher in pyosalpinx (10 to 40). The adjacent loops of the bowel are usually involved in the infection. An accompanying rind of ascites and masking of surrounding pelvic fat are characteristic signs of inflammation in surrounding tissue.

Contrast-enhanced scans: A bolus of contrast medium can demonstrate wall thickening or loculation associated with pyosalpinx, which is seen as a corresponding halo of enhancement.

Differential diagnosis: Inflamed conglomerate tumors can simulate the CT appearance of ovarian tumors. Proper contrast enhancement of the bowel is, therefore, a necessary prerequisite for obtaining an accurate diagnosis.

• CT

Plain scans: The different anatomical spaces can usually be readily differentiated, and the sites of exudative expansion can, therefore, be determined. In early stages, it is not possible to unequivocally differentiate between inflammatory and tumorous infiltrations because border surfaces are masked. Clinical findings must, therefore, be included in the diagnosis. The probable cause of extensive inflammatory processes can be determined rather well by computed tomography, because the paths of spread are oriented with respect to the retroperitoneal spaces, whereas the fascial borders are not penetrated.

Contrast-enhanced scans: Contrast medium enhances inflamed border surfaces. The enhancement of abscess membranes makes it possible to identify collections of purulent material.

Chapter 22
The Retroperitoneal Cavity

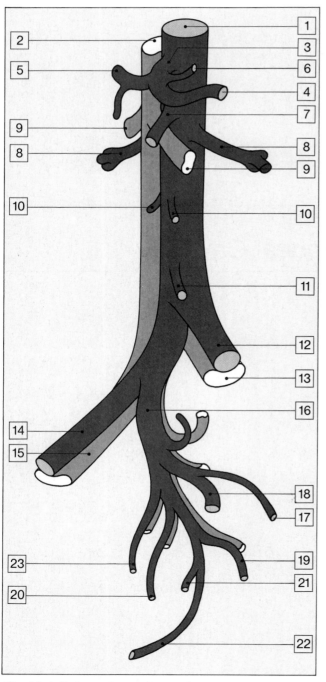

1a

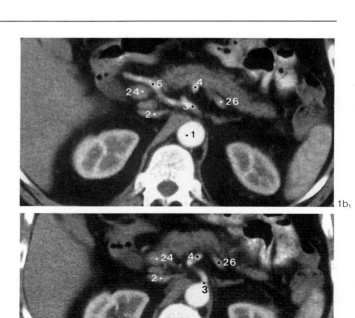

1b₁

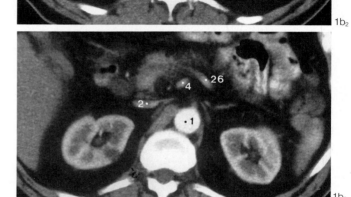

1b₂

1b₃

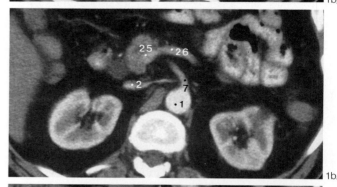

1b₄

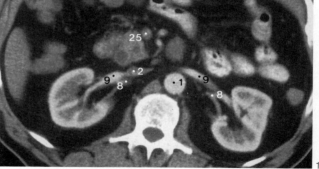

1b₅

Fig. 22-1. Retroperitoneal vessels.
a) Situs. **b, c)** Vessels as seen in CT. In the early bolus contrast medium phase (1 b), even small-caliber vessels are visible. Vascular courses are greatly variable.

Key to symbols:

1 Abdominal aorta	10 Testicular artery
2 Inferior vena cava	11 Inferior mesenteric artery
3 Celiac trunk	12 Common iliac artery
4 Splenic artery	13 Common iliac vein
5 Common hepatic artery	14 External iliac artery
6 Left gastric artery	15 External iliac vein
7 Superior mesenteric artery	16 Internal iliac artery
8 Renal artery	17 Lateral sacral artery
9 Renal vein	18 Superior gluteal artery

19 Inferior gluteal artery
20 Obturator artery
21 Medial rectal artery
22 Internal pudendal artery
23 Superior vesical artery
24 Portal vein
25 Superior mesenteric vein
26 Splenic vein

The Retroperitoneal Cavity

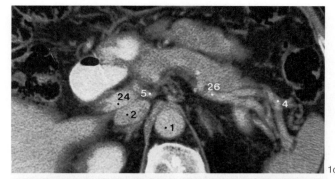

1c₁

Anatomy and Imaging

Retroperitoneal Vessels

The *abdominal aorta* lies just to the left of the midline, directly in front of the lumbar spine. The caliber of the abdominal aorta is age dependent, usually 2 to 3 cm wide, and decreases as the vessel extends caudally. The axial course of the vessel ensures optimum CT images with sharp delineation of borders. The *inferior vena cava* receives the three main hepatic veins just below the diaphragm. The intra-abdominal lumen of the inferior vena cava is usually a transverse oval. Depending on the amount of intra- abdominal pressure, it appears flat during inspiration and round during expiration. Directly below the aortic bifurcation (at the L4 level), the left common iliac vein crosses under the right common iliac artery and aligns dorsal to the left common iliac artery. The pelvic veins are usually located dorsal to their respective arteries. The site of branching of the *internal iliac* vessels is usually seen as a convolution near the piriformis muscle. With absence of arterial calcification, it is often necessary to administer intravenous contrast medium in order do perform a precise evaluation of these vessels.

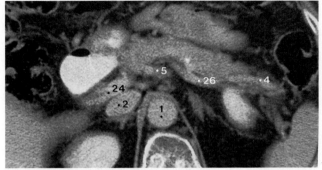

1c₂

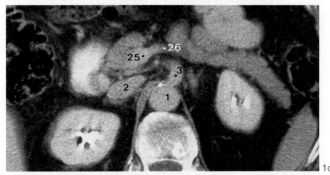

1c₃

The *celiac trunk* arises at the level of the ventral diaphragmatic aortic hiatus, where it branches from the abdominal artery at a variable angle to the axis of the body. This can be demonstrated well on plain scans. When its course is horizontal, the left gastric artery can often be traced to the dorsal gastric wall on a single section. The common hepatic artery can normally be traced up to the point where it gives off branches to the stomach and duodenum. It extends together with the portal vein to the porta hepatis, where it can be identified on CT scans only after administration of contrast medium.

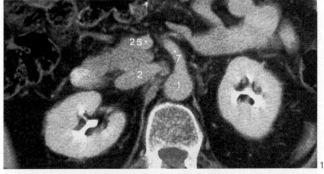

1c₄

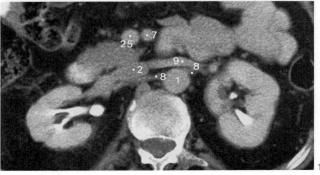

1c₅

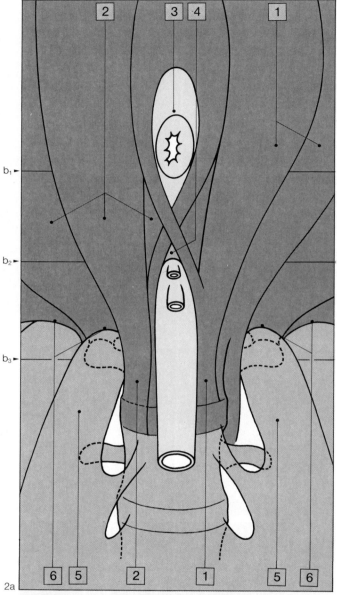

2a

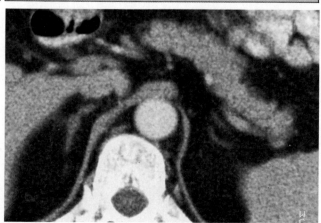

2c

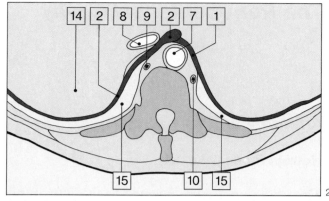

2b₁

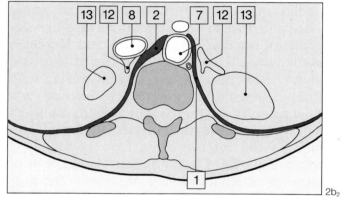

2b₂

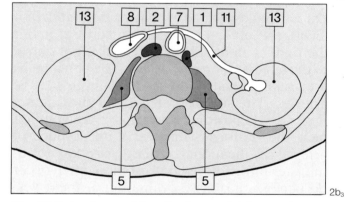

2b₃

Fig. 22-2. Anatomy of the diaphragm (lumbar part).

a) Situs.
b) Diaphragm in transverse section (see a) for level).
c) Normal retrocrural space as seen in CT.

Key to symbols:

1 Left crus	8 Inferior vena cava
2 Right crus (medial, inter-mediary, lateral)	9 Azygos vein
	10 Hemiazygos vein
3 Esophageal hiatus	11 Renal vein
4 Aortic hiatus	12 Adrenal gland
5 Psoas muscle	13 Kidney
6 Arcuate ligament	14 Liver
7 Aorta	15 Lung

The *splenic artery* has a serpentine course that makes it visible only in sections. It extends along the upper (and ventral) borders of the pancreas and branches out like a fan in the splenic hilum. The *splenic vein* is encased in surrounding pancreatic tissue and lies directly dorsal to the pancreas. Depending on the amount of retroperitoneal and intrapancreatic fat, the splenic vein can often be distinguished on plain CT scans.

The *superior mesenteric artery* is always demarcated by fat and is, therefore, a landmark that is always identifiable, even in cachetic patients. Since the *superior mesenteric vein* does not have a corresponding mantle of fat, it is less clearly visible on plain scans.

A targeted bolus of contrast medium often makes the primary and secondary sites of branching of the above mentioned veins plus the inferior mesenteric artery visible.

The *renal arteries* can often be seen on one section of plain scans, that is, if they do not branch caudally from the aorta at an acute angle. The left *renal vein* crosses over the abdominal aorta directly above the inferior part of the duodenum. The main renal vessels and any anomalies affecting them can be demonstrated in their entirety in only a few CT sections.

On contrast-enhanced scans, the external *perivertebral venous plexus* is demonstrated with variable intensity, whereas the origins of the lumbar arteries can be located only after painstaking search. The longitudinal structures of the *azygos* and *hemiazygos veins* can be found at the level of the diaphragmatic angle, where they appear as punctiform structures. These vessels are also visible on plain scans.

Retrocrural Space

This space is located between the angles of the diaphragm and the ventral circumference of the 11th and 12th thoracic vertebrae. The retrocrural space constitutes the lowest niche of the mediastinum. After emerging in the aortic

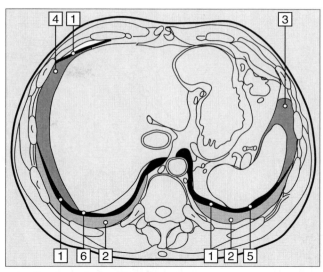

Fig. 22-3. The diaphragm is a landmark between the thoracic and abdominal spaces. When effusion fluid builds up on both sides of the diaphragm, careful evaluation of the diaphragmatic crura (1), the pleural cavity (2), left subphrenic space (3), and right subphrenic space (4) will be necessary. The fixed parts of both the spleen (5) and liver (6) bilaterally limit fluid accumulation in the subphrenic space. Fatty tissue can therefore be seen in front of the crura of the diaphragm.

hiatus, the abdominal aorta is accompanied on the right by the azygos vein and on the left by the hemiazygos vein (directly paravertebral). Non-tubular soft-tissue structures smaller than 6 mm in diameter probably correspond to enlarged lymph nodes. In questionable cases, it may be necessary to administer intravenous contrast medium in order to differentiate these structures from collateral venous channels. The *thoracic duct* extends along the right dorsal side of the aorta and can be identified on plains scans when its diameter is 2 mm or more. Retrocrural lymph nodes are considered to be normal as long as their transverse diameter is not larger than 7 mm.

Diaphragm

The diaphragm is attached to the lumbar spine on the anterior surfaces of L1–4 and the transverse processes of L1. The left median crus is less pronounced than the right crus, which extends deeper to the level of the 3rd and 4th lumbar vertebrae. The paravertebral muscle fibers can show cordlike thickening, and they

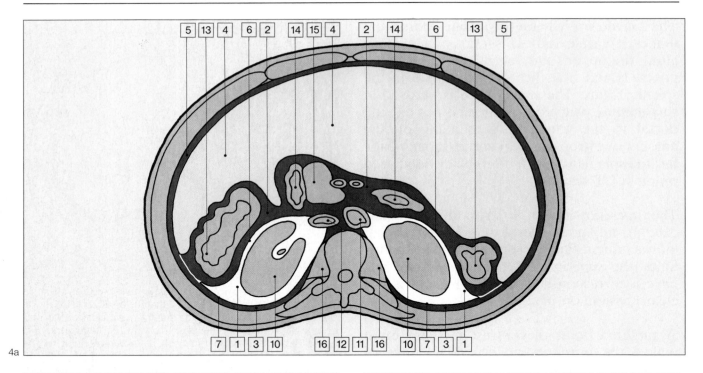

4a

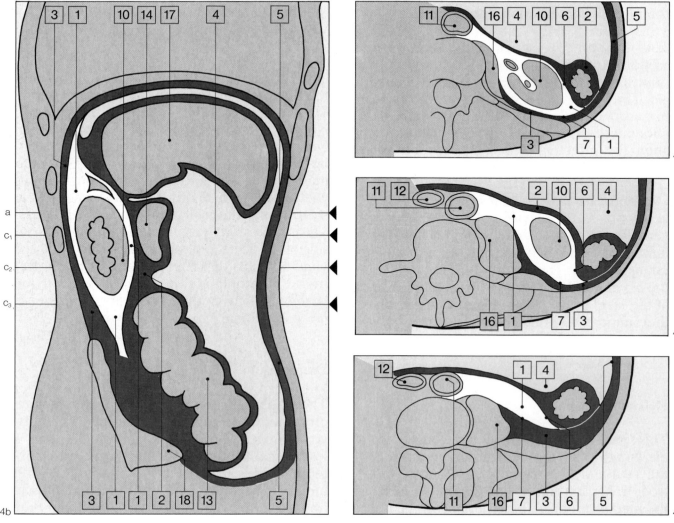

4b

4c₁

4c₂

4c₃

appear to have an increasingly nodular appearance on transverse scans taken with forced inspiration.

Fascial Spaces of the Retroperitoneum

The subperitoneal fascia lies laterally between the transversalis fascia and the peritoneal space. It is divided into anterior and posterior sections *(anterior and posterior renal fasciae)*. The posterior fascia fuses with the fasciae of the psoas muscle, and the anterior fuses with prevertebral, perivascular connective tissue, thus enclosing the *perirenal compartment*. The peritoneum extends across the colon and the pancreas and encloses the abdominal organs. The *anterior pararenal compartment* is limited ventrally by the peritoneum, laterally by the lateroconal fascia, and dorsally by the anterior renal fascia. The *posterior pararenal compartment* lies behind the posterior renal fascia and extends continuously throughout properitoneal fatty tissue. From a lateral projection, the perirenal compartment narrows caudally to a conical apex, and the posterior pararenal compartment increases in width. The conically shaped fascia, which is attached to the diaphragmatic fascia, is not sealed caudally, but both fasciae soon become adhesive when in-

◀

Fig. 22-4. Retrocrural fascial spaces.
a, c) Transverse sections (see b) for level.
b) Right paravertebral longitudinal section.

Key to symbols:
1 Perirenal space
2 Anterior pararenal space
3 Posterior pararenal space
4 Abdominal cavity
5 Properitoneal fat
6 Anterior renal fascia
7 Posterior renal fascia
8 Subperitoneal fascia
9 Peritoneum
10 Kidney
11 Aorta
12 Inferior vena cava
13 Colon
14 Duodenum
15 Pancreas
16 Psoas muscle
17 Liver
18 Pelvis

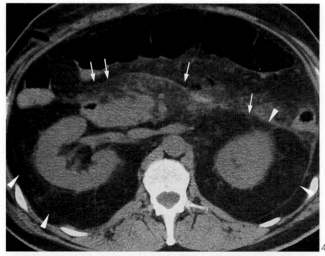

4d₁

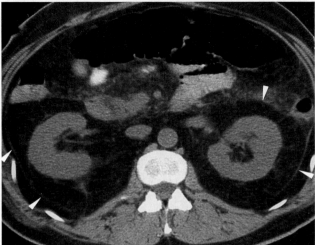

4d₂

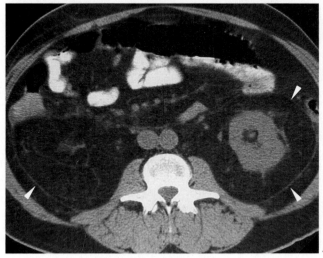

4d₃

Fig. 22-4d. Retroperitoneal fasciae. After regression of a pancreatitis, fascial borders within the retroperitoneal space become more clearly demarcated. The anterior and posterior renal fasciae (►) are easily identifiable in tangential scans. They communicate with the structurally honeycombed perirenal space. The transverse mesocolon (→), which attaches ventral to the pancreas, appears as a discrete linear structure that traverses the duodenum from the ventral, directly postpyloric aspect (⇉).

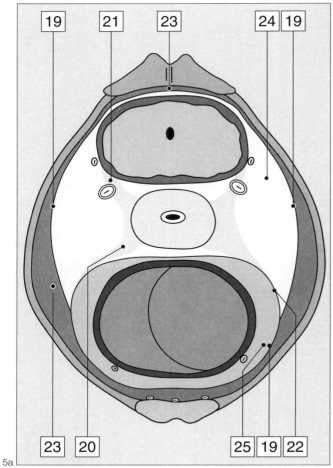

5a

Fig. 22-5. Subperitoneal fascial spaces.
a) Transverse section through the female pelvis at the level of the symphysis.

Key to symbols:
19 Umbilicovesical fascia
20 Recto-uterine ligament
21 Uterovesical ligament
22 Perirectal fascial coat
23 Prevesical space
24 Perivesical space
25 Perirectal space

The parametrium is formed by the supporting apparatus of the uterus, the vesicouterine and rectouterine ligaments, and the supplying vaso-nervous bundle. The structure of the male pelvis is basically the same, except that there are fewer ligaments surrounding the prostate.

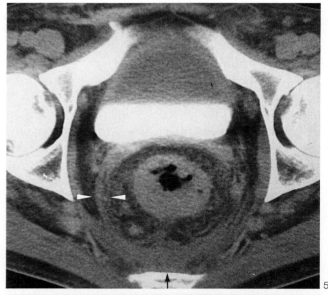

5b

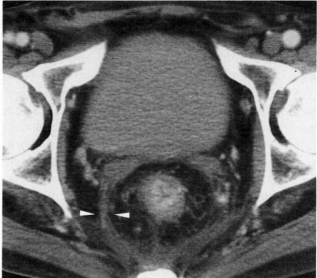

5c

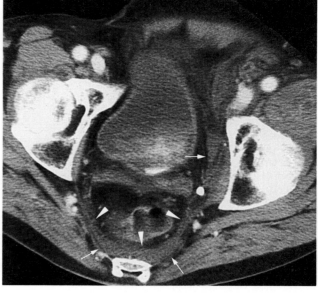

5d

Fig. 22-5b, c. Subperitoneal fasciae. After hemorrhoidectomy, the perirectal fascia is clearly thickened (b ►◄) and perirectal fat is slightly masked (b→). Three months later (c), the condition has improved: exudative processes are greatly regressed. Clear thickening (fibrosis) of the perirectal fascia (c►◄) remains persistent.

flammation develops. The anterior and posterior pararenal (and properitoneal) compartments communicate approximately at the level of the iliac crest. Communication between the right and left perirenal compartment has also been described. The possibility of connection between the retrocrural compartment and the posterior pararenal compartment is still being debated.

The individual fasciae are usually not more than 1 mm in thickness and are identifiable only if they pass vertically through the CT section. An adequate amount of fat must also be present for good demonstration of the fasciae. This usually is not the case for the *peritoneal* surface, which thus cannot be demonstrated in most cases. When thickening occurs due to exudative or hemorrhagic processes (irradiation, infection), the fasciae and the spaces surrounded by them are frequently demonstrable.

The described retroperitoneal compartments frequently contain substructures, so fluid collections are not evenly distributed throughout the compartments. The points of attachment of the mesocolon, the mesenteric root, and the splenorenal ligament prevent homogeneous fluid distribution in the anterior pararenal compartment. The perirenal compartment additionally contains fibrous renofascial and perirenal lamellae which form incomplete subcompartments. The posterior renal fascia is divided into anterior and posterior sections which may be pushed apart when effusion fluid collects. The strong fascia of the *psoas muscle* completely encases the muscle, although, communication with the perirenal compartment below the renal pedicle has been described.

Fig. 22-5d. Subperitoneal fasciae. After retroperitoneal bleeding, the blood descends along the fascial spaces, thereby demarcating the individual compartments. In this case, the perivesical space is filled (→), and perirectal fat is therefore demarcated (▶).

Subperitoneal Fascial Spaces

In the pelvis, the caudal continuation of the subperitoneal fascia is the *umbilicovesical fascia* that encases the urinary bladder. It continues dorsal in the true pelvis as the perirectal investment fascia. The *prevesical compartment* is a continuation of properitoneal fat on the anterior abdominal wall. It appears as a cleft that passes between the pelvic wall and the umbilicovesical fascia and extends dorsally to the sacrum. The umbilicovesical fascia encases the perivesical compartment and the uterine cervix and seminal vesicles, which are surrounded by a loose layer of fat. The rectum is enclosed in its own *perirectal fascia*, which is bilaterally reinforced by the recto-uterine folds. Mesosigmoid fat fuses with perirectal fat. The perivesical, prevesical, and perirectal compartments extend in a funnel-shaped configuration on the floor of the pelvis.

Lymph Nodes

Normal-sized lymph nodes have a diameter of 0.5 to 1 cm, and therefore lie in the lower range of CT capabilities of resolution. Their demonstration is, therefore, decisively influenced by the amount of fat that surrounds them.

Para and *peri-aortic* lymph nodes are organized around the abdominal aorta and the inferior vena cava. Both vessels extend axially throughout the scanning section, so their borders are sharply defined. Under these favorable scanning conditions, only a thin layer of fat is needed for demarcation of para-aortic lymph node enlargement. When enlargement of perivascular lymph nodes is more marked (sizes up to 10 mm are considered normal), the vessel wall is masked, i.e., fatty tissue is obliterated. The contours of the psoas muscles can ultimately become masked, which gives it the appearance of a large, homogeneous prevertebral soft-tissue mass.

Venous anomalies must be excluded from the diagnosis. Because of their variable course, they are not always recognized as tubular struc-

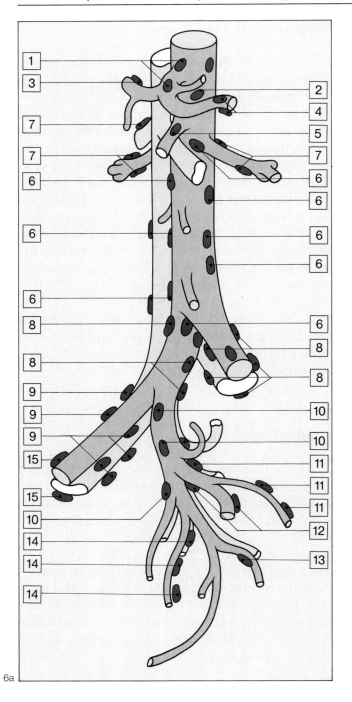

6a

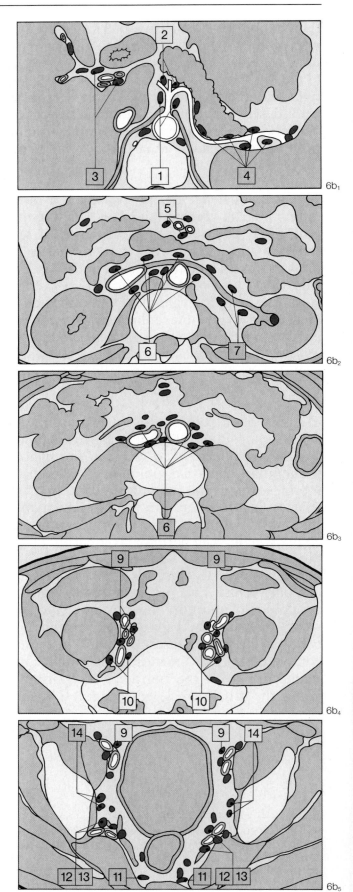

6b₁

6b₂

6b₃

6b₄

6b₅

Fig. 22-6. Topography of the retroperitoneal lymph nodes.
a) Situs.
b) Transverse section.

Key to symbols:

1 Celiac lymph nodes
2 Left gastric lymph nodes
3 Hepatic lymph nodes
4 Pancreatico-splenic lymph nodes
5 Superior mesenteric lymph nodes
6 Lumbar lymph nodes (periaortic, pericaval, subaortic)
7 Renal lymph nodes

8 Common iliac lymph nodes
9 External iliac lymph nodes
10 Internal iliac lymph nodes
11 Lateral sacral lymph nodes
12 Superior gluteal lymph nodes
13 Inferior gluteal lymph nodes
14 Obturator lymph nodes
15 Inguinal lymph nodes

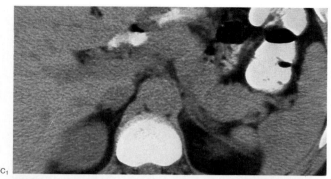

6c₁

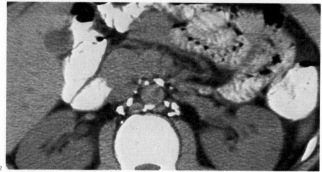

6c₂

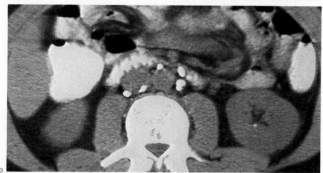

6c₃

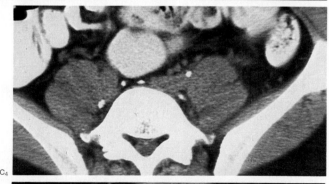

6c₄

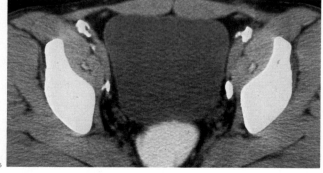

6c₅

ture. Intravenous contrast medium administration is, therefore, sometimes necessary.

Demonstration of *mesenteric* lymph node enlargement is also greatly dependent on the amount of delineating fat (in the mesenteric root). In some cases, lymph nodes as small as 0.5 cm in diameter can be seen when they are not too close to the loops of the bowel. Lymphatic spread can be traced from the mesenteric vessels to the region of the portal vein. When fat is insufficient for delineation of structures, optimum bowel opacification will be necessary to demonstrate enlarged lymph nodes (< 1.5 cm). The sensitivity for detection increases from the peripheral region towards the center.

Pelvic lymph node chains (> 1 cm) are difficult to visualize due to the course of their accompanying pelvic vessels, and can be seen only after vascular contrast enhancement. Structures in the niches of the aortic bifurcation and the area of branching of the internal iliac vessels must be carefully analyzed. Iliac lymph nodes are considered to be normal if their size is not larger than 12 mm.

Lymph node enlargement in the pedicles of organs can only be reliably and sensitively detected in the *renal hilum*. The narrow *porta hepatis* and the *splenic hilum* require considerable vascular opacification and, frequently, thin-section scanning before lymph node enlargement can be demonstrated.

In contrast to computed tomography, *lymphography* detects not only lymph node enlargement, but also structural changes in normal-sized lymph nodes. Proof of infiltrated, non-enlarged lymph nodes (incidence ca. 10%) can be obtained only by lymphography. However, lymphographic techniques cannot provide any diagnostic information on unopacified lymph node groups, especially those in the splenic and

Fig. 22-6c. Post-lymphography film. Only some of the lymph nodes enhance. The internal iliac group and epigastric nodes as well as the periaortic nodes do not become enhanced.

renal hila and para-aortal, retrocrural, mesenteric, and hypogastric lymph nodes. As a rule, large lymph node conglomerates are best demonstrated by CT. Lymphography can be dispensed with in most patients, provided the histology is known and CT is of good quality.

Peri- and Pararenal Lesions

Exudative Hemorrhagic Lesions of the Perirenal Space

Perirenal abscesses are the most common cause of renal inflammatory reactions, e.g., those seen in pyelonephritis or renal abscess. The perirenal compartment is filled with exudate and fatty tissue is ultimately broken down. Gas bubbles can be seen when gas-forming organisms are involved. The spread of infection from distant sites is a rarer occurrence, e.g. a pancreatic pseudocyst may drain into the perirenal compartment. In acute hemorrhagic, necrotizing pancreatitis, fatty tissue necrosis and accumulation of a gaseous exudate are not uncommon occurrences. Extensive, purulent perirenal processes can ultimately infiltrate the fascia of the psoas muscles.

• CT

Plain scans: The most common sign is a diffuse increase in attenuation throughout all perirenal fat. The perirenal cavity broadens in accordance with the amount of collected exudate. The renal fasciae, which are usually hardly visible, are then thickened and well demarcated. The attenuation can drop from 30 HU to 0 HU, depending on the protein content and the longevity of the process. There is usually complete restitution of fatty tissue after successful treatment.

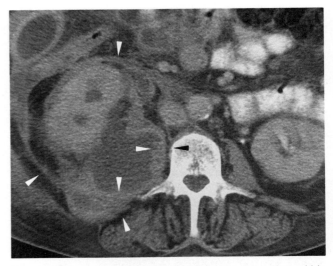

Fig. 22-7. Perirenal abscess. The kidney can be seen within a hypodense structure. It became encapsulated within the perirenal space because of increased granulation tissue (► ◄). Inflammatory thickening of perirenal fasciae (►).

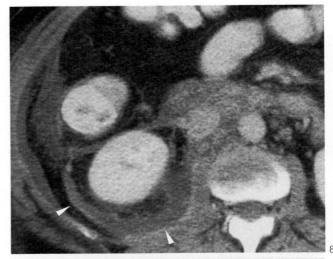

8

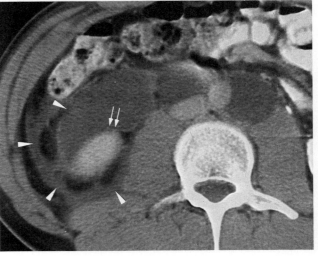

9

Fig. 22-8. After acute pancreatitis, the periphery of the perirenal fat space is permeated with exudation fluid (►). Due to fermentative exudates within, exudation has transmigrated the renal fascia.

Fig. 22-9. Lymphocele that extends into the perirenal space (►). Lower pole of the kidney (⇒).

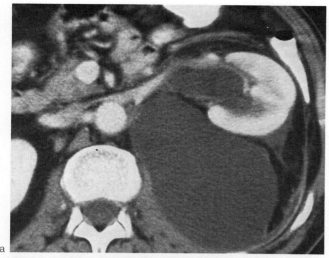

10a

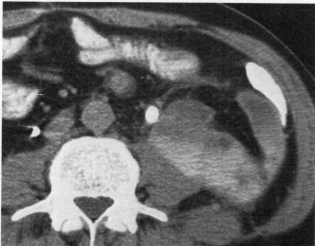

10b

Fig. 22-10. Urinoma. The collecting system of the left kidney exhibits slight dilatation, and the left kidney is ventrally displaced by perirenal fluid (a). This exhibits slight enhancement via the ureter 20 minutes later (b).

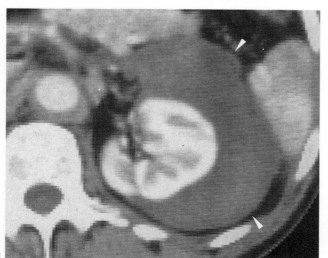

11

Contrast-enhanced scans: Contrast enhancement of fasciae, contiguous parenchymatous organs and, when applicable, the presence of pyogenic walls give additional diagnostic information for diagnosing the type and extent of the process.

Urinomas (Perirenal Pseudocysts)

After an injury to the efferent urinary passages (traumatic or iatrogenic), urine collects in perirenal fat, and the renal fascia becomes transformed into a wall. Three criteria must be met:
- the kidney must be functioning,
- the obstruction must be distal,
- urine must be sterile.

It may take weeks or years for symptoms to manifest after trauma. A perirenal abscess will develop if the extravasated fluid becomes infected.

• CT

Plain scans: A water-dense mass partially or completely fills the perirenal compartment. When chronic, the perirenal mass can extend as far as the pelvic inlet. Abscess formation due to urinoma must be evaluated clinically. Infection must be suspected if other retroperitoneal structures are affected (e.g. the psoas muscle). If the attenuation value increases to more than 30 HU, this must be taken as a further sign of an infected urinoma.

Contrast-enhanced scans: In acute stages, the leak in the renal collecting system causes visible leakage of contrast medium. A pyogenic membrane constitutes proof of abscess formation.

Fig. 22-11. Perirenal hematoma. The hematoma occupies a large portion of the perirenal space, thereby creating dilatation. It is bound by Gerota's fascia. The increased attenuation of fatty tissue is inhomogeneous because of the varying age of the hematoma.

Perirenal Hematoma

A perirenal hematoma can develop as the result or a renal hematoma or when an (aortic) aneurysm ruptures.

• CT

Plain scans: Hematomas usually fill the entire perirenal compartment, but localized blood accumulation is also possible.

The *attenuation* depends on the age and configuration of the hematoma. As compared with non-contrasted muscle and renal tissue, fresh hematomas form broad or focal hyperdense areas. The increased density values drop gradually in the following days.

Contrast-enhanced scans: The density of these avascular lesions is not changed by contrast medium administration. Hematomas usually appear hypodense as compared to the enhanced renal parenchyma.

Solid Perirenal Lesions

The perirenal compartment is only occasionally the primary site of neoplasms. The most frequent causes of solid perirenal processes are *renal malignancies*, fibrous organized *hematomas*, and *abscess formation*. Hypernephromas infiltrate into perirenal fat and spread up to the borders of the renal fascia, which they ultimately penetrate. Benign perirenal fibrosis respects the borders of the compartmental fascia. Extensive perirenal *fibrosis* is rare, since fatty tissue normally regenerates subsequent to inflammation or trauma. Frequently, the only signs of past infections (e.g. pyelonephritis) will be thickening and excrescences of the renal fascia.

• CT

Tumor-related soft-tissue lesions in the perirenal compartment can be demonstrated after the underlying (renal) tumor has been diagnosed. Depending on their age, benign fibrous tissue processes that thicken the renal fascia and partially or completely fill the perirenal

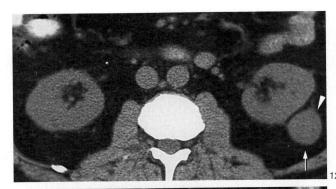
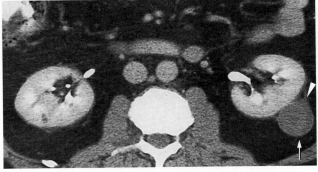

12a

12b

Fig. 22-12. Solid perirenal process (→) with one cordlike projection (►) that is contiguous with the renal capsule. It becomes slightly opaque-laden. Histological findings surprisingly included a renal cell carcinoma.

Fig. 22-13. Lymphocele after removal of lymph nodes. The lymphocele extends throughout the right anterior pararenal space (→) and extends caudally along the borders of the iliopsoas muscle.

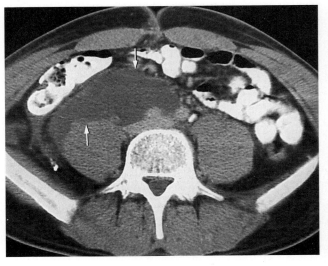

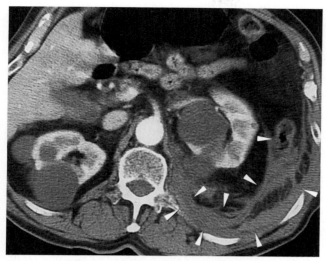

Fig. 22-14. Retroperitoneal bleeding that extends into the posterior pararenal space (►).

Fig. 22-15. Hematoma in the subperitoneal space after pelvic trauma. The hyperdense mass (→) displaces the bladder (►) (with catheter) to the right.

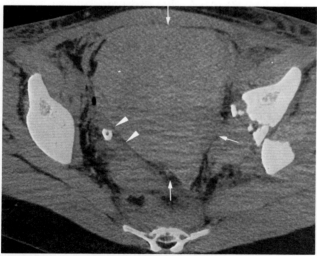

15

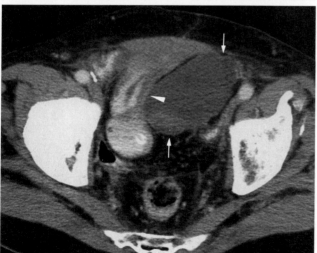

16

compartment show slight to moderate enhancement and can, thus, be differentiated from hematomas. Benign lesions in the perirenal compartment do not penetrate the borders of the compartmental fascia.

Lesions in the Anterior Pararenal Space

Exudative, hemorrhagic effusions in the anterior pararenal compartment arise due to extraperitoneal perforation of the gastrointestinal tract, pancreatic or renal infection or trauma and injuries or ruptures of the larger vessels. Gas bubbles that develop after perforation may come from either the intestines or aerobic bacteria.

• CT

Plain scans: Exudation and hemorrhage may be localized or may affect the entire retroperitoneal cavity. In focal fluid accumulation, it is possible to distinguish between hematomas and abscesses only when there is a high attenuation value attributable to fresh hematoma or gas as a result of infection. Diffuse effusion causes mixed attenuation values, which are caused by averaging of densities from retroperitoneal fat and blood or exudate. The latter values are, therefore, not as conclusive.

Differential diagnosis: The patient history, clinical symptoms, and, in some cases, followup examinations must be used to distinguish abscesses from hematomas.

Lesions in the Posterior Pararenal Space

These fluid collections are usually due to hemorrhage. Infection in the posterior pararenal compartment are usually secondary complications that arise from surgery or spondylitis. Exudates of acute pancreatitis spread to the pole of the renal conal fascia and penetrate from there into the posterior pararenal compartment.

Fig. 22-16. Lymphocele (→) lies in the subperitoneal region. It has formed a sac in the ileal conduit, which is displaced to the right (►).

• CT

Masses in the posterior pararenal compartment displace the perirenal compartment anteriorly. Properitoneal fat becomes involved in the process, so its attenuation value also rises. Most fluid collections are not isolated, so the anterior pararenal compartment (pancreatitis, aorta), the perirenal compartment and, if necessary, the pelvis must also be included in the examination. This is necessary in order to identify masses when patient's history and clinical findings are unclear.

When the lesion is cystic in nature, the possibility of lymphatic extravasation or a lymphocele must be considered in the diagnosis.

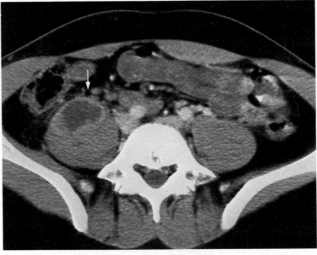

Fig. 22-17. Psoas abscess. Dilatation of the right psoas muscle after nephrectomy. After administration of contrast medium, hypodense, ringlike enhancement is observed.

Iliopsoas Muscle

The iliopsoas muscle is rarely the primary size of a pathological process (rhabdomyosarcoma, spontaneous hematoma due to excessive anticoagulation, hematogenous abscess formation). Inflammatory and neoplastic processes more frequently invade the muscle from the retroperitoneal cavity and spinal column. If the coarse muscle fascia is penetrated, the process can spread from the muscle to the groin. Tuberculosis has now become less prominent than pyogenic abscesses of the kidney, pancreas, spinal column, or intestine. When there is an aortic rupture, a peri-aortic hematoma will often spread within the muscle and may penetrate into the posterior pararenal compartment.

• CT

Abscesses can usually be seen on CT scans before and after contrast medium administration. Their appearance is typical, and there is usually a connection to other retroperitoneal processes.

Fig. 22-18. Psoas abscess. 5×6 cm mass in the region of the right iliopsoas muscle that extends downward to the inguinal ligament. After contrast medium administration, pronounced septal structures and loculation were detected (a→). Drainage and antibiotic treatment led to clear improvement within a week (b).

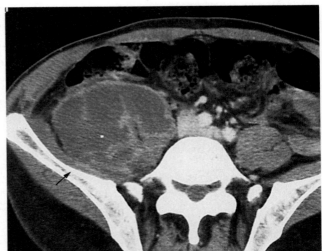

18a

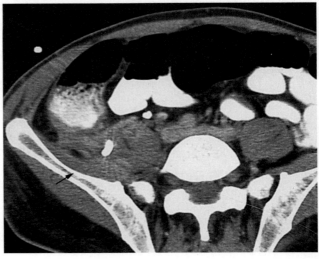

18b

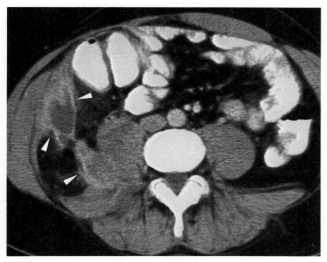

Fig. 22-19. Psoas abscess. After hemicolectomy, a shadow that extends down to the abdominal wall is detected in the psoas region. Peripheral enhancement is observed. Two months after treatment, the abscess transforms into a scarred cord.

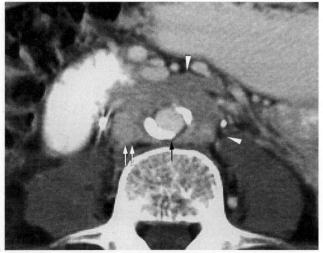

20a

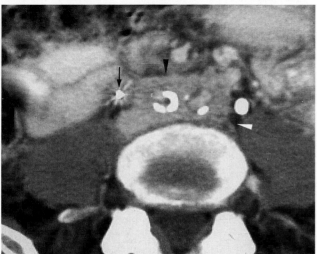

20b

Hematomas involving the psoas muscle often can be demonstrated only after contrast medium administration. Spontaneous muscle hematomas due to excessive anticoagulation generally enlarge the muscle without causing any clear increase in attenuation value. In most cases, neurological findings are required to secure the diagnosis.

Neoplastic infiltration arises from malignancies of the retroperitoneal cavity and spinal column. Masking of muscle structures does not necessarily mean that there is infiltration. This is proven, however, when there is evidence of a muscular defect (contrast medium can be administered as required).

Lesions in the Subperitoneal Space

As in the other retroperitoneal compartment, exudative hemorrhagic effusions in the subperitoneal compartment also develop along the fascial borders, which mainly include those associated with the uterus.

Lesions not Bound by Compartmental Fascia

Primary Retroperitoneal Fibrosis

Idiopathic retroperitoneal fibrosis (IRF) differs from the *secondary* type, which is induced by adjacent infection, trauma, irradiation damage, and carcinoma. On the whole, men are affected three times more often than women. Vasculitis of the vasa vasorum is debated to be a cause of IRF. The process infiltrates the fatty tissue surrounding the vessels, which would explain the perivascular development of fibrosis as well as localized vascular stenosis. In patients with IRF, a sclerotic fibrous tissue layer is most often located between the fourth

Fig. 22-20. Retroperitoneal fibrosis. Smoothly marginated cuff of soft tissue (▸) around the normal-calibered aorta (a→). On the right, at the level of the bifurcation, ureteral involvement can already be seen. The ureter must therefore be splinted (b→). The tissue becomes so opaque-laden that the veins are not clearly delineated. Inferior vena cava (⇒).

lumbar vertebra and the first sacral vertebra. The thickness of this layer can range from a several millimeters to a maximum of 6 cm. The fibrotic plate extends asymmetrically to the sides and encases, successively, the aorta, inferior vena cava, the ureters, and lymph vessels. The longitudinal extent of the plate is variable (maximum of 20 cm). Calcification within the zones of fibrosis has been described. The tentative diagnosis of IRF is usually made by urography, after signs of urinary obstruction with conical, bilateral stenosis and media deviation of both ureters in the middle or lower section.

Etiologically undefined perianeurysmatic fibrosis is also classified as a form of IRF. This occurs in 5 to 10% of all aorto-iliac aneurysms, preferentially in men over fifty.

• CT

Plain scans: Fibrosis appears as a homogeneous soft-tissue zone, usually at the level of the pelvic inlet. It surrounds the aorta, inferior vena cava and (possibly) the large pelvic vessels. The ventral and lateral boundaries are sharply delineated. The CT appearance can vary from strand-like to a broad confluent configuration. Renal obstruction can develop when there is involvement of the ureters. In perianeurysmatic forms, a variably wide soft-tissue ring can be seen around the external contours of the dilated aorta. The ring is delineated from adventitial calcification or thrombi.

Contrast-enhanced scans: Large vessels are demarcated by a bolus of contrast medium. These cuff-like lesions can show considerable enhancement in stages of fresh inflammation, but not in stages of fibrosis. Constriction of en-

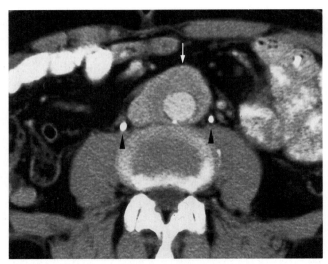

Fig. 22-21. Primary retroperitoneal fibrosis. A 2 cm large, circular soft-tissue structure (→) is detected in a normal aortic lumen with slightly calcified walls. The structure, which infiltrates the inferior vena cava, exhibits slight peripheral enhancement. The adjacent ureteral structures (►) are not involved in the process.

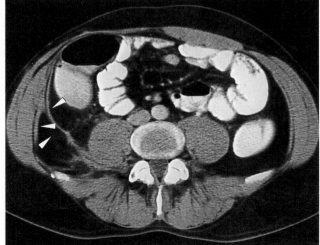

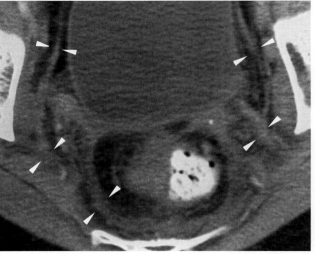

Fig. 22-22. Secondary retroperitoneal fibrosis. A scarred, cordlike structure is found on scans taken after hemicolectomy and postoperative abscess formation.

Fig. 22-23. Radiogenic fibrosis. Perirectal, perivesical fascia and fascia of the ligamentous apparatus (► ◄) are thickened. This characteristically strandlike appearance usually becomes more prominent after contrast medium administration, thereby making it easier to identify enlarged lymph nodes.

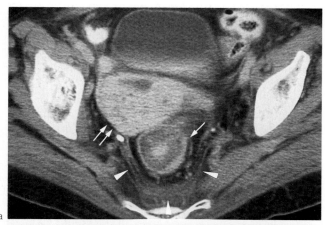

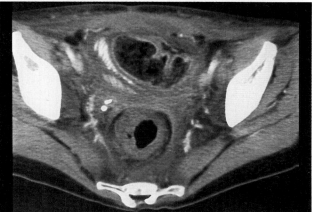

Fig. 22-24a, b. Radiogenic fibrosis. After completion of radiotherapy, CT revealed thickening of the perirectal fascia (a ►) and masking of the presacral perivesical space (a ►). The walls of the rectum are thickened and exhibit peripheral enhancement after the administration of contrast medium (→). Intense opacification of the uterus indicates reactive hyperemia (⇒). On a film taken 14 months after radiotherapy (b) and also after a hysterectomy, there is considerable thickening of the entire ligamentous apparatus of the pelvis.

Fig. 22-25. Pelvic fibrolipomatosis. Fatty tissue occupies the posterior portion of the pelvis (►). Fibrous cords are distributed throughout some of this tissue (→).

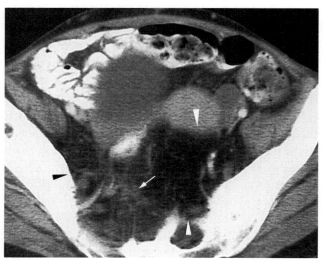

cased vessels and consecutive formation of collateral vascular channels can usually be detected on CT scans.

Differential diagnosis: The following diagnostic criteria speak in favor of idiopathic retroperitoneal fibrosis and against the possibility of compact lymph nodes.

– Demonstration of smooth, plate-like soft-tissue structures.
– Absence of displacement of the aorta and vena cava.
– Early signs of urinary obstruction.
– Often intense, localized enhancement.
– Absence of evidence of disseminated lymph node enlargement.

The intense contrast enhancement of perianeurysmatic fibrosis must be diagnostically differentiated from a dissection.

Secondary Retroperitoneal Fibrosis

Secondary retroperitoneal fibrosis (SRF) is often discovered incidentally, in absence of any typical clinical symptoms. Zones of fibrosis develop after trauma (surgery, injury, irradiation), infection (pancreatitis, abscessed appendicitis, ulcerative colitis, Crohn's disease), in association with primary retroperitoneal tumors, collagenosis, or a carcinoid tumor.

• CT

Areas of SRF can also be widespread, but usually appear as thickening of the fasciae (perirenal, perirectal). It is easier to make the diagnosis when one has a good knowledge of the patient's underlying condition and the paths of spread, and when the site of the primary process is known. Chronic inflammatory processes, which usually extend along the fascia borders, usually lead to the development of relatively smooth, non-nodular soft-tissue zones. The degree of contrast enhancement depends on the degree of inflammation.

Pelvic Fibrolipomatosis

Some authors see a close etiological connection between pelvic fibrolipomatosis and retroperitoneal fibrosis. In pelvic fibrolipomatosis, the amount of fibrous elements recedes in favor of fatty elements. The pelvis is entirely filled with fatty tissue, and symptoms of compression develop in the urinary bladder, the ureters, and the rectosigmoid. The clinical picture includes pains in the sides and symptoms of constipation, dysuria, and cystitis. Upon cystography, the urinary bladder displays a characteristically pear-shaped deformity.

• CT

The pelvis is entirely filled with hypodense fatty tissue that is readily demonstrable. The pelvic organs are symmetrically compromised.

Differential diagnosis: Retroperitoneal *lipoma* with asymmetrical displacement of the intestines and fatty infiltration of the mesentery associated with *Crohn's disease* must be considered in the diagnosis.

Malignant Lymphoma

Hodgkin's lymphomas (HL) have a pattern of attack and variable prognosis which distinguishes them from non-Hodgkin's lymphomas (NHL). Non-Hodgkin's lymphomas are further histopathologically classified as nodular or diffuse. Abdominal involvement is about half as likely to occur as in supradiaphragmatic manifestation of Hodgkin's disease than in all other malignant lymphomatous diseases. NHL shows equal involvement of para-aortic and mesenteric lymph nodes. The spleen is the most commonly affected abdominal organ in Hodgkin's disease, but is very rarely involved in diffuse non-Hodgkin's lymphomas. When splenomegaly is associated with NHL, the probability of splenic involvement is very high. In contrast, splenic enlargement is seen in only ca. 50 % of all Hodgkin's lymphomas. Hepatic involvement is relatively rare (5% in Hodgkin's disease, 15% in NHL;

Table 22-1. Staging of Hodgkin's disease and non-Hodgkin's lymphomas.

Stage		Sub-stage
Stage I	Involvement of a single lymph node chain	
	Localized involvement of a single extralymphatic organ or region	I E
Stage II	Involvement of two or more lymph node chains on the same side of the diaphragm	
	Localized involvement of a single extralymphatic organ or region including its regional lymph nodes with or without other lymph node chains on the same side of the diaphragm	II E
Stage III	Involvement of lymph node chains on both sides of the diaphragm with or without local involvement of a single extralymphatic organ or region	III E
	Splenic involvement	III S
	Both	III E + S
Stage IV	Diffuse infiltration of extralymphatic organs with or without regional lymph node involvement	
	Isolated involvement of an extralymphatic organ and non-regional lymph nodes	
All Stages are further divided into those:	Without weight loss, fever or sweating	A
	With weight loss, fever or sweating	B

for pattern of disease, see Chap. 6, Mediastinum).

• CT

Plain scans: Enlarged lymph nodes may be sharply marginated or fused together to form large, homogeneous conglomerates. Displacement of adjacent organs, which is sometimes severe, depends on the size of the lesion. Despite stretching of supply vessels, thrombosis is hardly ever observed. Diffuse lymphomas can lead to the development of soft-tissue zones that mask the retroperitoneal cavity and the mesenteric root. Retrocrural lymph nodes at the level of the diaphragm must be given careful attention. Evaluation of the status of the mesenteric root and the para-aortic region re-

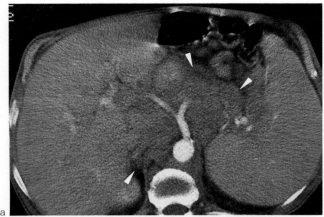

26a

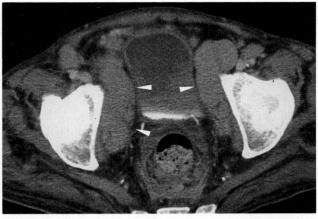

26e

Fig. 22-26. Lymph node enlargement due to chronic lymphatic leukemia. Enlarged lymph nodes of various sizes up to 2 cm (►) are distributed throughout the entire abdominal cavity. In the epigastric region beside the enlarged spleen, there is confluence of lymph node conglomerates. After administration of contrast medium, ventral displacement of vascular structures is clearly visible. (b) Splenic vein (→), portal vein (⇒); (c) renal vein (→), confluence of the superior mesenteric artery (⇒). The pancreas itself cannot be seen. One can only conclude that its position has changed in light of the displacement of vascular structures. Considerable enlargement of lymph nodes in the region of the mesenteric root and mesocolon (d) as well as in the region of the internal iliac chains, especially the internal obturator group.

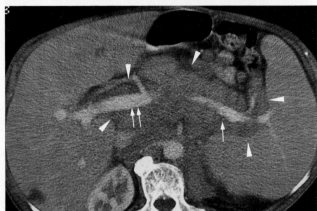

26b

quires uniform bowel opacification, which makes it possible to detect even slight lymph node enlargement. A lateral view should be used for comparison. Since lymphomas frequently adhere to the psoas muscle, lateral differences of the psoas muscle must also be taken into consideration, especially when its borders to the iliac muscle are obliterated or masked.

The *attenuation* of enlarged lymph nodes is equal to that of muscle tissue (40 to 60 HU).

Contrast-enhanced scans: Only moderate, sometimes inhomogeneous enhancement (ca. 20 HU) occurs after bolus contrast medium administration. However, in some cases, contrast enhancement may be significantly higher. Contrast medium is administered primarily to differentiate lymph node structures from vessels, to evaluate organ involvement in infiltrative processes, and to evaluate the status of the spleen and hepatic parenchyma.

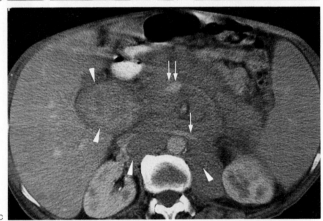

26c

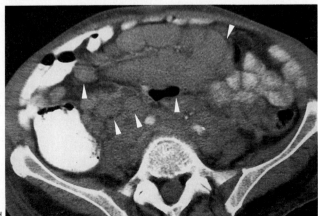

26d

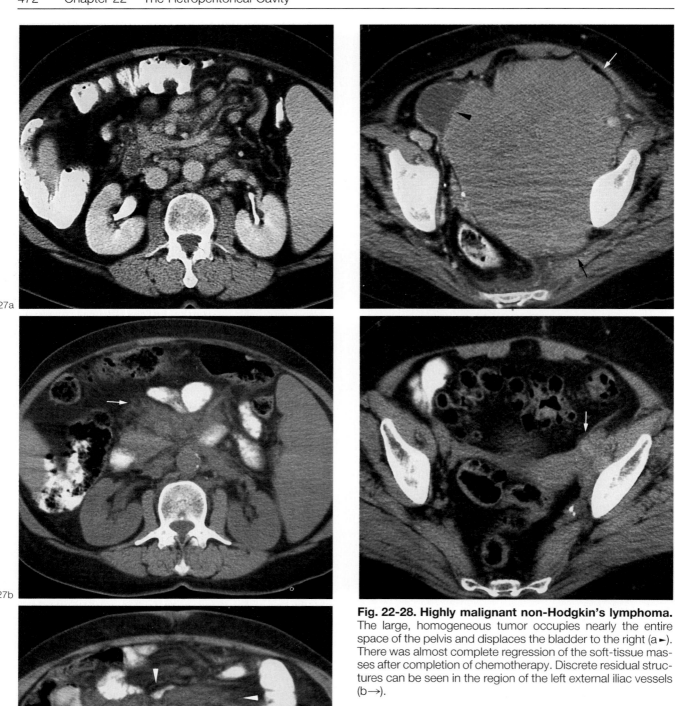

Fig. 22-28. Highly malignant non-Hodgkin's lymphoma. The large, homogeneous tumor occupies nearly the entire space of the pelvis and displaces the bladder to the right (a ►). There was almost complete regression of the soft-tissue masses after completion of chemotherapy. Discrete residual structures can be seen in the region of the left external iliac vessels (b→).

Fig. 22-27. Follow-up of a non-Hodgkin's lymphoma. Demonstration of multiple, well delineated, 1–2 cm large lymph nodes, predominantly in the mesenteric root in conjunction with splenomegaly (a). After remission, recidivation developed 4 years later. The lymph nodes have coalesced and are now grouped into a large, dense conglomerate in the region of the mesenteric root (b→). After completion of chemotherapy, the size of the soft-tissue mass was reduced, but not completely degenerated (c►). One must therefore conclude that there is still viable lymphomatous tissue.

Evaluation of the *liver* and *spleen* is a fundamental part of the examination. Although organ enlargement, itself, is an indication of organ involvement, it is not a reliable diagnostic criterion. The parenchymal density of an affected spleen may be moderately reduced, and localized infiltration is found on scans taken at narrow window widths in ca. 10% of all patients. The sensitivity for detection of focal lymphoma involvement can, in questionable cases, be increased significantly when sequential CT scans are taken after administration of a contrast medium bolus. In contrast, sequential scans are seldom able to demonstrate diffuse involvement of the spleen or liver, even though the absence of trabeculation of an enlarged spleen is frequently seen in the arterial phase in patients with lymph node involvement.

In order to prove that there is *involvement of the intestine*, the mesentery must be painstakingly examined. A reliable evaluation is possible only after optimum opacification of the bowel. Significant thickening of the intestinal wall (greater than 1 cm) is a suspicious sign suggestive of gastrointestinal involvement (see sections on lymphomas of the stomach, small intestine, colon, liver, and kidney).

At the end of *treatment*, the reduction in size of lymph nodes or lymphoma masses can be readily demonstrated on CT scans. There is often complete regeneration of retroperitoneal and mesenteric fatty tissues. Remnant structures frequently remain. When these show signs of retraction, the possibility of fibrosis must be taken into consideration, but this does not exclude the possibility of viable malignant tissue. When biopsy procedures have been forgone, quarterly follow-up examinations must be performed to check for recurrences.

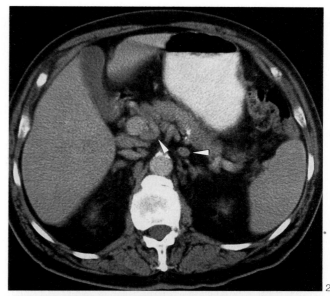

29a

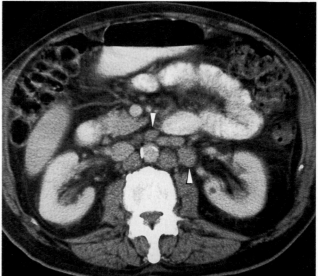

29b

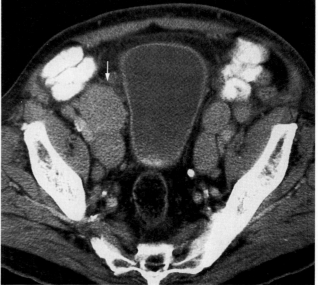

29c

Fig. 22-29. Non-Hodgkin's lymphoma. Lymphomas have primarily infiltrated the pelvis (c→). The mesenteric root has not been affected (b). Infiltration is seen primarily in the retroperitoneal cavity along the course of the large vessels. Splenomegaly was not found (a). In general, the lymph nodes are sharply delineated and do not coalesce.

Lymph Node Metastases

Lymph-borne spreading of malignancy is determined by the position and lymph drainage of the affected organ. The adjacent lymph nodes and distant lymph nodes must be evaluated for metastases, in order to determine the extent of tumor dissemination.

Malignant pancreatic, renal and stomach diseases in the epigastric region are the cause of regional lymph node enlargement, which can extend caudal to a point below the renal pedicle. In testicular, ovarian, and extensive uterine carcinoma, one must take into consideration that direct drainage paths extend bilaterally from the ovaries and testicles to the renal pedicle. Early involvement of para-aortic lymph nodes is observed with seminomas and ovarian carcinomas. Colon carcinomas are associated with early involvement of mesenteric lymph nodes, and uterine, prostate, and bladder tumors involve the iliac and, frequently, presacral lymph nodes in early stages.

• CT

Metastatic lymph node enlargement is less massive and frequently more nodular than that found in the malignant lymphomas, and the pattern of involvement is seldom generalized. Metastases from testicular tumors frequently form lymph node conglomerates (bulky masses). Precise, contiguous sections should be scanned when evaluating testicular tumors, and the first retroperitoneal lymph node chains in the region of the renal pedicle should be given special attention. Localization and precise evaluation of enlarged lymph nodes is possible only when there is good opacification of the intestine and of vessels, especially in the pelvis.

The *attenuation* of these lesions is equal to that of muscle. Hypodense areas (18 ± 7 HU) often appear subsequent to treatment of larger

Fig. 22-30a-d. Metastasizing ovarian carcinoma. Well delineated, slightly enlarged lymph nodes (▸) surround large vessels and can also be reliably demarcated in the porta hepatis (⇒) after administration of contrast medium.

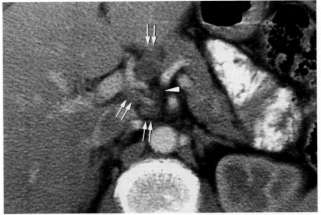

30a

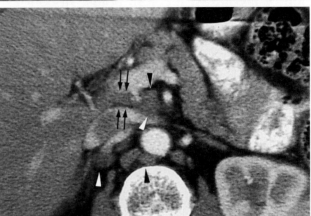

30b

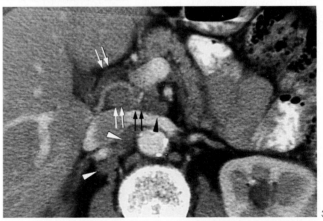

30c

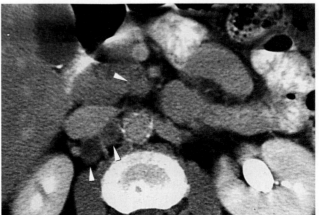

30d

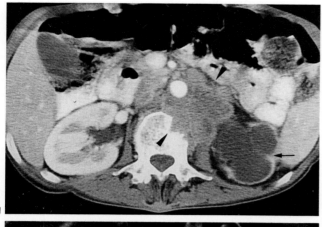

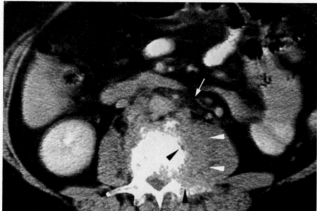

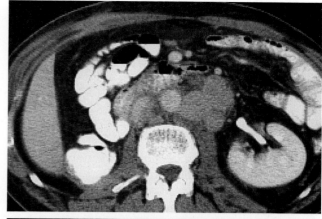

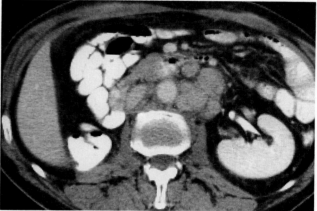

Fig. 22-31. Metastases from a carcinoma of the cervix in the para-aortic region. A large, para-aortic soft-tissue conglomerate at the level of the kidneys. The tumor tissue becomes moderately opaque-laden, primarily in peripheral regions (►). Demonstration of osseous destruction (►) and chronic hydronephrosis of the left kidney (→).

Fig. 22-34. Metastases from a renal cell carcinoma. Clear enhancement occurs after a bolus injection of contrast medium.

Fig. 22-32. Metastasizing bladder carcinoma. Perivertebral fat is masked, and external contours of the body of the vertebra are eroded (►). Additional findings include smaller nodular structures lying directly paravertebral in the periaortic region (→). Spread can be characterized as primarily micronodular and along the lymphatic vessels.

Fig. 22-33. Pelvic wall metastases from bladder carcinoma. After cystectomy, large soft-tissue masses are found on the pelvic wall. They exhibit peripheral enhancement and lower CT numbers in the tumor center (20 HU), an indication of tumor necrosis.

Fig. 22-35. Late metastases from a sigmoid carcinoma. A soft- tissue dense lesion is found at the level of the aortic bifurcation in the region of branching of the common iliac artery on the left. The lesion, which absorbs a moderate amount of contrast medium, causes hydronephrosis.

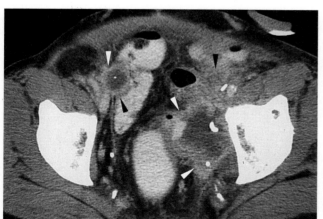

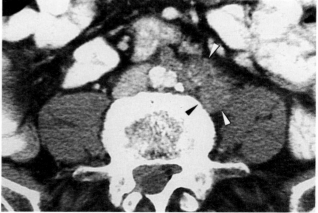

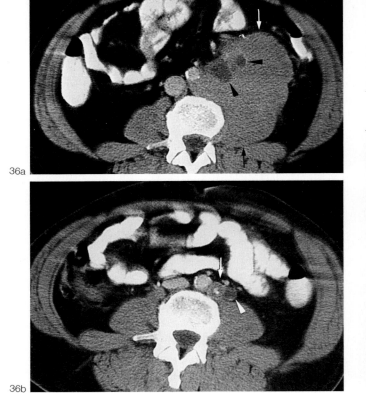

36a

36b

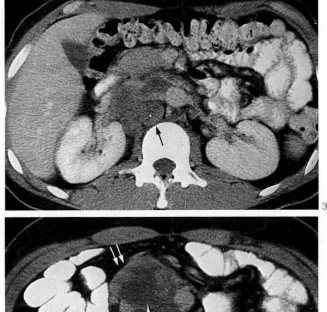

38a

38b

Fig. 22-36. Metastases from a seminoma. Large bulbous soft-tissue masses (a→) on retroperitoneal vessels contain focal areas of hypodensity (a►) representing necrosis. After completion of chemotherapy, a small, partially calcified soft-tissue structure (b→) persists as scar tissue. The hydronephrosis and ureteral dilatation (b►) found in the beginning do not regress.

Fig. 22-38. Metastases from embryonal testicular carcinoma with chorionic components. Enlarged lymph nodes ventrally displace the vessels (→) and display clearly hypodense centers (necrotic zones b►) after contrast medium administration. This demarcates viable tumor tissue (b⇛).

Fig. 22-37. Metastasizing embryonal testicular carcinoma with seminomal components. Retrocaval demonstration of a 1.5 to 2 cm broad, relatively hypodense nodule (►) that ventrally displaces the cava.

Fig. 22-39. Metastatic infiltration (►) from an ovarian carcinoma after multiple chemotherapy sessions.

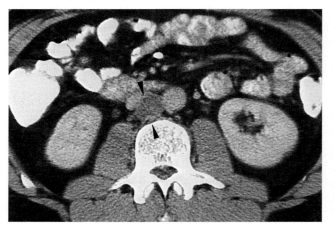

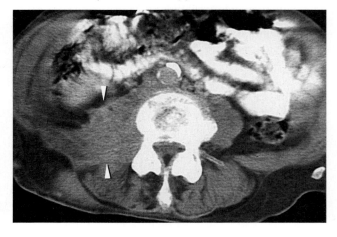

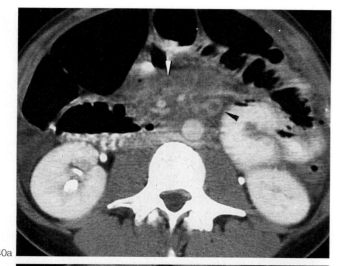

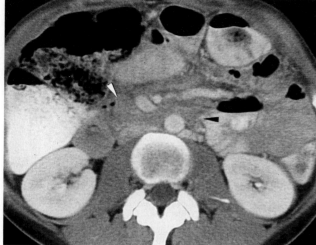

Fig. 22-40. Abscessed lymphadenitis. Fatty tissue of the mesenteric root is masked. After a bolus injection of contrast medium, several ringlike structures appear. They represent inflamed lymph nodes with central abscesses. These zones coalesce at the level of the pelvic inlet to form larger abscesses (a ►). After 14 days of antibiotic treatment, the abscess structures have disappeared. Fatty tissue of the mesenteric root is still masked by inflammatory granulomatous tissue that clearly enhances (b).

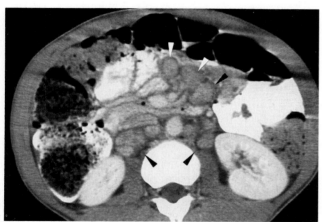

lymph node conglomerates. The attenuation value can even drop to the water range, giving the lesions a cystic appearance. As is the case with malignant lymphomas, bolus contrast medium administration leads to only slight contrast enhancement (10 to 20 HU).

Differential diagnosis: In individual cases, it may be impossible to distinguish these lesions from malignant lymphomas, i.e., if no other signs of lymphatic organ involvement (e.g. splenomegaly) are seen. Signs of bone destruction is more likely attributable to metastases than a malignant lymphoma. In most cases, the primary tumor has already been diagnosed, so CT usually is not required for differential diagnosis.

Benign Lymphadenopathies

Benign lymphadenopathies seldom occur in the retroperitoneal cavity, and they cause only ca. 6% of all lymph node enlargement. Reactively enlarged lymph nodes can reach a size of more than 2 cm, especially in immunosuppressed patients. It, therefore, is not possible to distinguish between lymphomas and metastases of Kaposi's sarcoma.

Lymph node enlargement associated with *sarcoidosis*, *tuberculosis*, and *mastocytosis* can be relatively generalized and may also cause diagnostic problems. Areas of liquefaction with reduced CT numbers have been reported in association with tuberculosis. Deposition of fat or fatty acids cause a constant reduction in attenuation value (10 to 30 HU) of slightly enlarged lymph nodes seen in *Whipple's disease*. *Amyloidosis* can lead to lymphoma-like lymph node enlargement.

Differential diagnosis: Malignant lymphomas and lymph node metastases must be considered in the diagnosis of benign lymphadenopathies.

Fig. 22-41. Mesenteric lymph node tuberculosis. The mesenteric root exhibits enlarged lymph nodes with a diameter of 1 to 2 cm. They clearly absorb contrast medium (►). Central areas of hypodensity representing caseation are not found.

Primary Retroperitoneal Tumors

Primary tumors of the retroperitoneum consist of neoplasms of various tissue types involving all three fasciae. Eighty-five percent of these tumors are malignant. All of them except the endocrine-secreting types are usually diagnosed very late. Embryonal rhabdomyosarcomas and neuroblastomas occur in pediatric patients, neurogenic and teratogenic tumors occur in patients under thirty, and mesenchymal and epithelial remnant tumors occur after the 4th decade. Patients with von Hippel-Lin-

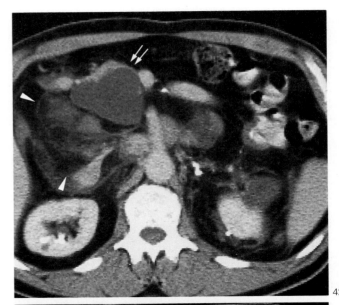

42a

Table 22-2. Relative frequency of primary retroperitoneal tumors.

		Benign types	Malign types
Mesodermal tumors	**50%** (40–60%)	**Lipoma** **Leiomyoma** Rhabdomyoma **Myxoma** Fibroma Lymphangioma Hemangioma Hemangiopericytoma Mesenchymoma	**Liposarcoma** Leiomyosarcoma Rhabdomyosarcoma **Myosarcoma** Fibrosarcoma Lymphangiosarcoma Angiosarcoma Malignant hemangiopericytoma **Malignant mesenchymoma**
Neurogenous tumors	**30%** (11–50%)	**Ganglioneuroma** Paraganglioma **Pheochromocytoma** **Neurofibroma** Neurolemmoma	**Neuroblastoma** (below age 6) Pheochromoblastoma Malignant schwannoma
Remnant tumors	**10%** (5–25%)	**Teratoma** (in children) Dermoid cystoma Chordoma	Teratocarcinoma Malignant chordoma
	10% (5–11%)	Adenoma Epithelial cysts	Carcinoma

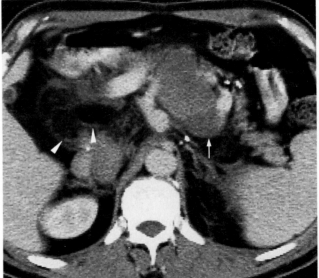

42b

Fig. 22-42. Extensive liposarcoma. Because it contains different tissue components, different tumor components are found. Their densities lie in the CT range of fat (►), water (⇒) and soft tissue (→).

Fig. 22-43. Liposarcoma (→) with reduced attenuation values (18 HU) and sharply delineated, fat-dense, narrow tissue zones (►).

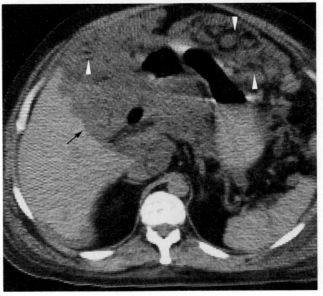

43

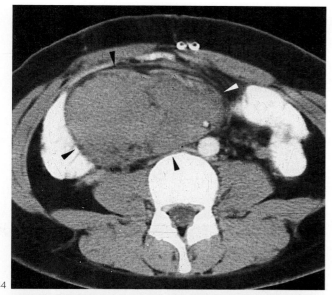

44

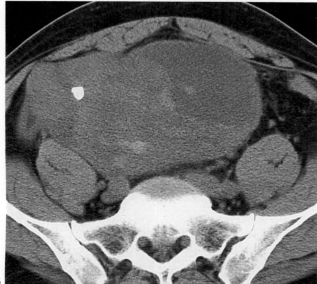

45

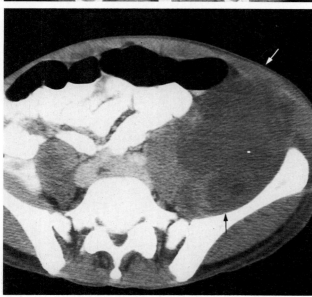

46

dau syndrome, tuberous sclerosis, or common neurofibromatosis have a genetic predisposition for neurogenic tumors.

Fatty tumors such as the lipoma and liposarcoma are relatively common (predominantly in females). Intratumoral *calcification* is frequently observed in neuroblastomas, ganglioneuromas, hemangiomas, and hemangiopericytomas. Larger tumors, particularly those with rapid growth, often show *cystic* degeneration.

Retroperitoneal sarcomas seldom display regional lymphogenous metastases. Bloodborne metastases spread to the lungs, liver, bone, peritoneum, skin and/or brain in advanced stages.

• CT

Plain scans: Findings usually include a solitary mass that may be bilateral if expansion has occurred. The mass is usually located in front of the spinal column and psoas muscle. Large masses may displace midline structures.

Good structural delineation due to the intact layer of fat and the absence of metastases is suggestive of a localized process, but does not exclude the possibility of malignancy. On the other hand, infiltrative growth that breaches anatomical boundaries, bone destruction, and evidence of metastases in the lungs, liver, mesentery, or soft-tissue are unequivocal malignancy criteria. Vessel erosion with a resultant hemorrhage is rare.

The malignancy of tumors is usually reflected as inhomogeneous density, which can be seen even on plain scans. The attenuation value reflects the nature of the tumor tissue, so it can help to distinguish the various sarcoma types, as described below.

Fig. 22-44. Fibroma in Gardner's syndrome.

Fig. 22-45. Neurogenic sarcoma with slightly lower, more inhomogeneous CT values than muscle tissue as well as isolated areas of calcification.

Fig. 22-46. Malignant hemangiopericytoma. As a result of necrosis, it exhibits only discrete enhancement after bolus contrast medium injection.

– *Fatty tumors:* Pure fatty values of -120 to -80 HU can be observed in *lipomas* and *liposarcomas*. The diagnosis of lipoma can be confidently made only if the mass contains homogeneously fat- dense tissue that is permeated with fine septa. Larger solid tumor components that surround the fat to form "islands" or broad areas of increased density are suggestive of liposarcoma. The changing composition of lipomatous, xanthomatous, and myxomatous tissue elements can also give rise to extremely variable tissue densities without identifiable areas of isolated fatty tissue. One can therefore find liposarcomas with a tissue density of over 30 HU (solid type), or with visible fatty components (mixed type), or pseudocystic types that are water-dense. Lipid deposits can lead to a significant drop in density of neurogenic tumors. Characteristic diagnostic features of *neurofibromas* include their hypodensity as compared with adjacent muscle tissue and their typical location near the courses of nerves.

– *Cystic tumors:* Cystic *lymphangiomas* differ from water-dense liposarcomas in that their delicate cyst wall absorbs a slight a small amount of contrast medium. Their configuration is generally unilocular or multilocular.

– *Soft-tissue tumors:* Differential diagnosis of an isolated mass is not possible if it has smooth borders and homogeneous attenuation values. Large masses, which usually contain areas of hypodensity, are suggestive of malignancy. Malignancy can be confidently diagnosed when signs of organ invasion or bone destruction are found. Large areas of necrosis, which develop especially in leiomyosarcomas and malignant histiocytomas, cause the CT numbers to drop to the water range (cystic degeneration).

Calcification is generally rare. This occurs preferentially in neurogenic (neuroblastomas) and angiomatous lesions (hemangiomas, hemangiopericytomas).

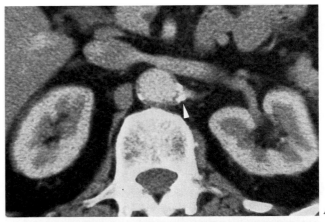

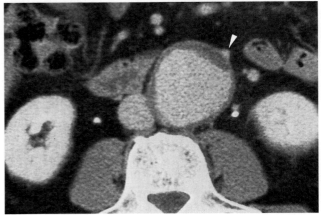

47a

47b

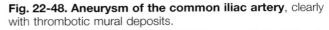

Fig. 22-47. Infrarenal aortic aneurysm. The appearance of the lumen is normal at the level of the renal arteries (a ►). Above the aortic bifurcation, the lumen then increases to a diameter of 5 cm and contains a few thrombotic mural deposits. Inferior mesenteric artery (b ►).

Fig. 22-48. Aneurysm of the common iliac artery, clearly with thrombotic mural deposits.

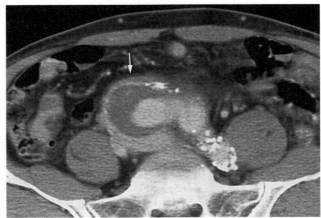

Contrast-enhanced scans: Viable tumor elements usually show clear enhancement after bolus contrast medium administration, and zones of necrosis and fatty deposits are clearly demarcated. Hemangiomas and hemangiopericytomas show especially strong contrast enhancement.

Differential diagnosis: It is often impossible to distinguish a solid sarcoma from a *lymphoma conglomerate*. Diagnostic signs of the latter include homogeneous attenuation, cuff-like growth around large vessels, and slight enhancement. Furthermore, *pheochromocytomas* (see Adrenal Glands), *dermoid cysts* (see Ovarian Tumors) must also be considered.

Vascular Lesions

Aneurysms

Large arteries in the retroperitoneal cavity can be seen on plain scans, and the smaller ones can be seen after a targeted bolus injection of contrast medium. Arteriosclerotic calcification further facilitates the demarcation of vessels. This must be differentiated from aneurysmatic calcification, which has a larger diameter than the corresponding supply vessel. As compared with aortic aneurysms, aneurysms of the organ arteries are rare and occur preferentially in the splenic artery (ca. 40%) and renal arteries (ca. 20%).

• *Aneurysm of the Abdominal Aorta*

About 98.5% of all aneurysms of the abdominal aorta are caused by arteriosclerosis. Syphilitic, mycotic, and traumatic types have become rare today. Only 5% of all arteriosclerotic, but 70% of all syphilitic aneurysms are cranial to the origins of the renal artery. Infrarenal aneurysms frequently extend to the pelvic arteries. Mural calcification is found over 75% of these lesions. An aneurysm involving the abdominal aorta is diagnosed when the outer diameter is 4 cm or larger. *Surgery is indicated* when the diameter is 5 cm or larger, but this is also dependent on the clinical course of the individual patient.

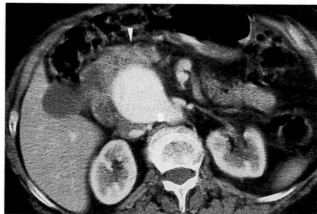

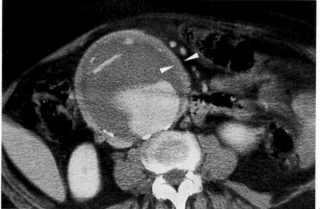

Fig. 22-49. Inflammatory aortic aneurysm. At the cranial attachment (a ►) as well as in infrarenal regions, not only the lumen, but also the external wall of the aneurysm (b ► ◄) enhances after bolus injection of contrast medium.

Fig. 22-50. Dissecting aneurysm. The thoracic dissection extends into the abdominal region (►). The left kidney is supplied by the left lumen.

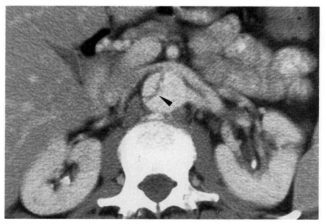

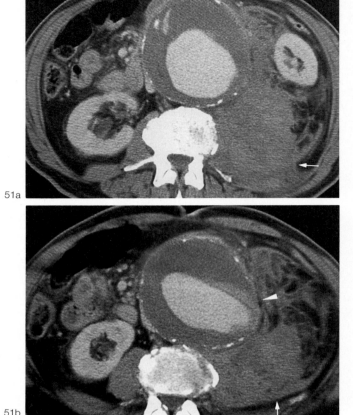

51a

51b

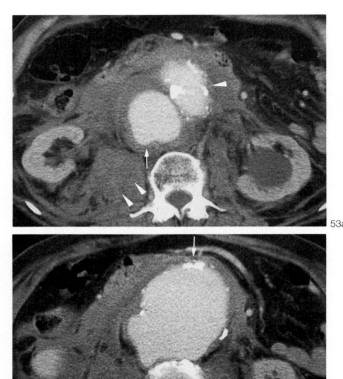

53a

53b

Fig. 22-51. Ruptured aortic aneurysm. Directly below the origins of the renal arteries (a), a large aortic aneurysm with a diameter of 9 cm can be seen. Above the left bifurcation, the eccentrically shaped lumen touches the external contours of the aorta, which contains no visible calcification in this region (b►). In the adjacent area, there are large soft-tissue structures (a, b→) of nonuniform radiodensity and a large retroperitoneal hematoma that infiltrates the perirenal space and ventrally displaces the left kidney (a).

Fig. 22-53. Spurious aneurysm. Right lateral to the aorta, which can be identified by mural calcification (a►), a second lumen is demonstrated (a→). It arises from a large abdominal aneurysm (b→) and extends from the caudal to cranial aspect. The spurious aneurysm lies inside a large, periaortic, hematoma that appears slightly hyperdense on plain scans. The hematoma is spread throughout the right retroperitoneal and perirenal spaces (►).

Fig. 22-52. Para-aortic hematoma in conjunction with aortic rupture. A small opaque-laden zone is detected inside the hematoma (→). This is attributable to aortic leakage.

Fig. 22-54. Perirenal hematoma in conjunction with a ruptured aortic aneurysm. Hemorrhage into the perirenal space is causing ventral displacement of the left kidney. For the most part, there is no encroachment of fascial boundaries (→).

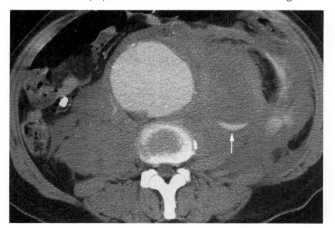

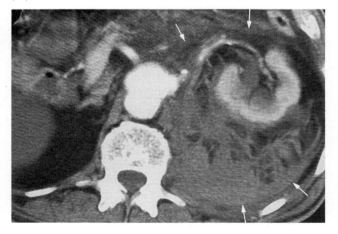

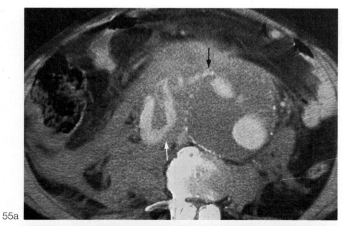

55a

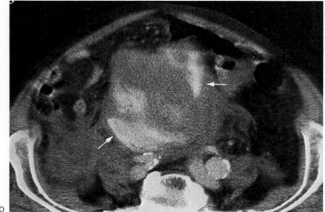

55b

Fig. 22-55. Ruptured aortic aneurysm. Leakage of contrast medium from the rupture can be demonstrated (a→). Blood forms a large hematoma in the pelvis (b→).

Fig. 22-56. Suture aneurysm. After implantation of a Y-shaped prosthesis, considerable dilatation of the iliac arteries (→) was found on both sides of the site of anastomosis. Thrombotic deposits were not found.

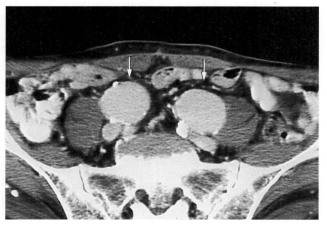

Dissecting aneurysms only rarely develop in the abdominal region, and they usually occur as a continuation of a thoracic dissection. Mycotic or infected aneurysms are rare and may develop in normal vessels, but also in arteriosclerotic vessels. Infection is either blood-borne or spreads from adjacent organs.

• CT

Plain scans: Arteriosclerotic changes can be seen in plain scans as areas of wall calcification. Thrombotic deposits in the vessel lumen can often be seen on plain scans as discreet, ring-shaped or semilunar internal areas of hypodensity. Erosion of adjacent vertebral bodies gives proof of long-standing, chronic effects of an aneurysm.

Contrast-enhanced scans: A bolus of contrast medium clearly delineates the lumen. Broadening of the outer diameter can be measured exactly via computed tomography. The outer diameter of a healthy aorta narrows from the cranial to caudal aspect. The absence of this narrowing is considered to be a sign of angiectasia in aortas with borderline outer diameters (ca. 4 cm), as well as dilatation of the iliac arteries.

Aneurysmatic *rupture* is demonstrated when outer margins are only diffusely distinguishable from perivascular fat. Depending on the location of blood leakage, extensive hemorrhages can spread to the anterior or posterior pararenal compartment, as well as to the perirenal compartment, and may lead to considerable organ displacement. Hyperdensity of around 70 HU is a sign of fresh hemorrhage. Evidence of blood in the peritoneal cavity is potentially fatal. The site of blood leakage can sometimes be identified after targeted *contrast medium administration*. When chronic, this condition can lead to the development of a peri- aortic hematoma with a fibrous tissue capsule (spurious aneurysm, *pseudoaneurysm*). A clue to this type of cause is provided when there is an interruption in the external aneurysmatic calcification at the location of the pseudoaneurysm.

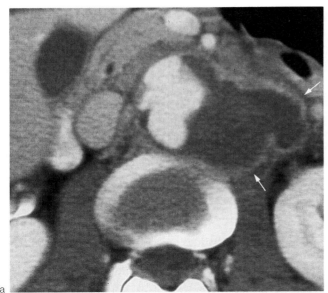

57a

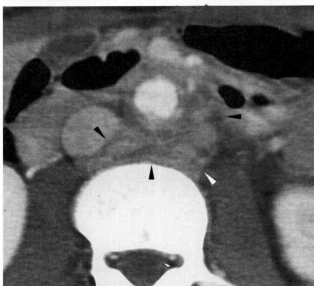

57b

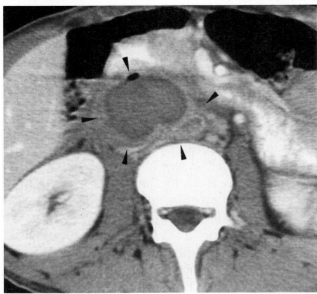

57c

Contrast enhancement of a usually smoothly marginated, peri-aortic soft-tissue zone is a sign of an inflammatory aortic aneurysm (see idiopathic retroperitoneal fibrosis).

Mycotic aneurysms are rare and are usually saccular. Although evidence of gas in the vessel wall is a pathognomonic sign, it is not a constant characteristic. Mural calcification can be "dissolved" by inflammation; calcification is usually completely absent in extensive lesions. An inflammatory process (osteomyelitis, abscess, empyema) in the immediate proximity is usually responsible for the aneurysm.

Arteriographic examination is now frequently dispensed with before aneurysm surgery. The CT examination must, therefore, precisely define the extent of the aneurysm and its location with respect to the renal arteries. If necessary, secondary image reconstruction techniques must be used.

Aortic dissections, which usually begin in the thoracic region, are demonstrated in a similar manner. The dissection membrane as well as the false and true lumina can be clearly demonstrated in a rapid scanning sequence when there is sufficient contrast enhancement. Questions concerning the supply of the visceral arteries from the respective lumina should be clarified before surgery, if necessary, by means of a separate CT sequence. If a long aortic segment demonstrates a hyperdense aortic wall on plain scans, this may be a sign of an underlying aortic dissection (fresh thrombosis in the dissection lumen).

Postoperative changes are also readily demonstrable by computed tomography. The im-

Fig. 22-57. Mycotic aneurysm. Below the renal arteries, the aortic lumen appears lobulated and its left external contour forms a broad arch. It clearly enhances after contrast medium administration (a→). Nodular structures (lymph nodes) are located in deeper layers; they become slightly enhanced (b►). Erosion of the adjacent vertebral body was not detected. Aneurysmic surgery triggered an attack of fever. 14 days later (c), air deposits representing a renewed infection were found in the aortic region. The opacifying granulation tissue (►) later degenerated.

planted prosthetic material (tubular or Y-shaped prosthesis) may be seen as a sharply marginated, discretely hyperdense, ringlike structure, depending on the material it is made from. When there is end-to-end anastomosis within the aneurysmal sac, a postoperative, sickle-shaped seam of fluid frequently develops around the prosthesis that was attached to the aortic sac. In end-to-side anastomosis, the region of anastomosis can be clearly visualized, because the distal aortic lumen and the bridged iliac arteries are usually thrombosed.

Possible postoperative *complications* include anastomotic hemorrhage leading to the development of a perivascular hematoma (false aneurysm, pseudoaneurysm) and thrombotic occlusion or *infection of the prosthesis*. A characteristic diagnostic feature of infection is a seam of fluid around the prosthesis. Bubbles of bacterial gas are unequivocal signs of infection. They are distinguishable from postoperative air deposits in that they remain visible more than ten days after the operation. Furthermore, they are often have a blister-like configuration that is oriented along the seams of fluid around the vessel prosthesis. Evidence of gas in a thrombotic vessel or prosthesis is also a clear sign of infection.

The later development of *stitch aneurysms* is diagnosed when there is evidence of lumen dilatation near sites of anastomosis.

Aortic Trauma

Blunt abdominal trauma or a piercing wound can cause injury to the aorta. This can lead to laceration of the aortic wall with extensive pararenal and perirenal hematomas.

Translumbar punctures usually lead to periaortic, localized hematoma.

Anomalies of the Inferior Vena Cava

During embryological development, the inferior vena cava (IVC) is derived from three sets of paired cardinal veins. Anomalies of the IVC

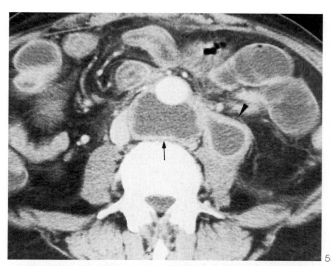

58

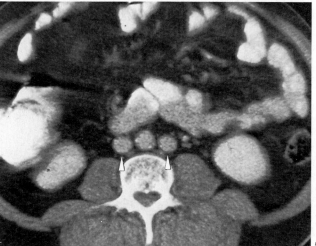

59

Fig. 22-58. Film taken after implantation of Y-shaped prosthesis. A hematoma has developed in the former aneurysmal sac (→) with sacculation of the left psoas muscle (►). Gas deposits, indicative of infection of the prosthesis, are not found.

Fig. 22-59. Double inferior vena cava. The aorta is accompanied by bilateral inferior vena cavae (►).

are rare and varied. If the hepatic segment fails to develop properly, the IVC is linked to the azygos vein, which becomes responsible for venous drainage of the abdominal cavity. Hemiazygos continuation is seen when there is duplication of the IVC.

• CT

Plain scans: When the azygos and hemiazygos veins are dilated (best seen in the retrocrural space), anomalies of the inferior vena cava

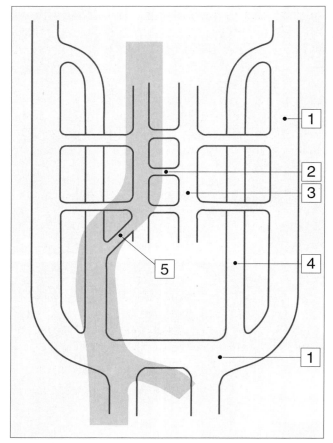

Fig. 22-60. Anomalies of the inferior vena cava (IVC). The embryological development of the IVC is very complex. Therefore, one may find extremely variable venous anomalies in the abdominal cavity. They may involve the azygos and hemiazygos venous systems (e.g. double IVC, left-sided IVC, periureteral venous ring, etc.).

Key to symbols:
1 Postcardinal vein
2 Supracardinal vein
3 Periureteral venous ring
4 Subcardinal vein
5 Subsupracardinal anastomosis

must be taken into consideration. Longitudinal strands beside the abdominal aorta generally are assumed to be vessels. Differentiation of enlarged lymph nodes becomes difficult when a venous plexus has developed. However, vascular structures are usually more sharply delineated than a lymphoma. Azygos vein continuation of the IVC can sometimes be diagnosed on the basis of plain scans when the contours of the vena cava are absent in the caudate lobe of the liver in conjunction with dilatation of the azygos vein.

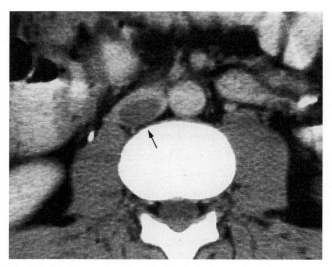

Fig. 22-61. Thrombosis of the inferior vena cava in a paraneoplastic syndrome. The filling defect is sharply marginated and surrounded by contrast medium. The defect arises from the right common iliac vein (→).

Contrast-enhanced scans: In order to secure the diagnose of vessel anomaly, a large and protracted dose of contrast medium is administered in order to achieve clear contrast enhancement, even when there is extensive collateral circulation.

Thrombosis of the Inferior Vena Cava (Including the Pelvic Veins)

Thrombosis of the inferior vena cava is most commonly caused by the extending effects of pelvic vein thrombosis. Less frequent causes include external compression, ingrowing of tumor thrombi, secondary vena cava inflammations. Primary vena cava thrombosis (seen, for example, in antithrombin deficiency) is a rarity.

In renal cell carcinoma, a tumor thrombus protrudes into the renal vein and partially displaces the inferior vena cava, the lumen of which then becomes increasingly dilated. A similar mechanism is found in adrenal carcinoma. Like hepatocellular carcinomas, it also causes direct infiltration that leads to vena cava thrombosis. Reorganization of the thrombus boundaries is seen four days after thrombus development. Centralized tissue softening is observed.

• CT

Plain scans: A dilated, hyperdense lumen is seen on CT scans of fresh thromboses of the inferior vena cava. In older occlusions, the dilated tube of the vena cava appears hypodense as compared with the aorta. Septic thrombi have inconsistent amounts of gas bubbles, and a CT-guided diagnostic biopsy may be necessary for clarification.

Contrast-enhanced scans: After contrast medium administration, a slightly hypervascular vena cava wall is often seen as a result of thrombus reorganization. When there is partial obstruction, a parietal thrombus can appear in the contrasted vessel lumen as a constant, sharply marginated filling defect. It can, therefore, be distinguished from low-density flow-related phenomena. A central area of enhancement inside the thrombus is suggestive of a tumor process, especially in clinically diagnosed hypernephromas. Even processes surrounding the vena cava (inflammation, tumor) can be demonstrated. Computed tomography can, therefore, help to find the underlying cause of the thrombus.

Differential diagnosis: Tumor thrombi in conjunction with renal (or adrenal) malignancies can usually be diagnosed with knowledge of the primary tumor. The thrombi often have a central area of enhancement. Although leiomyosarcomas of the inferior vena cava are rare, they have a tendency for intravascular growth which makes them difficult to distinguish from thrombi. It may be difficult to make a diagnosis when there is no clear evidence of tumor infiltration in surrounding structures.

Chapter 23
Muscle Tissue

Muscle Tissue

Atrophy

Muscle mass may be reduced due to inactivity, steroid treatment, and denervation. The diameter of the individual fibers of muscle is thereby decreased. In denervation of a muscular bundle, muscle tissue is increasingly replaced by fat. The amount of fat between muscular septa, which is normally moderate, is dependent upon the constitution of the patient.

• CT

Since muscle mass is extremely variable and dependent on the physical fitness of the patient, the degree of muscular atrophy can only be estimated. Localized atrophy due to injury can, however, be precisely assessed by comparison with the opposite side as can the pattern of spread of diseases leading to spinal atrophy. Implementation of CT for quantitative measurement has also been described.

Progressive Muscular Dystrophy

Most cases of progressive muscular dystrophy are categorized as Duchenne atrophy (progressive spinal muscular atrophy), which initially affects the muscles of the pelvic girdle. Pseudohypertrophy of the calf muscles is observed in 80% of these patients. Pseudohypertrophy of affected muscles occurs more infrequently in progressive limb girdle muscular atrophy and in only isolated cases of progressive fascioscapulohumeral types. The extent and intensity of metaplasia are the only histologic characteristics that differentiate the types of progressive muscular dystrophy. Hypertrophy of non-affected tissue elements compensates for focal necrosis of muscle fiber. In progressive disease, muscle tissue is continuously replaced by fat and connective tissue until almost complete atrophy of the muscle has occurred.

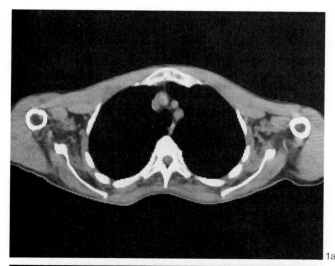

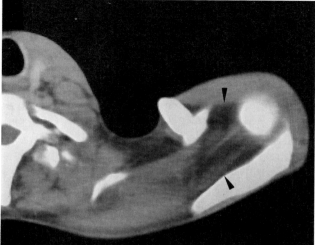

Fig. 23-1. Progressive muscular dystrophy (fascio-scapulo-humeral type). Symmetrical involvement of muscle groups, the attenuation values of which lie in the fat range. In this case, the subcapsular muscles and deep muscles of the back are affected.

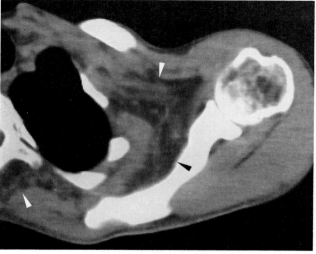

• CT

Plain scans: Progressive muscular dystrophy is characterized by fatty metaplasia; muscle septa usually appear as a distinct matrix. A homogeneous pattern of involvement of a muscle or muscle group may be demonstrated as well as an inhomogeneous, maculated pattern of fatty tissue distribution. In the calves, the peripheral muscle fibers become affected before the central fibers show signs of involvement. The extent of fatty metaplasia corresponds with the clinical severity of the disease.

Inflammatory Muscular Diseases

Pyogenic Myositis (Muscular Abscess)

Pyogenic myositis may develop due to post-traumatic or iatrogenic reasons, or due to metastatic and embolic reasons. In the latter case, common pus-forming organisms lead to liquefaction and encapsulation of muscle tissue and ultimate abscess formation. When infection is caused by Streptococcus pyogenes, gas may develop during liquefaction, which eventually leads to the development of gas phlegmons. The muscles of the paraspinal region and pelvic girdle are commonly affected.

• CT

Plain scans: The muscular septa and surrounding tissues are masked by a hypodense zone, and the affected region is frequently distended. Gas within the hypodense zone is considered a pathognomonic sign of bacterial involvement.

Fig. 23-2. Muscular atrophy. In a patient with a hip replacement, fatty infiltration of the gluteal muscles, a sign of atrophy, is detected. This has led to reduced attenuation values and broadening of intermuscular septa.

Fig. 23-3. Muscular abscess. After bolus injection of contrast medium, granulation tissue appears hyperdense as compared with the hypodense abscess cavity.

Fig. 23-4. Muscular hematoma. Within the greatly dilated psoas muscle (→), blotchy areas of hyperdensity (►) are demonstrated. These represent fresh hemorrhage. Atrophied back muscles (►), see Fig. 23-2.

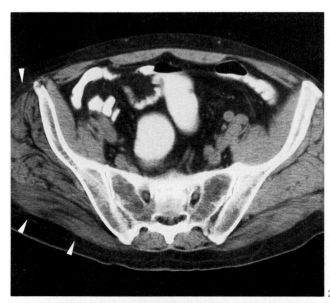

2

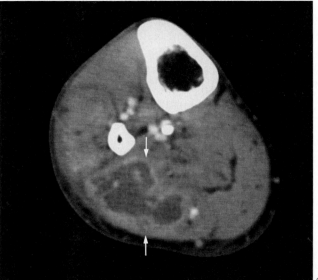

3

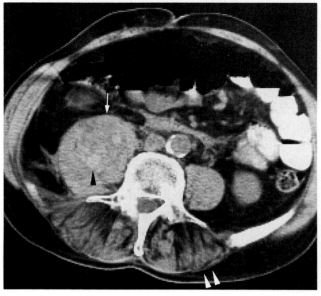

4

Contrast-enhanced scans: Especially in chronic pyogenic myositis, granulation tissue is demonstrated on CT scans as a hyperdense ring of variable intensity.

Differential diagnosis: If no liquefaction has occurred, circumscribed pyogenic myositis cannot be distinguished from infections caused by leukemic, plasma-cell, or other neoplastic infiltrates.

Sarcoidosis

Muscle tissue is affected in more than 50% of all patients with generalized sarcoidosis.

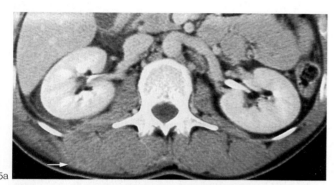

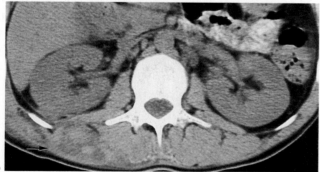

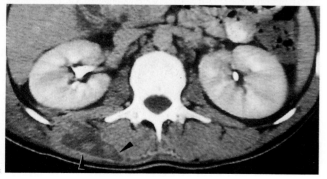

Granulomas can lead to muscle atrophy as a direct result of primary involvement of muscle fibers (rare) or indirectly as a result of changes in the motor nerves.

• CT

Atrophy cannot be demonstrated by CT until muscle fibres have been replaced by fatty tissue.

Polymyositis

In up to 80% of all cases, polymyositis initially manifests during the course of dermatomyositis. Acute polymyositis is characterized by extensive and rapidly developing muscular necrosis that may display fine, plaque-like calcification. Depending on the extent of muscle tissue necrosis, liposclerotic metaplasia can be observed more frequently in primary chronic polymyositis than in secondary chronic polymyositis.

• CT

The extent of fatty tissue transformation and atrophy can be assessed by computed tomography. The presence of fine, plaque-like calcification can be taken as an indication of polymyositis.

Muscular Hematoma

Blunt trauma can lead to the development of a hematoma, especially in hemophiliacs and patients receiving anticoagulants. The hematoma becomes encased in the surrounding fasciae and leads to swelling of the affected muscle. Vascular and neurologic function may frequently be disturbed as a result of muscular

Fig. 23-5. Muscular hematoma arising from blunt abdominal trauma. On the day of the accident, the only finding was dilatation of the erector spinae muscle, which exhibited homogeneous enhancement after a bolus injection of contrast medium (a→). Ten days later, plain scans revealed hypodense (30 HU) and slightly hyperdense (65 HU) zones in the muscular tissue (b→). A hypodense hematoma appears with a peripheral absorption zone appears after contrast medium administration (c►).

displacement. As the hematoma matures, it may be absorbed, liquefy, or transform into connective tissue that may calcify.

• CT

Plain scans: In an acute muscular hematoma, a maculated hyperdensity pattern is normally found within the swollen muscle, but this may be absent when the hematoma only diffusely permeates the muscle tissue. When the hematoma is still in subacute phases, the characteristically isodense or hypodense area of swelling is often demonstrable only when the opposite limb is scanned for comparison.

Localized subacute hematomas display inhomogeneous density and have ill-defined borders. Liquefaction is demarcated in chronic muscular hematoma as a hypodense, sharply marginated area that occasionally displays additional signs of sedimentation.

Contrast-enhanced scans: After the administration of contrast medium, the absorptive granulation tissue of a chronic hematoma displays a peripheral enhancement pattern that makes it difficult to distinguish from an abscess.

Myositis Ossificans

Myositis ossificans is characterized by the development of a localized, benign osseous mass within muscle tissue. Its development is either neurogenic, especially after severe cranio-cerebral trauma and peripheral paralysis, or the mass is a direct posttraumatic result of a muscle injury. A very rare form develops without trauma in adolescents, the preferential location of the mass being the iliohypogastric region.

Pluripotent, osteoid-forming connective tissue develops. It displays calcification and, ultimately, ossification. A neoplasm of myositis ossificans is said to be mature and resectable when the soft-tissue zone has given way to frank new bone formation.

• CT

Plain scans: Myositis ossificans usually appears as a ringlike structure with a variable degree of calcification or ossification. The center of the structure is isodense or hypodense as compared with surrounding muscle. It is not uncommon for the neoplasm to begin as a relatively sharply marginated mass that is hypodense as compared with muscle tissue. However, the degree of peripheral calcification continuously increases. The calcified structures may appear punctiform or cloudy, but are subtly radial. They may partially or completely fill the mass.

Differential diagnosis: The patient's history and location of the mass normally form the basis of the diagnosis. When located directly in the periosteum of a bone, it may be difficult to differentiate the mass from *reactive periostitis*, *osteochondroma*, or *chondrosarcoma*, since these lesions also have elements of soft-tissue and calcification. Symmetrical areas of muscular calcification in patients with acute renal failure are indicative of past *rhabdomyolysis*. Acute rhabdomyolysis is characterized by sharply marginated areas of hypodensity (especially after the administration of contrast medium and can give rise to the compartment syndrome in the extremities.

Chapter 24
Soft-Tissue Tumors

Table. 24-1. Histological classification of soft-tissue tumors.
(Simplified version based on Enzinger and Weiss, ref. 2573).

Tissue type	Benign tumors	Malign tumors
Connective tissue Fibrocytic structures	Fibroma nodular fasciitis, proliferating fasciitis, proliferative myositis, keloids Fibromatosis superficial, intra- and extra-abdominal, radiogenic fibromatosis in childhood	Adult fibrosarcoma congenital and infantile fibrosarcoma, fibrosarcoma after irradiation and scar formation
Fibrohistocytic structures	Fibrous histiocytoma xanthogranuloma, reticulohistiocytoma, xanthoma, fibroxanthoma	Maligant fibrous histiocytoma storiform/pleomorphic, myxoid, giant-cell, inflammatory, angiomatous
Fatty tissue	Lipoma angiolipoma, pleomorphic lipoma, lipoblastoma, angiomyelolipoma, myelolipoma, intramuscular lipoma, lipomatosis, hibernoma	Liposarcoma differentiated, myxoid, round-cell, pleomorphic, dedifferentiated
Muscle tissue	Rhabdomyoma adult, genital, fetal	Rhabdomyosarcoma embryonic (incl. botryoid), alveolar, pleomorphic, mixed-cell ectomesenchymoma
	Leiomyoma angiomyoma, leiomyomatosis, leiomyoblastoma	Leiomyosarcoma epithelial leiomyosarcoma, (malignant leiomyosarcoma)
Blood vessels	Hemangioma capillary, cavitary, arteriovenous, venous, epithelial, pyogenic, hemangiomatosis, glomous tumor, hemangiopericytoma, papillary endothelial hyperplasia Hemangioendothelioma (semimalignant)	Hemangiosarcoma, Kaposi's sarcoma, malignant angioendothelioma, proliferating angioendotheliomatosis, malignant glomous tumor, malignant hemangiopericytoma
Lymph vessels	Lymphangioma lymphangiomatosis, lymphangiomyomatosis	Lymphangiosarcoma
Synovial tissue	Giant cell tumor	Synovial sarcoma (biphasic, monophasic), malignant giant cell tumor of the nerve sheath
Mesothelial tissue	Localized mesothelioma epithelial, fibrous, biphasic, multicystic-peritoneal mesothelioma	Diffuse and localized mesothelioma epithelial, fibrous, biphasic
Mesenchymal tissue	Mesenchymoma	Malignant mesenchymoma
Bone and cartilage	Ossifying myositis ossifying panniculitis ossifying progressive fibrodysplasia, extraskeletal chondroma, extraskeletal osteoma	Extraskeletal chondrosarkoma Extraskeletal osteosarkoma
Autonomous ganglia	Ganglioneuroma	Neuroblastoma, ganglioneuroblastoma
Paraganglionic tissue	Paraganglioma	Malignant paraganglioma
Peripheral nerves	Neurilemoma (benign schwannoma) neurofibroma, neurofibromatosis, neuroma, neurilemma, ganglioma, neurothecoma	Malignant schwannoma malignant neuroepithelioma, olfactory neuroepithelioma

Soft-Tissue Tumors

A *lipoma* is the most common benign soft-tissue tumor. These tumors are localized preferentially in the shoulder, neck, and back, and seldom in the extremities. The majority of all lipomas originate in subcutaneous tissue. When the tumor is located in deeper tissue layers, intra- and intermuscular spreading may occur, possibly with local infiltration. Cellular atypia, however, is not demonstrable on histological sections.

Over half of all *liposarcomas* are located in the extremities. The amount of myxomatous and mucinous tissue elements will differ in accordance with the degree of tumor differentiation. The liposarcoma can mimic the appearance of a fibrosarcoma when it contains a disproportionately high amount of fibrotic elements. Cellular atypia is occasionally observed when the liposarcoma is well differentiated and composed primarily of mature fatty tissue components.

Fibromas originate in various connective tissue structures and are named accordingly. When musculo-aponeurotic fibromatosis becomes extensive, it invades surrounding tissues (including the bone) without forming metastases (aggressive fibromatosis). The transition from the fibroma stage to a *fibrosarcoma* is gradual and continuous.

Common soft-tissue tumors are, in order of frequency, the *rhabdomyosarcoma*, liposarcoma, and fibrosarcoma. All of these tumors, with the exception of botryoid embryonal rhabdomyosarcomas, occur preferentially in the extremities. Necrosis, hemorrhage, and cystic transformation can cause displacement phenomena in mature types. Benign *rhabdomyomas* are extremely rare.

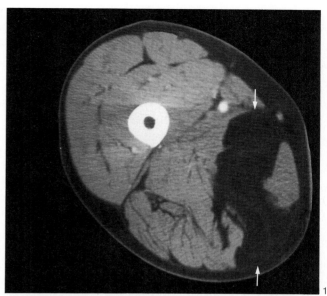

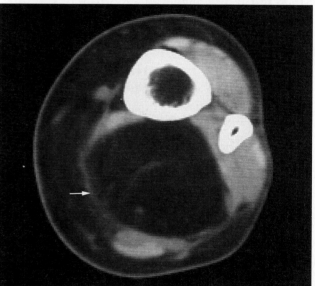

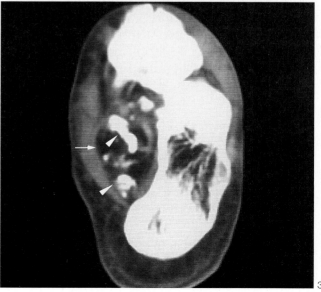

Fig. 24-1. Intermuscular lipoma in the thigh. The lipoferous tumor pushes apart the gracilis and adductor muscles. It is homogeneously fat-dense.

Fig. 24-2. Intramuscular lipoma in the lower leg. The lipoma completely distends a muscular space and displaces the surrounding muscle tissues.

Fig. 24-3. Lipoma (→) on the interior surface of the tarsal bone, with calcification (▶).

Leiomyomas not originating in the uterus develop within various intra-abdominal organs, usually in subcutaneous soft-tissue. Malignant *leiomyosarcomas* occur more frequently in deeper muscle layers than benign types.

Unlike lymphangiomas, lymphangiosarcomas, and angiosarcomas, the *hemangioma* (capillary and cavitary) is not uncommonly found in the soft-tissues of the extremities.

● CT

Soft-tissue tumors appear on CT scans as a mass causing displacement of contiguous structures. In the extremities, the amount of delineating fat determines how well the tumor will be demarcated from the muscular bundle. Since the shape, size and septation of the musculature is subject to individual variation, comparison with the opposite side is also necessary for proper diagnosis.

Sharply defined tumor borders and homogeneous CT numbers suggest that the tumor is *benign*. The *lipoma* appears as a fat-dense structure with smooth borders and an attenuation value of -70 to - 120 HU. Since soft-tissue dense tumors do not have a specific attenuation value, it is normally impossible to make a differential diagnosis on the basis of CT numbers. These tumors show homogeneous enhancement after bolus administration of contrast medium, which normally demarcates their smooth borders from the surrounding tissue, making them more easily identifiable. The blood cavities of *hemangiomas* and angiovenous dysplasias increase their enhancement; vascular structures can often be demonstrated in the bolus phase. Phleboliths should be interpreted as signs of hemangioma.

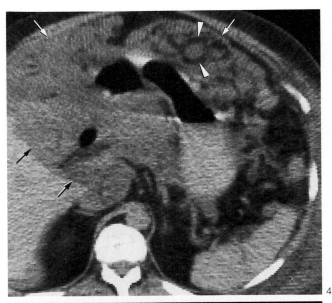

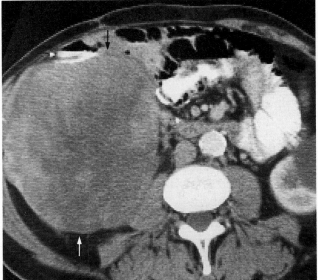

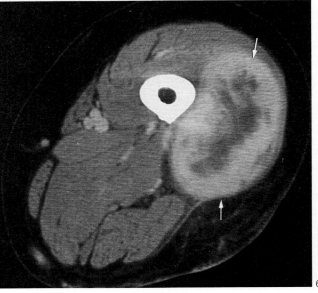

Fig. 24-4. Liposarcoma. Sharply marginated, fatty tumor components (►) can be seen within this intra-abdominal soft-tissue tumor that infiltrates adjacent organs (→).

Fig. 24-5. Liposarcoma. Homogeneous, expanding lesion in right mesogastrium. Because of its fatty tissue content, the attenuation value of the tumor, on the whole, is homogeneously reduced.

Fig. 24-6. Liposarcoma in the left thigh. Plain scans revealed a greatly pleomorphic tumor with an attenuation value of 30 HU. After contrast medium administration, it exhibited considerable, mainly peripheral enhancement.

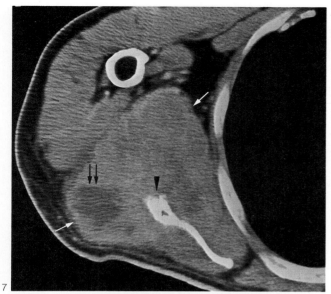

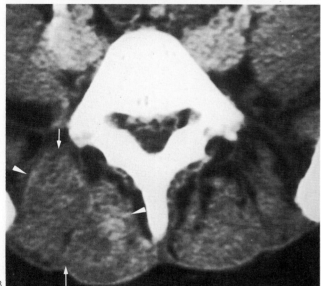

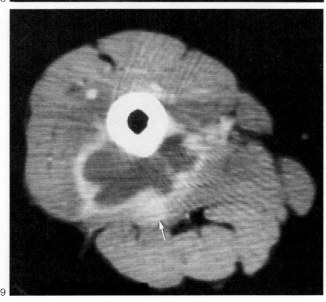

Since rapidly growing neoplasms are characterized by necrosis, edema and hemorrhage, ill-defined borders and inhomogeneous enhancement should be taken as signs of tumor *malignancy*. These tissue signs can usually be clearly demonstrated after intravenous administration of contrast medium. In addition to tissue regression, the attenuation of a malignant tumor can be reduced because of mixed tissue elements. Variation in the amount of fatty components leads to the appearance of homogeneous or inhomogeneous areas displaying CT numbers ranging from -50 to +20 HU. Myxomatous tissue appears hypodense as compared with muscle tissue.

The *malignant fibrous histiocytoma* is relatively common. It usually appears on CT scans as a lobulated, inhomogeneous mass with ill-defined margins and inhomogeneous contents. This inhomogeneous pattern becomes even more pronounced after contrast medium has been administered.

Most *fibrosarcomas* appear as an widespread, ill-defined, soft-tissue dense mass, but the attenuation of some fibrosarcomas can be inhomogeneously reduced due to myxomatous tissue elements.

Like retroperitoneal tumors, *liposarcomas* in the extremities also display extremely variable patterns of enhancement ranging from homogeneous low density to strandlike areas within fatty tissue (fibrotic, myxomatous, or mucinous components). Sarcomatous degeneration must be assumed when the normally homogeneous, transparent appearance of a lipoma is densified by localized soft-tissue dense strands of tissue. Smoothly marginated borders and homogeneous CT numbers do not necessarily

Fig. 24-7. Rhabdomyosarcoma. The teres major (→) and subcapsular (→) muscles are dilated. After contrast medium administration, hyperdense areas (⇒) representing tumor necrosis appear. The lateral scapular border is eroded (►).

Fig. 24-8. Ectosteal Ewing's sarcoma. On the right, the erector spinae muscle is slightly dilated (→), and there is slight, hypodense masking of muscular septa. Discrete peripheral enhancement occurs after bolus contrast medium administration (►). At this stage, tumorous infiltration cannot be differentiated from inflammatory infiltration.

Fig. 24-9. Malignant fibrous histiocytoma. The lesion lies parosteal and exhibits peripheral enhancement after contrast medium administration.

exclude the possibility of malignancy. In contrast, bone erosion, invasion of adjacent tissue and metastases provide positive evidence of malignancy.

The goal of the CT examination is to provide an exact pre- operative assessment of tumor extension. Not only the tumor itself, but also the borders of the affected compartment (muscle fasciae, periosteum, cortex of the bone) as well as the relationship of these structures to the larger vessels and the nerves must be adequately visualized for proper diagnosis. The size of the tumor is frequently overestimated when peritumoral edema is present. Targeted intravenous contrast medium administration usually makes the tumor borders more distinguishable from adjacent structures.

Magnetic resonance imaging (MRI), like computed tomography, is often unable to provide the necessary evidence for differential diagnosis. However, scanning in a longitudinal plane makes it easier to evaluate the tumor extent, especially since the corresponding pulse sequences can increase the tissue contrast difference of tumor tissue and surrounding tissue. On the other hand, computed tomography is superior to MRI in demonstrating slight amounts of bone erosion, calcification and gas.

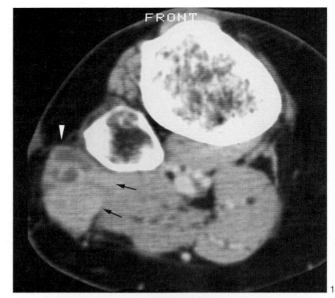

10

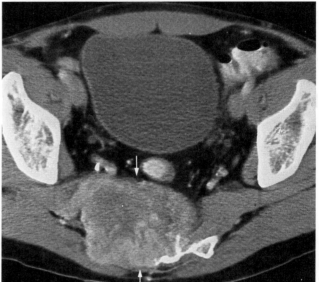

11

Fig. 24-10. Malignant schwannoma of the fibular nerve. The tumor is sharply delineated (→). It clearly enhances and contains areas of hypodensity, which correspond to hemorrhages (►). The nerve itself cannot be seen.

Fig. 24-12. Malignant fibrous histiocytoma in the thigh. On plain scans, the tumor exhibits an inhomogeneous range of attenuation values in areas that show greatly variable contrast enhancement: (a) plain scan, (b) early and (c) late bolus contrast medium phases.

Fig. 24-11. Malignant paraganglioma. The overall sharply marginated mass has obliterated the right sacrum and exhibits strong, nonuniform enhancement.

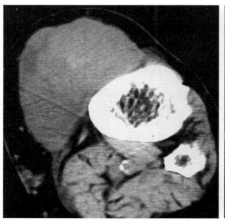

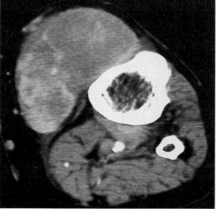

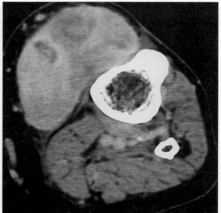

12a

12c

Chapter 25
Bone Tumors

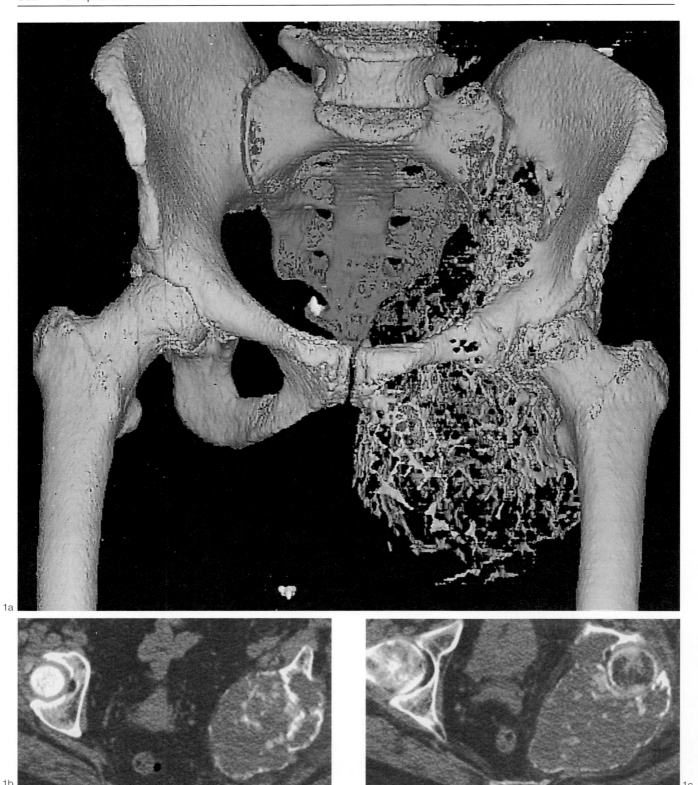

Fig. 25-1. Pelvic osteosarcoma.
a) 3D scan from ventral view. The bony tumor matrix is well demonstrated in the 3-dimensional image.
b, c) The CT scan demonstrates the positional relationship of the tumor to surrounding soft-tissue structures. The external borders of the tumor are surrounded by a delicate layer of bone.

Bone Tumors

Conventional radiographic techniques can provide images detailing the morphological appearance and localization of bone tumors, which can extensively narrow the diagnosis. Computed tomography may be required to provide additional diagnostic data such as:

- the extent of the tumor, especially along the internal and external contours of the cortex;
- clear images of the medullary space;
- proof of calcification;
- proof of soft-tissue elements;
- assessment of soft-tissue infiltration;
- differentiation of vascular, avascular, fatty, cystic and solid tissue types.

These factors all have an impact on the differential diagnosis. Magnetic resonance imaging (MRI) is usually the primary imaging modality.

Chondrogenous Tumors

Benign bone tumors *(chondroma, chondromyxoid fibroma, cartilaginous exostosis, osteochondroma)* are usually characterized by homogeneous distribution of calcium salts in the cartilaginous matrix. *Enchondromas* in long bones can be differentiated from bone infarcts on the basis of the "maplike" marginal calcification observed in the latter.

One must assume that an osteochondroma has malignant changed to a *chondrosarcoma* when inhomogeneous calcification is found within areas of increased chondrification. Chondrosarcomas of low malignancy are usually grow connected and eccentrically lobulated. They

Table 25-1. Classification of primary bone tumors

Type of Tissue	Age (years)	Benign Tumors	Age (years)	Malign Tumors
Cartilage	10–25	Chondro-blastoma	30–60	Chondro-sarcoma (primary, secondary)
	10–25	Chondro-myxoid fibroma		
	10–30	Osteo-chondroma	20–60	Mesen-chymal chondro-sarcoma
	10–40	Chondroma		
Bone	40–50	Osteoma	10–25	Osteo-sarcoma
	10–30	Osteoid osteoma		
	10–30	Osteo-blastoma	30–60	Parosteal osteosarcoma
Marrow Elements			40–60	Plasma-cell myeloma
			5–20	Ewing's sarcoma
			30–60	Reticulum cell sarcoma (histiocytic malignant lymphoma) (Liposarcoma)
		(Lipoma)		
Vessels	20–50	Hemangioma Glomes tumor Lymph-angioma		Angiosarcoma
Fibrous Tissue	20–30	Desmoplastic fibroma	20–60	Fibrosarcoma
Neurogenous Tissue		Neuro-fibromatous neurilemmoma Ganglio-neuroma		
	20–40	Giant-cell tumor	20–40	Giant-cell tumor Adamantinoma
			40–60	Chordoma

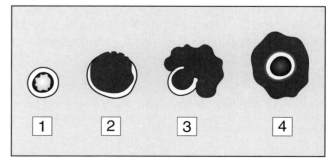

Fig. 25-2. Radiologic appearance of bone tumor growth. According to Brown as well as Lodwick's classification system, three tumor types can be distinguished via CT. In Type I tumors (2), expanding growth narrows the cortex (pseudocortex). In Type II (3), there is a cortical defect with asymmetrical tumor growth. In Type III (4), there is infiltrative, permeative tumor growth with finely porous transmigration of the cortical substance.

are further characterized by ringlike and arci-form calcification within tumor tissue with an attenuation value of more than 50 HU. Highly malignant chondrosarcomas, on the other hand, contain areas of necrosis with reduced CT numbers (lower than 50 HU) and subtly recognizable, amorphous calcification organized in a more concentric configuration. Clear signs of malignancy are bone erosion and bone destruction within the central chondrosarcoma.

Osteogenic Tumors

The *osteoma* appears on CT scans as a sharply defined and homogeneously dense bony structure. The typical nidus of an *osteoid osteoma* can be seen within dense bone and periosteal tissue; enhancement is observed after the administration of contrast medium. *Medullary osteosarcomas* are classified as lytic, sclerotic, or lytic-sclerotic. Infiltration of the medullary space (demonstrated as soft-tissue replacement of fatty tissue), expansion and permeation of the cortical substance and parosteal spreading can be readily demonstrated on CT scans. After the administration of contrast medium, these usually well vascularized tumors can be distinguished from surrounding soft-tissue. Pre- treatment assessment of fascial borders, vessels and nerve structures should also be performed during this examination. Immature osteosarcomas are frequently identifiable only as very discrete cortical lesions in the sites of predilection for tumor occurrence. Computed tomography can provide important evidence of discrete matrix calcification, which can significantly narrow the diagnosis. Parosteal matrix ossification is a typical sign of osteosarcoma. The soft-tissue components of

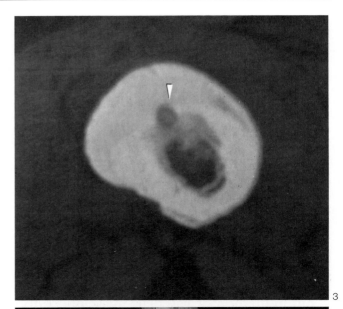

3

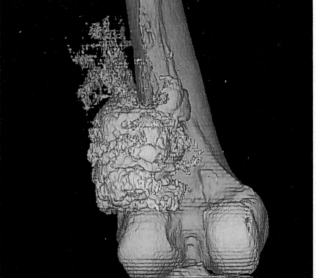

4a

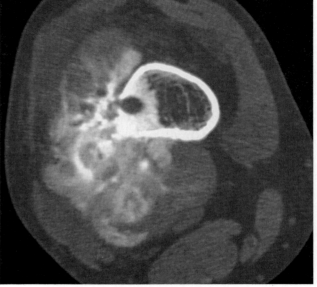

4b

Fig. 25-3. Osteoid osteoma. The clearly thickened femur shaft contains a translucent structure (►), corresponding to the typical nidus of an osteoid osteoma.

Fig. 25-4a, b. Femoral osteochondrosarcoma. Parosteal tumor ossification and calcification can be demonstrated on 3D images taken from the dorsal aspect (a). CT demonstrates the location of ossification and soft-tissue tumor constituents with respect to the surrounding muscles.

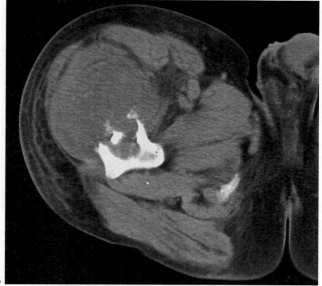

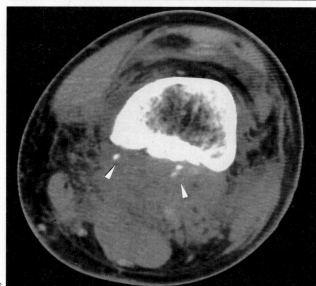

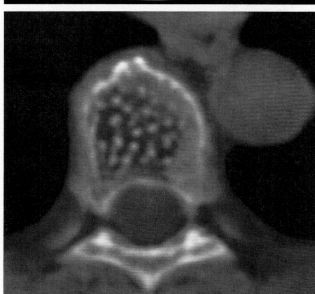

juxtacortical osteosarcomas (parosteal and periosteal osteosarcoma) can be assessed by computed tomography. In patients receiving chemotherapy, CT is a useful diagnostic tool for assessing reduction in tumor volume, especially of the soft-tissue components, and increase in tumor ossification, as well as for defining the limits of tumor borders.

Fibrous Tumors

Malignant fibrous histiocytomas and *fibrosarcomas* are typically ill-defined, osseous lesions which may demonstrate considerable intraosteal expansion as well as cortical breakthrough into surrounding soft-tissue structures. Even after the *administration of contrast medium*, the typical infiltrative growth of the tumor often makes it impossible to clearly distinguish the tumor from surrounding soft-tissue. Regressive calcification may occur, but cannot be differentiated from calcification of cartilaginous tissue on CT grounds. As compared with osteogenic and chondrosarcomas, periosteal reactions (lamellated and spiculated formations) are more uncommon.

Myelogenic Tumors

The *lipoma*, characterized by a delicate rim of sclerosis, can lead to swelling of bone due to osteolysis. Because of their fat-dense attenuation values, lipomas can be clearly identified on CT scans. Typical central areas of calcification are often seen. *Ewing's sarcoma* displays various patterns of destruction (Lodwick grades 2 and 3) on conventional scans. Ewing's sarcoma

Fig. 25-5. Chondrosarcoma. The tumor has spread beyond the cortical layer of the proximal femur shaft. It contains extraosseous soft-tissue constituents, which are sharply delineated from the surrounding muscles (false capsule).

Fig. 25-6. Osteosarcoma of the distal femur. Demonstration of primarily parosteal soft-tissue constituents with small areas of calcification proximal to the femur (▸).

Fig. 25-7. Hemangiomatous vertebral body. On CT scans, this can be identified as a coarsening of the vertical spongiosa structure, which can affect part of, or the entire vertebral body.

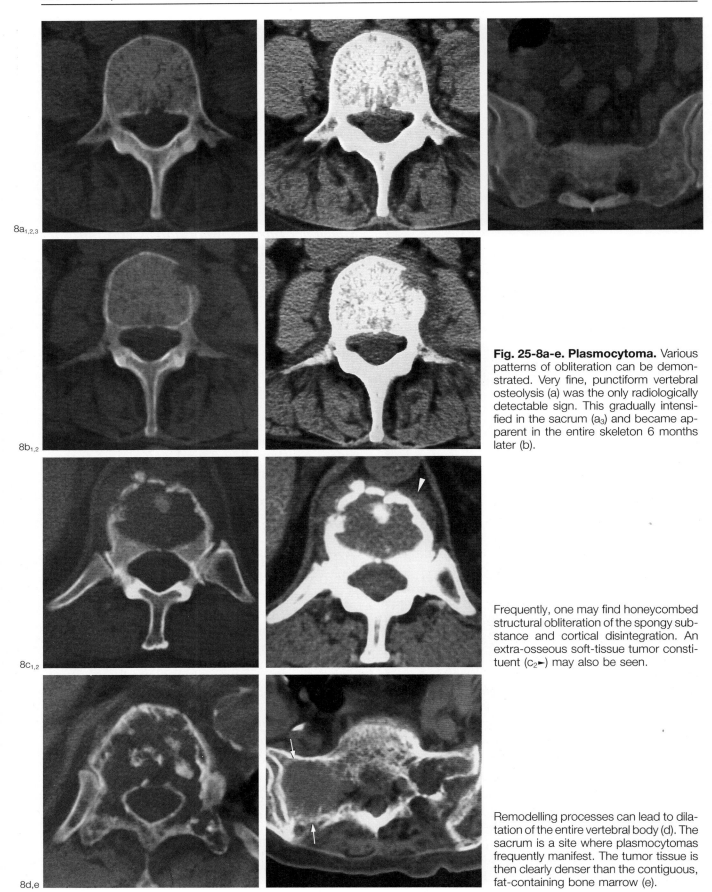

8a₁,₂,₃

8b₁,₂

8c₁,₂

8d,e

Fig. 25-8a-e. Plasmocytoma. Various patterns of obliteration can be demonstrated. Very fine, punctiform vertebral osteolysis (a) was the only radiologically detectable sign. This gradually intensified in the sacrum (a₃) and became apparent in the entire skeleton 6 months later (b).

Frequently, one may find honeycombed structural obliteration of the spongy substance and cortical disintegration. An extra-osseous soft-tissue tumor constituent (c₂►) may also be seen.

Remodelling processes can lead to dilatation of the entire vertebral body (d). The sacrum is a site where plasmocytomas frequently manifest. The tumor tissue is then clearly denser than the contiguous, fat-containing bone marrow (e).

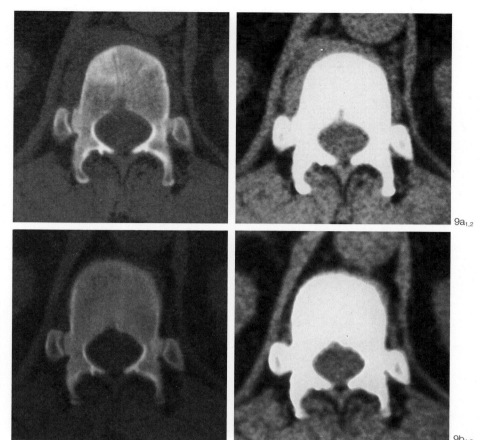

9a₁,₂

9b₁,₂

Fig. 25-9. Hodgkin's disease under chemotherapy. Structurally, the body of the vertebra is irregularly thickened (a_1). A perivertebral, soft-tissue tumor constituent is also visible (a_2). After the completion of chemotherapy, sclerosis of the spongiosa has increased (b_1). The disappearance of the soft-tissue component indicates the success of chemotherapy. Biopsy revealed osteomyelofibrosis of the medullary space.

usually produces lytic lesions that may contain a variable proportion of osteosclerotic elements. Even in early stages, extensive parosteal tumor areas are observed, which are more clearly demonstrated after bolus injection of contrast medium. Medullary infiltration is often extensive and can be demonstrated on CT scans as a soft- tissue dense structure within the normally fat-dense medullary space. It is often difficult to differentiate these tumors from osteomyelitis, but the diagnosis can be decisively narrowed with good knowledge of the CT appearance of the tumors.

The *reticulum cell sarcoma* is a type of *malignant lymphoma* that arises primarily in bone. It is a permeative destructive lesion which causes cortical destruction. Parosteal soft-tissue components of the tumor, which can be demonstrated on CT scans, can therefore be expected. Other types of malignant lymphoma (*Hodgkin's* and *non-Hodgkin's lymphomas*) are characterized by ill- defined margins of os-

teolysis (permeative, moth-eaten), reactive sclerosis and, thus, mixed structural changes. More severe signs of sclerosis are typical of Hodgkin's disease ("ivory whorl"). Computerized tomography is normally performed to demonstrate and assess soft-tissue components, especially in perivertebral and epidural regions. This data makes it possible to differentiate between secondary tumor growth that has spread to bone from a primary bone tumor (stage 4) when the type and pattern of tumor dissemination is known.

The *solid plasmocytoma*, which appears as an area of osteolysis on plain radiographs, can frequently be demonstrated on CT scans with clear swelling of (pseudo) cortical substance in the absence of visible periosteal reactions. Extraosseous soft-tissue components that develop after pathologic fractures are usually more pronounced than normal callus formations. *Generalized plasmocytomas* usually can be identified by morphological radiologic pat-

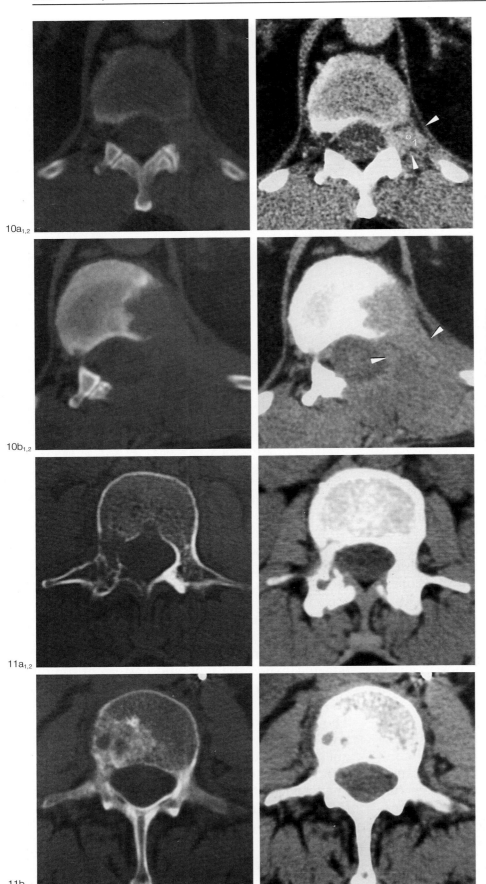

10a₁,₂

10b₁,₂

11a₁,₂

11b₁,₂

Fig. 25-10. Vertebral metastases. Metastasizing urothelial carcinoma. Bone destruction was not found at the bone window setting (a₁). With the soft-tissue window, however, thickening of the neuroforamen was revealed (a₂►). Six months later, extensive bone destruction was found. The soft-tissue constituent of the tumor has a massive appearance, but does not constrict the thecal sac (b₂).

Fig. 25-11. Metastasizing carcinoma of the breast. Discrete osteolysis in the region of the root of the arch at L2 (a₁), however, without signs of extraosseous tumor components. Metastasizing carcinoma of the breast during chemotherapy: clear recalcification of osteolytic structures (b₁), and reappearance of the original vertebral contours.

terns such as generalized osteoporosis in the form of multiple osteolyses or, very seldom, as diffuse osteosclerosis. CT is, however, a much more sensitive means of detecting osteolysis. When the pattern of invasion is homogeneous, computed tomography is even more sensitive than skeletal radionuclide imaging in detecting plasmocytomas. Within the fat-containing medullary space, the foci of plasmocytomas can be demonstrated as areas of soft-tissue shadowing, even when osseous destruction is minimal. Demonstration of extraosseous tumor components is another significant task of CT in the diagnosis of generalized plasmocytoma.

Hemangiomas of bone appear on CT scans as sharply marginated foci of osteolysis with a sclerotic or garland-like rim. They are usually discovered as an incidental finding inside vertebral bodies and display characteristically increasing coarseness of the vertical trabecular spongiosa. This appears on transverse scans as a densified, punctiform structure within a hypodense area of the medullary space. In these cases, only isolated osteoporosis of a vertebral body, which also can lead to a coarsening of the vertical spongiosa, must be considered in the differential diagnosis. After a substantial, protracted *bolus of contrast medium*, it is possible to differentiate hemangiotic blood-filled cavities (pooling) from the poorly vascularized medullary space of osteoporosis.

Most *giant cell tumors* are eccentrically located in the epiphysis of long bones. They are normally demarcated from bone without a sclerotic rim and frequently display parosteal expansion. These relatively well vascularized tumors have attenuation values ranging from 20 to 70 HU and display clear enhancement of ca. 50 HU in non-necrotic tumor areas. Giant cell tumors are therefore distinguishable from surrounding soft-tissue.

When a giant cell tumor is diagnosed, precise computer tomographic staging must be included in the pre-operative planning of the normally radical surgery. It is often difficult to distinguish between giant cell tumors and aneurysmal bone cysts. The two lesions can be distinguished computer tomographically, because eggshell-like areas of periosteal ossification and fluid fluid levels which are absent in giant cell tumor are found in bone cysts.

Chapter 26
The Spine

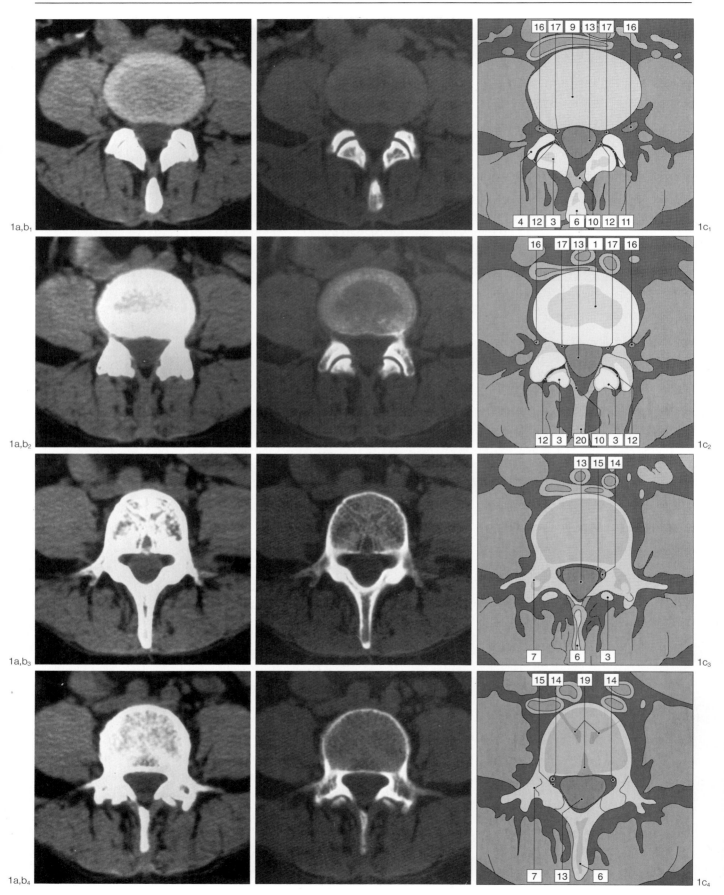

1a,b₁

16 17 9 13 17 16

4 12 3 6 10 12 11

1c₁

1a,b₂

16 17 13 1 17 16

12 3 20 10 3 12

1c₂

1a,b₃

13 15 14

7 6 3

1c₃

1a,b₄

15 14 19 14

7 13 6

1c₄

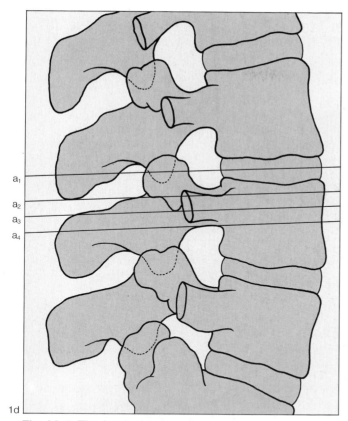

Fig. 26-1. The lumbar spine.

a) Transverse section at soft-tissue setting (window + 30 HU). See (d) for level.

b) The same transverse section at bone setting (window + 300 HU).

c) Diagram.

d) Lateral view.

Key to symbols:

 1 Vertebral body
 2 Root of the arch
 3 Superior articular process
 4 Inferior articular process
 5 Intervertebral joint
 6 Spinous process
 7 Transverse process
 8 Spondylophytes
 9 Intervertebral disk
10 Ligamentum flavum
11 Intervertebral joint
12 Intervertebral joint capsule
13 Thecal sac
14 Nerve root pocket
15 Lateral recess
16 Nerve root
17 Veins of the internal vertebral venous plexus
18 Paravertebral veins (external vertebral venous plexus)
19 Basovertebral vessels
20 Interspinal ligaments

The Spine

Anatomy and Imaging

By scanning a *vertebral body* parallel to its end plate, the center of the vertebral body can be accurately determined from the level of entry of the basivertebral vein along the posterior aspect. At this level, lower sections of the arch superior to the neural foramen are included in the scan, and the entire vertebral spinal canal appears as a closed structure due to demonstration of the arch, lateral mass with articular processes, lamina, and spinous process. Venous points of entry are usually marked by a small, bony spur. The veins run a y-shaped course throughout the corresponding bony channels, where they extend ventrally and enter the cortical substance. High-resolution scans taken at a bone window setting show the cortical substance and fine structures of the spongy substance. Even subtle lesions can therefore be detected early. Because the upper and lower plates frequently have a slight, sagging depression, disc-related partial volume effects often cause them to appear on CT scans as inhomogeneous structures with large, central areas of hypodensity.

When thin sections are scanned, *intervertebral discs* appear mostly homogeneous. A discrete, central low-density area is more likely to reflect partial volume effects than a true density reduction in the nucleus pulposus as compared to the annulus fibrosus. A healthy intervertebral disc has an attenuation value of 70 ± 5 HU. Its external contours conform to the boundaries of contiguous vertebral bodies. The dorsal edges of intervertebral discs in the cervical region are relatively rectilinear. Extending inferior to the lumbar region, the contours form a variably ventroconvex curvature. The configuration of intervertebral discs again becomes more rectilinear at the L4-5 level of the lumbar spine, and then more dorsoconvex at the L5-S1 level. The vertical height of lumbar intervertebral discs ranges from 8 to 12 mm. The height of

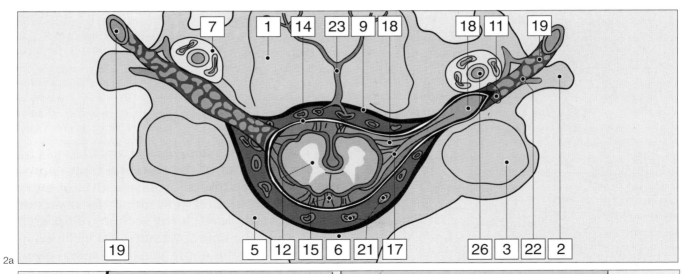

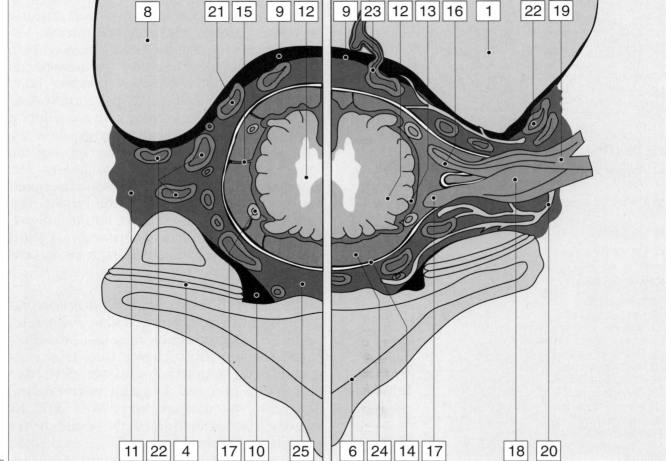

Fig. 26-2. Soft-tissue structures of the spinal canal.

a) At the level of the 4th cervical vertebra.

b) At the level of the 4th thoracic vertebra.

Key to symbols:

1 Vertebral body
2 Transverse process
3 Articular process
4 Intervertebral joint
5 Lamina
6 Spinous process
7 Vertebral foramen
8 Intervertebral disk
9 Posterior longitudinal ligament
10 Ligamentum flavum
11 Intervertebral foramen
12 Spinal cord
13 Pia mater

14 Dura mater (plus arachnoid mater and subdural space)
15 Ligamentum denticulatum
16 Anterior root (of the spinal nerves)
17 Posterior root (of the spinal nerves)
18 Spinal ganglion

19 Spinal nerve
20 Meningeal branch
21 Internal venous plexus
22 Intervertebral vein
23 Basivertebral vein
24 Subarachnoid space
25 Extradural space
26 Vertebral artery

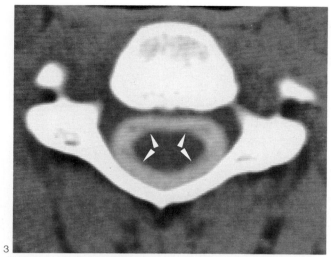

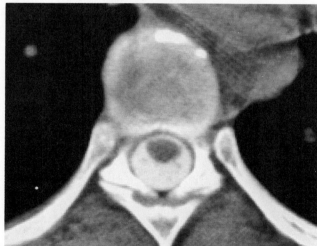

Fig. 26-3. Cervical spinal cord in postmyelographic CT scan. The contrast enhanced spinal cord is well delineated from spinal fluid. The exiting nerve roots (►) are discretely visible.

Fig. 26-4. Thoracic spinal cord in postmyelographic CT; demonstration of exiting nerve roots.

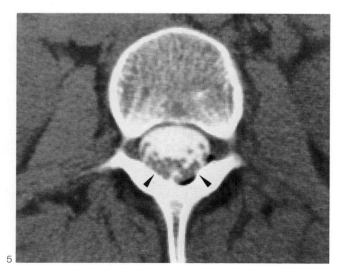

lumbosacral discs, on the other hand, is lower (often less than 5 mm). The height of cervical discs is greater than that of thoracic discs, but less than that of lumbar discs.

Sections taken at the level of the intervertebral disc show, dorsally, the *intervertebral articulations* of the vertebra and a section of the spinous process. The anterior articulating surface corresponds to the inferior articular process of the upper .vertebral body, and the posterior articulating surface belongs to the superior articular process of the lower vertebral body. The articular surfaces (facets) of the cervical spine are oriented along a frontal plane, whereas those in the lumbar region form a curvature with an open posterior angle of approximately 90°.

The *vertebral (spinal) canal* is not a simple cylindrical tube, but rather, is a rod of variable diameter. Because of the tile-shaped configuration of the vertebral (neural) arch, the vertebral canal is always narrowest at the upper borders of the lamina of a segment. It broadens slightly in its inferior, dorsal sections. The posterior *longitudinal ligament* covers the posterior side of the vertebral bodies and, thus, covers the ventral section of the spinal canal. The midline is reinforced by longitudinal fibers and is interlaced with transverse fibers at the level of the intervertebral discs. The transverse fibers, in turn, are attached in a belt-like fashion via the neural foramen to the fibers of the anterior longitudinal fibers. The posterior convexity of the spinal canal is closed by the ca. 3-mm-thick ligamenta flava, which are attached to the superior part of the lamina. They extend obliquely along the anterior aspect to the next spinous process. At the same time, the ligamenta flava form part of the articular capsule of small articulations. Since they are of higher density than the thecal sac and contiguous epidural fat, the ligamenta flava are always readily identifiable. Interspinous and supraspinous ligaments are located between the spinous processes.

Fig. 26-5. The cauda equina in postmyelographic CT. Individual nerve roots can be seen in detail.

Along the midline of the vertebral bodies, the posterior longitudinal ligament is slightly elevated by a pad of veins at the level of the point of entry of the basivertebral vein. The *veins* pass through the posterior longitudinal ligament and form a longitudinal pair of epidural veins on each side of the vertebral body (lateral and medial anterior veins). They form a rope-like ladder from the posterior to the longitudinal ligament to the anterior extradural space. In each neural foramen, they give off branches that create a plexiform structure around the nerves. The venous plexuses of the cervical region are especially prominent. The plexuses also communicate with the anterior epidural veins in a ringlike fashion. The entirety of epidural venous plexuses is called the *internal vertebral plexus*. Through the basivertebral vein and exiting intervertebral veins, it communicates reticularly with the *external vertebral plexus* (ascending paravertebral veins, inferior vena cava).

The center of the spinal canal is padded by the *thecal sac*, which contains the spinal cord and nerves and usually ends at the level of the second sacral vertebra at the point where the external filum terminale begins. The complementary space between the dura and the vertebral spinal column is filled with hypodense epidural fat (-50 to -100 HU), which delineates the external contours of the thecal sac and spinal nerve sheaths. Epidural fat is thickest in the lumbar region, where longitudinal epidural veins embedded in fat appear on the posterior contours of the vertebra as punctiform, 2 to 3 mm large densification structures on plain CT scans.

In adults, the *spinal cord* extends to the T12-L1 level. When scans are free of artifacts, the surrounding subarachnoid space is seen as a narrow, hypodense ring accompanied by vertebral arteries in the occipito-cervical junction. In the

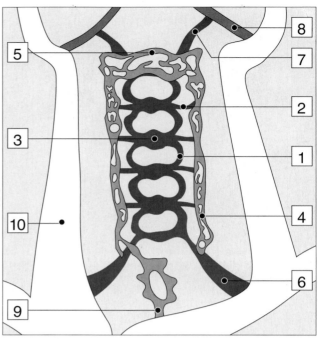

Fig. 26-6. Cervical epidural venous plexus (according to Theron).

Key to symbols:

1 Anterior longitudinal epidural veins	5 Occipital venous plexus
2 Intervertebral veins	6 Vertebral veins
3 Basivertebral veins	7 Condylar emissary veins
4 Vertebral venous plexus (around vertebral artery)	8 Inferior petrosal sinus
	9 Right intercostal vein
	10 Intervertebral vein

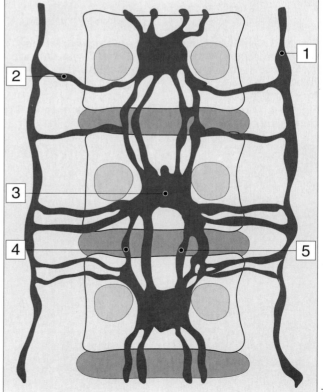

Fig. 26-7. Lumbar epidural venous plexus.

Key to symbols:

1 Ascending lumbar vein	4 Lateral anterior epidural veins
2 Intervertebral veins	5 Medial anterior epidural veins
3 Basivertebral veins	

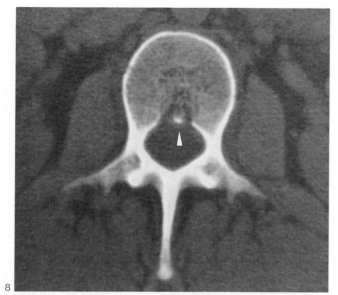

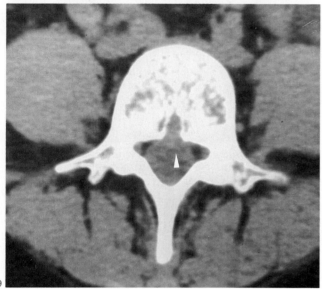

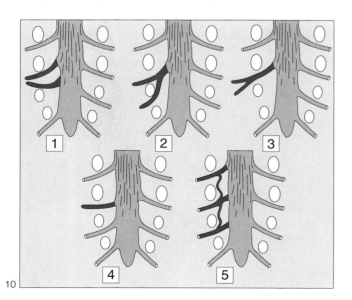

region of the cauda equina, the thecal sac and its branching nerve roots are usually homogeneously hypodense on CT scans. Bunched nerve fibers (hemicords) are sometimes discretely visible. High-resolution, detailed images of the sino-auricular cavity can be obtained after intrathecal contrast administration *(postmyelographic)*. The spinal cord as well as the dorsal and ventral nerve roots, including the fine ligamenta denticulata, can then be demonstrated. As in myelography, free nerve roots are opacified up to the level of the spinal ganglion on CT scans.

The *nerve roots* arise from a point just below the end plate of the corresponding vertebra. A small, lateral bony excavation (the lateral recess) can be seen on the vertebral body, especially near the last three lumbar segments. The nerve root passes through the *lateral recess* before it enters the intervertebral foramen from a point below the root of the arch. The superior dorsal boundary is formed by the ligamentum flavum and the superior articular process. The anteroposterior width of the recess is usually larger than 5 mm. It is assumed to be constricted at widths of 3 mm or less.

The internal vertebral plexus can be demonstrated after *intravenous contrast medium administration*. The longitudinal veins are then visible as punctiform structures. Intraforaminal veins are more prominent in the cervical region, where they form a cuff around nerve structures. A large dose of contrast medium will, therefore, enhance of most of the neural foramen. The nerves are then distinguishable

Fig. 26-8. Point of entry of the basivertebral vein. The configuration is variable, and it is sometimes covered by an osseous lamella.

Fig. 26-9. Basivertebral plexus at the point of entry of the basivertebral vein. This can protrude into the spinal canal as a prominent soft-tissue structure.

Fig. 26-10. Anomalies of the points of exit of the nerve roots.

Key to symbols:
1 Converging nerve root   4 Horizontal nerve root
2 Diverging nerve root   5 Nerve root anastomosis
3 Double nerve root

as hypodense structures. The lumbar neuroforamina are broader, and nerves make up 30% of the cross- sectional area. The remaining area is mainly filled by fatty tissue, which delineates the nerve roots. The visibility of foraminal lumbar veins is only slightly improved by contrast administration. The annulus fibrosus shows contrast enhancement in young patients, but not in adults.

Degenerative Spinal Diseases

Individual movement of vertebral bodies is restricted by strong articular connections. The intervertebral discs, the elastic anterior and posterior longitudinal ligaments which surround them, and the intervertebral articulations constitute three units of flexibility. Together with their contiguous vertebral structures, they constitute a *segment* of the spinal column. Spinal degeneration begins with dehydration of the intervertebral discs with consecutive reduction in the space of the discs. The latter condition leads to structural loosening of a spinal segment and, thus, to nonphysiologic stress on joints and ligaments. This, in turn, can ultimately lead to intervertebral arthrosis and spondylosis. Intervertebral disc degeneration, the primary cause of disc herniation, worsens after these degenerative processes set in.

Degenerative Processes in Intervertebral Discs

Increasing dehydration of the nucleus pulposus with consecutive changes in biochemical composition causes a reduction in height of the disc and bulging of the annulus fibrosus outside the external contours of the end plates of the vertebral body. Gas is a sign of dehydration and increased stress, whereas calcification of the fibrous ring is a sign of regressive or repair processes.

• CT

Intervertebral disc degeneration is characterized by a homogeneous, smoothly marginated,

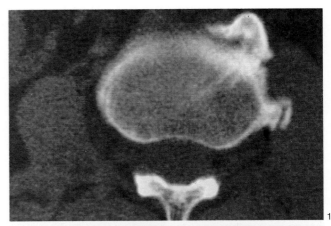
11

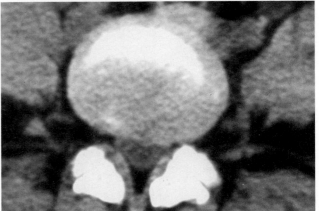
12

Fig. 26-11. Spondylophyte. Bony excresences along the edges of the vertebral bodies are sensitively detected via computed tomography.

Fig. 26-12. Disc protrusion. The disc protrudes beyond the rim of the vertebral body. It is smoothly marginated and eccentric.

Fig. 26-13. Disc degeneration with vacuum phenomena. The posterior edge of the disc exhibits dorsoconvex curvature. The external contours are somewhat wavey.

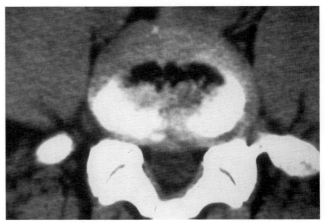

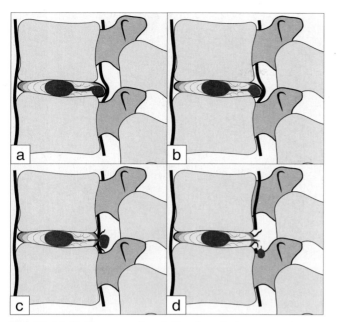

Fig. 26-14. Pathogenesis of disc herniation; examples illustrate subligamental (a,b) and transligamental (c,d) herniation, (b,d) each as a free fragment.

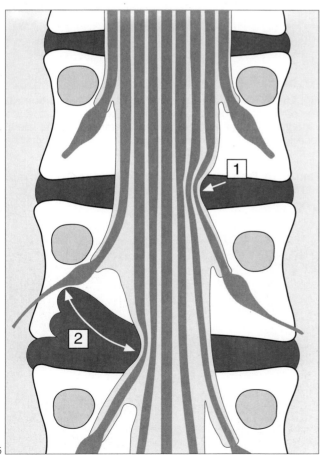

circular disc herniation that extends beyond the circumferential borders of a vertebral body. The dorsal disc contours, which conform to the structure of the contiguous vertebral bodies, are usually compromised. Unlike magnetic resonance imaging, the annulus fibrosus and the nucleus pulposus cannot be reliable differentiated on the basis of their attenuation value. Computed tomography is, however, a sensitive method of detecting calcification and vacuum phenomena.

Disc Herniation and Prolapse

As disc degeneration worsens, radial lacerations develop in the inner circular layers of the fibrous ring, and they are replaced by nucleus pulposus tissue (internal derangement). Local thinning of the annulus fibrosus then leads to minor bulging of the disc contours. Subligamental herniations are covered by the posterior longitudinal ligament and occur when the external layers of the fibrous ring have been compromised. In transligamental herniation, the longitudinal ligament is penetrated and the protruding tissue either forms a "buttonhole" configuration around the site of perforation or is found as a free fragment in the extradural space behind the vertebral bodies (sequestered fragment). The posterior longitudinal ligament is attached to the annular apophyses of the vertebral bodies and is stronger along the median plane. Therefore, when the prolapse is subligamentally located, tissue from the nucleus pulposus therefore usually migrates laterally. If the ligament is detached from the vertebral body, it may, instead, migrate longitudinally as a free fragment to a position behind the vertebral bodies.

Three basic types of disc herniation can be classified according to their location:
- *Medial herniation*, which compromises the spinal cord or cauda equina from a ventral aspect.

Fig. 26-15. Localization of disc herniation. Mediolateral location (1): irritation of nerve roots that emerge inferior to the disc. Lateral location (2): irritation of nerve roots at the level of the disc and inferior to it.

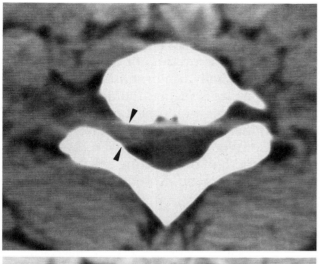

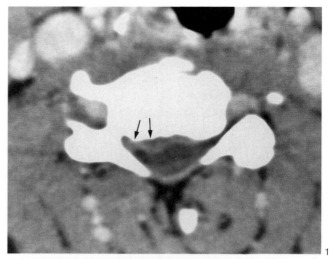

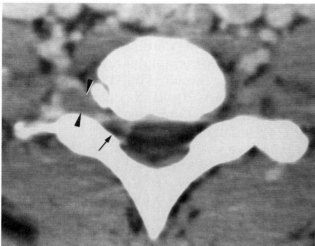

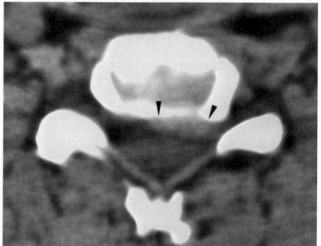

Fig. 26-16. Lateral disc herniation. In scan with slight arti-fact formation, a soft-tissue structure suggestive of disc her-niation is found at the site of entry of the neural foramen at C6-7 (a). Intravenous CM administration demarcates the disc se-questrum (b→) and the spinal ganglion (►). After intrathecal CM administration the same findings with richer contrast en-hancement are seen. The configuration is identical (c).

Fig. 26-17. Mediolateral, right-sided disc herniation. a) The edges of the disc protrude slightly beyond the rim of the vertebral body (→) and obstructs the entrance of the lateral recess (→). **b)** The sharp-edged contours of the disc can be seen left mediolateral, behind the vertebral body.

Fig. 26-18. Disc herniation. The broad contours of the disc (→) extend beyond the rim of the vertebral body.

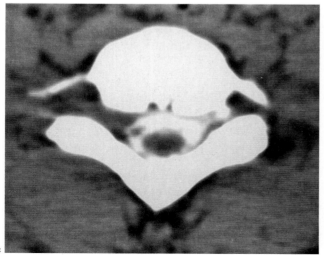

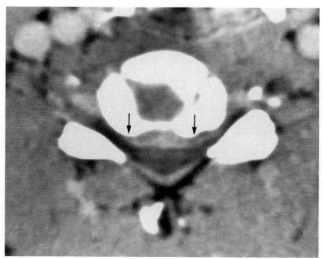

– *Mediolateral herniation*, which affects the spinal cord and/or the nerve root (more often affects nerve roots in the cauda region).

– *Lateral herniation* can be intraforaminal or extraforaminal and irritates the nerve roots seen at the same level.

• *Cervical Disc Herniation*

Cervical herniations usually occur at the C6-7 level of the spine, followed by herniations at the C7-T1 level. Because of the midline reinforcement provided by the dorsal longitudinal ligament, mediolateral disc herniation is most frequent. Herniation is usually transligamental and extends laterally and cranially to the corresponding neural foramen, thus compressing the nerve roots there. Since the extensive interspinal venous plexus drains via the intervertebral foramen, local venous stasis therefore occurs when it is obstructed.

• **CT**

Plain scans: *Soft-tissue* that bulges into the spinal canal or the neural foramen is a characteristic sign of disc herniation. Beam-hardening artifacts frequently lead to a reduction in the CT density of the spinal canal and make it more difficult to identify intraspinal structures. In order to reduce artifacts in the cervico-thoracic junction (caused by overshadowing from the shoulders), one should, if necessary, apply other techniques of patient positioning. Thin-section scanning reduces artifacts and provides highly detailed images, especially of the bony borders of the foramen.

Contrast-enhanced scans: Intravenous contrast medium can improve the differentiation of soft-tissue structures. The dorsal borders are formed by the dorsal annulus fibrosus, the posterior longitudinal ligament, the posterior spinal venous plexus and the ventral wall of the thecal sac. The latter appears as a small seam that is hypodense as compared with nucleus pulposus tissue or sequestered material. Venous stasis in the neural foramen is an indication of obstruction, which may be caused by lateral disc herniation or by a small, free fragment. The mass, itself, may not be visible.

Differential diagnosis: Evaluation of the status of cervical discs must include an examination of osseous structures at a wide window setting. Identification of osseous excrescences on the sides of vertebral bodies and the uncinate processes can be helpful in differentiating degenerative bony constriction of the nerve exits (*uncovertebral arthrosis*), *spinal stenosis*, and *disc herniation*.

• *Lumbosacral Disc Herniation*

The L5-S1 and L4-5 levels are involved in 95% of all disc herniations. Herniations at the L3-4 level are relatively infrequent (4%).

• **CT**

The characteristic sign of a herniation is focal bulging of the dorsal disc contours into the spinal canal, which can thus be differentiated from the uniform, broad bulge seen in patients with disc degeneration without prolapse. The bulge is often sharply marginated and aligns flatly along the disc contours. That configuration usually (ca. 75%) corresponds to a *subligamental* herniation with the center of protrusion at the level of the disc. A small or asymmetrical herniation at a sharp angle to the contours of the disc is seen in approximately 60% of all *transligamental* herniations. Serration or raggedness of disc borders is rare and arises due to underlying subligamental fragments. It may occur with or without degeneration of the longitudinal ligament.

Displacement of a *nerve root* can be demonstrated when there is sufficient epidural fat, and should be taken as a sign of compression. The degree of compression of the thecal sac depends on the amount of epidural fat and is often easier to evaluate from a sagittal reformatted image. A non-sequestered disc prolapse usually bulges a few millimeters caudal, out from behind the ridge of the vertebral body into the extradural space. With *sequestration*, discontinuity of the soft-tissue formation with respect to the space of the disc is seen. The fragment usually extends *caudal* and comes to lie in the inferior section of the lateral recess. In lumbosacral disc herniation, the sequestered fragment can migrate as far as the sacral fora-

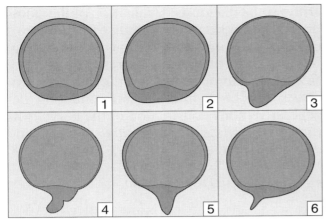
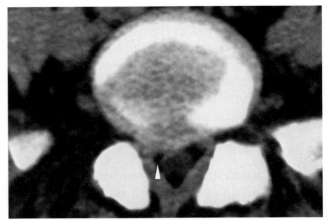

Fig. 26-19. Configuration of the intervertebral disc. Smooth, widely curved, concentric (1) and eccentric (2) protrusion is a sign of disc protrusion with an intact annulus fibrosus. Sharply angled, smooth protrusion (3) is indicative of subligamental prolapse. Irregularly margined, focal protrusion (4–6) is a sign of a transligamental prolapse.

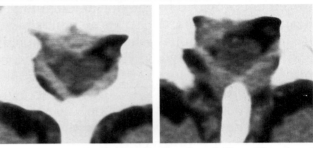

21a

21b,c

Fig. 26-21a-c. Mediolateral disc herniation. The dorsal contour of the disc is irregularly configurated, signalizing transligamental performation. It extends behind the upper rim of the 5th lumbar vertebra and masks the lateral recess as a free fragment (c).

Fig. 26-22. Medial herniation. The disc protrudes as a relatively sharp angle in the midline.

Fig. 26-23. Lateral intraforaminal herniation. The contours of the disc are not sharply marginated and form a broad curve (→) that masks the neural foramen. The emerging nerve root is masked by the disc tissue and venous stasis; it appears thickened (►).

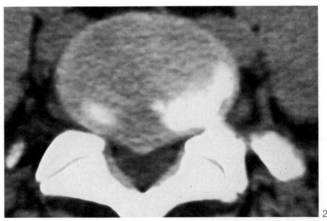

22

Fig. 26-20. Free sequester in the spinal canal (→) (medial prolapse).

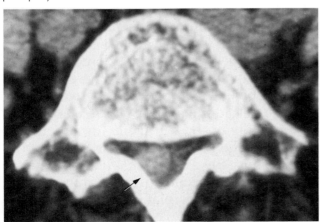

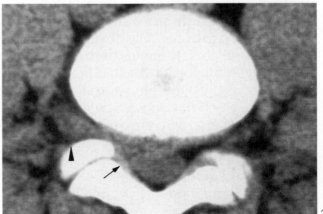

23

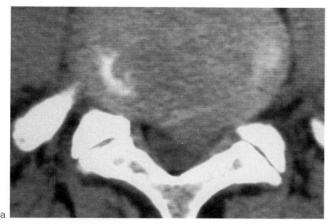

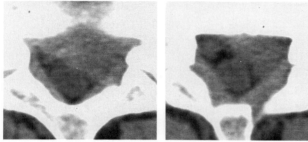

Fig. 26-24a-c. Mediolateral mass herniation. Sharp, left-sided delineation mediolateral (a). The tissue of the intervertebral disc occupies approximately two-thirds of the spinal canal behind the first sacral vertebra (b) and masks the lateral recess, from S1. This compresses the pocket of the nerve root (c).

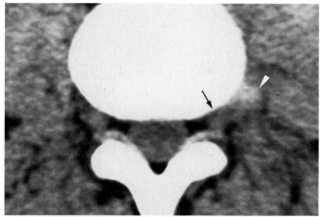

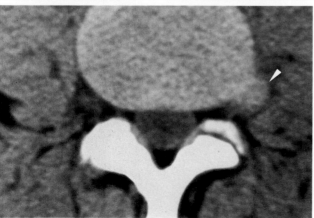

men. Approximately one quarter of all sequestered fragments *ascend* to the ipsilateral neural foramen or to the inferior part of the lateral recess of the vertebral body superior to it. A free fragment can also be attached to a site below the exit of a nerve root.

The *intervertebral foramen* is a structure that should be examined with care. Its exiting nerve roots are delineated by surrounding fat and are therefore identifiable. If the diagnosis is not complicated by narrow foramina, degenerative bone apposition, scoliosis, or generalized disc degeneration, masking of these structures can be taken as an indication of disc herniation.

Similarly, the *lateral recesses* should be carefully examined from their location behind the vertebral bodies to the root of the arch. When any masking or asymmetry caused by slightly hyperdense tissue is found, a free fragment must be suspected.

The *attenuation* of a normal intervertebral disc is greater than 50 HU and contrasts with the more hypodense thecal sac and its nerve roots. Free fragments are also more dense than their contiguous nerve root. For this reason, many hospitals now highlight their CT images to improve optical discrimination of individual disc structures. Calcification in sequestered fragments is a rare finding.

Differential diagnosis:
– *Lateral herniation:* A *conjoined nerve root* can simulate lateral disc herniation. When thin sections are scanned, however, it is usually possible to demonstrate two round (hypodense) structures which branch to form the root exiting from the foramen and a deeper root. Even a cystically dilated *nerve root* can lead to obliteration of the neural foramen. The nerve root then appears hypodense as compared with hyperdense, contrast-enriched *neurinomas*, which frequently lead to bony erosion of the foramen.

Fig. 26-25a, b. Extraforaminal herniation. The tissue has the attenuation value of disc tissue (▸). It constricts the emerging nerve roots (→).

– *Free segment:* Synovial cyst, basivertebral venous plexus, epidural tumor, focal fibrosis after previous surgery.

The Disc after Surgery – Recurrent Herniation

Postoperative processes complicate the identification of recurrent herniation. In a typical interlaminar fenestration, the prolapsed nucleus pulposus tissue is removed lateral to the thecal sac. A variable amount of epidural granular tissue develops and transforms into fibrosis in the postoperative phase. The fibrous tissue developing in the extradural space can fill the lateral recess and also lead to retraction of the nerve root and thecal sac. The extent of these changes depends on the surgical procedure and the individual response of the patient. The diagnosis of recurrent herniation is thereby problematic.

• CT

Plain scans: If only a small amount of epidural scar tissue develops after previous surgery, and if the dorsal limits of the discs can be satisfactorily identified, a recurrent, postoperative disc herniation can be diagnosed in the same manner as a pre-operative herniation.

Fibrotic tissue surrounds the thecal sac in variable widths and may also slightly displace it. Signs of displacement are more often observed in the immediate postoperative phase. Because of retraction, the thecal sac is usually drawn toward the operated side. In many cases, the lateral recess is masked, and the possibility of mediolateral disc herniation cannot be excluded.

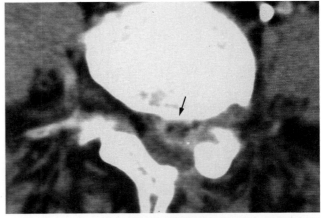
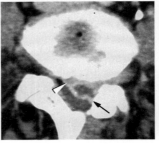
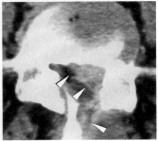

Fig. 26-26a-c. Recurring prolapse. Within an large region of scar tissue, which becomes richly opaque-laden (►), there is a highly visible hypodense zone (→) with discrete amounts of gas. At the same time, there are degenerative processes of the disc with vacuum phenomena.

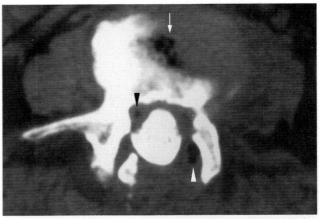

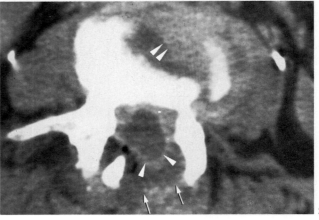

Fig. 26-27. Patient's condition after disc surgery and laminectomy. CT revealed postoperative vacuum phenomena in the intervertebral disc (a→), masking of peridural fat, with air inclusions (►). Seven days later, in a follow-up exam due to fever (b), contrast enhanced CT scans revealed fluid accumulations (b→), a hyperemic thecal sac (b►), and granulation tissue projecting into the disc (b⊨). The vacuum phenomenon disappeared during the onset of discitis.

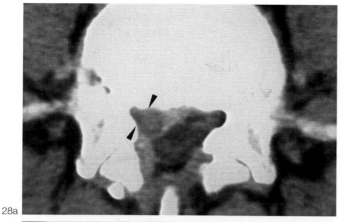

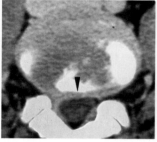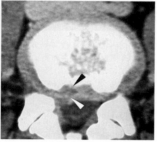

Fig. 26-28. Recurring prolapse. After intravenous contrast medium administration, scar tissue enhances around the thecal sac and the posterior contour of the disc (b ►) 4 mm caudal, a hypodense zone is demarcated inside the scar tissue (c ►). This zone, which can be traced deep into the lateral recess (a ►), corresponds to a recurrent disc prolapse.

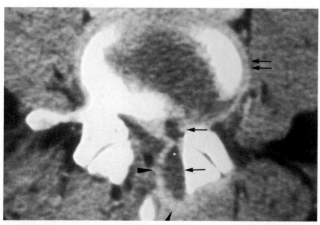

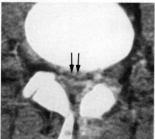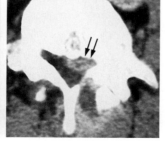

Contrast-enhanced scans: High-dose (prolonged) *intravenous administration of contrast medium* usually leads to homogeneous enhancement of fibrosis tissue. Depending on the degree of vascularisation of the fibrosis tissue, this (postoperative) reaction pattern may be demonstrable for years or may, alternatively, fail to occur even several months after surgery. Within an area of mostly homogeneous enhancement, the encased nerve root appears as a sharply marginated, hypodense figure and can be identified on the basis of its course.

Recurrent disc herniation appears on CT scans as a hypodense zone within contrast enhanced fibrosis tissue. Fatty tissue deposits sometimes create poorly marginated areas of hypodensity and may lead to a false-positive diagnosis.

Non-enhancing fibrosis is seen in approximately one quarter of all cases. The older the scar tissue, the higher the occurrence of non-enhancing recurrent herniations. Enhancement can, therefore, no longer serve as a differential diagnostic criterion. The diagnosis of recurrent herniation can then be made only when a mass is found near the scar. However, hypertrophic scar tissue may also have a similar, expansile appearance.

Differential diagnosis: A focal, soft-tissue mass can be found in the epidural region in the early *postoperative period*. It usually has the appearance of a hematoma, and follow-up examinations must be performed to secure the diagnosis and check progress. Hypodense, more dorsally located cystic formations occurring in postoperative patients are usually the result of the leakage of cerebrospinal fluid *(pseudomeningocele)*. In these stages, administration

Fig. 26-29. CT scan after surgery due to disc herniation. Three days after surgery, findings include enhanced granulation tissue (a ►), as well as collections of hypodense fluid (a →) along the surgical access route. Peripheral enhancement is seen along the edges of the disk as well as of the thecal sac as a result of an inflammatory reaction (a ⇉). The appearance of the granulation tissue resembles that of a mass lesion in the lateral recess (c ⇉) and in the spinal canal (b ⇉). This causes transitory symptoms.

of contrast medium will be helpful in delineating the strongly enhanced granular tissue that is more abundant along border surfaces (dura, periosteum).

Spondylarthrosis

Improper stress and disc degeneration lead to cartilage degeneration in the joints and later joint reduction and subchondral sclerosis. The articular surfaces may display bony excrescences as the condition progresses. This may become rather extensive and cause protrusion into the spinal canal and obstruction of the lateral recess from the dorsal aspect. The resulting structural loosening of that spinal segment leads to a simultaneous change in the capsular apparatus, which may become thickened or cystoid and bulge into the spinal canal (synovial cyst).

• CT

The signs of *arthrosis* described above can be precisely demonstrated when articular surfaces are virtually axial. The joint cavity can be visualized from a tangential view. Vacuum phenomena there are attributable to cartilaginous degeneration. Thickening of the articular capsule or ligamenta flava, deformity of articular surfaces, and subluxation can be demonstrated in addition to intra-articular fragments or fractures on the articular surfaces (facets).

Synovial cysts appear as small, hypodense protrusions that extend from the articular cavity. Because of their association to the joints, they can be distinguished from sequestered disc fragments.

Severe, degenerative articular deformation frequently occurs with osseous excrescences and *pseudospondylolisthesis* (degenerative form of spondylolisthesis). The joint cavity is often difficult to scan because of its non-axial course. Slipping of vertebral bodies is confirmed when the anterior side of the lower plate has been displaced parallel towards the front of the dorsal contours of the disc (ventral slip).

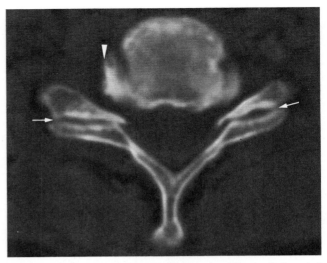

Fig. 26-30. Cervical spondylarthrosis. The subchondral border layers of the intervertebral joints show signs of sclerosis. The articular surfaces are incongruent and slightly extended (→). Also slight extension and deformity of the uncinate process (►).

Fig. 26-31. Spondylarthrosis. Excrescences on the articular surfaces of the intervertebral joint. Demonstration of vacuum phenomenon (→). Using the soft-tissue window, discrete protrusion of the articular capsule containing a central area of hypodensity, corresponding to a **synovial cyst**, can be seen (►).

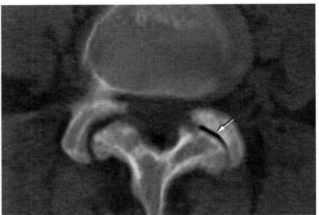

31a

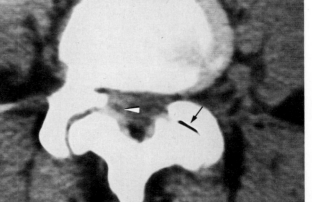

31b

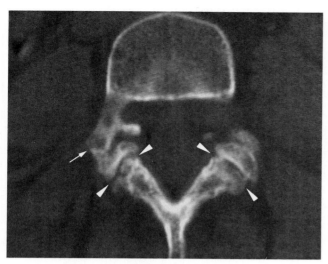

Fig. 26-32. **True spondylolisthesis.** The intervertebral joint (►) exhibits signs of arthrosis and narrowing of the joint cavity. Ventrally, there is irregularly configured, sclerotic interruption of the pars interarticularis (→).

Differential diagnosis: Very complex images are seen in patients with spinal pseudoarthrosis with ankylosing spondylitis. The deformed intervertebral articulations show bony bridging, and fissures are bridged by fibrous tissue.

Fig. 26-33. **True spondylolisthesis.** Differentiation between the joint and fissures is not always clearly demonstrable. Intervertebral joint (a ►), fissure (a →). Lateral reformatted image of ventral slip (b).

33a
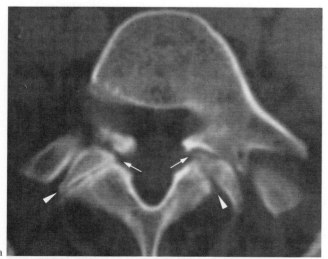
33b
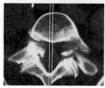
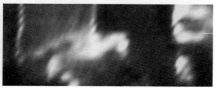

Spondylosis – True Spondylolisthesis

Symmetrical fissures along the articular processes (interarticular part) of the vertebrae leads to forward slip of the vertebrae with normal position of the facet joints. This usually affects the lumbosacral region. Depending on its extent, structural damage may cause constriction of the nerve paths and to disc protrusion.

• CT

Plain scans: Sites of fissures can be identified as a wavy or serrated area of increased translucence with an adjacent area of sclerosis in the inter-articular part. Soft-tissue is commonly found in broad gaps in the bone. This configuration usually makes them distinguishable from smoothly marginated facet joints, even in cases where the facet joints have been deformed by arthropathic changes. As in pseudospondylolisthesis, forward slip is characterized by parallel dislocation of the anterior half of the affected vertebral body as compared with the contiguous intervertebral disc. In order to avoid false interpretations, sections must be scanned exactly parallel to the discs.

Spinal Stenosis

Narrowing of the spinal canal due to osseous or ligamentous structures is often the cause of complex neurological complications. Spinal stenosis can be classified according to the system of Verbiest as follows:
- *Acquired:* in addition to trauma and surgery, Paget's disease, and discopathy, degenerative changes arising from intervertebral arthrosis and posterior spondylosis are also among the main causes of spinal stenosis.
- *Congenital:* chondroplasia and other chondrodysplasias, severe spinal deformity, meningoceles, spina bifida, vertebral dysgenesis.
- *Developmental:* usually dysplasias of the neural arch, e.g. shortened roots of the arch.

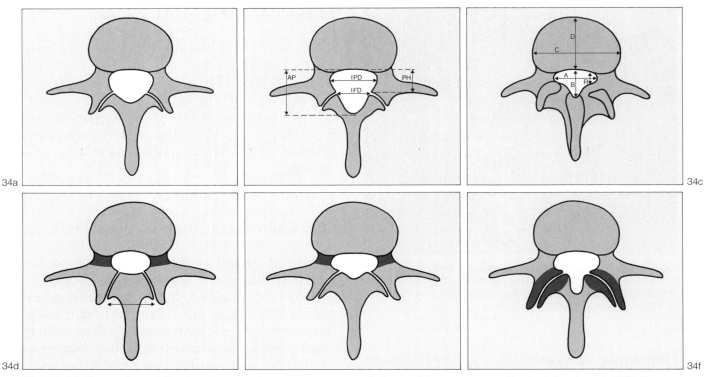

34a   34c
34d   34f

Fig. 26-34. Narrowing of the lumbar canal.
a) Normal width of the lumbar canal.
b) Dimensions of the lumbar canal.
   AP = sagittal diameter, i.e., antero-posterior distance
   IPD = Interpedicular distance
   IFD = Interfacet distance
   PH = Height of roots of the arch

c) Jones-Thompson quotient, defined as AxB/CxD, normally ranges from 1/2 and 1/4.5. Denominators greater than 4.5 indicate narrowness of the lumbar canal.
   R = Width of the radicular canal, i.e., the antero-lateral recess.
d) Concentric narrowing of the lumbar canal. Shortening of the roots of the arch and horizontal narrowing (medialization of the facet joints).
e) Shortened roots of the arch reduce the anterior-posterior distance of the lumen.
f) Arthrotic hypertrophy of the facet joints.

Fig. 26-35. Concentric narrowing of the spinal canal (AP = 10 mm; IPD = 18 mm).

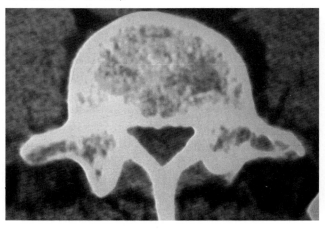

Fig. 26-36. Spinal stenosis due to intervertebral arthrosis. The sagittal diameter of the spinal canal is borderline (10 mm to the hypertrophied ligamentum flavum). Hypertrophy of the facet joints causes lateral narrowing.

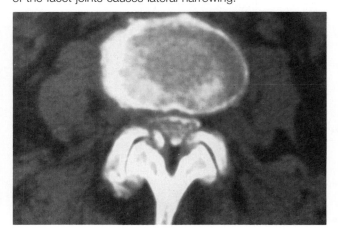

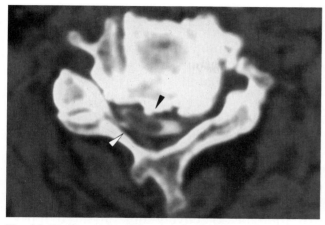

Fig. 26-37. Stenosis of the cervical spine arising from ossification of the posterior spinal ligament. The spinal cord and subarachnoid space are displaced to the right and compromised (►).

Fig. 26-38. Severe stenosis of the cervical spine arising from dorsal, bony excrescences on the rim (AP = 7 mm).

Fig. 26-39. Severe lumbar spinal stenosis due to massive intervertebral arthrosis and disc protrusion (contrast enhanced thecal sac →).

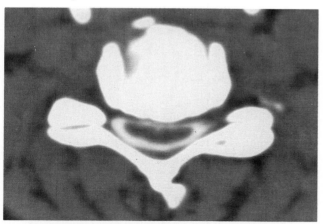

38

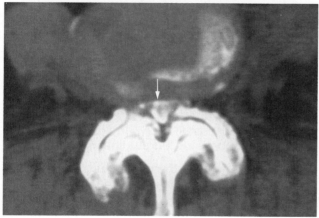

39

• CT

Computed tomography is superior to conventional techniques in demonstrating the lumen of the spinal canal, however, sections must be scanned exactly parallel to the intervertebral discs. In the cervical as well as lumbar regions, one speaks of *relative stenosis* when the anteroposterior distance equals a diameter of 12 to 15 mm. *Absolute stenosis* is characterized by a diameter of 10 mm. An additional sign is the reduction of the interpedicular distance to 20 mm. A further method of identification is the Jones-Thomson quotient.

The causes of stenosis can, at the same time, be demonstrated. In the region of the cervical spine, *central stenosis* frequently occurs when there are appositional dorsal osseous excrescences on the anterior half of the vertebral bodies, giving the lumen a flat, transverse oval appearance. Cervical intervertebral arthrosis combined with excrescences on the uncovertebral processes leads to *foraminal stenosis*. This can be demonstrated when a broad window setting is used, when a lateral view is used for comparison. Additional parasagittal reformatted images are sometimes needed for correct evaluation.

In the lumbar spine, spondylarthrosis leads to constriction of the spinal canal, especially in region of the lateral recess. This can ultimately cause constriction of the nerve root. Depending on the extent of the arthrotic articular excrescences, lateral constriction may lead to a slit-like or triangular appearance of the spinal canal on transverse images. Depending on the extent of the false vertebral posture which usually accompanies this, spinal stenosis may affect one or several segments of the spine. L3-4 and L4-5 are the segments most often affected in the lumbar spine.

Focal spinal stenosis is caused by pseudospondylolisthesis at the level of forward slip of the vertebral body. Thickening of the ligamentous apparatus, especially the ligamenta flava, to thicknesses of 5 mm and more and accompanying disc herniation or prolapse often lead to complex clinical constellations. The underlying factor of these is general degeneration of a segment of the spine.

Spinal Injuries

External trauma, now especially common in traffic accidents, cause various injuries to the spine. Subluxations, dislocations and fractures can lead to *instability* of the spinal column. Acute instability means that spinal cord and spinal nerve function is threatened immediately after trauma. Chronic instability leads to improper stress with a resulting increase in spinal deformity and neurological complications. A precise diagnosis which has taken into consideration the pathogenic mechanism is the key to successful therapy. After the clinical examination, a conventional x-ray examination is routinely performed. This usually gives important clues as to the nature of the trauma injuries. The task of CT is, then, to demonstrate critical regions, provide additional information for the evaluation of stability, and to provide images of regions that are inaccessible with conventional radiographic techniques.

The complementary nature of plain radiographs and computed tomography can be variably utilized in the different sections of the spinal column.

Plain radiographs are more sensitive than CT in demonstrating:
– posture of the spinal column,
– alignment of vertebral bodies,
– slight reduction in height of vertebral bodies and disc space narrowing,
– discrete deformation of vertebral bodies,
– discrete subluxations,
– complex fractures.

CT is more sensitive than plain radiographs in demonstrating:
– fractures in the vertebral circumference,
– disc deformity,
– deformity of the spinal canal,
– vertical fracture lines,
– surrounding soft-tissue processes (e.g. hematoma or leakage of cerebrospinal fluid).

Despite their limited spatial resolution, sagittal and frontal secondary *reformatted images* are a helpful supplement to plain radiographs. With them, bone contours and soft-tissues can be accurately evaluated.

In any examination of a traumatized spinal column, the *pathogenesis* of the trauma including the site affected by trauma and the type of movements which result (hyperflexion, hyperextension, compression, or rotation) should be taken into consideration. The examination can, then, be objectively supplemented, if necessary.

For better understanding of the fracture mechanism and for classification of spinal fractures, a *three-column model* was devised by

Fig. 26-40. Three-column model (according to Denis).

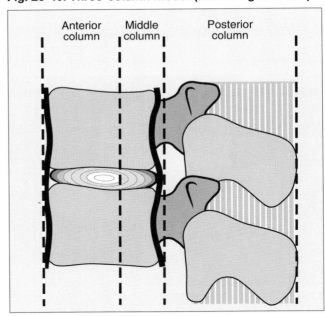

Anterior column:	Includes the anterior longitudinal ligament and the anterior two thirds of the vertebral body, including the disc.
Middle column:	Includes the posterior third of the vertebral body and disc, and the posterior longitudinal ligament.
Posterior column:	Includes the neural arch and articulations, including the ligamentous apparatus.

Denis (Fig. 26-40). Basically, any spinal fracture is considered to be stable as long as the middle column remains intact.

The classification system of McAfee and Magerl distinguishes six additional *types of injuries* (Fig. 26-41).

Fig. 26-41. Classification of spinal fractures (according to McAfee and Magerl).

Type 1: Impacted compression fracture (wedge fracture) involving the anterior column.

Type 2: Incomplete bursting fracture involving the anterior and middle columns.

Type 3: Complete bursting fracture involving all three columns.

Type 4: Chance fracture with hyperflexion in front of the vertebral body. Involves all three columns.

Type 5: Flexion-distraction injury with flexion behind the anterior longitudinal ligament. Involves all three columns.

Type 6: Translation injury. Fracture dislocation involves all three columns. May occur with or without axial rotation.

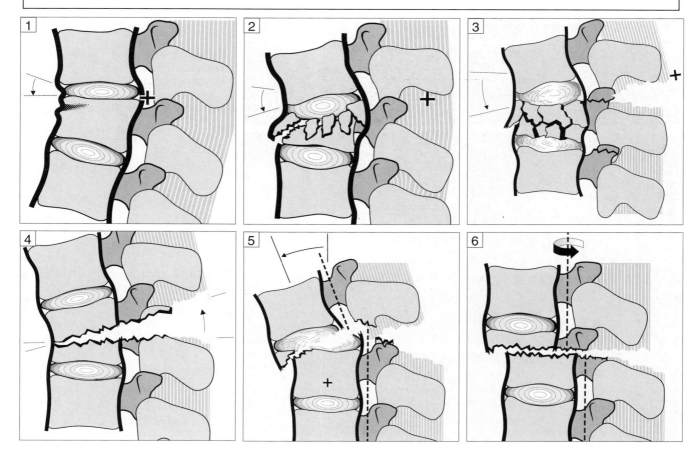

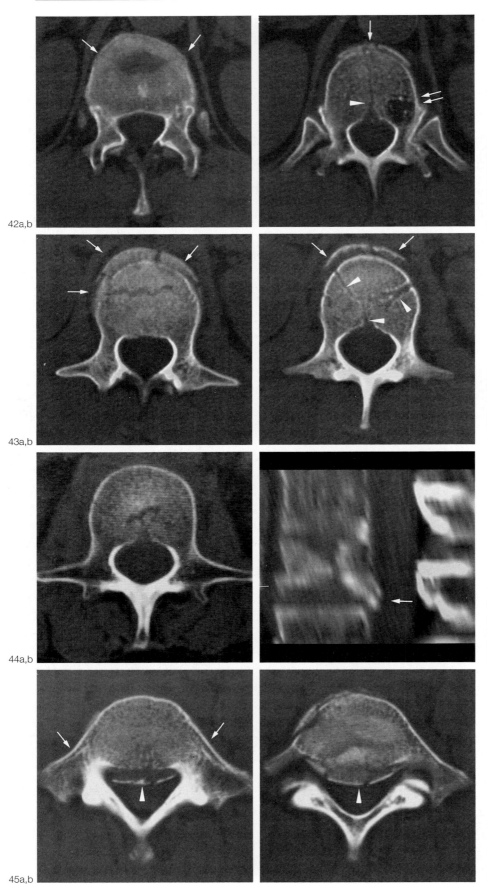

42a,b

Fig. 26-42. Impacted compression fracture. Wedging of the anterior aspect of the vertebra along the upper edge of the 12th thoracic vertebra. A ledge-shaped fragment is displaced 2 mm ventrally (b→). Additional findings: hemangioma (a⇒), venous channel (►).

43a,b

Fig. 26-43. Impacted compression fracture. Transverse fracture line below the upper plate of L1. A fragment is displaced 3 mm ventrally (→). The roots of the arch remain intact. Venous channels (b►).

44a,b

Fig. 26-44. Incomplete bursting fracture. The roots of the arch are intact, but the upper and lower plates are compromised. The reformatted image (b) demonstrates moderate dorsal displacement of a fragment (→).

45a,b

Fig. 26-45. Incomplete bursting fracture. The lower plate of L5 (b) is fragmented and protrudes into the spinal canal (►). The roots of the arch remain intact (a→).

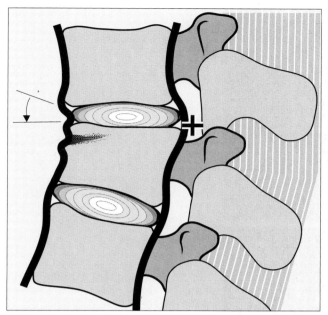

Fig. 26-46. Impacted compression fracture. The pivotal point of flexion forces lies in the anterior half of the body of the vertebra. The posterior rim of the vertebral body remains intact.

Fig. 26-47. Incomplete bursting fracture. The pivotal point of flexion forces lies in the middle and posterior third of the body of the vertebra. With the reduction in height of the entire vertebral body, the posterior aspect is usually also compromised. The roots of the arch remain intact.

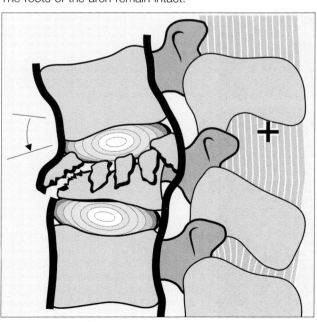

Impacted Compression Fracture

An impacted compression fracture usually has an etiology of an underlying hyperflexion trauma and involves preferentially the dorsolumbar section of the spinal column. The fracture occurs as the result of compression of the anterior sections of the vertebral body. The middle and posterior columns remain intact.

• CT

The fracture is usually visible on plain radiographs as a wedge- shaped deformity. The posterior half of the vertebral body is intact and the lateral, wedge-shaped interpedicular distance is normal. Usually, no CT examination is required. The fracture is seen on CT scans as an area of densification or irregularity in the plates of the vertebrae. The appearance of a double rim along the upper and lower edges of the vertebral body is characteristic. The spinal canal and the roots of the arch are not damaged.

Incomplete Burst Fracture

Axial compression affects the anterior and posterior halves of the vertebral body and, thus, involves the middle column. The intact posterior osteoligamentous column keeps the spinal canal extensively intact, but may be variably constricted ventrally, due to deformity of the posterior half of the vertebral body. The condition is, therefore, questionably stable.

• CT

Reduction in vertical height of the vertebral body, widening of anteroposterior and sagittal diameters, deformity of the sides and end plates of the vertebral body can be seen on plain radiographs. Computed tomography can supplement x-rays by providing better images of the spinal canal, which may be variably obstructed by fragments from the posterior side. The exclusion of complete burst fractures is often possible only by means of computed tomography.

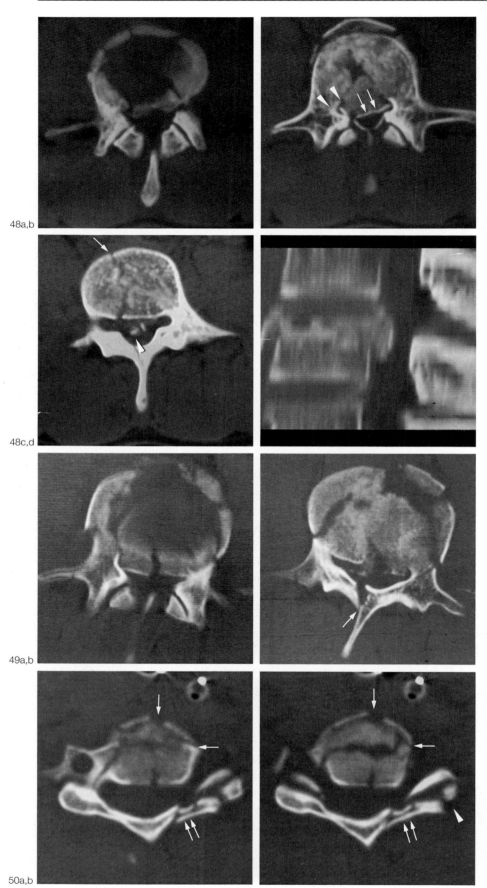

48a,b

48c,d

49a,b

50a,b

Fig. 26-48. Complete bursting fracture. The upper half of L4 is sprained, and there are signs of ventral and dorsal displacement (a). Detailed CT findings include: compromised roots of the arch (b▶), displacement of the anterior aspect, displacement of the posterior aspect into the spinal canal (b⇒), demonstration of intraspinal fragments (c▶), frontal fracture (c→), and slight torsion of the fracture towards the right. Sagittal image reconstruction (d) usually provides evidence of the fracture.

Fig. 26-49. Complete bursting fracture with severe narrowing of the spinal canal and a fractured arch (b→).

Fig. 26-50. Complete bursting fracture involving C6. The upper half of the vertebral body is fragmented (a, b→), the intervertebral joint is distracted (▶), and the lamina of the arch is interrupted (⇒). No intraspinal fragment was detected.

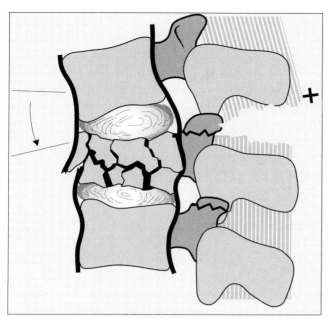

Fig. 26-51. Complete bursting fracture. In addition to predominantly axial compression, flexion leads to injury of the posterior osteoligamentous column.

Fig. 26-52. Chance fracture. The horizontal fracture breaks the vertebral body and its process horizontally, i.e., it lies in plane of the CT section. These fractures are, therefore, incompletely masked by partial volume artifacts.

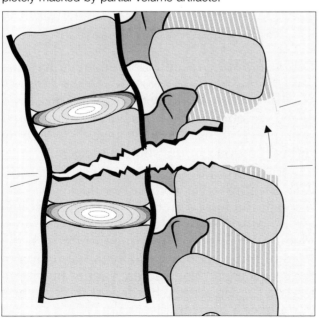

Complete Burst Fracture

These fractures, like the incomplete burst fracture, lead to axial compression. Additional shearing and flexion forces associated with these fractures also injure the posterior osteoligamentous column. In addition to height reduction and deformity of the vertebral body, an increase in interpedicular distance is often demonstrated on plain radiographs.

• CT

Computed tomography is able to demonstrate fractures of the vertebral arch, dislocation, and/or subluxation of the facet joints (naked facets). When effects of rotation are more severe, a similar dislocation of fragments can be seen in the vicinity of the vertebral body as well as in the arch. Constriction of the spinal canal via fragments from vertebral bodies or via traumatic disc herniation (possibly by means of secondary reformatting) as well as dislocated intracanalicular fragments can be precisely demonstrated by computed tomography.

Chance Fracture – Distraction Trauma

This very rare fracture arises due to hyperflexion with a pivotal point in front of the spinal column. Horizontal fractures involving all three columns develop, and a wedge-shaped fracture line is visible on the anterior side.

• CT

This fracture can usually be visualized best on a lateral view. It frequently leads to wedge-shaped deformation of a vertebral body. Since the fracture extends parallel to the sectional plane, the CT sections must be thin enough to adequately demonstrate the fracture. If the intervertebral articulations are burst, subluxation is recognizable as a bilateral lack of contact between articulations (naked facets).

Flexion – Distraction Trauma

The fracture mechanism of this trauma is also hyperflexion, which leads to compression of the anterior side of vertebral bodies and distraction in the regions of the middle and anterior columns.

• CT

This fracture type can be seen on lateral radiographs as a wedge- shaped deformation of a vertebral body accompanied by kyphosis of the spinal column and distraction of the spinous processes. The primary objective of a CT examination is to evaluate the anterior side of the

Fig. 26-53a, b. Flexion-distraction trauma.

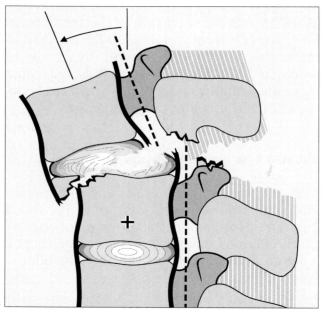

53a

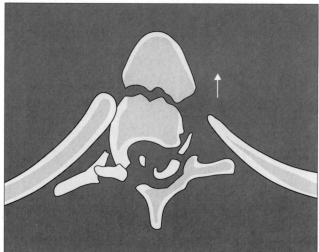

53b

vertebral bodies and, in particular, to determine whether any intracanalicular fragments are present. These frequently occur after the anterior longitudinal ligament has been damaged. Similar to chance injuries, injuries to the anterior column are characterized by dislocation of the facet joints and fractures in the spinous processes and arches. Fragmentation of the injured vertebral bodies can be demonstrated by computed tomography.

Translation Injuries

Laterally inflicted trauma injuries can damage the osteodiscoligamentous apparatus on one level. All three columns are involved and there is significant dislocation. Very severe neurological complications (paraplegia) may therefore occur.

• CT

On lateral scans, *subluxation* or dislocation frequently is demonstrated only as a slight ventral elevation at the level of the intervertebral space. It is easy to overlook this sign on CT scans, and one must, therefore, carefully evaluate the status of the facet joints. A lack of contact between intervertebral facets (naked facet) is indicative of type of subluxation with superposition of the articular surfaces. In the dorsolumbar region, a superior articular process is rarely displaced to a position in front of the inferior articular process.

Dislocations are usually accompanied by fractures of the articular processes in the sense of *fracture dislocation*. Ruptures in the processes of the vertebral arch are usually demonstrated well on CT scans. Sagittal image reformatting should be done in questionable cases.

The fracture zone sometimes does not pass through the intervertebral space, but through the vertebral body itself *(stratified fracture)*. Due to the course of the fracture through the level of the section, especially in the region of the spinal canal, the fracture cannot be visualized on CT scans if the borders of the vertebral body have not been displaced. When thicker sections are scanned, a double lumen of the spinal canal seems to appear because of underlying partial volume effects. The *rotary* effects of the fracture can be demonstrated well in computed tomography by evaluating the alignment of vertebral bodies above and below the level of the fracture.

In rotary translation injuries, the fracture is spiral-shaped in some places as it passes through the vertebral body. A synoptic view of all sectional planes is therefore necessary to evaluate the degree of dislocation of the intervertebral joint and to evaluate the total extent of the fracture.

Fig. 26-54. Translation injury.

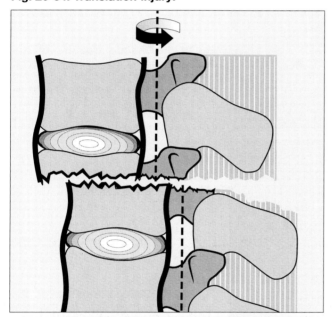

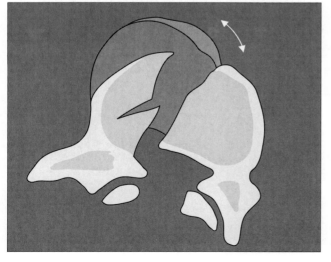

Atlanto-Occipital Dislocation

Atlanto-occipital dislocations usually have a fatal outcome. On plain radiographs, displaced occipital condyles are seen lying against the arches of the atlas. The distance between the base of the skull and the dorsal arch of the atlas is also increased. The severity of the lesion is further indicated by soft-tissue lesions in the occipito-cervical junction, hematomas, and leakage of cerebrospinal fluid.

Atlanto-Odontoid Subluxation

A forcible hyperflexion injury with an intact dens (odontoid process) can cause the transverse ligament to rupture. The dens is translocated dorsally into the spinal canal.

• CT

Widening of the anterior atlantoaxial joint space beyond 3 mm is a sign of subluxation that can also be demonstrated on plain radiographs. When computer tomographic demonstration of the arch of the atlas is free of shadows, the central location of the dens can be immediately identified.

Rotatory Atlantoaxial Dislocation

Forcible rotation of the head can lead to a rupture of the capsule of the anterior atlantoaxial joint with or without an accompanying avulsion fracture. If the site of trauma is located around the axis of the dens, bilateral dislocation of the lateral masses of the atlas will occur. If the effects of forced rotation were outside the axis of rotation of the dens, the transverse ligament will rupture and unilateral dislocation develops with rotation around one of the posterior atlantoaxial articulations.

• CT

On plain radiographs from an anteroposterior view, unilateral narrowing of the interval between atlas and its lateral mass or superposition of the lateral mass and the dens is often found. This rotational malposition is immediately vi-

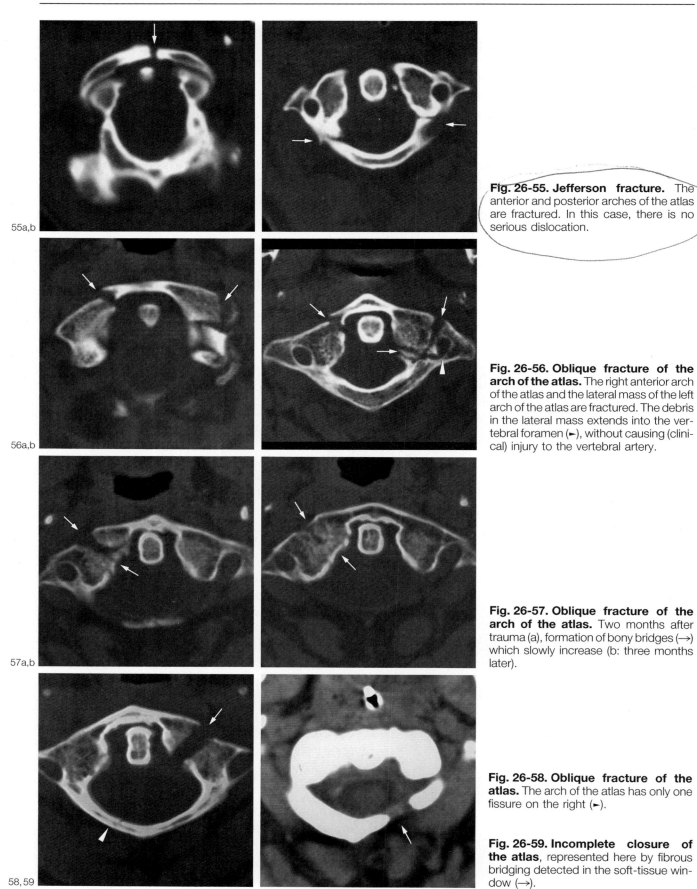

Fig. 26-55. Jefferson fracture. The anterior and posterior arches of the atlas are fractured. In this case, there is no serious dislocation.

Fig. 26-56. Oblique fracture of the arch of the atlas. The right anterior arch of the atlas and the lateral mass of the left arch of the atlas are fractured. The debris in the lateral mass extends into the vertebral foramen (►), without causing (clinical) injury to the vertebral artery.

Fig. 26-57. Oblique fracture of the arch of the atlas. Two months after trauma (a), formation of bony bridges (→) which slowly increase (b: three months later).

Fig. 26-58. Oblique fracture of the atlas. The arch of the atlas has only one fissure on the right (►).

Fig. 26-59. Incomplete closure of the atlas, represented here by fibrous bridging detected in the soft-tissue window (→).

sible on CT scans, especially when thick sections are scanned. The subluxation can be localized on functional scans taken at maximum left and right rotation of the head (the relative position of the atlas and axis remains unchanged). Increased mobility, on the other hand, must be concluded when there is more than 9° of rotation in the atlanto-occipital joint and over 50° of rotation in the atlantoaxial joint.

Fractures of the Atlas

The Jefferson fractures may occur as a true compression fracture involving both the anterior and posterior arches of the atlas or as a fracture of the posterior arch of the atlas due to compression and hyperextension. They are the most common types of atlas fractures. Horizontal fractures of the anterior arch are probably also a result of hyperextension. Fractures of the lateral mass, on the other hand, are compression fractures due to lateral flexion. Approximately 50% of these fractures are fractures of the atlas combined with an injury to the axis.

• CT

Plain radiographs show the lateral displacement of the lateral mass and fractures on a

lateral view. The corresponding CT images show clear, usually symmetrical fractures in the anterior and posterior arches of the atlas. The well defined fracture borders are usually clearly distinguishable from congenital fissures, which are also symmetrical. Fractures of the posterior arch and lateral mass are also easily identifiable on CT scans. Horizontal fractures, on the other hand, usually cannot be demonstrated.

Dens Fractures

The dens is involved in ca. 10% of all fractures of the cervical spine. Dens fractures are caused by extension or ventral or lateral flexion beyond the normal limits.

Fig. 26-60. Dens fractures.

Type 1: Usually characterized by oblique breakage of the apex in conjunction with rupture of the alar and apical ligaments (most uncommon).
Type 2: These are transverse, oblique or frontal fractures that extend through the neck of the dens.
Type 3: These fractures pass through the vertebral body and can involve the lateral atlantoaxial joints.

Fig. 26-61. Types of dens fractures, in a.-p. and lateral projections (b).

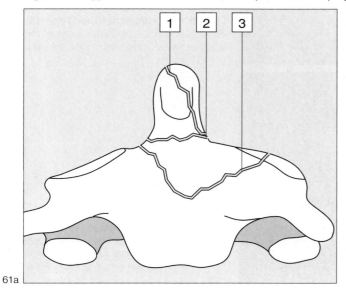

61a

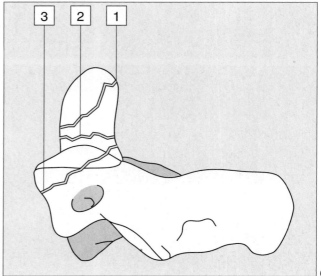

61b

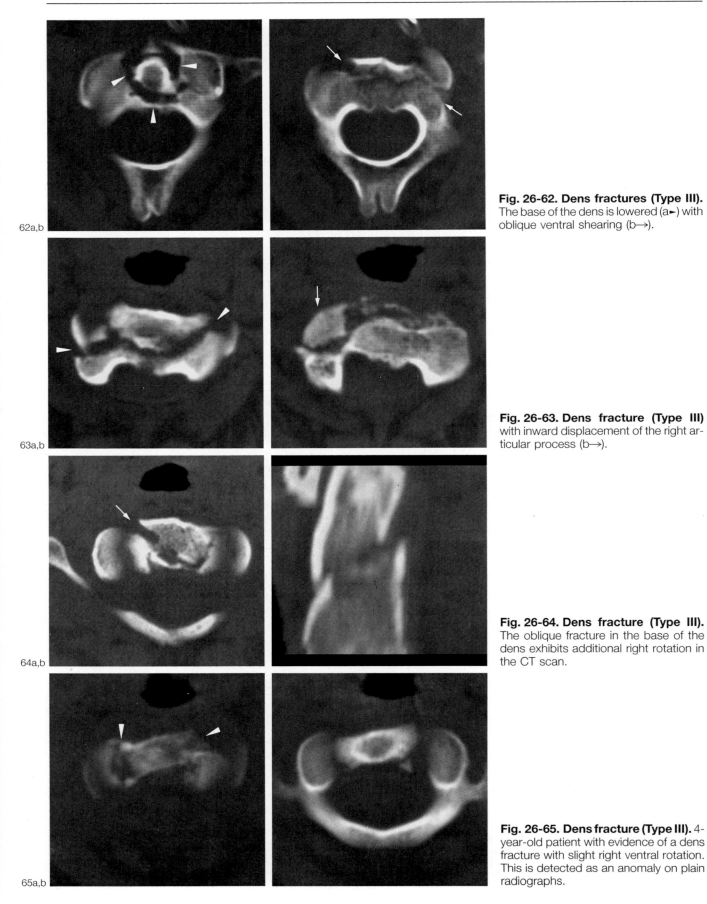

Fig. 26-62. Dens fractures (Type III).
The base of the dens is lowered (a►) with
oblique ventral shearing (b→).

Fig. 26-63. Dens fracture (Type III)
with inward displacement of the right articular process (b→).

Fig. 26-64. Dens fracture (Type III).
The oblique fracture in the base of the
dens exhibits additional right rotation in
the CT scan.

Fig. 26-65. Dens fracture (Type III). 4-
year-old patient with evidence of a dens
fracture with slight right ventral rotation.
This is detected as an anomaly on plain
radiographs.

• CT

Lateral and anteroposterior plain radiographs taken through the opened mouth usually provide satisfactory images of the fractures. In computed tomography, transverse fractures frequently can be demonstrated only when thin sections are carefully scanned. However, the size of the dislocation is usually several millimeters; there is only minor lateral deviation; and CT is a sensitive method of demonstrating bone fractures. Transverse dens fractures, therefore, are usually identifiable on CT scans.

Diagonal and dislocated dens fractures are easy to demonstrate. The occipito-cervical junction should therefore be examined as a prophylactic measure in the setting of any CT examination of cranial injuries. The imaging geometry for a questionable fracture can be improved by increasing the angulation of the scanning gantry.

Fractures of the Arch of the Axis

Bilateral fractures of the arches of the axis can occur due to hyperextension, especially in traffic accident victims. These fractures frequently occur in combination with additional injuries in the occipito-cervical junction. *Type 1* fractures consist of hairline fractures without dislocation. *Type 2* fractures are characterized by intervertebral disc injuries with ventral slip of the body of the axis. *Type 3* fractures have ad-

ditional dislocation of the intervertebral joints. Type 1 fractures are stable, whereas types 2 and 3 are unstable fractures.

• CT

Since the fractures run virtually perpendicular to the CT scanning plane, most of these fractures are readily demonstrable. This even applies to type 1 fractures, which have only discretely visible fracture lines.

Fractures of the Cervical Arches and Articular Processes of the Middle and Lower Cervical Spine (C3–7)

Due to the force of a violent trauma and the mobility of the cervical spine, including its elastic ligamentous apparatus, subluxations frequently occur in this section of the spinal column. Unilateral and bilateral subluxations

Fig. 26-66. Fracture of the arch of the axis (Type I). Discrete fissures (►) can be seen.

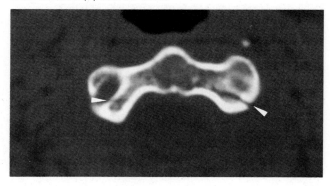

Fig. 26-67. Classification of fractures of the arch of the axis. (a) Type I, (b) Type II, (c) Type III.

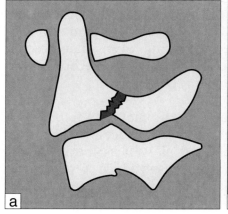
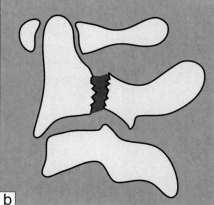
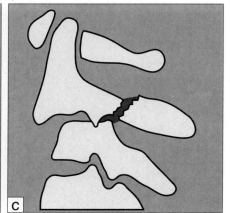

usually must be scanned on a lateral view for unequivocal demonstration. Frequent accompaniments are fractures of the articular processes and arches, the presence of which can only be suspected on plain radiographs and diagonal views with discrete dislocation and narrowing of the neuroforamina.

• CT

Fractures of the roots of the arch and the vertebral arch are results of compression that extend mostly frontal within the column of the joint and radiate dorsally into the arch. In distraction traumas, on the other hand, the entire articular process is usually separated. Because of their axial course, computed tomography can demonstrate these fractures in detail.

Fig. 26-68. Laminar fracture. Fracture of the right lamina in conjunction with a bursting fracture.

Fig. 26-69. Effect of shearing forces on the spinous process in a hyperflexion injury.

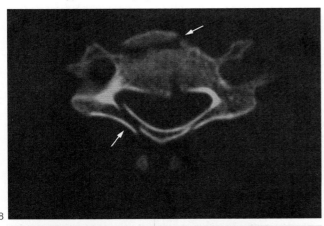

68

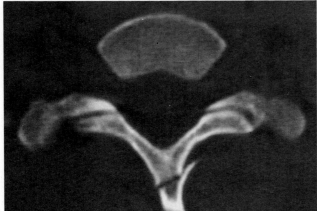

69

Fractures of the articular processes, usually caused by lateral flexion with or without rotation, frequently show only minor dislocations of the often multiply fragmented facets. Isolated lamina fractures are a rarity.

The same criteria used in other sections of the spine also apply for types 2 and 3 *burst fractures* and *translation injuries* of the cervical spine.

Vertebral Tumors and Tumor-Like Lesions

As compared with *metastasizing tumors*, *primary vertebral tumors* are rare (with the exception of *hemangiomas*). They include myelomas, chordomas, giant cell tumors, osteomas, osteoplastomas, osteoid osteomas, fibromas, osteochondromas, chondrosarcomas, osteosarcomas, fibrosarcomas, and Ewing's sarcomas. Spreading within the vertebral arch, constriction of the vertebral canal, erosion along the margins of vertebral bodies, and discrete, focal destruction of the vertebral arch and its processes can be demonstrated on CT scans better than on plain radiographs. CT is especially advantageous in defining the extent of *soft-tissue tumors* (myelomas, giant cell tumors, fibrosarcomas, etc.) in the spinal canal and paravertebral canal. Constriction of the vertebral canal by tumor-like lesions (Paget's disease, fibrous dysplasia) can be reliably evaluated.

Diffuse bone processes such as myeloma or myelofibrosis can often be demonstrated on CT scans, which provide structural images that are free of overshadowing, even when no evidence could be found by other methods (e.g. radionuclide imaging).

When searching for lytic metastases, obstruction of the compact substance of the bone should be evaluated as well as localized destruction of the spongy substance. *Osteoblastic* metastases must be differentiated from *islands of compact bone*, which are frequently visible

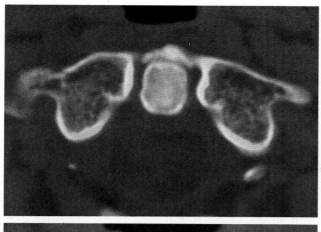

70a

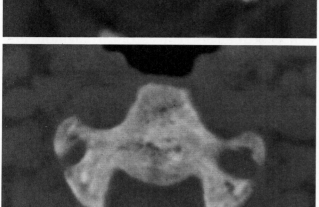

70b

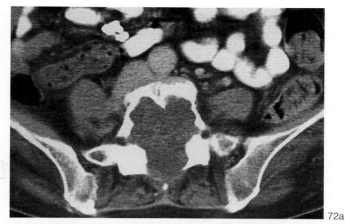

72a

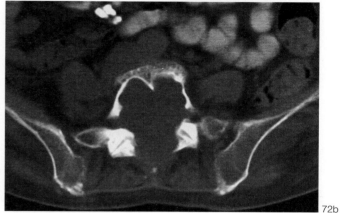

72b

Fig. 26-70. Paget's disease of C2. The vertebral body is dilated and exhibits irregular thickening of the bone structure (b), which extends into the dens (a).

Fig. 26-71. Osteoplastic metastases from a carcinoma of the breast. Inhomogeneous and irregular bone thickening can be seen throughout the body of the vertebra.

Fig. 26-72. Lumbosacral chordoma. The soft-tissue dense mass exhibits moderate, nonuniform enhancement after contrast medium administration. It expands the sacral canal and, due to peripheral enhancement, is demarcated from the vertebral body.

Fig. 26-73. Sacral metastases from bronchial carcinoma. Findings include obliteration of the sacrum, which is indistinctly demarcated from the soft-tissue dense mass.

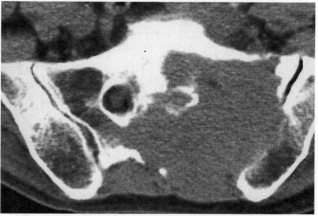

73a

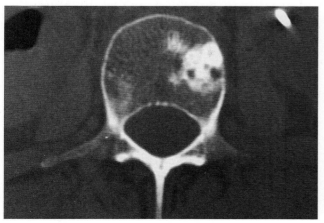

71

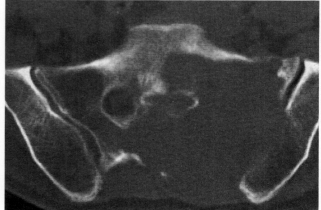

73b

on CT scans. Bone islands are sharply marginated structures without contour defects or local destruction.

Intraspinal Masses

Congenital Masses

Congenital tumors include lipomas, angiolipomas, dermoid cysts, epidermoid cysts, teratomas, meningoceles, and myelomeningoceles.

Lipomas are usually found in children under the age of 15. They are usually accompanied by defects of the neural arch (including the sacral canal), diastematomyelia, and other vertebral anomalies. Lipomas are usually extramedullary or secondary intramedullary (thoracic) occurrences with virtually equal frequency in each section of the vertebral canal. Extradural tumors can display an hourglass configuration in which the intraspinal and extraspinal segments communicate through the intervertebral foramen.

Dermoid cysts are usually encapsulated, round or oval masses with variably thick walls. They, too, are frequently associated with dysrhaphism. They may be intramedullary or extramedullary and lie predominantly in the lumbosacral dural sac.

Epidermoid cysts are slightly less common than dermoid cysts. They tend to occur late in life and are usually located in intradural extramedullary positions.

Teratomas are the most common sacrococcygeal tumors. When benign, these tumors can become very extensive, thereby lying inside and outside of the bony pelvis. They occur primarily in children and juveniles. Malignant teratomas, on the other hand, are found predominantly in adult men. They are usually highly aggressive and cause lymph-borne regional metastases.

The *(myelo-)meningocele* constitutes a congenital anomaly of the neural canal, which extends from the medullary plate to the closed vertebral canal. They are usually located in the lower lumbar region. Sacral meningoceles usually protrude ventrally or laterally through the sacral foramina. They are associated with variably severe bony malformations of the sacrum. (Myelo-) meningoceles are usually detected immediately after birth, whereas occult meningoceles, which lead to widening of the spinal canal, manifest later. A central spicule of bone is typically seen in a spinal canal affected by *diastematomyelia*. This division of the spinal cord can also consist of cartilaginous and fibrous septa.

Acquired Masses

• *Intramedullary Compartment*

Solid lesions primarily consist of gliomas and pargliomas (60 to 65 % are *ependymomas* and 25 to 30 % are *astrocytomas*. Rarer types include *oligodendrogliomas*, *melanomas*, *multiform glioblastomas*, and *angioblastomas*). Astrocytomas develop preferentially in thoracic and cervical regions, whereas ependymomas usually develop below the conus medullaris in the region of the filum terminale. They may, however, lie in other regions of the vertebral canal. Depending on their extent, ependymomas can lead to erosion of the vertebral body and to thinning and protrusion of the vertebral arch, which can ultimately break. Intramedullary *metastases* are very rare and usually occur in association with epidural metastases.

The *syringohydromyelia* is a *cystic* disease. Whereas hydromyelia is a developmental disease of the spinal cord that causes widening of the central canal (often in combination with type 1 Chiari malformations) syringomyelia is characterized by cystic, intramedullary formations. Although initially separated from the central canal, communication may develop later. Fusiform enlargement of the spinal cord is seen which can lead to secondary, focal enlargement of the vertebral canal. This enlargement usually is not found in postnecrotic cystic intramedullary lesions occurring after trauma or ischemia.

• Intradural Extramedullary Compartment

The most common intraspinal lesions are intradural extramedullary tumors (ca. 60%), of which the *meningioma* and *neurofibromas* are the most important types. Similar to intracranial meningiomas, intraspinal meningiomas often display psammomatous calcification and 80% are located in the thoracic region. The number of neurofibromas is approximately equal. They show no predilection for any particular segment of the spine. Approximately 15% of all meningiomas and 30% of all neurofibromas are extradural. These mostly small intraspinal tumors only later lead to osseous erosion after their size increases. In contrast, neurofibromas located peripherally in the root canal cause dilatation of the narrow, bony borders of the intervertebral foramen in the early stages of disease.

• Extradural Compartment

Extradural tumors, which usually invade the spinal canal from directly contiguous structures, are relatively common. They primarily consist of vertebral metastases from bronchial carcinoma or carcinoma of the breast. As they become more invasive, infiltration of the thecal sac occurs. Extradural metastases in the absence of bone destruction are rare, but occur more frequently in malignant lymphomas. Occasional primary extradural tumors include sarcomas and caudal chordomas.

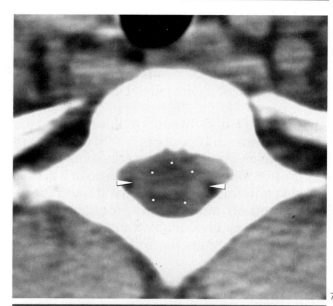
74

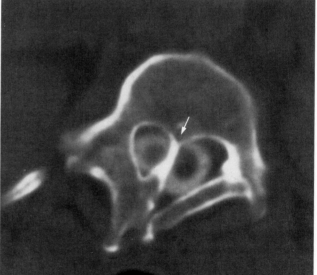
75

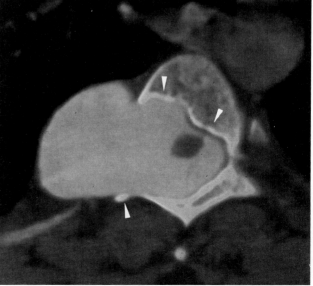
76

Fig. 26-74. Syringomyelia. The cervical spinal canal contains a discrete, ringlike structure (►) with a hypodense center (•).

Fig. 26-75. Diastematomyelia. The spinal canal is divided by a sagitally oriented osseous lamella. After intrathecal contrast medium administration, the hemicords inside the divided thecal sac can be demonstrated in both lumina.

Fig. 26-76. Thoracic meningocele. A hypodense mass was detected on plain scans. After intrathecal contrast medium administration, this enhances homogeneously. The contiguous vertebral body structures and the dilated neural foramen exhibit peripheral sclerosis as a result of the slow, expansive growth (►).

• CT

Congenital Masses

Congenital tumors with dysrhaphism are usually diagnosed clinically. The role of CT is, therefore, to define the *extent of bony changes* and the *size* and *extent* of lipomatous and cystic tumor components. When signs of dysrhaphism are discrete (occult spina bifida), CT is often able to provide evidence of a deeply seated conus medullaris or a fixed filum terminale. Ventrally and laterally emerging meningoceles are readily demonstrable on CT scans, as are the bony lamella of diastematomyelia.

Acquired Intradural Masses

Plain scan: As can be seen on plain radiographs, *enlargement* of the *spinal canal* is an important, though not very sensitive, radiographic sign of intraspinal lesions. Widening or narrowing of the spinal canal must be measured strictly perpendicular to the axis of the vertebral body. Thinning and convex deformity of the lamina can be demonstrated on CT scans while still in the early stages, and is indicative of an expansile intraspinal process.

Proof of an *intraspinal lesion* without enlargement of the vertebral canal can be obtained on plain radiographs only when there is a clear difference in density within the spinal canal. Thus, a meningioma can be sensitively detected when psammomatous *calcification* is present. Concentric, but more frequently well circumscribed, unilateral types are found. Focal regions of *fatty tissue density* may correspond to a lipoma, but must be differentiated from epidural fat or epidural lipomatosis. Dermoid and epidermoid cysts can often be diagnosed on the basis of their fat content,

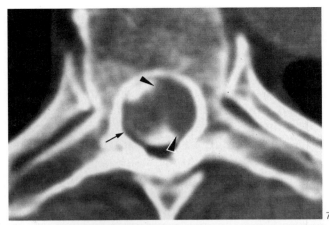

77

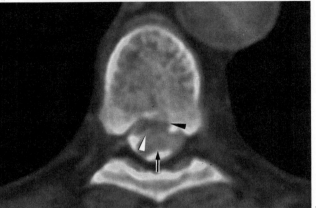

78

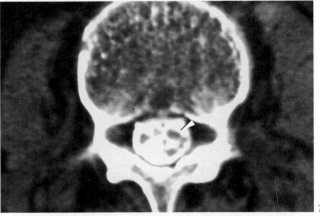

79a

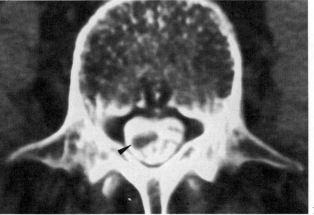

79b

Fig. 26-77. Spinal meningeoma. After intrathecal contrast medium administration, a lesion on the dura (→) is revealed as a filling defect. It displaces the spinal canal (►) laterally to the left.

Fig. 26-78. Intraspinal meningeoma. The meningeoma (→) ventrally displaces the atrophic spinal canal (►).

Fig. 26-79. Meningiosis carcinomatosa. After intrathecal contrast medium administration, the nerve roots of the cauda appear plump and thickened.

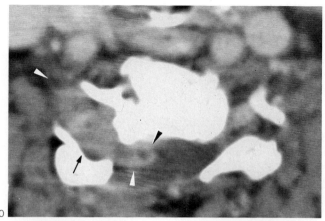

80

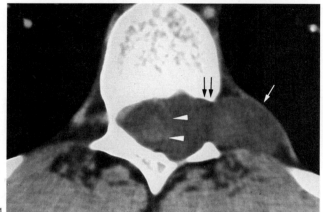

81

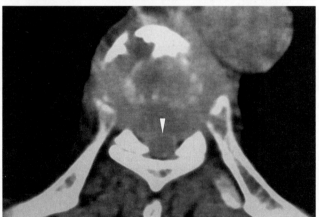

82a

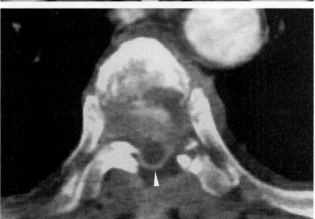

82b

their well-defined margins and, in some cases, calcified structures which they contain. On plain radiographs, the density of most intramedullary and extramedullary lesions is normally not clearly different from that of the spinal cord. Therefore, when the diameter of the spinal canal remains within normal limits, it is no longer possible to evaluate the size and extent of these tumors.

Contrast-enhanced scans: A bolus of contrast medium delineates only well vascularized lesions such as *angiomas*, *hemangioblastomas*, and *vascularized malformations*.

CT-assisted myelography: Intramedullary *cystic* changes in the cervical region can be demonstrated, and syringohydromyelia can sometimes be diagnosed on plain scans. As compared with MRT, however, computed tomography is not as conclusive in diagnosing these lesions. Communication between the subarachnoid space and the syrinx can be demonstrated by CT only after intrathecal contrast medium instillation.

Acquired Extradural Masses

Plain scans: Most processes attack the spinal canal from adjacent structures. Masking of the fat-containing peridural space must, therefore, be taken as a sign of infiltration. Invasion of the spinal canal by paravertebral lesions (frequently through the neural foramen) is frequently demonstrable, even in the absence of osseous destruction.

Fig. 26-80. Neurinoma. The intraspinal, extradural tumor (►) widens the neural foramen (→) and displaces the thecal sac to the left.

Fig. 26-81. Thoracic neurinoma. The hour-glass shape of the tumor (→) widens the neural foramen (⇉) and compromises the thecal sac (►).

Fig. 26-82. Metastasizing carcinoma of the breast. The vertebral body is partially obliterated by a soft-tissue mass, which also fills the spinal canal and dorsally displaces the thecal sac (►). Also, there is absence of contrast enhancement of the subarachnoid space after intrathecal contrast medium administration (a). A postoperative reduction in size of the tumor mass is demonstrated. The enhancement of the subarachnoid space indicates restored contrast medium passage (b ►).

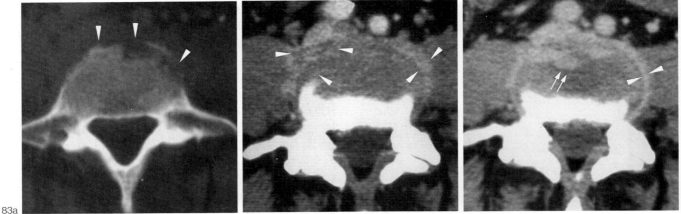

83a   83c

Fig. 26-83a-c. Spondylodiscitis. In the bone window, fine bone destruction can be seen on the lower edge of L5 (a ►). This was only discretly visible on plain radiographs. In the soft-tissue window, a peridiscal opacifying soft-tissue structure (granulation tissue ► ◄) is demonstrated. It extends caudally from the rim of the vertebral body. No signs of liquefaction. Four weeks after antibiotic treatment, the soft-tissue structure has slightly reduced in width. Granulation tissue protruding into the intervertebral space (c ⇒) can be differentiated from the slightly hpyodense intervertebral disc after contrast medium administration.

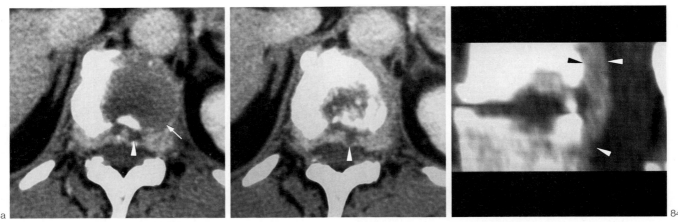

84a   84c

Fig. 26-84a-c. Spondylodiscitis. After contrast medium administration, clearly enhanced soft-tissue (granulation tissue) is detected behind the narrowed disc space at T12-L1. The disc (a→) as well as small, round zones (colliquation) are demarcated from this (a, b ►). Sagittal reformatting demonstrated the subligamentous expansion and mass-like nature of the granulation tissue (c ►).

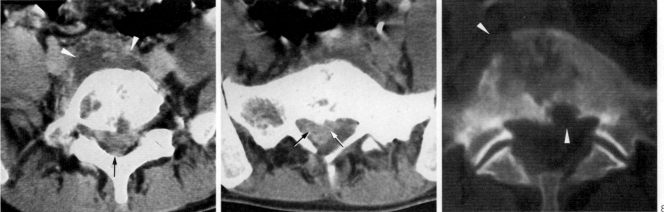

85a   85c

Fig. 26-85a-c. Spondylodiscitis. CT demonstration of a prevertebral soft-tissue structure (abscess), which becomes hypodensely delineated after contrast medium administration (a, b ►). Contrasting granulation tissue also lies inside the spinal canal (a→) and extends to the sacral canal (b→). Findings ten weeks after antibiotic therapy included regression of the soft-tissue structure, apparent sclerosis of the spongiosa of the vertebral body and bony defects (c ►).

Contrast-enhanced scans: A bolus of contrast medium usually clearly delineates the tumor tissue from the sharply marginated, hypodense thecal sac. Aggressive *hemangiomas* which show strong enhancement are seldom diagnosable.

Spondylitis – Spondylodiscitis

Infectious spondylitis, or spondylodiscitis, is more common in older patients. This is usually diagnosed in patients in the 5th to 6th decades, especially after pelvic infections and surgical intervention (disc operations). Staphylococcus aureus is the pyrogenic pathogen in 80 to 90% of all cases. More rare pathogens are streptococci, pneumococci, E. coli, pseudomonas, and klebsiella. Tuberculosis and fungal infections are less common. The preferential site of infection is the lumbar spine. These infections are usually spread by blood. Contagious spreading is infrequent, and travels from paravertebral abscesses or sites of disc surgery to a vertebral body. The induced focus of infection usually lies near the end plates of the vertebral body, because of the good arterial blood supply. As the infection progresses, the bone-cartilage border is penetrated and the disc is infiltrated. Contiguous vertebral bodies also become involved, and the typical constellation arises where one finds a reduced disc space with infection of the adjacent vertebral bodies. If liquefaction of the focus of inflammation occurs, an intravertebral abscess develops and spreads subligamentously to extravertebral locations in the longitudinal direction of the spinal column. This may also cause secondary infection of other sections of the spinal column.

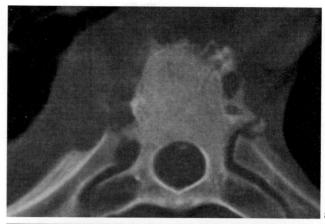

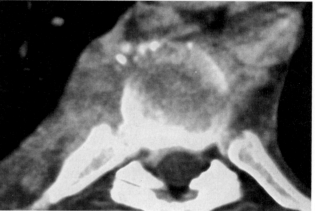

Fig. 26-86. Non-tuberculous spondylitis. The chronic nature of the disease is suggested by the sclerotic densification of the spongiosa of the vertebral body and the broad periosteal reaction in the vertebral body and ribs (a). Perivertebral, opaque-laden soft-tissue structure (granulation tissue) without clear demarcation suggestive of abscess formation (b).

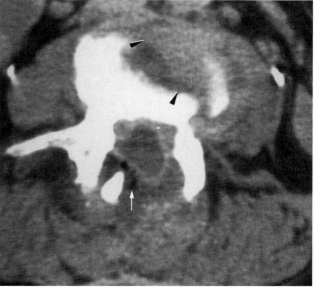

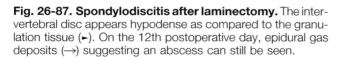

Fig. 26-87. Spondylodiscitis after laminectomy. The intervertebral disc appears hypodense as compared to the granulation tissue (►). On the 12th postoperative day, epidural gas deposits (→) suggesting an abscess can still be seen.

• CT

Plain scans: Early changes caused by spondylodiscitis, which basically take place in sites near the end plates of the vertebral body, cannot be demonstrated well on CT scans (not even on thin-section scans) because of artifacts caused by partial volume effects. Osteochondrotic changes in the end plates of the vertebral body often complicate the diagnosis. Hypodensity has been described as an indicator of disc involvement, but this is not always the case. Metaplastic bone changes which develop in the course of this disease usually occur in association with irregularly patterned sclerosis of the spongy substance and can be sensitively detected by computed tomography. They can be followed up in detail. These inflammatory processes frequently lead to obliteration of peridiscal fat. Perivertebral infiltrations, exudation, and abscesses are characterized by masking and displacement of surrounding soft tissues. Infiltration of the spinal canal can be recognized as a corresponding computer tomographic rise in attenuation of epidural fat. However, one must take physiological postoperative repair processes and scar tissue formation into consideration.

Contrast-enhanced scans: A bolus of contrast medium often enhances the margins of the affected intervertebral disc and increases, in some cases, the central hypodensity of the disc. Granular tissue, which absorbs contrast medium, can be computer tomographically differentiated from the disc. Spreading of inflammation to perivertebral soft tissues can often be clearly demonstrated after the administration of contrast medium. Infected granular tissue then becomes clearly opaque-laden. Zones of liquefaction are, thereby, clearly seen as areas of hypodensity.

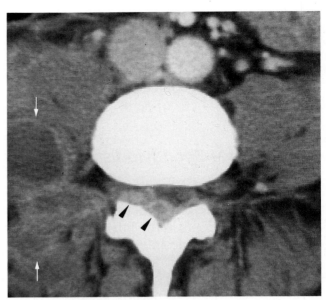

Fig. 26-88. Epidural abscess. Infection from a large psoas abscess (→) extends through the intervertebral foramen into the extradural space (►).

Fig. 26-89. Postoperative hygroma (►). The thecal sac is moderately displaced. Epidural fat is not masked, so there is no evidence of abscess formation.

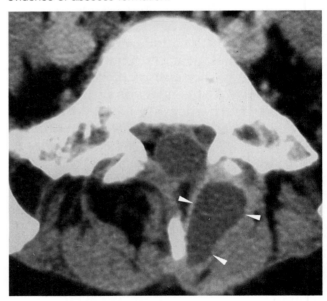

Chapter 27
The Bony Pelvis

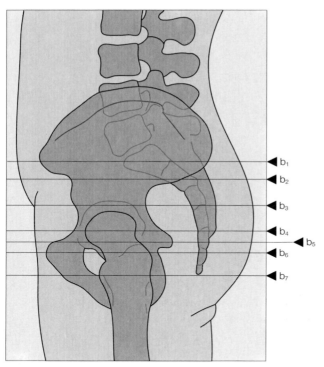

Fig. 27-1. Bony pelvis.
a) Lateral view.
b) In transverse sections. See (a) for the level of section.

Key to symbols:
  1 Wing of the ilium
  2 Promontory
  3 Sacral canal
  4 Sacro-iliac joints
  5 Sacral foramen of the pelvis
  6 Sacrum
  7 Head of the femur
  8 Anterior column of the acetabulum
  9 Posterior column of the acetabulum
10 Tuberosity of the pubis
11 Superior pubic ramus
12 Neck of the femur
13 Greater trochanter
14 Symphysis
15 Coccyx
16 Ischiadic foramen
17 Sacrospinal ligament
18 Anococcygeal ligament
19 Retroauricular space
20 Roof of the acetabulum
21 Anterior superior iliac spine
22 Posterior iliac spine
23 Femur
24 Inferior pubic ramus

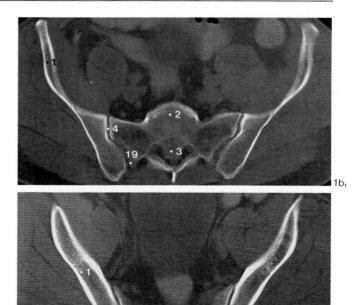

1b₁

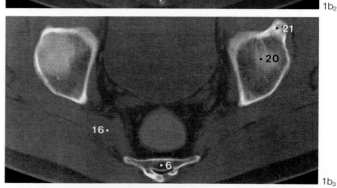

1b₂

1b₃

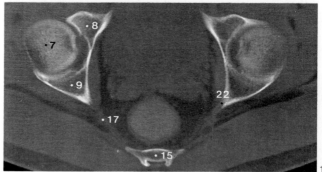

1b₄

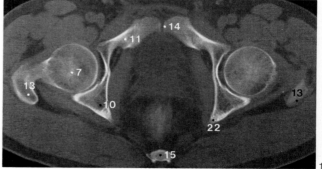

1b₅

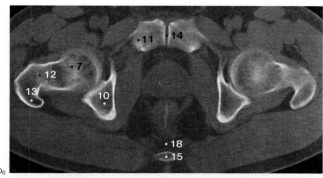

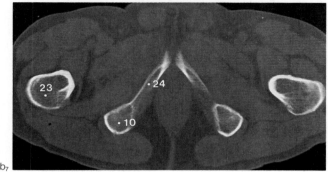

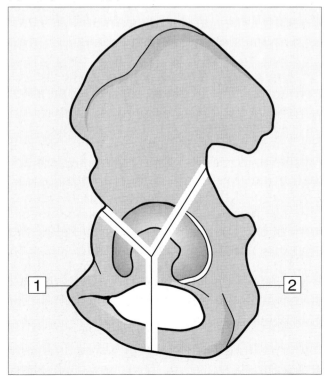

Fig. 27-2. Classification of pelvic structures into anterior (1) and posterior (2) column.

The Bony Pelvis

Anatomy and Imaging

The pelvis contains convex bony structures which form border surfaces that are difficult or impossible to demonstrate via the standard projections of conventional radiography. Computed tomography, with its transverse scanning plane, can provide additional images of structural contours that are essential for diagnosis.

The horizontal circumferences of the *acetabulum* and head of the hip joint, including the anterior and posterior borders of the hip joint, are demonstrated in detail, even in contiguous scans of 8 mm thickness. However, the roof of the acetabulum (which can be demonstrated well by pelvioradiography) and the upper joint space are masked by partial volume artifacts when scan sections are that thick. Sections of 2 mm thickness should therefore be scanned for better demonstration of these regions in patients with certain diagnostic problems. In contrast, detailed images of the joint cavity of the *sacro-iliac joint*, including its subchondral border lamella, can be obtained in nearly all CT scans, because of the virtually axial course of these pelvic structures. Depending on the degree of lordosis of the lumbar spine, the curved anterior surface of the sacrum is usually only indistinctly visible in the area directly below the sacral promontory. In more caudad sections, the image detail of cortical structures increases as the orientation of the structures becomes more axial, and a detailed evaluation of the sacrum is therefore possible. The anterior sacral foramina normally form unequivocal images.

The *relevant axes* of the pelvis can be clearly demonstrated on cross-sectional CT images. The acetabulum carries the entire weight of the body. It is surrounded by triangular bony reinforcements, the anterior (iliopubic) and posterior (ilioischial) pubic *columns*, which form the cranial convexity of the weight-bearing structure of the acetabular roof. The borders of the

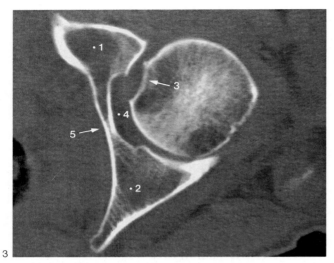

3

Fig. 27-3. The hip joint. (1) Anterior column, (2) posterior column, (3) fovea centralis, (4) acetabular fossa, (5) center of the acetabulum.

Fig. 27-4. Sacro-iliac joint in longitudinal scan. By tilting the gantry craniocaudally, the sacrum and its joints can be demonstrated in fewer sections with less radiation. Ventral view including pelvic foramen.

Fig. 27-5. Sacro-iliac joint in longitudinal scan. Dorsal view including sacral canal (→ synovial and ► ligamentous sections of the joint).

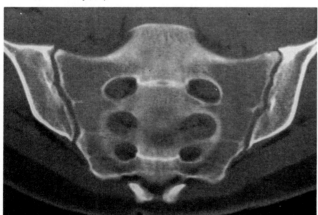

4

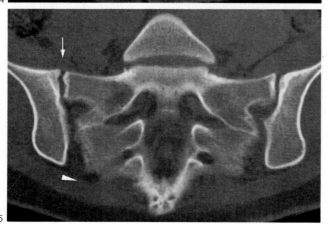

5

bony recess of the joint socket, the *acetabular fossa*, demarcate on each side the anterior and posterior columns and cranially mark the margins of the acetabular roof. The pelvic bone surface corresponding with the acetabular fossa marks the *center of the acetabulum*. The bony joint space is equally broad on both the anterior and posterior acetabular margins. It becomes incongruous in the middle segment due to the shapes of the recess of the acetabular fossa and the femoral fovea centralis. The weight of the body is transferred via the spine across the sacrum and posterior iliac spine to the hip joints. The rigid posterior *ligamental structure* (interosseous sacro-iliac ligaments) is usually only indistinctly visible within dorsal fatty tissue. The sacrospinous ligament, which extends from the ischial spine to the sacrum, can be identified. Sections of the sacrotuberous ligament can also be demonstrated. The anterior pelvic girdle is closed by the rami of the pubis. They extend diagonally through the scanning plane and can be demonstrated only in sections. The pubic symphyseal fissure can be precisely measured by computer tomographic techniques, and it should not be wider than 6 mm in adults.

The *capsule* of the hip joint appears on CT scans as a narrow strip of soft-tissue that extends from the anterior and posterior acetabular margins and ends directly contiguous with the head. In deeper sections near the neck of the femur, it extends to a point near the greater trochanter. These structures are sometimes masked by the contiguous iliopsoas and obturator internus muscles, but in most cases, they are demarcated by a fine layer of fat. Normal capsule thickness is 3 mm. Thickening greater than 6 mm must be considered pathological. The *bursa* of the psoas major tendon extends caudally from the iliopubic eminence and in front of the joint capsule to a point below the iliopsoas muscle. It can sometimes be seen when it is surrounded by or contains fat, but it is normally not visible on CT scans. It communicates with the hip joint cavity in 15% of all individuals.

The curvature of the *sacrum* is longitudinally and ventrally oriented. Therefore, only short segments of the synovial sacro- iliac joint, or the auricular surface of the sacrum, can be demonstrated on tangential scans at the level of the sacral promontory. Longer segments can be demonstrated in more caudal sections. The posterior ligamentous apparatus fills the open dorsal bony gap in cranial sections and becomes less prominent in caudal sections. The normal width of the joint space is 3 mm (2.5 to 4 mm).

Pelvic Trauma

Since most pelvic injuries are caused by external trauma (traffic accident, whiplash, fall from a great height), they are often associated with severe accompanying injuries to the skull and trunk of the body. Therapeutic and prognostic criteria are used to classify pelvic fractures as follows:

1. Fractures and injuries that do not compromise the pelvic girdle (stability is maintained);
2. Fractures and ruptures that compromise the pelvic girdle (loss of stability); and
3. Fractures (dislocations) of the acetabulum.

Fractures that do not cause a loss of *stability* therefore include isolated fractures of the superior pubis, isolated fractures of the ischium, strain fractures of the iliac spine, transverse fractures of the distal sacrum, fracture of the coccyx, fractures of the pelvic brim, and transverse fractures of the wing of the ilium. Destabilization is caused by unilateral or bilateral fractures of the anterior pelvic girdle (superior and inferior pubic rami), fractures of the posterior pelvic girdle (vertical ala fractures, ruptured sacro-iliac joint, vertical fracture of the sacrum) or a combination of these (on the same, or on opposite, sides). Instability may additionally be caused by fractures of the anzerior and posterior pelvic girdle as well as symphyseal ruptures. Various types of acetabular fractures lead to various fractures of the pelvic girdle and are only partially destabilizing.

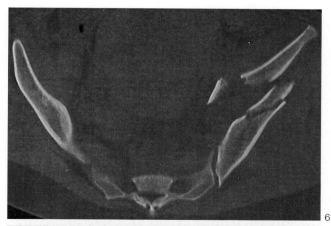

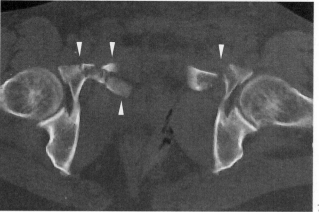

Fig. 27-6. Fracture involving the left wing of the ilium exhibits considerable dislocation.

Fig. 27-7. Bilateral anterior pelvic girdle fracture and superior pubic ramus fracture with no involvement of the acetabulum.

Fig. 27-8. Posterior pelvic girdle fracture. The sacrum clearly exhibits dehiscence (→). Demonstration of a small fragment proximal to the joint in the lateral mass (►). The left wing of the ilium is rotated outward because of the fracture.

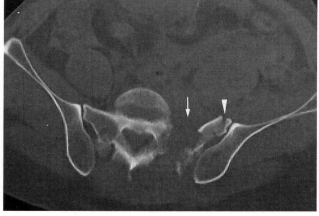

Most of the stable pelvic fractures listed above can be reliably demonstrated on plain radiographs. The same is true of fractures of the anterior pelvic girdle. Assessment of the posterior pelvic girdle and the acetabulum can, however, be much better and more reliably demonstrated by computerized tomography.

Fractures of the Posterior Pelvic Girdle

Most pelvic *fractures* are vertical, and vertical fractures in para-articular locations of the wing of the ilium and the sacrum are the most common. These fractures are followed, in order of frequency, by vertical fractures of the lateral mass and central segments of the sacrum. As compared with ridge fractures, the incidence of comminuted, horizontal and oblique fractures is much lower. *Ruptures* of the sacro-iliac joint occurring with or without ridge fractures of the sacrum occur with virtually the same frequency as vertical fractures of the posterior pelvic girdle.

• CT

Due to intra-articular vacuum phenomena, a lesion of the sacro- iliac joint can be detected when the joint cavity is not dilated. Clear ruptures of the anterior ligaments can be demonstrated due to expansion of the anterior joint space, and ruptures of the anterior and posterior ligaments will be visible due to general broadening of the joint space. More discrete dislocation or joint cavity distension is usually not detectable on plain radiographs.

With the combination of their predominantly vertical course and the mainly tangential scanning of the sacral cortical layers, fractures of the sacrum and para-articular iliac bone fractures can be sensitively detected and demonstrated by computed tomography.

The presacral and retrosacral spaces should also be carefully evaluated, since fatty tissue there can be masked by accompanying hematomas.

Differential diagnosis: In symmetrical fractures of the sacrum, fatigue fractures should be

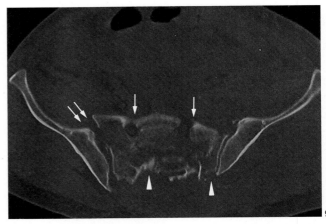
9

Fig. 27-9. Posterior pelvic girdle fracture. The comminuted fracture of the sacrum involves both lateral masses (→). On the right, luxation in the sacro-iliac joint is evident (⇉). The dorsal sections of the sacrum are also fractured (▸). The left wing of the ilium is rotated outwards.

Fig. 27-10. Posterior pelvic girdle fracture. A fracture involves the right lateral mass (a →). More caudally, the fracture is proximal to the joint (b →). The right wing of the ilium is rotated inwardly.

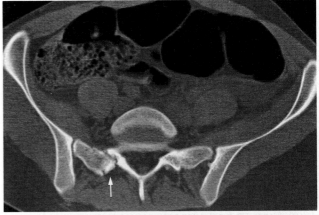
10a

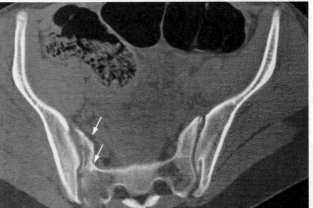
10b

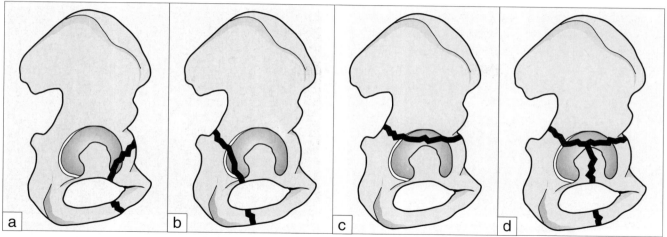

Fig. 27-11. Classification of acetabular fractures according to Letournel.
a) Anterior column fractures (anterior acetabular margin fractures).
b) Posterior column fractures (posterior acetabular margin fractures).
c) Transverse fractures.
d) Y-shaped fractures through both columns.

Fig. 27-12a, b. Posterior fracture of the roof of the acetabulum with clearly dorsal dislocation of the fragment (→). In the soft-tissue window, extensive hemarthrosis was detected (►).

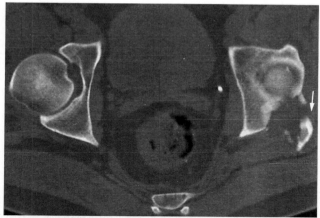

12a

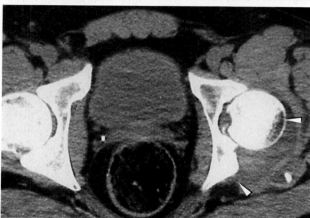

12b

considered in the diagnosis. They can occur due to osteoporosis and as a result of irradiation.

Acetabular Fractures

The force of the trauma causing the fracture is usually transferred via the condyle of the hip joint to the acetabulum. The most common isolated acetabular fractures are as follows:
– fractures of the posterior acetabular margin,
– fractures of the posterior column,
– true transverse fractures in both columns,
– fractures of the anterior column,
– fractures of the anterior acetabular margin.

Combined fractures occur with virtually the same frequency as the basic types. They include: T-shaped fractures, two-column fractures, fractures of the posterior acetabular margin and posterior column, transverse fracture plus fracture of the posterior column, fracture of the anterior acetabular margin and anterior column. The wing of the ilium is usually also severely injured in two-column fractures.

• CT

Because CT scans of the hip joint are free from overlapping structures, fractures in the anterior and posterior columns as well as the center of the acetabulum can be detected with sensi-

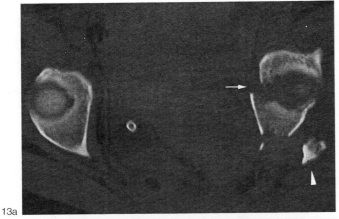

13a

13b

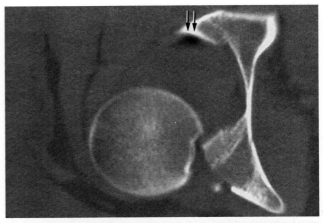

15a

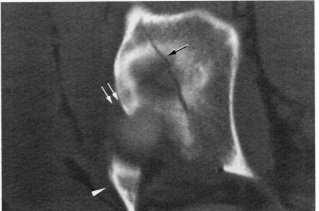

15b

Fig. 27-13a, b. Y-shaped fracture of the acetabulum with dehiscence of the anterior and posterior columns (→) as well as a fragmented anterior acetabular margin (►).

Fig. 27-15a, b. Fracture dislocation. The head of the femur exhibits dorsal subluxation. The posterior acetabular margin is craniodorsally dislocated (b ►). Demonstration of a fracture of the acetabular roof (b→). Head of the femur (⇒). A large effusion with raised CT numbers (70 HU) is found in the joint cavity. This corresponds to hemorrhage, not air (a ⇒).

Fig. 27-14a, b. Fracture of the anterior column (→), the posterior acetabular margin (⇒) and the intraarticular fragment (►). (b) Ventrocaudal three-dimensional image.

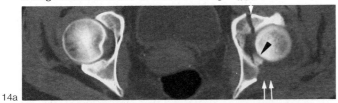

14a

Fig. 27-16. Central fracture dislocation (►). The center of the acetabulum is dislocated slightly into the true pelvis (→).

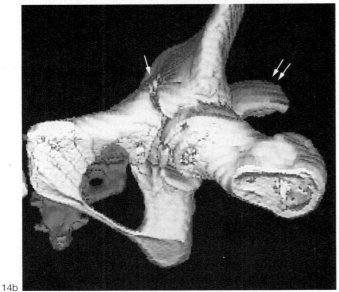

14b

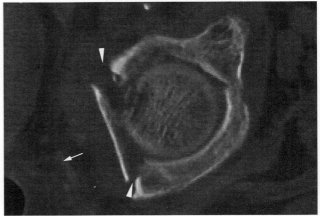

16

tivity. When the type of injury and fracture type are known, scans should be extended along the corresponding fracture lines, especially in the regions of the posterior column in the direction of the sacro-iliac joint. Non-dislocated transverse fractures can usually be identified, but thin-section scanning may be necessary to more clearly demonstrate questionable areas such as the region of the acetabular roof. It is especially important to verify the presence or absence of intra-articular fragments, which usually develop in the posterior compartment of the acetabulum. The width of the joint cavity in the region of the anterior and posterior acetabular margin should be carefully assessed for early identification of dislocation (or subluxation) injuries. High-resolution CT techniques should be used for detection of hair-line fractures.

Soft-tissues should always be assessed during CT examination of pelvic injuries. Unilateral thickening of the obturator internus muscle is an indirect sign of subperiosteal or parosteal hemorrhage and an indirect sign of a fracture. As fractures become more extensive, they tend to mask the fatty layers of periarticular muscles. Hemarthrosis can be identified as protrusion of the joint capsule, and it may lead to increased attenuation values near the head of the femur.

Coxitis

Bacterial infection usually develops hematogenously (staphylococcal or gonococcal infection), after a penetrating trauma, or iatrogeni-

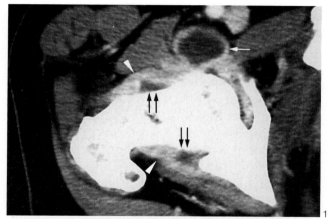
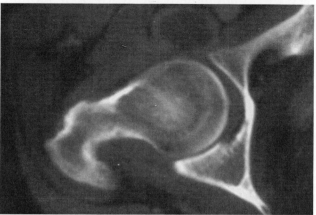
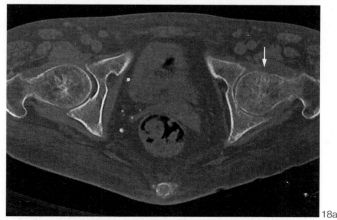
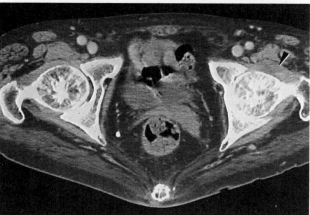

Fig. 27-17a, b. Coxitis. Inflammation of the joint caused by staphylococcal infection. Considerable thickening and opacification of the joint capsule (a ►) after contrast medium administration, with a small accumulation of effusion fluid (a ⇒). The bursa of the psoas major tendon is filled with fluid; it has inflamed, thickened walls (a→). The subchondral boundary layer of the femur head and the acetabular fossa at this stage is normal, with no evidence of erosion or decalcification (b).

Fig. 27-18a, b. Chronic coxitis. Findings include narrowing of the hip joint space, thinning of the subchondral boundary layer, and irregular bone structure in the entire femur head and neck, more so on the left than on the right (a). After contrast medium administration, the soft tissues show uniform enhancement of the thickened joint capsule (b ►).

cally. It leads to hydrarthrosis or hemarthrosis and inflammatory thickening of the synovial membrane and articular capsule. The surrounding soft-tissue and osseous tissue become inflamed as the disease progresses, and the communicating bursa of the psoas major tendon also becomes affected by inflammation. *Tuberculous infection* is insidious in nature. Its development is normally unilateral, and the occurrence of the disease is rising. Secondary juxta-articular osteoporosis is especially common in tuberculosis. Arthritides are characterized by broadening of the synovial membrane and successive absorption of cartilage. Erosion of bone occurs only along the edges. Osseous lesions (e.g. necrosis) mainly causes subchondral bone absorption that can eventually lead to the development of a fracture in the head of the hip joint.

• CT

Plain scans: Narrowing of the joint space, marginal and subchondral bone erosion and accompanying signs of demineralization can be detected early on high-resolution CT scans, especially when the other hip is used for comparison. Accompanying inflammation of the articular capsule leads to substantial broadening (greater than 6 mm).

Contrast-enhanced scans: Contrast medium can demonstrate a florid inflammation by enhancing the synovial membrane which, in turn, clearly demarcates the areas of joint effusion. Surrounding infiltrations and expanding abscesses can be better distinguished on contrast-mediated scans than on plain scans.

Sacroiliitis

Inflammation of the sacro-iliac joint sometimes occurs in patients with *rheumatic diseases*, including ankylosing spondylitis, Reiter's syndrome, juvenile rheumatoid arthritis, psoriatic arthritis, and inflammatory intestinal disease (enterocolic sacroiliitis). The inflammatory process is first limited to the joint space, but in florid stages, the disease can lead to extensive defects in the subchondral boundary lamella.

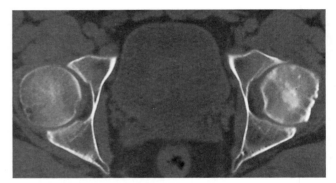

Fig. 27-19. Necrosis of the femoral head. Discretely stellate thickening of the bone structure in the head of the femur ("asterisk" sign; 2757, 2759, 2817).

Fig. 27-20. Sacroiliitis. The left sacro-iliac joint exhibits slight erosion (►) and a broad area of juxta-articular subchondral sclerosis. Bone erosion is also found in the dorsal section of the joint (b→).

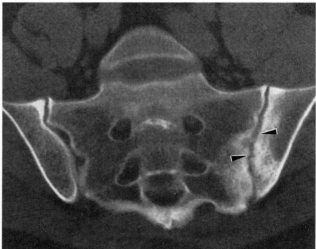

20a

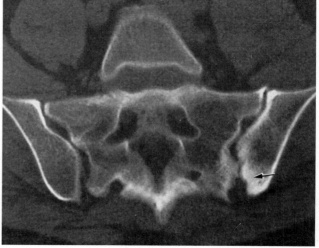

20b

Chronic forms of sacroiliitis can lead to sub-chondral sclerosis, narrowing of the joint space and, finally, to ankylosis. An *infectious cause* is rare and usually unilateral; the disease arises either hematogenously, by infiltration of puru-lent processes from the pelvis or surrounding muscle tissue into the joint, iatrogenically, or after a perforating injury. The course of the disease is usually acute. It leads to early lique-faction of cartilaginous tissue as well as contig-uous bony tissue, which shows increasing involvement in the inflammatory process in the form of osteomyelitis. When the disease is im-properly or insufficiently treated, abscesses may develop in surrounding soft-tissues.

• CT

Plain scans: Tangential scanning of articular surfaces affected by sacroiliitis, especially when utilizing high-resolution CT techniques, can provided detailed images of articular sur-faces and the surrounding bony tissue. Nar-rowing of the joint space to less than 2 mm, subchondral sclerosis, adjacent bony sclerosis and bony bridging can be demonstrated in de-tail. Early forms of sacroiliitis characterized by subtle erosion can be demonstrated and diag-nosed by CT when the findings of radionuclide imaging indicate abnormality.

Contrast-enhanced scans: The surrounding ex-udative components of infectious sacrociliitis can be demonstrated by CT after the adminis-tration of contrast medium. If necessary, nee-dle biopsy can be performed. Infiltration of adjacent organs, invasion of an infective pro-cess into the sacro-iliac joint, and involvement of osseous tissue via sclerosing osteomyelitis can be precisely demonstrated on contrast-en-hanced CT scans.

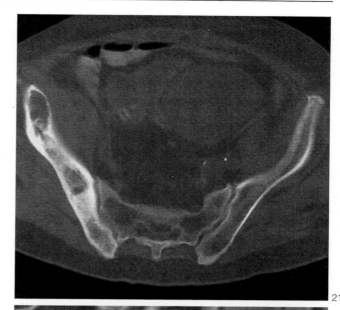

21

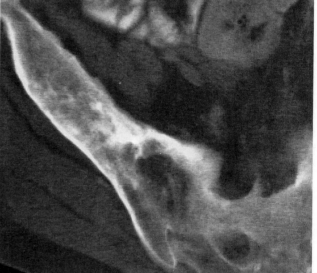

22a

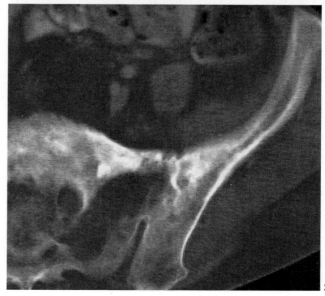

22b

Fig. 27-21. Paget's disease. Dilatation of the right wing of the ilium with irregular bone structure without evidence of soft-tissue components. Findings are limited to the wing of the ilium and end at the sacro-iliac joint.

Fig. 27-22a, b. Fibrous dysplasia. Dilatation of all pelvic bones, including the sacrum as well as the wings of the ilium. There is irregular strandlike or area thickening of bone structure and obliteration of cortical and spongiosa architecture.

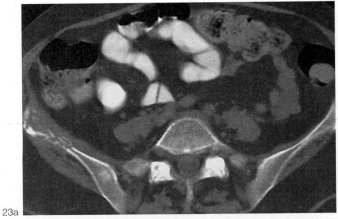

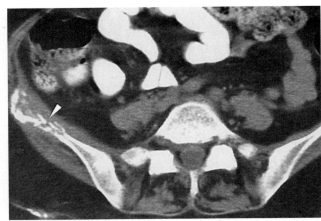

23a

23b

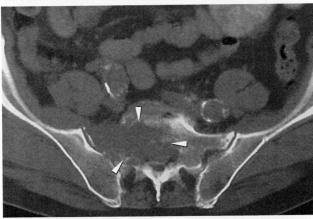

23c

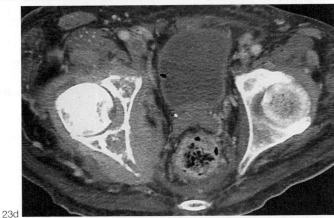

Fig. 27-23a-f. Patterns of osseous destruction in the bony pelvis.

a, b) Non-Hodgkin's lymphoma. At the bone-window setting, a "moth-eaten" pattern of disintegration of the cortical and spongy substance of the right wing of the ilium (a). At the soft-tissue window setting, the soft-tissue constituent of the non-Hodgkin's lymphoma can be seen on the interior surface of the wing of the ilium (b).

c)   Metastases from a bronchial carcinoma with osteolysis of the sacrum. The soft-tissue constituents of the tumor merge indistinctly into the disintegrated bone structure of the sacrum (►).

d-f) Metastasizing carcinoma of the bladder. Large soft-tissue masses in the region of the right hip joint with diffuse osseous permeation of the acetabulum extending into the joint space (d). Dilatation and disintegration of bone structure in the right wing of the ilium, which is surrounded by a large tumor (e, f).

23d

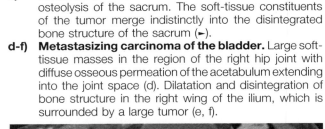

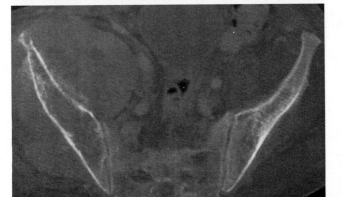

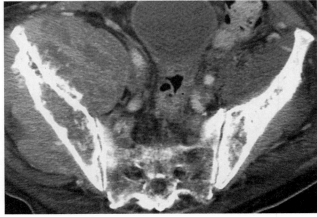

23e

23f

Chapter 28
CT Terminology

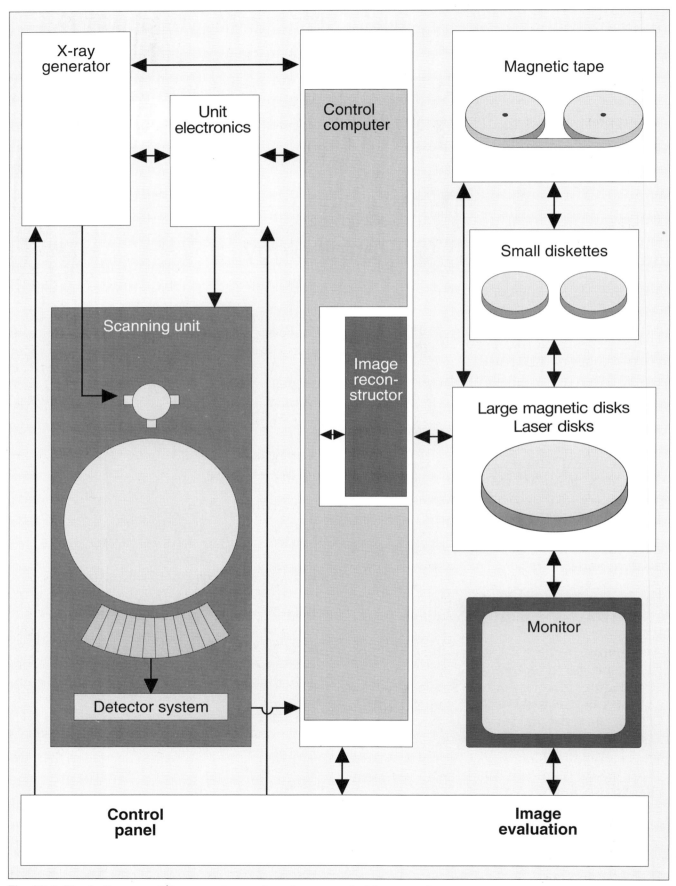

Fig. 28-1. Block diagram of the scanning system for computed tomography.

CT Terminology

Absorption of X-rays → Attenuation of X-rays.

Addition of image sections → Image analysis.

Algorithm = Set of rules for computation.

Angle measurement → Image analysis.

Archives → Documentation of images.

Artifacts: An artifact (artificial product) is a type of image disturbance. Several kinds of artifacts can develop in a diverse, complex imaging system such as computed tomography. Since the registration of attenuation values and electronic processing are subject to projection effects (→ Image reconstruction), image disturbance will often lead to the appearance of artifacts (linear, streak, etc.) that may extend throughout the entire image. Motion artifacts (see Fig. 28–3) are clinically relevant, and projections from the moving part of an organ cannot be exactly reconstructed. The result is not locally reduced resolution, but a stellate, striated pattern that radiates from the disturbed projection and tangentially intersects with the moving organ. Programs have been designed to correct many projection artifacts.

Attenuation of X-rays: Occurs when radiation passes through materials (e.g. tissues in CT). The degree of attenuation (absorption) depends on the intensity of the beam, scattering, and the physical characteristics of the tissue. Attenuation is quantitatively defined by the law of attenuation. The various tissues have quite precise ranges of attenuation values (see Hounsfield units).

Law of attenuation: $I = I_o e^{-\mu d}$

I_o = intensity on entrance
I = intensity on exit
μ = linear attenuation coefficient of the tissue
d = slice thickness.

Back projection → Image reconstruction.

Center → Display of images.

Cine-CT: Cinematographic imaging technique for rapid frame frequency. Used to produce dynamic CT images on the monitor.

Collimation: Controlling the beam. There are two types of collimation: primary (from the tube) and secondary (from the detector). Collimation affects the thickness and geometry of a section (→), the degree of contrast resolution (→), and the radiation dose (→).

Contrast resolution (= density resolution): This is limited by image noise, which is described as the standard deviation (SD) of CT numbers from a mean attenuation value (→ Image analysis, Histogram analysis). The lower the standard deviation, the better the contrast resolution. Depending on the X-ray intensity and dose, it can be less than 0.3% (≙ 3 HU).

Convolution (filtered back projection) → Image reconstruction.

Coordinates → Matrix.

Density profile → Image analysis.

Density resolution → Contrast resolution.

DEQCT = Dual energy quantitative CT: If a region of the body is scanned twice at two different tube voltages, substances containing elements with higher ordinal numbers (e.g. calcium, iodine, iron) will show greater attenuation differences as compared with elements with lower ordinal numbers (soft-tissue, fat). This reveals some clues as to the concentration of these substances. The technique is therefore used primarily in density measurement of bone among other things.

Detector: Detectors are used to detect and measure X-ray transmissions. Current detector systems for computed tomography use two types of materials: 1) highly pressurized gases

Fig. 28-2. Sources of artifacts.

Physical sources	Patient-related artifacts		
Beam-hardening	Patient movement	Metallic foreign body	Scanning beyond scanning circle
Classification			
Beam-hardening artifacts (shading, dishing)	Motion artifacts	Streak artifacts (high-density streaking)	
Appearance			
Shadowy artifacts adjacent to and inside high-contrast structures.	Linear artifacts, the extent of which depends on the level of contrast of the moving structure. The lines (tangentially) pass through the center of motion.	High-density (positive, negative) radial artifacts project from the mental object (see data blackout).	Widespread increase of attenuation values in areas of the image adjacent to the sections of the organ outside the boundaries of the scanning circle (field of measurement). This usually falsifies the attenuation values for the entire CT scan.
a, b) Teflon rod in water. The high attenuation values of teflon leads to the formation of shadowy artifacts (a) adjacent to and (b) within the image of the rod. **c)** Density gradient within image of a large renal cyst caused by adjacent high-contrast structures.	Linear artifacts caused by: **a)** brief linear motion. **b, c)** oscillating movements during the scanning process. **Contrast: a, b)** air in water, **c)** contrast medium (+ 150 HU) in water.	Streaking caused by: **a)** metal hip-joint replacement. **b, c)** metal clips.	**a)** Oval water phantom lying outside the scanning circle: Attenuation values increased by 14 HU and lateral (>) artifacts are visible. **b, c)** Analogous artifacts in a patient.

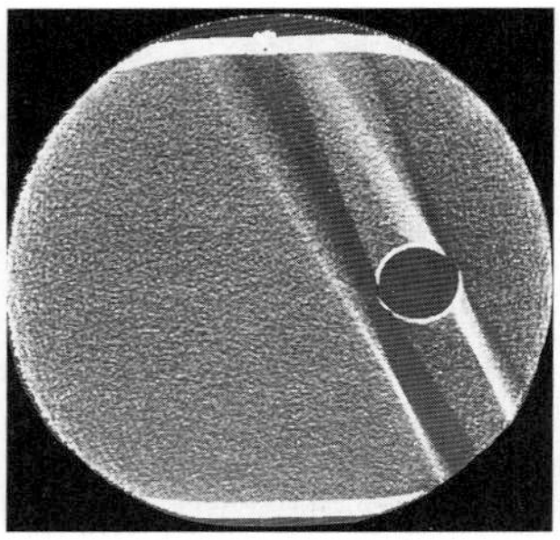

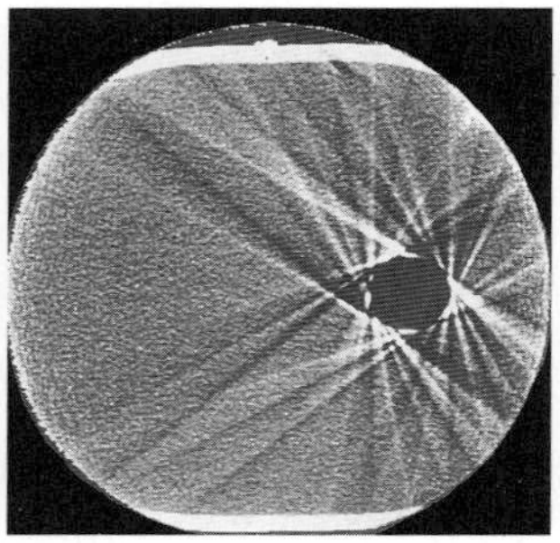

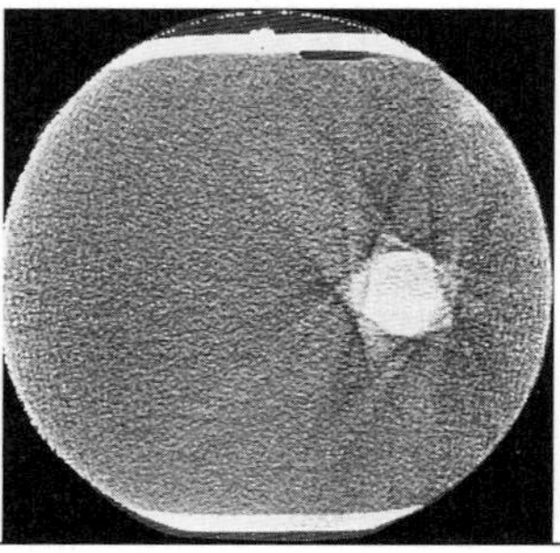

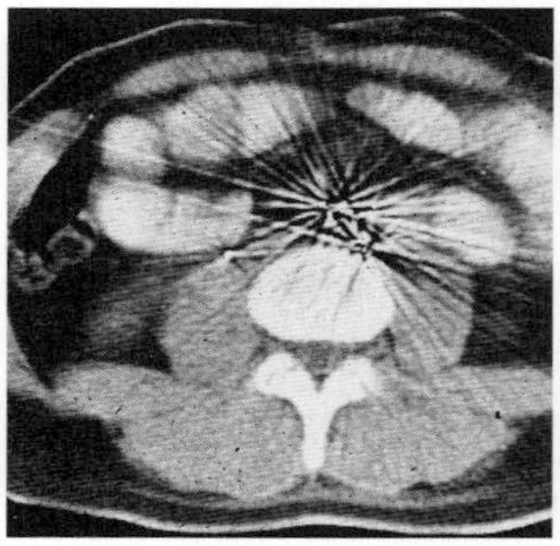

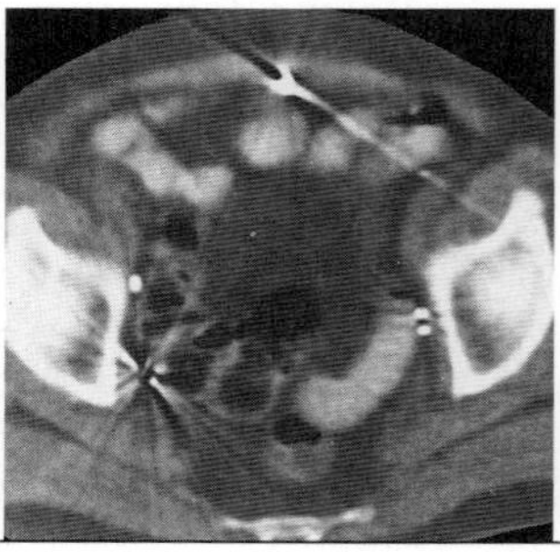

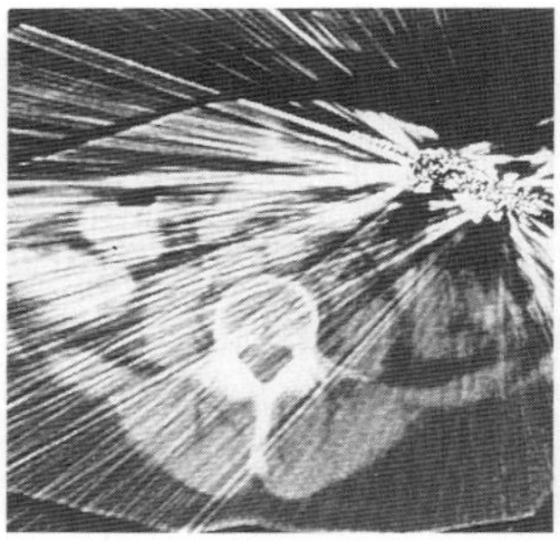

2a

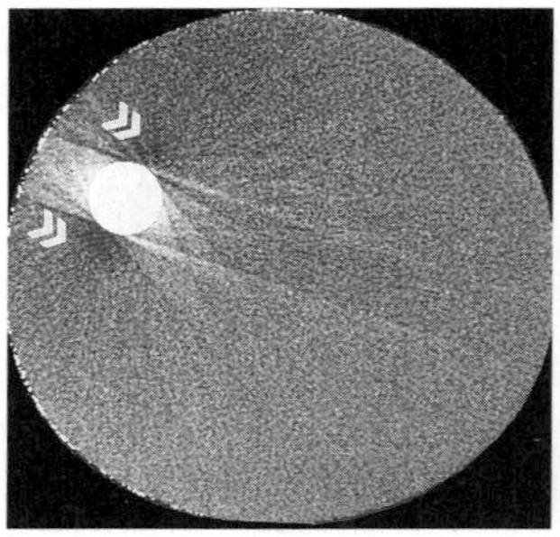

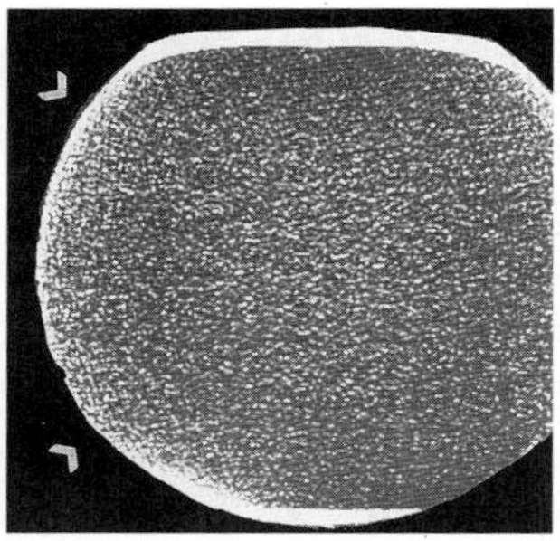

2b

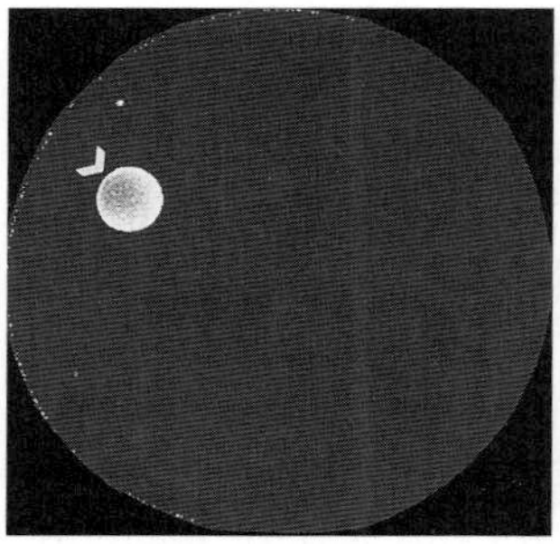

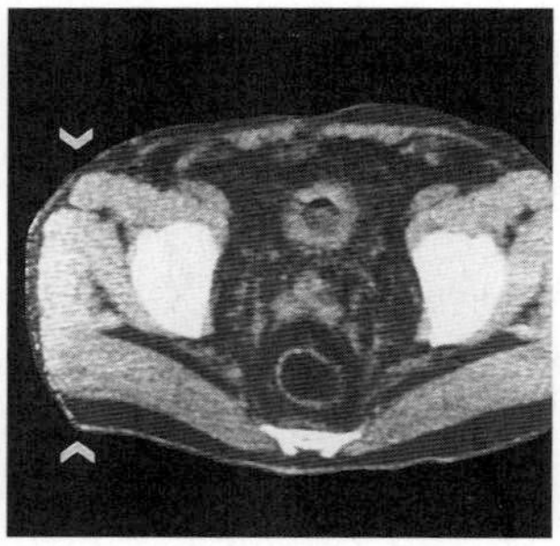

2c

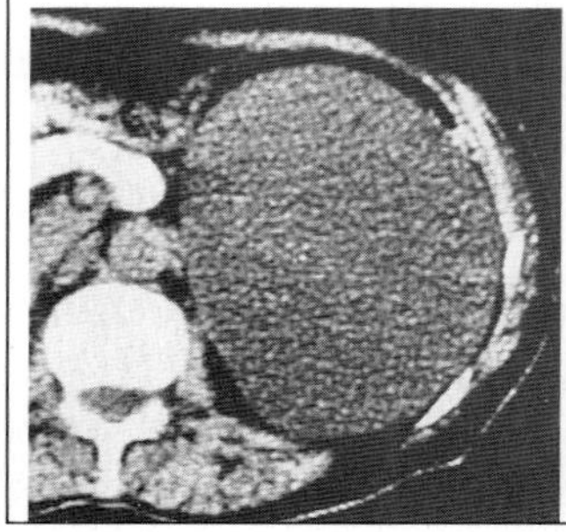

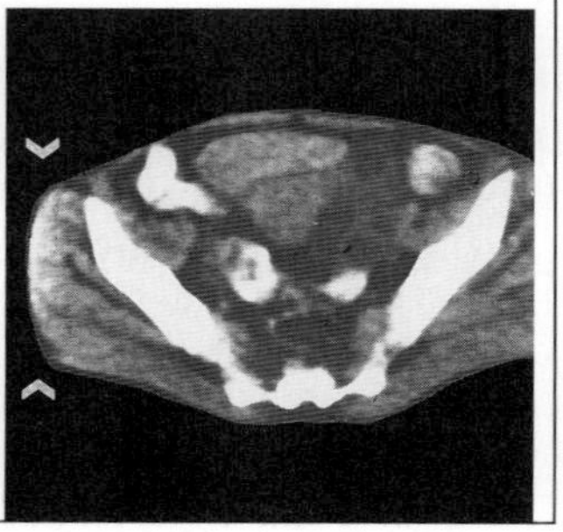

Fig. 28-2. Sources of artifacts (continued).

Equipment-related artifacts

Reconstruction filter	Overranging of scanner system	Dealignment of detectors (3rd generation scanners)	Data blackout due to defective equipment
Classification			
Edge effects	Overranging artifacts	Ringlike artifacts	Linear artifacts, etc.
Appearance			
"Raised" edges of contrast-rich organ borders (e.g. lung, bone) (simulating a subarachnoid space, pleural calcification, etc.).	Plateau-like artifacts in and surrounding regions of an organ where linear measurement was not possible due to overranging of the detector amplification system.	Linear round structures around the center of the image.	The missing projection is seen on CT scans as a diametrical, trilinear structure.
Edge effects causing: **a)** Simulation of a subarachnoid space. **b)** Simulation of pleural calcification.	**a)** Linear artifacts caused by overranging lung phantom. **b)** Patch of reduced density in ventral regions of the abdomen caused by overriding the scanning system.	**a, b)** Round artifacts arising from dealignment of detectors.	**a, b)** Blackout of single projections. **c)** Blackout of multiple projections from the same scanning direction.

2a

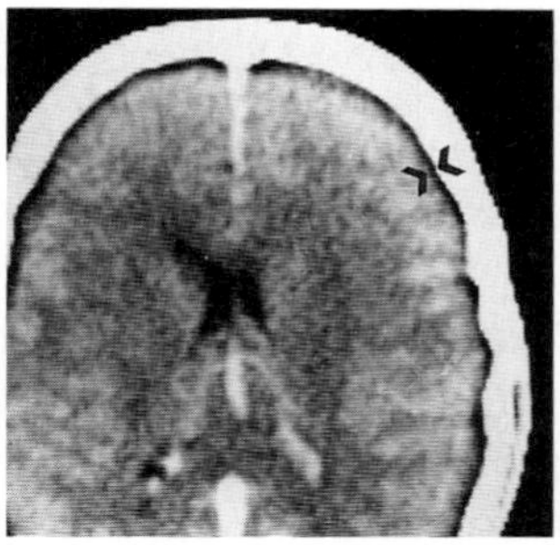

2a

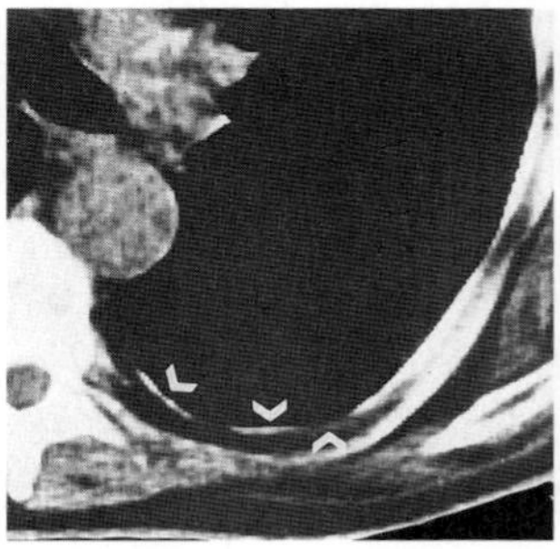

2a

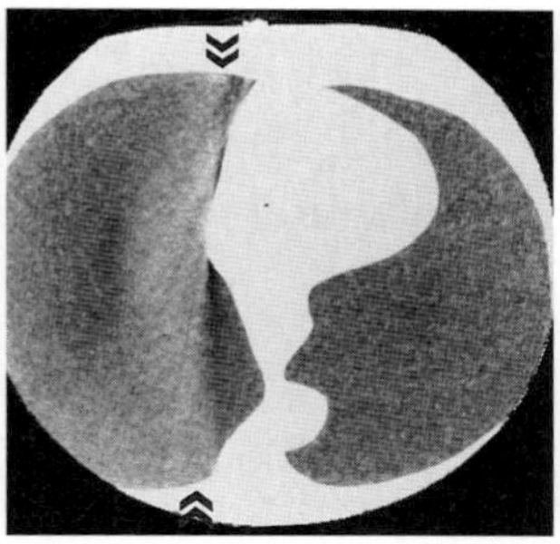

2a

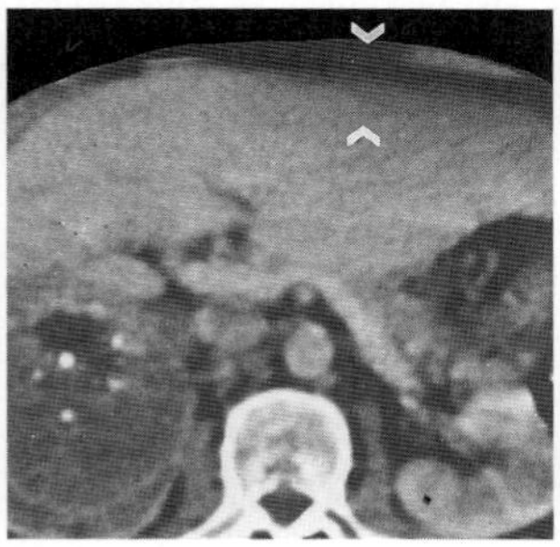

2b

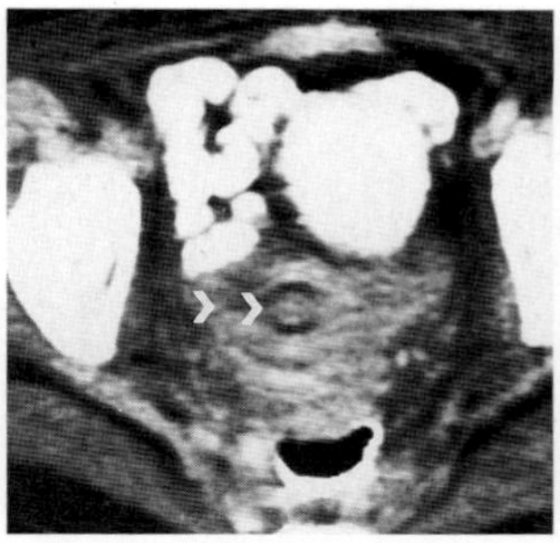

2b

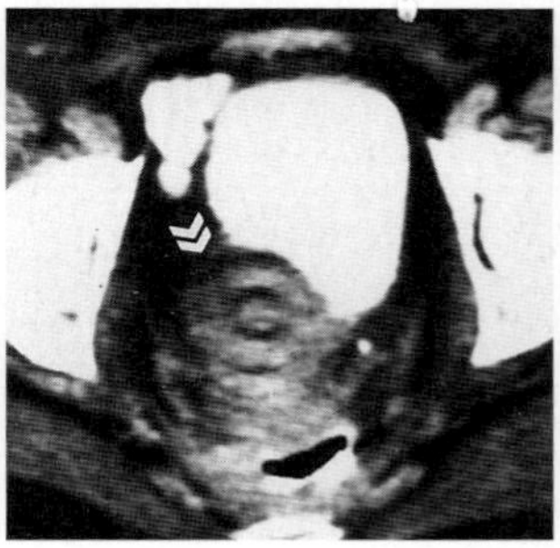

2b

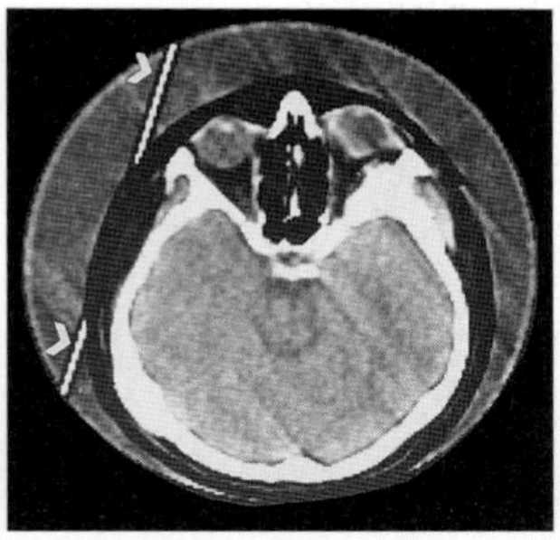

2b

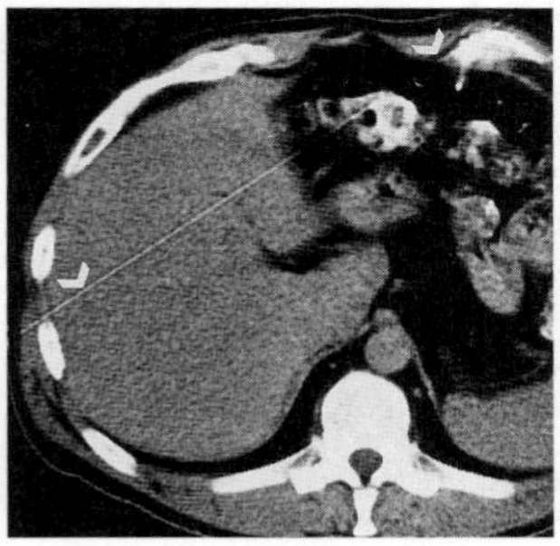

2c

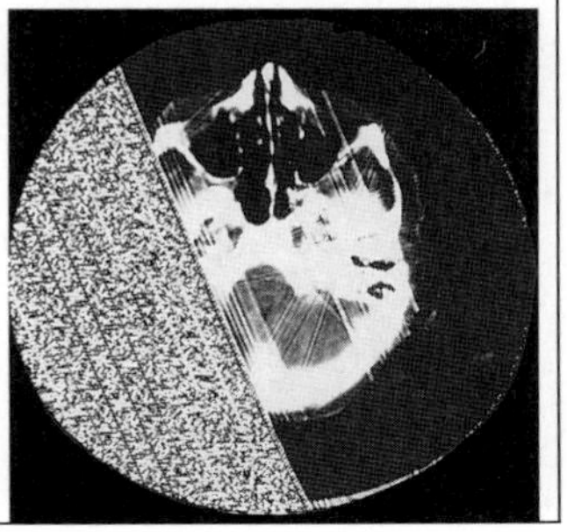

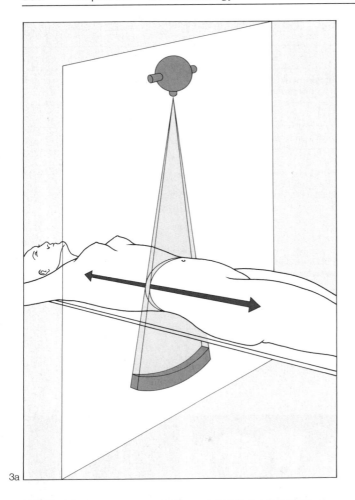

3a

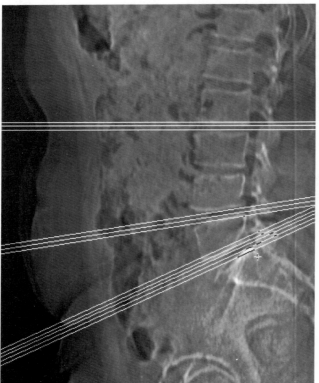

3b

such as xenon or 2) solid materials such as iodine or germanate crystals.

Digital image (scanogram, topogram, scout view, radiogram): In scanners with a fixed source and detector system, the patient is advanced longitudinally after each section has been scanned, until the entire scanning protocol has been covered. This creates a digital image matrix, the rows of which (height) correspond to the slice thickness. The number of pixels in each row corresponds to the number of detectors used for measurement. Depending on the orientation of the X-ray tube, lateral, anteroposterior, and oblique projections can be made, and the level of the slice can be reproducibly localized. Subsequent tilting of the gantry with respect to the axis of the body can be planned from a lateral digital image projection (of importance in spinal examinations).

Directory: Overview (list of contents) of stored files of CT images that can be called in for use.

Display device = Monitor.

Display of images: A computed tomogram consists of a matrix of numbers which covers a scale of 2000 Hounsfield units (-1000 to 1000 HU). The human eye can distinguish only 15 to 20 different *shades of grey*. Therefore, each shade would have to represent ca. 50 HU if an attempt were made to cover the entire scale with visible shades. The *image window* was therefore developed for better visualization of smaller density differences and to make contrasted structures more accessible to evaluation. The *window width* (WW) defines the range of CT numbers to be visualized, and the *window level* (WL) determines which attenuation values will be depicted at the center of the

Fig. 28-3. Digital X-ray image. A summated digital image is produced by maintaining a stationary scanning system and longitudinal table increment (a). By superimposing gantry gradient display (white lines) onto the X-ray image, it is possible to precisely position the level of each section (b).

grey scale. The window level is set in accordance with the tissue type(s) to be diagnosed. When narrow window widths are used, important structures outside the window range may be overlooked and omitted from the diagnosis. Broad window widths, on the other hand, tend to homogenize and mask slight density differences.

Distance, measurement of → Image analysis.

Documentation of images: Photographic documentation: The CT scan currently stored on a magnetic disk can be called up on the monitor and *photographically* documented. The window width (WW) and window level (WL) (→ Display of images) of the CT scan are then fixed. Magnetic storage: *Magnetic tapes* and *disks* preserve the electronic information about the CT scan and are suitable for long-term data storage. When re-read into the computer, the window width and level can be readjusted, and the CT images can be visualized and analyzed again (→ Image analysis).

Dose → Radiation dose.

Fan beam = Fan-shaped emission of X-rays.

Filter → Image reconstruction, → Filtration.

Filtered back projection → Image reconstruction.

Filtration: Each pixel is entered in a computation program that also analyzes its relationship and distance to surrounding pixels. Filters can reduce noise and improve image definition and contour sharpness for optimization of images. A filtered image can be filtered again as required (secondary filtration). However, primary filtration performed during image re-

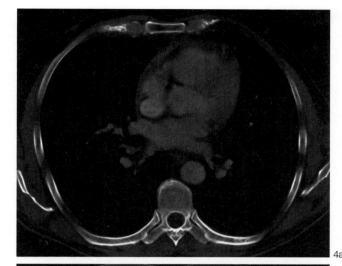
4a

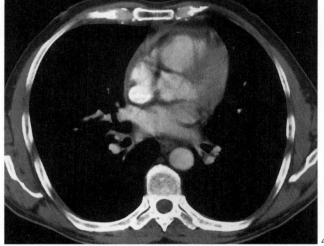
4b

Fig. 28-4. Window settings used in computed tomography. The level and range of the Hounsfield scale can be narrowed to create a "window" that can optimally utilize visible shades of grey for better visualization and analysis of body tissues of various types and densities. This can dramatically change the visual appearance of the image (see Chap. 1).

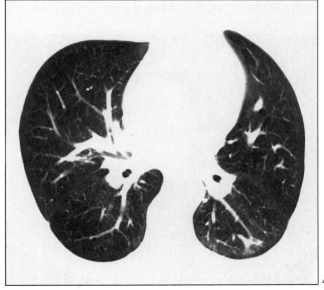
4c

construction (→) must be distinguished from secondary filtration.

Gantry (= scanning unit) → Imaging system.

Gonadal dose → Radiation dose.

HU = Hounsfield unit.

HRCT (high resolution computed tomography): By reducing the scan width, i.e. by reducing the distance between detectors, the pixel size in usually central areas of the image can be reduced, resulting in improvement of local resolution. At the present, pixel diameters as small as 0.25 mm have been achieved. Reduction of pixel or voxel size leads to an increase in image noise. Some structures, especially high-contrast objects such as bone, are particularly suitable for HRCT techniques. Longer scanning times must be used when scanning soft-tissue structures. Since the fields of measurement are usually small, the term *sector scanning* is often used.

High-contrast resolution: Ensures clear images of small structures on the CT scan with variably high object contrast (> 10% or 100 HU). Usually corresponds to an image contrast (MTF) of 2%.

Fig. 28-5. Highlighting. Picture elements within a certain (freely selectable) density range appear white (in this case, -850 to -1000 HU).

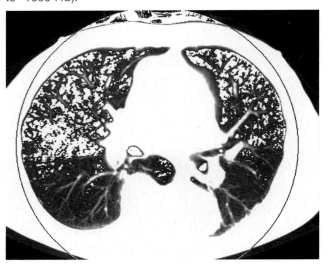

Highlighting: Highlighted attenuation values in a selected density range appear white in order to make them better distinguishable from surrounding morphological structures on the CT scan.

Hounsfield unit (HU): Unit on the CT scale. The CT number (attenuation value) of a given material is defined as the relative deviation of the effective linear attenuation coefficient of this material from the effective linear attenua-

Fig. 28-6. Contrast detail diagram describing resolution in CT.
K = Field for demonstrating fine, high-contrast structures (e.g. bone)
W = Field for differentiation inside soft-tissue range

1 = Scanning parameters:
    e.g., 7 s/700 projections/500 mAs/125 kV.
    Reformatting: high-resolution convolution method
2 = Scanning parameters:
    e.g., 14 s/1400 projections/1000 mAs/125 kV.
    Reformatting: conventional method.

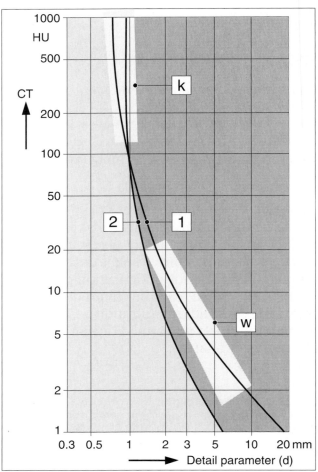

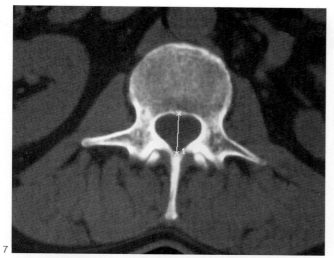

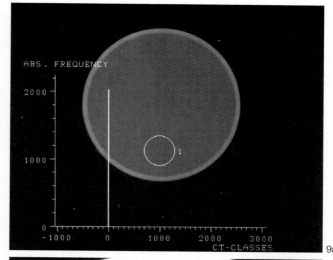

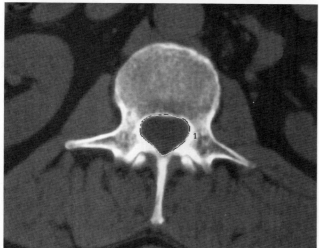

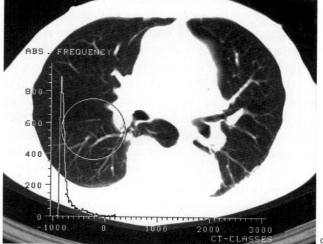

Fig. 28-7. Measurement of distance. Two picture points are marked (x). Distance is measured in millimeters.

Fig. 28-8. Spot measurement. The region of interest (ROI) is marked with a lightpen (trackball or mouse). The sum of all picture elements contained within it equals the cross-sectional area (mm²). The marked area also serves as the ROI for density measurements (see Figs. 28-7 and 28-8).

Fig. 28-9. Densitometry. Plotting the attenuation values of pixels in a region of interest (circular in this case) will result in (a) a symmetrical density curve in homogeneous media such as water, and (b) asymmetrical or irregular density curves in inhomogeneous media such as lung tissue.

tion coefficient of water multiplied by the factor 1000.

Image analysis: Objective data can be derived from the computer tomogram by utilizing simple computational operations. Imaging can be improved by interactive display functions (→).

Fig. 28-10. Density profile. The attenuation value of pixels on the selected line on the scan are not represented in grey tones. Instead, they are plotted on a scale with respect to their location.

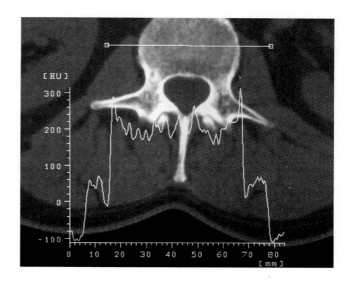

– *Measurement of distance*: The distance between two points in the body can be computed as the distance between the corresponding picture points on the CT image. *Angle measurement* can similarly be made by computing the angle between points in the coordinate system (x- and y-axis).

– *Measurement of area and volume*: The area of a region of interest *(ROI)* is equal to the sum of all picture elements within it. Similarly, the volume is the sum of all volume elements.

– *Histogram analysis:* A histogram shows the frequency distribution of a given variable, in this case, the attenuation value. The frequency distribution of the CT numbers in a given *ROI* (→) is usually represented as a column diagram spread across a density scale. A *normal histogram distribution* is considered to be a symmetrical bell-shaped (Gaussian) curve, the *standard deviation* (SD) of which can be computed with respect to the median value. The attenuation value of homogeneous material (e.g. water phantom) is usually characterized by a normal distribution pattern. The *mean value* and standard deviation can, therefore, be confidently calculated. The SD primarily represents the statistic variation of photon flux during scanning (quantum noise). Inhomogeneous materials (tissue, etc.) usually generate an asymmetrical histogram curve. Mixed tissue elements can create additional peaks on the histogram (plurimodal histogram). A median value then cannot be calculated, because it would be imprecise.

– *Subtraction, addition, density profile*: In *subtraction*, density difference is calculated by subtracting values from two different CT measurements at the *same site*. The subtraction method is especially suitable for contrast medium studies, where precontrast attenuation is subtracted from the contrast attenuation value. This provides a direct and graphic representation of contrast enhancement. In the *addition* method, CT numbers from contiguous sections are added to create larger sections of greater thickness. A grey scale is normally used to represent attenuation values on CT scans. On a *density profile*,

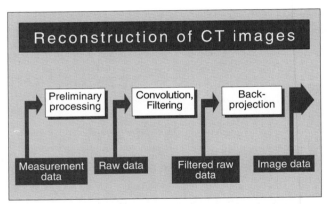

Fig. 28-11. Reconstruction (reformatting) of CT images.

attenuation values of a chosen length or diameter are represented on an (analogous) density curve on which the y-axis corresponds to the density scale.

Image reconstruction: In image reconstruction, a computation process is used to generate a computed tomogram of collected measurement data. Older algebraic methods have now been replaced by quicker convolution algorithms. In the convolution method, all attenuation data are filtered or *convolved* (convolution function, algorithm), before they are back projected. This method of filtered back projection is used to increase image sharpness around the edges of a scanned object and to produce images free of artifacts. It can be varied to make considerations for special problems. This, of course, changes the visual impression of the image. *Superimposition of edges* (edge effects) along the absorption borders may also create problems associated with artifacts.

Imaging system: An imaging system contains the following elements:
– *scanning unit* (recording unit, gantry), which consists of the X-ray source(s), detector system, and measurement registration system,
– *X-ray generator* and *electronic devices* that belong to the scanning unit,
– *table* (couch) for horizontal and vertical positioning of the patient,

– *computer console* (control panel) and *image reconstructor*, with which the individual functions can be called up after "dialogue" with the computer,
– *computer*, which is responsible for coordinating all system functions and calculating image reconstruction (→),
– *magnetic storage devices*: CT images can be stored on various storage devices. They include the fixed disk or magnetic core for short-term (primary) storage and magnetic disks, tapes and floppy diskettes for long-term (secondary) storage of patient scan images (→ Documentation of images).

Interactive display functions: Points on a computer matrix can be marked with a *track ball* or *mouse*. The picture point is then visually localized, which obviates the need for specification of the x and y coordinates (x_i, y_i). The marked area may represent the midpoint of a regular ROI (circle or square) of variable area. *Irregular ROI* can also be selected simply by marking them with the cursor.

Linear attenuation coefficient → Attenuation of X-rays.

Low-contrast resolution: Identification of small objects with slight contrast differences (> 1% or 10 HU).

Magnetic disk → Imaging system, Magnetic storage devices.

Matrix: A matrix (image matrix) is grid of individual picture elements (pixels) usually arranged as a two- dimensional square. Most scanners have matrices with 80 x 80, 160 x 160, 256 x 256, 320 x 320, and/or 512 x 512 pixels. These individual picture points can be taken as units in a *coordinate system* with an x- and y-axis. Enumeration of the individual coordinates begins in the upper left corner of the matrix. A pixel (x_1, y_1) can therefore be defined as the numeric pair of coordinates at a certain intercept (in this case, $x_1 = 10$ and $y_1 = 21$). X_1 can also be defined as the 10th *column*, and y_1 as the 21st *row*.

Memory → Imaging system, Magnetic storage devices.

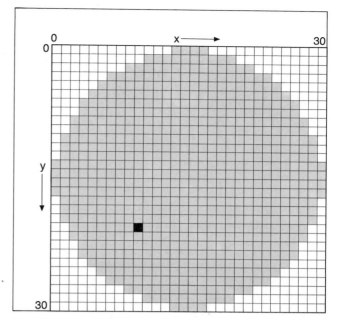

Fig. 28-12. Coordinates on the image matrix.

Modulation transfer function (MTF): Defines the relationship of image contrast to object contrast.

Monitor = Display device.

Mouse → Interactive display functions.

MTF = Modulation transfer function.

Noise: Statistical inaccuracy of the attenuation value of an individual picture element due to statistical fluctuation of photon flux. → Image analysis, Histogram analysis.

OSTEO-CT: Quantitative measurement of mineral content of bodies of the vertebra of the lumbar spine. → SEQCT, DEQCT.

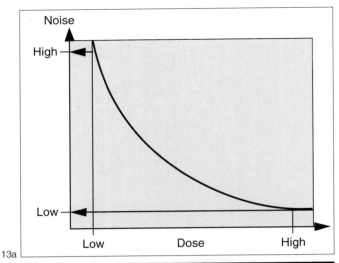

13a

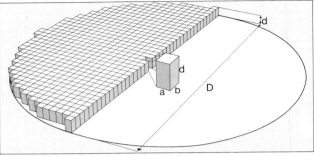

Fig. 28-14. Volume of a volume element. The area of the individual picture elements and the slice thickness (d) determine the volume of each individual volume element. (a) and (b) represent the edge length of the picture element. (D) is the diameter of the scanning circle, i.e., field of measurement.

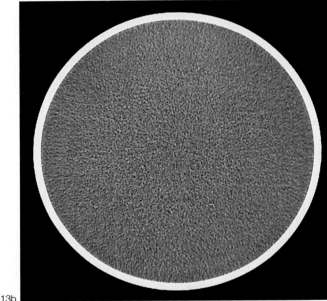

13b

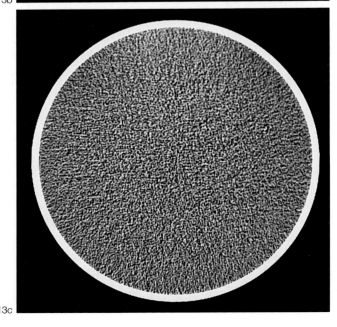

13c

Picture element: The smallest unit on a computer matrix (→), i.e. the individual picture point, called picture element or pixel for short.

Pixel = Picture element.

QCT = Quantitative computed tomography. Used for densitometry.

Radiation dose:
– *Somatic radiation dose*: With well collimated scanners, the somatic radiation dose for the *trunk of the body* is *2 to 3 rad*, which is comparable to that of other radiographic examinations (urography, colonic contrast enema).
Collimation of the X-ray beam restricts the dose to the imaged section of the body. According to McCullough (Ref. 361), the maximum surface dose is 3 to 13 rad per slice in the skull, 1.5 to 3.5 rad per slice in the trunk of the body. However, the trunk may receive doses greater than 10 rad when long scanning times (low noise scans) are utilized. Penumbra formation and scattered rays increases the dose in the individual slices by a factor of 1.2 to 1.9 (pile-up factor, multiple/single ratio) during a scan series. The total dose received in a whole-body examination

Fig. 28-13. Image noise. Image noise, which reduces the level of contrast resolution, is dose-dependent. b = high dose; c = low dose.

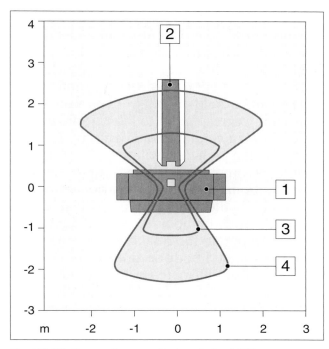

Fig. 28-15. Dose at scan site in a (rotary) CT scanner.

Table 28-1. Organ dose per slice on the axis of rotation, in the open air [91].

Organ	Mean value (mGy)	Range
Skull	35.8	7 – 207
Thorax	27.8	6.7 – 91.3
Abdomen	27.7	6.3 – 168
Pelvis	26.2	6.7 – 161.5
Spine	39.3	13 – 162

Table 28-2. Locational, personal, and total body dose.

In the terminology of radiation protection agencies, the following terms, based on the equivalent dose, are used to classify radiation dose:	
Site dose H$_P$	Equivalent dose for soft-tissues, measured at a specific site. It relates to the tube current, measured in mAs.
Unit of measurement	μSv/100 mAs
Personal dose H$_x$	Equivalent dose H for soft-tissues, measured at a site of the body surface with a representative radiation dose.
Unit of measurement	μSv
Terms relating to total body dose	
Total body dose H$_G$ (μSv)	Mean value of equivalent dose in head, trunk, upper arms, and thighs in uniform bodily radiation exposure.
Partial body dose H$_T$ (μSv)	Equivalent dose, averaged from the volume of one body part or organ or an area of skin.
Effective equivalent dose H$_E$ (μSv)	Sum of the mean equivalent dose (H$_T$) multiplied by applicable weighting factors (W$_T$) for the specific organ or tissue. $$H_E = \sum W_T \times H_T$$

The **site dose**, i.e. the dose distributed to the scanned region during scanning, is of significance for radiation protection. This is classified as isodense distribution (lines of equal dose), in one-millionth Sievert per 100 mAs tube current.
The site dose is directly proportional to scatter, slice thickness, the mAs product, and the kV value. The smaller the scatter, the thinner the slice, and the lower the mAs and kV, the lower the site dose during the scanning period.

Table 28-3. CT dose index (CTDI).

The **CT dose index (CTDI)** was established as an objective parameter of measurement of dose exposure in an area of 14 contiguous slices (with normed slice thickness). Data according to the Food and Drug Administration.	
CT dose index ("CTDI")	The CTDI is the quotient of the sum of the local radiation dose D(z) in 14 slices along the longitudinal axis of the scanning system z (socalled longitudinal dose product), divided by slice thickness h. $$CTDI = \frac{1}{h} \int_{-7h}^{+7h} D(z)\ dz;$$
Unit of measurement	mGy

The CTDI is measured with 16 and 32 cm plexiglass phantoms of 1 cm depth.
The CTDI value is measured in mGy, usually as relates to 100 mAs tube current. Because of radiation scatter and finite skirt selectivity of the dose profile, the CTDI is proportional to the slice thickness and kV value.

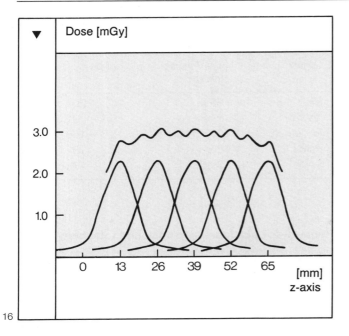

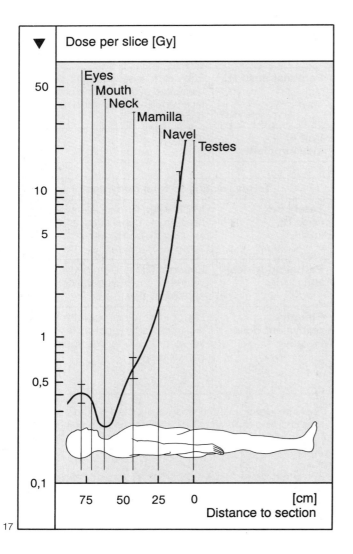

16

17

will therefore be at least 2 rad. The radiation exposure for the patient is more clearly described by the product of dose per unit area. This also allows for indirect conclusions about the integral dose of an examination. The entire field of entry of a scan series usually corresponds to the radiographic fields of conventional radiography. In other words, the radiated volume of a CT scan series is comparable to that of a large-format conventional radiograph. It is not admissible to multiply the dose of an individual section with the total number of scanned sections in order to obtain the total dose. As the number of scanned body sections increases, the volume dose will increase, but the amount of energy absorption per volume unit (measured in units of rad or mGy; 1 rad = 10 mGy) hardly increases.

– *Gonadal dose*: When the gonads are not included in the scanned section, they receive a variable degree of scatter radiation. This decreases considerably as the distance between the gonads and the section scanned increases. The scatter and transmission radiation is greater than that in intracorporal areas (ref. 361).

Reformatted (secondary) images: If a series of contiguous sections are scanned, the column formed by stacking the individual sections would represent a continuous volume divided into volume elements. For any given diameter, row, or column of the image matrix, analogous picture elements in contiguous sections can be found and imaged on the monitor. Secondary coronal and sagittal sections can therefore be created, which can be visualized only when thin sections have been scanned (2 to 5 mm, maximum of 8 mm). Complex interpolation programs will be necessary to reconstruct planes that deviate from the orthogonal coor-

Fig. 28-16. Increased radiation dose due to X-ray scattering and penumbra formation in contiguous sections (pile-up factor).

Fig. 28-17. Gonadal dose due to scatter varies in proportion with the proximity of the level of section to the gonads [753].

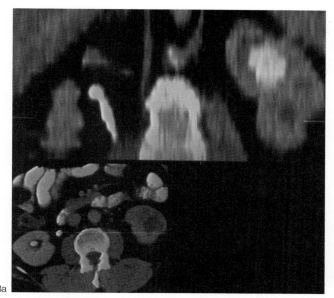

18a

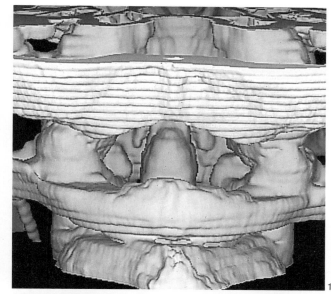

18c₁

Fig. 28-18. Secondary slices and three-dimensional reconstruction.

a) Frontal reconstruction of a carcinoma of the renal pelvis. The tumor and urinary obstruction are well demonstrated, despite limited vertical resolution.

b, c) In 3D reconstruction, the silhouettes of an anatomical structure are constructed from a series of sections, and the surface of the structure is reconstructed three-dimensionally. Then, spatial and perceptive impressions are made by shading the surface structures with a simulated light source. If this technique is to be utilized, there must be an adequate contrast difference between the target structure and surrounding tissues (e.g. bone, soft tissues) as well as total measurement of the structure's volume. (b) Three-dimensional image of a metastatic bone tumor and (c) of the occipito-cervical junction (dorsal scan) from different projections.

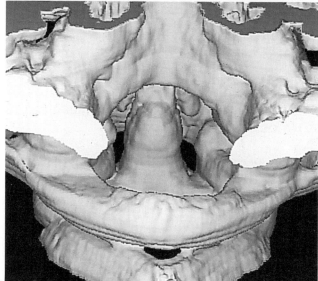

18c₂

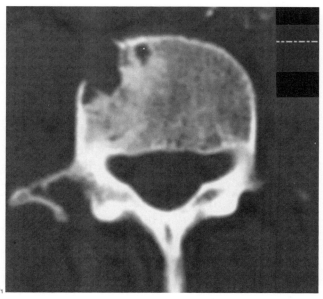

18b₁

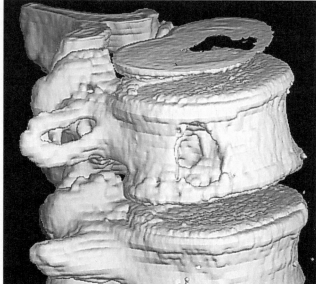

18b₂

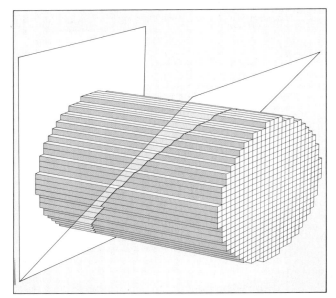

Fig. 28-19. Secondary slices. By interpolating the orthogonally arranged volume elements, freely selectable slices can be reconstructed. Different programs are available (multiplanar reconstruction).

dinates, i.e., x, y, and z (multiplanar reconstruction).

Region of interest (ROI): The region to be scanned, i.e. region of interest, can be freely selected by entering the corresponding coordinates (→ Matrix) or by marking them (→ Interactive display functions).

ROI = Region of interest.

Scanning: Imaging system in which a scanning gantry housing the X-ray tube and detectors is rotated around the patient. Various scanning modes and parameters that determine the quality of the CT scan can be freely selected:
– *Tube voltage*: The X-ray generator creates the tube voltage and, thus, the intensity of emitted X-rays. An increase in tube voltage leads to a corresponding increase in photon flux and a reduction in image noise due to reduced attenuation of X-rays. Increasing the tube voltage leads to a reduction in tissue contrast and the development of beam-hardening artifacts (→). Most scanning systems used in whole-body CT today operate with a tube voltage of 110 to 140 kV.

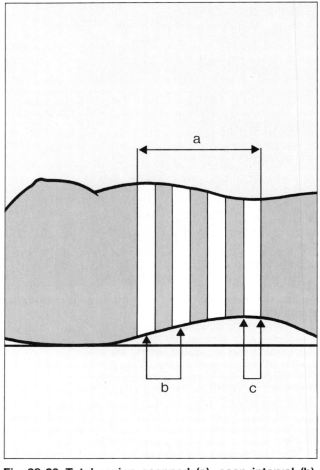

Fig. 28-20. Total region scanned (a), scan interval (b), slice thickness (c).

– *Scan field*: This refers to the circular field of measurement covered by the X-ray tube and detector array. Parts of an object that lie outside the scan field may not be imaged, which can lead to the generation of artifacts. The size of the scan field must, therefore, be large enough to include all important structures. The area of the scan field corresponds to the size of the image matrix (→). This, in turn, determines the pixel size. The diameter of the scan field (mm) divided by the number of pixels in a single row of the matrix determines the pixel size (mm).
– *Scanning protocol*: This is a longitudinally measured region of the body to be scanned in a series of CT scans. Contiguous sections (table advance = slice thickness), overlapping sections (table increment slice thick-

ness), or noncontiguous sections (table advance X slice thickness) may be scanned.

– *Scanning time*: A reduction in scanning time leads to a corresponding reduction in motion artifacts (→). This has certain restrictions, since tube capacity determines the radiation dose that is used during the scanning time. The radiation dose and image noise (→), i.e. contrast resolution, are closely related.

– *Slice thickness*: The width of the X-ray beam (on a z- axis) can be varied by collimation. Narrow collimation restricts the flow of photons, thereby increasing scan noise, and longer scanning times may be necessary.

Scoutview → Digital image processing.

SD = Standard deviation → Image analysis, Histogram analysis.

Slice (section), slice geometry: Measurement data collected by the different scanning techniques is obtained from a predominantly flat cross-sectional area of the body. Because of divergence of radiation from the focus of the beam:

– the CT section is not parallel, i.e., the slice thickness is not constant,
– the sensitivity of measurement within the slice thickness (longitudinal to the z-axis) is

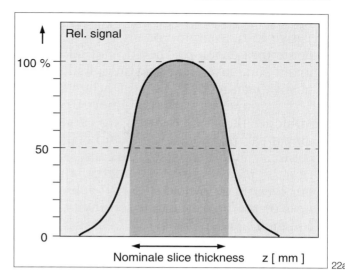

Fig. 28-22. Slice geometry.
a) The (nominal) slice thickness (NST) corresponds to the half-value of the dose profile in the center of the field of measurement.

b) The slice geometry is dependent upon slice thickness. The optimum goal of rectangular dose distribution cannot be achieved with very thin slices.

c) In spiral CT, the slice thickness increases in proportion with the table increment.

Fig. 28-21. Classification of plane of section. a = horizontal, transverse plane; b = sagittal plane; c = frontal plane.

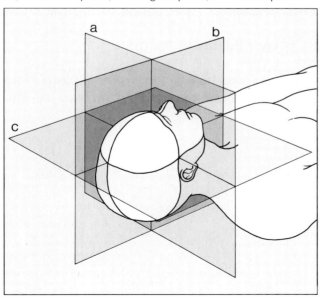

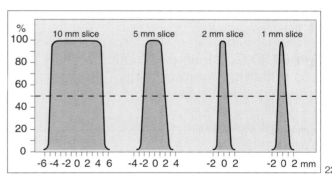

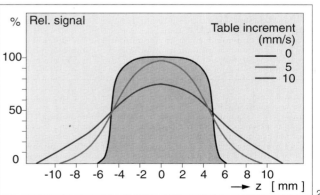

variable, i. e. the midsection of the slice is more sensitive to measurement,

– penumbra develop. They do not add to the image, but have an impact on radiation. Optically flat sections are best achieved with 360° scanning increments. Other effects that influence the slice geometry (to variable degrees) can be reduced by beam collimation (primary and secondary). Because of variation in measurement geometry, the *slice thickness* is defined as the half-value thickness of the measurement sensitivity profile (on the z-axis) in the middle of the scan field. The *level of the section*, which is determined by the imaging system, is usually set up so that it is vertical to the axis of the body (transverse sections, horizontal sections). The scanning gantry can be tilted slightly from the vertical position. Sections can be scanned in a *coronal plane* by repositioning the patient's head (hyperflexion) and tilting the gantry. In whole-body computed tomography, frontal and sagittal images can be generated by reformatting other images (→ Image reconstruction).

SEQCT = Single energy quantitative CT. In contrast to the dual energy method, density measurement of CT images is performed with only one tube voltage (conventional densitometry).

Spiral CT: Continuous volume recording with a continuously rotating X-ray tube and continuous table advance.

Standard deviation → Image analysis, Histogram analysis.

Superimposition of edges → Artifacts, Image reconstruction.

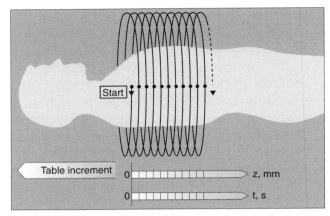

Fig. 28-23. Spiral CT. Continuous scanning during continuous table incrementation produces a spiral scan.

Table increment → Scanning.

Topogram → Digital image processing.

Voxel = Volume element of a scanned object.

Window → Display of images.

Window settings (level, width) → Display of images.

X-ray scatter → Attenuation of X-rays.

x-, y- coordinates → Matrix

z-axis: Axis vertical to the scanning plane. The z-axis is usually parallel to the axis of the body.

Table of Contents
Literature Section

Techniques and Image Analysis 583
Contrast Media 585
The Mediastinum 586
The Heart 591
The Lungs and the Pleura 593
The Chest Wall 599
The Liver 599
The Biliary System 605
The Pancreas 606
The Gastrointestinal Tract 609
The Peritoneal Cavity 612
The Spleen 616
The Kidney 617

The Adrenal Glands 620
The Urinary Bladder 622
The Prostate and Seminal Vesicles . . . 623
The Female Genital Organs 623
The Retroperitoneal Cavity 625
Muscle Tissue 626
Soft-Tissue Tumors and Bone Tumors . 627
Bones and Spine 629
Further Literature 639

Keyword Index 655

Author Index 661

Literature

Techniques and Image Analysis

1. Aichner F, Mayr U, Degenhart G
Eine neue dreidimensionale Bilddarstellung in der Computertomographie
A new 3-dimensional imaging method in computed tomography
RÖFO 1985 Apr, Vol. 142 (4), P. 395–8

2. Axel L
Cerebral blood flow determination by rapid-sequence computed tomography: theoretical analysis
Radiology 1980 Dec, Vol. 137 (3), P. 679–86

3. Ball W S, Wicks J D, Mettler F A Jr
Prone-supine change in organ position: CT demonstration
Am J Roentgenol 1980 Oct, Vol. 135 (4), P. 815–20

4. Bramble J M
Comparison of information-preserving and information-losing data-compression algorithms for CT images
Radiology 1989 Feb, Vol. 170 (2), P. 453–5

5. Breiman R S, Beck J W, Korobkin M, Glenny R, Akwari O E, Heaston D K, Moore A V, Ram P C
Volume determinations using computed tomography
Am J Roentgenol 1982 Feb, Vol. 138 (2), P. 329–33

6. Brisson L J, Zegel H G
Biopsy gun and sheath for CT-guided percutaneous biopsies letter
Am J Roentgenol 1991 Mar, Vol. 156 (3), P. 639

7. Brody A S, Saks B J, Field D R, Skinner S R, Capra R E
Artifacts seen during CT pelvimetry: implications for digital systems with scanning beams
Radiology 1986 Jul, Vol. 160 (1), P. 269–71

8. Brooks R A, Di Chiro G
Slice geometry in computer assisted tomography
J Comput Assist Tomogr 1977 Apr, Vol. 1 (2), P. 191–9

9. Brooks R D, Glover G H, Talbert A J, Eisner R L, DiBianca F A
Aliasing: a source of streaks in computed tomograms
J Comput Assist Tomogr 1979 Aug, Vol. 3 (4), P. 511–8

10. Burgess A E
Scatter radiation from abdominal CT examinations
J Comput Assist Tomogr 1985 Sep-Oct, Vol. 9 (5), P. 926–30

11. Castronovo F P Jr
A method for calculating linear attenuation coefficients for combinations of fat and muscle letter
Radiology 1983 Sep, Vol. 148 (3), P. 865–6

12. Chakraborty D P, Yester M V, Barnes G T, Lakshminarayanan A V
Self-masking subtraction tomosynthesis
Radiology 1984 Jan, Vol. 150 (1), P. 225–9

13. Charboneau J W, Reading C C, Welch T J
CT and sonographically guided needle biopsy: current techniques and new innovations
Am J Roentgenol 1990 Jan, Vol. 154 (1), P. 1–10

14. Chintapalli K, Wentworth W, Wilson C R
Simple radiation protection device for CT
Am J Roentgenol 1988 Jan, Vol. 150 (1), P. 199–200

15. Chopp M, Ewald L, Hartson M
The contribution of internal scatter to radiation dose during CT scan of the head
Neuroradiology 1981, Vol. 22 (3), P. 145–50

16. Cohan R H, Newman G E, Braun S D, Dunnick N R
CT assistance for fluoroscopically guided transthoracic needle aspiration biopsy
J Comput Assist Tomogr 1984 Dec, Vol. 8 (6), P. 1093–8

17. Conrad M R
Air-bolus technique for optimal contrast enhancement in abdominal CT studies letter
Am J Roentgenol 1988 Aug, Vol. 151 (2), P. 413

18. Correia J A, Davis K R, Kharasch M, Chesler D A, Taveras J M
Production of thin CT sections and coronal and sagittal images by spatial filtering
J Comput Assist Tomogr 1980 Feb, Vol. 4 (1), P. 83–90

19. Coscina W F, Arger P H, Mintz M C, Coleman B G
CT demonstration of pulmonary effects of tangential beam radiation
J Comput Assist Tomogr 1986 Jul-Aug, Vol. 10 (4), P. 600–2

20. Daffner R H
Visual illusions in computed tomography: phenomena related to Mach effect
Am J Roentgenol 1980 Feb, Vol. 134 (2), P. 261–4

21. de Geer G, Gamsu G, Cann C, Webb W R
Evaluation of a chest phantom for CT nodule densitometry
Am J Roentgenol 1986 Jul, Vol. 147 (1), P. 21–5

22. Dihlmann W
Lumbale Computertomographie im Bicolorbild-Modus
Lumbar computed tomography in a bicolor mode
RÖFO 1985 Mar, Vol. 142 (3), P. 263–6

23. Dohring W, Linke G
Modifizierte CT-Bildwiedergabe durch Schwächungswerttransformationen
Modified CT imaging by reduction factor transformations
RÖFO 1981 Apr, Vol. 134 (4), P. 343–52

24. Dohring W, Linke G
Ein Programmsystem zur quantitativen Auswertung von Computertomogrammen unter Anwendung einer digitalen Maskentechnik zur Isolierung interessierender Organe und Organbereiche aus der CT-Wertematrix
Program system for quantitative evaluation of computed tomograms using a digital masking technic for isolation of organs of interest and organ regions from the value matrix
RÖFO 1986 Feb, Vol. 144 (2), P. 135-48

25. Doi K, Rubin J
Evaluation of video-printer images as secondary CT images for clinical use
Radiology 1983 Jan, Vol. 146 (1), P. 233–6

26. Ell S R, Jolles H, Keyes W D, Galvin J R
Cine CT technique for dynamic airway studies
Am J Roentgenol 1985 Jul, Vol. 145 (1), P. 35–6

27. Elster A D, Jensen K M
Importance of sagittally reformatted images in CT evaluation of spondylolisthesis letter
AJNR 1986 Nov-Dec, Vol. 7 (6), P. 1102–3

28. Felmlee J P, Gray J E, Leetzow M L, Price J C
Estimated fetal radiation dose from multislice CT studies
Am J Roentgenol 1990 Jan, Vol. 154 (1), P. 185–90

29. Feuerbach S, Gmeinwieser J, Gerhardt P, Gossner W, Rotter M, Gossmann A
CT-gesteuerte Biopsie-Methoden, Resultate und Komplikationen
CT-guided biopsy: methods, results and complications
RÖFO 1989 Jul, Vol. 151 (1), P. 4–9

30. Fishman E K, Drebin R A, Hruban R H, Ney D R, Magid D
Three-dimensional reconstruction of the human body
Am J Roentgenol 1988 Jun, Vol. 150 (6), P. 1419–20

31. Foley W D, Jacobson D R, Taylor A J, Goodman L R, Stewart E T, Gurney J W, Stroka D
Display of CT studies on a two-screen electronic workstation versus a film panel alternator: sensitivity and efficiency among radiologists
Radiology 1990 Mar, Vol. 174 (3 Pt 1), P. 769–73

32. Frahm R, Fritz H, Drescher E
Winkelmessungen des Rückfußes im CT
Angular measurements of the hindfoot in CT
RÖFO 1989 Jul, Vol. 151 (1), P. 77–81

33. Frohlich H, Dohring W
A simple device for breath-level monitoring during CT
Radiology 1985 Jul, Vol. 156 (1), P. 235

34. Gluer C C, Reiser U J, Davis C A, Rutt B K, Genant H K
Vertebral mineral determination by quantitative computed tomography QCT: accuracy of single and dual energy measurements
J Comput Assist Tomogr 1988 Mar-Apr, Vol. 12 (2), P. 242–58

35. Gross S C, Kowalski J B, Lee S H, Terry B, Honickman S J
Surgical ligation clip artifacts on CT scans
Radiology 1985 Sep, Vol. 156 (3), P. 831–2

36. Haaga J R, Miraldi F, MacIntyre W, LiPuma J P, Bryan P J, Wiesen E
The effect of mAs variation upon computed tomography image quality as evaluated by in vivo and in vitro studies
Radiology 1981 Feb, Vol. 138 (2), P. 449–54

37. Helenon O, Chanin D S, Laval Jeantet M, Frija J
Artifacts on lung CT scans: removal with Fourier filtration
Radiology 1989 May, Vol. 171 (2), P. 572–4

38. Heller M, Grabbe E, Bucheler E
Serien-Computertomographie - Methodik und erste Erfahrungen
Serial computed tomography – methods and early experience
RÖFO 1981 Jan, Vol. 134 (1), P. 16–21

39. Hemmingsson A, Jung B, Ytterbergh C
Dual energy computed tomography: simulated monoenergetic and material-selective imaging
J Comput Assist Tomogr 1986 May-Jun, Vol. 10 (3), P. 490–9

40. Herman G T
Re: Three-dimensional display of computed tomographic scans letter
Radiology 1984 Jun, Vol. 151 (3), P. 805–6

41. Herman G T
Three-dimensional imaging on a CT or MR scanner
J Comput Assist Tomogr 1988 May-Jun, Vol. 12 (3), P. 450–8

42. Heuck F, Reiser U, Zieger M, Buck J
Informationswert dreidimensionaler Sekundärschnitt-Rekonstruktionen von Skelettbefunden bei der Röntgen-Computer-Tomographie
Informational value of 3-dimensional secondary section reconstruction of skeletal findings in roentgen computer tomography
Radiologe 1982 Nov, Vol. 22 (11), P. 512–23

43. Heuser L, Friedmann G
Technik der Kontrastmittelapplikation bei der Computertomographie des Herzens
Technique of application of contrast media in computed tomography of the heart
Radiologe 1982 Jan, Vol. 22 (1), P. 26–31

44. Hickey N M, Niklason L T, Sabbagh E, Fraser R G, Barnes G T
Dual-energy digital radiographic quantification of calcium in simulated pulmonary nodules
Am J Roentgenol 1987 Jan, Vol. 148 (1), P. 19–24

45. Hodapp N, Hinkelbein W, Slanina J, Wannenmacher M
Alternative Anwendung von Simulatormethode und Computertomographie bei der Bestrahlungsplanung des nicht metastasierten Prostatakarzinoms
Alternative use of the simulator method and computer tomography in planning radiotherapy for non-metastasizing prostatic cancer
Radiologe 1984 Jan, Vol. 24 (1), P. 19–23

46. Hounsfield G N
Potential uses of more accurate CT absorption values by filtering
Am J Roentgenol 1978 Jul, Vol. 131 (1), P. 103–6

47. Hounsfield G N
Computed medical imaging. Nobel lecture, December 8, 1979
J Comput Assist Tomogr 1980 Oct, Vol. 4 (5), P. 665–74

48. Hubener K H, Klott K J
"Statisches" und dynamisches Kontrastmittelenhancement der Körperstamm-Computertomographie (Ortsauflösung, Angio-CT, Sequenz-CT)
"Static" and dynamic contrast enhancement of the trunk – computer tomography
RÖFO 1980 Oct, Vol. 133 (4), P. 347–54

49. Hubener K H, Kalender W A, Metzger H O
Fast digital recording of X-ray dilution curves: a preliminary evaluation
Radiology 1982 Nov, Vol. 145 (2), P. 545−7

50. Ishigaki T, Sakuma S, Horikawa Y, Ikeda M, Yamaguchi H
One- shot dual-energy subtraction imaging
Radiology 1986 Oct, Vol. 161 (1), P. 271−3

51. Johnson G A, Korobkin M
Image techniques for multiplanar computed tomography
Radiology 1982 Sep, Vol. 144 (4), P. 829−34

52. Jones K R, Robinson P J
Organ volume determination by CT scanning: reduction of respiration- induced errors by feedback monitoring
J Comput Assist Tomogr 1986 Jan-Feb, Vol. 10 (1), P. 167−71

53. Joseph P M, Hilal S K, Schulz R A, Kelcz F
Clinical and experimental investigation of a smoothed CT reconstruction algorithm
Radiology 1980 Feb, Vol. 134 (2), P. 507−16

54. Joseph P M, Stockham C D
The influence of modulation transfer function shape on computed tomographic image quality
Radiology 1982 Oct, Vol. 145 (1), P. 179−85

55. Kaczmarek R G, Bednarek D R, Wong R, Kaczmarek R V, Rudin S, Alker G
Potential radiation hazards to personnel during dynamic CT letter
Radiology 1986 Dec, Vol. 161 (3), P. 853

56. Kaiser M C, Veiga Pires J A
Sitting position variation of direct longitudino-axial semi-coronal mode in CTT-scanning technical note
RÖFO 1981 Jan, Vol. 134 (1), P. 97−9

57. Kalender W A, Hebel R, Ebersberger J
Reduction of CT artifacts caused by metallic implants
Radiology 1987 Aug, Vol. 164 (2), P. 576−7

58. Kalender W A, Seissler W, Klotz E, Vock P
Spiral volumetric CT with single-breath-hold technique, continuous transport, and continuous scanner rotation
Radiology 1990 Jul, Vol. 176 (1), P. 181−3

59. Kaufman R A
Technical aspects of abdominal CT in infants and children
Am J Roentgenol 1989 Sep, Vol. 153 (3), P. 549−54

60. Keeter S, Benator R M, Weinberg S M, Hartenberg M A
Sedation in pediatric CT: national survey of current practice see comments
Radiology 1990 Jun, Vol. 175 (3), P. 745−52

61. Keller J M, Edwards F M, Rundle R
Automatic outlining of regions on CT scans
J Comput Assist Tomogr 1981 Apr, Vol. 5 (2), P. 240−5

62. Kogutt M S
Computed radiographic imaging: use in low-dose leg length radiography
Am J Roentgenol 1987 Jun, Vol. 148 (6), P. 1205−6

63. Kunin M, Phillips J J, Schwarz G
Visual contrast enhancement with a patterned overlay
Radiology 1988 Apr, Vol. 167 (1), P. 271- 3

64. Lange K, Carson R
EM reconstruction algorithms for emission and transmission tomography
J Comput Assist Tomogr 1984 Apr, Vol. 8 (2), P. 306−16

65. Lassen M N
Dedicated CT technique for scanning neonates
Radiology 1986 Nov, Vol. 161 (2), P. 363−6

66. Laval Jeantet A M, Cann C E, Roger B, Dallant P
A postprocessing dual energy technique for vertebral CT densitometry
J Comput Assist Tomogr 1984 Dec, Vol. 8 (6), P. 1164−7

67. Lee H C, Leung C H
Dynamic computed tomography through interpolation
J Comput Assist Tomogr 1982 Feb, Vol. 6 (1), P. 134−40

68. Lee J K, Barbier J Y, McClennan B L, Stanley R J
A support device for obtaining direct coronal computed-tomographic scans of the pelvis and lower abdomen
Radiology 1982 Oct, Vol. 145 (1), P. 209−10

69. Lehr J L
Truncated-view artifacts: clinical importance on CT
Am J Roentgenol 1983 Jul, Vol. 141 (1), P. 183−91

70. Lehr J L, Capek P
Histogram equalization of CT images
Radiology 1985 Jan, Vol. 154 (1), P. 163−9

71. Levin D N, Pelizzari C A, Chen G T, Chen C T, Cooper M D
Retrospective geometric correlation of MR, CT, and PET images
Radiology 1988 Dec, Vol. 169 (3), P. 817−23

72. Levine M L, Hall F M
Gantry angulation for CT-guided biopsy or aspiration letter
Am J Roentgenol 1989 Jun, Vol. 152 (6), P. 1345−6

73. Lohr H, Vogel H, Wroblewski H, Rehpenning W, Jantzen R
Strahlenexposition und Strahlenrisiko der Ganzkörpercomputertomographie
Radiation exposure and radiation risks from body scanners
RÖFO 1980 Jun, Vol. 132 (6), P. 667−71

74. Maravilla K R, Murry R C, Deck M, Horner S
Clinical application of digital tomosynthesis: a preliminary report
AJNR 1983 May-Jun, Vol. 4 (3), P. 277−80

75. Marshall W, Hall E, Doost Hoseini A, Alvarez R, Macovski A, Cassel D
An implementation of dual energy CT scanning
J Comput Assist Tomogr 1984 Aug, Vol. 8 (4), P. 745−9

76. Marshall W H Jr, Alvarez R E, Macovski A
Initial results with prereconstruction dual-energy computed tomography PREDECT
Radiology 1981 Aug, Vol. 140 (2), P. 421−30

77. Mayo J R, Muller N L, Henkelman R M
The double-fissure sign: a motion artifact on thin-section CT scans
Radiology 1987 Nov, Vol. 165 (2), P. 580−1

78. McCullough E C, Morin R L
CT-number variability in thoracic geometry
Am J Roentgenol 1983 Jul, Vol. 141 (1), P. 135−40

79. Meaney T F, Raudkivi U, McIntyre W J, Gallagher J H, Haaga J R, Havrilla T R, Reich N E
Detection of low-contrast lesions in computed body tomography: an experimental study of simulated lesions
Radiology 1980 Jan, Vol. 134 (1), P. 149−54

80. Miles S G, Rasmussen J F, Litwiller T, Osik A
Safe use of an intravenous power injector for CT: experience and protocol
Radiology 1990 Jul, Vol. 176 (1), P. 69−70

81. Moore M M, Shearer D R
Fetal dose estimates for CT pelvimetry
Radiology 1989 Apr, Vol. 171 (1), P. 265−7

82. Nakano Y, Hiraoka T, Togashi K, Nishimura K, Itoh K, Fujisawa I, Sagoh T, Minami S, Itoh H, Torizuka K
Direct radiographic magnification with computed radiography
Am J Roentgenol 1987 Mar, Vol. 148 (3), P. 569−73

83. Ney D R, Fishman E K, Magid D, Kuhlman J E
Interactive real- time multiplanar CT imaging
Radiology 1989 Jan, Vol. 170 (1 Pt 1), P. 275−6

84. Nikesch W
Using a radiation therapy simulator to localize the anatomical level of computed tomography slices
J Comput Assist Tomogr 1981 Aug, Vol. 5 (4), P. 593−5

85. Okudera H, Kobayashi S, Sugita K
Technical note: mobile CT scanner gantry for use in the operating room see comments
AJNR 1991 Jan-Feb, Vol. 12 (1), P. 131−2

86. Onik G, Cosman E R, Wells T H Jr, Goldberg H I, Moss A A, Costello P, Kane R A, Hoddick W I, Demas B
CT-guided aspirations for the body: comparison of hand guidance with stereotaxis
Radiology 1988 Feb, Vol. 166 (2), P. 389−94

87. Oon C L
A method of locating the plane of CT scans of the abdomen
J Comput Assist Tomogr 1980 Apr, Vol. 4 (2), P. 268−77

88. Oppenheimer D A, Young S W, Marmor J B
Work in progress: serial evaluation of tumor volume using computed tomography and contrast kinetics
Radiology 1983 May, Vol. 147 (2), P. 495−7

89. Oppenheimer D A, Young S W
Diatrizoate CT distribution kinetics: a study of human tissue characterization
J Comput Assist Tomogr 1983 Apr, Vol. 7 (2), P. 274−7

90. Palestrant A M
Comprehensive approach to CT-guided procedures with a hand-held guidance device
Radiology 1990 Jan, Vol. 174 (1), P. 270−2

91. Panzer W, Scheurer C, Drexler G, Regulla D
Feldstudie zur Ermittlung von Dosiswerten bei der Computertomographie
A field study to determine dosages in computed tomography
RÖFO 1988 Nov, Vol. 149 (5), P. 534−8

92. Pentlow K S, Rottenberg D A, Deck M D
Partial volume summation: a simple approach to ventricular volume determination from CT
Neuroradiology 1978, Vol. 16, P. 130−2

93. Pizer S M, Zimmerman J B, Staab E V
Adaptive grey level assignment in CT scan display
J Comput Assist Tomogr 1984 Apr, Vol. 8 (2), P. 300−5

94. Reese D F, McCullough E C, Baker H L Jr
Dynamic sequential scanning with table incrementation
Radiology 1981 Sep, Vol. 140 (3), P. 719−22

95. Reid M H
Organ and lesion volume measurements with computed tomography
J Comput Assist Tomogr 1983 Apr, Vol. 7 (2), P. 268−73

96. Reisner K, Fettig O, Bartscher K H, Knappschneider U
Die geburtshilfliche Beckenmessung mittels digitaler Radiographie (CT- Topogramm)
Obstetric pelvimetry using digital radiography CT topogram
RÖFO 1985 May, Vol. 142 (5), P. 566−9

97. Rigauts H, Marchal G, Baert A L, Hupke R
Initial experience with volume CT scanning
J Comput Assist Tomogr 1990 Jul-Aug, Vol. 14 (4), P. 675−82

98. Ritman E L, Kinsey J H, Robb R A, Harris L D, Gilbert B K
Physics and technical considerations in the design of the DSR: a high temporal resolution volume scanner
Am J Roentgenol 1980 Feb, Vol. 134 (2), P. 369−74

99. Robb W L
Technological seduction: diagnostic imaging technology facing new demands
Am J Roentgenol 1985 Dec, Vol. 145 (6), P. 1112−4

100. Robbins A H, Pugatch R D, Gerzof S G, Spira R, Rankin S C, Gale D R
An assessment of the role of scan speed in perceived image quality of body computed tomography
Radiology 1981 Apr, Vol. 139 (1), P. 139−46

101. Robertson D D, Weiss P J, Fishman E K, Magid D, Walker P S
Evaluation of CT techniques for reducing artifacts in the presence of metallic orthopedic implants
J Comput Assist Tomogr 1988 Mar-Apr, Vol. 12 (2), P. 236−41

102. Robertson J, Federle M P
Simple traction-immobilization device for CT scanners
Am J Roentgenol 1983 Dec, Vol. 141 (6), P. 1331

103. Robinson P J, Jones K R
Improved control of respiration during computed tomography by feedback monitoring
J Comput Assist Tomogr 1982 Aug, Vol. 6 (4), P. 802−6

104. Schmachtenberg A, Hundgen R, Zeumer H
Ein EDV-adaptiertes Rastermodell des Gehirns zur topographischen Analyse von Läsionen im kranialen Computertomogramm
EDP-adapted grid model of the brain for topographic analysis of lesions on the cranial computer tomogram
RÖFO 1983 Nov, Vol. 139 (5), P. 499−502

105. Schmitt W G
Zur Frage der Energieabhängigkeit der Hounsfield-Zahlen
Energy dependence of Hounsfield numbers
RÖFO 1986 Aug, Vol. 145 (2), P. 221−3

106. Schoppe W D, Hessel S J, Adams D F
Time requirements in performing body CT studies
J Comput Assist Tomogr 1981 Aug, Vol. 5 (4), P. 513−5

107. Shuman W P, Adam J L, Schoenecker S A, Tazioli P R, Moss A A
Use of a power injector during dynamic computed tomography
J Comput Assist Tomogr 1986 Nov-Dec, Vol. 10 (6), P. 1000−2

108. Silverman P M, Rosen A, Korobkin M, Genkins S
The "composite image": a photographic error in computed tomography with a multiformat camera
Am J Roentgenol 1984 May, Vol. 142 (5), P. 961–2

109. Singer P, Kober B
Dosimetrie in der Computertomographie
Dosimetry in computerized tomography
RÖFO 1985 Nov, Vol. 143 (5), P. 549–52

110. Smith D F, Rowberg A A
Data-base management system on a CT scanner computer: application to teaching file and procedure records
Am J Roentgenol 1984 Jun, Vol. 142 (6), P. 1219–23

111. Stimac G K, Burch D, Livingston R R, Anderson P, Dacey R G
A device for maintaining cervical spine stabilization and traction during CT scanning
Am J Roentgenol 1987 Aug, Vol. 149 (2), P. 345–6

112. Sundaram M, Wolverson M K, Heiberg E, Pilla T, Vas W G, Shields J B
Utility of CT-guided abdominal aspiration procedures
Am J Roentgenol 1982 Dec, Vol. 139 (6), P. 1111–5

113. Towbin R B, Strife J L
Percutaneous aspiration, drainage, and biopsies in children
Radiology 1985 Oct, Vol. 157 (1), P. 81–5

114. van Waes P F, Zonneveld F W
Direct coronal body computed tomography
J Comput Assist Tomogr 1982 Feb, Vol. 6 (1), P. 58–66

115. van Waes P F, Zonneveld F W
Patient positioning for direct coronal computed tomography of the entire body
Radiology 1982 Feb, Vol. 142 (2), P. 531–2

116. van Waes P F, Feldberg M A, Mali W P, Ruijs S H, Eenhoorn P C, Buijs P H, Kruis F J, Ramos L R
Management of loculated abscesses that are difficult to drain: a new approach
Radiology 1983 Apr, Vol. 147 (1), P. 57–63

117. Vannier M W, Gayou D E
Automated registration of multimodality images editorial
Radiology 1988 Dec, Vol. 169 (3), P. 860–1

118. Vogelzang R L, Gore R M, Neiman H L, Smith S J, Deschler T W, Vrla R F
Inferior vena cava CT pseudothrombus produced by rapid arm-vein contrast infusion
Am J Roentgenol 1985 Apr, Vol. 144 (4), P. 843–6

119. Wagner L K, Archer B R, Zeck O F
Conceptus dose from two state-of-the-art CT scanners
Radiology 1986 Jun, Vol. 159 (3), P. 787–92

120. Warren R C
Contrast and latitude of CT hard copy: an ROC study
Radiology 1981 Oct, Vol. 141 (1), P. 139–45

121. Wegener O H
Artefakte in der Computertomographie
Artefacts in computer tomography
RÖFO 1980 Jun, Vol. 132 (6), P. 643–51

122. Weidenmaier W, Christ G
Der Einfluß der Aufhärtung auf den CT- Wert
The effect of beam hardening on CT values
RÖFO 1985 Dec, Vol. 143 (6), P. 697–701

123. Wilbur A C, Kriz R J
Round CT film static artifacts: simulation of focal pathology
J Comput Assist Tomogr 1989 Jul-Aug, Vol. 13 (4), P. 730–1

124. Winter J
Edge enhancement of computed tomograms by digital unsharp masking
Radiology 1980 Apr, Vol. 135 (1), P. 234–5

125. Witte G, Hohne K H, Bocker F, Riemer M, Bucheler E
Anwendungsmöglichkeiten digitaler Methoden in der Röntgendiagnostik
Applicability of digital methods in X-ray diagnosis
RÖFO 1985 Jun, Vol. 142 (6), P. 600–10

126. Wolpert S M
Nuclear magnetic resonance vs. computed tomography
AJNR 1983 Jul-Aug, Vol. 4 (4), P. 996

127. Young S W, Muller H H, Marshall W H
Computed tomography: beam hardening and environmental density artifact
Radiology 1983 Jul, Vol. 148 (1), P. 279–83

128. Yueh N, Halvorsen R A Jr, Letourneau J G, Crass J R
Gantry tilt technique for CT-guided biopsy and drainage
J Comput Assist Tomogr 1989 Jan-Feb, Vol. 13 (1), P. 182–4

129. Zerhouni E A, Boukadoum M, Siddiky M A, Newbold J M, Stone D C, Shirey M P, Spivey J F, Hesselman C W, Leo F P, Stitik F P, et al
A standard phantom for quantitative CT analysis of pulmonary nodules
Radiology 1983 Dec, Vol. 149 (3), P. 767–73

130. Zwicker R D, Zamenhof R G, Wolpert S M
Comparative dosimetry of high-detail computed tomography using the Siemens Somatom-2 and complex motion tomography for examination of the sella turcica
AJNR 1982 May-Jun, Vol. 3 (3), P. 354–5

131. Zwirewich C V, Terriff B, Muller N L
High-spatial-frequency bone algorithm improves quality of standard CT of the thorax
Am J Roentgenol 1989 Dec, Vol. 153 (6), P. 1169–73

132. European Scientific User Conference SOMATOM Plus. 2–3 March 1990, Zurich
Radiologe 1990 May, Vol. 30 (5 (EUROP SCI)), P. 1–16

Contrast Media

133. Angelelli G, Macarini L, Fratello A
Use of water as an oral contrast agent for CT study of the stomach letter
Am J Roentgenol 1987 Nov, Vol. 149 (5), P. 1084

134. Angelelli G, Macarini L
CT of the bowel: use of water to enhance depiction
Radiology 1988 Dec, Vol. 169 (3), P. 848–9

135. Bloem J L, Wondergem J
Gd-DTPA as a contrast agent in CT
Radiology 1989 May, Vol. 171 (2), P. 578–9

136. Burgener F A, Hamlin D J
Contrast enhancement in abdominal CT: bolus vs. infusion
Am J Roentgenol 1981 Aug, Vol. 137 (2), P. 351- 8

137. Claussen C, Laniado M, Kazner E, Schorner W, Felix R
Application of contrast agents in CT and MRI NMR: their potential in imaging of brain tumors
Neuroradiology 1985, Vol. 27 (2), P. 164–71

138. Claussen C D, Linke G, Felix R, Lochner B, Weinmann H J, Wegener O H
Bolusgeometrie und -dynamik nach intravenöser Kontrastmittelinjektion. Studien mit Hilfe der Chronographie
Bolus geometry and dynamics after intravenous injections of contrast media. Studies using chronography
RÖFO 1982 Aug, Vol. 137 (2), P. 212–6

139. Claussen C D, Banzer D, Pfretzschner C, Kalender W A, Schorner W
Bolus geometry and dynamics after intravenous contrast medium injection
Radiology 1984 Nov, Vol. 153 (2), P. 365–8

140. Corrales M
Selective enhanced CT letter
AJNR 1986 May-Jun, Vol. 7 (3), P. 530

141. du Boulay G H, Teather D, Wills K
CT: to enhance or not to enhance: A computer-aided study
AJNR 1983 May-Jun, Vol. 4 (3), P. 421–4

142. Fischer H W
Contrast material for CT editorial
Am J Roentgenol 1981 Mar, Vol. 136 (3), P. 629

143. Fuchs W A, Vock P, Haertel M
Pharmakokinetik intravasaler Kontrastmittel bei der Computertomographie
Pharmacokinetics of intravascular contrast agents in computerized tomography
Radiologe 1979 Mar, Vol. 19 (3), P. 90–3

144. Galanski M, Cramer B M, Drewes G
Möglichkeiten der Kontrastmittelanwendung bei der Computertomographie
The use of contrast media in computer tomography
RÖFO 1980 Feb, Vol. 132 (2), P. 139–44

145. Gardeur D, Lautrou J, Millard J C, Berger N, Metzger J
Pharmacokinetics of contrast media: experimental results in dog and man with CT implications
J Comput Assist Tomogr 1980 Apr, Vol. 4 (2), P. 178–85

146. Garrett P R, Meshkov S L, Perlmutter G S
Oral contrast agents in CT of the abdomen
Radiology 1984 Nov, Vol. 153 (2), P. 545–6

147. Guinto F C Jr, Hashim H, Crofford M J, Mirfakhraee M
Dynamic CT using an arterial bolus
Radiology 1985 Nov, Vol. 157 (2), P. 529–30

148. Hasegawa B H, Cacak R K, Mulvaney J A, Hendee W R
Problems with contrast-detail curves for CT performance evaluation
Am J Roentgenol 1982 Jan, Vol. 138 (1), P. 135–8

149. Hayman L A, Evans R A, Fahr L M, Hinck V C
Renal consequences of rapid high dose contrast CT
Am J Roentgenol 1980 Mar, Vol. 134 (3), P. 553–5

150. Hildell J G, Nyman U R, Norlindh S T, Hellsten S F, Stenberg P B
New intravesical contrast medium for CT: preliminary studies with arachis peanut oil
Am J Roentgenol 1981 Oct, Vol. 137 (4), P. 777–80

151. Karasick S R, Magilner A D
Unintentional opacification of the stomach during computed tomography following ingestion of jelly candy
J Comput Assist Tomogr 1982 Feb, Vol. 6 (1), P. 184–5

152. Kendall B E, Pullicino P
Intravascular contrast injection in ischaemic lesions. II. Effect on prognosis
Neuroradiology 1980, Vol. 19 (5), P. 241–3

153. Leonardi M, Lavaroni A, Biasizzo E, Fabris G, Penco T, Zappoli F
High-dose contrast-enhanced computed tomography CECT with iopamidol in the detection of cerebral metastases. Tolerance of the contrast agent
Neuroradiology 1989, Vol. 31 (2), P. 148–50

154. Lewis E, AufderHeide J F, Bernardino M E, Barnes P A, Thomas J L
CT detection of hepatic metastases with Ethiodized Oil Emulsion 13
J Comput Assist Tomogr 1982 Dec, Vol. 6 (6), P. 1108–14

155. Lunderquist A, Ivancev K, Stridbeck H
Gastrografin-sorbitol solution for CT opacification of bowel letter
Am J Roentgenol 1988 Apr, Vol. 150 (4), P. 949

156. Maier W
Flow-gesteuerte Kontrastmittelapplikation zur Computertomographie
Flow-directed application of contrast media for computed tomography
RÖFO 1991 Feb, Vol. 154 (2), P. 187–91

157. Mattrey R F
Perfluorooctylbromide: a new contrast agent for CT, sonography, and MR imaging
Am J Roentgenol 1989 Feb, Vol. 152 (2), P. 247–52

158. Mattrey R F
Potential role of perfluorooctylbromide in the detection and characterization of liver lesions with CT published erratum appears in Radiology 1989 Apr; 1711:287
Radiology 1989 Jan, Vol. 170 (1 Pt 1), P. 18–20

159. McCarthy S, Moss A A
The use of a flow rate injector for contrast-enhanced computed tomography
Radiology 1984 Jun, Vol. 151 (3), P. 800

160. Megibow A J, Bosniak M A
Dilute barium as a contrast agent for abdominal CT
Am J Roentgenol 1980 Jun, Vol. 134 (6), P. 1273–4

161. Pagani J J, Hayman L A, Bigelow R H, Libshitz H I, Lepke R A, Wallace S
Diazepam prophylaxis of contrast media-induced seizures during computed tomography of patients with brain metastases
Am J Roentgenol 1983 Apr, Vol. 140 (4), P. 787–92

162. Palmieri A
Extravasation of contrast-enhanced blood in an epidural hematoma
Neuroradiology 1981, Vol. 21 (3), P. 163–4

163. Parvey L S, Grizzard M, Coburn T P
Use of infusion pump for intravenous enhanced computed tomography
J Comput Assist Tomogr 1983 Feb, Vol. 7 (1), P. 175–6

164. Passariello R, Salvolini U, Rossi P, Simonetti G, Pasquini U
Automatic contrast medium injector for computed tomography
J Comput Assist Tomogr 1980 Apr, Vol. 4 (2), P. 278–9

165. Platt J F, Glazer G M
IV contrast material for abdominal CT: comparison of three methods of administration
Am J Roentgenol 1988 Aug, Vol. 151 (2), P. 275–7

166. Polger M, Kuhlman J E, Hansen F C, Fishman E K
Computed tomography of angioedema of small bowel due to reaction to radiographic contrast
medium
J Comput Assist Tomogr 1988 Nov-Dec, Vol. 12 (6), P. 1044–6

167. Raininko R, Majurin M L, Virtama P, Kangasniemi P
Value of high contrast medium dose in brain CT
J Comput Assist Tomogr 1982 Feb, Vol. 6 (1), P. 54–7

168. Raptopoulos V, Davis M A, Davidoff A, Karellas A, Hays D, D Orsi C J, Smith E H
Fat-density oral contrast agent for abdominal CT
Radiology 1987 Sep, Vol. 164 (3), P. 653–6

169. Reiser U J
Study of bolus geometry after intravenous contrast medium injection: dynamic and quantitative
measurements Chronogram using an X-ray CT device
J Comput Assist Tomogr 1984 Apr, Vol. 8 (2), P. 251–62

170. Russell E J
Complete ring on noncontrast CT could indicate aging hemorrhage letter
AJNR 1983 Jul-Aug, Vol. 4 (4), P. 997–8

171. Sage M R
Blood-brain barrier: phenomenon of increasing importance to the imaging clinician
Am J Roentgenol 1982 May, Vol. 138 (5), P. 887–98

172. Schiffer M S
Use of contrast media in patients with hypovolemic shock letter
Radiology 1988 Feb, Vol. 166 (2), P. 579

173. Scotti G, Harwood Nash D C
Leakage of contrast into a postmeningitic subdural effusion: a CT finding
Neuroradiology 1980, Vol. 20 (2), P. 95–8

174. Shepp L A
Computerized tomography and nuclear magnetic resonance
J Comput Assist Tomogr 1980 Feb, Vol. 4 (1), P. 94–107

175. Sherwood T
Mobile CT, equity, and all those doxies
Am J Roentgenol 1983 May, Vol. 140 (5), P. 1035–6

176. Skalpe I O, Hordvik M
Comparison of side effects during cerebral computed tomography with a nonionic iohexol and an
ionic metrizoate contrast medium
AJNR 1983 May-Jun, Vol. 4 (3), P. 326- 8

177. Stellamor K, Hruby W, Assinger S, Luckner H
Vergleich der Nebenwirkungen nierengängiger Kontrastmittel (Jotalamat, Diatrizoat, Jodamid,
Jopamidol) im Rahmen der CT- Untersuchung
Comparison of the side effects of urographic contrast media iothalamate, diatrizoate, iodamide,
iopamidol within the scope of a CT study
Radiologe 1984 Oct, Vol. 24 (10), P. 488–90

178. Stork J
Intraperitoneal contrast agents for computed tomography
Am J Roentgenol 1985 Aug, Vol. 145 (2), P. 300

179. Suchato C, Osatavanichvong K, Pekanan P
Double-exposure technique for computed-tomographic imaging on x-ray film
Radiology 1982 Aug, Vol. 144 (3), P. 646

180. Vermess M, Doppman J L, Sugarbaker P, Fisher R I, Chatterji D C, Luetzeler J, Grimes G, Girton
M, Adamson R H
Clinical trials with a new intravenous liposoluble contrast material for computed tomography of the
liver and spleen
Radiology 1980 Oct, Vol. 137 (1 Pt 1), P. 217–22

181. Vermess M, Inscoe S, Sugarbaker P
Use of liposoluble contrast material to separate left renal and splenic parenchyma on computed
tomography
J Comput Assist Tomogr 1980 Aug, Vol. 4 (2), P. 540–2

182. Vermess M, Lau D H, Adams M D, Hopkins R M, Hoey G B, Grimes G, Chatterji D C, Girton M,
Doppman J L
Biodistribution study of Ethiodized Oil Emulsion 13 for computed tomography of the liver and
spleen
J Comput Assist Tomogr 1982 Dec, Vol. 6 (6), P. 1115–9

183. Vogelzang R L, Matalon T A, Neiman H L, Sakowicz B A
Lateral scout radiograph in CT-guided aspiration biopsy
Am J Roentgenol 1983 Jan, Vol. 140 (1), P. 164

184. Wende S, Speck U
Das Kontrastmittel-Risiko bei der Computertomographie
Risk of application of contrast medium in computed tomography
Radiologe 1981 Jun, Vol. 21 (6), P. 268–73

185. Wilmink J T, Roukema J G
Effects of i.v. contrast administration on intraspinal and paraspinal tissues: a CT study. 1. Mea-
surement of CT attenuation numbers
AJNR 1987 Jul-Aug, Vol. 8 (4), P. 703–9

186. Wilmink J T, Roukema J G, van den Burg W
Effects of i.v. contrast administration on intraspinal and paraspinal tissues: a CT study. 2. Visual
assessment
AJNR 1988 Jan-Feb, Vol. 9 (1), P. 191–3

187. Wood L P, Parisi M, Finch I J
Value of contrast enhanced CT scanning in the non-trauma emergency room patient
Neuroradiology 1990, Vol. 32 (4), P. 261–4

188. Woodring J H, Fried A M
Nonfatal venous air embolism after contrast-enhanced CT
Radiology 1988 May, Vol. 167 (2), P. 405–7

189. Young S W, Turner R J, Castellino R A
A strategy for the contrast enhancement of malignant tumors using dynamic computed tomography
and intravascular pharmacokinetics
Radiology 1980 Oct, Vol. 137 (1 Pt 1), P. 137–47

190. Yu Y L, du Boulay G H
Is there an increased risk of early side effects of metrizamide in post-myelogram computed to-
mography?
Neuroradiology 1984, Vol. 26 (5), P. 399–403

191. Zelenik M E, Mathis J M, McDaniel E C
An infusion system for improved vascular opacification during CT
Radiology 1984 Sep, Vol. 152 (3), P. 816

The Mediastinum

192. Adler O, Rosenberger A
Computed tomography in guiding of fine needle aspiration biopsy of the lung and medias-
tinum
RÖFO 1980 Aug, Vol. 133 (2), P. 135–7

193. Anda S, Roysland P, Fougner R, Stovring J
CT appearance of the diaphragm varying with respiratory phase and muscular tension
J Comput Assist Tomogr 1986 Sep-Oct, Vol. 10 (5), P. 744–5

194. Andonopoulos A P, Karadanas A H, Drosos A A, Acritidis N C, Katsiotis P, Moutsopoulos
H M
CT evaluation of mediastinal lymph nodes in primary Sjogren syndrome
J Comput Assist Tomogr 1988 Mar- Apr, Vol. 12 (2), P. 199–201

195. Aronberg D J, Glazer H S, Madsen K, Sagel S S
Normal thoracic aortic diameters by computed tomography
J Comput Assist Tomogr 1984 Apr, Vol. 8 (2), P. 247–50

196. Aronberg D J, Peterson R R, Glazer H S, Sagel S S
Superior diaphragmatic lymph nodes: CT assessment
J Comput Assist Tomogr 1986 Nov-Dec, Vol. 10 (6), P. 937–41

197. Aspestrand F
Demonstration of thoracic and abdominal fistulas by computed tomography
J Comput Assist Tomogr 1980 Aug, Vol. 4 (4), P. 536–7

198. Atlas S W, Vogelzang R L, Bressler E L, Gore R M, Bergan J J
CT diagnosis of a mycotic aneurysm of the thoracoabdominal aorta
J Comput Assist Tomogr 1984 Dec, Vol. 8 (6), P. 1211–2

199. Barnett S M
CT findings in tuberculous mediastinitis
J Comput Assist Tomogr 1986 Jan-Feb, Vol. 10 (1), P. 165–6

200. Baron R L, Levitt R G, Sagel S S, Stanley R J
Computed tomography in the evaluation of mediastinal widening
Radiology 1981 Jan, Vol. 138 (1), P. 107–13

201. Baron R L, Lee J K, Sagel S S, Levitt R G
Computed tomography of the abnormal thymus
Radiology 1982 Jan, Vol. 142 (1), P. 127–34

202. Baron R L, Lee J K, Sagel S S, Peterson R R
Computed tomography of the normal thymus
Radiology 1982 Jan, Vol. 142 (1), P. 121–5

203. Bashist B, Ellis K, Gold R P
Computed tomography of intrathoracic goiters
Am J Roentgenol 1983 Mar, Vol. 140 (3), P. 455–60

204. Carrol C L, Jeffrey R B Jr, Federle M P, Vernacchia R H
Superior vena caval obstruction: detection using CT
Radiology 1985 Nov, Vol. 157 (2), P. 485–7

205. Bennum R R, Costello P
CT findings in angioimmunoblastic lymphadenopathy
J Comput Assist Tomogr 1983 Jun, Vol. 7 (3), P. 454–6

206. Berger P E, Kuhn J P, Kuhns L R
Computed tomography and the occult tracheobronchial foreign body
Radiology 1980 Jan, Vol. 134 (1), P. 133–5

207. Bergin C, Castellino R A
Mediastinal lymph node enlargement on CT scans in patients with usual interstitial pneumoni-
tis
Am J Roentgenol 1990 Feb, Vol. 154 (2), P. 251–4

208. Berkmen Y M, Auh Y H
CT diagnosis of acquired tracheoesophageal fistula in adults
J Comput Assist Tomogr 1985 Mar-Apr, Vol. 9 (2), P. 302–4

209. Beyer Enke S A, Schmitteckert H, Gorich J
Computertomographie des tuberkulösen mediastinalen Senkungsabszesses
Computed tomography of a deep tuberculous mediastinal abscess
RÖFO 1988 Jul, Vol. 149 (1), P. 108–9

210. Binder R E, Pugatch R D, Faling L J, Kanter R A, Sawin C T
Diagnosis of posterior mediastinal goiter by computed tomography
J Comput Assist Tomogr 1980 Aug, Vol. 4 (4), P. 550–2

211. Black W C, Armstrong P, Daniel T M, Cooper P H
Computed tomography of aggressive fibromatosis in the posterior mediastinum
J Comput Assist Tomogr 1987 Jan-Feb, Vol. 11 (1), P. 153–5

212. Bottles K, Nyberg D A, Clark M, Hinchcliffe W A
CT diagnosis of tracheobronchopathia osteochondroplastica
J Comput Assist Tomogr 1983 Apr, Vol. 7 (2), P. 324–7

213. linger G, Thorsen M K, Lawson T L, Perret R, Smith T C
Plexiform neurofibromatosis of the mediastinum: CT appearance
Am J Roentgenol 1988 Sep, Vol. 151 (3), P. 461–3

214. Breatnach E, Stanley R J
CT diagnosis of segmental pulmonary artery embolus
J Comput Assist Tomogr 1984 Aug, Vol. 8 (4), P. 762–4

215. Brown B M, Oshita A K, Castellino R A
CT assessment of the adult extrathoracic trachea
J Comput Assist Tomogr 1983 Jun, Vol. 7 (3), P. 415–8

216. Brown B M
Computed tomography of mediastinal abscess secondary to post- traumatic esophageal lacera-
tion
J Comput Assist Tomogr 1984 Aug, Vol. 8 (4), P. 765–7

217. Buy J N, Ghossain M A, Poirson F, Bazot M, Meary E, Malbec L, Rochemaure J, Lebeau B,
Prudent J, Capron F, et al
Computed tomography of mediastinal lymph nodes in nonsmall cell lung cancer. A new approach
based on the lymphatic pathway of tumor spread
J Comput Assist Tomogr 1988 Jul-Aug, Vol. 12 (4), P. 545- 52

218. Carrol C L, Jeffrey R B Jr, Federle M P, Vernacchia F S
CT evaluation of mediastinal infections
J Comput Assist Tomogr 1987 May-Jun, Vol. 11 (3), P. 449–54

219. Casselman J W, Wilms G E, Baert A L
Computed tomography of bilateral carotid body tumours
RÖFO 1987 Apr, Vol. 146 (4), P. 381–6

220. Castellino R A, Hoppe R T, Blank N, Young S W, Neumann C, Rosenberg S A, Kaplan H S
Computed tomography, lymphography, and staging laparotomy: correlations in initial staging of
Hodgkin disease
Am J Roentgenol 1984 Jul, Vol. 143 (1), P. 37–41

221. Castellino R A, Blank N, Hoppe R T, Cho C
Hodgkin disease: contributions of chest CT in the initial staging evaluation
Radiology 1986 Sep, Vol. 160 (3), P. 603–5

222. Castellino R A
Hodgkin disease: imaging studies and patient management editorial
Radiology 1988 Oct, Vol. 169 (1), P. 269–70

223. Cayea P D, Seltzer S E
A new barium paste for computed tomography of the esophagus
J Comput Assist Tomogr 1985 Jan-Feb, Vol. 9 (1), P. 214–6

224. Chait S, Adler O B, Rosenberger A
Intramural dissection of the oesophagus after sclerotherapy. Value of CT
RÖFO 1990 Jan, Vol. 152 (1), P. 107–8

225. Chintapalli K, Thorsen M K, Olson D L, Goodman L R, Gurney J
Computed tomography of pulmonary thromboembolism and infarction
J Comput Assist Tomogr 1988 Jul-Aug, Vol. 12 (4), P. 553–9

226. Choyke P L, Zeman R K, Gootenberg J E, Greenberg J N, Hoffer F, Frank J A
Thymic atrophy and regrowth in response to chemotherapy: CT evaluation
Am J Roentgenol 1987 Aug, Vol. 149 (2), P. 269–72

227. Churchill R J, Wesbey G 3d, Marsan R E, Moncada R, Reynes C J, Love L
Computed tomographic demonstration of anomalous inferior vena cava with azygos continuation
J Comput Assist Tomogr 1980 Jun, Vol. 4 (3), P. 398–402

228. Cirimelli K M, Colletti P M, Beck S
Metastatic choriocarcinoma simulating an arteriovenous malformation on chest radiography and dynamic CT
J Comput Assist Tomogr 1988 Mar-Apr, Vol. 12 (2), P. 317–9

229. Clark K E, Foley W D, Lawson T L, Berland L L, Maddison F E
CT evaluation of esophageal and upper abdominal varices
J Comput Assist Tomogr 1980 Aug, Vol. 4 (4), P. 510–5

230. Cobb R J, Mendelson D S
CT findings in mediastinal extravasation of hyperalimentation fluid
J Comput Assist Tomogr 1987 Jan-Feb, Vol. 11 (1), P. 158–9

231. Cobet H, Richter K, Uhlich F, Waigand J
Seltene Gefäßbefunde im CT des oberen Mediastinums
Rare vascular findings in CT of the upper mediastinum
RÖFO 1988 Jun, Vol. 148 (6), P. 637–41

232. Cohen A M, Creviston S, LiPuma J P, Bryan P J, Haaga J R, Alfidi R J
NMR evaluation of hilar and mediastinal lymphadenopathy
Radiology 1983 Sep, Vol. 148 (3), P. 739–42

233. Cohen M I, Gore R M, Vogelzang R L, Rochester D, Neiman H L, Crampton A R
Accessory hemiazygos continuation of left inferior vena cava: CT demonstration
J Comput Assist Tomogr 1984 Aug, Vol. 8 (4), P. 777–9

234. Cohen M I, Gore R M, August C Z, Ossoff R H
Tracheal and bronchial stenosis associated with mediastinal adenopathy in Wegener granulomatosis: CT findings
J Comput Assist Tomogr 1984 Apr, Vol. 8 (2), P. 327–9

235. Conces D J Jr, Tarver R D, Lappas J C
The value of opacification of the esophagus by low density barium paste in computer tomography of the thorax
J Comput Assist Tomogr 1988 Mar- Apr, Vol. 12 (2), P. 202–5

236. Cornwell J, Walden C, Ghahremani G G
CT demonstration of fistula between esophageal carcinoma and spinal canal
J Comput Assist Tomogr 1986 Sep-Oct, Vol. 10 (5), P. 871–3

237. Cory D A, Cohen M D, Smith J A
Thymus in the superior mediastinum simulating adenopathy: appearance on CT
Radiology 1987 Feb, Vol. 162 (2), P. 457–9

238. Cramer M, Foley W D, Palmer T E, Werner P H, Ollinger G, Thorsen M K, Lawson T L, Perret R, Smith D F
Compression of the right pulmonary artery by aortic aneurysms: CT demonstration
J Comput Assist Tomogr 1985 Mar-Apr, Vol. 9 (2), P. 310–4

239. Crivello M S, Hayes C, Thurer R L, Kim D, Cahalane M
Traumatic pulmonary artery aneurysm: CT evaluation
J Comput Assist Tomogr 1986 May-Jun, Vol. 10 (3), P. 503–5

240. Cromwell L D, Mack L A, Loop J W
CT ScoutView for skull fracture: substitute for skull films?
AJNR 1982 Jul-Aug, Vol. 3 (4), P. 421–3

241. Danza F M, Fusco A, Falappa P
The role of computed tomography in the evaluation of dissecting aortic aneurysms letter
Radiology 1984 Sep, Vol. 152 (3), P. 827–9

242. Danza F M, Valentini A L, Colosimo C Jr, Vincenzoni M
Evolution of a mural thrombus in false aneurysm: CT demonstration
J Comput Assist Tomogr 1986 Jan-Feb, Vol. 10 (1), P. 126–9

243. Day D L, Warwick W J
Thoracic duct opacification for CT scanning
Am J Roentgenol 1985 Feb, Vol. 144 (2), P. 403–4

244. Day D L
Aortic arch in neonates with esophageal atresia: preoperative assessment using CT
Radiology 1985 Apr, Vol. 155 (1), P. 99–100

245. Daykin E L, Irwin G A, Harrison D A
CT demonstration of a traumatic aneurysm of the pulmonary artery
J Comput Assist Tomogr 1986 Mar-Apr, Vol. 10 (2), P. 323–4

246. De Boeck M, Potvliege R, Roels F, De Smedt E
The accessory costotransverse foramen: a radioanatomical study
J Comput Assist Tomogr 1984 Feb, Vol. 8 (1), P. 117–20

247. de Geer G, Webb W R, Gamsu G
Normal thymus: assessment with MR and CT
Radiology 1986 Feb, Vol. 158 (2), P. 313–7

248. Demos T C, Okrent D H, Studlo J D, Flisak M E
Spontaneous esophageal hematoma diagnosed by computed tomography
J Comput Assist Tomogr 1986 Jan-Feb, Vol. 10 (1), P. 133–5

249. Demos T C, Budorick N E, Posniak H V
Benign mediastinal cysts: pointed appearance on CT
J Comput Assist Tomogr 1989 Jan-Feb, Vol. 13 (1), P. 132–3

250. Dickey J E, Haaga J R
Benign iatrogenic cause of mediastinal gas seen on computed tomography
J Comput Assist Tomogr 1984 Apr, Vol. 8 (2), P. 330–1

251. Dobranowski J, Martin L F, Bennett W P
CT evaluation of posterior mediastinal teratoma
J Comput Assist Tomogr 1987 Jan- Feb, Vol. 11 (1), P. 156–7

252. Doppman J L, Krudy A G, Brennan M F, Schneider P, Lasker R D, Marx S J
CT appearance of enlarged parathyroid glands in the posterior superior mediastinum
J Comput Assist Tomogr 1982 Dec, Vol. 6 (6), P. 1099–102

253. Doppman J L, Shawker T H, Krudy A G, Miller D L, Marx S J, Spiegel A M, Norton J A, Brennan M F, Schaaf M, Aurbach G D
Parathymic parathyroid: CT, US, and angiographic findings
Radiology 1985 Nov, Vol. 157 (2), P. 419–23

254. Eftekhari F, Shirkhoda A, Cangir A
Cavitation of a mediastinal mass following chemotherapy for histiocytosis-X: CT demonstration
J Comput Assist Tomogr 1986 Jan-Feb, Vol. 10 (1), P. 130–2

255. Egan T J, Neiman H L, Herman R J, Malave S R, Sanders J H
Computed tomography in the diagnosis of aortic aneurysm dissection or traumatic injury
Radiology 1980 Jul, Vol. 136 (1), P. 141–6

256. Engel I A, Auh Y H, Rubenstein W A, Sniderman K, Whalen J P, Kazam E
CT diagnosis of mediastinal and thoracic inlet venous obstruction
Am J Roentgenol 1983 Sep, Vol. 141 (3), P. 521–6

257. English J T
Low-attenuation mediastinal masses on CT letter
Am J Roentgenol 1990 Jan, Vol. 154 (1), P. 199–200

258. Epstein D M, Kressel H, Gefter W, Axel L, Thickman D, Aronchick J, Miller W
MR imaging of the mediastinum: a retrospective comparison with computed tomography
J Comput Assist Tomogr 1984 Aug, Vol. 8 (4), P. 670–6

259. Fezoulidis I, Imhof H, Gritzmann N, Hajek P, Karnel F, Sieghart S
Mediastinales Lymphangiom – Wert der Computertomographie
Mediastinal lymphangioma – value of computed tomography
RÖFO 1985 Jul, Vol. 143 (1), P. 105–7

260. Fiore D, Biondetti P R, Calabro F, Rea F
CT demonstration of bilateral Castleman tumors in the mediastinum
J Comput Assist Tomogr 1983 Aug, Vol. 7 (4), P. 719–20

261. Fon G T, Bein M E, Mancuso A A, Keesey J C, Lupetin A R, Wong W S
Computed tomography of the anterior mediastinum in myasthenia gravis. A radiologic-pathologic correlative study
Radiology 1982 Jan, Vol. 142 (1), P. 135–41

262. Frey E E, Smith W L, Grandgeorge S, McCray P, Wagener J, Franken E A Jr, Sato Y
Chronic airway obstruction in children: evaluation with cine-CT
Am J Roentgenol 1987 Feb, Vol. 148 (2), P. 347–52

263. Frey E E, Sato Y, Smith W L, Franken E A Jr
Cine CT of the mediastinum in pediatric patients
Radiology 1987 Oct, Vol. 165 (1), P. 19–23

264. Frija J, Bellin M F, Laval Jeantet M
CT mediastinum examination in recurrent nerve paralysis
J Comput Assist Tomogr 1984 Oct, Vol. 8 (5), P. 901–5

265. Gamba J L, Heaston D K, Ling D, Korobkin M
CT diagnosis of an esophageal foreign body
Am J Roentgenol 1983 Feb, Vol. 140 (2), P. 289–90

266. Gamroth A, Gorich J
Diagnose der postoperativen mediastinalen Lymphozele
CT-Diagnose der postoperativen mediastinalen Lymphozele
RÖFO 1989 Mar, Vol. 150 (3), P. 356–7

267. Gaupp R J, Fagan C J, Davis M, Epstein N E
Pseudocoarctation of the aorta
J Comput Assist Tomogr 1981 Aug, Vol. 5 (4), P. 571–3

268. Genereux G P, Howie J L
Normal mediastinal lymph node size and number: CT and anatomic study
Am J Roentgenol 1984 Jun, Vol. 142 (6), P. 1095–100

269. Gerard P S, Lefkovitz Z, Golbey S H, Bryk D
Transient thoracic venous collaterals: an incidental CT finding
J Comput Assist Tomogr 1986 Jan-Feb, Vol. 10 (1), P. 75–7

270. Glanz S, Gordon D H
Right aortic arch with left descent
J Comput Assist Tomogr 1981 Apr, Vol. 5 (2), P. 256–8

271. Glazer G M, Orringer M B, Gross B H, Quint L E
The mediastinum in non-small cell lung cancer: CT-surgical correlation
Am J Roentgenol 1984 Jun, Vol. 142 (6), P. 1101–5

272. Glazer H S, Aronberg D J, Sagel S S
Pitfalls in CT recognition of mediastinal lymphadenopathy
Am J Roentgenol 1985 Feb, Vol. 144 (2), P. 267–74

273. Glazer H S, Siegel M J, Sagel S S
Low-attenuation mediastinal masses on CT
Am J Roentgenol 1989 Jun, Vol. 152 (6), P. 1173–7

274. Glazer H S, Kaiser L R, Anderson D J, Molina P L, Emami B, Roper C L, Sagel S S
Indeterminate mediastinal invasion in bronchogenic carcinoma: CT evaluation
Radiology 1989 Oct, Vol. 173 (1), P. 37–42

275. Glazer H S, Molina P L, Siegel M J, Sagel S S
High-attenuation mediastinal masses on unenhanced CT
Am J Roentgenol 1991 Jan, Vol. 156 (1), P. 45–50

276. Godwin J D, Herfkens R L, Skioldebrand C G, Federle M P, Lipton M J
Evaluation of dissections and aneurysms of the thoracic aorta by conventional and dynamic CT scanning
Radiology 1980 Jul, Vol. 136 (1), P. 125–33

277. Godwin J D, Herfkens R J, Brundage B H, Lipton M J
Evaluation of coarctation of the aorta by computed tomography
J Comput Assist Tomogr 1981 Apr, Vol. 5 (2), P. 153–6

278. Godwin J D, Breiman R S, Speckman J M
Problems and pitfalls in the evaluation of thoracic aortic dissection by computed tomography
J Comput Assist Tomogr 1982 Aug, Vol. 6 (4), P. 750–6

279. Godwin J D, Webb W R
Contrast-related flow phenomena mimicking pathology on thoracic computed tomography
J Comput Assist Tomogr 1982 Jun, Vol. 6 (3), P. 460–4

280. Godwin J D, MacGregor J M
Extension of ascites into the chest with hiatal hernia: visualization on CT
Am J Roentgenol 1987 Jan, Vol. 148 (1), P. 31–2

281. Goldberg R E, Haaga J R, Yulish B S
Serial CT scans in thymic hyperplasia
J Comput Assist Tomogr 1987 May-Jun, Vol. 11 (3), P. 539–40

282. Goodman L R, Kay H R, Teplick S K, Mundth E D
Complications of median sternotomy: computed tomographic evaluation
Am J Roentgenol 1983 Aug, Vol. 141 (2), P. 225–30

283. Goodman L R, Teplick S K, Kay H
Computed tomography of the normal sternum
Am J Roentgenol 1983 Aug, Vol. 141 (2), P. 219–23

284. Gorich J, Muller M, Beyer Enke S A, Zuna I, Probst G, van Kaick G
Computertomographische Befunde bei 36 Patienten mit Raumforderungen des Thymus
Computed tomographic findings in 36 patients with space-occupying lesions of the thymus
RÖFO 1988 Nov, Vol. 149 (5), P. 466–9

285. Gouliamos A, Striggaris K, Haliasos N, Vlahos L, Pontifex G
The diagnostic importance of the recognition of the inferior vena cava abnormalities on CT-examinations
Radiologe 1981 Sep, Vol. 21 (9), P. 437–40

286. Graen J, Dohring W, Grote R
Angiographische und computertomographische Diagnostik von Aortenaneurysemen
Angiographic and CT diagnosis of aortic aneurysms
RÖFO 1981 Mar, Vol. 134 (3), P. 273–8

287. Greene R, Miller S W
Cross-sectional imaging of silent pulmonary venous anomalies
Radiology 1986 Apr, Vol. 159 (1), P. 279–81

288. Griffin D J, Gross B H, McCracken S, Glazer G M
Observations on CT differentiation of pleural and peritoneal fluid
J Comput Assist Tomogr 1984 Feb, Vol. 8 (1), P. 24–8

289. Gross S C, Barr I, Eyler W R, Khaja F, Goldstein S
Computed tomography in dissection of the thoracic aorta
Radiology 1980 Jul, Vol. 136 (1), P. 135–9

290. Haertel M, Wiederkehr P, Zaunbauer W
Zur computertomographischen Diagnostik des Aneurysma dissecans aortae
Computed tomographic diagnosis of dissecting aneurysm of the aorta
RÖFO 1988 Sep, Vol. 149 (3), P. 267–70

291. Hahn C, Weiske R, Arlart I P
Kontrastmittel-CT des Mediastinums zur Lymphknotendiagnostik
Contrast-enhanced CT of the mediastinum in lymph node diagnosis
RÖFO 1990 Nov, Vol. 153 (5), P. 580–4

292. Halbsguth A, Schulze W, Ungeheuer E, Hoer P W
Pitfall in the CT diagnosis of pulmonary arteriovenous malformation
J Comput Assist Tomogr 1983 Aug, Vol. 7 (4), P. 710–2

293. Halden W J, Harnsberger H R, Mancuso A A
Computed tomography of esophageal varices after sclerotherapy
Am J Roentgenol 1983 Jun, Vol. 140 (6), P. 1195–6

294. Halvorsen R A Jr, Magruder Habib K, Foster W L Jr, Roberts L Jr, Postlethwait R W, Thompson W M
Esophageal cancer staging by CT: long-term follow-up study
Radiology 1986 Oct, Vol. 161 (1), P. 147–51

295. Hammerman A M, Susman N, Strzembosz A, Kaiser L R
The extrapleural fat sign: CT characteristics
J Comput Assist Tomogr 1990 May-Jun, Vol. 14 (3), P. 345–7

296. Hayward I, Forrest J V, Sagel S S
Hemiazygos vein aneurysm: CT documentation
J Comput Assist Tomogr 1989 Nov-Dec, Vol. 13 (6), P. 1072–4

297. Heiberg E, Wolverson M K, Hurd R N, Jagannadharao B, Sundaram M
CT recognition of traumatic rupture of the diaphragm
Am J Roentgenol 1980 Aug, Vol. 135 (2), P. 369–72

298. Heiberg E, Wolverson M, Sundaram M, Connors J, Susman N
CT findings in thoracic aortic dissection
Am J Roentgenol 1981 Jan, Vol. 136 (1), P. 13–7

299. Heiberg E
Standard for normal thickness of the thymus gland letter
Radiology 1983 Jun, Vol. 147 (3), P. 887

300. Heiberg E, Wolverson M K, Sundaram M, Shields J B
CT in aortic trauma
Am J Roentgenol 1983 Jun, Vol. 140 (6), P. 1119–24

301. Heiberg E, Wolverson M K, Sundaram M, Shields J B
CT characteristics of aortic atherosclerotic aneurysm versus aortic dissection
J Comput Assist Tomogr 1985 Jan-Feb, Vol. 9 (1), P. 78–83

302. Heron C W, Husband J E, Williams M P
Hodgkin disease: CT of the thymus
Radiology 1988 Jun, Vol. 167 (3), P. 647–51

303. Herter M, Harder T, Leipner N, Krahe T, Orellano L
Computertomographie und Angiographie bei der Aortendissektion
Computed tomography and angiography in aortic dissection
RÖFO 1987 Aug, Vol. 147 (2), P. 124–31

304. Higgins W L
Infiltrated retrocrural space following thoracic aorta trauma: CT evaluation
J Comput Assist Tomogr 1989 Nov-Dec, Vol. 13 (6), P. 949–51

305. Hirose J, Takashima T, Suzuki M, Matsui O
"Downhill" esophageal varices demonstrated by dynamic computed tomography
J Comput Assist Tomogr 1984 Oct, Vol. 8 (5), P. 1007–9

306. Hopper K D, Diehl L F, Cole B A, Lynch J C, Meilstrup J W, McCauslin M A
The significance of necrotic mediastinal lymph nodes on CT in patients with newly diagnosed Hodgkin disease
Am J Roentgenol 1990 Aug, Vol. 155 (2), P. 267–70

307. Hruby W, Stellamor K, Urban M, Tuchmann A
Prä- und postoperative Diagnostik des Aortenaneurysmas mittels dynamischer Computertomographie unter Verzicht auf die Angiographie
Pre- and postoperative diagnosis of an aortic aneurysm by dynamic computed tomography with omission of angiography
RÖFO 1985 Sep, Vol. 143 (3), P. 330–4

308. Hulnick D H, Naidich D P, Balthazar E J, Megibow A J, Bosniak M A
Lumbar artery pseudoaneurysm: CT demonstration
J Comput Assist Tomogr 1984 Jun, Vol. 8 (3), P. 570–2

309. Ikezoe J, Kadowaki K, Morimoto S, Takashima S, Kozuka T, Nakahara K, Kuwahara O, Takeuchi N, Yasumitsu T, Nakano N, et al
Mediastinal lymph node metastases from nonsmall cell bronchogenic carcinoma: reevaluation with CT
J Comput Assist Tomogr 1990 May-Jun, Vol. 14 (3), P. 340–4

310. Im J G, Song K S, Kang H S, Park J H, Yeon K M, Han M C, Kim C W
Mediastinal tuberculous lymphadenitis: CT manifestations
Radiology 1987 Jul, Vol. 164 (1), P. 115–9

311. Jardin M, Lemaitre L, Remy J
Narrow superior mediastinum and pseudomasses: CT features
J Comput Assist Tomogr 1986 Jul-Aug, Vol. 10 (4), P. 603–6

312. Kaiser M C, Capesius P, Petti M
Thoracic inlet mass due to cervical root avulsion diagnosed by CT- scanning
RÖFO 1983 Apr, Vol. 138 (4), P. 505–6

313. Kaplan I L, Swayne L C, Widmann W D, Wolff M
CT demonstration of "ectopic" thymoma
J Comput Assist Tomogr 1988 Nov-Dec, Vol. 12 (6), P. 1037–8

314. Karantanas A H
Low-attenuation mediastinal masses on CT letter
Am J Roentgenol 1990 Oct, Vol. 155 (4), P. 893

315. Kersjes W, Harder T, Nicolas V, Orellano L
CT-Befunde beim rupturierten abdominellen Aortenaneurysma
CT findings in ruptured abdominal aortic aneurysms
RÖFO 1987 Nov, Vol. 147 (5), P. 498–502

316. Kirks D R, Fram E K, Vock P, Effmann E L
Tracheal compression by mediastinal masses in children: CT evaluation
Am J Roentgenol 1983 Oct, Vol. 141 (4), P. 647–51

317. Koischwitz D
Computertomographische Diagnose eines monströsen gestielten Angiolipofibroms des Ösophagus
Computed tomographic diagnosis of a monstrous pedunculated angiolipofibroma of the esophagus
RÖFO 1988 Jul, Vol. 149 (1), P. 105–7

318. Konig R, van Kaick G, Vogt Moykopf I
Computertomographische Aspekte benigner intrathorakaler Raumforderungen
Computer tomography aspects of benign intrathoracic space-occupying lesions
Radiologe 1984 Mar, Vol. 24 (3), P. 101–10

319. Kormano M J, Dean P B, Hamlin D J
Upper extremity contrast medium infusion in computed tomography of upper mediastinal masses
J Comput Assist Tomogr 1980 Oct, Vol. 4 (5), P. 617–20

320. Kuhlman J E, Fishman E K, Wang K P, Siegelman S S
Esophageal duplication cyst: CT and transesophageal needle aspiration
Am J Roentgenol 1985 Sep, Vol. 145 (3), P. 531–2

321. Lee K S, Im J G, Han C H, Han M C, Kim C W, Kim W S
Malignant primary germ cell tumors of the mediastinum: CT features
Am J Roentgenol 1989 Nov, Vol. 153 (5), P. 947–51

322. Libshitz H I
CT of mediastinal lymph nodes in lung cancer: is there a "state of the art"?
Am J Roentgenol 1983 Nov, Vol. 141 (5), P. 1081–5

323. Machida K, Tasaka A
CT patterns of mural thrombus in aortic aneurysms
J Comput Assist Tomogr 1980 Dec, Vol. 4 (6), P. 840–2

324. Mantello M T, Panaccione J L, Moriarty P E, Esposito W J
Impending rupture of nonaneurysmal bacterial aortitis: CT diagnosis
J Comput Assist Tomogr 1990 Nov-Dec, Vol. 14 (6), P. 950–3

325. Mendelson D S, Berson B D, Janus C L, Gendal E S, Krellenstein D J
Computed tomography of mediastinal collaterals in SVC syndrome
J Comput Assist Tomogr 1988 Sep-Oct, Vol. 12 (5), P. 881–4

326. Miller G A Jr, Heaston D K, Moore A V Jr, Korobkin M, Braun S D, Dunnick N R
CT differentiation of thoracic aortic aneurysms from pulmonary masses adjacent to the mediastinum
J Comput Assist Tomogr 1984 Jun, Vol. 8 (3), P. 437–42

327. Mirvis S E, Dutcher J P, Haney P J, Whitley N O, Aisner J
CT of malignant pleural mesothelioma
Am J Roentgenol 1983 Apr, Vol. 140 (4), P. 665–70

328. Mirvis S E, Rodriguez A, Whitley N O, Tarr R J
CT evaluation of thoracic infections after major trauma
Am J Roentgenol 1985 Jun, Vol. 144 (6), P. 1183–7

329. Mirvis S E, Kostrubiak I, Whitley N O, Goldstein L D, Rodriguez A
Role of CT in excluding major arterial injury after blunt thoracic trauma
Am J Roentgenol 1987 Sep, Vol. 149 (3), P. 601–5

330. Mirvis S E, Tobin K D, Kostrubiak I, Belzberg H
Thoracic CT in detecting occult disease in critically ill patients
Am J Roentgenol 1987 Apr, Vol. 148 (4), P. 685–9

331. Mitsuoka A, Kitano M, Ishii S
Gas-contrasted computed tomography of the mediastinum
J Comput Assist Tomogr 1981 Aug, Vol. 5 (4), P. 588–90

332. Moncada R, Demos T C, Churchill R, Reynes C
Chronic stridor in a child: CT diagnosis of pulmonary vascular sling
J Comput Assist Tomogr 1983 Aug, Vol. 7 (4), P. 713–5

333. Moncada R, Demos T C, Marsan R, Churchill R J, Reynes C, Love L
CT diagnosis of idiopathic aneurysms of the thoracic systemic veins
J Comput Assist Tomogr 1985 Mar-Apr, Vol. 9 (2), P. 305–9

334. Moore A V, Korobkin M, Olanow W, Heaston D K, Ram P C, Dunnick N R, Silverman P M
Age-related changes in the thymus gland: CT- pathologic correlation
Am J Roentgenol 1983 Aug, Vol. 141 (2), P. 241–6

335. Moore E H, Farmer D W, Geller S C, Golden J A, Gamsu G
Computed tomography in the diagnosis of iatrogenic false aneurysms of the ascending aorta
Am J Roentgenol 1984 Jun, Vol. 142 (6), P. 1117–8

336. Moore E H, Greenberg R W, Merrick S H, Miller S W, McLoud T C, Shepard J A
Coronary artery calcifications: significance of incidental detection on CT scans
Radiology 1989 Sep, Vol. 172 (3), P. 711–6

337. Moss A A, Margulis A R, Schnyder P, Thoeni R F
A uniform, CT- based staging system for malignant neoplasms of the alimentary tube editorial
Am J Roentgenol 1981 Jun, Vol. 136 (6), P. 1251–2

338. Moss A A, Schnyder P, Thoeni R F, Margulis A R
Esophageal carcinoma: pretherapy staging by computed tomography
Am J Roentgenol 1981 Jun, Vol. 136 (6), P. 1051–6

339. Muhlberger V, Knapp E, zur Nedden D, Braunsteiner H
Vergleich zwischen angiographisch und computertomographisch dargestellten aortokoronaren Venenbrücken bei 100 Patienten
Comparison between angiographic and computed tomographic imaging of aortocoronary bypasses in 100 patients
RÖFO 1985 Apr, Vol. 142 (4), P. 406–10

340. Muhlberger V, Moes N, zur Nedden D, Knapp E
Quantitative computertomographische Flußmessungen in aortokoronaren Venenbrücken. Teil II: Korrelation mit angiographischen Messungen
Quantitative computed tomographic flow measurements of aortocoronary venous bypass grafts. II. Correlation with angiographic measurements
RÖFO 1989 Sep, Vol. 151 (3), P. 278–83

341. Muhlberger V, zur Nedden D, Knapp E
Quantitative computertomographische Flußmessungen in aortokoronaren Venenbrücken. Teil I: Varianzanalytische Untersuchungen
Quantitative computed tomographic flow measurements in aortocoronary venous bypass. I. Analysis of variance studies
RÖFO 1989 Aug, Vol. 151 (2), P. 163–6

342. Muhling T, Kuklinski M E, Hubsch T, Witte J
Computertomographie des Ösophaguskarzinoms. Korrelation computertomographischer und postoperativer Befunde
Computed tomography of esophageal carcinoma. Correlation between computed tomographic and postoperative findings
RÖFO 1985 Aug, Vol. 143 (2), P. 189–93

343. Muller N L
CT features of cystic teratoma of the diaphragm
J Comput Assist Tomogr 1986 Mar-Apr, Vol. 10 (2), P. 325–6

344. Munechika H, Cohan R H, Baker M E, Cooper C J, Dunnick N R
Hemiazygos continuation of a left inferior vena cava: CT appearance
J Comput Assist Tomogr 1988 Mar-Apr, Vol. 12 (2), P. 328–30

345. Munk P L, Muller N L
Pleural liposarcoma: CT diagnosis
J Comput Assist Tomogr 1988 Jul-Aug, Vol. 12 (4), P. 709–10

346. Murakami J, Russell W J, Hayabuchi N, Kimura S
Computed tomography of posterior longitudinal ligament ossification: its appearance and diagnostic value with special reference to thoracic lesions
J Comput Assist Tomogr 1982 Feb, Vol. 6 (1), P. 41–50

347. Murphy F B, Small W C, Wichman R D, Chalif M, Bernardino M E
CT and chest radiography are equally sensitive in the detection of pneumothorax after CT-guided pulmonary interventional procedures
Am J Roentgenol 1990 Jan, Vol. 154 (1), P. 45–6

348. Naidich D P, Khouri N F, Stitik F P, McCauley D I, Siegelman S S
Computed tomography of the pulmonary hila: 2. abnormal anatomy
J Comput Assist Tomogr 1981 Aug, Vol. 5 (4), P. 468–75

349. Naidich D P, Khouri N F, Scott W W Jr, Wang K P, Siegelman S S
Computed tomography of the pulmonary hila: 1. normal anatomy
J Comput Assist Tomogr 1981 Aug, Vol. 5 (4), P. 459–67

350. Nakata H, Nakayama C, Kimoto T, Nakayama T, Tsukamoto Y, Nobe T, Suzuki H
Computed tomography of mediastinal bronchogenic cysts
J Comput Assist Tomogr 1982 Aug, Vol. 6 (4), P. 733–8

351. Neff C C, vanSonnenberg E, Lawson D W, Patton A S
CT follow-up of empyemas: pleural peels resolve after percutaneous catheter drainage
Radiology 1990 Jul, Vol. 176 (1), P. 195–7

352. Nejatheim M, Strashun A M
CT vs. iodine scanning in diagnosis of mediastinal thyroid letter
Am J Roentgenol 1982 Oct, Vol. 139 (4), P. 834–5

353. Neufang K F, Theissen P, Deider S, Sechtem U
Thorakale Aortendissektion – Stellenwert von MRT und CT in der Verlaufskontrolle nach prothetischem Aortenersatz
Thoracic aorta dissection – the place of MRT and CT in the follow-up after prosthetic aortic replacement
RÖFO 1989 Dec, Vol. 151 (6), P. 659–65

354. Okada K, Lee M O, Hitomi S, Nagayama Y, Noma S
Sinus histiocytosis with massive lymphadenopathy and tracheobronchial lesions: CT and MR findings
J Comput Assist Tomogr 1988 Nov-Dec, Vol. 12 (6), P. 1039–40

355. Onitsuka H, Hirose N, Watanabe K, Nishitani H, Kawahira K, Matsuura K, Shigematsu N
Computed tomography of tracheopathia osteoplastica
Am J Roentgenol 1983 Feb, Vol. 140 (2), P. 268–70

356. Oppermann H C, Appell R G, Bostel F, Van Kaick G, Wahn U
Mediastinal hydatid disease in childhood: CT documentation of response to treatment with mebendazole
J Comput Assist Tomogr 1982 Feb, Vol. 6 (1), P. 175–6

357. Oudkerk M, Overbosch E, Dee P
CT recognition of acute aortic dissection
Am J Roentgenol 1983 Oct, Vol. 141 (4), P. 671–6

358. Owens G R, Arger P H, Mulhern C B Jr, Coleman B G, Gohel V
CT evaluation of mediastinal pseudocyst
J Comput Assist Tomogr 1980 Apr, Vol. 4 (2), P. 256–9

359. Pagani J J, Libshitz H I
CT manifestations of radiation- induced change in chest tissue
J Comput Assist Tomogr 1982 Apr, Vol. 6 (2), P. 243–8

360. Park C K, Webb W R, Klein J S
Inferior hilar window
Radiology 1991 Jan, Vol. 178 (1), P. 163–8

361. Patel S, Brennan J
Diagnosis of internal jugular vein thrombosis by computed tomography
J Comput Assist Tomogr 1981 Apr, Vol. 5 (2), P. 197–200

362. Pearlberg J L, Sandler M A, Madrazo B L
Computed tomographic features of esophageal intramural pseudodiverticulosis
Radiology 1983 Apr, Vol. 147 (1), P. 189–90

363. Pearlberg J L, Sandler M A, Kvale P, Beute G H, Madrazo B L
Computed-tomographic and conventional linear-tomographic evaluation of tracheobronchial lesions for laser photoresection
Radiology 1985 Mar, Vol. 154 (3), P. 759–62

364. Peterson I M, Guthaner D F
Aortic pseudoaneurysm complicating Takayasu disease: CT appearance
J Comput Assist Tomogr 1986 Jul- Aug, Vol. 10 (4), P. 676–8

365. Peterson M W, Austin J H, Yip C K, McManus R P, Jaretzki A 3d
CT findings in transdiaphragmatic empyema necessitatis due to tuberculosis
J Comput Assist Tomogr 1987 Jul-Aug, Vol. 11 (4), P. 704–6

366. Pezzulli F A, Aronson D, Goldberg N
Computed tomography of mediastinal hematoma secondary to unusual esophageal laceration: a Boerhaave variant
J Comput Assist Tomogr 1989 Jan-Feb, Vol. 13 (1), P. 129–31

367. Picus D, Balfe D M, Koehler R E, Roper C L, Owen J W
Computed tomography in the staging of esophageal carcinoma
Radiology 1983 Feb, Vol. 146 (2), P. 433–8

368. Pollack M S
Staphylococcal mediastinitis due to sternoclavicular pyarthrosis: CT appearance
J Comput Assist Tomogr 1990 Nov-Dec, Vol. 14 (6), P. 924–7

369. Pugatch R D, Faling L J, Robbins A H, Spira R
CT diagnosis of benign mediastinal abnormalities
Am J Roentgenol 1980 Apr, Vol. 134 (4), P. 685–94

370. Quint L E, Glazer G M, Orringer M B
Esophageal imaging by MR and CT: study of normal anatomy and neoplasms
Radiology 1985 Sep, Vol. 156 (3), P. 727–31

371. Quint L E, Glazer G M, Orringer M B, Francis I R, Bookstein F L
Mediastinal lymph node detection and sizing at CT and autopsy
Am J Roentgenol 1986 Sep, Vol. 147 (3), P. 469–72

372. Rankin S, Faling L J, Pugatch R D
CT diagnosis of pulmonary arteriovenous malformations
J Comput Assist Tomogr 1982 Aug, Vol. 6 (4), P. 746–9

373. Recht M P, Coleman B G, Barbot D J, Rosato E F, Aronchick J M, Epstein D M, Gefter W B, Miller W T
Recurrent esophageal carcinoma at thoracotomy incisions: diagnostic contributions of CT
J Comput Assist Tomogr 1989 Jan-Feb, Vol. 13 (1), P. 58–60

374. Reddy S C
Esophagopleural fistula
J Comput Assist Tomogr 1983 Apr, Vol. 7 (2), P. 376–7

375. Reinig J W, Stanley J H, Schabel S I
CT evaluation of thickened esophageal walls
Am J Roentgenol 1983 May, Vol. 140 (5), P. 931–4

376. Richardson P, Mirvis S E, Scorpio R, Dunham C M
Value of CT in determining the need for angiography when findings of mediastinal hemorrhage on chest radiographs are equivocal
Am J Roentgenol 1991 Feb, Vol. 156 (2), P. 273–9

377. Rieser R, Hauger W
Myxoider Primärtumor der Aorta – Diagnostik durch i.a. DSA und CT
A primary myxoid tumor of the aorta - diagnosis using i.a. DSA and CT
RÖFO 1990 Jan, Vol. 152 (1), P. 98–9

378. Rost R C Jr, Proto A V
Inferior pulmonary ligament: computed tomographic appearance
Radiology 1983 Aug, Vol. 148 (2), P. 479–83

379. Sakuma H, Takeda K, Hirano T, Okuda Y, Matsumura K, Yamaguchi N, Nakano T, Takano M
Plain chest radiograph with computed radiography: improved sensitivity for the detection of coronary artery calcification
Am J Roentgenol 1988 Jul, Vol. 151 (1), P. 27–30

380. Schild H, Gamstatter G, Teifke A, Heller M, Keller E
Aussagekraft des Ösophagogramms im Vergleich zur Computertomographie beim Ösophaguskarzinom
Significance of the esophagogram compared to computed tomography in esophageal cancer
RÖFO 1984 May, Vol. 140 (5), P. 551–5

381. Schumacher K A, Friedrich J M
Spontaner Chylothorax: Diagnostik durch Kombination von Lymphographie und CT
Spontaneous chylothorax: its diagnosis through a combination of lymphography and CT
RÖFO 1989 Jul, Vol. 151 (1), P. 108–9

382. Seibel D G, Hopper K D, Ghaed Ñ .
Mammographic and CT detection of extrathoracic lung herniation
J Comput Assist Tomogr 1987 May- Jun, Vol. 11 (3), P. 537–8

383. Seline T H, Gross B H, Francis I R
CT and MR imaging of mediastinal hemangiomas
J Comput Assist Tomogr 1990 Sep-Oct, Vol. 14 (5), P. 766–8

384. Seltzer S E, Herman P G, Sagel S S
Differential diagnosis of mediastinal fluid levels visualized on computed tomography
J Comput Assist Tomogr 1984 Apr, Vol. 8 (2), P. 244–6

385. Sens M, Brandt H, Dingler W, Kotterer O, Deininger H K
Untersuchung zur Bestimmung der Wertigkeit von konventioneller und computerunterstützter Tomographie bei der Untersuchung der Thoraxorgane
Determination of the value of conventional and computer-assisted tomography in examining the thoracic organs
RÖFO 1989 Oct, Vol. 151 (4), P. 423–7

386. Shapeero L G, Blank N, Young S W
Contrast enhancement in mediastinal and cervical lymph nodes
J Comput Assist Tomogr 1983 Apr, Vol. 7 (2), P. 242–4

387. Shapeero L G, Guthaner D F, Swerdlow C D, Wexler L
Rupture of a coronary bypass graft aneurysm: CT evaluation and coil occlusion therapy
Am J Roentgenol 1983 Nov, Vol. 141 (5), P. 1060–2

388. Shepard J O, Dedrick C G, Spizarny D L, McLoud T C
Dynamic incremental computed tomography of the pulmonary hila using a flow-rate injector
J Comput Assist Tomogr 1986 Mar-Apr, Vol. 10 (2), P. 369–71

389. Shin M S, Ceballos R, Bini R M, Ho K J
CT diagnosis of false aneurysm of the pulmonary artery not demonstrated by angiography
J Comput Assist Tomogr 1983 Jun, Vol. 7 (3), P. 524–6

390. Shin M S, Berland L L, Ho K J
Mediastinal cystic hygromas: CT characteristics and pathogenetic consideration
J Comput Assist Tomogr 1985 Mar-Apr, Vol. 9 (2), P. 297–301

391. Shin M S, Anderson S D, Myers J, Ho K J
Pitfalls in CT evaluation of chest wall invasion by lung cancer
J Comput Assist Tomogr 1986 Jan-Feb, Vol. 10 (1), P. 136–8

392. Shin M S, Jackson R M, Ho K J
Tracheobronchomegaly Mounier- Kuhn syndrome: CT diagnosis
Am J Roentgenol 1988 Apr, Vol. 150 (4), P. 777–9

393. Shipley R T, McLoud T C, Dedrick C G, Shepard J A
Computed tomography of the tracheal bronchus
J Comput Assist Tomogr 1985 Jan-Feb, Vol. 9 (1), P. 53–5

394. Sider L, Davis T M Jr
Hilar masses: evaluation with CT-guided biopsy after negative bronchoscopic examination
Radiology 1987 Jul, Vol. 164 (1), P. 107–9

395. Siegel M J, Sagel S S, Reed K
The value of computed tomography in the diagnosis and management of pediatric mediastinal abnormalities
Radiology 1982 Jan, Vol. 142 (1), P. 149–55

396. Siegel M J, Nadel S N, Glazer H S, Sagel S S
Mediastinal lesions in children: comparison of CT and MR
Radiology 1986 Jul, Vol. 160 (1), P. 241–4

397. Silverman P M, Baker M E, Mahony B S
Atelectasis and subpulmonic fluid: a CT pitfall in distinguishing pleural from peritoneal fluid
J Comput Assist Tomogr 1985 Jul-Aug, Vol. 9 (4), P. 763–6

398. Sinner W N
Zur computertomographischen Differentialdiagnostik von gut- und bösartigen lipoiden Raumforderungen des Mediastinums und deren Ausbreitung
The computer tomographic differential diagnosis of benign and malignant lipoid masses in the mediastinum and their spread
RÖFO 1980 Jun, Vol. 132 (6), P. 613–21

399. Sivit C J, Taylor G A, Eichelberger M R
Chest injury in children with blunt abdominal trauma: evaluation with CT
Radiology 1989 Jun, Vol. 171 (3), P. 815–8

400. Smathers R L, Buschi A J, Pope T L Jr, Brenbridge A N, Williamson B R
The azygous arch: normal and pathologic CT appearance
Am J Roentgenol 1982 Sep, Vol. 139 (3), P. 477–83401.Smathers R L, Lee J K, Heiken J P
Anomalous preaortic interazygous vein
J Comput Assist Tomogr 1983 Aug, Vol. 7 (4), P. 732–3

402. Smith T R, Khoury P T
Aneurysm of the proximal thoracic aorta simulating neoplasm: the role of CT and angiography
Am J Roentgenol 1985 May, Vol. 144 (5), P. 909–10

403. Som P M, Shugar J M, Sacher M, Lanzieri C F
Internal jugular vein phlebectasia and duplication: CT features
J Comput Assist Tomogr 1985 Mar-Apr, Vol. 9 (2), P. 390–2

404. Sone S, Higashihara T, Morimoto S, Ikezoe J, Arisawa J, Monden Y, Nahakara K
CT anatomy of hilar lymphadenopathy
Am J Roentgenol 1983 May, Vol. 140 (5), P. 887–92

405. Sones P J Jr, Torres W E, Colvin R S, Meier W L, Sprawls P, Rogers J V Jr
Effectiveness of CT in evaluating intrathoracic masses
Am J Roentgenol 1982 Sep, Vol. 139 (3), P. 469–75

406. Spizarny D L, Shepard J A, McLoud T C, Grillo H C, Dedrick C G
CT of adenoid cystic carcinoma of the trachea
Am J Roentgenol 1986 Jun, Vol. 146 (6), P. 1129–32

407. Spizarny D L, Gross B H, Shepard J A
CT findings in localized fibrous mesothelioma of the pleural fissure
J Comput Assist Tomogr 1986 Nov-Dec, Vol. 10 (6), P. 942–4

408. Spizarny D L, Rebner M, Gross B H
CT evaluation of enhancing mediastinal masses
J Comput Assist Tomogr 1987 Nov-Dec, Vol. 11 (6), P. 990–3

409. St Amour T E, Siegel M J, Glazer H S, Nadel S N
CT appearances of the normal and abnormal thymus in childhood
J Comput Assist Tomogr 1987 Jul-Aug, Vol. 11 (4), P. 645–50

410. St Amour T E, Gutierrez F R, Levitt R G, McKnight R C
CT diagnosis of type A aortic dissections not demonstrated by aortography
J Comput Assist Tomogr 1988 Nov-Dec, Vol. 12 (6), P. 963–7

411. Staples C A, Muller N L, Miller R R, Evans K G, Nelems B
Mediastinal nodes in bronchogenic carcinoma: comparison between CT and mediastinoscopy
Radiology 1988 May, Vol. 167 (2), P. 367–72

412. Stark D D, Federle M P, Goodman P C
CT and radiographic assessment of tube thoracostomy
Am J Roentgenol 1983 Aug, Vol. 141 (2), P. 253–8

413. Stark P
Die normale Anatomie der Lungenhili im Computertomogramm
The normal anatomy of the pulmonary hili on computed tomography
RÖFO 1982 Jul, Vol. 137 (1), P. 77–80

414. Stark P
CT of blunt chest trauma letter
Am J Roentgenol 1990 Jul, Vol. 155 (1), P. 194–5

415. Stein M G, Gamsu G, Webb W R, Stulbarg M S
Computed tomography of diffuse tracheal stenosis in Wegener granulomatosis
J Comput Assist Tomogr 1986 Sep-Oct, Vol. 10 (5), P. 868–70

416. Stein M G, Mayo J, Muller N, Aberle D R, Webb W R, Gamsu G
Pulmonary lymphangitic spread of carcinoma: appearance on CT scans
Radiology 1987 Feb, Vol. 162 (2), P. 371–5

417. Stricof D D, Gabrielsen T O, Latack J T, Gebarski S S, Chandler W F
CT demonstration of cavernous sinus fat
AJNR 1989 Nov-Dec, Vol. 10 (6), P. 1199–201

418. Strijk S P, Boetes C, Rosenbusch G, Ruijs J H
Lymphography and abdominal computed tomography in staging Hodgkin's disease
RÖFO 1987 Mar, Vol. 146 (3), P. 312–8

419. Suchato C, Pekanan P, Singjaroen T, Sereerat P
Indication of dissecting aortic aneurysm on noncontrast computed tomography
J Comput Assist Tomogr 1980 Feb, Vol. 4 (1), P. 115–6

420. Sullivan K L, Steiner R M, Wechsler R J
Lymphaticopleural fistula: diagnosis by computed tomography
J Comput Assist Tomogr 1984 Oct, Vol. 8 (5), P. 1005–6

421. Sullivan K L, Wechsler R J
CT diagnosis of mediastinal lymphocele
J Comput Assist Tomogr 1985 Nov-Dec, Vol. 9 (6), P. 1110–1

422. Sussman S K, Silverman P M, Donnal J F
CT demonstration of isolated mediastinal goiter
J Comput Assist Tomogr 1986 Sep-Oct, Vol. 10 (5), P. 863–4

423. Suzuki M, Takashima T, Itoh H, Choutoh S, Kawamura I, Watanabe Y
Computed tomography of mediastinal teratomas
J Comput Assist Tomogr 1983 Feb, Vol. 7 (1), P. 74–6

424. Swain M E, Coblentz C L
Tracheal chondroma: CT appearance
J Comput Assist Tomogr 1988 Nov-Dec, Vol. 12 (6), P. 1085–6

425. Takashima S, Takeuchi N, Shiozaki H, Kobayashi K, Morimoto S, Ikezoe J, Tomiyama N, Harada K, Shogen K, Kozuka T
Carcinoma of the esophagus: CT vs MR imaging in determining resectability
Am J Roentgenol 1991 Feb, Vol. 156 (2), P. 297–302

426. Takasugi J E, Godwin J D
CT appearance of the retroaortic anastomoses of the azygos system
Am J Roentgenol 1990 Jan, Vol. 154 (1), P. 41–4

427. Tarr R W, Page D L, Glick A G, Shaff M I
Benign hemangioendothelioma involving posterior mediastinum: CT findings
J Comput Assist Tomogr 1986 Sep-Oct, Vol. 10 (5), P. 865–7

428. ten Hove W, van Schaik J P
Saccular aneurysm of the aortic arch presenting as a nonenhancing mass on CT scanning. Case report
RÖFO 1989 Aug, Vol. 151 (2), P. 233–4

429. Teplick J G, Teplick S K, Goodman L, Haskin M E
The interface sign: a computed tomographic sign for distinguishing pleural and intra-abdominal fluid
Radiology 1982 Jul, Vol. 144 (2), P. 359–62

430. Thorsen M K, San Dretto M A, Lawson T L, Foley W D, Smith D F, Berland L L
Dissecting aortic aneurysms: accuracy of computed tomographic diagnosis
Radiology 1983 Sep, Vol. 148 (3), P. 773–7431.Thorsen M K, Goodman L R, Sagel S S, Olinger G N, Youker J E
Ascending aorta complications of cardiac surgery: CT evaluation
J Comput Assist Tomogr 1986 Mar-Apr, Vol. 10 (2), P. 219–25

432. Thorsen M K, Erickson S J, Mewissen M W, Youker J E
CT and MR imaging of partial anomalous pulmonary venous return to the azygos vein
J Comput Assist Tomogr 1990 Nov-Dec, Vol. 14 (6), P. 1007–9

433. Tocino I M, Miller M H, Frederick P R, Bahr A L, Thomas F
CT detection of occult pneumothorax in head trauma
Am J Roentgenol 1984 Nov, Vol. 143 (5), P. 987–90

434. Torres W E, Maurer D E, Steinberg H V, Robbins S, Bernardino M E
CT of aortic aneurysms: the distinction between mural and thrombus calcification
Am J Roentgenol 1988 Jun, Vol. 150 (6), P. 1317–9

435. Trigaux J P, Van Beers B
Thoracic collateral venous channels: normal and pathologic CT findings
J Comput Assist Tomogr 1990 Sep- Oct, Vol. 14 (5), P. 769–73

436. Triller J, Goldhirsch A, Fuchs W A
Wertigkeit der Computertomographie in der Beurteilung von Lymphknotenmetastasen beim Ovarialkarzinom
Value of computed tomography for the assessment of lymph node metastases in ovarian cancer
RÖFO 1984 Jul, Vol. 141 (1), P. 35–9

437. Triller J, Marincek B, Probst P, Stirnemann P, Nachbur B
Computertomographie des mykotischen Aortenaneurysmas
Radiologe 1984 Jan, Vol. 24 (1), P. 35–9

438. Unger J M, Peters M E, Hinke M L
Chest case of the day
Am J Roentgenol 1986 May, Vol. 146 (5), P. 1080–6

439. vanSonnenberg E, Lin A S, Deutsch A L, Mattrey R F
Percutaneous biopsy of difficult mediastinal, hilar, and pulmonary lesions by computed tomographic guidance and a modified coaxial technique
Radiology 1983 Jul, Vol. 148 (1), P. 300–2

440. vanSonnenberg E, Nakamoto S K, Mueller P R, Casola G, Neff C C, Friedman P J, Ferrucci J T Jr, Simeone J F
CT- and ultrasound- guided catheter drainage of empyemas after chest- tube failure
Radiology 1984 May, Vol. 151 (2), P. 349–53

441. vanSonnenberg E, Casola G, Ho M, Neff C C, Varney R R, Wittich G R, Christensen R, Friedman P J
Difficult thoracic lesions: CT- guided biopsy experience in 150 cases
Radiology 1988 May, Vol. 167 (2), P. 457–61

442. Vasile N, Mathieu D, Keita K, Lellouche D, Bloch G, Cachera J P
Computed tomography of thoracic aortic dissection: accuracy and pitfalls
J Comput Assist Tomogr 1986 Mar-Apr, Vol. 10 (2), P. 211- 5

443. Vilgrain V, Mompoint D, Palazzo L, Menu Y, Gayet B, Ollier P, Nahum H, Fekete F
Staging of esophageal carcinoma: comparison of results with endoscopic sonography and CT
Am J Roentgenol 1990 Aug, Vol. 155 (2), P. 277–81

444. Vint V C, Usselman J A, Warmath M A, Dilley R B
Aortic perianeurysmal fibrosis: CT density enhancement and ureteral obstruction
Am J Roentgenol 1980 Mar, Vol. 134 (3), P. 577–80

445. Vock P, Tillmann U, Fuchs W A
Computertomographie des Mediastinums
Computed tomography of the mediastinum
Radiologe 1981 Jul, Vol. 21 (7), P. 330–6

446. Vock P, Spiegel T, Fram E K, Effmann E L
CT assessment of the adult intrathoracic cross section of the trachea
J Comput Assist Tomogr 1984 Dec, Vol. 8 (6), P. 1076–82

447. Vogelzang R L, Sohaey R
Infected aortic aneurysms: CT appearance
J Comput Assist Tomogr 1988 Jan-Feb, Vol. 12 (1), P. 109–12

448. Waite R J, Carbonneau R J, Balikian J P, Umali C B, Pezzella A T, Nash G
Parietal pleural changes in empyema: appearances at CT
Radiology 1990 Apr, Vol. 175 (1), P. 145–50

449. Wall S D, Federle M P, Jeffrey R B, Brett C M
CT diagnosis of unsuspected pneumothorax after blunt abdominal trauma
Am J Roentgenol 1983 Nov, Vol. 141 (5), P. 919–21

450. Walter E, Hubener K H
Computertomographische Charakteristika raumfordernder Prozesse im vorderen Mediastinum und ihre Differentialdiagnose
Computer tomographic characteristics of space-occupying processes in the anterior mediastinum and their differential diagnosis
RÖFO 1980 Oct, Vol. 133 (4), P. 391–400

451. Wang A M, Jolesz F, Rumbaugh C L, Zamani A
CT assessment of thoracic extension and of concomitant lesions in syringohydromyelia
J Comput Assist Tomogr 1983 Feb, Vol. 7 (1), P. 18–24

452. Watanabe Y, Nishiyama Y, Kanayama H, Enomoto K, Kato K, Takeichi M
Congenital bronchiectasis due to cartilage deficiency: CT demonstration
J Comput Assist Tomogr 1987 Jul-Aug, Vol. 11 (4), P. 701–3

453. Webb W R, Gamsu G, Glazer G
Computed tomography of the abnormal pulmonary hilum
J Comput Assist Tomogr 1981 Aug, Vol. 5 (4), P. 485–90

454. Webb W R, Glazer G, Gamsu G
Computed tomography of the normal pulmonary hilum
J Comput Assist Tomogr 1981 Aug, Vol. 5 (4), P. 476–84

455. Webb W R, Gamsu G, Speckman J M, Kaiser J A, Federle M P, Lipton M J
CT demonstration of mediastinal aortic arch anomalies
J Comput Assist Tomogr 1982 Jun, Vol. 6 (3), P. 445–51

456. Webb W R, Gamsu G, Speckman J M, Kaiser J A, Federle M P, Lipton M J
Computed tomographic demonstration of mediastinal venous anomalies
Am J Roentgenol 1982 Jul, Vol. 139 (1), P. 157–61

457. Webb W R, Gamsu G, Speckman J M
Computed tomography of the pulmonary hilum in patients with bronchogenic carcinoma
J Comput Assist Tomogr 1983 Apr, Vol. 7 (2), P. 219–25

458. Webb W R, Gamsu G
Computed tomography of the left retrobronchial stripe
J Comput Assist Tomogr 1983 Feb, Vol. 7 (1), P. 65–9

459. Wechsler R J, Rao V M, Newman L M
The subclavian triangle: CT analysis
Am J Roentgenol 1989 Feb, Vol. 152 (2), P. 313–7

460. Wegener O H
Die Computertomographie des Mediastinums
Computer tomography of the mediastinum
RÖFO 1978 Dec, Vol. 129 (6), P. 727–35

461. Weinstein J B, Aronberg D J, Sagel S S
CT of fibrosing mediastinitis: findings and their utility
Am J Roentgenol 1983 Aug, Vol. 141 (2), P. 247–51

462. Weiss C, Dinkel E, Wimmer B, Schildge J, Grosser G
Der Thymus im Computertomogramm. Normalbefunde und Pathologie
The thymus gland in computerized tomography. Normal findings and pathology
Radiologe 1987 Sep, Vol. 27 (9), P. 414–21

463. Weiss L M, Fagelman D, Warhit J M
CT demonstration of an esophageal duplication cyst
J Comput Assist Tomogr 1983 Aug, Vol. 7 (4), P. 716–8

464. Wentz K U, Irngartinger G, Georgi P, van Kaick G, Kleckow M, Vollhaber H H
Malignes Pleuramesotheliom. Wertigkeit der 67Ga- Szintigraphie im Vergleich zur Computer-tomographie
Malignant pleural mesothelioma. Value of 67Ga scintigraphy compared to computerized tomography
RÖFO 1986 Jul, Vol. 145 (1), P. 61–6

465. Wernecke K, Vassallo P, Potter R, Luckener H G, Peters P E
Mediastinal tumors: sensitivity of detection with sonography compared with CT and radiography
Radiology 1990 Apr, Vol. 175 (1), P. 137–43

466. Westra D, Verbeeten B Jr
Left pulmonary venous indentation on the oesophagus confirmed by angio-CT. Case report
RÖFO 1983 Feb, Vol. 138 (2), P. 243–5

467. Whitley N O, Fuks J Z, McCrea E S, Whitacre M, Masler J A, Whitley J E, Aisner J
Computed tomography of the chest in small cell lung cancer: potential new prognostic signs
Am J Roentgenol 1984 May, Vol. 142 (5), P. 885–92

468. Whitman G J, Borkowski G P
Giant fibrovascular polyp of the esophagus: CT and MR findings
Am J Roentgenol 1989 Mar, Vol. 152 (3), P. 518–20

469. Williams M P, Husband J E, Heron C W
Intrathoracic manifestations of metastatic testicular seminoma: a comparison of chest radiographic and CT findings
Am J Roentgenol 1987 Sep, Vol. 149 (3), P. 473–5

470. Williams R A, Haaga J R, Karagiannis E
CT guided paravertebral biopsy of the mediastinum
J Comput Assist Tomogr 1984 Jun, Vol. 8 (3), P. 575–8

471. Williford M E, Hidalgo H, Putman C E, Korobkin M, Ram P C
Computed tomography of pleural disease
Am J Roentgenol 1983 May, Vol. 140 (5), P. 909–14

472. Wimbish K J, Agha F P, Brady T M
Bilateral pulmonary sequestration: computed tomographic appearance
Am J Roentgenol 1983 Apr, Vol. 140 (4), P. 689–90

473. Wolff P, Schweden F, Klose K, Kuhn F, Brost F, Thelen M
Die thorakale Computertomographie bei Intensivpatienten
Computerized tomography of the thorax in intensive care patients
RÖFO 1987 Jun, Vol. 146 (6), P. 646–53

474. Yamada T, Tada S, Harada J
Aortic dissection without intimal rupture: diagnosis with MR imaging and CT
Radiology 1988 Aug, Vol. 168 (2), P. 347–52

475. Yamaguchi T, Guthaner D F, Wexler L
Natural history of the false channel of type A aortic dissection after surgical repair: CT study
Radiology 1989 Mar, Vol. 170 (3 Pt 1), P. 743–7

476. Yeh H C, Gordon A, Kirschner P A, Cohen B A
Computed tomography and sonography of thymolipoma
Am J Roentgenol 1983 Jun, Vol. 140 (6), P. 1131–3

477. Yeoman L J, Dalton H R, Adam E J
Fat-fluid level in pleural effusion as a complication of a mediastinal dermoid: CT characteristics
J Comput Assist Tomogr 1990 Mar-Apr, Vol. 14 (2), P. 307–9

478. Zerhouni E A, Scott W W Jr, Baker R R, Wharam M D, Siegelman S S
Invasive thymomas: diagnosis and evaluation by computed tomography
J Comput Assist Tomogr 1982 Feb, Vol. 6 (1), P. 92–100

479. Ziegler K
Computertomographie des Thorax beim Poland- Syndrom
Computer tomography of the thorax in the Poland syndrome
RÖFO 1982 Nov, Vol. 137 (5), P. 597–9

480. Zinn W L, Naidich D P, Whelan C A, Litt A W, McCauley D I, Ettenger N A
Fluid within preexisting pulmonary air-spaces: a potential pitfall in the CT differentiation of pleural from parenchymal disease
J Comput Assist Tomogr 1987 May-Jun, Vol. 11 (3), P. 441–8

481. Zissin R, Shapiro M
Chest CT scan before transplantation letter
Am J Roentgenol 1990 Nov, Vol. 155 (5), P. 1136–7

The Heart

482. Aiello M R, Cohen W N
Inflammatory aneurysm of the abdominal aorta
J Comput Assist Tomogr 1980 Apr, Vol. 4 (2), P. 265–7

483. Aizenstein R, Wilbur A C
CT diagnosis of septic thrombus letter
Am J Roentgenol 1988 Aug, Vol. 151 (2), P. 409

484. Albrechtsson U, Stahl E, Tylen U
Evaluation of coronary artery bypass graft patency with computed tomography
J Comput Assist Tomogr 1981 Dec, Vol. 5 (6), P. 822–6

485. Andersen P E Jr, Lorentzen J E
Comparison of computed tomography and aortography in abdominal aortic aneurysms
J Comput Assist Tomogr 1983 Aug, Vol. 7 (4), P. 670–3

486. Aronberg D J, Peterson R R, Glazer H S, Sagel S S
The superior sinus of the pericardium: CT appearance
Radiology 1984 Nov, Vol. 153 (2), P. 489–92

487. Baim R S, MacDonald I L, Wise D J, Lenkel S C
Computed tomography of absent left pericardium
Radiology 1980 Vol.135 P. 127

488. Bilbey J H, Muller N L, Connell D G, Luoma A A, Nelems B
Thoracic outlet syndrome: evaluation with CT
Radiology 1989 May, Vol. 171 (2), P. 381–4

489. Borts F T, Rohatgi P K, Sehgal E
Bronchogenic cavoatrial tumor thrombus: CT demonstration
J Comput Assist Tomogr 1985 Nov-Dec, Vol. 9 (6), P. 1115–7

490. Bouchard A, Lipton M J, Farmer D W, Diethelm E, Killebrew E J, Garrett J, Dery R, Schiller N B
Evaluation of regional ventricular wall motion by ECG-gated CT
J Comput Assist Tomogr 1987 Nov-Dec, Vol. 11 (6), P. 969–74

491. Brecht G, Harder T
Aortenaneurysma und Aortendissektion. Computertomographie – Angiographie – Sonographie
Aortic aneurysms and aortic dissection. Computed tomography – angiography - sonography
RÖFO 1981 Oct, Vol. 135 (4), P. 388–98

492. Buck J, Heuck F, Both A, Seitz K H
Informationswert der Röntgencomputertomographie bei Vorhoftumoren des Herzens
The information value of roentgen computerized tomography in atrial tumors of the heart
RÖFO 1983 Jan, Vol. 138 (1), P. 36–41

493. Carlsson E, Lipton M J, Skioldebrand C G, Berninger W H, Redington R W
Erfahrungen mit der Computer-Tomographie bei der in vivo- Herzdiagnostik
Experience with computed transmission tomography of the heart in vivo
Radiologe 1980 Feb, Vol. 20 (2), P. 44–9

494. Chiles C, Baker M E, Silverman P M
Superior pericardial recess simulating aortic dissection on computed tomography
J Comput Assist Tomogr 1986 May-Jun, Vol. 10 (3), P. 421–3

495. Cipriano P R, Nassi M, Brody W R
Clinically applicable gated cardiac computed tomography
Am J Roentgenol 1983 Mar, Vol. 140 (3), P. 604–6

496. Conces D J Jr, Vix V A, Tarver R D
Diagnosis of a myocardial lipoma by using CT
Am J Roentgenol 1989 Oct, Vol. 153 (4), P. 725–6

497. Cornalba G, Dore R
Cardiac tumor associated with tuberous sclerosis: CT diagnosis
J Comput Assist Tomogr 1985 Jul-Aug, Vol. 9 (4), P. 809–11

498. Culham J A
The right heart border in infancy
Radiology 1981 May, Vol. 139 (2), P. 381–4

499. Daves M L, Groves B M
Computed tomography of absent left pericardium letter
Radiology 1981 Jun, Vol. 139 (3), P. 753

500. Dery R, Lipton M J, Garrett J S, Abbott J, Higgins C B, Schienman M M
Cine-computed tomography of arrhythmogenic right ventricular dysplasia
J Comput Assist Tomogr 1986 Jan-Feb, Vol. 10 (1), P. 120–3

501. Diethelm L, Simonson J S, Dery R, Gould R G, Schiller N B, Lipton M J
Determination of left ventricular mass with ultrafast CT and two- dimensional echocardiography
Radiology 1989 Apr, Vol. 171 (1), P. 213–7

502. Doppman J L, Rienmuller R, Lissner J, Cyran J, Bolte H D, Strauer B E, Hellwig H
Computed tomography in constrictive pericardial disease
J Comput Assist Tomogr 1981 Feb, Vol. 5 (1), P. 1–11

503. Doppman J L, Rienmuller R, Lissner J
The visualized interventricular septum on cardiac computed tomography: a clue to the presence of severe anemia
J Comput Assist Tomogr 1981 Apr, Vol. 5 (2), P. 157–60

504. Ehrlich C P, Goldberg R P
Paracardiac pseudotumor: a kymographic artifact of computed radiography
Am J Roentgenol 1984 May, Vol. 142 (5), P. 919–20

505. Engelstad B L, Wagner S, Herfkens R, Botvinick E, Brundage B, Lipton M
Evaluation of the post-coronary artery bypass patient by myocardial perfusion scintigraphy and computed tomography
Am J Roentgenol 1983 Sep, Vol. 141 (3), P. 507–12

506. Escarous A
CT findings of a posterior false aneurysm of the left ventricle letter
Am J Roentgenol 1989 Jun, Vol. 152 (6), P. 1339–40

507. Ewen K, Lackner K, Fischer P
Das somatische Strahlenrisiko bei Herzuntersuchungen mit der digitalen Angiographie und der EKG- getriggerten Computertomographie
Somatic radiation risk during heart examinations using digital angiography and ECG-triggered computed tomography
RÖFO 1983 Oct, Vol. 139 (4), P. 440–3

508. Farmer D W, Lipton M J, Webb W R, Ringertz H, Higgins C B
Computed tomography in congenital heart disease
J Comput Assist Tomogr 1984 Aug, Vol. 8 (4), P. 677–87

509. Felix R, Lackner K, Thurn P
Derzeitige und zukünftige Möglichkeiten des CT-Einsatzes am Herzen. Eine Übersicht
CT and the heart: present state of the art and its future. A review
Radiologe 1980 Feb, Vol. 20 (2), P. 50–5

510. Frey E E, Matherne G P, Mahoney L T, Sato Y, Stanford W, Smith W L
Coronary artery aneurysms due to Kawasaki disease: diagnosis with ultrafast CT
Radiology 1988 Jun, Vol. 167 (3), P. 725–6511.Gale M E, Kiwak M G, Gale D R
Pericardial fluid distribution: CT analysis
Radiology 1987 Jan, Vol. 162 (1 Pt 1), P. 171–4

512. Garrett J S, Schiller N B, Botvinick E H, Higgins C B, Lipton M J
Cine-computed tomography of Ebstein anomaly
J Comput Assist Tomogr 1986 Jul-Aug, Vol. 10 (4), P. 664–6

513. Glazer G M, Gross B H, Orringer M B, Buda A J, Francis I R, Shapiro B
Computed tomography of pericardial masses: further observations and comparison with echocardiography
J Comput Assist Tomogr 1984 Oct, Vol. 8 (5), P. 895–9

514. Godwin J D, Califf R M, Korobkin M, Moore A V, Breiman R S, Kong Y
Clinical value of coronary bypass graft evaluation with CT
Am J Roentgenol 1983 Apr, Vol. 140 (4), P. 649–55

515. Godwin J D, Moore A V, Ideker R E, Califf R M
Prospective demonstration of myocardial infarction by CT
Am J Roentgenol 1984 Nov, Vol. 143 (5), P. 985–6

516. Goldstein L, Mirvis S E, Kostrubiak I S, Turney S Z
CT diagnosis of acute pericardial tamponade after blunt chest trauma
Am J Roentgenol 1989 Apr, Vol. 152 (4), P. 739–41

517. Gooskens R H, Kaiser M C, Veiga Pires J A
Computed tomography in the management of complications due to ventricular shunting
Neuroradiology 1981 Feb, Vol. 21 (1), P. 47–9

518. Gorich J, Zuna I, Merle M, Beyer Enke I A, Merkle N, Weigelbaum K, van Kaick G
Aortenverkalkungen im CT. Korrelation zu Risikofaktoren und kardiovaskulären Erkrankungen
Aortic calcification in CT. Correlation with risk factors and cardiovascular diseases
Radiologe 1989 Dec, Vol. 29 (12), P. 614–9

519. Gouliamos A, Steriotis J, Kalovidouris A, Andreou J, Sandilos P, Michalis A, Papavasiliou C, Pontifex G
Computed tomography of water-like densities mimicking pericardial effusion in a case of a pericardial tumor
J Comput Assist Tomogr 1984 Apr, Vol. 8 (2), P. 343–4

520. Graeb D A, Robertson W D, Lapointe J S, Nugent R A, Harrison P B
Computed tomographic diagnosis of intraventricular hemorrhage. Etiology and prognosis
Radiology 1982 Apr, Vol. 143 (1), P. 91–6

521. Gross B H, Glazer G M, Francis I R
CT of intracardiac and intrapericardial masses
Am J Roentgenol 1983 May, Vol. 140 (5), P. 903–7

522. Guthaner D F, Wexler L, Harell G
CT demonstration of cardiac structures
Am J Roentgenol 1979 Jul, Vol. 133 (1), P. 75–81

523. Hackney D, Slutsky R A, Mattrey R, Peck W W, Abraham J L, Shabetai R, Higgins C B
Experimental pericardial inflammation evaluated by computed tomography
Radiology 1984 Apr, Vol. 151 (1), P. 145–8

524. Henry D A, Corcoran H L, Lewis T D, Barnhart G R, Szentpetery S, Lower R R
Orthotopic cardiac transplantation: evaluation with CT Radiology 1989 Feb, Vol. 170 (2), P. 343–50

525. Heuser L, Lackner K, Hauser H
Validität der Computertomographie bei der Darstellung offener und verschlossener aortokoronarer Venenbrücken (ACVB)
Validity of computed tomography for the demonstration of patent or occluded aortocoronary vein grafts. A multicenter study
RÖFO 1982 Dec, Vol. 137 (6), P. 619–26

526. Heuser L, Neufang K F, Jansen W
Computertomographische Befunde bei Mitralvitien
Computed tomographic findings in mitral valve disease
RÖFO 1984 Apr, Vol. 140 (4), P. 435–40

527. Hidalgo H, Korobkin M, Breiman R S, Kisslo J R
CT of intracardiac tumor
Am J Roentgenol 1981 Sep, Vol. 137 (3), P. 608–9

528. Higgins C B
Computed tomography of the heart editorial
Radiology 1981 Aug, Vol. 140 (2), P. 525–6

529. Higgins C B, Mattrey R F, Shea P
CT localization and aspiration of postoperative pericardial fluid collection
J Comput Assist Tomogr 1983 Aug, Vol. 7 (4), P. 734–6

530. Hodler J, Vock P
Die computertomographische Darstellung des vorderen kardiophrenischen Raumes
Computerized tomography imaging of the anterior cardiophrenic angle
RÖFO 1987 Jun, Vol. 146 (6), P. 654–7

531. Janson R, Lackner K, Grube E, Brecht G, Thurn P
Computerkardiotomographie der idiopathischen hypertrophen subvalvulären Aortenstenose (IHSS) – ein neuartiger Beitrag zur nicht-invasiven Diagnostik
Computer-cardio-tomography in idiopathic hypertrophic subvalvular aortic stenosis – a new contribution to non-invasive diagnosis
RÖFO 1979 May, Vol. 130 (5), P. 536–42

532. Jeffrey R B, Webb W R
CT appearance of rheumatoid pericarditis
J Comput Assist Tomogr 1980 Dec, Vol. 4 (6), P. 866–8

533. Johnson M A, Hirji M K, Hennig R C, Williams P
Pericardial abscess: diagnosis using two-dimensional echocardiography and CT
Radiology 1986 May, Vol. 159 (2), P. 419–21

534. Kirsch J D, Escarous A
CT diagnosis of traumatic pericardium rupture
J Comput Assist Tomogr 1989 May-Jun, Vol. 13 (3), P. 523–4

535. Klingensmith W C, Stern D, Spitzer V M
Single-composite image display of information from tomographic myocardial perfusion studies
Radiology 1981 Oct, Vol. 141 (1), P. 242–5

536. Korobkin M, Gasano V A
Intracaval and intracardiac extension of malignant thymoma: CT diagnosis
J Comput Assist Tomogr 1989 Mar-Apr, Vol. 13 (2), P. 348–50

537. Lackner K, Thurn P, Orellano L, Schuppan U, Simon H, Kirchhoff P G
Der aortokoronare Bypass im Computertomogramm
Computer tomography of aorto-coronary bypass
RÖFO 1980 Nov, Vol. 133 (5), P. 459–65

538. Lackner K, Thurn P
EKG-gesteuerte Kardiocomputertomographie
ECG-controlled cardio-computer tomography
RÖFO 1980 Feb, Vol. 132 (2), P. 164–9

539. Lackner K, Thurn P
Computed tomography of the heart: ECG-gated and continuous scans
Radiology 1981 Aug, Vol. 140 (2), P. 413–20

540. Lackner K, Landwehr P, von Uexkull V, Grube E, Biersack H J
Die Bestimmung der globalen Auswurffraktion des linken Ventrikels mit der EKG-gesteuerten Kardiocomputertomographie
Determination of left ventricular global ejection fraction using ECG-gated cardiac computed tomography
RÖFO 1985 Jun, Vol. 142 (6), P. 625–32

541. Laurent F, Drouillard J, Dorcier F, Choussat A, Tavernier J
CT appearance of coronary aneurysm in Kawasaki disease
J Comput Assist Tomogr 1987 Jan-Feb, Vol. 11 (1), P. 151–2

542. Lipton M J, Higgins C B, Farmer D, Boyd D P
Cardiac imaging with a high-speed Cine-CT Scanner: preliminary results
Radiology 1984 Sep, Vol. 152 (3), P. 579–82

543. Lipton M J, Farmer D W, Killebrew E J, Bouchard A, Dean P B, Ringertz H G, Higgins C B
Regional myocardial dysfunction: evaluation of patients with prior myocardial infarction with fast CT
Radiology 1985 Dec, Vol. 157 (3), P. 735–40

544. MacMillan R M, Rees M R, Maranhao V, Clark D L
Cine-computed tomography of cor triatriatum
J Comput Assist Tomogr 1986 Jan-Feb, Vol. 10 (1), P. 124–5

545. McAdams H P, Schaefer P S, Ghaed V N
Leukemic infiltrates of the heart: CT findings
J Comput Assist Tomogr 1989 May-Jun, Vol. 13 (3), P. 525–7

546. Meziane M A, Fishman E K, Siegelman S S
CT diagnosis of hemopericardium in acute dissecting aneurysm of the thoracic aorta
J Comput Assist Tomogr 1984 Feb, Vol. 8 (1), P. 10–4

547. Millward S F, Ramsewak W, Joseph G, Jones B, Zylak C J
Pericardial varices demonstrated by computed tomography
J Comput Assist Tomogr 1985 Nov-Dec, Vol. 9 (6), P. 1106–7

548. Modic M T, Janicki P C
Computed tomography of mass lesions of the right cardiophrenic angle
J Comput Assist Tomogr 1980 Aug, Vol. 4 (4), P. 521–6

549. Moncada R, Baliga K, Moguillansky S J, Subramanian R, Demos T C, Lozada C, Bianchi G, Ow E P
CT diagnosis of congenital intrapericardial masses
J Comput Assist Tomogr 1985 Jan-Feb, Vol. 9 (1), P. 56–9

550. Nebel G, Holzkamp J
Computertomographie und Angiographie bei Linkslage der Vena cava inferior
Computer tomography and angiography of left transposition of the inferior vena cava
RÖFO 1981 Feb, Vol. 134 (2), P. 206–7

551. Nickoloff E L, Perman W H, Esser P D, Bashist B, Alderson P O
Left ventricular volume: physical basis for attenuation corrections in radionuclide determinations
Radiology 1984 Aug, Vol. 152 (2), P. 511–5

552. O Callaghan J P, Heitzman E R, Somogyi J W, Spirt B A
CT evaluation of pulmonary artery size
J Comput Assist Tomogr 1982 Feb, Vol. 6 (1), P. 101–4

553. Oyama Y, Uji T, Hirayama T, Inada Y, Ishikawa T, Fujii M
Gated cardiac imaging using a continuously rotating CT scanner: clinical evaluation of 91 patients
Am J Roentgenol 1984 May, Vol. 142 (5), P. 865–76

554. Paling M R, Williamson B R
Epipericardial fat pad: CT findings
Radiology 1987 Nov, Vol. 165 (2), P. 335–9

555. Pugatch R D, Braver J H, Robbins A H, Faling L J
CT diagnosis of pericardial cysts
Am J Roentgenol 1978 Sep, Vol. 131 (3), P. 515–6

556. Rankin R N, Raval B, Finley R
Primary Chylopericardium: combined lymphangiographic and CT diagnosis
J Comput Assist Tomogr 1980 Dec, Vol. 4 (6), P. 869–70

557. Rees M R, MacMillan R M, Fender B, Clark D L
Cine-CT technique for evaluation of left ventricular function during supine exercise
Am J Roentgenol 1986 Nov, Vol. 147 (5), P. 916–8

558. Rees M R, Feiring A J, Rumberger J A, MacMillan R M, Clark D L
Heart evaluation by cine CT: use of two new oblique views
Radiology 1986 Jun, Vol. 159 (3), P. 804–6

559. Rienmuller R, Ontyd J, Krappel W, Strauer B E
Infarktbedingte Veränderungen des linksventrikulären Myokards in der kardialen Computertomographie
Infarct-induced changes in the left ventricular myocardium detected by cardiac computed tomography
RÖFO 1983 Apr, Vol. 138 (4), P. 403–11

560. Rogers C I, Seymour E Q, Brock J G
Atypical pericardial cyst location: the value of computed tomography
J Comput Assist Tomogr 1980 Oct, Vol. 4 (5), P. 683–4

561. Schlolaut K H, Lackner K, Becher H, Grube E, Orellano L
Treffsicherheit der Kardio-CT und Echokardiographie in der Diagnostik raumfordernder Prozesse des Herzens
Accuracy of cardiac CT and echocardiography in the diagnosis of space-occupying processes in the heart
RÖFO 1986 Nov, Vol. 145 (5), P. 527–35

562. Schorner W, Claussen C, Keilbach H, Hauer R
Computertomographischer Nachweis der abgekapselten perikardialen Raumforderung bei Pericarditis constrictiva calcarea
Computer tomographic demonstration of an encapsulated pericardial space- occupying lesion in pericarditis constrictiva calcarea
RÖFO 1983 Nov, Vol. 139 (5), P. 572–4

563. Shih T T, Huang K M
Acute stroke: detection of changes in cerebral perfusion with dynamic CT scanning
Radiology 1988 Nov, Vol. 169 (2), P. 469–74

564. Shin M S, Jolles P R, Ho K J
CT evaluation of distended pericardial recess presenting as a mediastinal mass
J Comput Assist Tomogr 1986 Sep-Oct, Vol. 10 (5), P. 860–2

565. Shin M S, Kirklin J K, Cain J B, Ho K J
Primary angiosarcoma of the heart: CT characteristics
Am J Roentgenol 1987 Feb, Vol. 148 (2), P. 267–8

566. Silver A J, Ganti S R, Hilal S K
Computed tomography of tumors involving the atria of the lateral ventricles
Radiology 1982 Oct, Vol. 145 (1), P. 71–8

567. Silverman P M, Harell G S, Korobkin M
Computed tomography of the abnormal pericardium
Am J Roentgenol 1983 Jun, Vol. 140 (6), P. 1125–9

568. Stosiek M, Klose K C, Rustige J
Computertomographischer Nachweis eines großen Pseudoaneurysmas des Herzens
Computed tomography diagnosis of a large pseudoaneurysm of the heart
RÖFO 1986 Dec, Vol. 145 (6), P. 728–30

569. Strasser S F, Matalon T A, Turner D A, Goldin M D, Eybel C E
Mycotic right coronary artery aneurysm: CT and MR diagnosis
J Comput Assist Tomogr 1986 Jul-Aug, Vol. 10 (4), P. 667–9

570. Sussman S K, Chiles C, Cooper C, Lowe J E
CT demonstration of myocardial perforation by a pacemaker lead
J Comput Assist Tomogr 1986 Jul-Aug, Vol. 10 (4), P. 670–2

571. Sussman S K, Halvorsen R A Jr, Silverman P M, Saeed M
Paracardiac adenopathy: CT evaluation
Am J Roentgenol 1987 Jul, Vol. 149 (1), P. 29–34

572. Thelen M, Duber C, Wolff P, Erbel R, Hoffmann T
Quantitative kardiale Computertomographie
Quantitative cardiac computed tomography
RÖFO 1985 Jun, Vol. 142 (6), P. 616–24

573. Tsuchiya F, Kohno A, Saitoh R, Shigeta A
CT findings of atrial myxoma
Radiology 1984 Apr, Vol. 151 (1), P. 139–43

574. Vestring T, Wahlers B, Halm H, Morgan J A, Achatzy R
Der computertomographische Nachweis einer Herzluxation nach linksseitiger erweiterter Pneu-
monektomie
Computed tomographic detection of cardiac luxation following left- sided extensive pneumonec-
tomy
RÖFO 1989 Nov, Vol. 151 (5), P. 632–3

575. Vogel H J, Wondergem J H, Falke T H
Mesothelioma of the pericardium: CT and MR findings
J Comput Assist Tomogr 1989 May-Jun, Vol. 13 (3), P. 543–4

576. Wolff P, Schreiner G, Duber C, Halbsguth A, Lochner R, Erbel R, Meyer J, Thelen M
Computertomographie, Magnetresonanztomographie und Echokardiographie bei der hyper-
trophen Kardiomyopathie
Computed tomography, magnetic resonance tomography and echocardiography in hypertrophic
cardiomyopathy
RÖFO 1985 Jun, Vol. 142 (6), P. 633–40

The Lungs and the Pleura

577. Aberle D R, Gamsu G, Ray C S
High-resolution CT of benign asbestos-related diseases: clinical and radiographic correlation
Am J Roentgenol 1988 Nov, Vol. 151 (5), P. 883–91

578. Aberle D R, Gamsu G, Ray C S, Feuerstein I M
Asbestos-related pleural and parenchymal fibrosis: detection with high-resolution CT
Radiology 1988 Mar, Vol. 166 (3), P. 729–34

579. Adam A, MacSweeney J E, Whyte M K, Smith P L, Ind P W
CT- guided extrapleural drainage of bronchogenic cyst
J Comput Assist Tomogr 1989 Nov-Dec, Vol. 13 (6), P. 1065–8

580. Adler O B, Rosenberger A
Localization of metallic foreign bodies in the chest by computed tomography
J Comput Assist Tomogr 1982 Oct, Vol. 6 (5), P. 955–7

581. Aggarwal S, Kumar A, Mukhopadhyay S, Berry M
A new radiologic sign of ruptured pulmonary hydatid cyst letter
Am J Roentgenol 1989 Feb, Vol. 152 (2), P. 431–2

582. Akira M, Kitatani F, Lee Y S, Kita N, Yamamoto S, Higashihara T, Morimoto S, Ikezoe J, Kozuka
T
Diffuse panbronchiolitis: evaluation with high-resolution CT
Radiology 1988 Aug, Vol. 168 (2), P. 433–8

583. Akira M, Higashihara T, Yokoyama K, Yamamoto S, Kita N, Morimoto S, Ikezoe J, Kozuka
T
Radiographic type p pneumoconiosis: high-resolution CT
Radiology 1989 Apr, Vol. 171 (1), P. 117–23

584. Akira M, Yamamoto S, Yokoyama K, Kita N, Morinaga K, Higashihara T, Kozuka T
Asbestosis: high-resolution CT-pathologic correlation
Radiology 1990 Aug, Vol. 176 (2), P. 389–94

585. Akira M, Yokoyama K, Yamamoto S, Higashihara T, Morinaga K, Kita N, Morimoto S, Ikezoe J,
Kozuka T
Early asbestosis: evaluation with high-resolution CT
Radiology 1991 Feb, Vol. 178 (2), P. 409–16

586. Alexander E, Clark R A, Colley D P, Mitchell S E
CT of malignant pleural mesothelioma
Am J Roentgenol 1981 Aug, Vol. 137 (2), P. 287–91

587. Altman N R, Purser R K, Post M J
Tuberous sclerosis: characteristics at CT and MR imaging
Radiology 1988 May, Vol. 167 (2), P. 527–32

588. Ang J G, Proto A V
CT demonstration of congenital pulmonary venolobar syndrome
J Comput Assist Tomogr 1984 Aug, Vol. 8 (4), P. 753–7

589. Aronberg D J, Sagel S S
High CT attenuation values of a benign pulmonary nodule
J Comput Assist Tomogr 1981 Aug, Vol. 5 (4), P. 563–4

590. Aronchick J M, Wexler J A, Christen B, Miller W, Epstein D, Gefter W B
Computed tomography of bronchial carcinoid
J Comput Assist Tomogr 1986 Jan-Feb, Vol. 10 (1), P. 71–4

591. Austin J H, Grimes M M, Carberry D
CT detection of calcified nodal metastases of lung adenocarcinoma
J Comput Assist Tomogr 1988 Mar-Apr, Vol. 12 (2), P. 314–6

592. Austin J H
Pulmonary sarcoidosis: what are we learning from CT?
Radiology 1989 Jun, Vol. 171 (3), P. 603–4

593. Ayuso M C, Gilabert R, Bombi J A, Salvador A
CT appearance of localized pulmonary amyloidosis
J Comput Assist Tomogr 1987 Jan- Feb, Vol. 11 (1), P. 197–9

594. Baber C E, Hedlund L W, Oddson T A, Putman C E
Differentiating empyemas and peripheral pulmonary abscesses: the value of computed tomo-
graphy
Radiology 1980 Jun, Vol. 135 (3), P. 755–8

595. Baker B K, Awwad E E
Computed tomography of fatal cerebral air embolism following percutaneous aspiration biopsy of
the lung
J Comput Assist Tomogr 1988 Nov-Dec, Vol. 12 (6), P. 1082–3

596. Baker E L, Gore R M, Moss A A
Retroperitoneal pulmonary sequestration: computed tomographic findings
Am J Roentgenol 1982 May, Vol. 138 (5), P. 956–7

597. Balakrishnan J, Meziane M A, Siegelman S S, Fishman E K
Pulmonary infarction: CT appearance with pathologic correlation
J Comput Assist Tomogr 1989 Nov-Dec, Vol. 13 (6), P. 941–5

598. Bankoff M S, Daly B D, Johnson H A, Carter B L
Bronchogenic cyst causing superior vena cava obstruction: CT appearance
J Comput Assist Tomogr 1985 Sep-Oct, Vol. 9 (5), P. 951–2

599. Bautz W, Hubener K H, Kurtz B
Wertigkeit der digitalen Projektionsradiographie mit einem CT-Gerät für die Thoraxdiagnostik
Value of digital projection radiography with a CT apparatus for thoracic diagnosis
RÖFO 1984 May, Vol. 140 (5), P. 579–84

600. Begin R, Bergeron D, Samson L, Boctor M, Cantin A
CT assessment of silicosis in exposed workers
Am J Roentgenol 1987 Mar, Vol. 148 (3), P. 509–14

601. Bennett L L, Lesar M S, Tellis C J
Multiple calcified chondrohamartomas of the lung: CT appearance
J Comput Assist Tomogr 1985 Jan-Feb, Vol. 9 (1), P. 180–2

602. Bergin C J, Muller N L
CT in the diagnosis of interstitial lung disease
Am J Roentgenol 1985 Sep, Vol. 145 (3), P. 505–10

603. Bergin C J, Muller N L
CT of interstitial lung disease: a diagnostic approach
Am J Roentgenol 1987 Jan, Vol. 148 (1), P. 9–15

604. Bergin C J, Coblentz C L, Chiles C, Bell D Y, Castellino R A
Chronic lung diseases: specific diagnosis by using CT
Am J Roentgenol 1989 Jun, Vol. 152 (6), P. 1183–8

605. Bergin C J, Bell D Y, Coblentz C L, Chiles C, Gamsu G, MacIntyre N R, Coleman R E, Putman
C E
Sarcoidosis: correlation of pulmonary parenchymal pattern at CT with results of pulmonary func-
tion tests
Radiology 1989 Jun, Vol. 171 (3), P. 619–24

606. Bergin C J, Wirth R L, Berry G J, Castellino R A
Pneumocystis carinii pneumonia: CT and HRCT observations
J Comput Assist Tomogr 1990 Sep-Oct, Vol. 14 (5), P. 756–9

607. Beyer Enke S A, Clorius J, Becker H, Goerich J, Probst G, van Kaick G
Synopsis von Computertomographie, Szintigraphie und Bronchoskopie bei der Diagnostik des
Bronchialkarzinoms
Synopsis of computed tomography, scintigraphy and bronchoscopy in the diagnosis of bronchial
carcinoma
RÖFO 1988 Aug, Vol. 149 (2), P. 147–51

608. Bhatt G M, Austin H M
CT demonstration of empyema necessitatis
J Comput Assist Tomogr 1985 Nov-Dec, Vol. 9 (6), P. 1108–9

609. Biondetti P R, Fiore D, Sartori F, Colognato A, Ravasini R, Romani S
Evaluation of post-pneumonectomy space by computed tomography
J Comput Assist Tomogr 1982 Apr, Vol. 6 (2), P. 238–42

610. Black W C, Armstrong P
Re: Role of CT in assessing mediastinal involvement in lung cancer letter
Radiology 1985 Aug, Vol. 156 (2), P. 552

611. Black W C, Armstrong P, Daniel T M
Cost effectiveness of chest CT in T1N0M0 lung cancer
Radiology 1988 May, Vol. 167 (2), P. 373–8

612. Bohndorf K, Calavreszos A, Koschel G, Husselmann H, Hain E
Computertomographische Befunde bei diffusem malignem Pleuramesotheliom
Computed tomographic findings in diffuse malignant pleural mesothelioma
RÖFO 1985 Sep, Vol. 143 (3), P. 279–84

613. Borkowski G P, O Donovan P B, Troup B R
Pulmonary varix: CT findings
J Comput Assist Tomogr 1981 Dec, Vol. 5 (6), P. 827–9

614. Brant Zawadzki M, Jeffrey R B Jr, Minagi H, Pitts L H
High resolution CT of thoracolumbar fractures
Am J Roentgenol 1982 Apr, Vol. 138 (4), P. 699–704

615. Brasch R C, Gould R G, Gooding C A, Ringertz H G, Lipton M J
Upper airway obstruction in infants and children: evaluation with ultrafast CT
Radiology 1987 Nov, Vol. 165 (2), P. 459–66

616. Brauner M W, Grenier P, Mompoint D, Lenoir S, de Cremoux H
Pulmonary sarcoidosis: evaluation with high-resolution CT
Radiology 1989 Aug, Vol. 172 (2), P. 467–71

617. Brauner M W, Grenier P, Mouelhi M M, Mompoint D, Lenoir S
Pulmonary histiocytosis X: evaluation with high-resolution CT
Radiology 1989 Jul, Vol. 172 (1), P. 255–8

618. Breatnach E S, Nath P H, McElvein R B
Preoperative evaluation of bronchiectasis by computed tomography
J Comput Assist Tomogr 1985 Sep-Oct, Vol. 9 (5), P. 949–50

619. Breckenridge J W, Kinlaw W B
Azygos continuation of inferior vena cava: CT appearance
J Comput Assist Tomogr 1980 Jun, Vol. 4 (3), P. 392–7

620. Bressler E L, Francis I R, Glazer G M, Gross B H
Bolus contrast medium enhancement for distinguishing pleural from parenchymal lung disease: CT
features
J Comput Assist Tomogr 1987 May-Jun, Vol. 11 (3), P. 436–40

621. Brion J P, Depauw L, Kuhn G, de Francquen P, Friberg J, Rocmans, Struyven J
Role of computed tomography and mediastinoscopy in preoperative staging of lung carcinoma
J Comput Assist Tomogr 1985 May-Jun, Vol. 9 (3), P. 480–4

622. Britt A R, Francis I R, Glazer G M, Ellis J H
Sarcoidosis: abdominal manifestations at CT
Radiology 1991 Jan, Vol. 178 (1), P. 91–4

623. Butler S, Smathers R L
Computed tomography of amiodarone pulmonary toxicity
J Comput Assist Tomogr 1985 Mar-Apr, Vol. 9 (2), P. 375–6

624. Checkley D R, Zhu X P, Antoun N, Chen S Z, Isherwood I
An investigation into the problems of attenuation and area measurements made from CT images of
pulmonary nodules
J Comput Assist Tomogr 1984 Apr, Vol. 8 (2), P. 237–43

625. Cho C S, Blank N, Castellino R A
CT evaluation of cardiophrenic angle lymph nodes in patients with malignant lymphoma
Am J Roentgenol 1984 Oct, Vol. 143 (4), P. 719–21

626. Choe K O, Jeong H J, Sohn H Y
Tuberculous bronchial stenosis: CT findings in 28 cases
Am J Roentgenol 1990 Nov, Vol. 155 (5), P. 971–6

627. Cohen M, Grosfeld J, Baehner R, Weetman R
Lung CT for detection of metastases: solid tissue neoplasms in children
Am J Roentgenol 1982 Nov, Vol. 139 (5), P. 895–8

628. Coleman B G, Arger P H, Stephenson L W
CT features of endobronchial granular cell myoblastoma
J Comput Assist Tomogr 1984 Oct, Vol. 8 (5), P. 998–1000

629. Cooper C, Moss A A, Buy J N, Stark D D
CT appearance of the normal inferior pulmonary ligament
Am J Roentgenol 1983 Aug, Vol. 141 (2), P. 237–40

630. Costello P, Rose R M
CT findings in pleural aspergillosis
J Comput Assist Tomogr 1985 Jul-Aug, Vol. 9 (4), P. 760–2

631. Curtis A M, Ravin C E, Deering T F, Putman C E, McLoud T C, Greenspan R H
The efficacy of full-lung tomography in the detection of early metastatic disease from melanoma
Radiology 1982 Jul, Vol. 144 (1), P. 27–9

632. Daly B D, Pugatch R D, Faling L J, Jung Legg Y, Gale M E, Snider G L
Computed-tomographic-guided minithoracotomy. A preliminary report of a new approach to open lung biopsy
Radiology 1983 Feb, Vol. 146 (2), P. 543–4

633. Davis S D, Berkmen Y M, King T
Peripheral bronchial involvement in relapsing polychondritis: demonstration by thin-section CT
Am J Roentgenol 1989 Nov, Vol. 153 (5), P. 953–4

634. Davis S D, Zirn J R, Govoni A F, Yankelevitz D F
Peripheral carcinoid tumor of the lung: CT diagnosis
Am J Roentgenol 1990 Dec, Vol. 155 (6), P. 1185–7

635. Dinkel E, Uhl H, Reinbold W D, Wimmer B, Wenz W
Computertomographie beim Thoraxtrauma
Computerized tomography in thoracic trauma
Radiologe 1987 Sep, Vol. 27 (9), P. 391–7

636. Dohring W, Linke G
Die Grundlagen der quantitativen pulmonalen Computertomographie
The basis of quantitative pulmonary computer tomography
RÖFO 1979 Feb, Vol. 130 (2), P. 133–43

637. Don C, Desmarais R
Peripheral upper lobe collapse in adults
Radiology 1989 Mar, Vol. 170 (3 Pt 1), P. 657–9

638. Doppman J L, Pass H I, Nieman L K, Findling J W, Dwyer A J, Feuerstein I M, Ling A, Travis W D, Cutler G B Jr, Chrousos G P, et al
Detection of ACTH-producing bronchial carcinoid tumors: MR imaging vs CT
Am J Roentgenol 1991 Jan, Vol. 156 (1), P. 39–43

639. Dore R, Alcerci M, D Andrea F, Di Giulio G, De Agostini A, Volpato G
Intracardiac extension of lung carcinoma via pulmonary veins: CT diagnosis
J Comput Assist Tomogr 1988 Jul-Aug, Vol. 12 (4), P. 565–8

640. Doyle T C, Lawler G A
CT features of rounded atelectasis of the lung
Am J Roentgenol 1984 Aug, Vol. 143 (2), P. 225–8

641. Dunnick N R, Ihde D C, Johnston Early A
Abdominal CT in the evaluation of small cell carcinoma of the lung
Am J Roentgenol 1979 Dec, Vol. 133 (6), P. 1085–8

642. Effmann E L, Ravin C E, Breiman R S, Hedlund L W
Comparison of CT localization radiography and high-kilovoltage chest radiography
Am J Roentgenol 1983 Jun, Vol. 140 (6), P. 1115–8

643. Epstein D M, Stephenson L W, Gefter W B, van der Voorde F, Aronchik J M, Miller W T
Value of CT in the preoperative assessment of lung cancer: a survey of thoracic surgeons
Radiology 1986 Nov, Vol. 161 (2), P. 423–7

644. Felson B
Scimitar syndrome: four new cases examined with CT letter
Radiology 1987 Feb, Vol. 162 (2), P. 581

645. Fink I, Gamsu G, Harter L P
CT-guided aspiration biopsy of the thorax
J Comput Assist Tomogr 1982 Oct, Vol. 6 (5), P. 958–62

646. Fiore D, Biondetti P R, Sartori F, Calabro F
The role of computed tomography in the evaluation of bullous lung disease
J Comput Assist Tomogr 1982 Feb, Vol. 6 (1), P. 105–8

647. Fishman E K, Gayler B W, Kashima H K, Harris A E, Siegelman S S
Computed tomography in the evaluation of cervical thorotrast granuloma
J Comput Assist Tomogr 1984 Apr, Vol. 8 (2), P. 224–8

648. Fitzgerald P M
Primary sarcoma of the pulmonary trunk: CT findings
J Comput Assist Tomogr 1983 Jun, Vol. 7 (3), P. 521–3

649. Flückinger F, Kullnig P, Jüttner-Smolle F, Melzer G
Intrapulmonale Pseudofehllage von Thoraxdrainagen im Computertomogramm (CT)
RÖFO 1991, Vol.155 , P.494–498

650. Foo S S, Weisbrod G L, Herman S J, Chamberlain D W
Wegener granulomatosis presenting on CT with atypical bronchovasocentric distribution
J Comput Assist Tomogr 1990 Nov-Dec, Vol. 14 (6), P. 1004–6

651. Foster W L Jr, Roberts L Jr, McLendon R E, Hill R C
Localized peribronchial thickening: a CT sign of occult bronchogenic carcinoma
Am J Roentgenol 1985 May, Vol. 144 (5), P. 906–8

652. Friedman A C, Fiel S B, Fisher M S, Radecki P D, Lev Toaff A S, Caroline D F
Asbestos-related pleural disease and asbestosis: a comparison of CT and chest radiography
Am J Roentgenol 1988 Feb, Vol. 150 (2), P. 269–75

653. Friedman A C, Radecki P D, Fiel S B
Detection of asbestosis with high-resolution CT letter
Radiology 1989 Jan, Vol. 170 (1 Pt 1), P. 278–9

654. Friedman P J
Limitations of CT in detecting bronchiectasis letter
Am J Roentgenol 1985 Mar, Vol. 144 (3), P. 650–1

655. Friedman P J
CT demonstration of tethering of the lung by the pulmonary ligament
J Comput Assist Tomogr 1985 Sep-Oct, Vol. 9 (5), P. 947–8

656. Frija J, Schmit P, Katz M, Vadrot D, Laval Jeantet M
Computed tomography of the pulmonary fissures: normal anatomy
J Comput Assist Tomogr 1982 Dec, Vol. 6 (6), P. 1069–74

657. Furuse M, Saito K, Kunieda E, Aihara T, Touei H, Ohara T, Fukushima K
Bronchial arteries: CT demonstration with arteriographic correlation
Radiology 1987 Feb, Vol. 162 (2), P. 393–8

658. Gale M E
Anterior diaphragm: variations in the CT appearance
Radiology 1986 Dec, Vol. 161 (3), P. 635–9

659. Gale M E, Greif W L
Intrafissural fat: CT correlation with chest radiography
Radiology 1986 Aug, Vol. 160 (2), P. 333–6

660. Gallagher S, Dixon A K
Streak artefacts of the thoracic aorta: pseudodissection
J Comput Assist Tomogr 1984 Aug, Vol. 8 (4), P. 688–93

661. Gamroth A, van Kaick G, Gorich J, Probst G, Eichberger D, Beyer Enke S, Tuengerthal S
Die Beurteilung intrapulmonaler Rundherde mit Hilfe der Dünnschichtcomputertomographie
Evaluation of intrapulmonary round foci using thin-layer computed tomography
RÖFO 1988 Jan, Vol. 148 (1), P. 21–7

662. Gatenby R A, Mulhern C B Jr, Broder G J, Moldofsky P J
Computed-tomographic-guided biopsy of small apical and peripheral upper-lobe lung masses
Radiology 1984 Feb, Vol. 150 (2), P. 591–2

663. Gilman M J, Laurens R G Jr, Somogyi J W, Honig E G
CT attenuation values of lung density in sarcoidosis
J Comput Assist Tomogr 1983 Jun, Vol. 7 (3), P. 407–10

664. Glazer G M, Francis I R, Gebarski K, Samuels B I, Sorensen K W
Dynamic incremental computed tomography in evaluation of the pulmonary hila
J Comput Assist Tomogr 1983 Feb, Vol. 7 (1), P. 59–64

665. Glazer G M
Evaluation of the pulmonary hila by CT letter
Radiology 1983 Jan, Vol. 146 (1), P. 261–2

666. Glazer G M, Gross B H, Aisen A M, Quint L E, Francis I R, Orringer M B
Imaging of the pulmonary hilum: a prospective comparative study in patients with lung cancer
Am J Roentgenol 1985 Aug, Vol. 145 (2), P. 245–8

667. Glazer H S, Aronberg D J, Sagel S S, Emami B
Utility of CT in detecting postpneumonectomy carcinoma recurrence
Am J Roentgenol 1984 Mar, Vol. 142 (3), P. 487–94

668. Glazer H S, Duncan Meyer J, Aronberg D J, Moran J F, Levitt R G, Sagel S S
Pleural and chest wall invasion in bronchogenic carcinoma: CT evaluation
Radiology 1985 Oct, Vol. 157 (1), P. 191–4

669. Gobien R P, Stanley J H, Vujic I, Gobien B S
Thoracic biopsy: CT guidance of thin-needle aspiration
Am J Roentgenol 1984 Apr, Vol. 142 (4), P. 827–30

670. Godwin J D, Webb W R, Gamsu G, Ovenfors C O
Computed tomography of pulmonary embolism
Am J Roentgenol 1980 Oct, Vol. 135 (4), P. 691–5

671. Godwin J D, Webb W R
Dynamic computed tomography in the evaluation of vascular lung lesions
Radiology 1981 Mar, Vol. 138 (3), P. 629–35

672. Godwin J D, Speckman J M, Fram E K, Johnson G A, Putman C E, Korobkin M, Breiman R S
Distinguishing benign from malignant pulmonary nodules by computed tomography
Radiology 1982 Jul, Vol. 144 (2), P. 349–51

673. Godwin J D, Fram E K, Cann C E, Gamsu G G
CT densitometry of pulmonary nodules: a phantom study
J Comput Assist Tomogr 1982 Apr, Vol. 6 (2), P. 254–8

674. Godwin J D, Vock P, Osborne D R
CT of the pulmonary ligament
Am J Roentgenol 1983 Aug, Vol. 141 (2), P. 231–6

675. Godwin J D, Muller N L, Takasugi J E
Pulmonary alveolar proteinosis: CT findings
Radiology 1988 Dec, Vol. 169 (3), P. 609–13

676. Goldberg A L, Tievsky A L, Jamshidi S
Wegener granulomatosis invading the cavernous sinus: a CT demonstration
J Comput Assist Tomogr 1983 Aug, Vol. 7 (4), P. 701–3

677. Goldstein M S, Rush M, Johnson P, Sprung C L
A calcified adenocarcinoma of the lung with very high CT numbers
Radiology 1984 Mar, Vol. 150 (3), P. 785–6

678. Goodman L R, Golkow R S, Steiner R M, Teplick S K, Haskin M E, Himmelstein E, Teplick J G
The right mid-lung window
Radiology 1982 Apr, Vol. 143 (1), P. 135–8

679. Goodman L R
Pulmonary metastatic disease: radiologic-surgical correlation letter
Radiology 1988 Apr, Vol. 167 (1), P. 284

680. Goralnik C H, O Connell D M, el Yousef S J, Haaga J R
CT- guided cutting-needle biopsies of selected chest lesions
Am J Roentgenol 1988 Nov, Vol. 151 (5), P. 903–7

681. Gorich J, Gamroth A, Beyer Enke S, Kayser K, van Kaick G
Computertomographische Differentialdiagnostik einschmelzender pulmonaler Raumforderungen
Differential computed tomographic diagnosis of cavity-forming space- occupying lesions of the lung
RÖFO 1987 Nov, Vol. 147 (5), P. 479–85

682. Gorich J, Beyer Enke S A, Kayser K, van Kaick G
Computertomographische Befunde beim Bronchialadenom
Computed tomographic findings in bronchial adenoma
RÖFO 1989 Feb, Vol. 150 (2), P. 147–50

683. Gorich J, Beyer Enke S A, Flentje M, Zuna I, Vogt Moykopf I, van Kaick G
Der Stellenwert der Computertomographie für die Erkennung von Rezidiven bei Patienten mit Bronchialkarzinomen
The place of computed tomography in the diagnosis of recurrences in patients with bronchogenic carcinoma
Radiologe 1990 Oct, Vol. 30 (10), P. 472–6

684. Grant D C, Seltzer S E, Antman K H, Finberg H J, Koster K
Computed tomography of malignant pleural mesothelioma
J Comput Assist Tomogr 1983 Aug, Vol. 7 (4), P. 626–32

685. Greene R, Anderson D J, Gefter W B, Levitt R G, McLoud T, Oestmann J, Schaefer C, Spirn P W, Stark P
Thoracic radiology
Radiology 1991 Mar, Vol. 178 (3), P. 916–8

686. Grenier P, Maurice F, Musset D, Menu Y, Nahum H
Bronchiectasis: assessment by thin-section CT
Radiology 1986 Oct, Vol. 161 (1), P. 95–9

687. Gross B H, Glazer G M, Bookstein F L
Multiple pulmonary nodules detected by computed tomography: diagnostic implications
J Comput Assist Tomogr 1985 Sep-Oct, Vol. 9 (5), P. 880–5

688. Gross B H, Glazer G M, Orringer M B, Spizarny D L, Flint A
Bronchogenic carcinoma metastatic to normal-sized lymph nodes: frequency and significance
Radiology 1988 Jan, Vol. 166 (1 Pt 1), P. 71–4

689. Guhl L, Heuck F
Diagnostische Möglichkeiten der Röntgencomputertomographie bei Thorotrastspeicherung
Diagnostic possibilities of computed x-ray tomography in thorotrast accumulation
RÖFO 1983 Feb, Vol. 138 (2), P. 225–30

690. Guhl L
Pulmonale Beteiligung bei Lymphangioleiomyomatose: Untersuchungen mit Hilfe der hochauf-
lösenden Computertomographie
Pulmonary involvement in lymphangioleiomyomatosis: studies using high-resolution computed
tomography
RÖFO 1988 Dec, Vol. 149 (6), P. 576–9

691. Guhl L, Schneider H, Weiske R
Diagnostik des Lungenbefalls bei der Wegenerschen Granulomatose mit hochauflösender
Computertomographie
The diagnosis of pulmonary manifestations of Wegener's granulomatosis using high-resolution
computed tomography
RÖFO 1990 Nov, Vol. 153 (5), P. 565–8

692. Gurtler K F, Riebel T, Beron G, Heller M, Euler A
Vergleich von Röntgenübersichtsaufnahmen, Röntgenschichtaufnahmen und Computertomo-
grammen bei pulmonalen Rundherden im Kindes- und Jugendalter
Comparison of x-ray plain films, x-ray tomograms and computed tomograms in lung nodules in
children and adolescents
RÖFO 1984 Apr, Vol. 140 (4), P. 416–20

693. Hajek P, Imhof H, Kumpan W, Schratter M, Klech H, Moritz E
Mediastinales CT-Staging von Bronchuskarzinomen
Mediastinal CT- staging of bronchial carcinomas
RÖFO 1985 Jan, Vol. 142 (1), P. 74–9

694. Hall F M
Abdominal CT in lung carcinoma letter
Am J Roentgenol 1980 May, Vol. 134 (5), P. 1092–3

695. Hamper U M, Fishman E K, Khouri N F, Johns C J, Wang K P, Siegelman S S
Typical and atypical CT manifestations of pulmonary sarcoidosis
J Comput Assist Tomogr 1986 Nov-Dec, Vol. 10 (6), P. 928–36

696. Harder T
Nachweis einer arteriovenösen Lungenfistel im CT
Detection of an arteriovenous lung fistula in CT
RÖFO 1982 Sep, Vol. 137 (3), P. 346–8

697. Hartshorne M F, Eisenberg B
CT diagnosis of a giant central pulmonary artery aneurysm arising quickly after pulmonary embolic
disease letter
Am J Roentgenol 1989 Jul, Vol. 153 (1), P. 190–1

698. Heaston D K, Putman C E, Rodan B A, Nicholson E, Ravin C E, Korobkin M, Chen J T, Seigler H
F
Solitary pulmonary metastases in high-risk melanoma patients: a prospective comparison of con-
ventional and computed tomography
Am J Roentgenol 1983 Jul, Vol. 141 (1), P. 169–74

699. Heater K, Revzani L, Rubin J M
CT evaluation of empyema in the postpneumonectomy space
Am J Roentgenol 1985 Jul, Vol. 145 (1), P. 39–40

700. Heavey L R, Glazer G M, Gross B H, Francis I R, Orringer M B
The role of CT in staging radiographic T1N0M0 lung cancer
Am J Roentgenol 1986 Feb, Vol. 146 (2), P. 285–90

701. Heelan R T, Martini N, Westcott J W, Bains M S, Watson R C, Caravelli J F, Berkmen Y M,
Henschke C I, McCormack P M, McCaughan B C, et al
Carcinomatous involvement of the hilum and mediastinum: computed tomographic and magnetic
resonance evaluation
Radiology 1985 Jul, Vol. 156 (1), P. 111–5

702. Heitzman E R
Fleischner Lecture. Computed tomography of the thorax: current perspectives
Am J Roentgenol 1981 Jan, Vol. 136 (1), P. 2–12

703. Henschke C I, Davis S D, Auh Y, Romano P, Westcott J, Berkmen Y M, Kazam E
Detection of bronchial abnormalities: comparison of CT and bronchoscopy
J Comput Assist Tomogr 1987 May-Jun, Vol. 11 (3), P. 432–5

704. Herold C J, Mostbeck G, Kramer J, Schwarzinger I, Wrba F, Haller J, Tschollakoff D
Invasive pulmonale Aspergillose: Radiologische und kernspintomographische Charakteristika
Invasive pulmonary aspergillosis: radiologic and magnetic resonance tomographic characteris-
tics
RÖFO 1990 Nov, Vol. 153 (5), P. 569–74

705. Hewer W, Grehn S
Computertomographischer Nachweis einer massiven intrathorakalen Blutung unter Phenprocou-
mon
Computed tomographic detection of massive intrathoracic hemorrhage due to phenprocoumon
RÖFO 1984 Jul, Vol. 141 (1), P. 113–4

706. Hidvegi R S
Efficacy of CT in evaluating intrathoracic masses letter
Am J Roentgenol 1983 Apr, Vol. 140 (4), P. 829

707. Hieckel H G, Muller S, Luning M
Computertomographische Befundmuster bei der exogen-allergischen Alveolitis. Ein Vergleich zur
konventionellen Röntgensymptomatik
Computed tomographic findings in extrinsic allergic alveolitis. Comparison with conventional x-ray
findings
RÖFO 1986 Oct, Vol. 145 (4), P. 402–6

708. Holbert B L, Holbert J M, Libshitz H I
CT of interpectoral lymph nodes
Am J Roentgenol 1987 Oct, Vol. 149 (4), P. 687–8

709. Horvath F, Nemeth L
Hartstrahlaufnahme der Lungen in leichter Dorsalflektion des Patienten bei Veränderungen in den
Oberlappen
High kv films of the lungs with slight dorsal flexion for lesions in the upper lobes
RÖFO 1980 Apr, Vol. 132 (4), P. 438–41

710. Horvath F, Csobaly S
Computertomographie bei der Caissonkrankheit
Computer tomography in Caisson's disease
RÖFO 1981 Jul, Vol. 135 (1), P. 16–9

711. Hruban R H, Meziane M A, Zerhouni E A, Wheeler P S, Dumler J S, Hutchins G M
Radiologic-pathologic correlation of the CT halo sign in invasive pulmonary aspergillosis
J Comput Assist Tomogr 1987 May-Jun, Vol. 11 (3), P. 534–6

712. Hruban R H, Ren H, Kuhlman J E, Fishman E K, Wheeler P S, Baumgartner W A, Reitz B A,
Hutchins G M
Inflation-fixed lungs: pathologic-radiologic CT correlation of lung transplantation
J Comput Assist Tomogr 1990 May-Jun, Vol. 14 (3), P. 329–35

713. Huang R M, Naidich D P, Lubat E, Schinella R, Garay S M, McCauley D I
Septic pulmonary emboli: CT-radiographic correlation
Am J Roentgenol 1989 Jul, Vol. 153 (1), P. 41–5

714. Hughes J J, Pollock W J, Schworm C P
Branching pattern in CT scans of mucin producing carcinoma metastases to the liver
J Comput Assist Tomogr 1984 Jun, Vol. 8 (3), P. 553–5

715. Huston J 3d, Muhm J R
Solitary pulmonary nodules: evaluation with a CT reference phantom
Radiology 1989 Mar, Vol. 170 (3 Pt 1), P. 653–6

716. Ikezoe J, Takashima S, Morimoto S, Kadowaki K, Takeuchi N, Yamamoto T, Nakanishi K, Isaza
M, Arisawa J, Ikeda H, et al
CT appearance of acute radiation-induced injury in the lung
Am J Roentgenol 1988 Apr, Vol. 150 (4), P. 765–70

717. Ikezoe J, Murayama S, Godwin J D, Done S L, Verschakelen J A
Bronchopulmonary sequestration: CT assessment
Radiology 1990 Aug, Vol. 176 (2), P. 375–9

718. Im J G, Choi B I, Park J H, Chang K H, Yeon K M, Han M C, Kim C W
CT findings of lobar bronchioloalveolar carcinoma
J Comput Assist Tomogr 1986 Mar-Apr, Vol. 10 (2), P. 320–2

719. Im J G, Chung J W, Han S K, Han M C, Kim C W
CT manifestations of tracheobronchial involvement in relapsing polychondritis
J Comput Assist Tomogr 1988 Sep-Oct, Vol. 12 (5), P. 792–3

720. Im J G, Webb W R, Rosen A, Gamsu G
Costal pleura: appearances at high-resolution CT
Radiology 1989 Apr, Vol. 171 (1), P. 125–31

721. Im J G, Han M C, Yu E J, Han J K, Park J M, Kim C W, Seo J W, Yoon Y, Lee J D, Lee
K S
Lobar bronchioloalveolar carcinoma: "angiogram sign" on CT scans
Radiology 1990 Sep, Vol. 176 (3), P. 749–53

722. Im J G, Webb W R, Han M C, Park J H
Apical opacity associated with pulmonary tuberculosis: high- resolution CT findings
Radiology 1991 Mar, Vol. 178 (3), P. 727–31

723. Ishigaki T, Sakuma S, Ikeda M, Itoh Y, Suzuki M, Iwai S
Clinical evaluation of irreversible image compression: analysis of chest imaging with computed
radiography
Radiology 1990 Jun, Vol. 175 (3), P. 739–43

724. Jardin M, Remy J
Segmental bronchovascular anatomy of the lower lobes: CT analysis
Am J Roentgenol 1986 Sep, Vol. 147 (3), P. 457–68

725. Jaschke W, Kempmann G, Wetzel E, Kihm W D
Computertomographischer Nachweis der zentralen Lungenembolie
CT detection of central pulmonary embolism
RÖFO 1981 Oct, Vol. 135 (4), P. 399–403

726. Jaspers M J, Bloem J L, Falke T H
Computed tomography of pulmonary blastoma in a child
RÖFO 1985 Jul, Vol. 143 (1), P. 104- 5

727. Joharjy I A, Bashi S A, Adbullah A K
Value of medium-thickness CT in the diagnosis of bronchiectasis
Am J Roentgenol 1987 Dec, Vol. 149 (6), P. 1133–7

728. Joshi R R, Cholankeril J V
Computed tomography in lipoid pneumonia
J Comput Assist Tomogr 1985 Jan-Feb, Vol. 9 (1), P. 211–3

729. Kalender W A, Rienmuller R, Seissler W, Behr J, Welke M, Fichte H
Measurement of pulmonary parenchymal attenuation: use of spirometric gating with quantitative
CT
Radiology 1990 Apr, Vol. 175 (1), P. 265–8

730. Karantanas A H
Imaging of pulmonary sequestration letter
Am J Roentgenol 1990 Dec, Vol. 155 (6), P. 1343

731. Kaufman R A
Calcified postinflammatory pseudotumor of the lung: CT features
J Comput Assist Tomogr 1988 Jul-Aug, Vol. 12 (4), P. 653–5

732. Kawashima A, Libshitz H I
Malignant pleural mesothelioma: CT manifestations in 50 cases
Am J Roentgenol 1990 Nov, Vol. 155 (5), P. 965–9

733. Kerns S R, Gay S B
CT of blunt chest trauma
Am J Roentgenol 1990 Jan, Vol. 154 (1), P. 55–60

734. Khan A, Gersten K C, Garvey J, Khan F A, Steinberg H
Oblique hilar tomography, computed tomography, and mediastinoscopy for prethoracotomy
staging of bronchogenic carcinoma
Radiology 1985 Aug, Vol. 156 (2), P. 295–8

735. Konig R, van Kaick G, Toomes H
Computertomographischer Beitrag zur Diagnostik der Bronchuskarzinoide
Contribution of computer tomography to the diagnosis of bronchial carcinoids
Radiologe 1984 Mar, Vol. 24 (3), P. 111–5

736. Konig R, Gademann G, van Kaick G, Zabel J, Lorenz W J, Vogt Moykopf I
Magnetresonanztomographie (MRT) und Computertomographie (CT) bei Bronchialkarzinomen.
Vergleich der Aussagekraft beider Untersuchungsmethoden im Rahmen des präoperativen Stag-
ings
Magnetic resonance tomography MRT and computed tomography CT of bronchial carcinoma.
Comparison of the value of both study methods for preoperative staging
RÖFO 1986 Apr, Vol. 144 (4), P. 377–83

737. Kormano M, Yrjana J
The posterior tracheal band: correlation between computed tomography and chest radiography
Radiology 1980 Sep, Vol. 136 (3), P. 689–94

738. Kowal L E, Goodman L R, Zarro V J, Haskin M E
CT diagnosis of broncholithiasis
J Comput Assist Tomogr 1983 Apr, Vol. 7 (2), P. 321–3

739. Kreipke D L, Lingeman R E
Cross-sectional imaging CT, NMR of branchial cysts: report of three cases
J Comput Assist Tomogr 1984 Feb, Vol. 8 (1), P. 114–6

740. Krestin G P, Bohndorf K, Walgenbach S, Mödder U, Junginger T
Pleurainfiltration bei peripheren Bronchialkarzinomen (BC). Ist die Computertomographie zuverlässig?
Pleural infiltration by peripheral bronchial carcinoma. Is computed tomography reliable?
RÖFO 1986 Apr, Vol. 144 (4), P. 384−7

741. Krestin G P, Friedmann G, Steinbrich W
Präoperatives Staging des Bronchialkarzinoms. Aussagekraft der magnetischen Resonanztomographie (MR) im Vergleich zur Computertomographie (CT)
Preoperative staging of bronchial carcinoma. Value of magnetic resonance in comparison with computed tomography
RÖFO 1986 Mar, Vol. 144 (3), P. 294−9

742. Krudy A G, Doppman J L, Herdt J R
Failure to detect a 1.5 centimeter lung nodule by chest computed tomography
J Comput Assist Tomogr 1982 Dec, Vol. 6 (6), P. 1178−80

743. Kruglik G D, Wayne K S
Occult lung cavity causing hemoptysis: recognition by computed tomography
J Comput Assist Tomogr 1980 Jun, Vol. 4 (3), P. 407−8

744. Kuhlman J E, Scatarige J C, Fishman E K, Zerhouni E A, Siegelman S S
CT demonstration of high attenuation pleural- parenchymal lesions due to amiodarone therapy
J Comput Assist Tomogr 1987 Jan-Feb, Vol. 11 (1), P. 160−2

745. Kuhlman J E, Fishman E K, Burch P A, Karp J E, Zerhouni E A, Siegelman S S
CT of invasive pulmonary aspergillosis
Am J Roentgenol 1988 May, Vol. 150 (5), P. 1015−20

746. Kuhlman J E, Fishman E K, Wang K P, Zerhouni E A, Siegelman S S
Mediastinal cysts: diagnosis by CT and needle aspiration
Am J Roentgenol 1988 Jan, Vol. 150 (1), P. 75−8

747. Kuhlman J E, Fishman E K, Kuhajda F P, Meziane M M, Khouri N F, Zerhouni E A, Siegelman S S
Solitary bronchioloalveolar carcinoma: CT criteria
Radiology 1988 May, Vol. 167 (2), P. 379−82

748. Kuhlman J E, Knowles M C, Fishman E K, Siegelman S S
Premature bullous pulmonary damage in AIDS: CT diagnosis
Radiology 1989 Oct, Vol. 173 (1), P. 23−6

749. Kuhlman J E, Kavuru M, Fishman E K, Siegelman S S Pneumocystis carinii pneumonia: spectrum of parenchymal CT findings
Radiology 1990 Jun, Vol. 175 (3), P. 711−4

750. Kuhlman J E, Fishman E K, Teigen C
Pulmonary septic emboli:diagnosis with CT
Radiology 1990 Vol. 174 ,P. 211−213

751. Kuhns L R, Borlaza G
The "twinkling star" sign: an aid in differentiating pulmonary vessels from pulmonary nodules on computed tomograms
Radiology 1980 Jun, Vol. 135 (3), P. 763−4

752. Kullnig P, Melzer G, Smolle Juttner F M
High-resolution- Computertomographie des Thorax bei Lymphangioleiomyomatose und tuberöser Sklerose
High-resolution computed tomography of the thorax in lymphangioleiomyomatosis and tuberous sclerosis
RÖFO 1989 Jul, Vol. 151 (1), P. 32−5

753. Kullnig P, Pongratz M, Kopp W, Ranner G
Die Computertomographie in der Diagnostik der allergischen bronchopulmonalen Aspergillose
Computerized tomography in the diagnosis of allergic bronchopulmonary aspergillosis
Radiologe 1989 May, Vol. 29 (5), P. 228−31

754. Kullnig P
High-Resolution-CT bei interstitiellen Lungenerkrankungen
High resolution CT of interstitial lung diseases
RÖFO 1990 Jan, Vol. 152 (1), P. 30−4

755. Kuriyama K, Tateishi R, Doi O, Kodama K, Tatsuta M, Matsuda M, Mitani T, Narumi Y, Fujita M
CT-pathologic correlation in small peripheral lung cancers
Am J Roentgenol 1987 Dec, Vol. 149 (6), P. 1139−43

756. Kurtz B, Konig H, Walter E
Computertomographische und sonographische Diagnostik von Zwerchfellhernien
Computer tomographic and sonographic diagnosis of diaphragmatic hernias
RÖFO 1983 Nov, Vol. 139 (5), P. 502−10

757. Kurtz B, Schmitt W G
Ultraschalldiagnostik pleuraler Verschattungen im Vergleich mit der Computertomographie
Ultrasonic diagnosis of pleural shadows compared to computer tomography
RÖFO 1983 May, Vol. 138 (5), P. 577−86

758. Lackner K, Brecht G, Janson R, Scherholz K, Lutzeler A, Thurn P
Wertigkeit der Computertomographie bei der Stadieneinteilung primärer Lymphknotenneoplasien
The value of computer tomography in the staging of primary lymph node neoplasms
RÖFO 1980 Jan, Vol. 132 (1), P. 21−30

759. Landay M J
Azygos vein abutting the posterior wall of the right main and upper lobe bronchi: a normal CT variant
Am J Roentgenol 1983 Mar, Vol. 140 (3), P. 461−2

760. Lang E V, Friedman P J
The anterior wall stripe of the left lower lobe bronchus on the lateral chest radiograph: CT correlative study
Am J Roentgenol 1990 Jan, Vol. 154 (1), P. 33−9

761. Larde D, Belloir C, Vasile N, Frija J, Ferrane J
Computed tomography of aortic dissection
Radiology 1980 Jul, Vol. 136 (1), P. 147−51

762. Lautin E M, Rosenblatt M, Friedman A C, Becker R D, Fromowitz F B, Neglia W
Calcification in non-Hodgkin lymphoma occurring before therapy: identification on plain films and CT
Am J Roentgenol 1990 Oct, Vol. 155 (4), P. 739−40

763. Layer G, van Kaick G
Staging des nichtkleinzelligen Bronchialkarzinoms mit CT und MRT
Staging of non-small cell bronchial carcinoma using CT and MRT
Radiologe 1990 Apr, Vol. 30 (4), P. 155−63

764. Lee J Y, Shank B, Bonfiglio P, Reid A
CT analysis of lung density changes in patients undergoing total body irradiation prior to bone marrow transplantation
J Comput Assist Tomogr 1984 Oct, Vol. 8 (5), P. 885−91

765. Lee K S, Im J G, Bae W K, Kim Y H, Jung S Y, Lee B H, Han M C, Kim C W
CT anatomy of the lingular segmental bronchi
J Comput Assist Tomogr 1991 Jan-Feb, Vol. 15 (1), P. 86−91

766. Leibman A J, Morehouse H T, Ziprkowski M
Spontaneous rupture of a thymic cyst demonstrated by computed tomography
J Comput Assist Tomogr 1984 Jun, Vol. 8 (3), P. 550−2

767. Leipner N, Brecht G, Holle J P, Lackner K, Ehlenz P, Magnussen H
Asbestose. Computertomographie im Vergleich mit der konventionellen Röntgendiagnostik
Asbestosis. Computed tomography in comparison with conventional roentgen diagnosis Asbestose.
RÖFO 1984 Sep, Vol. 141 (3), P. 275−84

768. Leipner N, Schuller H, von Uexkull Guldenband V, Schlolaut K H, Overlack A
Computertomographie und konventionelle Röntgendiagnostik bei interstitiellen Lungenerkrankungen
Computed tomography and conventional X-ray diagnosis of interstitial lung diseases
RÖFO 1988 Nov, Vol. 149 (5), P. 458−65

769. Leung A N, Muller N L, Miller R R
CT in differential diagnosis of diffuse pleural disease
Am J Roentgenol 1990 Mar, Vol. 154 (3), P. 487−92

770. Levine C
Cervical presentation of a large thymic cyst: CT appearance
J Comput Assist Tomogr 1988 Jul-Aug, Vol. 12 (4), P. 656−7

771. Levitt R G, Husband J E, Glazer H S
CT of primary germ-cell tumors of the mediastinum
Am J Roentgenol 1984 Jan, Vol. 142 (1), P. 73−8

772. Levitt R G, Glazer H S, Roper C L, Lee J K, Murphy W A
Magnetic resonance imaging of mediastinal and hilar masses: comparison with CT
Am J Roentgenol 1985 Jul, Vol. 145 (1), P. 9−14

773. Lewis E, Bernardino M E, Valdivieso M, Farha P, Barnes P A, Thomas J L
Computed tomography and routine chest radiography in oat cell carcinoma of the lung
J Comput Assist Tomogr 1982 Aug, Vol. 6 (4), P. 739−45

774. Libshitz H I, Shuman L S
Radiation-induced pulmonary change: CT findings
J Comput Assist Tomogr 1984 Feb, Vol. 8 (1), P. 15−9

775. Littleton J T, Durizch M L, Moeller G, Herbert D E
Pulmonary masses: contrast enhancement
Radiology 1990 Dec, Vol. 177 (3), P. 861−71

776. Lochner B, Loddenkemper R, Claussen C, Wegener O H
Thorakoskopische und computertomographische Befunde beim Pleuramesotheliom
Thoracoscopic and computer tomographic findings in pleural mesotheliomas
RÖFO 1983 May, Vol. 138 (5), P. 570−6

777. Long J A Jr, Doppman J L, Nienhuis A W
Computed tomographic studies of thoracic extramedullary hematopoiesis
J Comput Assist Tomogr 1980 Feb, Vol. 4 (1), P. 67−70

778. Lorcher U
Die Rundatelektase im computertomographischen Bild
Rounded atelectasis in the computerized tomographic image
RÖFO 1986 Jun, Vol. 144 (6), P. 662−4

779. Lynch D A, Gamsu G, Ray C S, Aberle D R
Asbestos-related focal lung masses: manifestations on conventional and high-resolution CT scans
Radiology 1988 Dec, Vol. 169 (3), P. 603−7

780. Lynch D A, Webb W R, Gamsu G, Stulbarg M, Golden J
Computed tomography in pulmonary sarcoidosis
J Comput Assist Tomogr 1989 May-Jun, Vol. 13 (3), P. 405−10

781. Lynch D A, Brasch R C, Hardy K A, Webb W R
Pediatric pulmonary disease: assessment with high-resolution ultrafast CT
Radiology 1990 Jul, Vol. 176 (1), P. 243−8

782. Magid D, Siegelman S S, Eggleston J C, Fishman E K, Zerhouni E A
Pulmonary carcinoid tumors: CT assessment
J Comput Assist Tomogr 1989 Mar-Apr, Vol. 13 (2), P. 244−7

783. Mah K, Poon P Y, Van Dyk J, Keane T, Majesky I F, Rideout D F
Assessment of acute radiation-induced pulmonary changes using computed tomography
J Comput Assist Tomogr 1986 Sep-Oct, Vol. 10 (5), P. 736−43

784. Maltby J D, Gouverne M L
CT findings in pulmonary venoocclusive disease
J Comput Assist Tomogr 1984 Aug, Vol. 8 (4), P. 758−61

785. Marks B W, Kuhns L R
Identification of the pleural fissures with computed tomography
Radiology 1982 Apr, Vol. 143 (1), P. 139−41

786. Marti Bonmati L, Ruiz Perales F, Catala F, Mata J M, Calonge E
CT findings in Swyer-James syndrome
Radiology 1989 Aug, Vol. 172 (2), P. 477−80

787. Martin J, Palacio A, Petit J, Martin C
Fatty transformation of thoracic extramedullary hematopoiesis following splenectomy: CT features
J Comput Assist Tomogr 1990 May-Jun, Vol. 14 (3), P. 477−8

788. Mata J M, Caceres J, Llauger J, Palmer J
CT demonstration of intrapulmonary right brachiocephalic vein associated with an azygos lobe
J Comput Assist Tomogr 1990 Mar-Apr, Vol. 14 (2), P. 305−6

789. Mathieson J R, Mayo J R, Staples C A, Muller N L
Chronic diffuse infiltrative lung disease: comparison of diagnostic accuracy of CT and chest radiography
Radiology 1989 Apr, Vol. 171 (1), P. 111−6

790. Mathieu D, Keita K, Loisance D, Cachera J P, Rousseau M, Vasile N
Postoperative CT follow-up of aortic dissection
J Comput Assist Tomogr 1986 Mar-Apr, Vol. 10 (2), P. 216−8

791. Matsumoto A H, Parker L A, Delany D J
CT demonstration of central pulmonary venous and arterial occlusive diseases
J Comput Assist Tomogr 1987 Jul-Aug, Vol. 11 (4), P. 640−4

792. Mayo J R, Webb W R, Gould R, Stein M G, Bass I, Gamsu G, Goldberg H I
High-resolution CT of the lungs: an optimal approach
Radiology 1987 May, Vol. 163 (2), P. 507−10

793. Mayo J R, Muller N L, Road J, Sisler J, Lillington G
Chronic eosinophilic pneumonia: CT findings in six cases
Am J Roentgenol 1989 Oct, Vol. 153 (4), P. 727−30

794. Mayr B, Heywang S H, Ingrisch H, Huber R M, Haussinger K, Lissner J
Comparison of CT with MR imaging of endobronchial tumors
J Comput Assist Tomogr 1987 Jan-Feb, Vol. 11 (1), P. 43−8

795. Mayr B, Ingrisch H, Haussinger K, Sunder Plassmann L, Huber R
Wertigkeit von konventioneller Tomographie und Computertomographie in der Diagnostik von Tumoren des Bronchialsystems

Value of conventional tomography and computerized tomography in the diagnosis of tumors of the bronchial system
RÖFO 1988 Apr, Vol. 148 (4), P. 347–52

796. Mayr B, Ingrisch H, Haussinger K, Huber R M, Sunder Plassmann L
Tumors of the bronchi: role of evaluation with CT
Radiology 1989 Sep, Vol. 172 (3), P. 647–52

797. McGahan J P
Carney syndrome: usefulness of computed tomography in demonstrating pulmonary chondromas
J Comput Assist Tomogr 1983 Feb, Vol. 7 (1), P. 137–9

798. McHugh K, Blaquiere R M
CT features of rounded atelectasis
Am J Roentgenol 1989 Aug, Vol. 153 (2), P. 257–60

799. McLoud T C
The use of CT in the examination of asbestos- exposed persons editorial
Radiology 1988 Dec, Vol. 169 (3), P. 862–3

800. Mendelsohn S L, Fagelman D, Zwanger Mendelsohn S
Endobronchial lipoma demonstrated by CT
Radiology 1983 Sep, Vol. 148 (3), P. 790

801. Mendelson D S, Rose J S, Efremidis S C, Kirschner P A, Cohen B A
Bronchogenic cysts with high CT numbers
Am J Roentgenol 1983 Mar, Vol. 140 (3), P. 463–5

802. Metzger R A, Mulhern C B Jr, Arger P H, Coleman B G, Epstein D M, Gefter W B
CT differentiation of solitary from diffuse bronchioloalveolar carcinoma
J Comput Assist Tomogr 1981 Dec, Vol. 5 (6), P. 830–3

803. Meyer J E, Linggood R M, Lindfors K K, McLoud T C, Stomper P C
Impact of thoracic computed tomography on radiation therapy planning in Hodgkin disease
J Comput Assist Tomogr 1984 Oct, Vol. 8 (5), P. 892–4

804. Miller D L, Schneider P D, Willis M, Vermess M, Doppman J L
Intraarterial administration of EOE-13 for the CT evaluation of hepatic artery infusion chemotherapy
J Comput Assist Tomogr 1984 Apr, Vol. 8 (2), P. 332–4

805. Miller P A, Williamson B R, Minor G R, Buschi A J
Pulmonary sequestration: visualization of the feeding artery by CT
J Comput Assist Tomogr 1982 Aug, Vol. 6 (4), P. 828–30

806. Mirvis S E, Whitley N O, Aisner J, Moody M, Whitacre M, Whitley J E
Abdominal CT in the staging of small-cell carcinoma of the lung: incidence of metastases and effect on prognosis
Am J Roentgenol 1987 May, Vol. 148 (5), P. 845–7

807. Moore A D, Godwin J D, Muller N L, Naidich D P, Hammar S P, Buschman D L, Takasugi J E, de Carvalho C R
Pulmonary histiocytosis X: comparison of radiographic and CT findings
Radiology 1989 Jul, Vol. 172 (1), P. 249–54

808. Mori K, Saitou Y, Tominaga K, Yokoi K, Miyazawa N, Okuyama A, Sasagawa M
Small nodular lesions in the lung periphery: new approach to diagnosis with CT
Radiology 1990 Dec, Vol. 177 (3), P. 843–9

809. Mori M, Galvin J R, Barloon T J, Gingrich R D, Stanford W
Fungal pulmonary infections after bone marrow transplantation: evaluation with radiography and CT
Radiology 1991 Mar, Vol. 178 (3), P. 721–6

810. Morris U L, Colletti P M, Ralls P W, Boswell W D, Lapin S A, Quinn M, Halls J M
CT demonstration of intrathoracic thyroid tissue
J Comput Assist Tomogr 1982 Aug, Vol. 6 (4), P. 821–4

811. Muller H A, van Kaick G, Schaaf J, Lullig H, Vogt Moykopf I, Delphendahl A
Präoperatives Staging des Bronchialkarzinoms: Wertigkeit der Computertomographie im Vergleich zur konventionellen Radiologie
Pre-operative staging of bronchial carcinomas: a comparison of computed tomography and conventional radiography
RÖFO 1981 Jun, Vol. 134 (6), P. 601–7

812. Muller N L, Bergin C J, Ostrow D N, Nichols D M
Role of computed tomography in the recognition of bronchiectasis
Am J Roentgenol 1984 Nov, Vol. 143 (5), P. 971–6

813. Muller N L, Gamsu G, Webb W R
Pulmonary nodules: detection using magnetic resonance and computed tomography
Radiology 1985 Jun, Vol. 155 (3), P. 687–90

814. Muller N L, Miller R R, Webb W R, Evans K G, Ostrow D N
Fibrosing alveolitis: CT-pathologic correlation
Radiology 1986 Sep, Vol. 160 (3), P. 585–8

815. Muller N L, Staples C A, Miller R R, Vedal S, Thurlbeck W M, Ostrow D N
Disease activity in idiopathic pulmonary fibrosis: CT and pathologic correlation
Radiology 1987 Dec, Vol. 165 (3), P. 731–4

816. Muller N L, Kullnig P, Miller R R
The CT findings of pulmonary sarcoidosis: analysis of 25 patients
Am J Roentgenol 1989 Jun, Vol. 152 (6), P. 1179–82

817. Muller N L, Mawson J B, Mathieson J R, Abboud R, Ostrow D N, Champion P
Sarcoidosis: correlation of extent of disease at CT with clinical, functional, and radiographic findings
Radiology 1989 Jun, Vol. 171 (3), P. 613–8

818. Muller N L, Chiles C, Kullnig P
Pulmonary lymphangiomyomatosis: correlation of CT with radiographic and functional findings
Radiology 1990 May, Vol. 175 (2), P. 335–9

819. Muller N L, Staples C A, Miller R R
Bronchiolitis obliterans organizing pneumonia: CT features in 14 patients
Am J Roentgenol 1990 May, Vol. 154 (5), P. 983–7

820. Munro N C, Currie D C, Cooke J C, Kerr I H, Strickland B, Cole P J
Value of medium-thickness CT in the diagnosis of bronchiectasis
Am J Roentgenol 1988 Aug, Vol. 151 (2), P. 411

821. Murata K, Itoh H, Todo G, Kanaoka M, Noma S, Itoh T, Furuta M, Asamoto H, Torizuka K
Centrilobular lesions of the lung: demonstration by high-resolution CT and pathologic correlation
Radiology 1986 Dec, Vol. 161 (3), P. 641–5

822. Murata K, Itoh H, Senda M, Yonekura Y, Nishimura K, Izumi T, Oshima S, Torizuka K
Stratified impairment of pulmonary ventilation in "diffuse panbronchiolitis:" PET and CT studies
J Comput Assist Tomogr 1989 Jan-Feb, Vol. 13 (1), P. 48–53

823. Murata K, Khan A, Herman P G
Pulmonary parenchymal disease: evaluation with high-resolution CT
Radiology 1989 Mar, Vol. 170 (3 Pt 1), P. 629–35

824. Musset D, Grenier P, Carette M F, Frija G, Hauuy M P, Desbleds M T, Girard P, Bigot J M, Lallemand D
Primary lung cancer staging: prospective comparative study of MR imaging with CT
Radiology 1986 Sep, Vol. 160 (3), P. 607–11

825. Nabawi P, Mantravadi R, Breyer D, Capek V
Computed tomography of radiation-induced lung injuries
J Comput Assist Tomogr 1981 Aug, Vol. 5 (4), P. 568–70

826. Naidich D P, McCauley D I, Siegelman S S
Computed tomography of bronchial adenomas
J Comput Assist Tomogr 1982 Aug, Vol. 6 (4), P. 725–32

827. Naidich D P, McCauley D I, Khouri N F, Stitik F P, Siegelman S S
Computed tomography of bronchiectasis
J Comput Assist Tomogr 1982 Jun, Vol. 6 (3), P. 437–44

828. Naidich D P, McCauley D I, Khouri N F, Leitman B S, Hulnick D H, Siegelman S S
Computed tomography of lobar collapse: 2. Collapse in the absence of endobronchial obstruction
J Comput Assist Tomogr 1983 Oct, Vol. 7 (5), P. 758–67

829. Naidich D P, McCauley D I, Khouri N F, Leitman B S, Hulnick D H, Siegelman S S
Computed tomography of lobar collapse: 1. Endobronchial obstruction
J Comput Assist Tomogr 1983 Oct, Vol. 7 (5), P. 745–57

830. Naidich D P, Megibow A J, Hilton S, Hulnick D H, Siegelman S S
Computed tomography of the diaphragm: peridiaphragmatic fluid localization
J Comput Assist Tomogr 1983 Aug, Vol. 7 (4), P. 641–9

831. Naidich D P, Megibow A J, Ross C R, Beranbaum E R, Siegelman S S
Computed tomography of the diaphragm: normal anatomy and variants
J Comput Assist Tomogr 1983 Aug, Vol. 7 (4), P. 633–40

832. Naidich D P, Lee J J, Garay S M, McCauley D I, Aranda C P, Boyd A D
Comparison of CT and fiberoptic bronchoscopy in the evaluation of bronchial disease
Am J Roentgenol 1987 Jan, Vol. 148 (1), P. 1–7

833. Naidich D P, Zinn W L, Ettenger N A, McCauley D I, Garay S M
Basilar segmental bronchi: thin-section CT evaluation
Radiology 1988 Oct, Vol. 169 (1), P. 11–6

834. Naidich D P
Pulmonary parenchymal high-resolution CT: to be or not to be
Radiology 1989 Apr, Vol. 171 (1), P. 22–4

835. Naidich D P, Funt S, Ettenger N A, Arranda C
Hemoptysis: CT- bronchoscopic correlations in 58 cases
Radiology 1990 Nov, Vol. 177 (2), P. 357–62

836. Naidich D P, Weinreb J C, Schinella R
MR imaging of pulmonary parenchyma: comparison with CT in evaluating cadaveric lung specimens
J Comput Assist Tomogr 1990 Jul-Aug, Vol. 14 (4), P. 595–9

837. Naidich D P, Marshall C H, Gribbin C, Arams R S, McCauley D I
Low-dose CT of the lungs: preliminary observations
Radiology 1990 Jun, Vol. 175 (3), P. 729–31

838. Nakata H, Kimoto T, Nakayama T, Kido M, Miyazaki N, Harada S
Diffuse peripheral lung disease: evaluation by high-resolution computed tomography
Radiology 1985 Oct, Vol. 157 (1), P. 181–5

839. Nakata H, Sato Y, Nakayama T, Yoshimatsu H, Kobayashi T
Bronchogenic cyst with high CT number: analysis of contents
J Comput Assist Tomogr 1986 Mar-Apr, Vol. 10 (2), P. 360

840. Neumayer K
Diagnostik der Lungensequestration – Stellenwert der Computertomographie
The diagnosis of pulmonary sequestration – the value of computed tomography
RÖFO 1989 Sep, Vol. 151 (3), P. 263–7

841. Ng S H, Ng K K, Pai S C, Tsai C C
Tuberous sclerosis with aortic aneurysm and rib changes: CT demonstration
J Comput Assist Tomogr 1988 Jul-Aug, Vol. 12 (4), P. 666–8

842. Nielsen M E Jr, Heaston D K, Dunnick N R, Korobkin M
Preoperative CT evaluation of adrenal glands in non-small cell bronchogenic carcinoma
Am J Roentgenol 1982 Aug, Vol. 139 (2), P. 317–20

843. Osborne D, Vock P, Godwin J D, Silverman P M
CT identification of bronchopulmonary segments: 50 normal subjects
Am J Roentgenol 1984 Jan, Vol. 142 (1), P. 47–52

844. Otsuji H, Hatakeyama M, Kitamura I, Yoshimura H, Iwasaki S, Ohishi H, Uchida H, Kitamura S, Narita N
Right upper lobe versus right middle lobe: differentiation with thin- section, high- resolution CT
Radiology 1989 Sep, Vol. 172 (3), P. 653–6

845. Pagani J J
Normal adrenal glands in small cell lung carcinoma: CT-guided biopsy
Am J Roentgenol 1983 May, Vol. 140 (5), P. 949–51

846. Paling M R, Griffin G K
Lower lobe collapse due to pleural effusion: a CT analysis
J Comput Assist Tomogr 1985 Nov-Dec, Vol. 9 (6), P. 1079–83

847. Paul D J, Mueller C F
Pulmonary sequestration
J Comput Assist Tomogr 1982 Feb, Vol. 6 (1), P. 163–5

848. Pearlberg J L, Sandler M A, Beute G H, Madrazo B L
T1N0M0 bronchogenic carcinoma: assessment by CT
Radiology 1985 Oct, Vol. 157 (1), P. 187–90

849. Pearlberg J L, Sandler M A, Lewis J W Jr, Beute G H, Alpern M B
Small-cell bronchogenic carcinoma: CT evaluation
Am J Roentgenol 1988 Feb, Vol. 150 (2), P. 265–8

850. Pedersen M L, LeQuire M H, Spies J B, Ladd W A
Computed tomography of intralobar bronchopulmonary sequestration supplied from the renal artery
J Comput Assist Tomogr 1988 Sep-Oct, Vol. 12 (5), P. 874–5

851. Peters J C, Desai K K
CT demonstration of postpneumonectomy tumor recurrence
Am J Roentgenol 1983 Aug, Vol. 141 (2), P. 259–62

852. Peuchot M, Libshitz H I
Pulmonary metastatic disease: radiologic-surgical correlation
Radiology 1987 Sep, Vol. 164 (3), P. 719–22

853. Pilate I, Marcelis S, Timmerman H, Beeckman P, Osteaux M J
Pulmonary asbestosis: CT study of subpleural curvilinear shadow letter
Radiology 1987 Aug, Vol. 164 (2), P. 584

854. Pinstein M L, Scott R L, Salazar J
Avoidance of negative percutaneous lung biopsy using contrast- enhanced CT
Am J Roentgenol 1983 Feb, Vol. 140 (2), P. 265–7

855. Platt J F, Glazer G M, Gross B H, Quint L E, Francis I R, Orringer M B
CT evaluation of mediastinal lymph nodes in lung cancer: influence of the lobar site of the primary neoplasm
Am J Roentgenol 1987 Oct, Vol. 149 (4), P. 683–6

856. Poon P Y, Feld R, Evans W K, Ege G, Yeoh J L, McLoughlin M L
Computed tomography of the brain, liver, and upper abdomen in the staging of small cell carcinoma of the lung
J Comput Assist Tomogr 1982 Oct, Vol. 6 (5), P. 963–5

857. Poon P Y, Bronskill M J, Henkelman R M, Rideout D F, Shulman H S, Weisbrod G L, Steinhardt M I, Dunlap H J, Ginsberg R J, Feld R, et al
Mediastinal lymph node metastases from bronchogenic carcinoma: detection with MR imaging and CT
Radiology 1987 Mar, Vol. 162 (3), P. 651–6

858. Proto A V, Thomas S R
Pulmonary nodules studied by computed tomography
Radiology 1985 Jul, Vol. 156 (1), P. 149–53

859. Pugatch R D, Gale M E
Obscure pulmonary masses: bronchial impaction revealed by CT
Am J Roentgenol 1983 Nov, Vol. 141 (5), P. 909–14

860. Quint L E, Glazer G M, Orringer M B
Central lung masses: prediction with CT of need for pneumonectomy versus lobectomy
Radiology 1987 Dec, Vol. 165 (3), P. 735–8

861. Radin D R, Ralls P W, Boswell W D, Lundell C, Halls J M
Alveolar soft part sarcoma: CT findings
J Comput Assist Tomogr 1984 Apr, Vol. 8 (2), P. 344–5

862. Rappaport D C, Weisbrod G L, Herman S J, Chamberlain D W
Pulmonary lymphangioleiomyomatosis: high-resolution CT findings in four cases
Am J Roentgenol 1989 May, Vol. 152 (5), P. 961–4

863. Reiser U, Heuck F, Pfeiler M
Einfluß und Quantifizierung der Atemverschieblichkeit von abdominellen Organen bei der Röntgencomputertomographie
Effect and quantification of respiratory movement of abdominal organs on X-ray computer tomography
RÖFO 1980 Jul, Vol. 133 (1), P. 9–17

864. Remy Jardin M, Remy J
Comparison of vertical and oblique CT in evaluation of bronchial tree
J Comput Assist Tomogr 1988 Nov-Dec, Vol. 12 (6), P. 956–62

865. Remy Jardin M, Degreef J M, Beuscart R, Voisin C, Remy J
Coal worker's pneumoconiosis: CT assessment in exposed workers and correlation with radiographic findings Radiology 1990 Nov, Vol. 177 (2), P. 363–71

866. Ren H, Hruban R H, Kuhlman J E, Fishman E K, Wheeler P S, Zerhouni E A, Hutchins G M
Computed tomography of rounded atelectasis
J Comput Assist Tomogr 1988 Nov-Dec, Vol. 12 (6), P. 1031–4

867. Ren H, Hruban R H, Kuhlman J E, Fishman E K, Wheeler P S, Zerhouni E A, Hutchins G M
Computed tomography of inflation-fixed lungs: the beaded septum sign of pulmonary metastases
J Comput Assist Tomogr 1989 May-Jun, Vol. 13 (3), P. 411–6

868. Ren H, Kuhlman J E, Hruban R H, Fishman E K, Wheeler P S, Hutchins G M
CT of inflation-fixed lungs: Wedge-density and vascular sign in diagnosis of infarction
J Comput Assist Tomogr 1990, Vol. 14 (1), P.82–6

869. Reuter M, Heller M, Triebel H J, Magnussen H
Computertomographie der Bronchiektasen
Computed tomography of bronchiectasis
RÖFO 1988 Aug, Vol. 149 (2), P. 152–7

870. Roberts C M, Citron K M, Strickland B
Intrathoracic aspergilloma: role of CT in diagnosis and treatment
Radiology 1987 Oct, Vol. 165 (1), P. 123–8

871. Rockoff S D
CT demonstration of interlobar fissure calcification due to asbestos exposure
J Comput Assist Tomogr 1987 Nov-Dec, Vol. 11 (6), P. 1066–8

872. Rosenblum L J, Mauceri R A, Wellenstein D E, Thomas F D, Bassano D A, Raasch B N, Chamberlain C C, Heitzman E R
Density patterns in the normal lung as determined by computed tomography
Radiology 1980 Nov, Vol. 137 (2), P. 409–16

873. Ross G J, Violi L, Friedman A C, Edmonds P R, Unger E
Intravascular bronchioloalveolar tumor: CT and pathologic correlation
J Comput Assist Tomogr 1989 Mar-Apr, Vol. 13 (2), P. 240–3

874. Rubinstein I, Hoffstein V
Pulmonary hamartoma: CT findings letter
Radiology 1987 Mar, Vol. 162 (3), P. 878

875. Sagel S S
The solitary pulmonary nodule: role of CT
Am J Roentgenol 1986 Jul, Vol. 147 (1), P. 26–7

876. Sakai F, Gamsu G, Im J G, Ray C S
Pulmonary function abnormalities in patients with CT-determined emphysema
J Comput Assist Tomogr 1987 Nov-Dec, Vol. 11 (6), P. 963–8

877. Saksouk F A, Fahl M H, Rizk G K
Computed tomography of pulmonary hydatid disease
J Comput Assist Tomogr 1986 Mar-Apr, Vol. 10 (2), P. 226–32

878. Schaefer C M, Greene R, Llewellyn H J, Mrose H E, Pile Spellman E A, Rubens J R, Lindemann S R
Interstitial lung disease: impact of postprocessing in digital storage phosphor imaging
Radiology 1991 Mar, Vol. 178 (3), P. 733–8

879. Scheid K F, Lissner J, Blaha H, Gebauer A
Densitometrische Analyse pulmonaler Rundherde im Computertomogramm
Computed tomography and densitometric pattern of pulmonary lesions
RÖFO 1981 Apr, Vol. 134 (4), P. 357–63

880. Schlolaut K H, Borre D, Leipner N, Koster O
Zur Wertigkeit der CT beim Lungenspitzenkarzinom
The value of CT in carcinoma of the lung apex
RÖFO 1989 Feb, Vol. 150 (2), P. 142–6

881. Schmitt W G H, Hübener K H
Verkalkte Pleuraschwarte und Pleuraempyem mit Wandverkalkung
RÖFO 1981, Vol. 134, P. 619–25

882. Schurawitzki H, Stiglbauer R, Graninger W, Herold C, Polzleitner D, Burghuber O C, Tscholakoff D
Interstitial lung disease in progressive systemic sclerosis: high- resolution CT versus radiography
Radiology 1990 Sep, Vol. 176 (3), P. 755–9

883. Scott I R, Muller N L, Miller R R, Evans K G, Nelems B
Resectable stage III lung cancer: CT, surgical, and pathologic correlation
Radiology 1988 Jan, Vol. 166 (1 Pt 1), P. 75–9

884. Shaer A H, Bashist B
Computed tomography of bronchial artery aneurysm with erosion into the esophagus
J Comput Assist Tomogr 1989 Nov-Dec, Vol. 13 (6), P. 1069–71

885. Shaffer K, Pugatch R D
Small pulmonary nodules: dynamic CT with a single-breath technique
Radiology 1989 Nov, Vol. 173 (2), P. 567–8

886. Shapiro M P, Gale M E, Carter B L
Variable CT appearance of plasma cell granuloma of the lung
J Comput Assist Tomogr 1987 Jan-Feb, Vol. 11 (1), P. 49–51

887. Sherrier R H, Chiles C, Roggli V
Pulmonary lymphangioleiomyomatosis: CT findings
Am J Roentgenol 1989 Nov, Vol. 153 (5), P. 937–40

888. Shin M S, Ho K J
Computed tomographic evaluation of solitary pulmonary nodules in chest roentgenograms
J Comput Assist Tomogr 1982 Oct, Vol. 6 (5), P. 947–54

889. Shin M S, Berland L L, Myers J L, Clary G, Zorn G L
CT demonstration of an ossifying bronchial carcinoid simulating broncholithiasis
Am J Roentgenol 1989 Jul, Vol. 153 (1), P. 51–2

890. Sider L, Mittal B B, Nemcek A A Jr, Bobba V S
CT-guided placement of iodine-125 seeds for unresectable carcinoma of the lung
J Comput Assist Tomogr 1988 May-Jun, Vol. 12 (3), P. 515–7

891. Siegelman S S, Zerhouni E A, Leo F P, Khouri N F, Stitik F P
CT of the solitary pulmonary nodule
Am J Roentgenol 1980 Jul, Vol. 135 (1), P. 1–13

892. Siegelman S S, Khouri N F, Leo F P, Fishman E K, Braverman R M, Zerhouni E A
Solitary pulmonary nodules: CT assessment
Radiology 1986 Aug, Vol. 160 (2), P. 307–12

893. Silver S F, Muller N L, Miller R R, Lefcoe M S
Hypersensitivity pneumonitis: evaluation with CT
Radiology 1989 Nov, Vol. 173 (2), P. 441–5

894. Silverman P M, Godwin J D
CT/bronchographic correlations in bronchiectasis
J Comput Assist Tomogr 1987 Jan-Feb, Vol. 11 (1), P. 52–6

895. Silverman S G, Mueller P R, Saini S, Hahn P F, Simeone J F, Forman B H, Steiner E, Ferrucci J T
Thoracic empyema: management with image-guided catheter drainage
Radiology 1988 Oct, Vol. 169 (1), P. 5–9

896. Singcharoen T, Silprasert W
CT findings in pulmonary paragonimiasis
J Comput Assist Tomogr 1987 Nov-Dec, Vol. 11 (6), P. 1101–2

897. Solomon A
A comparative study of mesothelioma and asbestosis using computed tomography and conventional chest radiography letter
Radiology 1983 Jul, Vol. 148 (1), P. 316

898. Solomon A, Burke M, Almog C, Stern D
Computerised tomographic demonstration of the "crescent sign" confirming gangrenous sloughing of the lung associated with a primary lung carcinoma
RÖFO 1986 Feb, Vol. 144 (2), P. 238–40

899. Sommer B, Walter P, Remberger K
Das Bronchuslipom. Diagnose durch die Computertomographie
Bronchial lipoma. Diagnosis by computer tomography
RÖFO 1982 May, Vol. 136 (5), P. 595–6

900. Spirt B A
Value of the prone position in detecting pulmonary nodules by computed tomography
J Comput Assist Tomogr 1980 Dec, Vol. 4 (6), P. 871–3

901. Staples C A, Muller N L, Vedal S, Abboud R, Ostrow D, Miller R R
Usual interstitial pneumonia: correlation of CT with clinical, functional, and radiologic findings
Radiology 1987 Feb, Vol. 162 (2), P. 377–81

902. Stark D D, Federle M P, Goodman P C, Podrasky A E, Webb W R
Differentiating lung abscess and empyema: radiography and computed tomography
Am J Roentgenol 1983 Jul, Vol. 141 (1), P. 163–7

903. Stark P, Greene R, Kott M M, Hall T, Vanderslice L
CT-findings in ARDS
Radiologe 1987 Aug, Vol. 27 (8), P. 367–9

904. Stark P, Wong V, Gold P
Solitary pulmonary granuloma with marked enhancement on dynamic CT scanning
Radiologe 1988 Oct, Vol. 28 (10), P. 489–90

905. Stark P, Robson D
CT of hemorrhagic lung infarction due to postoperative torsion
RÖFO 1991 Jan, Vol. 154 (1), P. 114

906. Steinbacher M, Konig R, van Kaick G, Schaaf J
Der Beitrag der Computertomographie zur Differentialdiagnostik entzündlicher und neoplastischer Lungenerkrankungen
Computed tomography in the differential diagnosis of inflammatory and neoplastic lung diseases
RÖFO 1984 May, Vol. 140 (5), P. 544–50

907. Steinbacher M, van Kaick G, Schaaf J, Vollhaber H H
Computertomographische und röntgenologische Befunde beim bronchiolo-alveolären Karzinom der Lunge
Computed tomographic and roentgenologic findings in bronchiolo-alveolar carcinoma of the lung
RÖFO 1985 Mar, Vol. 142 (3), P. 267–9

908. Steinberg D L, Webb W R
CT appearances of rheumatoid lung disease
J Comput Assist Tomogr 1984 Oct, Vol. 8 (5), P. 881–4

909. Tarver R D, Holden R W, Ellis J H
Experimental lung nodule model: CT numbers, nodule size, and actual calcium content
J Comput Assist Tomogr 1983 Jun, Vol. 7 (3), P. 402–6

910. Tarver R D, Richmond B D, Klatte E C
Cerebral metastases from lung carcinoma: neurological and CT correlation. Work in progress
Radiology 1984 Dec, Vol. 153 (3), P. 689–92

911. Tarver R D, Conces D J Jr, Godwin J D
Motion artifacts on CT simulate bronchiectasis
Am J Roentgenol 1988 Dec, Vol. 151 (6), P. 1117–9

912. Templeton P A, McLoud T C, Muller N L, Shepard J A, Moore E H
Pulmonary lymphangioleiomyomatosis: CT and pathologic findings
J Comput Assist Tomogr 1989 Jan-Feb, Vol. 13 (1), P. 54–7

913. Triebel H J, Kanzow G, Heller M, Magnussen H, Bucheler E
Zur Bedeutung der Thorax-CT für die Diagnose der Lungensarkoidose
The importance of thoracic CT in the diagnosis of pulmonary sarcoidosis
RÖFO 1990 Nov, Vol. 153 (5), P. 557–64

914. Triller J, Stirnemann P, Greiner R
Computertomographie bei Lungenspitzenkarzinom
Computed tomography of apical lung cancer
RÖFO 1985 Jun, Vol. 142 (6), P. 658–63

915. Tylen U, Nilsson U
Computed tomography in pulmonary pseudotumors and their relation to asbestos exposure
J Comput Assist Tomogr 1982 Apr, Vol. 6 (2), P. 229–37

916. Van Dyke J A, Sagel S S
Calcified pulmonary sequestration: CT demonstration
J Comput Assist Tomogr 1985 Mar-Apr, Vol. 9 (2), P. 372–4

917. van Kaick G, Siegert A, Luhrs H, Liebermann D
Der Beitrag der Computertomographie zur Quantifizierung der Thorotrastose und zur Erkennung thorotrastinduzierter Lebertumoren
Use of computed tomography for quantifying Thorotrast and detecting Thorotrast- induced liver tumors
Radiologe 1986 Mar, Vol. 26 (3), P. 123–8

918. vanSonnenberg E, D Agostino H B, Casola G, Wittich G R, Varney R R, Harker C
Lung abscess: CT-guided drainage
Radiology 1991 Feb, Vol. 178 (2), P. 347–51

919. Vas W, Zylak C J, Mather D, Figueredo A
The value of abdominal computed tomography in the pre-treatment assessment of small cell carcinoma of the lung
Radiology 1981 Feb, Vol. 138 (2), P. 417–8

920. Vock P, Haertel M
Die Computertomographie zur Stadieneinteilung des Bronchuskarzinoms
Computer tomography for staging of bronchial carcinomas
RÖFO 1981 Feb, Vol. 134 (2), P. 131–5

921. Vock P, Soucek M, Daepp M, Kalender W A
Lung: spiral volumetric CT with single-breath-hold technique
Radiology 1990 Sep, Vol. 176 (3), P. 864–7

922. Wagner R B, Crawford W O Jr, Schimpf P P
Classification of parenchymal injuries of the lung
Radiology 1988 Apr, Vol. 167 (1), P. 77–82

923. Webb W R, Gamsu G, Birnberg F A
CT appearance of bronchial carcinoid with recurrent pneumonia and hyperplastic hilar lymphadenopathy
J Comput Assist Tomogr 1983 Aug, Vol. 7 (4), P. 707–9

924. Webb W R, Hirji M, Gamsu G
Posterior wall of the bronchus intermedius: radiographic-CT correlation
Am J Roentgenol 1984 May, Vol. 142 (5), P. 907–11

925. Webb W R, Stein M G, Finkbeiner W E, Im J H, Lynch D, Gamsu G
Normal and diseased isolated lungs: high-resolution CT
Radiology 1988 Jan, Vol. 166 (1 Pt 1), P. 81–7

926. Webb W R, Gatsonis C, Zerhouni E A, Heelan R T, Glazer G M, Francis I R, McNeil B J
CT and MR imaging in staging non-small cell bronchogenic carcinoma: report of the Radiologic Diagnostic Oncology Group
Radiology 1991 Mar, Vol. 178 (3), P. 705–13

927. Wegener O H, Koeppe P, Oeser H
Measurement of lung density by computed tomography
J Comput Assist Tomogr 1978 Jul, Vol. 2 (3), P. 263–73

928. Weir I H, Muller N L, Connell D G
CT diagnosis of bronchial rupture
J Comput Assist Tomogr 1988 Nov-Dec, Vol. 12 (6), P. 1035–6

929. Winer Muram H T, Gavant M L
Pulmonary CT findings in Behcet disease
J Comput Assist Tomogr 1989 Mar-Apr, Vol. 13 (2), P. 346–7

930. Winzelberg G G, Boller M, Sachs M, Weinberg J
CT evaluation of pulmonary alveolar microlithiasis
J Comput Assist Tomogr 1984 Oct, Vol. 8 (5), P. 1029–31

931. Woodring J H
Determining the cause of pulmonary atelectasis: a comparison of plain radiography and CT
Am J Roentgenol 1988 Apr, Vol. 150 (4), P. 757–63

932. Wouters E F, Oei T K, Van Engelshoven J M, Lemmens H A, Greve L H
Evaluation of the contribution of computed tomography to the staging of non-oat-cell primary bronchogenic carcinoma. A retrospective study
RÖFO 1982 Nov, Vol. 137 (5), P. 540–3

933. Wurche K D, Kubale R, Vallee D, Ostertag H
Quantifizierung der pulmonalen alveolären Mikrolithiasis im CT
Quantification of pulmonary alveolar microlithiasis in the CT
RÖFO 1987 Jul, Vol. 147 (1), P. 36–8

934. Yoshikawa J, Takashima T, Miyata S, Kitagawa M
CT demonstration of calcification in an adenoid cystic carcinoma of the lung letter
Am J Roentgenol 1990 Feb, Vol. 154 (2), P. 419

935. Zaunbauer W, Robotti G C, Probst P, Haertel M, Schopf R
Zur Computertomographie der Lungenaplasie
Computer tomography of pulmonary aplasia
RÖFO 1981 Dec, Vol. 135 (6), P. 682–6

936. Zerhouni E A, Spivey J F, Morgan R H, Leo F P, Stitik F P, Siegelman S S
Factors influencing quantitative CT measurements of solitary pulmonary nodules
J Comput Assist Tomogr 1982 Dec, Vol. 6 (6), P. 1075–87

937. Zerhouni E A, Stitik F P, Siegelman S S, Naidich D P, Sagel S S, Proto A V, Muhm J R, Walsh J W, Martinez C R, Heelan R T, et al
CT of the pulmonary nodule: a cooperative study
Radiology 1986 Aug, Vol. 160 (2), P. 319–27

938. Zwirewich C V, Miller R R, Muller N L
Multicentric adenocarcinoma of the lung: CT-pathologic correlation
Radiology 1990 Jul, Vol. 176 (1), P. 185–90

939. Zwirewich C V, Muller N L, Lam S C
Photodynamic laser therapy to alleviate complete bronchial obstruction: comparison of CT and bronchoscopy to predict outcome
Am J Roentgenol 1988 Nov, Vol. 151 (5), P. 897–901

The Chest Wall

940. Bahren W, Sigmund G, Lenz M
Wertigkeit der Computertomographie im Vergleich zu Mediastinoskopie und Probethorakotomie bei intrathorakalen Raumforderungen mit mediastinaler Beteiligung
Value of computer tomography in comparison to mediastinoscopy and test thoracotomy in intrathoracic space- occupying lesions with mediastinal involvement
RÖFO 1982 Sep, Vol. 137 (3), P. 269–74

941. Beyer Enke S A, Gorich J, van Kaick G, Vogt Moykopf I
CT- Morphologie und klinische Diagnose thorakaler Raumforderungen bei unter 40jährigen Patienten
CT morphology and clinical diagnosis of thoracic space-occupying lesions in patients under 40 years of age
RÖFO 1989 Jun, Vol. 150 (6), P. 674–9

942. Bhalla M, McCauley D I, Golimbu C, Leitman B S, Naidich D P
Counting ribs on chest CT
J Comput Assist Tomogr 1990 Jul-Aug, Vol. 14 (4), P. 590–4

943. Bittner R, Schorner W, Sander B, Weiss T, Loddenkemper R, Kaiser D, Felix R
Maligne Thoraxwandinfiltration in der MR: Vergleich mit CT- und operativen Befunden
Malignant chest wall infiltration in MR: comparison with CT and surgical findings
RÖFO 1989 Nov, Vol. 151 (5), P. 590–6

944. Buxton R C, Tan C S, Khine N M, Cuasay N S, Shor M J, Spigos D G
Atypical transmural thoracic lipoma: CT diagnosis
J Comput Assist Tomogr 1988 Mar-Apr, Vol. 12 (2), P. 196–8

945. Caskey C I, Zerhouni E A, Fishman E K, Rahmouni A D
Aging of the diaphragm: a CT study
Radiology 1989 May, Vol. 171 (2), P. 385–9

946. Edelstein G, Levitt R G, Slaker D P, Murphy W A
Computed tomography of Tietze syndrome
J Comput Assist Tomogr 1984 Feb, Vol. 8 (1), P. 20–3

947. Faer M J, Burnam R E, Beck C L
Transmural thoracic lipoma: demonstration by computed tomography
Am J Roentgenol 1978 Jan, Vol. 130 (1), P. 161–3

948. Gouliamos A D, Carter B L, Emami B
Computed tomography of the chest wall
Radiology 1980 Feb, Vol. 134 (2), P. 433–6

949. Lackner K, Weiand G, Koster O
Erweiterung der Röntgendiagnostik raumfordernder Prozesse der Thoraxwand durch die Computertomographie
Improved radiographic diagnosis of expanding lesions of the thoracic wall by computer tomography
RÖFO 1981 Jun, Vol. 134 (6), P. 607–13

950. Pearlberg J L, Sandler M A, Beute G H, Lewis J W Jr, Madrazo B L
Limitations of CT in evaluation of neoplasms involving chest wall
J Comput Assist Tomogr 1987 Mar-Apr, Vol. 11 (2), P. 290–3

951. Pennes D R, Glazer G M, Wimbish K J, Gross B H, Long R W, Orringer M B
Chest wall invasion by lung cancer: limitations of CT evaluation
Am J Roentgenol 1985 Mar, Vol. 144 (3), P. 507–11

952. Press G A, Glazer H S, Wasserman T H, Aronberg D J, Lee J K, Sagel S S
Thoracic wall involvement by Hodgkin disease and non- Hodgkin lymphoma: CT evaluation
Radiology 1985 Oct, Vol. 157 (1), P. 195–8

953. Shea W J Jr, de Geer G, Webb W R
Chest wall after mastectomy. Part II. CT appearance of tumor recurrence
Radiology 1987 Jan, Vol. 162 (1 Pt 1), P. 162–4

954. Shea W J Jr, de Geer G, Webb W R
Chest wall after mastectomy. Part I. CT appearance of normal postoperative anatomy, postirradiation changes, and optimal scanning techniques
Radiology 1987 Jan, Vol. 162 (1 Pt 1), P. 157–61

955. Webb W R, Sagel S S
Actinomycosis involving the chest wall: CT findings
Am J Roentgenol 1982 Nov, Vol. 139 (5), P. 1007–9

The Liver

956. Adkins M C, Halvorsen R A Jr, duCret R P
CT evaluation of atypical hepatic fatty metamorphosis
J Comput Assist Tomogr 1990 Nov-Dec, Vol. 14 (6), P. 1013–5

957. Adler J
Venous calcifications associated with cavernous transformation of the portal vein: computed tomographic and angiographic correlations
Radiology 1979 Jul, Vol. 132 (1), P. 27–8

958. Ahmadi J, Miller C A, Segall H D, Park S H, Zee C S, Becker R L
CT patterns in histopathologically complex cavernous hemangiomas
AJNR 1985 May-Jun, Vol. 6 (3), P. 389–93

959. Alderson P O, Adams D F, McNeil B J, Sanders R, Siegelman S S, Finberg H J, Hessel S J, Abrams H L
Computed tomography, ultrasound, and scintigraphy of the liver in patients with colon or breast carcinoma: a prospective comparison
Radiology 1983 Oct, Vol. 149 (1), P. 225–30

960. Alpern M B, Lawson T L, Foley W D, Perlman S J, Reif L J, Arevalos E, Rimm A A
Focal hepatic masses and fatty infiltration detected by enhanced dynamic CT
Radiology 1986 Jan, Vol. 158 (1), P. 45–9

961. Alspaugh J P, Bernardino M E, Sewell C W, Sones P J Jr, Berkman W A, Price R B
CT directed hepatic biopsies: increased diagnostic accuracy with low patient risk
J Comput Assist Tomogr 1983 Dec, Vol. 7 (6), P. 1012–7

962. Amendola M A, Blane C E, Amendola B E, Glazer G M
CT findings in hepatoblastoma
J Comput Assist Tomogr 1984 Dec, Vol. 8 (6), P. 1105–9

963. Ament A E, Haaga J R, Wiedenmann S D, Barkmeier J D, Morrison S C
Primary sclerosing cholangitis: CT findings
J Comput Assist Tomogr 1983 Oct, Vol. 7 (5), P. 795–800

964. Andoh K, Tanohata K, Asakura K, Katsumata Y, Nagashima T, Kitoh F
CT demonstration of portal vein aneurysm
J Comput Assist Tomogr 1988 Mar-Apr, Vol. 12 (2), P. 325–7

965. Ashida C, Fishman E K, Zerhouni E A, Herlong F H, Siegelman S S
Computed tomography of hepatic cavernous hemangioma
J Comput Assist Tomogr 1987 May-Jun, Vol. 11 (3), P. 455–60

966. Auh Y H, Rubenstein W A, Zirinsky K, Kneeland J B, Pardes J C, Engel I A, Whalen J P, Kazam E
Accessory fissures of the liver: CT and sonographic appearance
Am J Roentgenol 1984 Sep, Vol. 143 (3), P. 565–72

967. Axel L, Moss A A, Berninger W
Dynamic computed tomography demonstration of hepatic arteriovenous fistula
J Comput Assist Tomogr 1981 Feb, Vol. 5 (1), P. 95–8

968. Baert A L, Wilms G, Marchal G, de Somer P, de Maeyer P, Ponette E
Die Aussage der Computer-Tomographie bei der Leberzirrhose
CT of the liver in cirrhosis
Radiologe 1980 Jul, Vol. 20 (7), P. 343–6

969. Baker M E, Silverman P M
Nodular focal fatty infiltration of the liver: CT appearance
Am J Roentgenol 1985 Jul, Vol. 145 (1), P. 79–80

970. Baker M E, Silverman P M, Halvorsen R A Jr, Cohan R H
Computed tomography of masses in periportal/hepatoduodenal ligament
J Comput Assist Tomogr 1987 Mar-Apr, Vol. 11 (2), P. 258–63

971. Bankoff M S, Tuckman G A, Scarborough D
CT appearance of liver metastases from medullary carcinoma of the thyroid
J Comput Assist Tomogr 1987 Nov-Dec, Vol. 11 (6), P. 1102–3

972. Barnes P A, Thomas J L, Bernardino M E
Pitfalls in the diagnosis of hepatic cysts by computed tomography
Radiology 1981 Oct, Vol. 141 (1), P. 129–33

973. Barnett P H, Zerhouni E A, White R I Jr, Siegelman S S
Computed tomography in the diagnosis of cavernous hemangioma of the liver
Am J Roentgenol 1980 Mar, Vol. 134 (3), P. 439–47

974. Bashist B, Hecht H L, Harley W D
Computed tomographic demonstration of rapid changes in fatty infiltration of the liver
Radiology 1982 Mar, Vol. 142 (3), P. 691–2

975. Bechtold R E, Karstaedt N, Wolfman N T, Glass T A
Prolonged hepatic enhancement on computed tomography in a case of hepatic lymphoma
J Comput Assist Tomogr 1985 Jan-Feb, Vol. 9 (1), P. 186–9

976. Belton R L, VanZandt T F
Congenital absence of the left lobe of the liver: a radiologic diagnosis
Radiology 1983 Apr, Vol. 147 (1), P. 184

977. Berland L L, Lawson T L, Foley W D, Melrose B L, Chintapalli K N, Taylor A J
Comparison of pre- and postcontrast CT in hepatic masses
Am J Roentgenol 1982 May, Vol. 138 (5), P. 853–8

978. Bernardino M E
Computed tomography of calcified liver metastases
J Comput Assist Tomogr 1979 Feb, Vol. 3 (1), P. 32–5

979. Bernardino M E, Berkman W A, Plemmons M, Sones P J Jr, Price R B, Casarella W J
Percutaneous drainage of multiseptated hepatic abscess
J Comput Assist Tomogr 1984 Feb, Vol. 8 (1), P. 38–41

980. Biondetti P R, Fiore D, Muzzio P C
Computed tomography of the liver in von Gierke's disease
J Comput Assist Tomogr 1980 Oct, Vol. 4 (5), P. 685–6

981. Boechat M I, Kangarloo H, Ortega J, Hall T, Feig S, Stanley P, Gilsanz V
Primary liver tumors in children: comparison of CT and MR imaging
Radiology 1988 Dec, Vol. 169 (3), P. 727–32

982. Brandt J, Schaffstein J, Schafer K, Eickhoff U
Arterioportale Fistel im CT
RÖFO 1989 Mar, Vol. 150 (3), P. 354–5

983. Brendel A J, Leccia F, Drouillard J, San Galli F, Eresue J, Wynchank S, Barat J L, Ducassou D
Single photon emission computed tomography SPECT, planar scintigraphy, and transmission computed tomography: a comparison of accuracy in diagnosing focal hepatic disease
Radiology 1984 Nov, Vol. 153 (2), P. 527–32

984. Bressler E L, Alpern M B, Glazer G M, Francis I R, Ensminger W D
Hypervascular hepatic metastases: CT evaluation
Radiology 1987 Jan, Vol. 162 (1 Pt 1), P. 49–51

985. Brick S H, Hill M C, Lande A
The mistaken or indeterminate CT diagnosis of hepatic metastases: the value of sonography
Am J Roentgenol 1987 Apr, Vol. 148 (4), P. 723–6

986. Brick S H, Taylor G A, Potter B M, Eichelberger M R
Hepatic and splenic injury in children: role of CT in the decision for laparotomy
Radiology 1987 Dec, Vol. 165 (3), P. 643–6

987. Burgener F A, Hamlin D J
Contrast enhancement of focal hepatic lesions in CT: effect of size and histology
Am J Roentgenol 1983 Feb, Vol. 140 (2), P. 297–301

988. Burgener F A, Hamlin D J
Contrast enhancement of hepatic tumors in CT: comparison between bolus and infusion techniques
Am J Roentgenol 1983 Feb, Vol. 140 (2), P. 291–5

989. Callen P W, Filly R A, Marcus F T
Ultrasonography and computed tomography in the evaluation of hepatic microabscesses in the immunosuppressed patient
Radiology 1980 Aug, Vol. 136 (2), P. 433–4

990. Cates J D, Thorsen M K, Foley W D, Lawson T L
CT diagnosis of massive hemorrhage from hepatocellular carcinoma
J Comput Assist Tomogr 1987 Jan-Feb, Vol. 11 (1), P. 81–2

991. Choi B I, Kim H J, Han M C, Do Y S, Han M H, Lee S H
CT findings of clonorchiasis
Am J Roentgenol 1989 Feb, Vol. 152 (2), P. 281–4

992. Choi B I, Han M C, Park J H, Kim S H, Han M H, Kim C W
Giant cavernous hemangioma of the liver: CT and MR imaging in 10 cases
Am J Roentgenol 1989 Jun, Vol. 152 (6), P. 1221–6

993. Couanet D, Shirkhoda A, Wallace S
Computed tomography after partial hepatectomy
J Comput Assist Tomogr 1984 Jun, Vol. 8 (3), P. 453–7

994. Cunningham D G, Churchill R J, Reynes C J
Computed tomography in the evaluation of liver disease in cystic fibrosis patients
J Comput Assist Tomogr 1980 Apr, Vol. 4 (2), P. 151–4

995. Cutillo D P, Swayne L C, Fasciano M G, Schwartz J R
Absence of fatty replacement in radiation damaged liver: CT demonstration
J Comput Assist Tomogr 1989 Mar-Apr, Vol. 13 (2), P. 259–61

996. Danielson K S, Sheedy P F, Stephens D H, Hattery R R, LaRusso N F
Computed tomography and peritoneoscopy for detection of liver metastases: review of Mayo Clinic experience
J Comput Assist Tomogr 1983 Apr, Vol. 7 (2), P. 230–4

997. de Diego Choliz J, Lecumberri Olaverri F J, Franquet Casas T, Ostiz Zubieta S
Computed tomography in hepatic echinococcosis
Am J Roentgenol 1982 Oct, Vol. 139 (4), P. 699–702

998. Demaerel P, Marchal G, Van Steenbergen W, Fevery J, Van Damme B, Baert A L
CT demonstration of right hepatic lobe atrophy
J Comput Assist Tomogr 1989 Mar-Apr, Vol. 13 (2), P. 351–3

999. Dick L, Parker L A, Mauro M A
Chronic arsenic poisoning as a cause of increased hepatic density with CT
J Comput Assist Tomogr 1990 Sep-Oct, Vol. 14 (5), P. 828–9

1000. Didier D, Weiler S, Rohmer P, Lassegue A, Deschamps J P, Vuitton D, Miguet J P, Weill F
Hepatic alveolar echinococcosis: correlative US and CT study
Radiology 1985 Jan, Vol. 154 (1), P. 179–86

1001. Dixon A K, Walshe J M
Computed tomography of the liver in Wilson disease
J Comput Assist Tomogr 1984 Feb, Vol. 8 (1), P. 46–9

1002. Dixon G D
Combined CT and fluoroscopic guidance for liver abscess drainage
Am J Roentgenol 1980 Aug, Vol. 135 (2), P. 397–9

1003. Djang W T, Young S W, Castellino R A, Lantieri R
Computed tomography of the liver: evaluating focal defects on radionuclide liver-spleen scans
Am J Roentgenol 1984 May, Vol. 142 (5), P. 937–40

1004. Donaldson J S, Fabian T M, Billimoria P E
CT appearance of hepatic oil embolization following lymphangiography
J Comput Assist Tomogr 1984 Oct, Vol. 8 (5), P. 1012–4

1005. Doppman J L, Cornblath M, Dwyer A J, Adams A J, Girton M E, Sidbury J
Computed tomography of the liver and kidneys in glycogen storage disease
J Comput Assist Tomogr 1982 Feb, Vol. 6 (1), P. 67–71

1006. Doppman J L, Dwyer A, Vermess M, Girton M, Sugarbaker P, Miller D, Cornblath M
Segmental hyperlucent defects in the liver
J Comput Assist Tomogr 1984 Feb, Vol. 8 (1), P. 50–7

1007. DuBrow R A, David C L, Libshitz H I, Lorigan J G
Detection of hepatic metastases in breast cancer: the role of nonenhanced and enhanced CT scanning
J Comput Assist Tomogr 1990 May-Jun, Vol. 14 (3), P. 366–9

1008. Duewell S, Marincek B, von Schulthess G K, Ammann R
MRT und CT bei alveolärer Echinokokkose der Leber
MRT and CT in alveolar echinococcosis of the liver
RÖFO 1990 Apr, Vol. 152 (4), P. 441–5

1009. Dunnick N R, Ihde D C, Doppman J L, Bates H R
Computed tomography in primary hepatocellular carcinoma
J Comput Assist Tomogr 1980 Feb, Vol. 4 (1), P. 59–62

1010. Eising E G, Montag M, Mayer J
Unklarer Prozeß im CT der Leber. Caroli-Syndrom
An unclear process in CT of the liver. Caroli syndrome
Radiologe 1989 Nov, Vol. 29 (11), P. 577–9

1011. Fahrendorf G, Fischedick A R
Aneurysma der Vena portae. Sonographische und computertomographische Diagnostik
Portal vein aneurysm. Sonographic and computerized tomographic diagnosis
RÖFO 1986 Jun, Vol. 144 (6), P. 732–4

1012. Fataar S, Bassiony H, Satyanath S, Rudwan M A, Khaffaji S, el Magdy W, Al Ansari A G, Hanna R
CT of hepatic schistosomiasis mansoni
Am J Roentgenol 1985 Jul, Vol. 145 (1), P. 63–6

1013. Federle M P, Filly R A, Moss A A
Cystic hepatic neoplasms: complementary roles of CT and sonography
Am J Roentgenol 1981 Feb, Vol. 136 (2), P. 345–8

1014. Feuerbach S, Rupp N, Reiser M, Emmerich B
Lipiodolembolie der Leber im Computertomogramm
Lipiodol embolism of the liver on a computer tomogram
RÖFO 1981 Nov, Vol. 135 (5), P. 604–5

1015. Fiegler W, Schutz H, Claussen C, Schorner W, Felix R
Herdförmige Lebererkrankungen. Vergleichsstudie Computertomographie, konventioneller Ultraschall, automatisierter Multisektorscanner (Octoson)
Focal liver diseases. Comparative study of computed tomography, conventional ultrasound and the automated multisector scanner Octoson
RÖFO 1984 Jul, Vol. 141 (1), P. 71–4

1016. Fischedick A R, Rosler H
Zur Diagnostik des Caroli- Syndroms mit hepatobiliärer Sequenzszintigraphie
Diagnosis of Caroli syndrome with hepatobiliary sequence scintigraphy
RÖFO 1980 Nov, Vol. 133 (5), P. 547–9

1017. Fischedick A R, Peters P E, Muller R P
Computertomographische Diagnostik des Caroli-Syndroms
Computer tomographic diagnosis of Caroli's syndrome
RÖFO 1982 Jan, Vol. 136 (1), P. 74–7

1018. Fishman E K, Farmlett E, Kadir S, Siegelman S S
Computed tomography of benign hepatic tumors
J Comput Assist Tomogr 1982 Jun, Vol. 6 (3), P. 472–81

1019. Flentje M, Hohenberger P, Adolph J, Kober B
Intraarterielle dynamische Computertomographie in der Charakterisierung von Lebermetastasen kolorektaler Karzinome
Intra-arterial dynamic computed tomography in characterizing liver metastases of colorectal cancer
RÖFO 1986 Sep, Vol. 145 (3), P. 263–7

1020. Flournoy J G, Potter J L, Sullivan B M, Gerza C B, Ramzy I
CT appearance of multifocal hepatic steatosis
J Comput Assist Tomogr 1984 Dec, Vol. 8 (6), P. 1192–4

1021. Fobbe F, Hamm B, Schwarting R
Angiomyolipoma of the liver: CT, MR, and ultrasound imaging
J Comput Assist Tomogr 1988 Jul-Aug, Vol. 12 (4), P. 658–9

1022. Foley W D, Berland L L, Lawson T L, Smith D F, Thorsen M K
Contrast enhancement technique for dynamic hepatic computed tomographic scanning
Radiology 1983 Jun, Vol. 147 (3), P. 797–803

1023. Foley W D, Varma R R, Lawson T L, Berland L L, Smith D F, Thorsen K
Dynamic computed tomography and duplex ultrasonography: adjuncts to arterial portography
J Comput Assist Tomogr 1983 Feb, Vol. 7 (1), P. 77–82

1024. Foley W D, Cates J D, Kellman G M, Langdon T, Aprahamian C, Lawson T L, Middleton W D
Treatment of blunt hepatic injuries: role of CT
Radiology 1987 Sep, Vol. 164 (3), P. 635–8

1025. Foley W D
Dynamic hepatic CT scanning
Am J Roentgenol 1989 Feb, Vol. 152 (2), P. 272–4

1026. Foley W D
Dynamic hepatic CT
Radiology 1989 Mar, Vol. 170 (3 Pt 1), P. 617–22

1027. Freeny P C
Portal vein tumor thrombus: demonstration by computed tomographic ateriography
J Comput Assist Tomogr 1980 Apr, Vol. 4 (2), P. 263–4

1028. Freeny P C, Marks W M
Computed tomographic arteriography of the liver
Radiology 1983 Jul, Vol. 148 (1), P. 193–7

1029. Freeny P C, Marks W M
Hepatic hemangioma: dynamic bolus CT
Am J Roentgenol 1986 Oct, Vol. 147 (4), P. 711–9

1030. Freeny P C, Marks W M
Patterns of contrast enhancement of benign and malignant hepatic neoplasms during bolus dynamic and delayed CT
Radiology 1986 Sep, Vol. 160 (3), P. 613–8

1031. Freeny P C, Marks W M
Hepatic perfusion abnormalities during CT angiography: detection and interpretation
Radiology 1986 Jun, Vol. 159 (3), P. 685–91

1032. Freeny P C
Hepatic CT: state of the art
Radiology 1988 Aug, Vol. 168 (2), P. 319–23

1033. Fretz C J, Stark D D, Metz C E, Elizondo G, Weissleder R, Shen J H, Wittenberg J, Simeone J, Ferrucci J T
Detection of hepatic metastases: comparison of contrast-enhanced CT, unenhanced MR imaging, and iron oxide-enhanced MR imaging
Am J Roentgenol 1990 Oct, Vol. 155 (4), P. 763–70

1034. Friedrich M, Ziegler U, Albrecht A
Toxocariasis (visceral larva migrans) der Leber. Computertomographische Aspekte
Toxocariasis visceral larva migrans of the liver. The computed tomographic aspects
RÖFO 1987 May, Vol. 146 (5), P. 600–2

1035. Fritschy P, Schneekloth G
Praktische Probleme der Lebervolumenbestimmung aus computertomographischen Transversalschnitten
Practical problems of determining liver volume from computed tomographic transverse sections
RÖFO 1983 Apr, Vol. 138 (4), P. 453–7

1036. Ginaldi S, Chuang V P, Wallace S
Absence of hepatic segment of the inferior vena cava with azygous continuation
J Comput Assist Tomogr 1980 Feb, Vol. 4 (1), P. 112–4

1037. Giyanani V L, Meyers P C, Wolfson J J
Mesenchymal hamartoma of the liver: computed tomography and ultrasonography
J Comput Assist Tomogr 1986 Jan-Feb, Vol. 10 (1), P. 51–4

1038. Goldberg H I, Moss A A
CT of noncystic liver lesions letter
Am J Roentgenol 1981 Mar, Vol. 136 (3), P. 635

1039. Gonzalez L R, Marcos J, Illanas M, Hernandez Mora M, Pena F, Picouto J P, Cienfuegos J A, Alvarez J L
Radiologic aspects of hepatic echinococcosis. Value of the intravenous viscerogram and computed tomography
Radiology 1979 Jan, Vol. 130 (1), P. 21–7

1040. Goodman A, Harries Jones E P, Lipinski J K
Two unusual causes of jaundice with similar ultrasound and CT findings
J Comput Assist Tomogr 1984 Dec, Vol. 8 (6), P. 1110–3

1041. Gostner P, Fugazzola C, Martin F, Marzoli G P
Der Pfortaderkreislauf nach der Warrenschen Operation. Langzeitkontrollen mit der Computertomographie
Portal circulation following Warren's operation. Long-term control using computerized tomography
RÖFO 1986 Jun, Vol. 144 (6), P. 711–6

1042. Grabbe E, Brockmann W P, Klapdor R
Tumorthrombus in der V. portae. Diagnostik durch Sonographie und CT
Tumor thrombus in the portal vein. Diagnosis by sonography and CT
RÖFO 1981 Mar, Vol. 134 (3), P. 330–2

1043. Grabenwoger F, Dock W, Pichler W, Farres M T, Metz V
Diagnostik des Lebertraumas: Ultraschall versus Computertomographie
RÖFO 1989 Feb, Vol. 150 (2), P. 163–6

1044. Grant T, Brandt T D
Use of the cluster sign in the diagnosis of small pyogenic hepatic abscesses letter; comment
Am J Roentgenol 1989 Aug, Vol. 153 (2), P. 429–30

1045. Grote R, Schmoll E, Rosenthal H, Bokemeier B
Chemoembolisation hepatozellulärer Karzinome – computertomographische Verlaufsbeobachtung
Chemoembolisation of hepatocellular carcinoma – computed tomographic follow-up observation
RÖFO 1989 Jul, Vol. 151 (1), P. 15–22

1046. Haaga J R, Weinstein A J
CT-guided percutaneous aspiration and drainage of abscesses
Am J Roentgenol 1980 Dec, Vol. 135 (6), P. 1187–94

1047. Haertel M
Das kavernöse Leberhämangiom im Computertomogramm
Computer tomographic findings in cavernous haemangiomas of the liver
RÖFO 1980 Oct, Vol. 133 (4), P. 379–81

1048. Hall F M, Hurwitz E F, Royal H D
Radionuclide and CT diagnosis: cavernous hemangioma of liver letter
Am J Roentgenol 1980 Aug, Vol. 135 (2), P. 424–5

1049. Halvorsen R A, Korobkin M, Ram P C, Thompson W M
CT appearance of focal fatty infiltration of the liver
Am J Roentgenol 1982 Aug, Vol. 139 (2), P. 277–81

1050. Halvorsen R A, Korobkin M, Foster W L, Silverman P M, Thompson W M
The variable CT appearance of hepatic abscesses
Am J Roentgenol 1984 May, Vol. 142 (5), P. 941–6

1051. Hamm B, Romer T, Friedrich M, Felix R, Wolf K J
Magnetische Resonanztomographie fokaler Leberläsionen im Vergleich zur Computertomographie und Sonographie
Magnetic resonance tomography of focal liver lesions in comparison with computed tomography and sonography
RÖFO 1986 Mar, Vol. 144 (3), P. 278–86

1052. Hammerman A M, Kotner L M Jr, Doyle T B
Periportal contrast enhancement on CT scans of the liver
Am J Roentgenol 1991 Feb, Vol. 156 (2), P. 313–5

1053. Haney P J, Whitley N O, Brotman S, Cunat J S, Whitley J
Liver injury and complications in the postoperative trauma patient: CT evaluation
Am J Roentgenol 1982 Aug, Vol. 139 (2), P. 271–5

1054. Harbin W P, Robert N J, Ferrucci J T Jr
Diagnosis of cirrhosis based on regional changes in hepatic morphology: a radiological and pathological analysis
Radiology 1980 May, Vol. 135 (2), P. 273–83

1055. Harter L P, Gross B H, St Hilaire J, Filly R A, Goldberg H I
CT and sonographic appearance of hepatic vein obstruction
Am J Roentgenol 1982 Jul, Vol. 139 (1), P. 176–8

1056. Hauenstein K H, Wimmer B, Friedburg H, Hennig J
Aussagekraft der Kernspintomographie im Vergleich zur Sonographie und Computertomographie in der Diagnostik fokaler Leberläsionen
Predictive value of magnetic resonance tomography in comparison with sonography and computed tomography in the diagnosis of focal liver lesions
Radiologe 1988 Aug, Vol. 28 (8), P. 362–9

1057. Hayashi N, Yamamoto K, Tamaki N, Shibata T, Itoh K, Fujisawa I, Nakano Y, Yamaoka Y, Kobayashi N, Mori K, et al
Metastatic nodules of hepatocellular carcinoma: detection with angiography, CT, and US
Radiology 1987 Oct, Vol. 165 (1), P. 61–3

1058. Heiken J P, Lee J K, Glazer H S, Ling D
Hepatic metastases studied with MR and CT
Radiology 1985 Aug, Vol. 156 (2), P. 423–7

1059. Heiken J P, Weyman P J, Lee J K, Balfe D M, Picus D, Brunt E M, Flye M W
Detection of focal hepatic masses: prospective evaluation with CT, delayed CT, CT during arterial portography, and MR imaging
Radiology 1989 Apr, Vol. 171 (1), P. 47–51

1060. Herman T E, Siegel M J
Central dot sign on CT of liver cysts
J Comput Assist Tomogr 1990 Nov-Dec, Vol. 14 (6), P. 1019–21

1061. Hodler J, Meier P
Leberbefall bei Fasciola hepatica: Sonographie und CT
Liver involvement by Fasciola hepatica: sonography and CT
RÖFO 1989 Dec, Vol. 151 (6), P. 740–1

1062. Hoevels J, Saeger H D
Computertomographische Studie der portalvenösen Kontrastmittelperfusion der Leber
Computed tomographic study of portal venous contrast medium perfusion of the liver
RÖFO 1986 Jan, Vol. 144 (1), P. 52–6

1063. Holley H C, Koslin D B, Berland L L, Stanley R J
Inhomogeneous enhancement of liver parenchyma secondary to passive congestion: contrast-enhanced CT
Radiology 1989 Mar, Vol. 170 (3 Pt 1), P. 795–800

1064. Honda H, Franken E A Jr, Barloon T J, Smith J L
Hepatic lymphoma in cyclosporine-treated transplant recipients: sonographic and CT findings
Am J Roentgenol 1989 Mar, Vol. 152 (3), P. 501–3

1065. Hosoki T, Chatani M, Mori S
Dynamic computed tomography of hepatocellular carcinoma
Am J Roentgenol 1982 Dec, Vol. 139 (6), P. 1099–106

1066. Hosoki T, Toyonaga Y, Araki Y, Mori S
Dynamic computed tomography of isodense hepatocellular carcinoma
J Comput Assist Tomogr 1984 Apr, Vol. 8 (2), P. 263–8

1067. Hruby W, Traxler M, Wassipaul M, Stellamor K
Vergleich zwischen Ultraschall- und CT-Diagnostik solider Lebertumoren
Comparison of ultrasonic and CT diagnosis of solid liver tumors
RÖFO 1988 Apr, Vol. 148 (4), P. 378–83

1068. Hubener K H
Computertomographische Densitometrie von Leber, Milz und Nieren bei intravenös verabreichten lebergängigen Kontrastmitteln in Bolusform
Densitometry via CT scan of liver, spleen and kidneys with bolus-shaped liver contrast media by the intravenous route
RÖFO 1978 Sep, Vol. 129 (3), P. 289–97

1069. Imaeda T, Yamawaki Y, Hirota K, Suzuki M, Seki M, Doi H
Tumor thrombus in the branches of the distal portal vein: CT demonstration
J Comput Assist Tomogr 1989 Mar-Apr, Vol. 13 (2), P. 262–8

1070. Inamoto K, Sugiki K, Yamasaki H, Miura T
CT of hepatoma: effects of portal vein obstruction
Am J Roentgenol 1981 Feb, Vol. 136 (2), P. 349–53

1071. Ishikawa I, Tateishi K, Shinoda A, Onouchi Z, Saito Y, Asato T
Changes of the hepatic CT absorption value in hemodialysis patients
J Comput Assist Tomogr 1984 Aug, Vol. 8 (4), P. 701–3

1072. Ishikawa I, Masuzaki S, Saito T, Tateishi K, Kitada H, Yuri T, Shinoda A, Onouchi Z, Saito Y, Futyu Y
Dynamic computed tomography in acute renal failure: analysis of time-density curve
J Comput Assist Tomogr 1985 Nov-Dec, Vol. 9 (6), P. 1097–102

1073. Ishikawa I, Saito Y, Onouchi Z, Matsuura H, Saito T, Suzuki M, Futyu Y
Delayed contrast enhancement in acute focal bacterial nephritis: CT features
J Comput Assist Tomogr 1985 Sep-Oct, Vol. 9 (5), P. 894–7

1074. Ishikawa N, Nakagawa K, Hirata K, Takizawa Y, Hayashi S, Obara T, Ishikawa T
Long-term follow-up of hepatitis using computed tomography
J Comput Assist Tomogr 1989 Jul-Aug, Vol. 13 (4), P. 645–9

1075. Ishikawa T, Tsukune Y, Ohyama Y, Fujikawa M, Sakuyama K, Fujii M
Venous abnormalities in portal hypertension demonstrated by CT
Am J Roentgenol 1980 Feb, Vol. 134 (2), P. 271–6

1076. Ishikawa T, Clark R A, Tokuda M, Ashida H
Focal contrast enhancement on hepatic CT in superior vena caval and brachiocephalic vein obstruction
Am J Roentgenol 1983 Feb, Vol. 140 (2), P. 337–8

1077. Ishikawa T
"Hot spot" in liver may represent collateral blood flow letter
Am J Roentgenol 1984 Mar, Vol. 142 (3), P. 649–50

1078. Itai Y, Furui S, Araki T, Yashiro N, Tasaka A
Computed tomography of cavernous hemangioma of the liver
Radiology 1980 Oct, Vol. 137 (1 Pt 1), P. 149–55

1079. Itai Y, Araki T, Furui S, Tasaka A, Atomi Y, Kuroda A
Computed tomography and ultrasound in the diagnosis of intrahepatic calculi
Radiology 1980 Aug, Vol. 136 (2), P. 399–405

1080. Itai Y, Araki T, Furui S, Tasaka A
Differential Diagnosis of hepatic masses on computed tomography, with particular reference to hepatocellular carcinoma
J Comput Assist Tomogr 1981, Vol.5(6) P.834–42

1081. Itai Y, Moss A A, Goldberg H I
Transient hepatic attenuation difference of lobar or segmental distribution detected by dynamic computed tomography
Radiology 1982 Sep, Vol. 144 (4), P. 835–9

1082. Itai Y, Ohtomo K, Araki T, Furui S, Iio M, Atomi Y
Computed tomography and sonography of cavernous hemangioma of the liver
Am J Roentgenol 1983 Aug, Vol. 141 (2), P. 315–20

1083. Itai Y, Furui S, et al
Dynamic CT features of arterioportal shunts in hepatocellular carcinoma
Am J Roentgenol 1986, Vol. 146, P.723–7

1084. Itai Y, Ohtomo K, Kokubo T, Yamauchi T, Okada Y, Makita K
CT demonstration of fluid-fluid levels in nonenhancing hemangiomas of the liver
J Comput Assist Tomogr 1987 Sep-Oct, Vol. 11 (5), P. 763–5

1085. Itai Y, Hachiya J, Makita K, Ohtomo K, Kokubo T, Yamauchi T
Transient hepatic attenuation differences on dynamic computed tomography
J Comput Assist Tomogr 1987 May-Jun, Vol. 11 (3), P. 461–5

1086. Itai Y, Ohtomo K, Kokubo T, Makita K, Okada Y, Machida T, Yashiro N
CT and MR imaging of fatty tumors of the liver
J Comput Assist Tomogr 1987 Mar-Apr, Vol. 11 (2), P. 253–7

1087. Itai Y
Peripheral low-density area of hepatic tumors: CT-pathologic correlation letter
Radiology 1987 Mar, Vol. 162 (3), P. 876

1088. Itai Y, Ohtomo K, Kokubo T, Minami M, Yoshida H
CT and MR imaging of postnecrotic liver scars
J Comput Assist Tomogr 1988 Nov-Dec, Vol. 12 (6), P. 971–5

1089. Itai Y, Araki T, Ohtomo K, Kokubo T, Yoshida H, Minami M, Yashiro N
Well-defined, dense and continuously spreading enhancement on single level dynamic CT of the liver: a characteristic sign of hepatic cavernous haemangioma
RÖFO 1989 Dec, Vol. 151 (6), P. 697–701

1090. Janson R, Lackner K, Paquet K J, Thelen M, Thurn P
Computertomographische und angiographische Synopsis histologisch gesicherter intrahepatischer Raumforderungen
Computer tomographic and angiographic studies of histologically confirmed intrahepatic masses
RÖFO 1980 Jun, Vol. 132 (6), P. 658–65

1091. Jeffrey R B Jr, Tolentino C S, Chang F C, Federle M P
CT of small pyogenic hepatic abscesses: the cluster sign see comments
Am J Roentgenol 1988 Sep, Vol. 151 (3), P. 487–9

1092. Jeffrey R B Jr
CT diagnosis of blunt hepatic and splenic injuries: a look to the future editorial
Radiology 1989 Apr, Vol. 171 (1), P. 17–8

1093. Johnson C M, Sheedy P F, Stanson A W, Stephens D H, Hattery R R, Adson M A
Computed tomography and angiography of cavernous hemangiomas of the liver
Radiology 1981 Jan, Vol. 138 (1), P. 115–21

1094. Kaplan S B, Sumkin J H, Campbell W L, Zajko A B, Demetris A J
Periportal low-attenuation areas on CT: value as evidence of liver transplant rejection
Am J Roentgenol 1989 Feb, Vol. 152 (2), P. 285–7

1095. Kathrein H, Judmaier G, Vogel W
Lymphadenopathy in primary biliary cirrhosis: CT observations letter
Radiology 1990 Apr, Vol. 175 (1), P. 285–6

1096. Kaurich J D, Coombs R J, Zeiss J
Myelolipoma of the liver: CT features
J Comput Assist Tomogr 1988 Jul-Aug, Vol. 12 (4), P. 660–1

1097. Kawashima A, Suehiro S, Murayama S, Russell W J
Focal fatty infiltration of the liver mimicking a tumor: sonographic and CT features
J Comput Assist Tomogr 1986 Mar-Apr, Vol. 10 (2), P. 329–31

1098. Kier R, Rosenfield A T
Focal nodular hyperplasia of the liver on delayed enhanced CT letter
Am J Roentgenol 1989 Oct, Vol. 153 (4), P. 885–6

1099. Kimura A, Makuuchi M, Takayasu K, Sakamoto M, Hirohashi S
Ciliated hepatic foregut cyst with solid tumor appearance on CT
J Comput Assist Tomogr 1990 Nov-Dec, Vol. 14 (6), P. 1016–8

1100. Klose K C, Skora T
Mastozytom der Leber – Computertomographische Verlaufsbeobachtung und Biopsie
A mastocytoma of the liver – computed tomographic follow-up and biopsy
Radiologe 1990 Feb, Vol. 30 (2), P. 81–3

1101. Knopf D R, Torres W E, Fajman W J, Sones P J Jr
Liver lesions: comparative accuracy of scintigraphy and computed tomography
Am J Roentgenol 1982 Apr, Vol. 138 (4), P. 623–7

1102. Kobayashi A, Sugihara M, Kurosaki M, Ishida Y, Takayanagi N, Matsui O, Takashima T
CT characteristics of intrahepatic, periportal, extramedullary hematopoiesis
J Comput Assist Tomogr 1989 Mar-Apr, Vol. 13 (2), P. 354–6

1103. Kober B, Gamroth A, Hermann H J, zum Winkel K, Mende U, Kimmig B
Angio-CT: Eine Erweiterung der Diagnostik maligner Leberprozesse
Angio-CT: an improvement in the diagnosis of malignant liver diseases
RÖFO 1983 Sep, Vol. 139 (3), P. 260–6

1104. Kober B, Flentje M, Adolph J, Rieden K, Bieber J, zum Winkel K
Funktionelle Heterogenität von Lebermetastasen im Dreiphasen-Computertomogramm
Functional heterogeneity of liver metastases in 3-phase computerized tomograms
RÖFO 1986 Jun, Vol. 144 (6), P. 707–12

1105. Kokubo T, Itoh K, Kondoh S, Kojima K, Ohtomo K
CT demonstration of a bizarre intrahepatic portal branch
J Comput Assist Tomogr 1987 Mar-Apr, Vol. 11 (3), P. 365–7

1106. Koppenhofer H, van Kaick G
Sonographischer und computertomographischer Nachweis eines Cruveilhier-von Baumgarten-Syndroms
Cruveilhier-von Baumgarten-syndrom. Evaluation by ultrasound and computerized tomography
Radiologe 1980 Jan, Vol. 20 (1), P. 35–7

1107. Koslin D B, Stanley R J, Berland L L, Shin M S, Dalton S C
Hepatic perivascular lymphedema: CT appearance
Am J Roentgenol 1988 Jan, Vol. 150 (1), P. 111–3

1108. Koster O, Lelbach W K, Leipner N, Distelmaier W
Maligne mesenchymale Lebertumoren im Computertomogramm
Malignant mesenchymal liver tumors in the computed tomogram
RÖFO 1983 Oct, Vol. 139 (4), P. 394–9

1109. Koster O, Fischer P, Lindecken K D, Lackner K
Computertomographische Befunde bei portaler Hypertension infolge Leberzirrhose. Teil 3: Hämodynamische Veränderungen – Angio- CT
Computed tomographic findings in portal hypertension secondary to liver cirrhosis. 3. Hemodynamic changes – angio-CT
RÖFO 1984 Mar, Vol. 140 (3), P. 308–13

1110. Koster O, Rau W, Lackner K, Koischwitz D
Sonographie und Computertomographie vor und nach Leberresektion und - transplantation
Sonography and computed tomography before and after liver resection and transplantation
RÖFO 1986 Jan, Vol. 144 (1), P. 56–62

1111. Koster O, Harder T, Steudel A, Sommer H J
CT-Portographie bei malignen Raumforderungen der Leber
CT portography in malignant space-occupying lesions of the liver
RÖFO 1989 Feb, Vol. 150 (2), P. 156–62

1112. Krahe T, Harder T, Lackner K
Seriencomputertomographie. Wertigkeit densitometrischer Messungen in der Diagnostik benigner und maligner Läsionen von Leber, Pankreas und Niere
Serial computed tomography. Value of densitometric measurements in the diagnosis of benign and malignant lesions of the liver, pancreas and kidney
RÖFO 1985 Jul, Vol. 143 (1), P. 28–35

1113. Kriegshauser J S, Reading C C, King B F, Welch T J
Combined systemic and portal venous gas: sonographic and CT detection in two cases
Am J Roentgenol 1990 Jun, Vol. 154 (6), P. 1219–21

1114. Kuhns L R, Borlaza G
Normal roentgen variant: aberrant right hepatic artery on computed tomography
Radiology 1980 May, Vol. 135 (2), P. 392

1115. Kunstlinger F, Federle M P, Moss A A, Marks W
Computed tomography of hepatocellular carcinoma
Am J Roentgenol 1980 Mar, Vol. 134 (3), P. 431–7

1116. Kurtz B
Dynamische CT bei Lymphommanifestationen von Leber und Milz
Dynamic CT of lymphoma manifestations of the liver and spleen
RÖFO 1986 Feb, Vol. 144 (2), P. 149–53

1117. Kurtz B, Plauth M, Metzger H
Bedeutung der schnellen sequentiellen Computertomographie für die Diagnostik der Leberzirrhose
Value of rapid sequential computed tomography for the diagnosis of liver cirrhosis
RÖFO 1986 Jan, Vol. 144 (1), P. 46–51

1118. Kvicala V, Vymazal J, Nevsimalova S
Computed tomography of Wilson disease
AJNR 1983 May-Jun, Vol. 4 (3), P. 429–30

1119. Letourneau J G, Day D L, Maile C W, Crass J R, Ascher N L, Frick M P
Liver allograft transplantation: postoperative CT findings
Am J Roentgenol 1987 Jun, Vol. 148 (4), P. 1099–103

1120. Lev Toaff A S, Friedman A C, Cohen L M, Radecki P D, Caroline D F
Hepatic infarcts: new observations by CT and sonography
Am J Roentgenol 1987 Jul, Vol. 149 (1), P. 87–90

1121. Lewis E, Bernardino M E, Barnes P A, Parvey H R, Soo C S, Chuang V P
The fatty liver: pitfalls of the CT and angiographic evaluation of metastatic disease
J Comput Assist Tomogr 1983 Apr, Vol. 7 (2), P. 235–41

1122. Liddell R M, Baron R L, Ekstrom J E, Varnell R M, Shuman W P
Normal intrahepatic bile ducts: CT depiction
Radiology 1990 Sep, Vol. 176 (3), P. 633–5

1123. Lim G M, Jeffrey R B Jr, Ralls P W, Marn C S
Septic thrombosis of the portal vein: CT and clinical observations
J Comput Assist Tomogr 1989 Jul-Aug, Vol. 13 (4), P. 656–8

1124. Lin G, Gustafson T, Hagerstrand I, Lunderquist A
CT demonstration of low density ring in liver metastases
J Comput Assist Tomogr 1984 Jun, Vol. 8 (3), P. 450–2

1125. Long J A Jr, Doppman J L, Nienhus A W, Mills S R
Computed tomographic analysis of beta-thalassemic syndromes with hemochromatosis: pathologic findings with clinical and laboratory correlations
J Comput Assist Tomogr 1980 Apr, Vol. 4 (2), P. 159–65

1126. Longmaid H E, Seltzer S E, Costello P, Gordon P
Hepatocellular carcinoma presenting as primary extrahepatic mass on CT
Am J Roentgenol 1986 May, Vol. 146 (5), P. 1005–9

1127. Lopez Rasines G J, Alonso J R, Longo J M, Pagola M A
Aneurysmal dilatation of the superior mesenteric vein: CT findings
J Comput Assist Tomogr 1985 Jul-Aug, Vol. 9 (4), P. 830–2

1128. Luburich P, Bru C, Ayuso M C, Azon A, Condom E
Hepatic Kaposi sarcoma in AIDS: US and CT findings
Radiology 1990 Apr, Vol. 175 (1), P. 172–4

1129. Luning M, Wolff H, Simon C, Dewey C, Decker T
CT- Diagnostik der fokalen nodulären Hyperplasie
CT diagnosis of focal nodular hyperplasia
RÖFO 1986 Oct, Vol. 145 (4), P. 456–63

1130. Macrander S J, Lawson T L, Foley W D, Dodds W J, Erickson S J, Quiroz F A
Periportal tracking in hepatic trauma: CT features
J Comput Assist Tomogr 1989 Nov-Dec, Vol. 13 (6), P. 952–7

1131. Majewski A, Hendrickx P, Brolsch C, Wiese H
Computertomographische Densitometrie primärer Lebertumoren
Computer tomographic densitometry of primary liver tumors
RÖFO 1983 Jan, Vol. 138 (1), P. 8–14

1132. Marchal G J, Baert A L, Wilms G E
CT of noncystic liver lesions: bolus enhancement
Am J Roentgenol 1980 Jul, Vol. 135 (1), P. 57–65

1133. Marincek B, Barbier P A, Becker C D, Mettler D, Ruchti C
CT appearance of impaired lymphatic drainage in liver transplants
Am J Roentgenol 1986 Sep, Vol. 147 (3), P. 519–23

1134. Marincek B, Thurnher S, Decurtins M, von Schulthess G K, Largiader F
CT und MRT nach Lebertransplantation
CT and MRT following liver transplantation
Radiologe 1988 Dec, Vol. 28 (12), P. 544–8

1135. Martino C R, Haaga J R, Bryan P J, LiPuma J P, El Yousef S J, Alfidi R J
CT-guided liver biopsies: eight years' experience. Work in progress
Radiology 1984 Sep, Vol. 152 (3), P. 755–7

1136. Mathieu D, Larde D, Vasile N
CT features of iatrogenic hepatic arterioportal fistulae
J Comput Assist Tomogr 1983 Oct, Vol. 7 (5), P. 810–4

1137. Mathieu D, Grenier P, Larde D, Vasile N
Portal vein involvement in hepatocellular carcinoma: dynamic CT features
Radiology 1984 Jul, Vol. 152 (1), P. 127–32

1138. Mathieu D, Vasile N, Fagniez P L, Segui S, Grably D, Larde D
Dynamic CT features of hepatic abscesses
Radiology 1985 Mar, Vol. 154 (3), P. 749–52

1139. Mathieu D, Vasile N, Dibie C, Grenier P
Portal cavernoma: dynamic CT features and transient differences in hepatic attenuation
Radiology 1985 Mar, Vol. 154 (3), P. 743–8

1140. Mathieu D, Vasile N, Grenier P
Portal thrombosis: dynamic CT features and course
Radiology 1985 Mar, Vol. 154 (3), P. 737- 41

1141. Mathieu D, Ladeb M F, Guigui B, Rousseau M, Vasile N
Periportal tuberculous adenitis: CT features
Radiology 1986 Dec, Vol. 161 (3), P. 713–5

1142. Mathieu D, Elouaer Blanc L, Divine M, Rene E, Vasile N
Hepatic plasmocytoma: sonographic and CT findings
J Comput Assist Tomogr 1986 Jan-Feb, Vol. 10 (1), P. 144–5

1143. Mathieu D, Vasile N, Menu Y, Van Beers B, Lorphelin J M, Pringot J
Budd-Chiari syndrome: dynamic CT
Radiology 1987 Nov, Vol. 165 (2), P. 409–13

1144. Matsui O, Kadoya M, Suzuki M, Inoue K, Itoh H, Ida M, Takashima T
Work in progress: dynamic sequential computed tomography during arterial portography in the detection of hepatic neoplasms
Radiology 1983 Mar, Vol. 146 (3), P. 721–7

1145. Matsui O, Takashima T, Kadoya M, Ida M, Suzuki M, Kitagawa K, Kamimura R, Inoue K, Konishi H, Itoh H
Dynamic computed tomography during arterial portography: the most sensitive examination for small hepatocellular carcinomas
J Comput Assist Tomogr 1985 Jan-Feb, Vol. 9 (1), P. 19–24

1146. Matsui O, Takashima T, Kadoya M, Suzuki M, Hirose J, Kameyama T, Choto S, Konishi H, Ida M, Yamaguchi A, et al
Liver metastases from colorectal cancers: detection with CT during arterial portography
Radiology 1987 Oct, Vol. 165 (1), P. 65–9

1147. Matsui O
Hepatic metastasis detection: comparison of three CT contrast enhancement methods letter
Radiology 1988 Jul, Vol. 168 (1), P. 283–4

1148. McCain A H, Bernardino M E, Sones P J Jr, Berkman W A, Casarella W J
Varices from portal hypertension: correlation of CT and angiography
Radiology 1985 Jan, Vol. 154 (1), P. 63–9

1149. McDonnell C H, Fishman E K, Zerhouni E A
CT demonstration of calcified liver metastases in medullary thyroid carcinoma
J Comput Assist Tomogr 1986 Nov-Dec, Vol. 10 (6), P. 976–8

1150. Menu Y, Lorphelin J M, Scherrer A, Grenier P, Nahum H
Sonographic and computed tomographic evaluation of intrahepatic calculi
Am J Roentgenol 1985 Sep, Vol. 145 (3), P. 579–83

1151. Merine D, Fishman E K, Sitzmann J V, Kuhlman J E, Order S, Pessar M, Zerhouni E A
Vascular abnormalities following radio- and chemotherapy of hepatic neoplasms: CT angiographic findings
J Comput Assist Tomogr 1988 Jul-Aug, Vol. 12 (4), P. 584–7

1152. Merine D, Takayasu K, Wakao F
Detection of hepatocellular carcinoma: comparison of CT during arterial portography with CT after intraarterial injection of iodized oil
Radiology 1990 Jun, Vol. 175 (3), P. 707–10

1153. Mikulis D J, Costello P, Clouse M E
Hepatic hemangioma: atypical appearance
Am J Roentgenol 1985 Jul, Vol. 145 (1), P. 77–8

1154. Miller D L, Rosenbaum R C, Sugarbaker P H, Vermess M, Willis M, Doppman J L
Detection of hepatic metastases: comparison of EOE-13 computed tomography and scintigraphy
Am J Roentgenol 1983 Nov, Vol. 141 (5), P. 931–5

1155. Miller D L, Schneider P D, Gianola F J, Willis M, Vermess M, Doppman J L
Assessment of perfusion patterns during hepatic artery infusion chemotherapy: EOE-13 CT and 99mTc-MAA scintigraphy
Am J Roentgenol 1984 Oct, Vol. 143 (4), P. 827–31

1156. Miller D L, Vermess M, Doppman J L, Simon R M, Sugarbaker P H, O Leary T J, Grimes G, Chatterji D G, Willis M
CT of the liver and spleen with EOE-13: review of 225 examinations
Am J Roentgenol 1984 Aug, Vol. 143 (2), P. 235–43

1157. Miller D L, Simmons J T, Chang R, Ward B A, Shawker T H, Doppman J L, Chang A E
Hepatic metastasis detection: comparison of three CT contrast enhancement methods
Radiology 1987 Dec, Vol. 165 (3), P. 785–901158.Miller D L, Carrasquillo J A, Lutz R J, Chang A E
Hepatic perfusion during hepatic artery infusion chemotherapy: evaluation with perfusion CT and perfusion scintigraphy
J Comput Assist Tomogr 1989 Nov-Dec, Vol. 13 (6), P. 958–64

1159. Mirvis S E, Whitley N O, Vainwright J R, Gens D R
Blunt hepatic trauma in adults: CT-based classification and correlation with prognosis and treatment
Radiology 1989 Apr, Vol. 171 (1), P. 27–32

1160. Mitnick J S, Bosniak M A, Megibow A J, Karpatkin M, Feiner H D, Kutin N, Van Natta F, Piomelli S
CT in B-thalassemia: iron deposition in the liver, spleen, and lymph nodes
Am J Roentgenol 1981 Jun, Vol. 136 (6), P. 1191–4

1161. Moon K L Jr, Federle M P
Computed tomography in hepatic trauma
Am J Roentgenol 1983 Aug, Vol. 141 (2), P. 309–14

1162. Morehouse H, Leibman A J, Biempica L, Hoffman J
Infiltrating periductal neoplasm mimicking biliary dilatation on computed tomography
J Comput Assist Tomogr 1983 Aug, Vol. 7 (4), P. 721–3

1163. Mori H, Hayashi K, Uetani M, Matsuoka Y, Iwao M, Maeda H
High-attenuation recent thrombus of the portal vein: CT demonstration and clinical significance
Radiology 1987 May, Vol. 163 (2), P. 353–6

1164. Mori H, Aikawa H, Hirao K, Futagawa S, Fukuda T, Maeda H, Hayashi K
Exophytic spread of hepatobiliary disease via perihepatic ligaments: demonstration with CT and US
Radiology 1989 Jul, Vol. 172 (1), P. 41–6

1165. Mori H, Maeda H, Fukuda T, Miyake H, Aikawa H, Maeda T, Nakashima A, Isomoto I, Hayashi K
Acute thrombosis of the inferior vena cava and hepatic veins in patients with Budd-Chiari syndrome: CT demonstration
Am J Roentgenol 1989 Nov, Vol. 153 (5), P. 987- 91

1166. Moss A A, Cann C E, Friedman M A, Marcus F S, Resser K J, Berninger W
Volumetric CT analysis of hepatic tumors
J Comput Assist Tomogr 1981 Oct, Vol. 5 (5), P. 714–8

1167. Moss A A, Dean P B, Axel L, Goldberg H I, Glazer G M, Friedman M A
Dynamic CT of hepatic masses with intravenous and intraarterial contrast material
Am J Roentgenol 1982 May, Vol. 138 (5), P. 847–52

1168. Moss A A, Goldberg H I, Stark D B, Davis P L, Margulis A R, Kaufman L, Crooks L E
Hepatic tumors: magnetic resonance and CT appearance
Radiology 1984 Jan, Vol. 150 (1), P. 141–7

1169. Moulton J S, Miller B L, Dodd G D, Vu D N
Passive hepatic congestion in heart failure: CT abnormalities
Am J Roentgenol 1988 Nov, Vol. 151 (5), P. 939–42

1170. Muhler A, Luning M
Frequenzanalyse und Wertbestimmung von Kriterien der dynamischen CT und Test zur CT-Diagnostik von Leberraumforderungen
A frequency analysis and evaluation of the criteria for dynamic CT and a test of the CT diagnosis of space- occupying lesions of the liver
RÖFO 1990 Dec, Vol. 153 (6), P. 637–44

1171. Mukai J K, Stack C M, Turner D A, Matalon T A, Gould R J, Petasnick J P, Doolas A M, Murakami M
Imaging of surgically relevant hepatic vascular and segmental anatomy. Part 2. Extent and resectability of hepatic neoplasms
Am J Roentgenol 1987 Aug, Vol. 149 (2), P. 293–7

1172. Mukai J K, Stack C M, Turner D A, Gould R J, Petasnick J P, Matalon T A, Doolas A M, Murakami M
Imaging of surgically relevant hepatic vascular and segmental anatomy. Part 1. Normal anatomy
Am J Roentgenol 1987 Aug, Vol. 149 (2), P. 287–92

1173. Muramatsu Y, Takajasu K, Moriyama N, et al
Peripheral low-density area of hepatic tumors:CT-pathologic correlation
Radiology 1986, Vol.160 ,P. 49–52

1174. Murayama S, Tsukamoto Y, Watanabe H, Nakata H
Computed tomography of residual hepatomas following transcatheter arterial embolization
J Comput Assist Tomogr 1986 Nov-Dec, Vol. 10 (6), P. 969–72

1175. Murphy F B, Barefield K P, Steinberg H V, Bernardino M E
CT- or sonography-guided biopsy of the liver in the presence of ascites: frequency of complications
Am J Roentgenol 1988 Sep, Vol. 151 (3), P. 485–6

1176. Nakao N, Miura K, Takayasu Y, Wada Y, Miura T
CT angiography in hepatocellular carcinoma
J Comput Assist Tomogr 1983 Oct, Vol. 7 (5), P. 780–7

1177. Nakao N, Miura K, Takahashi H, Miura T, Ashida H, Ishikawa Y, Utsunomiya J
Hepatic perfusion in cavernous transformation of the portal vein: evaluation by using CT angiography
Am J Roentgenol 1989 May, Vol. 152 (5), P. 985–6

1178. Nakata K, Iwata K, Kojima K, Kanai K
Computed tomography of liver sarcoidosis
J Comput Assist Tomogr 1989 Jul-Aug, Vol. 13 (4), P. 707–8

1179. Nakayama T, Hiyama Y, Ohnishi K, Tsuchiya S, Kohno K, Nakajima Y, Okuda K
Arterioportal shunts on dynamic computed tomography
Am J Roentgenol 1983 May, Vol. 140 (5), P. 953–7

1180. Nelson R C, Chezmar J L, Sugarbaker P H, Bernardino M E
Hepatic tumors: comparison of CT during arterial portography, delayed CT, and MR imaging for preoperative evaluation
Radiology 1989 Jul, Vol. 172 (1), P. 27–34

1181. Nelson R C, Chezmar J L, Peterson J E, Bernardino M E
Contrast-enhanced CT of the liver and spleen: comparison of ionic and nonionic contrast agents
Am J Roentgenol 1989 Nov, Vol. 153 (5), P. 973–6

1182. Nelson R C, Chezmar J L, Sugarbaker P H, Murray D R, Bernardino M E
Preoperative localization of focal liver lesions to specific liver segments: utility of CT during arterial portography
Radiology 1990 Jul, Vol. 176 (1), P. 89–94

1183. Nelson R C, Moyers J H, Chezmar J L, Hoel M J, Jones E C, Peterson J E, Cork R D, Bernardino M E
Hepatic dynamic sequential CT: section enhancement profiles with a bolus of ionic and nonionic contrast agents
Radiology 1991 Feb, Vol. 178 (2), P. 499–502

1184. Nino Murcia M, Kurtz A, Wechsler R J
Inferior mesenteric artery aneurysm: demonstration by computed tomography
J Comput Assist Tomogr 1984 Jun, Vol. 8 (3), P. 564–6

1185. Nomura F, Ohnishi K, Ochiai T, Okuda K
Obesity-related nonalcoholic fatty liver: CT features and follow-up studies after low-calorie diet
Radiology 1987 Mar, Vol. 162 (3), P. 845–7

1186. Noon M A, Young S W, Castellino R A
Leiomyosarcoma metastatic to the liver: CT appearance
J Comput Assist Tomogr 1980 Aug, Vol. 4 (4), P. 527–30

1187. Oei T K, van Engelshoven J M
Ultrasonographic and computed tomographic findings of thromboembolism of the portal system by superior mesenteric vein thrombosis as a complication of appendicitis
RÖFO 1984 Apr, Vol. 140 (4), P. 473–5

1188. Outwater E, Kaplan M M, Bankoff M S
Lymphadenopathy in primary biliary cirrhosis: CT observations
Radiology 1989 Jun, Vol. 171 (3), P. 731–3

1189. Pagani J J
Intrahepatic vascular territories shown by computed tomography CT. The value of CT in determining resectability of hepatic tumors
Radiology 1983 Apr, Vol. 147 (1), P. 173–8

1190. Pagola Serrano M A, Vega A, Ortega E, Gonzalez A
Computed tomography of hepatic fascioliasis
J Comput Assist Tomogr 1987 Mar-Apr, Vol. 11 (2), P. 269–72

1191. Pandolfo I, Blandino G, Scribano E, Longo M, Certo A, Chirico G
CT findings in hepatic involvement by Echinococcus granulosus
J Comput Assist Tomogr 1984 Oct, Vol. 8 (5), P. 839–45

1192. Pardes J G, Haaga J R, Borkowski G
Focal hepatic fatty metamorphosis secondary to trauma
J Comput Assist Tomogr 1982 Aug, Vol. 6 (4), P. 769–71

1193. Parienty R
Computed tomography in the diagnostic approach to cavernous hemangioma of the liver
Radiology 1980 Feb, Vol. 134 (2), P. 553–4

1194. Parienty R
Computed tomography in venoocclusive liver disorders letter
Am J Roentgenol 1981 Apr, Vol. 136 (4), P. 842–4

1195. Parikh V P, Iyer G N
Pedunculated hepatic hemangioma: CT findings letter
Am J Roentgenol 1990 Nov, Vol. 155 (5), P. 1137–8

1196. Parizel P, Van Gijsegem D, Vereycken H, De Schepper A
CT demonstration of mobile echinococcal daughter cysts
J Comput Assist Tomogr 1984 Feb, Vol. 8 (1), P. 179–80

1197. Patel S, Sandler C M, Rauschkolb E N, McConnell B J
133xe uptake in focal hepatic fat accumulation: CT correlation
Am J Roentgenol 1982 Mar, Vol. 138 (3), P. 541–4

1198. Paushter D M, Zeman R K, Scheibler M L, Choyke P L, Jaffe M H, Clark L R
CT evaluation of suspected hepatic metastases: comparison of techniques for i.v. contrast enhancement
Am J Roentgenol 1989 Feb, Vol. 152 (2), P. 267–71

1199. Perkerson R B Jr, Erwin B C, Baumgartner B R, Phillips V M, Torres W E, Clements J L Jr, Gedgaudas McClees K, Bernardino M E
CT densities in delayed iodine hepatic scanning
Radiology 1985 May, Vol. 155 (2), P. 445–6

1200. Phillips V M, Erwin B C, Bernardino M E
Delayed iodine scanning of the liver: a promising CT technique
J Comput Assist Tomogr 1985 Mar-Apr, Vol. 9 (2), P. 415–6

1201. Piekarski J, Goldberg H I, Royal S A, Axel L, Moss A A
Difference between liver and spleen CT numbers in the normal adult: its usefulness in predicting the presence of diffuse liver disease
Radiology 1980 Dec, Vol. 137 (3), P. 727–9

1202. Quinn S F, Bodne D J, Clark R A, Karl R C, Nicosia S V
Upper abdomen: CT findings following partial hepatectomy letter
Radiology 1988 Sep, Vol. 168 (3), P. 879–80

1203. Radin D R, Ralls P W, Colletti P M, Halls J M
CT of amebic liver abscess
Am J Roentgenol 1988 Jun, Vol. 150 (6), P. 1297–301

1204. Radin D R, Craig J R, Colletti P M, Ralls P W, Halls J M
Hepatic epithelioid hemangioendothelioma
Radiology 1988 Oct, Vol. 169 (1), P. 145–8

1205. Reinig J W, Sanchez F W, Vujic I
Hemodynamics of portal blood flow shown by CT portography. Work in progress
Radiology 1985 Feb, Vol. 154.(2), P. 473–6

1206. Reinig J W, Dwyer A J, Miller D L, White M, Frank J A, Sugarbaker P H, Chang A E, Doppman J L
Liver metastasis detection: comparative sensitivities of MR imaging and CT scanning
Radiology 1987 Jan, Vol. 162 (1 Pt 1), P. 43–7

1207. Roesler P J Jr, Wills J S
Hepatic actinomycosis: CT features
J Comput Assist Tomogr 1986 Mar-Apr, Vol. 10 (2), P. 335–7

1208. Rossi S, Sposito M, Simonetti G, Sposato S, Cusumano G
CT diagnosis of Budd-Chiari syndrome
J Comput Assist Tomogr 1981 Jun, Vol. 5 (3), P. 366–9

1209. Roth J, Wallner B, Safi F
Arterial perfusion abnormalities of the liver after hepatic arterial infusion chemotherapy and their correlation with changes in the metastases: evaluation with CT and angiography
Am J Roentgenol 1989 Oct, Vol. 153 (4), P. 751–4

1210. Rubenstein W A, Auh Y H, Whalen J P, Kazam E
The perihepatic spaces: computed tomographic and ultrasound imaging
Radiology 1983 Oct, Vol. 149 (1), P. 231–9

1211. Sanders L M, Botet J F, Straus D J, Ryan J, Filippa D A, Newhouse J H
CT of primary lymphoma of the liver
Am J Roentgenol 1989 May, Vol. 152 (5), P. 973–6

1212. Savolaine E R, Grecos G P, Howard J, White P
Evolution of CT findings in hepatic hematoma
J Comput Assist Tomogr 1985 Nov- Dec, Vol. 9 (6), P. 1090–6

1213. Scatarige J C, Fishman E K, Saksouk F A, Siegelman S S
Computed tomography of calcified liver masses
J Comput Assist Tomogr 1983 Feb, Vol. 7 (1), P. 83–9

1214. Scatarige J C, Kenny J M, Fishman E K, Herlong F H, Siegelman S S
CT of giant cavernous hemangioma
Am J Roentgenol 1987 Jul, Vol. 149 (1), P. 83–5

1215. Schild H, Kreitner K F, Thelen M, Grönninger J, Weber M, Börner N, et al
Fokal-noduläre Hyperplasie der Leber bei 930 Patienten
RÖFO 1987 Dec, Vol. 147 (6), P. 612–18

1216. Schild H, Mildenberger P, Schweden F, Eckmann A, Nagel K, Knuth A, Borner N, Thelen M, Junginger T
Liver CT with portal vein administration of a contrast medium Leber-CT mit portal-venöser Kontrastmittelgabe
RÖFO 1987 Dec, Vol. 147 (6), P. 623–8

1217. Schnyder P A, Candardjis G
Case report. Extreme hydronephrosis versus echinococcal cyst of the liver: computed tomography evaluation
J Comput Assist Tomogr 1979 Feb, Vol. 3 (1), P. 126–7

1218. Schopf R, Fretz C, Haertel M
Computertomographie bei Leber- und Milzverletzungen
Computed tomography for injuries of the liver and spleen
RÖFO 1982 Jun, Vol. 136 (6), P. 681–4

1219. Schulze K, Hubener K H, Klott K, Jenss H, Bahr R
Computertomographische und sonographische Diagnostik der Echinokokkose
Computer tomographic and sonographic diagnosis of echinococcus
RÖFO 1980 May, Vol. 132 (5), P. 514–21

1220. Schurawitzki H, Barton P, Stiglbauer R, Karnel F, Gritzmann N, Muhlbacher F
CT vor und nach Lebertransplantation
CT before and after liver transplantation
RÖFO 1988 Oct, Vol. 149 (4), P. 349–53

1221. Schwartz A M, Dorkin H L, Carter B L
CT appearance of the liver in a patient with biliary cirrhosis and cystic fibrosis
J Comput Assist Tomogr 1983 Jun, Vol. 7 (3), P. 530–3

1222. Sexton C C, Zeman R K
Correlation of computed tomography, sonography, and gross anatomy of the liver
Am J Roentgenol 1983 Oct, Vol. 141 (4), P. 711–8

1223. Shapiro M P, Gale M E
Tertiary syphilis of the liver: CT appearance
J Comput Assist Tomogr 1987 May-Jun, Vol. 11 (3), P. 546–7

1224. Shirkhoda A, Fallone B G
CT diagnosis of hepatic metastases letter
Am J Roentgenol 1987 Nov, Vol. 149 (5), P. 1080–1

1225. Shirkhoda A
CT findings in hepatosplenic and renal candidiasis
J Comput Assist Tomogr 1987 Sep-Oct, Vol. 11 (5), P. 795–8

1226. Silverman P M, Ram P C, Korobkin M
CT appearance of abdominal thorotrast deposition and Thorotrast- induced angiosarcoma of the liver
J Comput Assist Tomogr 1983 Aug, Vol. 7 (4), P. 655–8

1227. Siskind B N, Malat J, Hammers L, Rigsby C M, Taylor C, Radin D R, Rosenfield A T
CT features of hemorrhagic malignant liver tumors
J Comput Assist Tomogr 1987 Sep-Oct, Vol. 11 (5), P. 766–70

1228. Smathers R L, Heiken J P, Lee J K, Press G A, Balfe D M
Computed tomography of fatal hepatic rupture due to peliosis hepatis
J Comput Assist Tomogr 1984 Aug, Vol. 8 (4), P. 768–9

1229. Stalker H P, Kaufman R A, Towbin R
Patterns of liver injury in childhood: CT analysis
Am J Roentgenol 1986 Dec, Vol. 147 (6), P. 1199–205

1230. Stark D D, Wittenberg J, Butch R J, Ferrucci J T Jr
Hepatic metastases: randomized, controlled comparison of detection with MR imaging and CT
Radiology 1987 Nov, Vol. 165 (2), P. 399–406

1231. Stephens D H, Mckusick M A
Retention of contrast material in focal nodular hyperplasia of the liver on delayed CT: another case letter
Am J Roentgenol 1990 Feb, Vol. 154 (2), P. 422–3

1232. Suzuki S, Takizawa K, Nakajima Y, Katayama S, Sagawa F
CT findings in hepatic and splenic amyloidosis
J Comput Assist Tomogr 1986 Mar-Apr, Vol. 10 (2), P. 332–4

1233. Takayasu K, Ikeya S, Mukai K, Muramatsu Y, Makuuchi M, Hasegawa H
CT of hilar cholangiocarcinoma: late contrast enhancement in six patients
Am J Roentgenol 1990 Jun, Vol. 154 (6), P. 1203–6

1234. Titelbaum D S, Burke D R, Meranze S G, Saul S H
Fibrolamellar hepatocellular carcinoma:pitfalls in nonoperative diagnosis
Radiology 1988 Apr, Vol.167 (1), P.25–34

1235. Toombs B D, Sandler C M, Rauschkolb E N, Strax R, Harle T S
Assessment of hepatic injuries with computed tomography
J Comput Assist Tomogr 1982 Feb, Vol. 6 (1), P. 72–5

1236. Torres W E, Whitmire L F, Gedgaudas McClees K, Bernardino M E
Computed tomography of hepatic morphologic changes in cirrhosis of the liver
J Comput Assist Tomogr 1986 Jan-Feb, Vol. 10 (1), P. 47–50

1237. Tyrrel R T, Kaufman S L, Bernardino M E
Straight line sign: appearance and significance during CT portography
Radiology 1989 Dec, Vol. 173 (3), P. 635–7

1238. Unger E C, Lee J K, Weyman P J
CT and MR imaging of radiation hepatitis
J Comput Assist Tomogr 1987 Mar-Apr, Vol. 11 (2), P. 264–8

1239. Vasile N, Larde D, Zafrani E S, Berard H, Mathieu D
Hepatic angiosarcoma
J Comput Assist Tomogr 1983 Oct, Vol. 7 (5), P. 899–901

1240. Vogelzang R L, Anschuetz S L, Gore R M
Budd-Chiari syndrome: CT observations
Radiology 1987 May, Vol. 163 (2), P. 329–33

1241. Vujic I, Rogers C I, LeVeen H H
Computed tomographic detection of portal vein thrombosis
Radiology 1980 Jun, Vol. 135 (3), P. 697–8

1242. Wechsler R J, Munoz S J, Needleman L, Kurtz A B, Miller C L, Yang S L, Maddrey W C, Jarrell B E
The periportal collar: a CT sign of liver transplant rejection
Radiology 1987 Oct, Vol. 165 (1), P. 57–60

1243. Wernecke K, Peters P E
Sonographische und computertomographische Diagnostik von Lebermetastasen. Eine Übersicht
Sonographic and computed tomographic diagnosis of liver metastases. A review
Radiologe 1985 Apr, Vol. 25 (4), P. 141–51

1244. Whalen E
Liver Imaging – Current Trends in MRI, CT, and US: international symposium and course, June 1990 news
Am J Roentgenol 1990 Nov, Vol. 155 (5), P. 1125–32

1245. Wimmer B, Hauenstein K H
Grenzen der computertomographischen Differentialdiagnostik bei fokalen Leberveränderungen
Limitations of computed tomographic differential diagnosis of focal liver changes
Radiologe 1988 Aug, Vol. 28 (8), P. 356–61

1246. Yamamoto S, Kojoh K, Saito I, Yamamoto R, Ideguchi K, Ohmoto K, Ohumi T, Hino K, Yamamoto M, Wada A, et al
Computer tomography of congenital absence of the left lobe of the liver
J Comput Assist Tomogr 1988 Mar-Apr, Vol. 12 (2), P. 206–8

1247. Yang N C, Leichner P K, Fishman E K, Siegelman S S, Frenkel T L, Wallace J R, Loudenslager D M, Hawkins W G, Order S E
CT volumetrics of primary liver cancers
J Comput Assist Tomogr 1986 Jul-Aug, Vol. 10 (4), P. 621–8

1248. Yang P J, Glazer G M, Bowerman R A
Budd-Chiari syndrome: computed tomographic and ultrasonographic findings
J Comput Assist Tomogr 1983 Feb, Vol. 7 (1), P. 148–50

1249. Yasumori K, Tamura S, Hasuo K, Kudo S, Uchino A, Nishitani H, Onitsuka H, Kawanami T, Kawahira K, Ono M, et al
Posttranscatheter embolization computed tomography in hepatocellular carcinoma. Evaluation of embolization effects
RÖFO 1984 Dec, Vol. 141 (6), P. 649–53

1250. Yoshikawa J, Matsui O, Takashima T, Sugiura H, Katayama K, Nishida Y, Tsuji M
Focal fatty change of the liver adjacent to the falciform ligament: CT and sonographic findings in five surgically confirmed cases
Am J Roentgenol 1987 Sep, Vol. 149 (3), P. 491–4

1251. Yoshikawa J, Matsui O, Takashima T, Ida M, Takanaka T, Kawamura I, Kakuda K, Miyata S
Fatty metamorphosis in hepatocellular carcinoma: radiologic features in 10 cases
Am J Roentgenol 1988 Oct, Vol. 151 (4), P. 717–20

1252. Yoshimatsu S, Inoue Y, Ibukuro K, Suzuki S
Hypovascular hepatocellular carcinoma undetected at angiography and CT with iodized oil
Radiology 1989 May, Vol. 171 (2), P. 343–7

1253. Zeman R K, Clements L A, Silverman P M, Paushter D M, Garra B, Jaffe M H, Clark L R
CT of the liver: a survey of prevailing methods for administration of contrast material
Am J Roentgenol 1988 Jan, Vol. 150 (1), P. 107–9

1254. Zeman R K, Dritschilo A, Silverman P M, Clark L R, Garra B S, Thomas D S, Ahlgren J D, Smith F P, Korec S M, Nauta R J, et al
Dynamic CT vs 0.5 T MR imaging in the detection of surgically proven hepatic metastases
J Comput Assist Tomogr 1989 Jul-Aug, Vol. 13 (4), P. 637–44

1255. Zocholl G, Kuhn F P, Augustin N, Thelen M
Diagnostische Aussagekraft von Sonographie und Computertomographie bei Lebermetastasen
Diagnostic value of sonography and computed tomography in liver metastases
RÖFO 1988 Jan, Vol. 148 (1), P. 8–14

1256. Zornoza J, Ginaldi S
Computed tomography in hepatic lymphoma
Radiology 1981 Feb, Vol. 138 (2), P. 405–10

1257. Zwicker C, Langer M, Langer R, Steffen R, Bradaczek M, Astinet F, Felix R
Dynamische CT und Angio-CT nach Lebertransplantation
Dynamic CT and angio-CT following liver transplantation
RÖFO 1990 Oct, Vol. 153 (4), P. 362–8

1258. Zwicker C, Langer M, Astinet F, Langer R, Urich V, Felix R
Differenzierung maligner Lebertumoren mit schneller dynamischer CT
Differentiation of malignant liver tumors using rapid dynamic CT
RÖFO 1990 Mar, Vol. 152 (3), P. 293–302

The Biliary System

1259. Araki T, Itai Y, Tasaka A
CT of choledochal cyst
Am J Roentgenol 1980 Oct, Vol. 135 (4), P. 729–34

1260. Barakos J A, Ralls P W, Lapin S A, Johnson M B, Radin D R, Colletti P M, Boswell W D Jr, Halls J M
Cholelithiasis: evaluation with CT
Radiology 1987 Feb, Vol. 162 (2), P. 415–8

1261. Baron R L, Stanley R J, Lee J K, Koehler R E, Melson G L, Balfe D M, Weyman P J
A prospective comparison of the evaluation of biliary obstruction using computed tomography and ultrasonography
Radiology 1982 Oct, Vol. 145 (1), P. 91–8

1262. Baron R L, Stanley R J, Lee J K, Koehler R E, Levitt R G
Computed tomographic features of biliary obstruction
Am J Roentgenol 1983 Jun, Vol. 140 (6), P. 1173–8

1263. Baron R L
Common bile duct stones: reassessment of criteria for CT diagnosis
Radiology 1987 Feb, Vol. 162 (2), P. 419–24

1264. Baron R L, Rohrmann C A Jr, Lee S P, Shuman W P, Teefey S A
CT evaluation of gallstones in vitro: correlation with chemical analysis
Am J Roentgenol 1988 Dec, Vol. 151 (6), P. 1123–8

1265. Baron R L
Role of CT in characterizing gallstones: an unsettled issue comment
Radiology 1991 Mar, Vol. 178 (3), P. 635–6

1266. Becker C D, Hassler H, Terrier F
Preoperative diagnosis of the Mirizzi syndrome: limitations of sonography and computed tomography
Am J Roentgenol 1984 Sep, Vol. 143 (3), P. 591–6

1267. Berland L L, Doust B D, Foley W D
Acute hemorrhage into the gallbladder diagnosed by computed tomography and ultrasonography
J Comput Assist Tomogr 1980 Apr, Vol. 4 (2), P. 260–2

1268. Berland L L, Lawson T L, Stanley R J
CT appearance of Mirizzi syndrome
J Comput Assist Tomogr 1984 Feb, Vol. 8 (1), P. 165–6

1269. Boukadoum M, Siddiky M A, Zerhouni E A, Stitik F P
CT demonstration of adenomyomatosis of the gallbladder
J Comput Assist Tomogr 1984 Feb, Vol. 8 (1), P. 177

1270. Brakel K, Lameris J S, Nijs H G, Terpstra O T, Steen G, Blijenberg B C
Predicting gallstone composition with CT: in vivo and in vitro analysis
Radiology 1990 Feb, Vol. 174 (2), P. 337–41

1271. Brink J A, Ferrucci J T
Use of CT for predicting gallstone composition: a dissenting view see comments
Radiology 1991 Mar, Vol. 178 (3), P. 633–4

1272. Brodey P A, Fisch A E, Fertig S, Roberts G S
Computed tomography of choledochocele
J Comput Assist Tomogr 1984 Feb, Vol. 8 (1), P. 162–4

1273. Carr D H, Hadjis N S, Banks L M, Hemingway A P, Blumgart L H
Computed tomography of hilar cholangiocarcinoma: a new sign
Am J Roentgenol 1985 Jul, Vol. 145 (1), P. 53–6

1274. Chan F L, Man S W, Leong L L, Fan S T
Evaluation of recurrent pyogenic cholangitis with CT: analysis of 50 patients
Radiology 1989 Jan, Vol. 170 (1 Pt 1), P. 165–9

1275. Choi B I, Park J H, Kim Y I, Yu E S, Kim S H, Kim W H, Kim C Y, Han M C
Peripheral cholangiocarcinoma and clonorchiasis: CT findings
Radiology 1988 Oct, Vol. 169 (1), P. 149–53

1276. Choi B I, Lee J H, Han M C, Kim S H, Yi J G, Kim C W
Hilar cholangiocarcinoma: comparative study with sonography and CT
Radiology 1989 Sep, Vol. 172 (3), P. 689–92

1277. Choi B I, Lim J H, Han M C, Lee D H, Kim S H, Kim Y I, Kim C W
Biliary cystadenoma and cystadenocarcinoma: CT and sonographic findings
Radiology 1989 Apr, Vol. 171 (1), P. 57–61

1278. Co C S, Shea W J Jr, Goldberg H I
Evaluation of common bile duct diameter using high resolution computed tomography
J Comput Assist Tomogr 1986 May-Jun, Vol. 10 (3), P. 424–7

1279. Crone Munzebrock W, Rowedder A, Meyer Pannwitt U, Kremer B
Leistungsvergleich von Sonographie, Computertomographie, ERCP und Angiographie in der Diagnostik primärer Gallenwegskarzinome
A comparison of the efficacy of sonography, computed tomography, ERCP and angiography in the diagnosis of primary bile duct carcinoma
RÖFO 1989 Nov, Vol. 151 (5), P. 523–6

1280. Dennis M A, Pretorius D, Manco Johnson M L, Bangert Burroughs K
CT detection of portal venous gas associated with suppurative cholangitis and cholecystitis
Am J Roentgenol 1985 Nov, Vol. 145 (5), P. 1017–8

1281. Duber C, Storkel S, Wagner P K, Muller J
Xanthogranulomatous cholecystitis mimicking carcinoma of the gallbladder: CT findings
J Comput Assist Tomogr 1984 Dec, Vol. 8 (6), P. 1195–8

1282. Dunne M G, Johnson M L
Gas within gallstones on CT
Am J Roentgenol 1980 May, Vol. 134 (5), P. 1065–6

1283. Eisenberg D, Hurwitz L, Yu A C
CT and sonography of multiple bile-duct hamartomas simulating malignant liver disease case report
Am J Roentgenol 1986 Aug, Vol. 147 (2), P. 279–80

1284. Engels J T, Balfe D M, Lee J K
Biliary carcinoma: CT evaluation of extrahepatic spread
Radiology 1989 Jul, Vol. 172 (1), P. 35–40

1285. Farman J, Javors B, Chao P, Fagelman D, Collins R, Glanz S
CT demonstration of giant choledochal cysts in adults
J Comput Assist Tomogr 1987 Sep-Oct, Vol. 11 (5), P. 771–4

1286. Ferris R A, Kirschner L P, Mero J H, Chung D H
Increased attenuation value in a hydropic gallbladder
J Comput Assist Tomogr 1979 Aug, Vol. 3 (4), P. 545–6

1287. Foley W D, Wilson C R, Quiroz F A, Lawson T L
Demonstration of the normal extrahepatic biliary tract with computed tomography
J Comput Assist Tomogr 1980 Feb, Vol. 4 (1), P. 48–52

1288. Fork F T, Nyman U, Sigurjonsson S
Recognition of gas in gallstones in routine computed tomograms of the abdomen
J Comput Assist Tomogr 1983 Oct, Vol. 7 (5), P. 805–9

1289. Friedburg H, Kirchner R, Bohm N, Ruf G
Cholecystitis emphysematosa durch Clostridium perfringens. Sonographische und computer-tomographische Befunde
Emphysematous cholecystitis caused by Clostridium perfringens. Sonographic and computer tomographic findings
RÖFO 1983 Mar, Vol. 138 (3), P. 357–60

1290. Gerard P S, Berman D, Zafaranloo S
CT and ultrasound of gallbladder adenomyomatosis mimicking carcinoma
J Comput Assist Tomogr 1990 May-Jun, Vol. 14 (3), P. 490–1

1291. Gibson R N
Suprapancreatic biliary obstruction: CT evaluation letter
Radiology 1987 Dec, Vol. 165 (3), P. 875–6

1292. Goldberg R P
Distal bile duct "septum". A computed tomographic finding with a dilated retained cystic duct remnant
Radiology 1982 Apr, Vol. 143 (1), P. 142

1293. Goldstein R B, Wing V W, Laing F C, Jeffrey R B
Computed tomography of thick-walled gallbladder mimicking pericholecystic fluid
J Comput Assist Tomogr 1986 Jan-Feb, Vol. 10 (1), P. 55–6

1294. Greenberg M, Rubin J M, Greenberg B M
Appearance of the gallbladder and biliary tree by CT cholangiography
J Comput Assist Tomogr 1983 Oct, Vol. 7 (5), P. 788–94

1295. Grumbach K, Levine M S, Wexler J A
Gallstone ileus diagnosed by computed tomography
J Comput Assist Tomogr 1986 Jan- Feb, Vol. 10 (1), P. 146–8

1296. Haertel M, Fischedick A R, Zaunbauer W, Triller J
Computertomographie bei biliären Karzinomen
Computer tomography in biliary carcinoma
RÖFO 1981 Mar, Vol. 134 (3), P. 278–83

1297. Havrilla T R, Reich N E, Haaga J R, Seidelmann F E, Cooperman A M, Alfidi R J
Computed tomography of the gallbladder
Am J Roentgenol 1978 Jun, Vol. 130 (6), P. 1059–67

1298. Heuck F, Buck J
Der Informationswert der Röntgen- Computer-Tomographie für die Beurteilung von Gallenwegen und Gallenblase
The value of CT in the evaluation of bile ducts and gallbladder
Radiologe 1980 Jan, Vol. 20 (1), P. 6–15

1299. Inamoto K, Tanaka S, Yamazaki H, Suzuki E, Ishikawa Y
Computed tomography of carcinoma of the ampulla of Vater
RÖFO 1982 Jun, Vol. 136 (6), P. 689–93

1300. Itai Y, Araki T, Yoshikawa K, Furui S, Yashiro N, Tasaka A
Computed tomography of gallbladder carcinoma
Radiology 1980 Dec, Vol. 137 (3), P. 713–8

1301. Itai Y, Araki T, Furui S, Yashiro N, Ohtomo K, Iio M
Computed tomography of primary intrahepatic biliary malignancy
Radiology 1983 May, Vol. 147 (2), P. 485–90

1302. Jeffrey R B, Federle M P, Laing F C, Wall S, Rego J, Moss A A
Computed tomography of choledocholithiasis
Am J Roentgenol 1983 Jun, Vol. 140 (6), P. 1179–83

1303. Jeffrey R B Jr, Federle M P, Laing F C, Wing V W
Computed tomography of blunt trauma to the gallbladder
J Comput Assist Tomogr 1986 Sep-Oct, Vol. 10 (5), P. 756–8

1304. Jenkins M, Golding R H, Cooperberg P L
Sonography and computed tomography of hemorrhagic cholecystitis
Am J Roentgenol 1983 Jun, Vol. 140 (6), P. 1197–8

1305. Kane R A, Costello P, Duszlak E
Computed tomography in acute cholecystitis: new observations
Am J Roentgenol 1983 Oct, Vol. 141 (4), P. 697–701

1306. Kane R A, Jacobs R, Katz J, Costello P
Porcelain gallbladder: ultrasound and CT appearance
Radiology 1984 Jul, Vol. 152 (1), P. 137–41

1307. Korobkin M, Stephens D H, Lee J K, Stanley R J, Fishman E K, Francis I R, Alpern M B, Rynties M
Biliary cystadenoma and cystadenocarcinoma: CT and sonographic findings
Am J Roentgenol 1989 Sep, Vol. 153 (3), P. 507–11

1308. Krudy A G, Doppman J L, Bissonette M B, Girton M
Hemobilia: computed tomographic diagnosis
Radiology 1983 Sep, Vol. 148 (3), P. 785–9

1309. Lee J K, McClennan B L, Stanley R J, Levitt R G, Sagel S S
Use of CT in evaluation of postcystectomy patients
Am J Roentgenol 1981 Mar, Vol. 136 (3), P. 483–7

1310. Leekam R N, Ilves R, Shankar L
Inversion of gallbladder secondary to traumatic herniation of liver: CT findings
J Comput Assist Tomogr 1987 Jan-Feb, Vol. 11 (1), P. 163–4

1311. Lorenz R, Beyer D, Friedmann G, Eisenhardt H J
Bedeutung von Sonographie und Computertomographie für die Diagnose intraperitonealer Galleansammlungen (Galleaszites-Biliom)
Value of sonography and computerized tomography for the diagnosis of intraperitoneal bile accumulations bile ascites bilioma
RÖFO 1983 Jan, Vol. 138 (1), P. 14–8

1312. Luska G, Elgeti H, Wanner K, Rumpf K D, Gerber R
Computertomographie (CT) beim tumorbedingten Verschlußikterus zur Therapieentscheidung und zur Planung der perkutantranshepatischen Gallenwegsdrainage (PTCD)
Computer tomography CT in the choice of treatment and the planning of percutaneous transhepatic biliary drainage in obstructive jaundice due to tumour
RÖFO 1981 Jan, Vol. 134 (1), P. 28–34

1313. McMillin K
Computed tomography of emphysematous cholecystitis
J Comput Assist Tomogr 1985 Mar-Apr, Vol. 9 (2), P. 330–2

1314. Merine D, Meziane M, Fishman E K
CT diagnosis of gallbladder torsion
J Comput Assist Tomogr 1987 Jul-Aug, Vol. 11 (4), P. 712–3

1315. Middleton W D, Thorsen M K, Lawson T L, Foley W D
False- positive CT diagnosis of gallstones due to thickening of the gallbladder wall
Am J Roentgenol 1987 Nov, Vol. 149 (5), P. 941–4

1316. Mirvis S E, Whitley N O, Miller J W
CT diagnosis of acalculous cholecystitis
J Comput Assist Tomogr 1987 Jan-Feb, Vol. 11 (1), P. 83–7

1317. Mitchell S E, Clark R A
A comparison of computed tomography and sonography in choledocholithiasis
Am J Roentgenol 1984 Apr, Vol. 142 (4), P. 729–33

1318. Miyake H, Takeda H, Mori H, Hayashi K, Muta T, Ohshima T, Matsuo T
CT findings in lipomatosis of the gallbladder
J Comput Assist Tomogr 1987 Jan-Feb, Vol. 11 (1), P. 165–6

1319. Morehouse H T, Roush G, Deshmukh S, Baker S
Milk of calcium in the common bile duct
J Comput Assist Tomogr 1984 Feb, Vol. 8 (1), P. 177–9

1320. Moss A A, Filly R A, Way L W
In vitro investigation of gallstones with computed tomography
J Comput Assist Tomogr 1980 Dec, Vol. 4 (6), P. 827–31

1321. Musante F, Derchi L E, Bonati P
CT cholangiography in suspected Caroli's disease
J Comput Assist Tomogr 1982 Jun, Vol. 6 (3), P. 482–5

1322. Nardi P M, Yaghoobian J, Ruchman R B
CT demonstration of retrohepatic gallbladder in severe cirrhosis
J Comput Assist Tomogr 1988 Nov-Dec, Vol. 12 (6), P. 968–70

1323. Nesbit G M, Johnson C D, James E M, MacCarty R L, Nagorney D M, Bender C E
Cholangiocarcinoma: diagnosis and evaluation of resectability by CT and sonography as procedures complementary to cholangiography
Am J Roentgenol 1988 Nov, Vol. 151 (5), P. 933–8

1324. Pedrosa C S, Casanova R, Rodriguez R
CT cholangiography: multiplanar reconstruction in obstructive jaundice
J Comput Assist Tomogr 1981 Aug, Vol. 5 (4), P. 503–8

1325. Pedrosa C S, Casanova R, de la Torre S, Villacorta J
CT findings in Mirizzi syndrome
J Comput Assist Tomogr 1983 Jun, Vol. 7 (3), P. 419–25

1326. Pollack M, Shirkhoda A, Charnsangavej C
Computed tomography of choledochocele
J Comput Assist Tomogr 1985 Mar-Apr, Vol. 9 (2), P. 360–2

1327. Quinn S F, Fazzio F, Jones E
Torsion of the gallbladder: findings on CT and sonography and role of percutaneous cholecystostomy
Am J Roentgenol 1987 May, Vol. 148 (5), P. 881–2

1328. Radin D R, Vachon L A
CT findings in biliary and pancreatic ascariasis
J Comput Assist Tomogr 1986 May-Jun, Vol. 10 (3), P. 508–9

1329. Rahn N H, Koehler R E, Weyman P J, Truss C D, Sagel S S, Stanley R J
CT appearance of sclerosing cholangitis
Am J Roentgenol 1983 Sep, Vol. 141 (3), P. 549–52

1330. Rebner M, Ruggieri P M, Gross B H, Glazer G M
CT evaluation of intracholecystic bile
Am J Roentgenol 1985 Aug, Vol. 145 (2), P. 237–40

1331. Schulte S J, Baron R L, Teefey S A, Rohrmann C A Jr, Freeny P C, Shuman W P, Foster M A
CT of the extrahepatic bile ducts: wall thickness and contrast enhancement in normal and abnormal ducts
Am J Roentgenol 1990 Jan, Vol. 154 (1), P. 79–85

1332. Schumacher K A, Zoller A, Swobodnik W, Janowitz P
Morphologische Veränderungen in der Gallenblase nach extrakorporaler Stoßwellenlithotripsie
Morphological changes in the gallbladder after extracorporeal shock- wave lithotripsy
RÖFO 1990 Jul, Vol. 153 (1), P. 76–8

1333. Shimizu H, Ida M, Takayama S, Seki T, Yoneda M, Nakaya S, Yanagi T, Bando B, Sato H, Uchiyama M, Okumura T, Miura S, Fujisawa M
The diagnostic accuracy of computed tomography in obstructive biliary disease: a comparative evaluation with direct cholangiography
Radiology 1981 Feb, Vol. 138 (2), P. 411–6

1334. Smathers R L, Lee J K, Heiken J P
Differentiation of complicated cholecystitis from gallbladder carcinoma by computed tomography
Am J Roentgenol 1984 Aug, Vol. 143 (2), P. 255–9

1335. Solomon A, Rubinstein Z J
Carcinoma of the gall bladder: a CT diagnosis
RÖFO 1981 Nov, Vol. 135 (5), P. 622–3

1336. Sorensen K W, Glazer G M, Francis I R
Diagnosis of cystic ectasia of intrahepatic bile ducts by computed tomography
J Comput Assist Tomogr 1982 Jun, Vol. 6 (3), P. 486–9

1337. Strax R, Toombs B D, Kam J, Rauschkolb E N, Patel S, Sandler C M
Gallbladder enhancement following angiography: a normal CT finding
J Comput Assist Tomogr 1982 Aug, Vol. 6 (4), P. 766–8

1338. Teefey S A, Baron R L, Rohrmann C A, Shuman W P, Freeny P C
Sclerosing cholangitis: CT findings
Radiology 1988 Dec, Vol. 169 (3), P. 635–9

1339. Terrier F, Becker C D, Stoller C, Triller J K
Computed tomography in complicated cholecystitis
J Comput Assist Tomogr 1984 Feb, Vol. 8 (1), P. 58–62

1340. Thomas J L, Bernardino M E
Segmental biliary obstruction: its detection and significance
J Comput Assist Tomogr 1980 Apr, Vol. 4 (2), P. 155–8

1341. Thorsen M K, Quiroz F, Lawson T L, Smith D F, Foley W D, Stewart E T
Primary biliary carcinoma: CT evaluation
Radiology 1984 Aug, Vol. 152 (2), P. 479–83

1342. Toombs B D, Sandler C M, Conoley P M
Computed tomography of the nonvisualizing gallbladder
J Comput Assist Tomogr 1981 Apr, Vol. 5 (2), P. 164–8

1343. Triller J, Coray T, Kappeler M, Scheurer U
CT und ERCP als Kombinationsuntersuchung bei Erkrankungen der Gallenwege
CT and ERCP for the combined study of biliary tract diseases
RÖFO 1985 Feb, Vol. 142 (2), P. 138–45

1344. Ueda J, Hara K, Ohishi H, Uchida H
High density bile in the gallbladder observed by computed tomography
J Comput Assist Tomogr 1983 Oct, Vol. 7 (5), P. 801–4

1345. Warren L P, Kadir S, Dunnick N R
Percutaneous cholecystostomy: anatomic considerations
Radiology 1988 Sep, Vol. 168 (3), P. 615–6

1346. Weiner S N, Koenigsberg M, Morehouse H, Hoffman J
Sonography and computed tomography in the diagnosis of carcinoma of the gallbladder
Am J Roentgenol 1984 Apr, Vol. 142 (4), P. 735–9

1347. Weinerman P M, Arger P H, Coleman B G, Pollack H M, Banner M P, Wein A J
Pelvic adenopathy from bladder and prostate carcinoma: detection by rapid-sequence computed tomography
Am J Roentgenol 1983 Jan, Vol. 140 (1), P. 95–9

1348. Wimmer B, Lausen M
Computertomographie bei Komplikationen der Cholezystitis
Computed tomography of complications of cholecystitis
Radiologe 1989 Jul, Vol. 29 (7), P. 349–53

1349. Woerner H, Scherer K, Kramann B
Gallenblasenperforation im Computertomogramm
Gallbladder perforation on the computed tomogram
RÖFO 1987 Dec, Vol. 147 (6), P. 629–31

1350. Yeh H C
Ultrasonography and computed tomography of carcinoma of the gallbladder
Radiology 1979 Oct, Vol. 133 (1), P. 167–73

The Pancreas

1351. Andriole J G, Haaga J R, Bolwell B J
Spontaneous pancreatic decalcification
J Comput Assist Tomogr 1983 Jun, Vol. 7 (3), P. 534–5

1352. Arndt R D, Joyce P W, Gray R K, Haveson S B, Bos C J
Iodipamide-enhanced computed tomography of the pancreas
Radiology 1981 May, Vol. 139 (2), P. 491–3

1353. Baker M E, Cohan R H, Nadel S N, Leder R A, Dunnick N R
Obliteration of the fat surrounding the celiac axis and superior mesenteric artery is not a specific CT finding of carcinoma of the pancreas
Am J Roentgenol 1990 Nov, Vol. 155 (5), P. 991–4

1354. Balthazar E J, Subramanyam B R, Lefleur R S, Barone C M
Solid and papillary epithelial neoplasm of the pancreas. Radiographic, CT, sonographic, and angiographic features
Radiology 1984 Jan, Vol. 150 (1), P. 39–40

1355. Balthazar E J, Ranson J H, Naidich D P, Megibow A J, Caccavale R, Cooper M M
Acute pancreatitis: prognostic value of CT
Radiology 1985 Sep, Vol. 156 (3), P. 767–72

1356. Balthazar E J
Prognostic value of CT in acute pancreatitis: is the early CT examination indicated? letter
Radiology 1987 Mar, Vol. 162 (3), P. 876–8

1357. Balthazar E J, Robinson D L, Megibow A J, Ranson J H
Acute pancreatitis: value of CT in establishing prognosis
Radiology 1990 Feb, Vol. 174 (2), P. 331–6

1358. Bernardino M, Fernandez M, Neylan J, Hertzler G, Whelchel J, Olson R
Pancreatic transplants: CT-guided biopsy
Radiology 1990 Dec, Vol. 177 (3), P. 709–11

1359. Borlaza G S, Kuhns L R, Seigel R, Pozderac R, Eckhauser F
Computed tomographic and angiographic demonstration of gastroduodenal artery pseudoaneurysm in a pancreatic pseudocyst
J Comput Assist Tomogr 1979 Oct, Vol. 3 (5), P. 612–4

1360. Brachlow J, Zaunbauer W, Haertel M
Zur Computertomographie der zystischen Pankreasfibrose
Computed tomography of pancreatic cystic fibrosis
RÖFO 1984 Feb, Vol. 140 (2), P. 145–6

1361. Brambs H J, Schutz B, Wimmer B, Hoppe Seyler P
Das Pancreas divisum als mögliche Ursache von Fehlinterpretationen bei ERCP, Computertomographie, Sonographie und MDP
Pancreas divisum as a possible cause of misinterpretation in ERCP, computed tomography, sonography and MDP
RÖFO 1986 Mar, Vol. 144 (3), P. 273–7

1362. Breatnach E S, Han S Y, Rahatzad M T, Stanley R J
CT evaluation of glucagonomas
J Comput Assist Tomogr 1985 Jan-Feb, Vol. 9 (1), P. 25–9

1363. Buck J, Binder J P
Nachweis des Insulinoms im Pankreas durch die Röntgen- Computertomographie
Diagnosis of insulinoma of the pancreas by computed tomography
Radiologe 1982 Jun, Vol. 22 (6), P. 279–82

1364. Burke J W, Erickson S J, Kellum C D, Tegtmeyer C J, Williamson B R, Hansen M F
Pseudoaneurysms complicating pancreatitis: detection by CT
Radiology 1986 Nov, Vol. 161 (2), P. 447–50

1365. Bydder G M, Kreel L
Pleural calcification in pancreatitis demonstrated by computed tomography
J Comput Assist Tomogr 1981 Apr, Vol. 5 (2), P. 161–3

1366. Callen P W, Breiman R S, Korobkin M, De Martini W J, Mani J R
Carcinoma of the tail of the pancreas: an unusual CT appearance
Am J Roentgenol 1979 Jul, Vol. 133 (1), P. 135–7

1367. Callen P W, London S S, Moss A A
Computed tomographic evaluation of the dilated pancreatic duct: the value of thin- section collimation
Radiology 1980 Jan, Vol. 134 (1), P. 253–5

1368. Choi B I, Kim K W, Han M C, Kim Y I, Kim C W
Solid and papillary epithelial neoplasms of the pancreas: CT findings
Radiology 1988 Feb, Vol. 166 (2), P. 413–6

1369. Claussen C, Lochner B
Pankreaskarzinomdiagnostik durch Einsatz der dynamischen Computertomographie (Serien-CT)
Diagnosis of pancreatic carcinoma using dynamic computed tomography serial CT
RÖFO 1983 Oct, Vol. 139 (4), P. 389–93

1370. Cohen D J, Fagelman D
Pancreas islet cell carcinoma with complete fatty replacement: CT characteristics
J Comput Assist Tomogr 1986 Nov-Dec, Vol. 10 (6), P. 1050–1

1371. Daneman A, Gaskin K, Martin D J, Cutz E
Pancreatic changes in cystic fibrosis: CT and sonographic appearances
Am J Roentgenol 1983 Oct, Vol. 141 (4), P. 653–5

1372. DelMaschio A, Vanzulli A, Sironi S, Castrucci M, Mellone R, Staudacher C, Carlucci M, Zerbi A, Parolini D, Faravelli A, et al
Pancreatic cancer versus chronic pancreatitis: diagnosis with CA 19–9 assessment, US, CT, and CT-guided fine-needle biopsy
Radiology 1991 Jan, Vol. 178 (1), P. 95–9

1373. Dembner A G, Jaffe C C, Simeone J, Walsh J
A new computed tomographic sign of pancreatitis
Am J Roentgenol 1979 Sep, Vol. 133 (3), P. 477–9

1374. deSantos L A, Bernardino M E, Paulus D D, Martin R E
Case report: computed tomography of cystadenoma of the pancreas
J Comput Assist Tomogr 1978 Apr, Vol. 2 (2), P. 222–5

1375. Dodds W J, Taylor A J, Erickson S J, Lawson T L
Traumatic fracture of the pancreas: CT characteristics
J Comput Assist Tomogr 1990 May-Jun, Vol. 14 (3), P. 375–8

1376. Eelkema E A, Stephens D H, Ward E M, Sheedy P F
CT features of nonfunctioning islet cell carcinoma
Am J Roentgenol 1984 Nov, Vol. 143 (5), P. 943–8

1377. Elbrechtz F, Albrecht A, Renner P
Gas im Pankreas: Bedeutung der Computertomographie
Gas in the pancreas: value of computed tomography
RÖFO 1986 Jan, Vol. 144 (1), P. 63–6

1378. Ellis J H
Superior location of pancreas letter
Am J Roentgenol 1982 Dec, Vol. 139 (6), P. 1242–3

1379. Federle M P, Jeffrey R B, Crass R A, Van Dalsem V
Computed tomography of pancreatic abscesses
Am J Roentgenol 1981 May, Vol. 136 (5), P. 879–82

1380. Ferrucci J T, Wittenberg J, Black E B, Kirkpatrick R H, Hall D A
Computed body tomography in chronic pancreatitis
Radiology 1979 Jan, Vol. 130 (1), P. 175–82

1381. Fink I J, Krudy A G, Shawker T H, Norton J A, Gorden P, Doppman J L
Demonstration of an angiographically hypovascular insulinoma with intraarterial dynamic CT
Am J Roentgenol 1985 Mar, Vol. 144 (3), P. 555–6

1382. Fischedick A R, Muller R P
Computertomographische und angiographische Diagnostik eines innerhalb einer Pankreaspseudozyste rupturierten Pseudoaneurysms
Computer tomographic and angiographic diagnosis of a ruptured pseudoaneurysm within a pancreatic pseudocyst
RÖFO 1983 Mar, Vol. 138 (3), P. 360–2

1383. Fishman A, Isikoff M B, Barkin J S, Friedland J T
Significance of a dilated pancreatic duct on CT examination
Am J Roentgenol 1979 Aug, Vol. 133 (2), P. 225–7

1384. Freeny P C, Marks W M, Ball T J
Impact of high-resolution computed tomography of the pancreas on utilization of endoscopic retrograde cholangiopancreatography and angiography
Radiology 1982 Jan, Vol. 142 (1), P. 35–9

1385. Freeny P C, Marks W M, Ryan J A, Traverso L W
Pancreatic ductal adenocarcinoma: diagnosis and staging with dynamic CT
Radiology 1988 Jan, Vol. 166 (1 Pt 1), P. 125–33

1386. Frick M P, O Leary J F, Salomonowitz E, Stoltenberg P, Hutton S, Gedgaudas E
Pancreas imaging by computed tomography after endoscopic retrograde pancreatography
Radiology 1984 Jan, Vol. 150 (1), P. 191–4

1387. Fricke M, Zick R, Mitzkat H J
Das Insulinom im Computer- Tomogramm
Insulinoma in the computer-tomogram
Radiologe 1978 Jul, Vol. 18 (7), P. 252–4

1388. Galiber A K, Reading C C, Charboneau J W, Sheedy P F, James E M, Gorman B, Grant C S, van Heerden J A, Telander R L
Localization of pancreatic insulinoma: comparison of pre- and intraoperative US with CT and angiography
Radiology 1988 Feb, Vol. 166 (2), P. 405–8

1389. Gamroth A, Hirning T, Rosenthal R
Pankreaspseudoaneurysma und Aneurysma spurium der Arteria lienalis – Diagnostik durch Angio-CT und Ultraschall
Pancreatic pseudoaneurysm and spurious aneurysm of the splenic artery – diagnosis by angio-CT and ultrasound

Radiologe 1986 Feb, Vol. 26 (2), P. 73–5

1390. Gmelin E, Weiss H D, Fuchs H D, Reiser M
Vergleich der diagnostischen Treffsicherheit von Ultraschall, Computertomographie und ERPC bei der chronischen Pankreatitis und beim Pankreaskarzinom
A comparison of the diagnostic accuracy of ultrasound, computer tomography and ERPC in chronic pancreatitis and carcinoma of the pancreas
RÖFO 1981 Feb, Vol. 134 (2), P. 136–41

1391. Gmelin E, Burmester E, Thies E
Blutung in eine Pankreaspseudozyste: Diagnose durch Arteriocomputertomographie
Bleeding into a pancreatic pseudocyst: diagnosis by arterial computed tomography
RÖFO 1984 Aug, Vol. 141 (2), P. 231–2

1392. Grabbe E, Dammann H G, Heller M
Wert der Computertomographie für die Prognose der akuten Pankreatitis
Prognostic value of computed tomography in acute pancreatitis
RÖFO 1982 May, Vol. 136 (5), P. 534–7

1393. Greenberg M, Greenberg B M, Rubin J M, Greenberg I M
Computed-tomographic cholangiography: a new technique for evaluating the head of the pancreas and distal biliary tree
Radiology 1982 Jul, Vol. 144 (2), P. 363–8

1394. Gunther R W, Klose K J, Ruckert K, Kuhn F P, Beyer J, Klotter H J, Cordes U
Islet-cell tumors: detection of small lesions with computed tomography and ultrasound
Radiology 1983 Aug, Vol. 148 (2), P. 485–8

1395. Gustafson K D, Karnaze G C, Hattery R R, Scheithauer B W
Pseudomyxoma peritonei associated with mucinous adenocarcinoma of the pancreas: CT findings and CT-guided biopsy
J Comput Assist Tomogr 1984 Apr, Vol. 8 (2), P. 335–8

1396. Haaga J R, Highman L M, Cooperman A V, Owens F J
Percutaneous CT-guided pancreatography and pseudocystography
Am J Roentgenol 1979 May, Vol. 132 (5), P. 829–30

1397. Haaga J R, Owens D B, Kellermeyer R W, Shina D, Pilai K, Began N
CT guided interstitial therapy of pancreatic carcinoma
J Comput Assist Tomogr 1987 Nov-Dec, Vol. 11 (6), P. 1077–8

1398. Haertel M, Zaunbauer W, Fuchs W A
Die computertomographische Morphologie des Pankreaskarzinoms
The computer tomographic appearances of carcinoma of the pancreas
RÖFO 1980 Jul, Vol. 133 (1), P. 1–5

1399. Hauser H, Battikha J G, Wettstein P
Computed tomography of the dilated main pancreatic duct
J Comput Assist Tomogr 1980 Feb, Vol. 4 (1), P. 53–8

1400. Heiken J P, Balfe D M, Picus D, Scharp D W
Radical pancreatectomy: postoperative evaluation by CT
Radiology 1984 Oct, Vol. 153 (1), P. 211–5

1401. Hertzanu Y, Bar Ziv J, Freund U
Computed tomography of unusual calcified pancreatic tumors
J Comput Assist Tomogr 1989 Jan-Feb, Vol. 13 (1), P. 75–6

1402. Hessel S J, Siegelman S S, McNeil B J, Sanders R, Adams D F, Alderson P O, Finberg H J, Abrams H L
A prospective evaluation of computed tomography and ultrasound of the pancreas
Radiology 1982 Apr, Vol. 143 (1), P. 129–33

1403. Heuck A, Feuerbach S, Reiser M, Anacker H
Computertomographische Morphometrie des normalen Pankreas bei Erwachsenen
Computed tomographic morphometry of the normal pancreas in adults
RÖFO 1985 May, Vol. 142 (5), P. 519–23

1404. Hill M C, Barkin J, Isikoff M B, Silverstein W, Kalser M
Acute pancreatitis: clinical vs. CT findings
Am J Roentgenol 1982 Aug, Vol. 139 (2), P. 263–9

1405. Hosoki T
Dynamic CT of pancreatic tumors
Am J Roentgenol 1983 May, Vol. 140 (5), P. 959–65

1406. Itai Y, Moss A A, Goldberg H I
Pancreatic cysts caused by carcinoma of the pancreas: a pitfall in the diagnosis of pancreatic carcinoma
J Comput Assist Tomogr 1982 Aug, Vol. 6 (4), P. 772–6

1407. Itai Y, Araki T, Tasaka A, Maruyama M
Computed tomographic appearance of resectable pancreatic carcinoma
Radiology 1982 Jun, Vol. 143 (3), P. 719–26

1408. Itai Y, Ohtomo K, Kokubo T, Nagai H, Atomi Y, Kuroda A
CT demonstration of gas in dilated pancreatic duct
J Comput Assist Tomogr 1986 Nov-Dec, Vol. 10 (6), P. 1052–3

1409. Itai Y, Ohhashi K, Furui S, Araki T, Murakami Y, Ohtomo K, Atomi Y
Microcystic adenoma of the pancreas: spectrum of computed tomographic findings
J Comput Assist Tomogr 1988 Sep-Oct, Vol. 12 (5), P. 797–803

1410. Jaffe M H, Glazer G M, Amendola M A, Nostrant T, Wilson J A
Endoscopic retrograde computed tomography of the pancreas
J Comput Assist Tomogr 1984 Feb, Vol. 8 (1), P. 63–6

1411. Jafri S Z, Aisen A M, Glazer G M, Weiss C A
Comparison of CT and angiography in assessing resectability of pancreatic carcinoma
Am J Roentgenol 1984 Mar, Vol. 142 (3), P. 525–9

1412. Jeffrey R B, Federle M P, Laing F C
Computed tomography of mesenteric involvement in fulminant pancreatitis
Radiology 1983 Apr, Vol. 147 (1), P. 185–8

1413. Jeffrey R B Jr, Federle M P, Crass R A
Computed tomography of pancreatic trauma
Radiology 1983 May, Vol. 147 (2), P. 491–4

1414. Johnson C D, Stephens D H, Charboneau J W, Carpenter H A, Welch T J
Cystic pancreatic tumors: CT and sonographic assessment
Am J Roentgenol 1988 Dec, Vol. 151 (6), P. 1133–8

1415. Johnson C D, Stephens D H, Sarr M G
CT of acute pancreatitis: correlation between lack of contrast enhancement and pancreatic necrosis
Am J Roentgenol 1991 Jan, Vol. 156 (1), P. 93–5

1416. Kaplan J O, Isikoff M B, Barkin J, Livingstone A S
Necrotic carcinoma of the pancreas: "the pseudo-pseudocyst"
J Comput Assist Tomogr 1980 Apr, Vol. 4 (2), P. 166–7

1417. Karasawa E, Goldberg H I, Moss A A, Federle M P, London S S
CT pancreatogram in carcinoma of the pancreas and chronic pancreatitis
Radiology 1983 Aug, Vol. 148 (2), P. 489–93

1418. Kim S Y, Lim J H, Lee J D
Papillary carcinoma of the pancreas: findings of US and CT
Radiology 1985 Feb, Vol. 154 (2), P. 338

1419. Kivisaari L, Kormano M, Rantakokko V
Contrast enhancement of the pancreas in computed tomography
J Comput Assist Tomogr 1979 Dec, Vol. 3 (6), P. 722–6

1420. Kivisaari L, Makela P, Aarimaa M
Pancreatic mobility: an important factor in pancreatic computed tomography
J Comput Assist Tomogr 1982 Aug, Vol. 6 (4), P. 854–6

1421. Kolmannskog F, Kolbenstvedt A, Aakhus T
Computed tomography in inflammatory mass lesions following acute pancreatitis
J Comput Assist Tomogr 1981 Apr, Vol. 5 (2), P. 169–72

1422. Konig H, Walter E, Heitland W
Aneurysmatische Pankreaspseudozyste. Angiographie und dynamische Computertomographie
Aneurysmatic pancreatic pseudocyst. Angiography and dynamic computed tomography
RÖFO 1985 Mar, Vol. 142 (3), P. 338–9

1423. Krudy A G, Doppman J L, Jensen R T, Norton J A, Collen M J, Shawker T H, Gardner J D, McArthur K, Gorden P
Localization of islet cell tumors by dynamic CT: comparison with plain CT, arteriography, sonography, and venous sampling
Am J Roentgenol 1984 Sep, Vol. 143 (3), P. 585–9

1424. Kursawe R, Luning M, Wolff H, Mai A
Ergebnisse der computertomographischen Diagnostik zur Differenzierung des Schweregrades der akuten Pankreatitis
Results of computed tomographic diagnosis in the grading of acute pancreatitis
RÖFO 1987 Jan, Vol. 146 (1), P. 27–33

1425. Lackner K, Frommhold H, Grauthoff H, Mödder U, Heuser L, Braun G, Buurman R, Scherer K
Wertigkeit der Computertomographie und der Sonographie innerhalb der Pankreasdiagnostik
The value of computer tomography and sonography in the investigation of the pancreas
RÖFO 1980 May, Vol. 132 (5), P. 509–13

1426. Lepke R A, Pagani J J
Pancreatic Castleman disease simulating pancreatic carcinoma on computed tomography
J Comput Assist Tomogr 1982 Dec, Vol. 6 (6), P. 1193–5

1427. Levin D C
Pancreatic angiography: two views letter
Am J Roentgenol 1980 Mar, Vol. 134 (3), P. 618–9

1428. Levin D C, Wilson R, Abrams H L
The changing role of pancreatic arteriography in the era of computed tomography
Radiology 1980 Jul, Vol. 136 (1), P. 245–9

1429. Levitt R G, Stanley R J, Sagel S S, Lee J K, Weyman P J
Computed tomography of the pancreas: three second scanning versus 18 second scanning
J Comput Assist Tomogr 1982 Apr, Vol. 6 (2), P. 259–67

1430. Longley D G, Dunn D L, Gruessner R, Halvorsen R A Jr, Sutherland D E, Letourneau J G
Detection of pancreatic fluid and urine leakage after pancreas transplantation: value of CT and cystography
Am J Roentgenol 1990 Nov, Vol. 155 (5), P. 997–1000

1431. Luetmer P H, Stephens D H, Fischer A P
Obliteration of periarterial retropancreatic fat on CT in pancreatitis: an exception to the rule
Am J Roentgenol 1989 Jul, Vol. 153 (1), P. 63–4

1432. Luetmer P H, Stephens D H, Ward E M
Chronic pancreatitis: reassessment with current CT
Radiology 1989 May, Vol. 171 (2), P. 353–7

1433. Magnuson J E, Stephens D H
CT demonstration of pancreatic atrophy following acute pancreatitis
J Comput Assist Tomogr 1988 Nov-Dec, Vol. 12 (6), P. 1050–3

1434. Maier W
Frühdiagnose und Staging der akuten Pankreatitis durch Computertomographie
Early diagnosis and staging of acute pancreatitis using computed tomography
RÖFO 1988 Mar, Vol. 148 (3), P. 251–4

1435. Maier W
Zur Wertigkeit der Nativ-Computertomographie bei der akuten Pankreatitis
The value of non-contrast computed tomography in acute pancreatitis
RÖFO 1989 Apr, Vol. 150 (4), P. 458–61

1436. Manelfe C, Louvet J P
Computed tomography in diabetes insipidus
J Comput Assist Tomogr 1979 Jun, Vol. 3 (3), P. 309–16

1437. McCarthy S, Pellegrini C A, Moss A A, Way L W
Pleuropancreatic fistula: endoscopic retrograde cholangiopancreatography and computed tomography
Am J Roentgenol 1984 Jun, Vol. 142 (6), P. 1151–4

1438. McCowin M J, Federle M P
Computed tomography of pancreatic pseudocysts of the duodenum
Am J Roentgenol 1985 Nov, Vol. 145 (5), P. 1003–7

1439. Minami M, Itai Y, Ohtomo K, Yoshida H, Yoshikawa K, Iio M
Cystic neoplasms of the pancreas: comparison of MR imaging with CT
Radiology 1989 Apr, Vol. 171 (1), P. 53–6

1440. Mitchell D G, Hill M C
Obstructive jaundice due to multiple myeloma of the pancreatic head: CT evaluation
J Comput Assist Tomogr 1985 Nov-Dec, Vol. 9 (6), P. 1118–9

1441. Mödder U, Friedmann G, Rosenberger J
Wert der Angio-CT für Stadieneinteilung, Verlaufsbeobachtung und Therapie bei akuter Pankreatitis
The value of angio-CT for staging, observation and treatment of acute pancreatitis
RÖFO 1981 Jan, Vol. 134 (1), P. 22–7

1442. Moss A A, Federle M, Shapiro H A, Ohto M, Goldberg H, Korobkin M, Clemett A
The combined use of computed tomography and endoscopic retrograde cholangiopancreatography in the assessment of suspected pancreatic neoplasm: a blind clinical evaluation
Radiology 1980 Jan, Vol. 134 (1), P. 159–63

1443. Moss G D, Malvar T C
CT demonstration of an ectopic pancreatic tail causing a renal pseudotumor
J Comput Assist Tomogr 1983 Aug, Vol. 7 (4), P. 724–6

1444. Moulton J S, Munda R, Weiss M A, Lubbers D J
Pancreatic transplants: CT with clinical and pathologic correlation
Radiology 1989 Jul, Vol. 172 (1), P. 21–6

1445. Munk P L, Muller N L
CT diagnosis of oil-induced granuloma secondary to diabetes insipidus therapy
J Comput Assist Tomogr 1985 Nov-Dec, Vol. 9 (6), P. 1147–8

1446. Nacianceno S E, Gross S C, Raju J S, Song S H, Joseph R R
Pancreatic pseudocyst simulating dilated biliary duct system on computed tomography
Radiology 1980 Jan, Vol. 134 (1), P. 165–6

1447. Nakata H, Nakayama T, Kimoto T, Kimura N
Dynamic computed tomography of the pancreas
J Comput Assist Tomogr 1982 Jun, Vol. 6 (3), P. 646–9

1448. Neumann C H, Hessel S J
CT of the pancreatic tail
Am J Roentgenol 1980 Oct, Vol. 135 (4), P. 741–5

1449. Novetsky G J, Berlin L, Smith C, Epstein A J
CT diagnosis of annular pancreas
J Comput Assist Tomogr 1984 Oct, Vol. 8 (5), P. 1031–2

1450. Ormson M J, Charboneau J W, Stephens D H
Sonography in patients with a possible pancreatic mass shown on CT
Am J Roentgenol 1987 Mar, Vol. 148 (3), P. 551–5

1451. Pandolfo I, Scribano E, Gaeta M, Fiumara F, Longo M
Cystic lymphangioma of the pancreas: CT demonstration
J Comput Assist Tomogr 1985 Jan-Feb, Vol. 9 (1), P. 209–10

1452. Parienty R A, Ducellier R, Lubrano J M, Picard J D, Pradel J, Smolarski N
Cystadenomas of the pancreas: diagnosis by computed tomography
J Comput Assist Tomogr 1980 Jun, Vol. 4 (3), P. 364–7

1453. Pombo F, Soler R, Martin R, Castro J M
Periportal- peripancreatic tuberculous adenitis. US and CT findings
RÖFO 1990 Feb, Vol. 152 (2), P. 142–6

1454. Radin D R, Santiago E M
Cholecystoduodenal fistula due to pancreatic carcinoma: CT diagnosis
J Comput Assist Tomogr 1986 Jan-Feb, Vol. 10 (1), P. 149–50

1455. Raptopoulos V, Davidoff A, Karellas A, Davis M A, Coolbaugh B L, Smith E H
CT of the pancreas with a fat-density oral contrast regimen
Am J Roentgenol 1988 Jun, Vol. 150 (6), P. 1303–6

1456. Raval B
A new computed tomographic sign of pancreatitis letter
Am J Roentgenol 1980 Jan, Vol. 134 (1), P. 210

1457. Reiman T H, Balfe D M, Weyman P J
Suprapancreatic biliary obstruction: CT evaluation
Radiology 1987 Apr, Vol. 163 (1), P. 49–56

1458. Roberts L Jr, Dunnick N R, Foster W L Jr, Halvorsen R A, Gibbons R G, Meyers W C, Feldman J M, Thompson W M
Somatostatinoma of the endocrine pancreas: CT findings
J Comput Assist Tomogr 1984 Oct, Vol. 8 (5), P. 1015–7

1459. Rossi P, Baert A, Marchal W, Tipaldi L, Wilms W, Pavone P
Multiple bolus technique vs. single bolus or infusion of contrast medium to obtain prolonged contrast enhancement of the pancreas
Radiology 1982 Sep, Vol. 144 (4), P. 929–31

1460. Rossi P, Baert A, Passariello R, Simonetti G, Pavone P, Tempesta P
CT of functioning tumors of the pancreas
Am J Roentgenol 1985 Jan, Vol. 144 (1), P. 57–60

1461. Rumancik W M, Megibow A J, Bosniak M A, Hilton S
Metastatic disease to the pancreas: evaluation by computed tomography
J Comput Assist Tomogr 1984 Oct, Vol. 8 (5), P. 829–34

1462. Scatarige J C, Fishman E K, Crist D W, Cameron J L, Siegelman S S
Diverticulitis of the right colon: CT observations
Am J Roentgenol 1987 Apr, Vol. 148 (4), P. 737–9

1463. Shah K K, DeRidder P H, Schwab R E, Alexander T J
CT diagnosis of dorsal pancreas agenesis
J Comput Assist Tomogr 1987 Jan-Feb, Vol. 11 (1), P. 170–1

1464. Shirkhoda A, Mittelstaedt C A
Demonstration of pancreatic cysts in adult polycystic disease by computed tomography and ultrasound
Am J Roentgenol 1978 Dec, Vol. 131 (6), P. 1074–6

1465. Silverman P M, McVay L, Zeman R K, Garra B S, Grant E G, Jaffe M H
Pancreatic pseudotumor in pancreas divisum: CT characteristics
J Comput Assist Tomogr 1989 Jan-Feb, Vol. 13 (1), P. 140–1

1466. Silverstein W, Isikoff M B, Hill M C, Barkin J
Diagnostic imaging of acute pancreatitis: prospective study using CT and sonography
Am J Roentgenol 1981 Sep, Vol. 137 (3), P. 497–502

1467. Smith T R, Koenigsberg M
Low-density insulinoma on dynamic CT
Am J Roentgenol 1990 Nov, Vol. 155 (5), P. 995–6

1468. Stark D D, Moss A A, Goldberg H I, Deveney C W
CT of pancreatic islet cell tumors
Radiology 1984 Feb, Vol. 150 (2), P. 491–4

1469. Stark D D, Moss A A, Goldberg H I, Davis P L, Federle M P
Magnetic resonance and CT of the normal and diseased pancreas: a comparative study
Radiology 1984 Jan, Vol. 150 (1), P. 153–62

1470. Steiner E, Stark D D, Hahn P F, Saini S, Simeone J F, Mueller P R, Wittenberg J, Ferrucci J T
Imaging of pancreatic neoplasms: comparison of MR and CT
Am J Roentgenol 1989 Mar, Vol. 152 (3), P. 487–91

1471. Strax R, Toombs B D, Rauschkolb E N
Correlation of barium enema and CT in acute pancreatitis
Am J Roentgenol 1981 Jun, Vol. 136 (6), P. 1219–20

1472. Stuck K J, Kuhns L R
Improved visualization of the pancreatic tail after maximum distension of the stomach
J Comput Assist Tomogr 1981 Aug, Vol. 5 (4), P. 509–12

1473. Tremmel K, Zimmer P, Barth V
Differentialdiagnose der chronischen peripankreatischen Pseudozyste im Computertomogramm. Fehlermöglichkeiten und Fallgruben
Differential diagnosis of chronic peripancreatic pseudocysts on the computerized tomogram. Possibility of error and pitfalls
RÖFO 1987 Mar, Vol. 146 (3), P. 284–90

1474. Triller J, Kappeler M, Coray T, Halter F
CT und ERCP als Kombinationsuntersuchung bei Erkrankungen des Pankreas
CT and ERCP as a combination research method in pancreatic diseases
RÖFO 1984 Nov, Vol. 141 (5), P. 483–90

1475. Vernacchia F S, Jeffrey R B Jr, Federle M P, Grendell J H, Laing F C, Wing V W, Wall S D
Pancreatic abscess: predictive value of early abdominal CT
Radiology 1987 Feb, Vol. 162 (2), P. 435–8

1476. White E M, Wittenberg J, Mueller P R, Simeone J F, Butch R J, Warshaw A L, Neff C C, Nardi G L, Ferrucci J T Jr
Pancreatic necrosis: CT manifestations
Radiology 1986 Feb, Vol. 158 (2), P. 343–6

1477. Williford M E, Foster W L Jr, Halvorsen R A, Thompson W M
Pancreatic pseudocyst: comparative evaluation by sonography and computed tomography
Am J Roentgenol 1983 Jan, Vol. 140 (1), P. 53–7

1478. Wilson T E, Korobkin M, Francis I R
Pancreatic plasmacytoma: CT findings
Am J Roentgenol 1989 Jun, Vol. 152 (6), P. 1227–8

1479. Wolfman N T, Karstaedt N, Kawamoto E H
Pleomorphic carcinoma of the pancreas: computed-tomographic, sonographic, and pathologic findings
Radiology 1985 Feb, Vol. 154 (2), P. 329–32

1480. Yoshikai T, Murakami J, Nishihara H, Oshiumi Y
Hemosuccus pancreaticus: CT manifestations
J Comput Assist Tomogr 1986 May- Jun, Vol. 10 (3), P. 510–2

1481. Zeman R K, McVay L V, Silverman P M, Cattau E L, Benjamin S B, Fleischer D F, Garra B S, Jaffe M H
Pancreas divisum: thin- section CT
Radiology 1988 Nov, Vol. 169 (2), P. 395–8

The Gastrointestinal Tract

1482. Adolph J M, Kimmig B N, Georgi P, zum Winkel K
Carcinoid tumors: CT and I-131 meta-iodo-benzylguanidine scintigraphy
Radiology 1987 Jul, Vol. 164 (1), P. 199–203

1483. Agostini S, Grimaud J C, Salducci J, Clement J P
Idiopathic muscular hypertrophy of the esophagus: CT features
J Comput Assist Tomogr 1988 Nov-Dec, Vol. 12 (6), P. 1041–3

1484. Allen K S, Siskind B N, Burrell M I
Perforation of distal esophagus with lesser sac extension: CT demonstration
J Comput Assist Tomogr 1986 Jul-Aug, Vol. 10 (4), P. 612–4

1485. Angelelli G, Macarini L, Lupo L, Caputi Jambrenghi O, Pannarale O, Memeo V
Rectal carcinoma: CT staging with water as contrast medium
Radiology 1990 Nov, Vol. 177 (2), P. 511–4

1486. Baert A L, Roex L, Marchal G, Hermans P, Dewilde D, Wilms G
Computed tomography of the stomach with water as an oral contrast agent: technique and preliminary results
J Comput Assist Tomogr 1989 Jul-Aug, Vol. 13 (4), P. 633–6

1487. Balfe D M, Koehler R E, Karstaedt N, Stanley R J, Sagel S S
Computed tomography of gastric neoplasms
Radiology 1981 Aug, Vol. 140 (2), P. 431–6

1488. Balfe D M, Mauro M A, Koehler R E, Lee J K, Weyman P J, Picus D, Peterson R R
Gastrohepatic ligament: normal and pathologic CT anatomy
Radiology 1984 Feb, Vol. 150 (2), P. 485–90

1489. Balthazar E J, Megibow A, Naidich D, LeFleur R S
Computed tomographic recognition of gastric varices
Am J Roentgenol 1984 Jun, Vol. 142 (6), P. 1121–5

1490. Balthazar E J, Bauman J S, Megibow A J
CT diagnosis of closed loop obstruction
J Comput Assist Tomogr 1985 Sep-Oct, Vol. 9 (5), P. 953–5

1491. Balthazar E J, Hulnick D, Megibow A J, Opulencia J F
Computed tomography of intramural intestinal hemorrhage and bowel ischemia
J Comput Assist Tomogr 1987 Jan-Feb, Vol. 11 (1), P. 67–72

1492. Balthazar E J, Naidich D P, Megibow A J, Lefleur R S
CT evaluation of esophageal varices
Am J Roentgenol 1987 Jan, Vol. 148 (1), P. 131–5

1493. Balthazar E J, Megibow A J, Gordon R B, Hulnick D
Cecal diverticulitis: evaluation with CT
Radiology 1987 Jan, Vol. 162 (1 Pt 1), P. 79–81

1494. Balthazar E J, Megibow A J, Hulnick D, Naidich D P
Carcinoma of the colon: detection and preoperative staging by CT
Am J Roentgenol 1988 Feb, Vol. 150 (2), P. 301–6

1495. Balthazar E J, Megibow A J, Gordon R B, Whelan C A, Hulnick D
Computed tomography of the abnormal appendix
J Comput Assist Tomogr 1988 Jul-Aug, Vol. 12 (4), P. 595–601

1496. Balthazar E J, Gordon R, Hulnick D
Ileocecal tuberculosis: CT and radiologic evaluation
Am J Roentgenol 1990 Mar, Vol. 154 (3), P. 499–503

1497. Balthazar E J, Megibow A, Schinella R A, Gordon R
Limitations in the CT diagnosis of acute diverticulitis: comparison of CT, contrast enema, and pathologic findings in 16 patients
Am J Roentgenol 1990 Feb, Vol. 154 (2), P. 281–5

1498. Balthazar E J
CT of the gastrointestinal tract: principles and interpretation
Am J Roentgenol 1991 Jan, Vol. 156 (1), P. 23–32 20 Refs

1499. Bank E R, Hernandez R J, Byrne W J
Gastrointestinal hemangiomatosis in children: demonstration with CT
Radiology 1987 Dec, Vol. 165 (3), P. 657–8

1500. Barakos J A, Jeffrey R B Jr, Federle M P, Wing V W, Laing F C, Hightower D R
CT in the management of periappendiceal abscess
Am J Roentgenol 1986 Jun, Vol. 146 (6), P. 1161–4

1501. Becker C D, Barbier P, Porcellini B
CT evaluation of patients undergoing transhiatal esophagectomy for cancer
J Comput Assist Tomogr 1986 Jul-Aug, Vol. 10 (4), P. 607–11

1502. Benson M, Bree R L, Schwab R E, Ouimette M
Computed tomographic studies of the painful abdomen
Radiology 1985 May, Vol. 155 (2), P. 443–4

1503. Berger P E, Kuhn J P
CT of blunt abdominal trauma in childhood
Am J Roentgenol 1981 Jan, Vol. 136 (1), P. 105–10

1504. Bernardino M E, Jing B S, Wallace S
Computed tomography diagnosis of mesenteric masses
Am J Roentgenol 1979 Jan, Vol. 132 (1), P. 33–6

1505. Berry D F, Willing S J, Beers G J
Small bowel obstruction due to enterolith: CT appearance
J Comput Assist Tomogr 1987 Jul- Aug, Vol. 11 (4), P. 707–8

1506. Billimoria P E, Fabian T M, Schulz E E
Computed tomography of intussusception in the bypassed jejunoileal segment
J Comput Assist Tomogr 1982 Feb, Vol. 6 (1), P. 86–8

1507. Bonatti G P, Ortore P G
Computertomographischer Nachweis eines Dünndarmkarzinoids
Computed tomography detection of a small bowel carcinoid
Radiologe 1987 May, Vol. 27 (5), P. 229–31

1508. Bowen B, Ros P R, McCarthy M J, Olmsted W W, Hjermstad B M
Gastrointestinal teratomas: CT and US appearance with pathologic correlation
Radiology 1987 Feb, Vol. 162 (2), P. 431–3

1509. Brown B M, Federle M P, Jeffrey R B
Gastric wall thickening and extragastric inflammatory processes: a retrospective CT study
J Comput Assist Tomogr 1982 Aug, Vol. 6 (4), P. 762–5

1510. Bulas D I, Taylor G A, Eichelberger M R
The value of CT in detecting bowel perforation in children after blunt abdominal trauma
Am J Roentgenol 1989 Sep, Vol. 153 (3), P. 561–4

1511. Butch R J, Stark D D, Wittenberg J, Tepper J E, Saini S, Simeone J F, Mueller P R, Ferrucci J T Jr
Staging rectal cancer by MR and CT
Am J Roentgenol 1986 Jun, Vol. 146 (6), P. 1155–60

1512. Buy J N, Moss A A
Computed tomography of gastric lymphoma
Am J Roentgenol 1982 May, Vol. 138 (5), P. 859–65

1513. Callen P W
Computed tomographic evaluation of abdominal and pelvic abscesses
Radiology 1979 Apr, Vol. 131 (1), P. 171–5

1514. Carvalho P, Bannerjee A K, Goodman A
Computed tomography of rectal lymphoma
J Comput Assist Tomogr 1990 May-Jun, Vol. 14 (3), P. 379–80

1515. Chen Y M, Ott D J, Wolfman N T, Gelfand D W, Karstaedt N, Bechtold R E
Recurrent colorectal carcinoma: evaluation with barium enema examination and CT
Radiology 1987 May, Vol. 163 (2), P. 307–10

1516. Cho K C, Hoffman Tretin J C, Alterman D D
Closed-loop obstruction of the small bowel: CT and sonographic appearance
J Comput Assist Tomogr 1989 Mar-Apr, Vol. 13 (2), P. 256–8

1517. Cho K C, Morehouse H T, Alterman D D, Thornhill B A
Sigmoid diverticulitis: diagnostic role of CT-comparison with barium enema studies
Radiology 1990 Jul, Vol. 176 (1), P. 111–5

1518. Clark R A
Computed tomography of bowel infarction
J Comput Assist Tomogr 1987 Sep-Oct, Vol. 11 (5), P. 757–62

1519. Cranston P E
Colon opacification by oral water-soluble contrast medium administration the night prior to CT examination
J Comput Assist Tomogr 1982 Apr, Vol. 6 (2), P. 413–5

1520. Crass J R, Simmons R L, Frick M P, Maile C W
Percutaneous decompression of the colon using CT guidance in Ogilvie syndrome
Am J Roentgenol 1985 Mar, Vol. 144 (3), P. 475–6

1521. Crone Munzebrock W, Brockmann W P
Computertomographische und sonographische Diagnostik und Verlaufskontrolle beim malignen Lymphom des Magens
Computer tomographic and sonographic diagnosis and control in malignant lymphoma of the stomach
RÖFO 1983 Dec, Vol. 139 (6), P. 676–80

1522. Curcio C M, Feinstein R S, Humphrey R L, Jones B, Siegelman S S
Computed tomography of entero-enteric intussusception
J Comput Assist Tomogr 1982 Oct, Vol. 6 (5), P. 969–74

1523. de Lange E E, Slutsky V S, Swanson S, Shaffer H A Jr
Computed tomography of emphysematous gastritis
J Comput Assist Tomogr 1986 Jan-Feb, Vol. 10 (1), P. 139–41

1524. Dey C, Duvoisin B
CT findings in primary amyloidosis of the colon
J Comput Assist Tomogr 1989 Nov-Dec, Vol. 13 (6), P. 1094–5

1525. Donaldson J S, Gilsanz V
CT findings in rectal cuff abscess following surgery for Hirschsprung disease
J Comput Assist Tomogr 1986 Jan-Feb, Vol. 10 (1), P. 151–3

1526. Donovan A T, Goldman S M
Computed tomography of ileocecal intussusception: mechanism and appearance
J Comput Assist Tomogr 1982 Jun, Vol. 6 (3), P. 630–2

1527. Doringer E, Watzinger F
Computertomographie des Magenwandneurinoms
Computed tomography of a neurinoma of the gastric wall
RÖFO 1989 Aug, Vol. 151 (2), P. 235–6

1528. Doringer E, Ferner R
Computertomographie der Kolondivertikulitis
Computed tomography of colonic diverticulitis
RÖFO 1990 Jan, Vol. 152 (1), P. 76–9

1529. Dudiak K M, Johnson C D, Stephens D H
Primary tumors of the small intestine: CT evaluation
Am J Roentgenol 1989 May, Vol. 152 (5), P. 995–8

1530. Duvoisin B, Schnyder P
Die Computertomographie des Dünndarms
Computerized tomography of the small bowel
Radiologe 1990 Jun, Vol. 30 (6), P. 280–5

1531. Fagelman D, Warhit J M, Reiter J D, Geiss A C
CT diagnosis of fecaloma
J Comput Assist Tomogr 1984 Jun, Vol. 8 (3), P. 559–61

1532. Farah M C, Jafri S Z, Schwab R E, Mezwa D G, Francis I R, Noujaim S, Kim C
Duodenal neoplasms: role of CT
Radiology 1987 Mar, Vol. 162 (3), P. 839–43

1533. Federle M P, Chun G, Jeffrey R B, Rayor R
Computed tomographic findings in bowel infarction
Am J Roentgenol 1984 Jan, Vol. 142 (1), P. 91–5

1534. Fisher J K
Normal colon wall thickness on CT
Radiology 1982 Nov, Vol. 145 (2), P. 415–8

1535. Fisher J K
Abnormal colonic wall thickening on computed tomography
J Comput Assist Tomogr 1983 Feb, Vol. 7 (1), P. 90–7

1536. Fisher J K
Computed tomography of colonic pneumatosis intestinalis with mesenteric and portal venous air
J Comput Assist Tomogr 1984 Jun, Vol. 8 (3), P. 573–4

1537. Fishman E K, Wolf E J, Jones B, Bayless T M, Siegelman S S
CT evaluation of Crohn's disease: effect on patient management
Am J Roentgenol 1987 Mar, Vol. 148 (3), P. 537–40

1538. Frager D H, Goldman M, Beneventano T C
Computed tomography in Crohn disease
J Comput Assist Tomogr 1983 Oct, Vol. 7 (5), P. 819–24

1539. Francis I R, Glazer G M, Shapiro B, Sisson J C, Gross B H
Complementary roles of CT and 131I-MIBG scintigraphy in diagnosing pheochromocytoma
Am J Roentgenol 1983 Oct, Vol. 141 (4), P. 719–25

1540. Freeny P C, Marks W M, Ryan J A, Bolen J W
Colorectal carcinoma evaluation with CT: preoperative staging and detection of postoperative recurrence
Radiology 1986 Feb, Vol. 158 (2), P. 347–53

1541. Frick M P, Maile C W, Crass J R, Goldberg M E, Delaney J P
Computed tomography of neutropenic colitis
Am J Roentgenol 1984 Oct, Vol. 143 (4), P. 763–5

1542. Fruauff A, Irwin G A, Williams H C, Gold B
CT demonstration of gastric carcinoid letter
Am J Roentgenol 1987 Jun, Vol. 148 (6), P. 1276–7

1543. Gaa J, Deininger H K
Computertomographie kolorektaler Tumoren mit Wasser als Kontrastmittel
The computed tomography of colorectal tumors with water as the contrast medium
RÖFO 1990 Jun, Vol. 152 (6), P. 723–6

1544. Glazer G M, Buy J N, Moss A A, Goldberg H I, Federle M P
CT detection of duodenal perforation
Am J Roentgenol 1981 Aug, Vol. 137 (2), P. 333–6

1545. Glick S N, Levine M S, Teplick S K, Gasparaitis A
Splenic penetration by benign gastric ulcer: preoperative recognition with CT
Radiology 1987 Jun, Vol. 163 (3), P. 637–9

1546. Goldberg H I, Gore R M, Margulis A R, Moss A A, Baker E L
Computed tomography in the evaluation of Crohn disease
Am J Roentgenol 1983 Feb, Vol. 140 (2), P. 277–82

1547. Goldman S M, Fishman E K, Gatewood O M, Jones B, Brendler C, Siegelman S S
CT demonstration of colovesical fistulae secondary to diverticulitis
J Comput Assist Tomogr 1984 Jun, Vol. 8 (3), P. 462–8

1548. Gonzalez J G, Gonzalez R R, Patino J V, Garcia A T, Alvarez C P, Pedrosa C S
CT findings in gastrointestinal perforation by ingested fish bones
J Comput Assist Tomogr 1988 Jan-Feb, Vol. 12 (1), P. 88–90

1549. Goodman P C, Federle M P
Pseudomembranous colitis
J Comput Assist Tomogr 1980 Jun, Vol. 4 (3), P. 403–4

1550. Gore R M, Marn C S, Kirby D F, Vogelzang R L, Neiman H L
CT findings in ulcerative, granulomatous, and indeterminate colitis
Am J Roentgenol 1984 Aug, Vol. 143 (2), P. 279–84

1551. Grabbe E, Lierse W, Winkler R
Die Hüllfaszien des Rektums. Anatomische und computertomographische Korrelation
The fascial planes round the rectum. Anatomic and computer tomographic correlations
RÖFO 1982 Jun, Vol. 136 (6), P. 653–9

1552. Grabbe E, Winkler R
Local recurrence after sphincter- saving resection for rectal and rectosigmoid carcinoma
Radiology 1985 Vol. 155 ,P. 305–310

1553. Greenstein S, Jones B, Fishman E K, Cameron J L, Siegelman S S
Small-bowel diverticulitis: CT findings
Am J Roentgenol 1986 Aug, Vol. 147 (2), P. 271–4

1554. Grosser G, Wimmer B, Ruf G
Diagnostischer Wert der Computertomographie beim Magenkarzinom
Diagnostic value of computed tomography in stomach cancer
RÖFO 1985 May, Vol. 142 (5), P. 514–9

1555. Grote R, Dohring W, Meyer H J, Schmied W, Lohlein D
Computertomographie bei malignen Tumoren des Magens
Computed tomography of malignant stomach tumors
RÖFO 1984 Dec, Vol. 141 (6), P. 654–60

1556. Guillaumin E, Jeffrey R B Jr, Shea W J, Asling C W, Goldberg H I
Perirectal inflammatory disease: CT findings
Radiology 1986 Oct, Vol. 161 (1), P. 153–7

1557. Hall F M
Computed tomography in the evaluation of diverticulitis letter
Radiology 1985 Mar, Vol. 154 (3), P. 835–6

1558. Hall F M
Cecal diverticulitis: evaluation with CT letter
Radiology 1987 Jun, Vol. 163 (3), P. 832

1559. Hamlin D J, Burgener F A, Sischy B
New technique to stage early rectal carcinoma by computed tomography
Radiology 1981 Nov, Vol. 141 (2), P. 539–40

1560. Hendricks P J, Keefe B, Wechsler R J
The value of CT in rectal villous tumors
J Comput Assist Tomogr 1989 Mar-Apr, Vol. 13 (2), P. 269–72

1561. Hoddick W K, Demas B E, Moss A A
CT-guided percutaneous bowel loopogram
Am J Roentgenol 1984 Nov, Vol. 143 (5), P. 1098–100

1562. Hodgman C G, Lantz E J, Maus T P, Conley C R
Computed tomography of intussusception due to colon lipoma
J Comput Assist Tomogr 1987 Jul-Aug, Vol. 11 (4), P. 740–1

1563. Hollmann J P, Goebel N
Computertomographie (CT) und Sonographie (US) in der Rezidivdiagnostik kolorektaler Tumoren
Computerized tomography and sonography in the diagnosis of recurrent colorectal tumors
RÖFO 1985 Dec, Vol. 143 (6), P. 665–71

1564. Hughes J J, Blunck C E
CT demonstration of gastropancreatic fistula due to penetrating gastric ulcer
J Comput Assist Tomogr 1987 Jul-Aug, Vol. 11 (4), P. 709–11

1565. Hulnick D H, Megibow A J, Balthazar E J, Naidich D P, Bosniak M A
Computed tomography in the evaluation of diverticulitis
Radiology 1984 Aug, Vol. 152 (2), P. 491–5

1566. Hulnick D H, Megibow A J, Balthazar E J
Diverticulitis: evaluation by CT and contrast enema letter
Am J Roentgenol 1987 Sep, Vol. 149 (3), P. 644–6

1567. Iko B O, Teal J S, Siram S M, Chinwuba C E, Roux V J, Scott V F
Computed tomography of adult colonic intussusception: clinical and experimental studies
Am J Roentgenol 1984 Oct, Vol. 143 (4), P. 769–72

1568. Jacobs J M, Hill M C, Steinberg W M
Peptic ulcer disease: CT evaluation
Radiology 1991 Mar, Vol. 178 (3), P. 745–8

1569. James S, Balfe D M, Lee J K, Picus D
Small-bowel disease: categorization by CT examination
Am J Roentgenol 1987 May, Vol. 148 (5), P. 863–8

1570. Jaramillo D, Raval B
CT diagnosis of primary small-bowel volvulus
Am J Roentgenol 1986 Nov, Vol. 147 (5), P. 941–2

1571. Jeffrey R B, Federle M P, Wall S
Value of computed tomography in detecting occult gastrointestinal perforation
J Comput Assist Tomogr 1983 Oct, Vol. 7 (5), P. 825–7

1572. Jeffrey R B, Federle M P, Laing F C
Computed tomography of silent abdominal abscesses
J Comput Assist Tomogr 1984 Feb, Vol. 8 (1), P. 67–70

1573. Johnson C D, Baker M E, Rice R P, Silverman P, Thompson W M
Diagnosis of acute colonic diverticulitis: comparison of barium enema and CT
Am J Roentgenol 1987 Mar, Vol. 148 (3), P. 541–6

1574. Jones B, Fishman E K, Siegelman S S
Ischemic colitis demonstrated by computed tomography
J Comput Assist Tomogr 1982 Dec, Vol. 6 (6), P. 1120–3

1575. Jones B, Bayless T M, Fishman E K, Siegelman S S
Lymphadenopathy in celiac disease: computed tomographic observations
Am J Roentgenol 1984 Jun, Vol. 142 (6), P. 1127–32

1576. Jones B, Fishman E K, Hamilton S R, Rubesin S E, Bayless T M, Cameron J C, Siegelman S S
Submucosal accumulation of fat in inflammatory bowel disease: CT /pathologic correlation
J Comput Assist Tomogr 1986 Sep-Oct, Vol. 10 (5), P. 759–63

1577. Kampmann H
Pitfall bei der Abdomencomputertomographie. Pseudotumor durch extrem dilatiertes Colon ascendens
Pitfalls in computer tomography of the abdomen. Pseudotumor due to an extremely dilated ascending colon RÖFO 1982 Nov, Vol. 137 (5), P. 603–5

1578. Kane V G, Silverstein G S
CT demonstration of hernia through an iliac crest defect
J Comput Assist Tomogr 1986 May-Jun, Vol. 10 (3), P. 432–4

1579. Kanehann L B, Caroline D F, Friedman A C, Lev Toaff A S, Radecki P D
CT findings in venous intravasation complicating diverticulitis
J Comput Assist Tomogr 1988 Nov-Dec, Vol. 12 (6), P. 1047–9

1580. Karnaze G C, Sheedy P F, Stephens D H, McLeod R A
Computed tomography in duodenal rupture due to blunt abdominal trauma
J Comput Assist Tomogr 1981 Apr, Vol. 5 (2), P. 267–9

1581. Kleinhaus U, Weich Y
Computed tomography of Crohn's disease – reevaluation
RÖFO 1987 Dec, Vol. 147 (6), P. 607–11

1582. Klooster N J, Goei R, Baeten C G
Sigmoido-rectal invagination secondary to carcinoma: findings on CT
RÖFO 1989 Nov, Vol. 151 (5), P. 623–4

1583. Klose K C, Persigehl M
Computertomographische Darstellung eines Trichobezoars
Computed tomographic image of a trichobezoar
RÖFO 1985 May, Vol. 142 (5), P. 585–6

1584. Klose K J, Duber C, Kempf P, Gunther R, Schweden F
Stellenwert der Computertomographie in der Diagnostik des lokalen Rektumkarzinomrezidivs
The value of computer tomography in the diagnosis of local recurrences of carcinoma of the rectum
RÖFO 1982 May, Vol. 136 (5), P. 538–42

1585. Knowles M C, Fishman E K, Kuhlman J E, Bayless T M
Transient intussusception in Crohn disease: CT evaluation
Radiology 1989 Mar, Vol. 170 (3 Pt 1), P. 814

1586. Komaki S
Normal or benign gastric wall thickening demonstrated by computed tomography
J Comput Assist Tomogr 1982 Dec, Vol. 6 (6), P. 1103–7

1587. Koster O, Harder T
Computertomographische und sonographische Therapiekontrolle beim Non-Hodgkin-Lymphom des Magens
Computed tomographic and sonographic control of the treatment of non-Hodgkin's lymphoma of the stomach
RÖFO 1982 Dec, Vol. 137 (6), P. 727–9

1588. Kramer E L, Noz M E, Sanger J J, Megibow A J, Maguire G Q
CT-SPECT fusion to correlate radiolabeled monoclonal antibody uptake with abdominal CT findings
Radiology 1989 Sep, Vol. 172 (3), P. 861–5

1589. Krestin G P, Steinbrich W, Friedmann G
Recurrent rectal cancer: diagnosis with MR imaging versus CT
Radiology 1988 Aug, Vol. 168 (2), P. 307–11

1590. Krestin G P, Steinbrich W, Friedmann G
Rezidivdiagnostik der Rektumkarzinome: Vergleich CT/MR
Diagnosis of recurrent rectal cancer: Comparison of CT and MR
RÖFO 1988 Jan, Vol. 148 (1), P. 28–33

1591. Kuper K, Bautz W, Gnann H
Wertigkeit der MR-Tomographie für die Diagnostik des Rektumkarzinoms und dessen Rezidiv im Vergleich zur CT
Value of MR tomography vs. CT in the diagnosis of rectal carcinoma and its recurrence
RÖFO 1985 Sep, Vol. 143 (3), P. 301–6

1592. Kuwabara Y, Nishitani H, Numaguchi Y, Kamoi I, Matsuura K, Saito S
Afferent loop syndrome
J Comput Assist Tomogr 1980 Oct, Vol. 4 (5), P. 687–9

1593. Lackner K, Weiand G, Koster O, Engel K
Computertomographie bei Tumoren des Ösophagus und Magens
Computer tomography for tumours of the oesophagus and stomach
RÖFO 1981 Apr, Vol. 134 (4), P. 364–70

1594. Larsson S G, Lufkin R B
Anomalies of digastric muscles: CT and MR demonstration
J Comput Assist Tomogr 1987 May-Jun, Vol. 11 (3), P. 422–5

1595. Lee K R, Levine E, Moffat R E, Bigongiari L R, Hermreck A S
Computed tomographic staging of malignant gastric neoplasms
Radiology 1979 Oct, Vol. 133 (1), P. 151–5

1596. Leyman P, Ponette E, Marchal G, Vercruyssen J, Timmermans G, Ceulemans R, Baert A L
Computed tomography of acute jejunogastric intussusception
J Comput Assist Tomogr 1989 May-Jun, Vol. 13 (3), P. 531–3

1597. Lieberman J M, Haaga J R
Computed tomography of diverticulitis
J Comput Assist Tomogr 1983 Jun, Vol. 7 (3), P. 431–3

1598. Lo J, Sage M R, Paterson H S, Hamilton D W
Gastric duplication in an adult
J Comput Assist Tomogr 1983 Apr, Vol. 7 (2), P. 328–30

1599. Lorenz R, Zankovich R, Mödder U, Beyer D
Primäres malignes Lymphom des Magens. MDP, Sonographie, Computertomographie
Primary malignant lymphoma of the stomach. Barium meal, sonography and computed tomography
RÖFO 1987 Aug, Vol. 147 (2), P. 156–60

1600. Low R N, Wall S D, Jeffrey R B Jr, Sollitto R A, Reilly L M, Tierney L M Jr
Aortoenteric fistula and perigraft infection: evaluation with CT
Radiology 1990 Apr, Vol. 175 (1), P. 157–62

1601. Madrazo B L, Halpert R D, Sandler M A, Pearlberg J L
Computed tomographic findings in penetrating peptic ulcer
Radiology 1984 Dec, Vol. 153 (3), P. 751–4

1602. Marn C S, Yu B F, Nostrant T T, Ellis J H
Idiopathic cecal ulcer: CT findings
Am J Roentgenol 1989 Oct, Vol. 153 (4), P. 761–3

1603. Megibow A J, Redmond P E, Bosniak M A, Horowitz L
Diagnosis of gastrointestinal lipomas by CT
Am J Roentgenol 1979 Oct, Vol. 133 (4), P. 743–5

1604. Megibow A J, Balthazar E J, Naidich D P, Bosniak M A
Computed tomography of gastrointestinal lymphoma
Am J Roentgenol 1983 Sep, Vol. 141 (3), P. 541–7

1605. Megibow A J, Zerhouni E A, Hulnick D H, Beranbaum E R, Balthazar E J
Air insufflation of the colon as an adjunct to computed tomography of the pelvis
J Comput Assist Tomogr 1984 Aug, Vol. 8 (4), P. 797–800

1606. Megibow A J, Streiter M L, Balthazar E J, Bosniak M A
Pseudomembranous colitis: diagnosis by computed tomography
J Comput Assist Tomogr 1984 Apr, Vol. 8 (2), P. 281–3

1607. Megibow A J, Balthazar E J, Hulnick D H, Naidich D P, Bosniak M A
CT evaluation of gastrointestinal leiomyomas and leiomyosarcomas
Am J Roentgenol 1985 Apr, Vol. 144 (4), P. 727–31

1608. Merine D, Fishman E K, Jones B, Siegelman S S
Enteroenteric intussusception: CT findings in nine patients
Am J Roentgenol 1987 Jun, Vol. 148 (6), P. 1129–32

1609. Merine D, Fishman E K, Jones B
Pseudomembranous colitis: CT evaluation
J Comput Assist Tomogr 1987 Nov-Dec, Vol. 11 (6), P. 1017–20

1610. Meyer J E, Dosoretz D E, Gunderson L L, Stark P, Kopans D B
CT evaluation of locally advanced carcinoma of the distal colon and rectum
J Comput Assist Tomogr 1983 Apr, Vol. 7 (2), P. 265–7

1611. Meyers M A, (Ed.)
Computed Tomographie of the Gastrointestinal Tract
1986, Springer, New York-Berlin-Heidelberg- Tokyo

1612. Miyake H, Maeda H, Kurauchi S, Watanabe H, Kawaguchi M, Tsuji K
Thickened gastric walls showing diffuse low attenuation on CT
J Comput Assist Tomogr 1989 Mar-Apr, Vol. 13 (2), P. 253–5

1613. Monteferrante M, Shimkin P
CT diagnosis of emphysematous gastritis letter
Am J Roentgenol 1989 Jul, Vol. 153 (1), P. 191–2

1614. Moody A R, Haddock J A, Given Wilson R, Adam E J
CT monitoring of therapy for meconium ileus
J Comput Assist Tomogr 1990 Nov-Dec, Vol. 14 (6), P. 1010–2

1615. Moss A A, Thoeni R F, Schnyder P, Margulis A R
Value of computed tomography in the detection and staging of recurrent rectal carcinomas
J Comput Assist Tomogr 1981 Dec, Vol. 5 (6), P. 870–4

1616. Mullin D, Shirkhoda A
Computed tomography after gastrectomy in primary gastric carcinoma
J Comput Assist Tomogr 1985 Jan-Feb, Vol. 9 (1), P. 30–3

1617. Niethammer J G, Gould H R, Nelson H S Jr
Anorectal actinomycosis: CT evaluation
J Comput Assist Tomogr 1990 Sep-Oct, Vol. 14 (5), P. 838–9

1618. Nishimura K, Togashi K, Tohdo G, Dodo Y, Tanada S, Nakano Y, Torizuka K
Computed tomography of calcified gastric carcinoma
J Comput Assist Tomogr 1984 Oct, Vol. 8 (5), P. 1010–1

1619. Orel S G, Rubesin S E, Jones B, Fishman E K, Bayless T M, Siegelman S S
Computed tomography vs barium studies in the acutely symptomatic patient with Crohn disease
J Comput Assist Tomogr 1987 Nov-Dec, Vol. 11 (6), P. 1009–16

1620. Pagani J J, Bernardino M E
CT-radiographic correlation of ulcerating small bowel lymphomas
Am J Roentgenol 1981 May, Vol. 136 (5), P. 998–1000

1621. Pandolfo I, Scribano E, Blandino A, Salvi L, de Francesco F, Picciotto M, Bottari M
Tumors of the ampulla diagnosed by CT hypotonic duodenography
J Comput Assist Tomogr 1990 Mar-Apr, Vol. 14 (2), P. 199–200

1622. Parienty R A, Smolarski N, Pradel J, Ducellier R, Lubrano J M
Computed tomography of the gastrointestinal tract: lesion recognition and pitfalls
J Comput Assist Tomogr 1979 Oct, Vol. 3 (5), P. 615–9

1623. Parienty R A, Lepreux J F, Gruson B
Sonographic and CT features of ileocolic intussusception
Am J Roentgenol 1981 Mar, Vol. 136 (3), P. 608–10

1624. Picus D, Glazer H S, Levitt R G, Husband J E
Computed tomography of abdominal carcinoid tumors
Am J Roentgenol 1984 Sep, Vol. 143 (3), P. 581–4

1625. Plojoux O, Hauser H, Wettstein P
Computed tomography of intramural hematoma of the small intestine: a report of 3 cases
Radiology 1982 Aug, Vol. 144 (3), P. 559–61

1626. Pupols A, Ruzicka F F
Hiatal hernia causing a cardia pseudomass on computed tomography
J Comput Assist Tomogr 1984 Aug, Vol. 8 (4), P. 699–700

1627. Reh T E, Srivisal S, Schmidt E H
Portal venous thrombosis in ulcerative colitis: CT diagnosis with angiographic correlation
J Comput Assist Tomogr 1980 Aug, Vol. 4 (4), P. 545–7

1628. Rifkin M D, Ehrlich S M, Marks G
Staging of rectal carcinoma: prospective comparison of endorectal US and CT
Radiology 1989 Feb, Vol. 170 (2), P. 319–22

1629. Rodl W, Nebel G, Harms D
Computertomographie bei juvenilem malignem Gastrinom
Computer tomography in juvenile malignant gastrinoma
RÖFO 1983 Aug, Vol. 139 (2), P. 206–8

1630. Samuels T, Hamilton P, Shaw P
Whipple disease of the mediastinum
Am J Roentgenol 1990 Jun, Vol. 154 (6), P. 1187–8

1631. Scatarige J C, Fishman E K, Jones B, Cameron J L, Sanders R C, Siegelman S S
Gastric leiomyosarcoma: CT observations
J Comput Assist Tomogr 1985 Mar-Apr, Vol. 9 (2), P. 320–7

1632. Schepke P, Haubner W, Hager T
CT nach Rektumamputation. Eine radiologisch-klinische Nachuntersuchung
Computed Axial tomography in patients with abdomino-perineal excision. A radiological and clinical control
Radiologe 1982 Apr, Vol. 22 (4), P. 162–5

1633. Seigel R S, Kuhns L R, Borlaza G S, McCormick T L, Simmons J L
Computed tomography and angiography in ileal carcinoid tumor and retractile mesenteritis
Radiology 1980 Feb, Vol. 134 (2), P. 437–40

1634. Shaff M I, Himmelfarb E, Sacks G A, Burks D D, Kulkarni M V
The whirl sign: a CT finding in volvulus of the large bowel
J Comput Assist Tomogr 1985 Mar-Apr, Vol. 9 (2), P. 410

1635. Sherman J L, Hopper K D, Greene A J, Johns T T
The retrorenal colon on computed tomography: a normal variant
J Comput Assist Tomogr 1985 Mar-Apr, Vol. 9 (2), P. 339–41

1636. Sheward S E, Williams A G Jr, Mettler F A Jr, Lacey S R
CT appearance of a surgically retained towel gossypiboma
J Comput Assist Tomogr 1986 Mar-Apr, Vol. 10 (2), P. 343–5

1637. Shirkhoda A, Biggers W P
Choanal atresia: a case report illustrating the use of computed tomography
Radiology 1982 Jan, Vol. 142 (1), P. 93–4

1638. Shirkhoda A, Staab E V, Bunce L A, Herbst C A, McCartney W H
Computed tomography in recurrent or metastatic colon cancer: relation to rising serum carcinoembryonic antigen
J Comput Assist Tomogr 1984 Aug, Vol. 8 (4), P. 704–8

1639. Siegel M J, Evans S J, Balfe D M
Small bowel disease in children: diagnosis with CT
Radiology 1988 Oct, Vol. 169 (1), P. 127–30

1640. Sigurjonsson S V, Ekberg O, Hjelmquist B, Nyman U
Acute afferent loop syndrome simulating pancreatic pseudocysts. Diagnostic pitfall with CT
RÖFO 1983 Dec, Vol. 139 (6), P. 699–701

1641. Silverman P M
Gastric diverticulum mimicking adrenal mass: CT demonstration
J Comput Assist Tomogr 1986 Jul-Aug, Vol. 10 (4), P. 709–10

1642. Silverman P M, Baker M E, Cooper C, Kelvin F M
CT appearance of diffuse mesenteric edema
J Comput Assist Tomogr 1986 Jan-Feb, Vol. 10 (1), P. 67–70

1643. Siskind B N, Burrell M I, Klein M L, Princenthal R A
Toxic dilatation in Crohn disease with CT correlation
J Comput Assist Tomogr 1985 Jan-Feb, Vol. 9 (1), P. 193–5

1644. Siskind B N, Burrell M I, Richter J O, Radin D R
CT appearance of giant sigmoid diverticulum
J Comput Assist Tomogr 1986 May-Jun, Vol. 10 (3), P. 543–4

1645. Skaane P, Aasen A O
Sonographic and CT appearance of exogastric leiomyoma
Radiologe 1989 Aug, Vol. 29 (8), P. 394–5

1646. Skaane P
Primary adenocarcinoma of the vermiform appendix: ultrasound and CT demonstration
RÖFO 1990 May, Vol. 152 (5), P. 613–4

1647. Skaane P, Sandbaek G
Ultrasound and CT evaluation of pedunculated gastrointestinal lipomas
Radiologe 1990 Jan, Vol. 30 (1), P. 12–4

1648. Smerud M J, Johnson C D, Stephens D H
Diagnosis of bowel infarction: a comparison of plain films and CT scans in 23 cases
Am J Roentgenol 1990 Jan, Vol. 154 (1), P. 99–103

1649. Soulen M C, Fishman E K, Scatarige J C, Hutchins D, Zerhouni E A
Cryptosporidiosis of the gastric antrum: detection using CT
Radiology 1986 Jun, Vol. 159 (3), P. 705–6

1650. Spring D B, Moss A A
Computed tomography of ileal loop urinary diversion in adults
J Comput Assist Tomogr 1984 Oct, Vol. 8 (5), P. 866–70

1651. Stone E E, Brant W E, Smith G B
Computed tomography of duodenal diverticula
J Comput Assist Tomogr 1989 Jan-Feb, Vol. 13 (1), P. 61–3

1652. Strauss J E, Balthazar E J, Naidich D P
Jejunal perforation by a toothpick: CT demonstration
J Comput Assist Tomogr 1985 Jul-Aug, Vol. 9 (4), P. 812–4

1653. Strunk H, Zocholl G, Schweden F, Schild H, Heintz A, Braunstein S
Hochauflösende Dünnschicht-CT zum präoperativen Staging beim Rektumtumor: Vergleich mit der endoluminalen Sonographie und der Histologie
High-resolution thin-section CT in the preoperative staging of rectal tumors: a comparison with endoluminal sonography and histology
RÖFO 1990 Nov, Vol. 153 (5), P. 591–4

1654. Styles R A, Larsen C R
CT appearance of adult intussusception
J Comput Assist Tomogr 1983 Apr, Vol. 7 (2), P. 331–3

1655. Sussman S K, Halvorsen R A Jr, Illescas F F, Cohan R H, Saeed M, Silverman P M, Thompson W M, Meyers W E
Gastric adenocarcinoma: CT versus surgical staging Radiology 1988 May, Vol. 167 (2), P. 335–40

1656. Thoeni R F, Moss A A, Schnyder P, Margulis A R
Detection and staging of primary rectal and rectosigmoid cancer by computed tomography
Radiology 1981 Oct, Vol. 141 (1), P. 135–8

1657. Thompson W M, Halvorsen R A, Foster W L Jr, Williford M E, Postlethwait R W, Korobkin M
Computed tomography for staging esophageal and gastroesophageal cancer: reevaluation
Am J Roentgenol 1983 Nov, Vol. 141 (5), P. 951–8

1658. Thompson W M, Halvorsen R A, Foster W Jr, Roberts L, Korobkin M
Computed tomography of the gastroesophageal junction: value of the left lateral decubitus view
J Comput Assist Tomogr 1984 Apr, Vol. 8 (2), P. 346–9

1659. Van Beers B, Trigaux J P, De Ronde T, Melange M
CT findings of perforated duodenal diverticulitis
J Comput Assist Tomogr 1989 May-Jun, Vol. 13 (3), P. 528–30

1660. van Waes P F, Koehler P R, Feldberg M A
Management of rectal carcinoma: impact of computed tomography
Am J Roentgenol 1983 Jun, Vol. 140 (6), P. 1137–42

1661. Vanarthos W J, Aizpuru R N, Lerner H H
CT demonstration of ingested cocaine packets letter
Am J Roentgenol 1990 Aug, Vol. 155 (2), P. 419–20

1662. Wojtowycz M M, Arata J A Jr, Micklos T J, Miller F J Jr
CT findings after uncomplicated percutaneous gastrostomy
Am J Roentgenol 1988 Aug, Vol. 151 (2), P. 307–9

1663. Yeh H C, Rabinowitz J G
Ultrasonography and computed tomography of gastric wall lesions
Radiology 1981 Oct, Vol. 141 (1), P. 147–55

1664. Yeh H C, Rabinowitz J G
Granulomatous enterocolitis: findings by ultrasonography and computed tomography
Radiology 1983 Oct, Vol. 149 (1), P. 253–9

1665. Yoshimitsu K, Fukuya T, Onitsuka H, Kitagawa S, Masuda K, Adachi Y, Haraguchi Y
Computed tomography of ileoileocolic intussusception caused by a lipoma
J Comput Assist Tomogr 1989 Jul-Aug, Vol. 13 (4), P. 704–6

1666. Yousem D M, Fishman E K, Jones B
Crohn disease: perirectal and perianal findings at CT
Radiology 1988 May, Vol. 167 (2), P. 331–4

The Peritoneal Cavity

1667. Alterman D D, Cho K C
Histoplasmosis involving the omentum in an AIDS patient: CT demonstration
J Comput Assist Tomogr 1988 Jul-Aug, Vol. 12 (4), P. 664–5

1668. Amato M, Levitt R
Abdominal wall endometrioma: CT findings
J Comput Assist Tomogr 1984 Dec, Vol. 8 (6), P. 1213–4

1669. Applegate G R, Cohen A J
Dynamic CT in superior mesenteric artery syndrome
J Comput Assist Tomogr 1988 Nov-Dec, Vol. 12 (6), P. 976–80

1670. Araki T, Itai Y, Iio M
CT features of calcification in abdominal neuroblastoma
J Comput Assist Tomogr 1982 Aug, Vol. 6 (4), P. 789–91

1671. Aronberg D J, Stanley R J, Levitt R G, Sagel S S
Evaluation of abdominal abscess with computed tomography
J Comput Assist Tomogr 1978 Sep, Vol. 2 (4), P. 384–7

1672. Auh Y H, Rubenstein W A, Markisz J A, Zirinsky K, Whalen J P, Kazam E
Intraperitoneal paravesical spaces: CT delineation with US correlation
Radiology 1986 May, Vol. 159 (2), P. 311–7

1673. Ball D S, Radecki P D, Friedman A C, Caroline D F, Mayer D P
Contrast medium precipitation during abdominal CT
Radiology 1986 Jan, Vol. 158 (1), P. 258–60

1674. Banyoczki G, Goebel N, Antonucci F, Zollikofer C, Stuckmann G
CT-Diagnostik bei idiopathischer Thrombose der Vena mesenterica superior
CT diagnosis in idiopathic thrombosis of the superior mesenteric vein
RÖFO 1990 Aug, Vol. 153 (2), P. 192–6

1675. Becker W, Fischer H J
Computertomographische Darstellung einer tuberkulösen Peritonitis
Computed tomographic image of tuberculous peritonitis
RÖFO 1984 Jan, Vol. 140 (1), P. 104–5

1676. Blair R H, Resnik M D, Polga J P
CT appearance of mycotic abdominal aortic aneurysms
J Comput Assist Tomogr 1989 Jan-Feb, Vol. 13 (1), P. 101–4

1677. Bostel F, Deininger H K
Die computertomographische Diagnose des extraabdominellen Desmoids
Computed tomographic diagnosis of extra-abdominal desmoids
RÖFO 1987 Jan, Vol. 146 (1), P. 109–11

1678. Brachlow M, Zaunbauer W, Haertel M
Computertomographie bei rupturiertem Bauchaortenaneurysma
Computed tomography in ruptured abdominal aortic aneurysms
RÖFO 1984 Jul, Vol. 141 (1), P. 61–3

1679. Brasch R C, Abols I B, Gooding C A, Filly R A
Abdominal disease in children: a comparison of computed tomography and ultrasound
Am J Roentgenol 1980 Jan, Vol. 134 (1), P. 153–8

1680. Brown D L, Johnson J B Jr, Kraus A P Jr, Duke R A, Barrett M R
Computed tomography with intraperitoneal contrast medium for localization of peritoneal dialysis leaks
J Comput Assist Tomogr 1987 Mar-Apr, Vol. 11 (2), P. 276–8

1681. Bydder G M, Kreel L
Attenuation values of fluid collections within the abdomen
J Comput Assist Tomogr 1980 Apr, Vol. 4 (2), P. 145–50

1682. Callen P W, Filly R A, Korobkin M
Ascitic fluid in the anterior paravesical fossa: misleading appearance on CT scans
Am J Roentgenol 1978 Jun, Vol. 130 (6), P. 1176–7

1683. Castellino R A
Lymph nodes of the posterior iliac crest: CT and lymphographic observations
Radiology 1990 Jun, Vol. 175 (3), P. 687–9

1684. Catsikis B D, French W M, Norcus G, Brotman S, Smith J L, Harris R D
CT diagnosis of bowel herniation at pelvic fracture site
J Comput Assist Tomogr 1989 Jan-Feb, Vol. 13 (1), P. 148–9

1685. Ceuterick L, Baert A L, Marchal G, Kerremans R, Geboes K
CT diagnosis of primary torsion of greater omentum
J Comput Assist Tomogr 1987 Nov-Dec, Vol. 11 (6), P. 1083–4

1686. Chan F L, Tso W K, Wong L C, Ngan H
Barium intravasation: radiographic and CT findings in a nonfatal case
Radiology 1987 May, Vol. 163 (2), P. 311–2

1687. Cheng J, Castellino R A
Post-treatment calcification of mesenteric non-Hodgkin lymphoma: CT findings
J Comput Assist Tomogr 1989 Jan-Feb, Vol. 13 (1), P. 64–6

1688. Chezmar J L, Rumancik W M, Megibow A J, Hulnick D H, Nelson R C, Bernardino M E
Liver and abdominal screening in patients with cancer: CT versus MR imaging
Radiology 1988 Jul, Vol. 168 (1), P. 43–7

1689. Chintapalli K, Thorsen M K, Foley W D, Unger G F
Abdominal abscesses with enteric communications: CT findings
Am J Roentgenol 1983 Jul, Vol. 141 (1), P. 27–8

1690. Choi B I, Lee W J, Chi J G, Han J K
CT manifestations of peritoneal leiomyosarcomatosis
Am J Roentgenol 1990 Oct, Vol. 155 (4), P. 799–801

1691. Chui M, Tucker W, Hudson A, Bayer N
High resolution CT of Meckel's cave
Neuroradiology 1985, Vol. 27 (5), P. 403–9

1692. Clarke P D
Computed tomography of gangrenous appendicitis
J Comput Assist Tomogr 1987 Nov-Dec, Vol. 11 (6), P. 1081–2

1693. Cockey B M, Fishman E K, Jones B, Siegelman S S
Computed tomography of abdominal carcinoid tumor
J Comput Assist Tomogr 1985 Jan-Feb, Vol. 9 (1), P. 38–42

1694. Cohan R H, Silverman P M, Thompson W M, Halvorsen R A, Baker M E
Computed tomography of epithelial neoplasms of the anal canal
Am J Roentgenol 1985 Sep, Vol. 145 (3), P. 569–73

1695. Cohen J M, Weinreb J C, Maravilla K R
Fluid collections in the intraperitoneal and extraperitoneal spaces: comparison of MR and CT
Radiology 1985 Jun, Vol. 155 (3), P. 705–8

1696. Connor R, Jones B, Fishman E K, Siegelman S S
Pneumatosis intestinalis: role of computed tomography in diagnosis and management
J Comput Assist Tomogr 1984 Apr, Vol. 8 (2), P. 269–75

1697. Cooper C, Jeffrey R B, Silverman P M, Federle M P, Chun G H
Computed tomography of omental pathology
J Comput Assist Tomogr 1986 Jan-Feb, Vol. 10 (1), P. 62–6

1698. Corbetti F, Vigo M, Bulzacchi A, Angelini F, Burigo E, Thiene G
CT diagnosis of spontaneous dissection of the superior mesenteric artery
J Comput Assist Tomogr 1989 Nov-Dec, Vol. 13 (6), P. 965–7

1699. Cubillo E
Obturator hernia diagnosed by computed tomography
Am J Roentgenol 1983 Apr, Vol. 140 (4), P. 735–6

1700. Cutillo D P, Swayne L C, Cucco J, Dougan H
CT and MR imaging in cystic abdominal lymphangiomatosis
J Comput Assist Tomogr 1989 May-Jun, Vol. 13 (3), P. 534–6

1701. Dahlene D H Jr, Stanley R J, Koehler R E, Shin M S, Tishler J M
Abdominal tuberculosis: CT findings
J Comput Assist Tomogr 1984 Jun, Vol. 8 (3), P. 443–5

1702. Danielson K, Chernin M M, Amberg J R, Goff S, Durham J R
Epiploic appendicitis: CT characteristics
J Comput Assist Tomogr 1986 Jan-Feb, Vol. 10 (1), P. 142–3

1703. Demaerel P, Wilms G, Suy R, Nevelsteen A, Penninckx F, Baert A L
Computed tomography in paraprosthetic sigmoid fistula
J Comput Assist Tomogr 1988 Sep-Oct, Vol. 12 (5), P. 888–90

1704. Demas B E, Moss A A
Computed tomography of visceral infarction due to coagulopathy
J Comput Assist Tomogr 1984 Jun, Vol. 8 (3), P. 556–8

1705. Demirci A, Cengiz K, Baris S, Karagoz F
CT and ultrasound of abdominal hemorrhage in Henoch-Schonlein purpura
J Comput Assist Tomogr 1991 Jan-Feb, Vol. 15 (1), P. 143–5

1706. Denath F M
Congenital aneurysm of the superior mesenteric artery: CT diagnosis letter
Am J Roentgenol 1990 Jul, Vol. 155 (1), P. 199–200

1707. Deutch S J, Sandler M A, Alpern M B
Abdominal lymphadenopathy in benign diseases: CT detection
Radiology 1987 May, Vol. 163 (2), P. 335–8

1708. Didier D, Racle A, Etievent J P, Weill F
Tumor thrombus of the inferior vena cava secondary to malignant abdominal neoplasms: US and CT evaluation
Radiology 1987 Jan, Vol. 162 (1 Pt 1), P. 83–9

1709. Dooms G C, Hricak H, Crooks L E, Higgins C B
Magnetic resonance imaging of the lymph nodes: comparison with CT
Radiology 1984 Dec, Vol. 153 (3), P. 719–28

1710. Dooms G C, Hricak H, Sollitto R A, Higgins C B
Lipomatous tumors and tumors with fatty component: MR imaging potential and comparison of MR and CT results
Radiology 1985 Nov, Vol. 157 (2), P. 479–83

1711. Dore R, Alerci M, Cornalba G, Vadala G, De Agostini A
Unusual CT features in ruptures of abdominal aortic aneurysms
RÖFO 1988 Feb, Vol. 148 (2), P. 127–30

1712. Druy E M, Rubin B E
Computed tomography in the evaluation of abdominal trauma
J Comput Assist Tomogr 1979 Feb, Vol. 3 (1), P. 40–4

1713. DuBrow R A, Rubin J M
Intraabdominal metastatic carcinoma: unusual presentation and potential pitfall in CT evaluation
J Comput Assist Tomogr 1982 Oct, Vol. 6 (5), P. 966–8

1714. Enzi G, Biondetti P R, Fiore D, Mazzoleni F
Computed tomography of deep fat masses in multiple symmetrical lipomatosis
Radiology 1982 Jul, Vol. 144 (1), P. 121–4

1715. Epstein B M, Mann J H
CT of abdominal tuberculosis
Am J Roentgenol 1982 Nov, Vol. 139 (5), P. 861–6

1716. Fakhri A, Fishman E K, Jones B, Kuhajda F, Siegelman S S
Primary intestinal lymphangiectasia: clinical and CT findings
J Comput Assist Tomogr 1985 Jul-Aug, Vol. 9 (4), P. 767–70

1717. Farmlett E J, Fishman E K, Jones B, Siegelman S S
Torsion of lipoma of appendix epiploica: CT evaluation
J Comput Assist Tomogr 1985 Mar-Apr, Vol. 9 (2), P. 366–8

1718. Fataar S, Bassiony H, Satyanath S, Rudwan M, Hebbar G, Khalifa A, Cherian M J
CT of schistosomal calcification of the intestine
Am J Roentgenol 1985 Jan, Vol. 144 (1), P. 75–6

1719. Federle M P, Goldberg H I, Kaiser J A, Moss A A, Jeffrey R B Jr, Mall J C
Evaluation of abdominal trauma by computed tomography
Radiology 1981 Mar, Vol. 138 (3), P. 637–44

1720. Federle M P, Jeffrey R B Jr
Hemoperitoneum studied by computed tomography
Radiology 1983 Jul, Vol. 148 (1), P. 187–92

1721. Feldberg M A, van Waes P F, ten Haken G B
CT diagnosis of perianeurysmal fibrotic reactions in aortoiliac aneurysm
J Comput Assist Tomogr 1982 Jun, Vol. 6 (3), P. 465–71

1722. Fernandez Sanchez J, Bucklein W
Mukozele der Appendix. Sonographische, computertomographische und radiologische Eigen-schaften
Mucocele of the appendix. Sonographic, computed tomographic and radiologic characteristics
Radiologe 1990 Jan, Vol. 30 (1), P. 15–8

1723. Ferreiros J, Gomez Leon N, Mata M I, Casanova R, Pedrosa C S, Cuevas A
Computed tomography in abdominal Castleman's disease
J Comput Assist Tomogr 1989 May-Jun, Vol. 13 (3), P. 433–6

1724. Feuerbach S, Gullotta U, Reiser M, Ingianni G
Röntgensymptomatik intraabdomineller Abszesse im Computertomogramm
Computer tomographic appearances of intra-abdominal abscesses
RÖFO 1980 Sep, Vol. 133 (3), P. 296–8

1725. Feuerstein I M, Shawker T H, Savarese D M
CT demonstration of calcifying sludge balls
J Comput Assist Tomogr 1990 Mar-Apr, Vol. 14 (2), P. 325–6

1726. Fezoulidis I, Schadlbauer E, Traxler M, Schurawitzki H, Kalavritinos M, Alexiadis I
Retinierte und verlagerte Zähne in der Computertomographie
Retained and displaced teeth detected by computed tomography
RÖFO 1989 Dec, Vol. 151 (6), P. 729–31

1727. Fiegler W, Wegener O H, Hartmann K, Felix R
Computertomographie und Sonographie – Vergleichsstudie bei Erkrankungen des Oberbauches und des Retroperitonealraumes
Computed tomorgraphy and ultrasound; comparative study in diseases of the upper abdomen and retroperitoneal space
RÖFO 1980 Mar, Vol. 132 (3), P. 262–71

1728. Fisher J K
Computed tomographic diagnosis of volvulus in intestinal malrotation
Radiology 1981 Jul, Vol. 140 (1), P. 145–6

1729. Fishman E K, Jones B, Magid D, Siegelman S S
Intraabdominal abscesses in pseudomyxoma peritonei: the value of computed tomography
J Comput Assist Tomogr 1983 Jun, Vol. 7 (3), P. 449–53

1730. Fletcher T B, Setiawan H, Harrell R S, Redman H C
Posterior abdominal stab wounds: role of CT evaluation
Radiology 1989 Dec, Vol. 173 (3), P. 621–5

1731. Frick M P, Feinberg S B
Deceptions in localizing extrahepatic right-upper-quadrant abdominal masses by CT
Am J Roentgenol 1982 Sep, Vol. 139 (3), P. 501–4

1732. Frick M P, Salomonowitz E, Hanto D W, Gedgaudas McClees K
CT of abdominal lymphoma after renal transplantation
Am J Roentgenol 1984 Jan, Vol. 142 (1), P. 97–9

1733. Friedman A C, Hartman D S, Sherman J, Lautin E M, Goldman M
Computed tomography of abdominal fatty masses
Radiology 1981 May, Vol. 139 (2), P. 415–29

1734. Friedman A C, Pyatt R S, Hartman D S, Downey E F Jr, Olson W B
CT of benign cystic teratomas
Am J Roentgenol 1982 Apr, Vol. 138 (4), P. 659–65

1735. Friedmann G, Mödder U
Computertomographie bei Bauchtraumen
Computed tomography of abdominal trauma
Radiologe 1982 Mar, Vol. 22 (1), P. 112–6

1736. Furukawa T, Yamada T, Mori Y, Shibakiri I, Fukakusa S, Jitsukawa K, Ihori M, Tamaki M
Idiopathic aneurysm of inferior vena cava: CT demonstration
J Comput Assist Tomogr 1986 Nov-Dec, Vol. 10 (6), P. 1076–7

1737. Gale M E, Birnbaum S, Gerzof S G, Sloan G, Johnson W C, Robbins A H
CT appearance of appendicitis and its local complications
J Comput Assist Tomogr 1985 Jan-Feb, Vol. 9 (1), P. 34–7

1738. Gale M E, Johnson W C, Gerzof S G, Robbins A H
Problems in CT diagnosis of ruptured abdominal aortic aneurysms
J Comput Assist Tomogr 1986 Jul-Aug, Vol. 10 (4), P. 637–41

1739. Gamroth A, Schmitteckert H, Beyer Enke S A, Gorich J
Computertomographischer Aspekt des Empyema necessitatis
Computerized tomography aspect of empyema necessitatis
Radiologe 1987 Sep, Vol. 27 (9), P. 422–4

1740. Gentry L R, Gould H R, Alter A J, Wegenke J D, Atwell D T
Hemorrhagic angiomyolipoma: demonstration by computed tomography
J Comput Assist Tomogr 1981 Dec, Vol. 5 (6), P. 861–5

1741. Geoffray A, Shirkhoda A, Wallace S
Abdominal and pelvic computed tomography in leukemic patients
J Comput Assist Tomogr 1984 Oct, Vol. 8 (5), P. 857–60

1742. Ginaldi S, Long W D
Concurrent dissection and intracaval rupture of an abdominal aortic aneurysm: CT findings
J Comput Assist Tomogr 1985 Mar-Apr, Vol. 9 (2), P. 369–71

1743. Goldberg H I, Cann C E, Moss A A, van Waes P F
Device for performing direct coronal CT scanning of the abdomen and pelvis
Am J Roentgenol 1984 Oct, Vol. 143 (4), P. 900–2

1744. Goodman P, Raval B
CT of the abdominal wall
Am J Roentgenol 1990 Jun, Vol. 154 (6), P. 1207–11

1745. Gore R M, Callen P W, Filly R A
Lesser sac fluid in predicting the etiology of ascites: CT findings
Am J Roentgenol 1982 Jul, Vol. 139 (1), P. 71–4

1746. Gorich J, Flentje M, Guckel F, Beyer Enke S A, van Kaick G
Computertomographische Darstellung von Kollateralbahnen bei Stenosen großer Mediastinal-venen
Computed tomographic imaging of collateral pathways in stenoses of the large mediastinal veins
RÖFO 1988 May, Vol. 148 (5), P. 560–5

1747. Grabbe E
Methodik und Wert der Darmkontrastierung bei der abdominellen Computertomographie
Method and value of the opacified intestine in the computed tomography of abdomen
RÖFO 1979 Dec, Vol. 131 (6), P. 588–94

1748. Gurney J, Harrison W L, Anderson J C
Omental fat simulating pleural fluid in traumatic diaphragmatic hernia: CT characteristics
J Comput Assist Tomogr 1985 Nov-Dec, Vol. 9 (6), P. 1112–4

1749. Halvorsen R A, Jones M A, Rice R P, Thompson W M
Anterior left subphrenic abscess: characteristic plain film and CT appearance
Am J Roentgenol 1982 Aug, Vol. 139 (2), P. 283–9

1750. Handel D B, Heaston D K, Korobkin M, Silverman P M, Dunnick N R
Circumaortic left renal vein with tumor thrombus: CT diagnosis with angiographic and pathologic correlation
Am J Roentgenol 1983 Jul, Vol. 141 (1), P. 97–8

1751. Haney P J, Whitley N O
CT of benign cystic abdominal masses in children
Am J Roentgenol 1984 Jun, Vol. 142 (6), P. 1279–81

1752. Hanson R D, Hunter T B
Tuberculous peritonitis: CT appearance
Am J Roentgenol 1985 May, Vol. 144 (5), P. 931–2

1753. Hemminghytt S, Kalkhoff R K, Daniels D L, Williams A L, Grogan J P, Haughton V M
Computed tomographic study of hormone- secreting microadenomas
Radiology 1983 Jan, Vol. 146 (1), P. 65–9

1754. Hirsch M
Enhanced ascites: CT sign of ureteral fistula
J Comput Assist Tomogr 1985 Jul-Aug, Vol. 9 (4), P. 825–6

1755. Hofer G A, Cohen A J
CT signs of duodenal perforation secondary to blunt abdominal trauma
J Comput Assist Tomogr 1989 May-Jun, Vol. 13 (3), P. 430–2

1756. Hoffer F A, Kozakewich H, Colodny A, Goldstein D P
Peritoneal inclusion cysts: ovarian fluid in peritoneal adhesions
Radiology 1988 Oct, Vol. 169 (1), P. 189–91

1757. Horejs D, Gilbert P M, Burstein S, Vogelzang R L
Normal aortoiliac diameters by CT
J Comput Assist Tomogr 1988 Jul-Aug, Vol. 12 (4), P. 602–3

1758. Horgan J G, Chow P P, Richter J O, Rosenfield A T, Taylor K J
CT and sonography in the recognition of mucocele of the appendix
Am J Roentgenol 1984 Nov, Vol. 143 (5), P. 959–62

1759. Hulnick D H, Megibow A J, Naidich D P, Hilton S, Cho K C, Balthazar E J
Abdominal tuberculosis: CT evaluation
Radiology 1985 Oct, Vol. 157 (1), P. 199–204

1760. Jaques P, Mauro M, Safrit H, Yankaskas B, Piggott B
CT features of intraabdominal abscesses: prediction of successful percutaneous drainage
Am J Roentgenol 1986 May, Vol. 146 (5), P. 1041–5

1761. Jeffrey R B Jr
CT demonstration of peritoneal implants
Am J Roentgenol 1980 Aug, Vol. 135 (2), P. 323–6

1762. Jeffrey R B Jr, Nyberg D A, Bottles K, Abrams D I, Federle M P, Wall S D, Wing V W, Laing F C
Abdominal CT in acquired immunodeficiency syndrome
Am J Roentgenol 1986 Jan, Vol. 146 (1), P. 7–13

1763. Jeffrey R B Jr, Federle M P, Tolentino C S
Periappendiceal inflammatory masses: CT-directed management and clinical outcome in 70 patients published erratum appears in Radiology 1988 Jul; 1681:286
Radiology 1988 Apr, Vol. 167 (1), P. 13–6

1764. Johnson A R, Ros P R, Hjermstad B M
Tailgut cyst: diagnosis with CT and sonography
Am J Roentgenol 1986 Dec, Vol. 147 (6), P. 1309–11

1765. Jolles H, Coulam C M
CT of ascites: differential diagnosis
Am J Roentgenol 1980 Aug, Vol. 135 (2), P. 315–22

1766. Jones B, Fishman E K, Siegelman S S
Computed tomography and appendiceal abscess: special applicability in the elderly
J Comput Assist Tomogr 1983 Jun, Vol. 7 (3), P. 434–8

1767. Kahn T, Reiser M, Wackerle B, Bader M
Computertomographie des Pseudomyxoma peritonei
Computed tomography of pseudomyxoma peritonei
RÖFO 1986 Apr, Vol. 144 (4), P. 468–9

1768. Kane N M, Dorfman G S, Cronan J J
Efficacy of CT following peritoneal lavage in abdominal trauma
J Comput Assist Tomogr 1987 Nov-Dec, Vol. 11 (6), P. 998–1002

1769. Kapila A, Chakeres D W, Blanco E
The Meckel cave: computed tomographic study. Part I: Normal anatomy; Part II: Pathology
Radiology 1984 Aug, Vol. 152 (2), P. 425–33

1770. Kapila A, Steinbaum S, Chakeres D W
Meckel's cave epidermoid with trigeminal neuralgia: CT findings
J Comput Assist Tomogr 1984 Dec, Vol. 8 (6), P. 1172–4

1771. Kaufman R A, Towbin R, Babcock D S, Gelfand M J, Guice K S, Oldham K T, Noseworthy J
Upper abdominal trauma in children: imaging evaluation
Am J Roentgenol 1984 Mar, Vol. 142 (3), P. 449–60

1772. Kelly J, Raptopoulos V, Davidoff A, Waite R, Norton P
The value of non-contrast-enhanced CT in blunt abdominal trauma
Am J Roentgenol 1989 Jan, Vol. 152 (1), P. 41–8

1773. Kelly R B, Mahoney P D, Johnson J F
CT demonstration of an unusual enteric duplication cyst
J Comput Assist Tomogr 1986 May-Jun, Vol. 10 (3), P. 506–7

1774. Kelvin F M, Korobkin M, Rauch R F, Rice R P, Silverman P M
Computed tomography of pneumatosis intestinalis
J Comput Assist Tomogr 1984 Apr, Vol. 8 (2), P. 276–80

1775. Kittredge R D, Gordon R B
CT demonstration of dissecting hematoma originating in abdominal aorta
J Comput Assist Tomogr 1987 Mar-Apr, Vol. 11 (2), P. 279–81

1776. Kleinhaus U, Goldsher D, Kaftori J K
Computed tomographic diagnosis of abdominal abscesses
Radiologe 1982 May, Vol. 22 (5), P. 230–4

1777. Kniffert T, Kohler D, Langer M, Fiegler W
CT-Befunde bei frischer Beckenvenenthrombose
CT findings in fresh pelvic vein thrombosis
RÖFO 1985 Mar, Vol. 142 (3), P. 342–3

1778. Kopp W, Becker H, Kullnig P, Fotter R
Spontaninfarkt des Omentum majus: computertomographische Darstellung
Spontaneous infarct of the omentum majus: visualization by computed tomography
Radiologe 1987 Jul, Vol. 27 (7), P. 303–5

1779. Kumpan W
Computertomographische Analyse postoperativer abdomineller Kompartments. Eine Vergleichsstudie an 100 Patienten mit abdominellen Abszessen
Computed tomographic analysis of postoperative abdominal compartments. A comparative study of 100 patients with abdominal abscesses
Radiologe 1987 May, Vol. 27 (5), P. 203–15

1780. Lamorgese B
Aneurysms of superior mesenteric artery: CT demonstration
J Comput Assist Tomogr 1988 Nov-Dec, Vol. 12 (6), P. 1059–60

1781. Lawate P S, Singh S P, Jasper M P, William R, Bharathi M V, Rolston D D
CT and sonographic features of pseudomyxoma peritonei letter
Am J Roentgenol 1989 Feb, Vol. 152 (2), P. 429

1782. Lee H, Bellon E M, Vibhakar S D
The confluence of common iliac veins: a pitfall on computed tomography
J Comput Assist Tomogr 1982 Feb, Vol. 6 (1), P. 89–91

1783. Lee J K, Stanley R J, Sagel S S, Melson G L, Koehler R E
Limitations of the post-lymphangiogram plain abdominal radiograph as an indicator of recurrent lymphoma: comparison to computed tomography
Radiology 1980 Jan, Vol. 134 (1), P. 155–8

1784. Lee J T, Kim M J, Yoo K S, Suh J H, Leong H J
Primary leiomyosarcoma of the greater omentum: CT findings
J Comput Assist Tomogr 1991 Jan-Feb, Vol. 15 (1), P. 92–4

1785. Letourneau J G, Steely J W, Crass J R, Goldberg M E, Grage T, Day D L
Upper abdomen: CT findings following partial hepatectomy
Radiology 1988 Jan, Vol. 166 (1 Pt 1), P. 139–41

1786. Levine E, Collins D L, Horton W A, Schimke R N
CT screening of the abdomen in von Hippel-Lindau disease
Am J Roentgenol 1982 Sep, Vol. 139 (3), P. 505–10

1787. Levine E, Wetzel L H, Neff J R
MR imaging and CT of extrahepatic cavernous hemangiomas
Am J Roentgenol 1986 Dec, Vol. 147 (6), P. 1299–304

1788. Levitt R G, Sagel S S, Stanley R J
Detection of neoplastic involvement of the mesentery and omentum by computed tomography
Am J Roentgenol 1978 Nov, Vol. 131 (5), P. 835–8

1789. Lewin J R, Patterson E A
CT recognition of spontaneous intraperitoneal hemorrhage complicating anticoagulant therapy
Am J Roentgenol 1980 Jun, Vol. 134 (6), P. 1271–2

1790. Lewin J R
Femoral hernia with upward extension into abdominal wall: CT diagnosis
Am J Roentgenol 1981 Jan, Vol. 136 (1), P. 206–7

1791. Li D K, Rennie C S
Abdominal computed tomography in Whipple's disease
J Comput Assist Tomogr 1981 Apr, Vol. 5 (2), P. 249–52

1792. Lorenz R, Krestin G P, Schmitz Rixen T, Arnold G
Bedeutung von Sonographie und Computertomographie für die Diagnostik intraperitonealer Tumorausbreitungen. Befunde bei 307 Peritonealkarzinosen
The significance of sonography and computed tomography for the diagnosis of the intraperitoneal spread of tumors. Findings in 307 cases of peritoneal carcinosis
RÖFO 1990 May, Vol. 152 (5), P. 516–22

1793. Love L, Meyers M A, Churchill R J, Reynes C J, Moncada R, Gibson D
Computed tomography of extraperitoneal spaces
Am J Roentgenol 1981 Apr, Vol. 136 (4), P. 781–9

1794. Lubat E, Gordon R B, Birnbaum A, Megibow A J
CT diagnosis of posterior perineal hernia
Am J Roentgenol 1990 Apr, Vol. 154 (4), P. 761–2

1795. Lubbers P R, Goff W B, Lichtman D, Gottlieb R
CT diagnosis of celiac artery aneurysm
J Comput Assist Tomogr 1988 Mar-Apr, Vol. 12 (2), P. 352–4

1796. Lupetin A R, Beckman I, Daffner R H
CT diagnosis of traumatic abdominal aortic rupture
J Comput Assist Tomogr 1990 Mar-Apr, Vol. 14 (2), P. 313–4

1797. Lynch M A, Cho K C, Jeffrey R B Jr, Alterman D D, Federle M P
CT of peritoneal lymphomatosis
Am J Roentgenol 1988 Oct, Vol. 151 (4), P. 713–5

1798. Magid D, Fishman E K, Charache S, Siegelman S S
Abdominal pain in sickle cell disease: the role of CT
Radiology 1987 May, Vol. 163 (2), P. 325–8

1799. Magill H L, Roy S 3d, Stapleton F B
CT peritoneography in evaluation of pediatric dialysis complications
Am J Roentgenol 1986 Aug, Vol. 147 (2), P. 325–8

1800. Marchal G, Wilms G, Baert A, Ponette E
Applications of specific vascular opacification in CT of the upper abdomen
RÖFO 1980 Jan, Vol. 132 (1), P. 45–8

1801. Marin Grez M, Kauczor H U, Kuppers S, Delorme S
Posttraumatischer abdomineller Aortenverschluß. Computertomographischer Nachweis
Posttraumatic abdominal aortic occlusion. Computed tomographic detection
RÖFO 1991 Feb, Vol. 154 (2), P. 209–10

1802. Marincek B, Nachbur B
Computertomographie beim aortoiliakalen Aneurysma mit Ureterstenose
Computed tomography of an aortoiliac aneurysm with ureteral stenosis
RÖFO 1986 Sep, Vol. 145 (3), P. 256–62

1803. Mark A S, McCarthy S M, Moss A A, Price D
Detection of abdominal aortic graft infection: comparison of CT and in-labeled white blood cell scans
Am J Roentgenol 1985 Feb, Vol. 144 (2), P. 315–8

1804. Marks W M, Callen P W, Moss A A
Gastroesophageal region: source of confusion on CT
Am J Roentgenol 1981 Feb, Vol. 136 (2), P. 359–62

1805. Mata J M, Inaraja L, Martin J, Olazabal A, Castilla M T
CT features of mesenteric panniculitis
J Comput Assist Tomogr 1987 Nov-Dec, Vol. 11 (6), P. 1021–3

1806. Mauro M A, Vincent L M, Mandell V S, Guilford W B
Gas within hemophiliac pelvic pseudotumors: CT demonstration
J Comput Assist Tomogr 1984 Jun, Vol. 8 (3), P. 473–5

1807. McCarthy S M, Stark D D, Moss A A, Goldberg H I
Computed tomography of malignant carcinoid disease
J Comput Assist Tomogr 1984 Oct, Vol. 8 (5), P. 846–50

1808. McLeod A J, Zornoza J, Shirkhoda A
Leiomyosarcoma: computed tomographic findings
Radiology 1984 Jul, Vol. 152 (1), P. 133–6

1809. Megibow A J, Wagner A G
Obturator hernia
J Comput Assist Tomogr 1983 Apr, Vol. 7 (2), P. 350–2

1810. Melnick G S
Post-CT abdominal film: a radiologist's obligation editorial
Am J Roentgenol 1981 Jun, Vol. 136 (6), P. 1252–3

1811. Meshkov S L, Seltzer S E, Finberg H J
CT detection of intraabdominal disease in patients with lower extremity signs and symptoms
J Comput Assist Tomogr 1982 Jun, Vol. 6 (3), P. 497–501

1812. Miller D L, Udelsman R, Sugarbaker P H
Calcification of pseudomyxoma peritonei following intraperitoneal chemotherapy: CT demonstration
J Comput Assist Tomogr 1985 Nov-Dec, Vol. 9 (6), P. 1123–4

1813. Minutoli A, Volta S, Gaeta M
Delayed enhancement of ascites following high-dose contrast CT for liver metastases
J Comput Assist Tomogr 1989 Sep-Oct, Vol. 13 (5), P. 916–7

1814. Mirich D R, Gray R R, Grosman H
Abdominal plexiform neurofibromatosis simulating pseudomyxoma peritonei on computed tomography
J Comput Assist Tomogr 1989 Jul-Aug, Vol. 13 (4), P. 709–11

1815. Mödder U, Fiedler V, Lorenz R
Computertomographische Zeichen der Peritonealkarzinose
Computer tomographic features of peritoneal carcinosis
RÖFO 1982 Jan, Vol. 136 (1), P. 60–3

1816. Mueller P R, Ferrucci J T Jr, Harbin W P, Kirkpatrick R H, Simeone J F, Wittenberg J
Appearance of lymphomatous involvement of the mesentery by ultrasonography and body computed tomography: the "sandwich sign"
Radiology 1980 Feb, Vol. 134 (2), P. 467–73

1817. Mueller P R, vanSonnenberg E, Ferrucci J T Jr
Percutaneous drainage of 250 abdominal abscesses and fluid collections. Part II: Current procedural concepts
Radiology 1984 May, Vol. 151 (2), P. 343–7

1818. Nakamura H, Hashimoto T, Akashi H, Mizumoto S
Distinctive CT-findings of unusual mesenteric cysts
J Comput Assist Tomogr 1987 Nov-Dec, Vol. 11 (6), P. 1024–5

1819. Nardi P M, Ruchman R B
CT appearance of diffuse peritoneal endometriosis
J Comput Assist Tomogr 1989 Nov-Dec, Vol. 13 (6), P. 1075–7

1820. Neumann C H, Robert N J, Canellos G, Rosenthal D
Computed tomography of the abdomen and pelvis in non-Hodgkin lymphoma
J Comput Assist Tomogr 1983 Oct, Vol. 7 (5), P. 846–50

1821. Neumann C H, Robert N J, Rosenthal D, Canellos G
Clinical value of ultrasonography for the management of non-Hodgkin lymphoma patients as compared with abdominal computed tomography
J Comput Assist Tomogr 1983 Aug, Vol. 7 (4), P. 666–9

1822. Neumann D R, Pearlstein A E
Retracted testis mimicking lymphomatous recurrence: CT demonstration
J Comput Assist Tomogr 1986 Jan-Feb, Vol. 10 (1), P. 159–60

1823. Nichols D M, Li D K
Superior mesenteric vein rotation: a CT sign of midgut malrotation
Am J Roentgenol 1983 Oct, Vol. 141 (4), P. 707–8

1824. Nyberg D A, Federle M P, Jeffrey R B, Bottles K, Wofsy C B
Abdominal CT findings of disseminated Mycobacterium avium- intracellulare in AIDS
Am J Roentgenol 1985 Aug, Vol. 145 (2), P. 297–9

1825. Oliphant M, Berne A S
Computed tomography of the subperitoneal space: demonstration of direct spread of intra-abdominal disease
J Comput Assist Tomogr 1982 Dec, Vol. 6 (6), P. 1127–37

1826. Orwig D, Federle M P
Localized clotted blood as evidence of visceral trauma on CT: the sentinel clot sign
Am J Roentgenol 1989 Oct, Vol. 153 (4), P. 747–9

1827. Orwig D S, Jeffrey R B Jr
CT of false-negative peritoneal lavage following blunt abdominal trauma
J Comput Assist Tomogr 1987 Nov-Dec, Vol. 11 (6), P. 1079–80

1828. Osborn A G, Koehler P R, Gibbs F A, Leavitt D D, Anderson R E, Lee T G, Ferris D T
Direct sagittal computed tomographic scans in the radiographic evaluation of the pelvis
Radiology 1980 Jan, Vol. 134 (1), P. 255–7

1829. Pandolfo I, Racchiusa S, Giunta A, Freni O F
CT demonstration of pelvic hydatid cysts
J Comput Assist Tomogr 1984 Jun, Vol. 8 (3), P. 479–81

1830. Pandolfo I, Blandino A, Gaeta M, Racchiusa S, Chirico G
CT findings in palpable lesions of the anterior abdominal wall
J Comput Assist Tomogr 1986 Jul-Aug, Vol. 10 (4), P. 629–33

1831. Papanicolaou N, Wittenberg J, Ferrucci J T Jr, Stauffer A E, Waltman A C, Simeone J F, Mueller P R, Brewster D C, Darling R C
Preoperative evaluation of abdominal aortic aneurysms by computed tomography
Am J Roentgenol 1986 Apr, Vol. 146 (4), P. 711–5

1832. Parikh V P, Jain C, Desai M B
CT of pseudomyxoma peritonei letter
Am J Roentgenol 1987 Nov, Vol. 149 (5), P. 1077–8

1833. Passariello R, Simonetti G, Rovighi L, Ciolina A
Characteristic CT pattern of giant superior mesenteric artery aneurysms
J Comput Assist Tomogr 1980 Oct, Vol. 4 (5), P. 621–6

1834. Passas V, Karavias D, Grilias D, Birbas A
Computed tomography of left paraduodenal hernia
J Comput Assist Tomogr 1986 May-Jun, Vol. 10 (3), P. 542–3

1835. Pastakia B, Horvath K, Kurtz D, Udelsman R, Doppman J L
Giant rectus sheath hematomas of the pelvis complicating anticoagulant therapy: CT findings
J Comput Assist Tomogr 1984 Dec, Vol. 8 (6), P. 1120–3

1836. Pera A, Capek M, Shirkhoda A
Lymphangiography and CT in the follow-up of patients with lymphoma
Radiology 1987 Sep, Vol. 164 (3), P. 631–3

1837. Peters J C, Reinertson J S, Polansky S M, Lamont B M, Fortune J B
CT demonstration of traumatic ventral hernia
J Comput Assist Tomogr 1988 Jul-Aug, Vol. 12 (4), P. 710–1

1838. Picus D, Siegel M J, Balfe D M
Abdominal computed tomography in children with unexplained prolonged fever
J Comput Assist Tomogr 1984 Oct, Vol. 8 (5), P. 851–6

1839. Piechowiak H, Fuessl H S, Sommer B
Sonographischer und computertomographischer Befund nach kongenitalem Bauchwandbruch mit Malrotation
Sonographic and computer tomographic findings in congenital hernia of the abdominal wall with malrotation
RÖFO 1983 Nov, Vol. 139 (5), P. 580–1

1840. Quinn M J, Sheedy P F, Stephens D H, Hattery R R
Computed tomography of the abdomen in evaluation of patients with fever of unknown origin
Radiology 1980 Aug, Vol. 136 (2), P. 407–11

1841. Radin D R
Intraabdominal Mycobacterium tuberculosis vs Mycobacterium avium- intracellulare infections in patients with AIDS: distinction based on CT findings
Am J Roentgenol 1991 Mar, Vol. 156 (3), P. 487–91

1842. Ralls P W, Hartman B, White W, Radin D R, Halls J
Computed tomography of benign cystic teratoma of the omentum
J Comput Assist Tomogr 1987 May-Jun, Vol. 11 (3), P. 548–9

1843. Rao B K, Scanlan K A, Hinke M L
Abdominal case of the day
Am J Roentgenol 1986 May, Vol. 146 (5), P. 1074–9

1844. Rao B K, Brodell G K, Haaga J R, Whitlatch S, Chiu L C
Visceral CT findings associated with Thorotrast
J Comput Assist Tomogr 1986 Jan-Feb, Vol. 10 (1), P. 57–61

1845. Raptopoulos V
On the value of non-contrast-enhanced CT in blunt abdominal trauma letter
Am J Roentgenol 1989 Mar, Vol. 152 (3), P. 651–2

1846. Reuter K, Raptopoulos V, Reale F, Krolikowski F J, D Orsi C J, Graham S, Smith E H
Diagnosis of peritoneal mesothelioma: computed tomography, sonography, and fine-needle aspiration biopsy
Am J Roentgenol 1983 Jun, Vol. 140 (6), P. 1189–94

1847. Reuther G, Vogel J, Wallner B
MRT und CT bei Zwerchfell- Lipomen
MRT and CT of diaphragmatic lipomas
RÖFO 1989 Jun, Vol. 150 (6), P. 691–3

1848. Richmond T, Virapongse C, Sarwar M, Kier E L, Rothman S
Intraparenchymal blood-fluid levels: new CT sign of arteriovenous malformation rupture
AJNR 1981 Nov-Dec, Vol. 2 (6), P. 577–9

1849. Rizzo M J, Federle M P, Griffiths B G
Bowel and mesenteric injury following blunt abdominal trauma: evaluation with CT
Radiology 1989 Oct, Vol. 173 (1), P. 143–8

1850. Rosen A, Korobkin M, Silverman P M, Moore A V Jr, Dunnick N R
CT diagnosis of ruptured abdominal aortic aneurysm
Am J Roentgenol 1984 Aug, Vol. 143 (2), P. 265–8

1851. Rosen A, Korobkin M, Silverman P M, Dunnick N R, Kelvin F M
Mesenteric vein thrombosis: CT identification
Am J Roentgenol 1984 Jul, Vol. 143 (1), P. 83–6

1852. Rubenstein W A, Auh Y H, Zirinsky K, Kneeland J B, Whalen J P, Kazam E
Posterior peritoneal recesses: assessment using CT
Radiology 1985 Aug, Vol. 156 (2), P. 461–8

1853. Russ P D, Friefeld G D, Nauck C J, Wilmouth R J
Infarcted Meckel diverticulum detected by CT
Am J Roentgenol 1988 Feb, Vol. 150 (2), P. 299–300

1854. Salerno M D, Rose B S
CT diagnosis of traumatic mesenteric venous thrombosis letter
Am J Roentgenol 1990 Feb, Vol. 154 (2), P. 425

1855. Sanders R C, McNeil B J, Finberg H J, Hessel S J, Siegelman S S, Adams D F, Alderson P O, Abrams H L
A prospective study of computed tomography and ultrasound in the detection and staging of pelvic masses
Radiology 1983 Feb, Vol. 146 (2), P. 439–42

1856. Sandler C M, Jackson H, Kaminsky R I
Right perirenal hematoma secondary to a leaking abdominal aortic aneurysm
J Comput Assist Tomogr 1981 Apr, Vol. 5 (2), P. 264–6

1857. Schmid P, Haertel M
Zur computertomographischen Diagnose und Differentialdiagnose des Leiomyosarkoms der Vena cava inferior
Computed tomographic diagnosis and differential diagnosis of leiomyosarcoma of the inferior vena cava
RÖFO 1987 Mar, Vol. 146 (3), P. 263–6

1858. Schulman A, Fataar S
CT in diaphragmatic rupture? letter
Am J Roentgenol 1981 Jun, Vol. 136 (6), P. 1256

1859. Sefczek R J, Lupetin A R, Beckman I, Dash N
CT appearance of omental packs
Radiology 1985 Aug, Vol. 156 (2), P. 472

1860. Shah H R, Williamson M R, Boyd C M, Balachandran S, Angtuaco T L, Mc Connell J R
CT findings in abdominal actinomycosis
J Comput Assist Tomogr 1987 May-Jun, Vol. 11 (3), P. 466–9

1861. Shapir J, Rubin J
CT appearance of the inferior mesenteric vein
J Comput Assist Tomogr 1984 Oct, Vol. 8 (5), P. 877–80

1862. Shin M S, Berland L L
Computed tomography of retrocrural spaces: normal, anatomic variants, and pathologic conditions
Am J Roentgenol 1985 Jul, Vol. 145 (1), P. 81–6

1863. Shirkhoda A, Albin J
Malignant melanoma: correlating abdominal and pelvic CT with clinical staging
Radiology 1987 Oct, Vol. 165 (1), P. 75–8

1864. Siegel M J, Glasier C M, Sagel S S
CT of pelvic disorders in children
Am J Roentgenol 1981 Dec, Vol. 137 (6), P. 1139–43

1865. Silverman P M, Kelvin F M, Korobkin M, Dunnick N R
Computed tomography of the normal mesentery
Am J Roentgenol 1984 Nov, Vol. 143 (5), P. 953–7

1866. Sivit C J, Peclet M H, Taylor G A
Life-threatening intraperitoneal bleeding: demonstration with CT
Radiology 1989 May, Vol. 171 (2), P. 430

1867. Sivit C J, Taylor G A, Bulas D I, Bowman L M, Eichelberger M R
Blunt trauma in children: significance of peritoneal fluid
Radiology 1991 Jan, Vol. 178 (1), P. 185–8

1868. Smevik B, Swensen T, Kolbenstvedt A, Trygstad O
Computed tomography and ultrasonography of the abdomen in congenital generalized lipodystrophy
Radiology 1982 Mar, Vol. 142 (3), P. 687–9

1869. Somers J M, Pollard S G, Dixon A K
The recognition of previous abdominal surgery by computed tomography
J Comput Assist Tomogr 1991 Jan-Feb, Vol. 15 (1), P. 95–100

1870. Sommer B, Mayr B, Sunder Plassmann L, Lissner J
Isolierte Aneurysmen der Iliakalarterien im Computertomogramm
Isolated aneurysms of the iliac arteries in computer tomograms
RÖFO 1981 Feb, Vol. 134 (2), P. 204–5

1871. Sones P J
Percutaneous drainage of abdominal abscesses
Am J Roentgenol 1984 Jan, Vol. 142 (1), P. 35–9

1872. Spring D B, Vandeman F, Watson R A
Computed tomographic demonstration of ureterosciatic hernia
Am J Roentgenol 1983 Sep, Vol. 141 (3), P. 579–80

1873. Steinberg A W, Lloyd R, Wood B P
Ingested raisins simulating abdominal calcifications letter
Radiology 1990 Feb, Vol. 174 (2), P. 576–7

1874. Steinbrich W, Friedmann G
CT der Organe des kleinen Beckens – normale und pathologische Anatomie, Indikationen, Ergebnisse
CT of the lesser pelvis – normal and abnormal anatomy, indications, results
RÖFO 1981 Feb, Vol. 134 (2), P. 115–22

1875. Straub W H, Gur D, Good W F, Campbell W L, Davis P L, Hecht S T, Skolnick M L, Thaete F L, Rosenthal M S, Sashin D
Primary CT diagnosis of abdominal masses in a PACS environment see comments
Radiology 1991 Mar, Vol. 178 (3), P. 739–43

1876. Takehara Y, Takahashi M, Fukaya T, Kaneko M, Koyano K, Sakaguchi S
Computed tomography of isolated dissecting aneurysm of superior mesenteric artery
J Comput Assist Tomogr 1988 Jul-Aug, Vol. 12 (4), P. 678–80

1877. Taneja K, Gothi R, Kumar K, Jain S, Mani R K
Peritoneal Echinococcus multilocularis infection: CT appearance
J Comput Assist Tomogr 1990 May-Jun, Vol. 14 (3), P. 493–4

1878. Taylor G A, Fallat M E, Eichelberger M R
Hypovolemic shock in children: abdominal CT manifestations
Radiology 1987 Aug, Vol. 164 (2), P. 479–81

1879. Taylor G A, Fishman E K, Kramer S S, Siegelman S S
CT demonstration of the phrenic nerve
J Comput Assist Tomogr 1983 Jun, Vol. 7 (3), P. 411–4

1880. Taylor G A, Guion C J, Potter B M, Eichelberger M R
CT of blunt abdominal trauma in children
Am J Roentgenol 1989 Sep, Vol. 153 (3), P. 555–9

1881. Teefey S A, Baron R L, Schulte S J, Shuman W P
Differentiating pelvic veins and enlarged lymph nodes: optimal CT techniques
Radiology 1990 Jun, Vol. 175 (3), P. 683–5

1882. Thoeni R F, Filson R G
Abdominal and pelvic CT: use of oral metoclopramide to enhance bowel opacification
Radiology 1988 Nov, Vol. 169 (2), P. 391–3

1883. Tisnado J, Amendola M A, Walsh J W, Jordan R L, Turner M A, Krempa J
Computed tomography of the perineum
Am J Roentgenol 1981 Mar, Vol. 136 (3), P. 475–81

1884. Triller J, Kraft R, Marincek B
Computertomographisch gezielte Feinnadelaspirationspunktion pelviner Raumforderungen
Computer tomographic guided fine needle puncture of abdominal masses
RÖFO 1982 Oct, Vol. 137 (4), P. 422–7

1885. Triller J, Schneekloth G, Marincek B, Kraft R
Computertomographisch gezielte Feinnadelpunktion abdominaler Raumforderungen
Computer tomographic guided fine needle puncture of abdominal masses
Radiologe 1982 Nov, Vol. 22 (11), P. 484–92

1886. Triller J, Robotti G
Computertomographie bei primären mesenterialen Tumoren
Computed tomography in primary mesenteric tumors
RÖFO 1984 Jan, Vol. 140 (1), P. 40–5

1887. Tschakert H, Will C H
Was leistet die Computertomographie für die Differentialdiagnose von Raumforderungen im Bereich des linken Oberbauches?
The value of CT in the differential diagnostic evaluation of masses in the left upper abdominal quadrant
Radiologe 1980 Jul, Vol. 20 (7), P. 373–8

1888. Turner R J, Young S W, Castellino R A
Dynamic continuous computed tomography: study of retroaortic left renal vein
J Comput Assist Tomogr 1980 Feb, Vol. 4 (1), P. 109–11

1889. Tyrrel R T, Montemayor K A, Bernardino M E
CT density of mesenteric, retroperitoneal, and subcutaneous fat in cirrhotic patients: comparison with control subjects
Am J Roentgenol 1990 Jul, Vol. 155 (1), P. 73–5

1890. Tyrrel R T, Baumgartner B R, Montemayor K A
Blue rubber bleb nevus syndrome: CT diagnosis of intussusception
Am J Roentgenol 1990 Jan, Vol. 154 (1), P. 105–6

1891. van Sonnenberg E, Mueller P R, Ferrucci J T Jr
Percutaneous drainage of 250 abdominal abscesses and fluid collections. Part 1: Results, failures, and complications
Radiology 1984 May, Vol. 151 (2), P. 337–41

1892. van Zanten T E, Golding R P
CT and MR demonstration of leiomyosarcoma of inferior vena cava
J Comput Assist Tomogr 1987 Jul-Aug, Vol. 11 (4), P. 670–4

1893. Vas W, Bilotta W, Sundaram M, Wolverson M, Markivee C
Computed tomography of omental liver packs
J Comput Assist Tomogr 1988 Jul-Aug, Vol. 12 (4), P. 592–4

1894. Vigo M, De Faveri D, Biondetti P R Jr, Benedetti L
CT demonstration of portal and superior mesenteric vein thrombosis in hepatocellular carcinoma
J Comput Assist Tomogr 1980 Oct, Vol. 4 (5), P. 627–9

1895. Voegeli E, Ayer G, Hofer B
Sonographie und Computertomographie bei postoperativen, abdominellen Abszedierungen
Sonography and computed tomography in postoperative abdominal abscesses
Radiologe 1984 Feb, Vol. 24 (2), P. 90–4

1896. Vogel J, Haberle H J, Friedrich J M, Schumacher K A, Bargon G
Kongenitale und erworbene Anomalien der Vena cava inferior. Differentialdiagnose durch digitale Subtraktionsangiographie (DSA) und Computertomographie (CT)
Congenital and acquired anomalies of the inferior vena cava. Differential diagnosis using digital subtraction angiography and computed tomography
RÖFO 1991 Feb, Vol. 154 (2), P. 180–6

1897. Vujic I, Stanley J, Tyminski L J
Computed tomography of suspected caval thrombosis secondary to proximal extension of phlebitis from the leg
Radiology 1981 Aug, Vol. 140 (2), P. 437–41

1898. Wagner Manslau C, Reiser M, Lukas P
Computertomographische Befunde bei der Amöbiasis
Computed tomographic findings in amebiasis
Radiologe 1985 Dec, Vol. 25 (12), P. 597–4

1899. Waligore M P, Stephens D H, Soule E H, McLeod R A
Lipomatous tumors of the abdominal cavity: CT appearance and pathologic correlation
Am J Roentgenol 1981 Sep, Vol. 137 (3), P. 539–45

1900. Walkey M M, Friedman A C, Sohotra P, Radecki P D
CT manifestations of peritoneal carcinomatosis
Am J Roentgenol 1988 May, Vol. 150 (5), P. 1035–41

1901. Walter E, Petersen D
Röntgenbefunde bei der Lipoidproteinose
Radiological findings in lipoid proteinosis
RÖFO 1981 Aug, Vol. 135 (2), P. 156–60

1902. Watts R W, Spellacy E, Kendall B E, du Boulay G, Gibbs D A
Computed tomography studies on patients with mucopolysaccharidoses
Neuroradiology 1981 Feb, Vol. 21 (1), P. 9–23

1903. Weiand G, Lackner K, Koischwitz D
CT-Nachweis des venösen Umgehungskreislaufs bei Verschluß oder Agenesie der Vena cava
CT demonstration of venous collaterals with occlusion or agenesis of the vena cava
RÖFO 1980 Sep, Vol. 133 (3), P. 250–8

1904. Weigert F, Lindner P, Rohde U
Computed tomography and magnetic resonance of pseudomyxoma peritonei
J Comput Assist Tomogr 1985 Nov-Dec, Vol. 9 (6), P. 1120–2

1905. Whitley N O, Bohlman M E, Baker L P
CT patterns of mesenteric disease
J Comput Assist Tomogr 1982 Jun, Vol. 6 (3), P. 490–6

1906. Whitley N O, Shatney C H
Diagnosis of abdominal abscesses in patients with major trauma: the use of computed tomography
Radiology 1983 Apr, Vol. 147 (1), P. 179–83

1907. Widlus D M
Inguinal hernia: CT appearance after injection therapy
Radiology 1984 Apr, Vol. 151 (1), P. 156

1908. Williams M P, Dixon A K
Aortic graft abscess with duodenal communication
J Comput Assist Tomogr 1983 Oct, Vol. 7 (5), P. 916

1909. Wilms G, Storme L, Vandaele L, De Baets M
CT demonstration of aneurysm of a persistent sciatic artery
J Comput Assist Tomogr 1986 May-Jun, Vol. 10 (3), P. 524–5

1910. Wilms G, Oyen R, Waer M, Baert A L, Michielsen P
CT demonstration of aneurysms in polyarteritis nodosa
J Comput Assist Tomogr 1986 May-Jun, Vol. 10 (3), P. 513–5

1911. Wimmer B, Hauenstein K
Hernien im Computertomogramm des Abdomens
Hernias in the computed tomogram of the abdomen
RÖFO 1985 Oct, Vol. 143 (4), P. 443–9

1912. Wimmer B, Hillesheimer W
Präoperativer Einsatz der Computertomographie bei Fremdkörpern
Preoperative use of computed tomography for foreign bodies
Radiologe 1985 Mar, Vol. 25 (3), P. 135–8

1913. Wing V W, Federle M P, Morris J A Jr, Jeffrey R B, Bluth R
The clinical impact of CT for blunt abdominal trauma
Am J Roentgenol 1985 Dec, Vol. 145 (6), P. 1191–4

1914. Wise R H Jr, Retterbush D W, Stanley R J
CT findings in acute thrombosis of superior mesenteric vein aneurysm
J Comput Assist Tomogr 1987 Jan-Feb, Vol. 11 (1), P. 172–4

1915. Wojtowicz J, Rzymski K, Czarnecki R
A CT evaluation of the intraperitoneal fluid distribution
RÖFO 1982 Jul, Vol. 137 (1), P. 95–9

1916. Wolverson M K, Jagannadharao B, Sundaram M, Joyce P F, Riaz M A, Shields J B
CT as a primary diagnostic method in evaluating intraabdominal abscess
Am J Roentgenol 1979 Dec, Vol. 133 (6), P. 1089–95

1917. Wolverson M K, Crepps L F, Sundaram M, Heiberg E, Vas W G, Shields J B
Hyperdensity of recent hemorrhage at body computed tomography: incidence and morphologic variation
Radiology 1983 Sep, Vol. 148 (3), P. 779–84

1918. Yeh H C, Chahinian A P
Ultrasonography and computed tomography of peritoneal mesothelioma
Radiology 1980 Jun, Vol. 135 (3), P. 705–12

1919. Yeh H C, Rabinowitz J G
Ultrasonography and computed tomography of inflammatory abdominal wall lesions
Radiology 1982 Sep, Vol. 144 (4), P. 859–63

1920. Young R, Friedman A C, Hartman D S
Computed tomography of leiomyosarcoma of the inferior vena cava
Radiology 1982 Oct, Vol. 145 (1), P. 99–103

1921. Zirinsky K, Auh Y H, Kneeland J B, Rubenstein W A, Kazam E
Computed tomography, sonography, and MR imaging of abdominal tuberculosis
J Comput Assist Tomogr 1985 Sep-Oct, Vol. 9 (5), P. 961–3

1922. Zirinsky K, Auh Y H, Rubenstein W A, Kneeland J B, Whalen J P, Kazam E
The portacaval space: CT with MR correlation
Radiology 1985 Aug, Vol. 156 (2), P. 453–60

1923. Zwicker C, Langer M, Astinet F
Computertomographische Befunde bei der Lymphangioleiomyomatose
Computed tomographic findings in lymphangioleiomyomatosis
RÖFO 1990 Apr, Vol. 152 (4), P. 478–9

The Spleen

1924. Balcar I, Seltzer S E, Davis S, Geller S
CT patterns of splenic infarction: a clinical and experimental study
Radiology 1984 Jun, Vol. 151 (3), P. 723–9

1925. Balthazar E J, Hilton S, Naidich D, Megibow A, Levine R
CT of splenic and perisplenic abnormalities in septic patients
Am J Roentgenol 1985 Jan, Vol. 144 (1), P. 53–6

1926. Berland L L, VanDyke J A
Decreased splenic enhancement on CT in traumatized hypotensive patients
Radiology 1985 Aug, Vol. 156 (2), P. 469–71

1927. Bottger E, Semerak M, Jaschke W
Computertomographische Befunde bei Milzruptur, subkapsulärem Milzhämatom und perisplenitischem Abszeß
Computer tomographic findings in splenic ruptures, subcapsular haematomas of the spleen and perisplenic abscesses
RÖFO 1980 Mar, Vol. 132 (3), P. 282–6

1928. Brody A S, Seidel F G, Kuhn J P
CT evaluation of blunt abdominal trauma in children: comparison of ultrafast and conventional CT
Am J Roentgenol 1989 Oct, Vol. 153 (4), P. 803–6

1929. Brunet W G, Greenberg H M
CT demonstration of a ruptured splenic artery aneurysm
J Comput Assist Tomogr 1991 Jan-Feb, Vol. 15 (1), P. 177–8

1930. Cohen B A, Mitty H A, Mendelson D S
Computed tomography of splenic infarction
J Comput Assist Tomogr 1984 Feb, Vol. 8 (1), P. 167–8

1931. Conrad M R
Splenic trauma: false-negative CT diagnosis in cases of delayed rupture letter
Am J Roentgenol 1988 Jul, Vol. 151 (1), P. 200–1

1932. Conrad M R
Blunt hepatic/splenic trauma in adults: CT- based classification and correlation with prognosis and treatment letter
Radiology 1989 Oct, Vol. 173 (1), P. 285–6

1933. Cools L, Osteaux M, Divano L, Jeanmart L
Prediction of splenic volume by a simple CT measurement: a statistical study
J Comput Assist Tomogr 1983 Jun, Vol. 7 (3), P. 426–30

1934. Cordes M, Muller C
Radiographischer Aspekt eines großen Milzarterienaneurysmas -Magendarmpassage und Computertomographie
Radiographic aspects of a large splenic artery aneurysm – gastrointestinal radiography and computed tomography
RÖFO 1985 Aug, Vol. 143 (2), P. 234–6

1935. Darling J D, Flickinger F W
Splenosis mimicking neoplasm in the perirenal space: CT characteristics
J Comput Assist Tomogr 1990 Sep-Oct, Vol. 14 (5), P. 839–41

1936. Dautenhahn L W, Rona G, Saperstein M L, Williams C D, Vermess M
Lymphoma in a pelvic spleen: CT features
J Comput Assist Tomogr 1989 Nov-Dec, Vol. 13 (6), P. 1081–2

1937. Fagelman D, Hertz M A, Ross A S
Delayed development of splenic subcapsular hematoma: CT evaluation
J Comput Assist Tomogr 1985 Jul-Aug, Vol. 9 (4), P. 815–6

1938. Federle M P, Griffiths B, Minagi H, Jeffrey R B Jr
Splenic trauma: evaluation with CT
Radiology 1987 Jan, Vol. 162 (1 Pt 1), P. 69–71

1939. Foley W D, Gleysteen J J, Lawson T L, Berland L L, Smith D F, Thorsen M K, Unger G F
Dynamic computed tomography and pulsed Doppler ultrasonography in the evaluation of splenorenal shunt patency
J Comput Assist Tomogr 1983 Feb, Vol. 7 (1), P. 106–12

1940. Franquet T, Montes M, Lecumberri F J, Esparza J, Bescos J M
Hydatid disease of the spleen: imaging findings in nine patients
Am J Roentgenol 1990 Mar, Vol. 154 (3), P. 525–8

1941. Gentry L R, Brown J M, Lindgren R D
Splenosis: CT demonstration of heterotopic autotransplantation of splenic tissue
J Comput Assist Tomogr 1982 Dec, Vol. 6 (6), P. 1184–7

1942. Glazer G M, Axel L, Goldberg H I, Moss A A
Dynamic CT of the normal spleen
Am J Roentgenol 1981 Aug, Vol. 137 (2), P. 343–6

1943. Gooding G A
The ultrasonic and computed tomographic appearance of splenic lobulations: a consideration in the ultrasonic differential of masses adjacent to the left kidney
Radiology 1978 Mar, Vol. 126 (3), P. 719–20

1944. Goodman L R, Aprahamian C
Changes in splenic size after abdominal trauma
Radiology 1990 Sep, Vol. 176 (3), P. 629–32

1945. Goodman P C, Federle M P
Splenorrhaphy: CT appearance
J Comput Assist Tomogr 1980 Apr, Vol. 4 (2), P. 251–2

1946. Herman T E, Siegel M J
CT of acute splenic torsion in children with wandering spleen
Am J Roentgenol 1991 Jan, Vol. 156 (1), P. 151–3

1947. Lehar S C, Zajko A B, Koneru B, Stevenson W, Sumkin J
Splenic infarction complicating pediatric liver transplantation: incidence and CT appearance
J Comput Assist Tomogr 1990 May-Jun, Vol. 14 (3), P. 362–5

1948. Lorenz R, Beyer D, Friedmann G, Mödder U
Grenzen der Differenzierung fokaler Milzläsionen durch Sonographie und Computertomographie
Limits of differentiation of focal splenic lesions by sonography and computed tomography
RÖFO 1983 Apr, Vol. 138 (4), P. 447–52

1949. Magid D, Fishman E K, Siegelman S S
Computed tomography of the spleen and liver in sickle cell disease
Am J Roentgenol 1984 Aug, Vol. 143 (2), P. 245–9

1950. Mahony B, Jeffrey R B, Federle M P
Spontaneous rupture of hepatic and splenic angiosarcoma demonstrated by CT
Am J Roentgenol 1982 May, Vol. 138 (5), P. 965–6

1951. Mall J C, Kaiser J A
CT diagnosis of splenic laceration
Am J Roentgenol 1980 Feb, Vol. 134 (2), P. 265–9

1952. Marn C S, Glazer G M, Williams D M, Francis I R
CT- angiographic correlation of collateral venous pathways in isolated splenic vein occlusion: new observations
Radiology 1990 May, Vol. 175 (2), P. 375–80

1953. Mata J, Alegret X, Llauger J
Splenic pseudocyst as a complication of ventriculoperitoneal shunt: CT features
J Comput Assist Tomogr 1986 Mar-Apr, Vol. 10 (2), P. 341–2

1954. Mathieu D, Vanderstigel M, Schaeffer A, Vasile N
Computed tomography of splenic sarcoidosis
J Comput Assist Tomogr 1986 Jul- Aug, Vol. 10 (4), P. 679–80

1955. Mendelson D S, Cohen B A, Armas R R
CT appearance of splenosis
J Comput Assist Tomogr 1982 Dec, Vol. 6 (6), P. 1188–90

1956. Meyer J E, Harris N L, Elman A, Stomper P C
Large-cell lymphoma of the spleen: CT appearance
Radiology 1983 Jul, Vol. 148 (1), P. 199–201

1957. Mirvis S E, Whitley N O, Gens D R
Blunt splenic trauma in adults: CT-based classification and correlation with prognosis and treatment
Radiology 1989 Apr, Vol. 171 (1), P. 33–9

1958. Mitnick J S, Bosniak M A, Rothberg M, Megibow A J, Raghavendra B N, Subramanyam B R
Metastatic neoplasm to the kidney studied by computed tomography and sonography
J Comput Assist Tomogr 1985 Jan-Feb, Vol. 9 (1), P. 43–9

1959. Nino Murcia M, Kurtz A, Brennan R E, Shaw E, Peiken S R, Weiss S M
CT diagnosis of a splenic artery pseudoaneurysm: a complication of chronic pancreatitis and pseudocyst formation
J Comput Assist Tomogr 1983 Jun, Vol. 7 (3), P. 527–9

1960. Pakter R L, Fishman E K, Nussbaum A, Giargiana F A, Zerhouni E A
CT findings in splenic hemangiomas in the Klippel- Trenaunay-Weber syndrome
J Comput Assist Tomogr 1987 Jan-Feb, Vol. 11 (1), P. 88–91

1961. Pappas D, Mirvis S E, Crepps J T
Splenic trauma: false- negative CT diagnosis in cases of delayed rupture
Am J Roentgenol 1987 Oct, Vol. 149 (4), P. 727–8

1962. Parker L A, Mittelstaedt C A, Mauro M A, Mandell V S, Jaques P F
Torsion of a wandering spleen: CT appearance
J Comput Assist Tomogr 1984 Dec, Vol. 8 (6), P. 1201–4

1963. Pastakia B, Shawker T H, Thaler M, O Leary T, Pizzo P A
Hepatosplenic candidiasis: wheels within wheels
Radiology 1988 Feb, Vol. 166 (2), P. 417–21

1964. Piekarski J, Federle M P, Moss A A, London S S
Computed tomography of the spleen
Radiology 1980 Jun, Vol. 135 (3), P. 683–9

1965. Pistoia F, Markowitz S K
Splenic lymphangiomatosis: CT diagnosis
Am J Roentgenol 1988 Jan, Vol. 150 (1), P. 121–2

1966. Rauch R F, Korobkin M, Silverman P M, Moore A V
CT detection of iatrogenic percutaneous splenic injury
J Comput Assist Tomogr 1983 Dec, Vol. 7 (6), P. 1018–21

1967. Scatamacchia S A, Raptopoulos V, Fink M P, Silva W E
Splenic trauma in adults: impact of CT grading on management
Radiology 1989 Jun, Vol. 171 (3), P. 725–9

1968. Stiris M G
Accessory spleen versus left adrenal tumor: computed tomographic and abdominal angiographic evaluation
J Comput Assist Tomogr 1980 Aug, Vol. 4 (4), P. 543–4

1969. Stiris M G
Computed tomography of the spleen letter
Radiology 1981 Jul, Vol. 140 (1), P. 249

1970. Strijk S P, Wagener D J, Bogman M J, de Pauw B E, Wobbes T
The spleen in Hodgkin disease: diagnostic value of CT
Radiology 1985 Mar, Vol. 154 (3), P. 753–7

1971. Sutton C S, Haaga J R
CT evaluation of limited splenic trauma
J Comput Assist Tomogr 1987 Jan-Feb, Vol. 11 (1), P. 167–9

1972. Taylor C R, Rosenfield A T
Limitations of computed tomography in the recognition of delayed splenic rupture
J Comput Assist Tomogr 1984 Dec, Vol. 8 (6), P. 1205–7

1973. Triller J, Bona E, Barbier P
Der Milzinfarkt im Computertomogramm
Splenic infarct in the computed tomogram
RÖFO 1985 Apr, Vol. 142 (4), P. 374–9

1974. Umlas S L, Cronan J J
Splenic trauma: can CT grading systems enable prediction of successful nonsurgical treatment?
Radiology 1991 Feb, Vol. 178 (2), P. 481–7

1975. van der Laan R T, Verbeeten B Jr, Smits N J, Lubbers M J
Computed tomography in the diagnosis and treatment of solitary splenic abscesses
J Comput Assist Tomogr 1989 Jan-Feb, Vol. 13 (1), P. 71–4

1976. Vibhakar S D, Bellon E M
The bare area of the spleen: a constant CT feature of the ascitic abdomen
Am J Roentgenol 1984 May, Vol. 142 (5), P. 953–5

The Kidney

1977. Abeln E L, Paushter D M, Mehta A
Computed tomography of renal lymphomatoid granulomatosis
J Comput Assist Tomogr 1988 Jul- Aug, Vol. 12 (4), P. 671–3

1978. Araki T
Leukemic involvement of the kidney in children: CT features
J Comput Assist Tomogr 1982 Aug, Vol. 6 (4), P. 781–4

1979. Arenson A M, Graham R T, Shaw P, Srigley J, Herschorn S
Angiomyolipoma of the kidney extending into the inferior vena cava: sonographic and CT findings
Am J Roentgenol 1988 Dec, Vol. 151 (6), P. 1159–61

1980. Baert A L, Wilms G, Marchal G, De Mayer P, De Somer F
Contrast enhancement by bolus technique in the CT examination of the kidney
Radiologe 1980 Jun, Vol. 20 (6), P. 279–87

1981. Barth V, Eisenberger F, Buck J
Angiographie und Computertomographie bei seltenen Nierenerkrankungen
Angiography and CT in rare types of renal disease
Radiologe 1981 Jan, Vol. 21 (1), P. 52–7

1982. Boijsen E, Lin G
Lateral displacement of the right kidney by the ascending colon
J Comput Assist Tomogr 1983 Apr, Vol. 7 (2), P. 344–6

1983. Bosniak M A, Megibow A J, Hulnick D H, Horii S, Raghavendra B N
CT diagnosis of renal angiomyolipoma: the importance of detecting small amounts of fat
Am J Roentgenol 1988 Sep, Vol. 151 (3), P. 497–501

1984. Braedel H U, Rzehak L, Schindler E, Polsky M S, Dohring W
Computertomographische Untersuchungen bei Nierenverletzungen
Computer tomography in the investigation of renal trauma
RÖFO 1980 Jan, Vol. 132 (1), P. 49–54

1985. Brasch R C, Randel S B, Gould R G
Follow-up of Wilms tumor: comparison of CT with other imaging procedures
Am J Roentgenol 1981 Nov, Vol. 137 (5), P. 1005–9

1986. Breatnach E, Stanley R J, Carpenter J T Jr
Intrarenal chloroma causing obstructive nephropathy: CT characteristics
J Comput Assist Tomogr 1985 Jul-Aug, Vol. 9 (4), P. 822–4

1987. Breatnach E, Stanley R J, Bueschen A J
CT demonstration of spontaneous extrusion of staghorn calculus
J Comput Assist Tomogr 1986 Mar-Apr, Vol. 10 (2), P. 346–8

1988. Breatnach E S, Stanley R J, Lloyd K
Focal obstructive nephrogram: an unusual CT appearance of a transitional cell carcinoma
J Comput Assist Tomogr 1984 Oct, Vol. 8 (5), P. 1019–22

1989. Bree R L, Schultz S R, Hayes R
Large infiltrating renal transitional cell carcinomas: CT and ultrasound features
J Comput Assist Tomogr 1990 May-Jun, Vol. 14 (3), P. 381–5

1990. Brennan R P, Pearlstein A E, Miller S A
Computed tomography of the kidneys in a patient with methoxyflurane abuse
J Comput Assist Tomogr 1988 Jan-Feb, Vol. 12 (1), P. 155–6

1991. Bruna J
The renovertebral index in kidney size estimation using computerised tomography
RÖFO 1985 May, Vol. 142 (5), P. 587

1992. Chilcote W A, Borkowski G P
Computed tomography in renal lymphoma
J Comput Assist Tomogr 1983 Jun, Vol. 7 (3), P. 439–43

1993. Claussen C, Ludwigsen B, Knipper H, Weiss T, Fiegler W
Computertomographische Stadieneinteilung des hypernephroiden Karzinoms
Computed tomographic staging of hypernephroid carcinoma
RÖFO 1984 Oct, Vol. 141 (4), P. 390–4

1994. Cohan R H, Dunnick N R, Degesys G E, Korobkin M
Computed tomography of renal oncocytoma
J Comput Assist Tomogr 1984 Apr, Vol. 8 (2), P. 284–7

1995. Cohan R H, Dunnick N R, Leder R A, Baker M E
Computed tomography of renal lymphoma
J Comput Assist Tomogr 1990 Nov-Dec, Vol. 14 (6), P. 933–8

1996. Coleman B G, Arger P H, Mintz M C, Pollack H M, Banner M P
Hyperdense renal masses: a computed tomographic dilemma
Am J Roentgenol 1984 Aug, Vol. 143 (2), P. 291–4

1997. Coleman B G, Arger P H, Pollack H M, Banner M, Grossman R A
Contrast medium pooling in cystic renal carcinoma: CT findings
J Comput Assist Tomogr 1984 Dec, Vol. 8 (6), P. 1208–10

1998. Coleman C C, Saxena K M, Johnson K W
Renal vein thrombosis in a child with the nephrotic syndrome: CT diagnosis
Am J Roentgenol 1980 Dec, Vol. 135 (6), P. 1285–6

1999. Cormier P J, Donaldson J S, Gonzalez Crussi F
Nephroblastomatosis: missed diagnosis
Radiology 1988 Dec, Vol. 169 (3), P. 737–8

2000. Cramer B C, Twomey B P, Katz D
CT findings in obstructed upper moieties of duplex kidneys
J Comput Assist Tomogr 1983 Apr, Vol. 7 (2), P. 251–3

2001. Cronan J J, Amis E S, Zeman R K, Dorfman G S
Obstruction of the upper-pole moiety in renal duplication in adults: CT evaluation
Radiology 1986 Oct, Vol. 161 (1), P. 17–21

2002. Curry N S, Gobien R P, Schabel S I
Minimal-dilatation obstructive nephropathy
Radiology 1982 May, Vol. 143 (2), P. 531–4

2003. Curry N S, Schabel S I, Garvin A J, Fish G
Intratumoral fat in a renal oncocytoma mimicking angiomyolipoma
Am J Roentgenol 1990 Feb, Vol. 154 (2), P. 307–8

2004. Davis J M, McLaughlin A P
Spontaneous renal hemorrhage due to cyst rupture: CT findings
Am J Roentgenol 1987 Apr, Vol. 148 (4), P. 763–4

2005. Demos T C, Malone A J Jr
Computed tomography of a giant renal oncocytoma
J Comput Assist Tomogr 1988 Sep-Oct, Vol. 12 (5), P. 899–900

2006. Derouet H, Braedel H U, Mast G J, Ziegler M
Computertomographie bei akuten bakteriellen Nierenentzündungen
Computed tomography of acute bacterial nephritis
RÖFO 1988 Jan, Vol. 148 (1), P. 54–7

2007. Dunnick N R, Long J A Jr, Javadpour N
Perirenal extravasation of urographic contrast medium demonstrated by computed tomography
J Comput Assist Tomogr 1980 Aug, Vol. 4 (4), P. 538–9

2008. Dunnick N R, Korobkin M, Clark W M
CT demonstration of hyperdense renal carcinoma
J Comput Assist Tomogr 1984 Oct, Vol. 8 (5), P. 1023–4

2009. Dunnick N R, Korobkin M, Silverman P M, Foster W L Jr
Computed tomography of high density renal cysts
J Comput Assist Tomogr 1984 Jun, Vol. 8 (3), P. 458–61

2010. Ehrman K O, Kopecky K K, Wass J L, Thomalla J V
Parapelvic lymph cyst in a renal allograft mimicking hydronephrosis: CT diagnosis
J Comput Assist Tomogr 1987 Jul-Aug, Vol. 11 (4), P. 714–6

2011. Engelstad B L, McClennan B L, Levitt R G, Stanley R J, Sagel S S
The role of pre-contrast images in computed tomography of the kidney
Radiology 1980 Jul, Vol. 136 (1), P. 153–5

2012. Fajardo L L, Hillman B J, Hunter T B, Claypool H R, Westerman B R, Mockbee B
Excretory urography using computed radiography
Radiology 1987 Feb, Vol. 162 (2), P. 345–51

2013. Falkoff G E, Rigsby C M, Rosenfield A T
Partial, combined cortical and medullary nephrocalcinosis: US and CT patterns in AIDS-associated MAI infection
Radiology 1987 Feb, Vol. 162 (2), P. 343–4

2014. Federle M P, Kaiser J A, McAninch J W, Jeffrey R B, Mall J C
The role of computed tomography in renal trauma
Radiology 1981 Nov, Vol. 141 (2), P. 455–60

2015. Federle M P, Brown T R, McAninch J W
Penetrating renal trauma: CT evaluation
J Comput Assist Tomogr 1987 Nov-Dec, Vol. 11 (6), P. 1026–30

2016. Fein A B, Lee J K, Balfe D M, Heiken J P, Ling D, Glazer H S, Mc Clennan B L
Diagnosis and staging of renal cell carcinoma: a comparison of MR imaging and CT
Am J Roentgenol 1987 Apr, Vol. 148 (4), P. 749–53

2017. Fernbach S K, Feinstein K A, Donaldson J S, Baum E S
Nephroblastomatosis: comparison of CT with US and urography
Radiology 1988 Jan, Vol. 166 (1 Pt 1), P. 153–6

2018. Fischedick A R, Peters P E
CT-Untersuchungen nach Äthanolembolisation maligner Nierentumoren
CT studies following ethanol embolization of malignant kidney tumors
RÖFO 1986 Jan, Vol. 144 (1), P. 76–9

2019. Fischer H J, Becker W
Computertomographische Untersuchung einer akuten Nierentuberkulose
Computer tomographic study of acute renal tuberculosis
RÖFO 1983 May, Vol. 138 (5), P. 619–21

2020. Fishman E K, Hartman D S, Goldman S M, Siegelman S S
The CT appearance of Wilms tumor
J Comput Assist Tomogr 1983 Aug, Vol. 7 (4), P. 659–65

2021. Forbes W S, Isherwood I, Fawcitt R A
Computed tomography in the evaluation of the solitary or unilateral nonfunctioning kidney
J Comput Assist Tomogr 1978 Sep, Vol. 2 (4), P. 389–94

2022. Fretz C, Haertel M
Computertomographie nach Nierentrauma
Computer tomography following renal trauma
RÖFO 1981 Dec, Vol. 135 (6), P. 653–6

2023. Frija J, Larde D, Belloir C, Botto H, Martin N, Vasile N
Computed tomography diagnosis of renal angiomyolipoma
J Comput Assist Tomogr 1980 Dec, Vol. 4 (6), P. 843–6

2024. Fund G, Fischedick A R, Muller R P, Langenbruch K, Muller Rensing R
Die Bedeutung der Computertomographie in der Stufendiagnostik von Nierenbeckentumoren
Significance of computed tomography in the staging of renal pelvic tumors
RÖFO 1983 Apr, Vol. 138 (4), P. 473–6

2025. Gavant M L, Salazar J E, Ellis J
Intrarenal rupture of the abdominal aorta: CT features
J Comput Assist Tomogr 1986 May- Jun, Vol. 10 (3), P. 516–8

2026. Glazer G M, London S S
CT appearance of global renal infarction
J Comput Assist Tomogr 1981 Dec, Vol. 5 (6), P. 847–50

2027. Glazer G M, Francis I R, Brady T M, Teng S S
Computed tomography of renal infarction: clinical and experimental observations
Am J Roentgenol 1983 Apr, Vol. 140 (4), P. 721–7

2028. Glazer G M, Francis I R, Gross B H, Amendola M A
Computed tomography of renal vein thrombosis
J Comput Assist Tomogr 1984 Apr, Vol. 8 (2), P. 288–93

2029. Gold R P, McClennan B L, Rottenberg R R
CT appearance of acute inflammatory disease of the renal interstitium
Am J Roentgenol 1983 Aug, Vol. 141 (2), P. 343–9

2030. Goldman S M, Hartman D S, Fishman E K, Finizio J P, Gatewood O M, Siegelman S S
CT of xanthogranulomatous pyelonephritis: radiologic-pathologic correlation
Am J Roentgenol 1984 May, Vol. 142 (5), P. 963–9

2031. Goldman S M, Fishman E K, Hartman D S, Kim Y C, Siegelman S S
Computed tomography of renal tuberculosis and its pathological correlates
J Comput Assist Tomogr 1985 Jul-Aug, Vol. 9 (4), P. 771–6

2032. Gourtsoyiannis N, Prassopoulos P, Cavouras D, Pantelidis N
The thickness of the renal parenchyma decreases with age: a CT study of 360 patients
Am J Roentgenol 1990 Sep, Vol. 155 (3), P. 541–4

2033. Grote R, Dohring W, Aeikens B
Computertomographischer und sonographischer Nachweis von renalen und perirenalen Veränderungen nach einer extrakorporalen Stoßwellenlithotripsie
Computed tomographic and sonographic detection of renal and perirenal changes following shockwave lithotripsy
RÖFO 1986 Apr, Vol. 144 (4), P. 434–9

2034. Haaga J R, Morrison S C
CT appearance of renal infarct
J Comput Assist Tomogr 1980 Apr, Vol. 4 (2), P. 246–7

2035. Hansen G C, Hoffman R B, Sample W F, Becker R
Computed tomography diagnosis of renal angiomyolipoma
Radiology 1978 Sep, Vol. 128 (3), P. 789–91

2036. Hartman D S, Davidson A J, Davis C J Jr, Goldman S M
Infiltrative renal lesions: CT-sonographic-pathologic correlation
Am J Roentgenol 1988 May, Vol. 150 (5), P. 1061–4

2037. Hata Y, Tada S, Kato Y, Onishi T, Masuda F, Machida T
Staging of renal cell carcinoma by computed tomography
J Comput Assist Tomogr 1983 Oct, Vol. 7 (5), P. 828–32

2038. Haynes J W, Walsh J W, Brewer W H, Vick C W, Allen H A
Traumatic renal artery occlusion: CT diagnosis with angiographic correlation
J Comput Assist Tomogr 1984 Aug, Vol. 8 (4), P. 731–3

2039. Haynes J W, Miller P R, Zingas A P
Computed tomography and lymphangiography in chyluria
J Comput Assist Tomogr 1984 Apr, Vol. 8 (2), P. 341–2

2040. Heiken J P, Gold R P, Schnur M J, King D L, Bashist B, Glazer H S
Computed tomography of renal lymphoma with ultrasound correlation
J Comput Assist Tomogr 1983 Apr, Vol. 7 (2), P. 245–50

2041. Hekali P, Kivisaari L, Standerskjold Nordenstam C G, Pajari R, Turto H
Renal complications of polyarteritis nodosa: CT findings
J Comput Assist Tomogr 1985 Mar-Apr, Vol. 9 (2), P. 333–8

2042. Hill S C, Hoeg J M, Avila N A
Nephrocalcinosis in homozygous familial hypercholesterolemia: ultrasound and CT findings
J Comput Assist Tomogr 1991 Jan-Feb, Vol. 15 (1), P. 101–3

2043. Hillman B J, Drach G W, Tracey P, Gaines J A
Computed tomographic analysis of renal calculi
Am J Roentgenol 1984 Mar, Vol. 142 (3), P. 549–52

2044. Hoddick W, Jeffrey R B, Goldberg H I, Federle M P, Laing F C
CT and sonography of severe renal and perirenal infections
Am J Roentgenol 1983 Mar, Vol. 140 (3), P. 517–20

2045. Hoffman E P, Mindelzun R E, Anderson R U
Computed tomography in acute pyelonephritis associated with diabetes
Radiology 1980 Jun, Vol. 135 (3), P. 691–5

2046. Honda H, McGuire C W, Barloon T J, Hashimoto K
Replacement lipomatosis of the kidney: CT features
J Comput Assist Tomogr 1990 Mar-Apr, Vol. 14 (2), P. 229–31

2047. Hughes J J, Wilder W M
Computed tomography of renal sarcoidosis
J Comput Assist Tomogr 1988 Nov-Dec, Vol. 12 (6), P. 1057–8

2048. Hulnick D H, Bosniak M A
"Faceless kidney": CT sign of renal duplicity
J Comput Assist Tomogr 1986 Sep-Oct, Vol. 10 (5), P. 771–2

2049. Ishikawa I, Matsuura H, Onouchi Z, Suzuki M
CT appearance of the kidney in traumatic renal artery occlusion
J Comput Assist Tomogr 1982 Oct, Vol. 6 (5), P. 1021–4

2050. Jafri S Z, Ellwood R A, Amendola M A, Farah J
Therapeutic angioinfarction of renal carcinoma: CT follow-up
J Comput Assist Tomogr 1989 May-Jun, Vol. 13 (3), P. 443–7

2051. Jansen O, Gmelin E, Burmester E, Rob P, Weiss H D
Analyse von dynamischen CT-Kurven bei Nierentransplantaten mit Abstoßungsreaktion und Cyclosporin-A-Intoxikation
Analysis of dynamic CT curves in kidney transplants with rejection reaction and cyclosporin A poisoning
RÖFO 1989 Oct, Vol. 151 (4), P. 473–6

2052. Jaschke W, van Kaick G, Palmtag H
Vergleich der Wertigkeit von Echographie und Computertomographie bei der Diagnostik raumfordernder Prozesse der Nieren
A comparison of echography and computer tomography for the diagnosis of space- occupying lesions in the kidney
RÖFO 1980 Feb, Vol. 132 (2), P. 145–51

2053. Jeffrey R B Jr
Bacterial renal infection: role of CT letter
Radiology 1989 Nov, Vol. 173 (2), P. 574–5

2054. Kim W S, Goldman S M, Gatewood O M, Marshall F F, Siegelman S S
Computed tomography in calcified renal masses
J Comput Assist Tomogr 1981 Dec, Vol. 5 (6), P. 855–60

2055. Klose K C, Schwartz R, Karstens J H
Computertomographie renaler maligner Lymphome
Computer tomography of malignant renal lymphomas
RÖFO 1983 Nov, Vol. 139 (5), P. 515–20

2056. Kneeland J B, Auh Y H, Rubenstein W A, Zirinsky K, Morrison H, Whalen J P, Kazam E
Perirenal spaces: CT evidence for communication across the midline
Radiology 1987 Sep, Vol. 164 (3), P. 657–64

2057. Kolbenstvedt A, Lien H H
Isolated renal hilar lip on computed tomography
Radiology 1982 Apr, Vol. 143 (1), P. 150

2058. Kothari K, Segal A J, Spitzer R M, Peartree R J
Preoperative radiographic evaluation of hypernephroma
J Comput Assist Tomogr 1981 Oct, Vol. 5 (5), P. 702–4

2059. Kratz H W, Hamper P
Präoperative radiologische Diagnostik des renalen Angiomyolipoms. Bedeutung von Angiographie und Computertomographie
Preoperative radiologic diagnosis of renal angiomyolipoma. Significance of angiography and computerized tomography
RÖFO 1982 Aug, Vol. 137 (2), P. 183–9

2060. Krudy A G, Dunnick N R, Magrath I T, Shawker T H, Doppman J L, Spiegel R
CT of American Burkitt lymphoma
Am J Roentgenol 1981 Apr, Vol. 136 (4), P. 747–54

2061. Kunin M
Renal masses considered indeterminate on computed tomography letter
Radiology 1983 Jan, Vol. 146 (1), P. 260–1

2062. Lackner K, Koischwitz D, Molitor B, Vogel J, Schmidt S
Treffsicherheit in der Diagnostik renaler Raumforderungen. CT, Sonographie, Urographie, Angiographie.
Accuracy in the diagnosis of renal masses. Computed tomography, sonography, urography, angiography
RÖFO 1984 Apr, Vol. 140 (4), P. 363–72

2063. Lang E K
Angio-computed tomography and dynamic computed tomography in staging of renal cell carcinoma
Radiology 1984 Apr, Vol. 151 (1), P. 149–55

2064. Lautin E M, Gordon P M, Friedman A C, McCormick J F, Fromowitz F B, Goldman M J, Sugarman L A
Radionuclide imaging and computed tomography in renal oncocytoma
Radiology 1981 Jan, Vol. 138 (1), P. 185–90

2065. Levine L, Vrlenich L
Renal lymphoma in ataxia- telangiectasia: CT contribution
J Comput Assist Tomogr 1989 May- Jun, Vol. 13 (3), P. 537–9

2066. Levine C, Levine E
Small pediatric renal neoplasms detected by CT
J Comput Assist Tomogr 1990 Jul-Aug, Vol. 14 (4), P. 615–8

2067. Levine E, Lee K R, Weigel J
Preoperative determination of abdominal extent of renal cell carcinoma by computed tomography
Radiology 1979 Aug, Vol. 132 (2), P. 395–8

2068. Levine E, Lee K R, Weigel J W, Farber B
Computed tomography in the diagnosis of renal carcinoma complicating Hippel-Lindau syndrome
Radiology 1979 Mar, Vol. 130 (3), P. 703–6

2069. Levine E, Huntrakoon M
Computed tomography of renal oncocytoma
Am J Roentgenol 1983 Oct, Vol. 141 (4), P. 741–6

2070. Levine E, Grantham J J, Slusher S L, Greathouse J L, Krohn B P
CT of acquired cystic kidney disease and renal tumors in long-term dialysis patients
Am J Roentgenol 1984 Jan, Vol. 142 (1), P. 125–31

2071. Levine E, Grantham J J
High-density renal cysts in autosomal dominant polycystic kidney disease demonstrated by CT
Radiology 1985 Feb, Vol. 154 (2), P. 477–82

2072. Levine E, Grantham J J
Perinephric hemorrhage in autosomal dominant polycystic kidney disease: CT and MR findings
J Comput Assist Tomogr 1987 Jan-Feb, Vol. 11 (1), P. 108–11

2073. Levine E
Computed tomography of renal abscesses complicating medullary sponge kidney
J Comput Assist Tomogr 1989 May-Jun, Vol. 13 (3), P. 440–2

2074. Levine E, Huntrakoon M
Unilateral renal cystic disease: CT findings
J Comput Assist Tomogr 1989 Mar-Apr, Vol. 13 (2), P. 273–6

2075. Levine E, Slusher S L, Grantham J J, Wetzel L H
Natural history of acquired renal cystic disease in dialysis patients: a prospective longitudinal CT study
Am J Roentgenol 1991 Mar, Vol. 156 (3), P. 501–6

2076. Lim T H, Lee J S, Choi B I, Kim I O, Suh C H, Han M C, Kim C W
An explanation of renal hemodynamics in acute renal failure based on sequential CT in patients with Korean hemorrhagic fever
J Comput Assist Tomogr 1987 May-Jun, Vol. 11 (3), P. 474–9

2077. Love L, Yedlicka J
Computed tomography of internally calcified renal cysts
Am J Roentgenol 1985 Dec, Vol. 145 (6), P. 1225–7

2078. Love L, Demos T C, Posniak H
CT of retrorenal fluid collections
Am J Roentgenol 1985 Jul, Vol. 145 (1), P. 87–91

2079. Love L, Lind J A Jr, Olson M C
Persistent CT nephrogram: significance in the diagnosis of contrast nephropathy
Radiology 1989 Jul, Vol. 172 (1), P. 125–9

2080. Lupetin A R, Mainwaring B L, Daffner R H
CT diagnosis of renal artery injury caused by blunt abdominal trauma
Am J Roentgenol 1989 Nov, Vol. 153 (5), P. 1065–8

2081. Mangano F A, Zaontz M, Pahira J J, Clark L R, Jaffe M H, Choyke P L, Zeman R K
Computed tomography of acute renal failure secondary to rhabdomyolysis
J Comput Assist Tomogr 1985 Jul-Aug, Vol. 9 (4), P. 777–9

2082. Mansfeld L, Boitz F, Marciniak H, Schnorr H, Harzendorf E, Poehls C, Cimanowski N, Cobet H
CT-gezielte Nierenzystenverödung. Erfahrungsbericht über 100 Patienten
CT- guided sclerosing therapy of kidney cysts. Report of experience with 100 patients
RÖFO 1987 Jun, Vol. 146 (6), P. 674–80

2083. Mastrodomenico L, Korobkin M, Silverman P M, Dunnick N R
Perinephric hemorrhage from metastatic carcinoma to the kidney
J Comput Assist Tomogr 1983 Aug, Vol. 7 (4), P. 727–9

2084. Mauro M A, Wadsworth D E, Stanley R J, McClennan B L
Renal cell carcinoma: angiography in the CT era
Am J Roentgenol 1982 Dec, Vol. 139 (6), P. 1135–8

2085. Mayer D P, Baron R L, Pollack H M
Increase in CT attenuation values of parapelvic renal cysts after retrograde pyelography
Am J Roentgenol 1982 Nov, Vol. 139 (5), P. 991–3

2086. McClennan B L, Lee J K, Peterson R R
Anatomy of the perirenal area
Radiology 1986 Feb, Vol. 158 (2), P. 555–7

2087. Meziane M A, Fishman E K, Goldman S M, Friedman A C, Siegelman S S
Computed tomography of high density renal cysts in adult polycystic kidney disease
J Comput Assist Tomogr 1986 Sep- Oct, Vol. 10 (5), P. 767–70

2088. Mindell H J
CT of the renal cyst letter
Am J Roentgenol 1980 Mar, Vol. 134 (3), P. 620–1

2089. Mindell H J
Imaging studies for screening native kidneys in long-term dialysis patients
Am J Roentgenol 1989 Oct, Vol. 153 (4), P. 768–9

2090. Morag B, Rubinstein Z J, Hertz M, Solomon A
Computed tomography in the diagnosis of renal parapelvic cysts
J Comput Assist Tomogr 1983 Oct, Vol. 7 (5), P. 833–6

2091. Nakstad P, Kolmannskog F, Kolbenstvedt A, Sodal G
Computed tomography in surgical complications following renal transplantation
J Comput Assist Tomogr 1982 Apr, Vol. 6 (2), P. 286–9

2092. Nebel G, Lingg G, Berg E, Fischer R
Zum computertomographischen und sonographischen Nachweis von renalen Hämatomen nach perkutaner Nierenbiopsie
Computer tomographic and sonographic demonstration of renal haematomas following percutaneous renal biopsy
RÖFO 1982 Apr, Vol. 136 (4), P. 413–6

2093. Nishitani H, Onitsuka H, Kawahira K, Ono M, Jinnouchi Y, Ohba T, Matsuura K
Computed tomography of renal metastases
J Comput Assist Tomogr 1984 Aug, Vol. 8 (4), P. 727–30

2094. Novetsky G J, Berlin L, Epstein A J, Lobo N, Miller S H
CT diagnosis of renal cyst wall tumor
J Comput Assist Tomogr 1983 Jun, Vol. 7 (3), P. 539–40

2095. Nussbaum A, Hunter T B, Stables D P
Spontaneous cyst rupture on renal CT
Am J Roentgenol 1984 Apr, Vol. 142 (4), P. 751–2

2096. Nyman U, Hildell J, Husberg B, Molde A, Treugut H
Computed tomography in the diagnosis of complications following renal allograft surgery
RÖFO 1982 Feb, Vol. 136 (2), P. 138–43

2097. Olson M, Posniak H
CT characteristics of a hyperdense renal mass due to Richter syndrome
J Comput Assist Tomogr 1988 Jul-Aug, Vol. 12 (4), P. 669–70

2098. Pagani J J
Solid renal mass in the cancer patient: second primary renal cell carcinoma versus renal metastasis
J Comput Assist Tomogr 1983 Jun, Vol. 7 (3), P. 444–8

2099. Papanicolaou N, Harbury O L, Pfister R C
Fat-filled postoperative renal cortical defects: sonographic and CT appearance
Am J Roentgenol 1988 Sep, Vol. 151 (3), P. 503–5

2100. Parienty R A, Pradel J, Imbert M C, Picard J D, Savart P
Computed tomography of multilocular cystic nephroma
Radiology 1981 Jul, Vol. 140 (1), P. 135–9

2101. Parienty R A, Pradel J, Picard J D, Ducellier R, Lubrano J M, Smolarski N
Visibility and thickening of the renal fascia on computed tomograms
Radiology 1981 Apr, Vol. 139 (1), P. 119–24

2102. Parvey L S, Warner R M, Callihan T R, Magill H L
CT demonstration of fat tissue in malignant renal neoplasms: atypical Wilms' tumors
J Comput Assist Tomogr 1981 Dec, Vol. 5 (6), P. 851–4

2103. Pazmino P, Pyatt R, Williams E, Bohan L
Computed tomography in renal ischemia
J Comput Assist Tomogr 1983 Feb, Vol. 7 (1), P. 102–5

2104. Peretz G S, Lam A H
Distinguishing neuroblastoma from Wilms tumor by computed tomography
J Comput Assist Tomogr 1985 Sep-Oct, Vol. 9 (5), P. 889–93

2105. Pollack H M, Arger P H, Banner M P, Mulhern C B Jr, Coleman B G
Computed tomography of renal pelvic filling defects
Radiology 1981 Mar, Vol. 138 (3), P. 645–51

2106. Pope T L Jr, Buschi A J, Moore T S, Williamson B R, Brenbridge A N
CT features of renal polyarteritis nodosa
Am J Roentgenol 1981 May, Vol. 136 (5), P. 986–7

2107. Press G A, McClennan B L, Melson G L, Weyman P J, Mauro M A, Lee J K
Papillary renal cell carcinoma: CT and sonographic evaluation
Am J Roentgenol 1984 Nov, Vol. 143 (5), P. 1005–9

2108. Probst P, Kruker T, Hoogewoud H M
Cavographie und Computertomographie zum Nachweis der Tumorinfiltration in die Vena cava bei malignen Nierentumoren
Cavography and CT for demonstration of canalicular spread of renal neoplasms into the inferior vena cava
Radiologe 1982 Jun, Vol. 22 (6), P. 272–8

2109. Raghavendra B N, Bosniak M A, Megibow A J
Small angiomyolipoma of the kidney: sonographic-CT evaluation
Am J Roentgenol 1983 Sep, Vol. 141 (3), P. 575–8

2110. Rausch H P, Hanefeld F, Kaufmann H J
Medullary nephrocalcinosis and pancreatic calcifications demonstrated by ultrasound and CT in infants after treatment with ACTH
Radiology 1984 Oct, Vol. 153 (1), P. 105–7

2111. Rauschkolb E N, Sandler C M, Patel S, Childs T L
Computed tomography of renal inflammatory disease
J Comput Assist Tomogr 1982 Jun, Vol. 6 (3), P. 502–6

2112. Reed M D, Friedman A C, Nealey P
Anomalies of the left renal vein: analysis of 433 CT scans
J Comput Assist Tomogr 1982 Dec, Vol. 6 (6), P. 1124–6

2113. Reiman T A, Siegel M J, Shackelford G D
Wilms tumor in children: abdominal CT and US evaluation
Radiology 1986 Aug, Vol. 160 (2), P. 501–5

2114. Rhodes R A, Fried A M, Lorman J G, Kryscio R J
Tomographic levels for intravenous urography: CT-determined guidelines
Radiology 1987 Jun, Vol. 163 (3), P. 673–5

2115. Rhyner P, Federle M P, Jeffrey R B
CT of trauma to the abnormal kidney
Am J Roentgenol 1984 Apr, Vol. 142 (4), P. 747–50

2116. Rigsby C M, Rosenfield A T, Glickman M G, Hodson J
Hemorrhagic focal bacterial nephritis: findings on gray-scale sonography and CT
Am J Roentgenol 1986 Jun, Vol. 146 (6), P. 1173–7

2117. Robsen C J, Churchill B M, Anderson W
The results of radical nephrectomy for renal cell carcinoma
J.Urol.1969 Vol.101, P.297

2118. Rofsky N M, Bosniak M A, Weinreb J C, Coppa G F
Giant renal cell carcinoma: CT and MR characteristics
J Comput Assist Tomogr 1989 Nov-Dec, Vol. 13 (6), P. 1078–80

2119. Rothenberg D M, Brandt T D, D Cruz I
Computed tomography of renal angiomyolipoma presenting as right atrial mass
J Comput Assist Tomogr 1986 Nov-Dec, Vol. 10 (6), P. 1054–6

2120. Rubin B E
Computed tomography in the evaluation of renal lymphoma
J Comput Assist Tomogr 1979 Dec, Vol. 3 (6), P. 759–64

2121. Schild H, Riedmiller H
Computertomographischer Nachweis einer seltenen Mesonephronmißbildung
Computerized tomographic demonstration of a rare mesonephron abnormality
RÖFO 1983 Jan, Vol. 138 (1), P. 104–6

2122. Schumacher R, Klingmuller V, Reither M
Stellenwert der Sonographie gegenüber Röntgen und Computertomographie bei der Diagnose von Nephrokalzinosen
Status of sonography versus roentgen and computed tomography in the diagnosis of nephrocalcinosis
RÖFO 1984 Jul, Vol. 141 (1), P. 75–9

2123. Schurawitzki H, Karnel F, Mostbeck G, Langle F, Watschinger B, Hubsch P
Radiologische Therapie von symptomatischen Lymphozelen nach Nierentransplantation
Radiologic therapy of symptomatic lymphoceles following kidney transplantation
RÖFO 1990 Jan, Vol. 152 (1), P. 71–5

2124. Schweden F, Klose K J, Schild H, Engelmann U, Riedmiller H, Weber M
Computertomographie des renalen Angiomyolipoms
Computed tomography of renal angiomyolipomas
RÖFO 1983 Sep, Vol. 139 (3), P. 269–73

2125. Schweden F, Duber C, Schild H, Storkel S, Engelmann U, Thelen M
Das Onkozytom der Niere. 1. Computertomographie
Oncocytoma of the kidney. 1. Computed tomography
RÖFO 1988 Feb, Vol. 148 (2), P. 137–42

2126. Segal A J, Spitzer R M
Pseudo thick-walled renal cyst by CT
Am J Roentgenol 1979 May, Vol. 132 (5), P. 827–8

2127. Shah M, Haaga J R
Focal xanthogranulomatous pyelonephritis simulating a renal tumor: CT characteristics
J Comput Assist Tomogr 1989 Jul-Aug, Vol. 13 (4), P. 712–3

2128. Shirkhoda A
Computed tomography of perirenal metastases
J Comput Assist Tomogr 1986 May-Jun, Vol. 10 (3), P. 435–8

2129. Shirkhoda A, Lewis E
Renal sarcoma and sarcomatoid renal cell carcinoma: CT and angiographic features
Radiology 1987 Feb, Vol. 162 (2), P. 353–7

2130. Siegel M J, Sagel S S
Computed tomography as a supplement to urography in the evaluation of suspected neuro-blastoma
Radiology 1982 Feb, Vol. 142 (2), P. 435–8

2131. Siegel M J, Balfe D M
Blunt renal and ureteral trauma in childhood: CT patterns of fluid collections
Am J Roentgenol 1989 May, Vol. 152 (5), P. 1043–7

2132. Siegel S C, Sandler M A, Alpern M B, Pearlberg J L
CT of renal cell carcinoma in patients on chronic hemodialysis
Am J Roentgenol 1988 Mar, Vol. 150 (3), P. 583–5

2133. Silverman P M, Kelvin F M, Korobkin M
Lateral displacement of the right kidney by the colon: an anatomic variation demonstrated by CT
Am J Roentgenol 1983 Feb, Vol. 140 (2), P. 313–4

2134. Skolnick L
Renal imaging in long-term dialysis patients: a comparison of CT and sonography letter
Am J Roentgenol 1990 May, Vol. 154 (5), P. 1125–6

2135. Smith W P, Levine E
Sagittal and coronal CT image reconstruction: application in assessing the inferior vena cava in renal cancer
J Comput Assist Tomogr 1980 Aug, Vol. 4 (4), P. 531–5

2136. Soffer O, Miller L R, Lichtman J B
CT findings in complications of acquired renal cystic disease
J Comput Assist Tomogr 1987 Sep-Oct, Vol. 11 (5), P. 905–8

2137. Som P M, Norton K I, Shugar J M, Reede D L, Norton L, Biller H F, Som M L
Metastatic hypernephroma to the head and neck
AJNR 1987 Nov-Dec, Vol. 8 (6), P. 1103–6

2138. Soulen M C, Fishman E K, Goldman S M, Gatewood O M
Bacterial renal infection: role of CT
Radiology 1989 Jun, Vol. 171 (3), P. 703–7

2139. Soulen M C, Fishman E K, Goldman S M
Sequelae of acute renal infections: CT evaluation
Radiology 1989 Nov, Vol. 173 (2), P. 423–6

2140. Starinsky R, Graif M, Lotan D, Kessler A
Thrombus calcification of renal vein in neonate: ultrasound and CT diagnosis
J Comput Assist Tomogr 1989 May-Jun, Vol. 13 (3), P. 545–6

2141. Steinberg H V, Nelson R C, Murphy F B, Chezmar J L, Baumgartner B R, Delaney V B, Whelchel J D, Bernardino M E
Renal allograft rejection: evaluation by Doppler US and MR imaging
Radiology 1987 Feb, Vol. 162 (2), P. 337–42

2142. Subramanyam B R, Bosniak M A, Horii S C, Megibow A J, Balthazar E J
Replacement lipomatosis of the kidney: diagnosis by computed tomography and sonography
Radiology 1983 Sep, Vol. 148 (3), P. 791–2

2143. Sussman S K, Cochran S T, Pagani J J, McArdle C, Wong W, Austin R, Curry N, Kelly K M
Hyperdense renal masses: a CT manifestation of hemorrhagic renal cysts
Radiology 1984 Jan, Vol. 150 (1), P. 207–11

2144. Sussman S K, Goldberg R P, Griscom N T
Milk-of-calcium hydronephrosis in patients with paraplegia and urinary-enteric diversion: CT demonstration
J Comput Assist Tomogr 1986 Mar-Apr, Vol. 10 (2), P. 257–9

2145. Sussman S K, Gallmann W H, Cohan R H, Saeed M, Lawton J S
CT findings in xanthogranulomatous pyelonephritis with coexistent renocolic fistula
J Comput Assist Tomogr 1987 Nov-Dec, Vol. 11 (6), P. 1088–90

2146. Takahashi M, Tamakawa Y, Shibata A, Fukushima Y
Case report: computed tomography of "Page" kidney
J Comput Assist Tomogr 1977 Jul, Vol. 1 (3), P. 344–8

2147. Takao R, Amamoto Y, Matsunaga N, Tasaki T, Kakimoto S, Ito M, Fujii H, Futagawa S, Sekine I
Computed tomography of multicystic kidney
J Comput Assist Tomogr 1980 Aug, Vol. 4 (4), P. 548–9

2148. Taylor A J, Cohen E P, Erickson S J, Olson D L, Foley W D
Renal imaging in long-term dialysis patients: a comparison of CT and sonography
Am J Roentgenol 1989 Oct, Vol. 153 (4), P. 765–7

2149. Thierman D, Haaga J R, Anton P, LiPuma J P
Renal replacement lipomatosis
J Comput Assist Tomogr 1983 Apr, Vol. 7 (2), P. 341–3

2150. Totty W G, McClennan B L, Melson G L, Patel R
Relative value of computed tomography and ultrasonography in the assessment of renal angio-myolipoma
J Comput Assist Tomogr 1981 Apr, Vol. 5 (2), P. 173–8

2151. Treugut H, Nyman U, Hildell J
Sequenz-CT: Frühe Dichteveränderungen der gesunden Niere nach Kontrastmittelapplikation
Sequence-CT: early enhancement – curves of the healthy kidney
Radiologe 1980 Nov, Vol. 20 (11), P. 558–62

2152. Treugut H, Andersson I, Hildell J, Nyman U, Weibull H
Diagnostik renaler Perfusionsstörungen durch Sequenz-CT
The diagnosis of renal perfusion abnormalities by sequential CT
RÖFO 1981 Oct, Vol. 135 (4), P. 381–8

2153. Treugut H, Nyman U, Hildell J, Molde A
Funktionskontrolle des Nierentransplantats durch Sequenz-CT. Erste Ergebnisse
Functional control of the renal transplant via sequential computerized tomography. First results
RÖFO 1981 Aug, Vol. 135 (2), P. 133–42

2154. Ueda J, Kobayashi Y, Itoh H, Itatani H
Angiomyolipoma and renal cell carcinoma occurring in same kidney: CT evaluation
J Comput Assist Tomogr 1987 Mar-Apr, Vol. 11 (2), P. 340–1

2155. Uhlenbrock D, Fischer C, Ruhl G, Beyer H K, Hummelsheim P
Kernspintomographie und Computertomographie des malignen Hypernephroms
Nuclear spin tomography and computerized tomography in malignant hypernephroma
RÖFO 1987 Jun, Vol. 146 (6), P. 664–74

2156. Weinberger E, Rosenbaum D M, Pendergrass T W
Renal involvement in children with lymphoma: comparison of CT with sonography
Am J Roentgenol 1990 Aug, Vol. 155 (2), P. 347–9

2157. Winfield A C, Gerlock A J Jr, Shaff M I
Perirenal cobwebs: a CT sign of renal vein thrombosis
J Comput Assist Tomogr 1981 Oct, Vol. 5 (5), P. 705–8

2158. Wong W S, Moss A A, Federle M P, Cochran S T, London S S
Renal infarction: CT diagnosis and correlation between CT findings and etiologies
Radiology 1984 Jan, Vol. 150 (1), P. 201–5

2159. Yale Loehr A J, Kramer S S, Quinlan D M, La France N D, Mitchell S E, Gearhart J P
CT of severe renal trauma in children: evaluation and course of healing with conservative therapy
Am J Roentgenol 1989 Jan, Vol. 152 (1), P. 109–13

2160. Yashiro N, Yoshida H, Araki T
Bilateral "milk of calcium" renal cysts: CT findings
J Comput Assist Tomogr 1985 Jan-Feb, Vol. 9 (1), P. 199–200

2161. Yokoyama M, Watanabe K, Inatsuki S, Ochi K, Takeuchi M
Measurement of renal parenchymal volume using computed tomography
J Comput Assist Tomogr 1982 Oct, Vol. 6 (5), P. 975–7

2162. Zagoria R J, Dyer R B
Computed tomography of primary renal osteosarcoma
J Comput Assist Tomogr 1991 Jan-Feb, Vol. 15 (1), P. 146–8

2163. Zeman R K, Cronan J J, Rosenfield A T, Lynch J H, Jaffe M H, Clark L R
Renal cell carcinoma: dynamic thin-section CT assessment of vascular invasion and tumor vascularity
Radiology 1988 May, Vol. 167 (2), P. 393–6

2164. Zieger M, Treugut H
Computertomographische Diagnostik renaler Tumoren ohne Anwendung von Kontrastmittel
Computed tomographic diagnosis of renal tumors without using contrast media
RÖFO 1984 Mar, Vol. 140 (3), P. 290–4

2165. Zimmer W D, Williamson B Jr, Hartman G W, Hattery R R, O Brien P C
Changing patterns in the evaluation of renal masses: economic implications
Am J Roentgenol 1984 Aug, Vol. 143 (2), P. 285–9

2166. Zirinsky K, Auh Y H, Rubenstein W A, Williams J J, Pasmantier M W, Kazam E
CT of the hyperdense renal cyst: sonographic correlation
Am J Roentgenol 1984 Jul, Vol. 143 (1), P. 151–6

2167. Zirinsky K, Auh Y H, Hartman B J, Rubenstein W A, Morrison H S, Sherman S J, Kazam E
Computed tomography of renal aspergillosis
J Comput Assist Tomogr 1987 Jan-Feb, Vol. 11 (1), P. 177–8

2168. Zissin R, Hertz M, Apter S, Madgar I
Focal renal infarction after retroperitoneal lymph-node dissection: CT diagnosis
Am J Roentgenol 1989 Aug, Vol. 153 (2), P. 325–6

The Adrenal Glands

2169. Abrams H L, Siegelman S S, Adams D F, Sanders R, Finberg H J, Hessel S J, McNeil B J
Computed tomography versus ultrasound of the adrenal gland: a prospective study
Radiology 1982 Apr, Vol. 143 (1), P. 121–8

2170. Behan M, Martin E C, Muecke E C, Kazam E
Myelolipoma of the adrenal: two cases with ultrasound and CT findings
Am J Roentgenol 1977 Dec, Vol. 129 (6), P. 993–6

2171. Berland L L, Koslin D B, Kenney P J, Stanley R J, Lee J Y
Differentiation between small benign and malignant adrenal masses with dynamic incremented CT
Am J Roentgenol 1988 Jul, Vol. 151 (1), P. 95–101

2172. Berliner L, Bosniak M A, Megibow A
Adrenal pseudotumors on computed tomography
J Comput Assist Tomogr 1982 Apr, Vol. 6 (2), P. 281–5

2173. Bernardino M E, Walther M M, Phillips V M, Graham S D Jr, Sewell C W, Gedgaudas McClees K, Baumgartner B R, Torres W E, Erwin B C
CT-guided adrenal biopsy: accuracy, safety, and indications
Am J Roentgenol 1985 Jan, Vol. 144 (1), P. 67–9

2174. Bernardino M E
Management of the asymptomatic patient with a unilateral adrenal mass
Radiology 1988 Jan, Vol. 166 (1 Pt 1), P. 121–3

2175. Brownlie K, Kreel L
Computer assisted tomography of normal suprarenal glands
J Comput Assist Tomogr 1978 Jan, Vol. 2 (1), P. 1–10

2176. Derchi L E, Rapaccini G L, Banderali A, Danza F M, Grillo F
Ultrasound and CT findings in two cases of hemangioma of the adrenal gland
J Comput Assist Tomogr 1989 Jul-Aug, Vol. 13 (4), P. 659–61

2177. Doppman J L, Gill J R Jr, Nienhuis A W, Earll J M, Long J A Jr
CT findings in Addison's disease
J Comput Assist Tomogr 1982 Aug, Vol. 6 (4), P. 757–61

2178. Doppman J L, Miller D L, Dwyer A J, Loughlin T, Nieman L, Cutler G B, Chrousos G P, Oldfield E, Loriaux D L
Macronodular adrenal hyperplasia in Cushing disease
Radiology 1988 Feb, Vol. 166 (2), P. 347–52

2179. Doppman J L, Travis W D, Nieman L, Miller D L, Chrousos G P, Gomez M T, Cutler G B Jr, Loriaux D L, Norton J A
Cushing syndrome due to primary pigmented nodular adrenocortical disease: findings at CT and MR imaging
Radiology 1989 Aug, Vol. 172 (2), P. 415–20

2180. Doppman J L, Nieman L, Miller D L, Pass H I, Chang R, Cutler G B Jr, Schaaf M, Chrousos G P, Norton J A, Ziessman H A, et al
Ectopic adrenocorticotropic hormone syndrome: localization studies in 28 patients
Radiology 1989 Jul, Vol. 172 (1), P. 115–24

2181. Drouineau J, De Verbizier G
CT discriminators of malignant from benign adrenal masses letter
Am J Roentgenol 1986 Jun, Vol. 146 (6), P. 1316–7

2182. Dunnick N R, Schaner E G, Doppman J L, Strott C A, Gill J R, Javadpour N
Computed tomography in adrenal tumors
Am J Roentgenol 1979 Jan, Vol. 132 (1), P. 43–6

2183. Dunnick N R, Heaston D, Halvorsen R, Moore A V, Korobkin M
CT appearance of adrenal cortical carcinoma
J Comput Assist Tomogr 1982 Oct, Vol. 6 (5), P. 978–82

2184. Eghrari M, McLoughlin M J, Rosen I E, St Louis E L, Wilson S R, Yeung H P
The role of computed tomography in assessment of tumoral pathology of the adrenal glands
J Comput Assist Tomogr 1980 Feb, Vol. 4 (1), P. 71–7

2185. Falke T H, te Strake L, Shaff M I, Sandler M P, Kulkarni M V, Partain C L, Nieuwenhuizen Kruseman A C, James A E Jr
MR imaging of the adrenals: correlation with computed tomography
J Comput Assist Tomogr 1986 Mar-Apr, Vol. 10 (2), P. 242–53

2186. Fink D W, Wurtzebach L R
Symptomatic myelolipoma of the adrenal: report of a case with computed tomographic evaluation
Radiology 1980 Feb, Vol. 134 (2), P. 451–2

2187. Fishman E K, Deutch B M, Hartman D S, Goldman S M, Zerhouni E A, Siegelman S S
Primary adrenocortical carcinoma: CT evaluation with clinical correlation
Am J Roentgenol 1987 Mar, Vol. 148 (3), P. 531–5

2188. Geisinger M A, Zelch M G, Bravo E L, Risius B F, O Donovan P B, Borkowski G P
Primary hyperaldosteronism: comparison of CT, adrenal venography, and venous sampling
Am J Roentgenol 1983 Aug, Vol. 141 (2), P. 299–302

2189. Georgi M, Jaschke W, Trede M, von Mittelstaedt G, Cordes U, Sinterhauf K, Magin E
Erfahrungen mit der Computertomographie und der Nebennierenphlebographie in der Diagnostik hormonaktiver Nebennierenprozesse
Experience with CT and adrenal venography in the diagnosis of adrenal disease with endocrine activity
Radiologe 1980 Apr, Vol. 20 (4), P. 172–80

2190. Georgi M, Hofbauer J, Weiss H, Keller W, Wunschik F, von Mittelstaedt G, Linder M
Wertigkeit von Sonographie, Computertomographie und Angiographie in der Nebennierendiagnostik
Value of sonography, computed tomography and angiography in adrenal diagnosis
RÖFO 1984 Apr, Vol. 140 (4), P. 373–9

2191. Glazer H S, Weyman P J, Sagel S S, Levitt R G, McClennan B L
Nonfunctioning adrenal masses: incidental discovery on computed tomography
Am J Roentgenol 1982 Jul, Vol. 139 (1), P. 81–5

2192. Gmelin E, Wagner T, Babaian E, Weiss H D
Optimierte Diagnostik eines exzentrisch wachsenden Nebennierentumors durch simultane Katheterangiographie und Computertomographie
Optimized diagnosis of an eccentrically growing adrenal tumor by simultaneous catheter angiography and computer tomography
RÖFO 1982 May, Vol. 136 (5), P. 603–5

2193. Goldman S M, Gatewood O M, Walsh P C, Dornhorst A, Siegelman S S
CT configuration of the enlarged adrenal gland
J Comput Assist Tomogr 1982 Apr, Vol. 6 (2), P. 276–80

2194. Greene K M, Brantly P N, Thompson W R
Adenocarcinoma metastatic to the adrenal gland simulating myelolipoma: CT evaluation
J Comput Assist Tomogr 1985 Jul-Aug, Vol. 9 (4), P. 820–1

2195. Gross B H, Goldberg H I, Moss A A, Harter L P
CT demonstration and guided aspiration of unusual adrenal metastases
J Comput Assist Tomogr 1983 Feb, Vol. 7 (1), P. 98–101

2196. Haertel M, Probst P, Bollmann J, Zingg E, Fuchs W A
Computertomographische Nebennierendiagnostik
Computer tomography in the investigation of the suprarenal gland
RÖFO 1980 Jan, Vol. 132 (1), P. 31–6

2197. Halvorsen R A Jr, Heaston D K, Johnston W W, Ashton P R, Burton G M
Case report. CT guided thin needle aspiration of adrenal blastomycosis
J Comput Assist Tomogr 1982 Apr, Vol. 6 (2), P. 389–91

2198. Hauser H, Gurret J P
Miliary tuberculosis associated with adrenal enlargement: CT appearance
J Comput Assist Tomogr 1986 Mar-Apr, Vol. 10 (2), P. 254–6

2199. Heiberg E, Wolverson M K
Ipsilateral decubitus position for percutaneous CT-guided adrenal biopsy
J Comput Assist Tomogr 1985 Jan-Feb, Vol. 9 (1), P. 217–8

2200. Heuck F, Buck J, Reiser U
Die gesunde und kranke Nebenniere im Röntgen-Computer-Tomogramm
Computer assisted tomography of the normal and abnormal adrenal gland
Radiologe 1980 Apr, Vol. 20 (4), P. 158–71

2201. Hubener K H, Grehn S, Schulze K
Indikationen zur computertomographischen Nebennierenuntersuchung; Leistungsfähigkeit, Stellenwert und Differentialdiagnostik
Indications for the computer tomographic investigation of the suprarenal gland
RÖFO 1980 Jan, Vol. 132 (1), P. 37–44

2202. Huebener K H, Treugut H
Adrenal cortex dysfunction: CT findings
Radiology 1984 Jan, Vol. 150 (1), P. 195–9

2203. Hussain S, Belldegrun A, Seltzer S E, Richie J P, Gittes R F, Abrams H L
Differentiation of malignant from benign adrenal masses: predictive indices on computed tomography
Am J Roentgenol 1985 Jan, Vol. 144 (1), P. 61–5

2204. Jafri S Z, Francis I R, Glazer G M, Bree R L, Amendola M A
CT detection of adrenal lymphoma
J Comput Assist Tomogr 1983 Apr, Vol. 7 (2), P. 254–6

2205. Johnson C D, Baker M E, Dunnick N R
CT demonstration of an adrenal pseudocyst
J Comput Assist Tomogr 1985 Jul-Aug, Vol. 9 (4), P. 817–9

2206. Kaiser R
Bilaterales malignes Phäochromozytom mit Metastasen. Diagnostische Wertigkeit der Computertomographie
Bilateral malignant pheochromocytoma with metastases. Diagnostic value of computed tomography
RÖFO 1987 Oct, Vol. 147 (4), P. 461–2

2207. Karstaedt N, Sagel S S, Stanley R J, Melson G L, Levitt R G
Computed tomography of the adrenal gland
Radiology 1978 Dec, Vol. 129 (3), P. 723–30

2208. Kenney P J, Robbins G L, Ellis D A, Spirt B A
Adrenal glands in patients with congenital renal anomalies: CT appearance
Radiology 1985 Apr, Vol. 155 (1), P. 181–2

2209. Kimmig B, Bihl H, Adolph J, zum Winkel K
Computertomographie und Szintigraphie beim malignen Phäochromozytom
Computed tomography and scintigraphy in malignant pheochromocytoma
RÖFO 1984 Aug, Vol. 141 (2), P. 144–8

2210. Korobkin M, White E A, Kressel H Y, Moss A A, Montagne J P
Computed tomography in the diagnosis of adrenal disease
Am J Roentgenol 1979 Feb, Vol. 132 (2), P. 231–8

2211. Krestin G P, Freidmann G, Fishbach R, Neufang K F, Allolio B
Evaluation of adrenal masses in oncologic patients: dynamic contrast-enhanced MR vs CT
J Comput Assist Tomogr 1991 Jan-Feb, Vol. 15 (1), P. 104–10

2212. Laursen K, Damgaard Pedersen K
CT for pheochromocytoma diagnosis
Am J Roentgenol 1980 Feb, Vol. 134 (2), P. 277–80

2213. Liebman R, Srikantaswamy S
Adrenal myelolipoma demonstrated by computed tomography
J Comput Assist Tomogr 1981 Apr, Vol. 5 (2), P. 262–3

2214. Ling D, Korobkin M, Silverman P M, Dunnick N R
CT demonstration of bilateral adrenal hemorrhage
Am J Roentgenol 1983 Aug, Vol. 141 (2), P. 307–8

2215. Luning M, Hoppe E, Schopke W
Ergebnisse der Diagnostik von Nebennierenraumforderungen durch perkutane CT-gestützte Feinnadelbiopsien
Results of the diagnosis of adrenal masses using percutaneous CT-guided fine needle biopsy
RÖFO 1986 Feb, Vol. 144 (2), P. 154–9

2216. McMillan J H, Levine E, Stephens R H
Computed tomography in the evaluation of metastatic adenocarcinoma from an unknown primary site. A retrospective study
Radiology 1982 Apr, Vol. 143 (1), P. 143–6

2217. Mitnick J S, Bosniak M A, Megibow A J, Naidich D P
Non-functioning adrenal adenomas discovered incidentally on computed tomography
Radiology 1983 Aug, Vol. 148 (2), P. 495–9

2218. Mitty H A, Cohen B A, Sprayregen S, Schwartz K
Adrenal pseudotumors on CT due to dilated portosystemic veins
Am J Roentgenol 1983 Oct, Vol. 141 (4), P. 727–30

2219. Miyake H, Maeda H, Tashiro M, Suzuki K, Nagatomo H, Aikawa H, Ashizawa A, Iechika S, Moriuchi A
CT of adrenal tumors: frequency and clinical significance of low-attenuation lesions
Am J Roentgenol 1989 May, Vol. 152 (5), P. 1005–7

2220. Musante F, Derchi L E, Zappasodi F, Bazzocchi M, Riviezzo G C, Banderali A, Cicio G R
Myelolipoma of the adrenal gland: sonographic and CT features
Am J Roentgenol 1988 Nov, Vol. 151 (5), P. 961–4

2221. Neumann G, Mödder U, Friedmann G
Morphologie atypischer und metastasierender Phäochromozytome in der Computertomographie
Morphology of atypical and metastatic pheochromocytoma in computed tomography
Radiologe 1984 Dec, Vol. 24 (12), P. 568–72

2222. Nicolas V, Eichler H, Franken T
Die Bedeutung der Computertomographie bei der Diagnose und Differentialdiagnose primärer Nebennierentumoren
Importance of computed tomography in the diagnosis and differential diagnosis of primary adrenal tumors
RÖFO 1985 Oct, Vol. 143 (4), P. 437–43

2223. O Brien W M, Choyke P L, Copeland J, Klappenbach R S, Lynch J H
Computed tomography of adrenal abscess
J Comput Assist Tomogr 1987 May-Jun, Vol. 11 (3), P. 550–1

2224. Pillari G, Mandon V, Cruz V, Chen M
Foot vein contrast medium infusion useful in computed tomography of right adrenal gland
J Comput Assist Tomogr 1982 Feb, Vol. 6 (1), P. 169–71

2225. Pojunas K W, Daniels D L, Williams A L, Thorsen M K, Haughton V M
Pituitary and adrenal CT of Cushing syndrome
Am J Roentgenol 1986 Jun, Vol. 146 (6), P. 1235–8

2226. Quint L E, Glazer G M, Francis I R, Shapiro B, Chenevert T L
Pheochromocytoma and paraganglioma: comparison of MR imaging with CT and I-131 MIBG scintigraphy
Radiology 1987 Oct, Vol. 165 (1), P. 89–93

2227. Radin D R, Rosenstein H, Boswell W D, Ralls P W, Lundell C, Halls J M
Computed tomography of Sipple syndrome
J Comput Assist Tomogr 1984 Feb, Vol. 8 (1), P. 169–70

2228. Radin D R, Ralls P W, Boswell W D Jr, Colletti P M, Lapin S A, Halls J M
Pheochromocytoma: detection by unenhanced CT
Am J Roentgenol 1986 Apr, Vol. 146 (4), P. 741–4

2229. Rzymski K, Sobieszczyk S, Kosowicz J
Computed tomography of the adrenal glands in Addison's disease
RÖFO 1984 Jan, Vol. 140 (1), P. 48–9

2230. Schwartz J M, Bosniak M A, Megibow A J, Hulnick D H
Right adrenal pseudotumor by colon: CT demonstration
J Comput Assist Tomogr 1988 Jan-Feb, Vol. 12 (1), P. 153–4

2231. Scotti G, Scialfa G, Pieralli S, Chiodini P G, Spelta B, Dallabonzana D
Macroprolactinomas: CT evaluation of reduction of tumor size after medical treatment
Neuroradiology 1982, Vol. 23 (3), P. 123–6

2232. Shah H R, Love L, Williamson M R, Buckner B C, Ferris E J
Hemorrhagic adrenal metastases: CT findings
J Comput Assist Tomogr 1989 Jan-Feb, Vol. 13 (1), P. 77–81

2233. Solomon N, Sumkin J
Right adrenal gland hemorrhage as a complication of liver transplantation: CT appearance
J Comput Assist Tomogr 1988 Jan-Feb, Vol. 12 (1), P. 95–7

2234. Tisnado J, Amendola M A, Konerding K F, Shirazi K K, Beachley M C
Computed tomography versus angiography in the localization of pheochromocytoma
J Comput Assist Tomogr 1980 Dec, Vol. 4 (6), P. 853–9

2235. Vlahos L, Strigaris K, Aliferopoulos D, Pontifex G
Cushing's syndrome with an apparently normal CT scan
Radiologe 1981 Aug, Vol. 21 (8), P. 396–7

2236. Welch T J, Sheedy P F, van Heerden J A, Sheps S G, Hattery R R, Stephens D H
Pheochromocytoma: value of computed tomography
Radiology 1983 Aug, Vol. 148 (2), P. 501–3

2237. Whaley D, Becker S, Presbrey T, Shaff M
Adrenal myelolipoma associated with Conn syndrome: CT evaluation
J Comput Assist Tomogr 1985 Sep-Oct, Vol. 9 (5), P. 959–60

2238. Wilms G, Marchal G, Baert A, Adisoejoso B, Mangkuwerdojo S
CT and ultrasound features of post-traumatic adrenal hemorrhage
J Comput Assist Tomogr 1987 Jan-Feb, Vol. 11 (1), P. 112–5

2239. Wilson D A, Muchmore H G, Tisdal R G, Fahmy A, Pitha J V
Histoplasmosis of the adrenal glands studied by CT
Radiology 1984 Mar, Vol. 150 (3), P. 779–83

The Urinary Bladder

2240. Aisen A M, Gross B H, Glazer G M
Computed tomography of ureterovesical schistosomiasis
J Comput Assist Tomogr 1983 Feb, Vol. 7 (1), P. 161–3

2241. Amendola M A, Glazer G M, Grossman H B, Aisen A M, Francis I R
Staging of bladder carcinoma: MRI-CT-surgical correlation
Am J Roentgenol 1986 Jun, Vol. 146 (6), P. 1179–83

2242. Apter S, Rubinstein Z J, Hertz M
CT demonstration of urinary bladder displacement causing medial deviation of the distal ureter
J Comput Assist Tomogr 1984 Apr, Vol. 8 (2), P. 294–5

2243. Baum M L, Baum R D, Plaine L, Bosniak M A
Computed tomography in the diagnosis of fistula between the ureter and iliac artery
J Comput Assist Tomogr 1987 Jul-Aug, Vol. 11 (4), P. 719–21

2244. Bidwell J K, Dunne M G
Computed tomography of bladder malakoplakia
J Comput Assist Tomogr 1987 Sep-Oct, Vol. 11 (5), P. 909–10

2245. Brant W E, Williams J L
Computed tomography of bladder leiomyoma
J Comput Assist Tomogr 1984 Jun, Vol. 8 (3), P. 562–3

2246. Bryan P J, Butler H E, LiPuma J P, Resnick M I, Kursh E D
CT and MR imaging in staging bladder neoplasms
J Comput Assist Tomogr 1987 Jan-Feb, Vol. 11 (1), P. 96–101

2247. Burgener F A, Hamlin D J
Intravenous contrast enhancement in computed tomography of pelvic malignancies
RÖFO 1981 Jun, Vol. 134 (6), P. 656–61

2248. Chen H H, Panella J S, Rochester D, Ignatoff J M, McVary K T
Non-Hodgkin lymphoma of ureteral wall: CT findings
J Comput Assist Tomogr 1988 Jan-Feb, Vol. 12 (1), P. 157–8

2249. Crone Munzebrock W, Brockmann W P, Brassow F, Meyer W H
Computertomographie und Sonographie bei Uretertumoren
Computerized tomography and sonography in ureter tumors
RÖFO 1983 Jan, Vol. 138 (1), P. 19–21

2250. Duvoisin B, Fournier D
Inverted layering of contrast material and urine in the bladder on CT: sonographic correlation
letter
Am J Roentgenol 1990 Nov, Vol. 155 (5), P. 1139

2251. Epstein B M, Patel V, Porteous P H
CT appearance of bladder malakoplakia
J Comput Assist Tomogr 1983 Jun, Vol. 7 (3), P. 541–3

2252. Federle M P, McAninch J W, Kaiser J A, Goodman P C, Roberts J, Mall J C
Computed tomography of urinary calculi
Am J Roentgenol 1981 Feb, Vol. 136 (2), P. 255–8

2253. Frennby B, Aspelin P, Uden P, Nyman U
Computed tomography of malignant pheochromocytoma of the bladder. A case report
RÖFO 1990 Aug, Vol. 153 (2), P. 225–7

2254. Goff W B
Cystitis cystica and cystitis glandularis: cause of bladder mass
J Comput Assist Tomogr 1983 Apr, Vol. 7 (2), P. 347–9

2255. Greiner K G, Jacob F, Klose K C, Schwartz R
Sicherung der T-Klassifikation von Harnblasentumoren durch transkutane Sonographie, intra-vesikale Sonographie und Computertomographie
Confirmation of the T classification of bladder tumors by transcutaneous sonography, intra-vesical sonography and computer tomography
RÖFO 1983 Nov, Vol. 139 (5), P. 510–5

2256. Hamlin D J, Cockett A T, Burgener F A
Computed tomography of the pelvis: sagittal and coronal image reconstruction in the evaluation of infiltrative bladder carcinoma
J Comput Assist Tomogr 1981 Feb, Vol. 5 (1), P. 27–33

2257. Hattori N, Fujikawa J, Kubo K, Saga T, Nagata Y, Kohno S, Tanabe M
CT diagnosis of periureteric venous ring
J Comput Assist Tomogr 1986 Nov-Dec, Vol. 10 (6), P. 1078–9

2258. Healy M E, Teng S S, Moss A A
Uriniferous pseudocyst: computed tomographic findings
Radiology 1984 Dec, Vol. 153 (3), P. 757–62

2259. Hidalgo H, Dunnick N R, Rosenberg E R, Ram P C, Korobkin M
Parapelvic cysts: appearance on CT and sonography
Am J Roentgenol 1982 Apr, Vol. 138 (4), P. 667–71

2260. Husband J E, Olliff J F, Williams M P, Heron C W, Cherryman G R
Bladder cancer: staging with CT and MR imaging
Radiology 1989 Nov, Vol. 173 (2), P. 435–40

2261. Jaffe J, Friedman A C, Seidmon E J, Radecki P D, Lev Toaff A S, Caroline D F
Diagnosis of ureteral stump transitional cell carcinoma by CT and MR imaging
Am J Roentgenol 1987 Oct, Vol. 149 (4), P. 741–2

2262. Jeffrey R B, Palubinskas A J, Federle M P
CT evaluation of invasive lesions of the bladder
J Comput Assist Tomogr 1981 Feb, Vol. 5 (1), P. 22–6

2263. Kalovidouris A, Pissiotis C, Pontifex G, Gouliamos A, Pentea S, Papavassiliou C
CT characterization of multivesicular hydatid cysts
J Comput Assist Tomogr 1986 May-Jun, Vol. 10 (3), P. 428–31

2264. Kane N M, Francis I R, Ellis J H
The value of CT in the detection of bladder and posterior urethral injuries
Am J Roentgenol 1989 Dec, Vol. 153 (6), P. 1243–6

2265. Kelvin F M, Korobkin M, Heaston D K, Grant J P, Akwari O
The pelvis after surgery for rectal carcinoma: serial CT observations with emphasis on nonneoplastic features
Am J Roentgenol 1983 Nov, Vol. 141 (5), P. 959–64

2266. Kenney P J, Panicek D M, Witanowski L S
Computed tomography of ureteral disruption
J Comput Assist Tomogr 1987 May-Jun, Vol. 11 (3), P. 480–4

2267. Kenney P J, Stanley R J
Computed tomography of ureteral tumors
J Comput Assist Tomogr 1987 Jan-Feb, Vol. 11 (1), P. 102–7

2268. Korobkin M, Cambier L, Drake J
Computed tomography of urachal carcinoma
J Comput Assist Tomogr 1988 Nov-Dec, Vol. 12 (6), P. 981–7

2269. Kossol J M, Patel S K
Suburothelial hemorrhage: the value of preinfusion computed tomography
J Comput Assist Tomogr 1986 Jan-Feb, Vol. 10 (1), P. 157–8

2270. Kwok Liu J P, Zikman J M, Cockshott W P
Carcinoma of the urachus: the role of computed tomography
Radiology 1980 Dec, Vol. 137 (3), P. 731–4

2271. Lautin E M, Becker R D, Fromowitz F B, Bezahler G H
Computed tomography of the lower urinary tract in schistosomiasis
J Comput Assist Tomogr 1983 Feb, Vol. 7 (1), P. 164–5

2272. Lautin E M, Haramati N, Frager D, Friedman A C, Gold K, Kurtz A, Self J
CT diagnosis of circumcaval ureter
Am J Roentgenol 1988 Mar, Vol. 150 (3), P. 591–4

2273. Lee S H, Kitchens H H, Kim B S
Adenocarcinoma of the urachus: CT features
J Comput Assist Tomogr 1990 Mar-Apr, Vol. 14 (2), P. 232–5

2274. Lis L E, Cohen A J
CT cystography in the evaluation of bladder trauma
J Comput Assist Tomogr 1990 May-Jun, Vol. 14 (3), P. 386–9

2275. Lorenz R, Beyer D, Allhoff E, Mödder U
Möglichkeiten und Grenzen der computertomographischen Stadieneinteilung beim Blasenkarzinom
Possibilities and limitations of computed tomographic staging of bladder carcinoma
RÖFO 1984 Jun, Vol. 140 (6), P. 660–5

2276. Lutgemeier J, Wunschik F, Horst M
Die Rolle der Computertomographie beim Staging von Harnblasenkarzinomen
The role of computer tomography in staging of carcinomas of the bladder
RÖFO 1981 Jun, Vol. 134 (6), P. 661–5

2277. McMillin K I, Gross B H
CT demonstration of peripelvic and periureteral non-Hodgkin lymphoma
Am J Roentgenol 1985 May, Vol. 144 (5), P. 945–6

2278. Merine D, Fishman E K, Kuhlman J E, Jones B, Bayless T M, Siegelman S
Bladder involvement in Crohn disease: role of CT in detection and evaluation
J Comput Assist Tomogr 1989 Jan-Feb, Vol. 13 (1), P. 90–3

2279. Mieza M, Rotstein J M, Geffen A
CT demonstration of periureteral fibrosis of malignant etiology
J Comput Assist Tomogr 1982 Apr, Vol. 6 (2), P. 290–3

2280. Mitty H A
CT for diagnosis and management of urinary extravasation
Am J Roentgenol 1980 Mar, Vol. 134 (3), P. 497–501

2281. Narumi Y, Sato T, Kuriyama K, Fujita M, Saiki S, Kuroda M, Miki T, Kotake T
Vesical dome tumors: significance of extravesical extension on CT
Radiology 1988 Nov, Vol. 169 (2), P. 383–5

2282. Narumi Y, Sato T, Hori S, Kuriyama K, Fujita M, Kadowaki K, Inoue E, Maeshima S, Fujino Y, Saiki S, et al
Squamous cell carcinoma of the uroepithelium: CT evaluation
Radiology 1989 Dec, Vol. 173 (3), P. 853–6

2283. Newhouse J H, Prien E L, Amis E S Jr, Dretler S P, Pfister R C
Computed tomographic analysis of urinary calculi
Am J Roentgenol 1984 Mar, Vol. 142 (3), P. 545–8

2284. Ney C, Kumar M, Billah K, Doerr J
CT demonstration of cystitis emphysematosa
J Comput Assist Tomogr 1987 May-Jun, Vol. 11 (3), P. 552–3

2285. Nicolas V, Spielmann R, Maas R, Bressel M, Wagner B, Porst H, Bucheler E
Diagnostische Aussagekraft der MR-Tomographie nach Gadolinium-DTPA im Vergleich zur Computertomographie bei Harnblasentumoren
The diagnostic value of MR tomography following gadolinium-DTPA compared to computed tomography in bladder tumors
RÖFO 1990 Aug, Vol. 153 (2), P. 197–203

2286. Noto A M, Ragosin R J, Beltran J
CT demonstration of a ureteroinguinal hernia causing hydronephrosis
J Comput Assist Tomogr 1985 Jul-Aug, Vol. 9 (4), P. 832–3

2287. Oliva L, Cariati M, Reggiani L, Romanzi F
CT evaluation of the pelvic cavity after cystectomy: observation in 40 cases
J Comput Assist Tomogr 1984 Aug, Vol. 8 (4), P. 734–8

2288. Pillari G
Computed tomographic cavo-urography: lower-extremity contrast infusion simultaneous with computed tomography of the retroperitoneum
Radiology 1979 Mar, Vol. 130 (3), P. 797

2289. Premkumar A, Lattimer J, Newhouse J H
CT and sonography of advanced urinary tract tuberculosis
Am J Roentgenol 1987 Jan, Vol. 148 (1), P. 65–9

2290. Ryan K G, Hoch W H, Craven R M
Intraureteral tumor demonstrated by computed tomography
J Comput Assist Tomogr 1979 Aug, Vol. 3 (4), P. 474–7

2291. Sager E M, Talle K, Fossa S, Ous S, Stenwig A E
The role of CT in demonstrating perivesical tumor growth in the preoperative staging of carcinoma of the urinary bladder
Radiology 1983 Feb, Vol. 146 (2), P. 443–6

2292. Sarno R C, Klauber G, Carter B L
Computer assisted tomography of urachal abnormalities
J Comput Assist Tomogr 1983 Aug, Vol. 7 (4), P. 674–6

2293. Sasai K, Sano A, Imanaka K, Nishizawa S, Nagae T, Mizutani M, Sadatoh N, Hatabu H, Kuroda Y
Right periureteric venous ring detected by computed tomography
J Comput Assist Tomogr 1986 Mar-Apr, Vol. 10 (2), P. 349–51

2294. Savit R M, Udis D S
"Upside-down" contrast-urine level in glycosuria: CT features
J Comput Assist Tomogr 1987 Sep-Oct, Vol. 11 (5), P. 911–2

2295. Schnyder P, Candardjis G
Vesicourachal diverticulum: CT diagnosis in two adults
Am J Roentgenol 1981 Nov, Vol. 137 (5), P. 1063–5

2296. Thickman D, Mintz M, Arger P, Coleman B
CT imaging of the unusually shaped bladder
J Comput Assist Tomogr 1984 Aug, Vol. 8 (4), P. 801–3

2297. Zingas A P, Kling G A, Crotte E, Shumaker E, Vazquez P M
Computed tomography of nephrogenic adenoma of the urinary bladder
J Comput Assist Tomogr 1986 Nov-Dec, Vol. 10 (6), P. 979–82

The Prostate and Seminal Vesicles

2298. Baker M E, Silverman P M, Korobkin M
Computed tomography of prostatic and bladder rhabdomyosarcomas
J Comput Assist Tomogr 1985 Jul-Aug, Vol. 9 (4), P. 780-3

2299. Bland P H, DiPietro M A, Chenevert T L, Hutchinson R J, Carson P L
Tissue characterization of the testes using ultrasonic CT. Work in progress
Radiology 1986 Apr, Vol. 159 (1), P. 101-5

2300. Burkhalter J L, Morano J U
Partial priapism: the role of CT in its diagnosis
Radiology 1985 Jul, Vol. 156 (1), P. 159

2301. Burney B T, Klatte E C
Ultrasound and computed tomography of the abdomen in the staging and management of testicular carcinoma
Radiology 1979 Aug, Vol. 132 (2), P. 415-9

2302. Cordes M, Tunn U W, Neidl K, Haasner E
Prostatakarzinom. Stadieneinteilung durch transrektale Prostatasonographie und Computertomographie mit histopathologischer Korrelation
Prostatic cancer. Staging via transrectal prostatic sonography and computed tomography with histopathological correlation
RÖFO 1987 Apr, Vol. 146 (4), P. 412-4

2303. Dennis M A, Donohue R E
Computed tomography of prostatic abscess
J Comput Assist Tomogr 1985 Jan-Feb, Vol. 9 (1), P. 201-2

2304. Derouet H, Braedel H U, Ziegler M, Zwergel T, Khorsandian C
Computertomographische Untersuchungen des Scrotalinhaltes, insbesondere des Hodens
Computed tomographic studies of the scrotal contents, particularly the testis
RÖFO 1988 May, Vol. 148 (5), P. 566-71

2305. Emory T H, Reinke D B, Hill A L, Lange P H
Use of CT to reduce understaging in prostatic cancer: comparison with conventional staging techniques
Am J Roentgenol 1983 Aug, Vol. 141 (2), P. 351-4

2306. Freedy R M, Miller K D Jr
Small-cell carcinoma of the prostate: metastases to the brain as shown by CT and MR with pathologic correlation
AJNR 1990 Sep-Oct, Vol. 11 (5), P. 947-8

2307. Gore R M, Moss A A
Value of computed tomography in interstitial 125I brachytherapy of prostatic carcinoma
Radiology 1983 Feb, Vol. 146 (2), P. 453-8

2308. Hales E D, Rosser S B
Computed tomography of testicular feminization
J Comput Assist Tomogr 1984 Aug, Vol. 8 (4), P. 772-3

2309. Hricak H, Dooms G C, Jeffrey R B, Avallone A, Jacobs D, Benton W K, Narayan P, Tanagho E A
Prostatic carcinoma: staging by clinical assessment, CT, and MR imaging
Radiology 1987 Feb, Vol. 162 (2), P. 331-6

2310. Husband J E, Hawkes D J, Peckham M J
CT estimations of mean attenuation values and volume in testicular tumors: a comparison with surgical and histologic findings
Radiology 1982 Aug, Vol. 144 (3), P. 553-8

2311. Husband J E, Bellamy E A
Unusual thoracoabdominal sites of metastases in testicular tumors
Am J Roentgenol 1985 Dec, Vol. 145 (6), P. 1165-71

2312. Kneeland J B, Auh Y H, McCarron J P, Zirinsky K, Rubenstein W A, Kazam E
Computed tomography, sonography, vesiculography, and MR imaging of a seminal vesicle cyst
J Comput Assist Tomogr 1985 Sep-Oct, Vol. 9 (5), P. 964-6

2313. Kullmann G, Lien H H
Intraabdominal hematoma following orchiectomy: a potential pitfall in using CT for staging of testicular cancer
Radiology 1987 Apr, Vol. 163 (1), P. 129-30

2314. Lee J K, McClennan B L, Stanley R J, Sagel S S
Computed tomography in the staging of testicular neoplasms
Radiology 1979 Feb, Vol. 130 (2), P. 387-90

2315. Levine M S, Arger P H, Coleman B G, Mulhern C B Jr, Pollack H M, Wein A J
Detecting lymphatic metastases from prostatic carcinoma: superiority of CT
Am J Roentgenol 1981 Aug, Vol. 137 (2), P. 207-11

2316. Lutgemeier J, Wunschik F, Horst M
Computertomographisches Staging des Prostatakarzinoms
Computer tomographic staging of prostatic carcinomas
RÖFO 1981 May, Vol. 134 (5), P. 503-6

2317. Parienty R A, Vallancien G, Pradel J, Veillon B
CT features of perirectal fascia thickening after transurethral resection of prostatic adenoma
J Comput Assist Tomogr 1987 Jan- Feb, Vol. 11 (1), P. 92-5

2318. Patel P S, Wilbur A C
Cystic seminal vesiculitis: CT demonstration
J Comput Assist Tomogr 1987 Nov-Dec, Vol. 11 (6), P. 1103-4

2319. Platt J F, Bree R L, Schwab R E
The accuracy of CT in the staging of carcinoma of the prostate
Am J Roentgenol 1987 Aug, Vol. 149 (2), P. 315-8

2320. Poskitt K J, Cooperberg P L, Sullivan L D
Sonography and CT in staging nonseminomatous testicular tumors
Am J Roentgenol 1985 May, Vol. 144 (5), P. 939-44

2321. Premkumar A, Newhouse J H
Seminal vesicle tuberculosis: CT appearance
J Comput Assist Tomogr 1988 Jul-Aug, Vol. 12 (4), P. 676-7

2322. Rebner M, Gross B H, Korobkin M, Ruiz J
CT appearance of right gonadal vein
J Comput Assist Tomogr 1989 May-Jun, Vol. 13 (3), P. 460-2

2323. Scatarige J C, Fishman E K, Kuhajda F P, Taylor G A, Siegelman S S
Low attenuation nodal metastases in testicular carcinoma
J Comput Assist Tomogr 1983 Aug, Vol. 7 (4), P. 682-7

2324. Schwartz J M, Bosniak M A, Hulnick D H, Megibow A J, Raghavendra B N
Computed tomography of midline cysts of the prostate
J Comput Assist Tomogr 1988 Mar-Apr, Vol. 12 (2), P. 215- 8

2325. Soo C S, Bernardino M E, Chuang V P, Ordonez N
Pitfalls of CT findings in post-therapy testicular carcinoma
J Comput Assist Tomogr 1981 Feb, Vol. 5 (1), P. 39-41

2326. Stomper P C, Fung C Y, Socinski M A, Jochelson M S, Garnick M B, Richie J P
Detection of retroperitoneal metastases in early-stage nonseminomatous testicular cancer: analysis of different CT criteria
Am J Roentgenol 1987 Dec, Vol. 149 (6), P. 1187-90

2327. Sukov R J, Scardino P T, Sample W F, Winter J, Confer D J
Computed tomography and transabdominal ultrasound in the evaluation of the prostate
J Comput Assist Tomogr 1977 Jul, Vol. 1 (3), P. 281-9

2328. Sussman S K, Dunnick N R, Silverman P M, Cohan R H
Carcinoma of the seminal vesicle: CT appearance
J Comput Assist Tomogr 1986 May-Jun, Vol. 10 (3), P. 519-20

2329. Thomas J L, Bernardino M E, Bracken R B
Staging of testicular carcinoma: comparison of CT and lymphangiography
Am J Roentgenol 1981 Nov, Vol. 137 (5), P. 991-6

2330. Thornhill B A, Morehouse H T, Coleman P, Hoffman Tretin J C
Prostatic abscess: CT and sonographic findings
Am J Roentgenol 1987 May, Vol. 148 (5), P. 899-900

2331. Triller J, Fuchs W A
Die computertomographische Stadieneinteilung beim Prostatakarzinom
Computed tomographic staging of prostatic cancer
RÖFO 1982 Dec, Vol. 137 (6), P. 669-74

2332. Triller J, Fuchs W A, Helzel M V
Die computertomographische Stadieneinteilung beim Prostatakarzinom
Computer tomographic staging of prostatic cancers
RÖFO 1983 Dec, Vol. 139 (6), P. 691-2

2333. Van Engelshoven J M, Kreel L
Computed tomography of the prostate
J Comput Assist Tomogr 1979 Feb, Vol. 3 (1), P. 45-51

2334. Wilbur A C, Mostowfi K, Heydemann J, Daza R C
Infarcted undescended testis appearing as a calcified abdominal mass in an adult
Am J Roentgenol 1990 Sep, Vol. 155 (3), P. 547-8

2335. Wolverson M K, Jagannadharao B, Sundaram M, Riaz M A, Nalesnik W J, Houttuin E
CT in localization of impalpable cryptorchid testes
Am J Roentgenol 1980 Apr, Vol. 134 (4), P. 725-9

2336. Wolverson M K, Houttuin E, Heiberg E, Sundaram M, Shields J B
Comparison of computed tomography with high-resolution real- time ultrasound in the localization of the impalpable undescended testis
Radiology 1983 Jan, Vol. 146 (1), P. 133-6

2337. Zagoria R J, Papanicolaou N, Pfister R C, Stafford S A, Young H H
Seminal vesicle abscess after vasectomy: evaluation by transrectal sonography and CT
Am J Roentgenol 1987 Jul, Vol. 149 (1), P. 137-8

2338. Zwanger Mendelsohn S, Shreck E H, Doshi V
Burkitt lymphoma involving the epididymis and spermatic cord: sonographic and CT findings
Am J Roentgenol 1989 Jul, Vol. 153 (1), P. 85-6

The Female Genital Organs

2339. Amendola M A, Walsh J W, Amendola B E, Tisnado J, Hall D J, Goplerud D R
Computed tomography in the evaluation of carcinoma of the ovary
J Comput Assist Tomogr 1981 Apr, Vol. 5 (2), P. 179-86

2340. Balfe D M, Van Dyke J, Lee J K, Weyman P J, McClennan B L
Computed tomography in malignant endometrial neoplasms
J Comput Assist Tomogr 1983 Aug, Vol. 7 (4), P. 677-81

2341. Barzen G, Cordes M, Langer M, Friedman W, Mayr A C, Felix R
Wertigkeit der Radioimmunszintigraphie im Vergleich zur Computertomographie in der Diagnostik und Verlaufskontrolle des primären Ovarialkarzinoms
Value of radioimmunoscintigraphy compared to computed tomography in the diagnosis and follow-up of primary ovarian carcinoma
RÖFO 1990 Jul, Vol. 153 (1), P. 85-91

2342. Bellah R D, Griscom N T
Torsion of normal uterine adnexa before menarche: CT appearance
Am J Roentgenol 1989 Jan, Vol. 152 (1), P. 123-4

2343. Bernardy M O, Umer M A, Flanigan R C
Computed tomography of hydrocele of the tunica vaginalis
J Comput Assist Tomogr 1985 Jan-Feb, Vol. 9 (1), P. 203-4

2344. Bierman S M, Reuter K L, Hunter R E
Meigs syndrome and ovarian fibroma: CT findings
J Comput Assist Tomogr 1990 Sep-Oct, Vol. 14 (5), P. 833-4

2345. Buy J N, Moss A A, Ghossain M A, Sciot C, Malbec L, Vadrot D, Paniel B J, Decroix Y
Peritoneal implants from ovarian tumors: CT findings
Radiology 1988 Dec, Vol. 169 (3), P. 691-4

2346. Buy J N, Ghossain M A, Moss A A, Bazot M, Doucet M, Hugol D, Truc J B, Poitout P, Ecoiffier J
Cystic teratoma of the ovary: CT detection
Radiology 1989 Jun, Vol. 171 (3), P. 697-701

2347. Casillas J, Joseph R C, Guerra J J
CT appearance of uterine leiomyomas
Radiographics 1990 , Vol.10 ,P. 999-1007

2348. Cho K C, Gold B M
Computed tomography of Krukenberg tumors
Am J Roentgenol 1985 Aug, Vol. 145 (2), P. 285-8

2349. Davis M C, Fishman E K, Cameron J L, Magid D, Siegelman S S
Computed tomography of vaginal cuff cyst: a late complication of hysterectomy
J Comput Assist Tomogr 1986 Mar-Apr, Vol. 10 (2), P. 354-6

2350. Davis W K, McCarthy S, Moss A A, Braga C
Computed tomography of gestational trophoblastic disease
J Comput Assist Tomogr 1984 Dec, Vol. 8 (6), P. 1136-9

2351. Dolinskas C A, Simeone F A
Transsphenoidal hypophysectomy: postsurgical CT findings
Am J Roentgenol 1985 Mar, Vol. 144 (3), P. 487-92

2352. Epstein D M, Arger P H, LaRossa D, Mintz M C, Coleman B G
CT evaluation of gracilis myocutaneous vaginal reconstruction after pelvic exenteration
Am J Roentgenol 1987 Jun, Vol. 148 (6), P. 1143-6

2353. Federle M P, Cohen H A, Rosenwein M F, Brant Zawadzki M N, Cann C E
Pelvimetry by digital radiography: a low-dose examination
Radiology 1982 Jun, Vol. 143 (3), P. 733-5

2354. Feldberg M A, van Waes P F, Hendriks M J
Direct multiplanar CT findings in cystic teratoma of the ovary
J Comput Assist Tomogr 1984 Dec, Vol. 8 (6), P. 1131–5

2355. Feuerbach S, Gullotta U, Reiser M, Allgayer B, Ingianni G
Computertomographische Symptomatologie des Becken- und Bauchtraumas
Computer tomographic findings in pelvic and abdominal trauma
RÖFO 1981 Mar, Vol. 134 (3), P. 293–6

2356. Fishman E K, Scatarige J C, Saksouk F A, Rosenshein N B, Siegelman S S
Computed tomography of endometriosis
J Comput Assist Tomogr 1983 Apr, Vol. 7 (2), P. 257–64

2357. Fukuda T, Ikeuchi M, Hashimoto H, Shakudo M, Oonishi M, Saiwai S, Nakazima H, Miyamoto
T, Takashima E, Inoue Y
Computed tomography of ovarian masses
J Comput Assist Tomogr 1986 Nov-Dec, Vol. 10 (6), P. 990–6

2358. Gale M E
Hermaphroditism demonstrated by computed tomography
Am J Roentgenol 1983 Jul, Vol. 141 (1), P. 99–100

2359. Garagiola D M, Tarver R D, Gibson L, Rogers R E, Wass J L
Anatomic changes in the pelvis after uncomplicated vaginal delivery: a CT study on 14
women
Am J Roentgenol 1989 Dec, Vol. 153 (6), P. 1239–41

2360. Ginaldi S, Wallace S, Jing B S, Bernardino M E
Carcinoma of the cervix: lymphangiography and computed tomography
Am J Roentgenol 1981 Jun, Vol. 136 (6), P. 1087–91

2361. Goldman S M, Fishman E K, Rosenshein N B, Gatewood O M, Siegelman S S
Excretory urography and computed tomography in the initial evaluation of patients with cervical
cancer: are both examinations necessary?
Am J Roentgenol 1984 Nov, Vol. 143 (5), P. 991–6

2362. Gross B H, Jafri S Z, Glazer G M
Significance of intrauterine gas demonstrated by computed tomography
J Comput Assist Tomogr 1983 Oct, Vol. 7 (5), P. 842–5

2363. Gross B H, Moss A A, Mihara K, Goldberg H I, Glazer G M
Computed tomography of gynecologic diseases
Am J Roentgenol 1983 Oct, Vol. 141 (4), P. 765–73

2364. Haertel M
Zur Computertomographie gynäkologischer Karzinome
Computer tomography for gynaecological carcinomas
RÖFO 1980 Jun, Vol. 132 (6), P. 652–7

2365. Hamlin D J, Burgener F A, Beecham J B
CT of intramural endometrial carcinoma: contrast enhancement is essential
Am J Roentgenol 1981 Sep, Vol. 137 (3), P. 551–4

2366. Hamm B, Albig M, Romer T, Felix R, Wolf K J
Bildgebende Diagnostik der Ovarialtumoren. Magnetische Resonanztomographie im Vergleich
zur Computertomographie und Sonographie
Imaging diagnosis of ovarian tumors. Magnetic resonance tomography in comparison with com-
puterized tomography and sonography
RÖFO 1987 Jun, Vol. 146 (6), P. 684–8

2367. Huber D J
Die puerperale Thrombophlebitis der Ovarialvenen – Diagnose mittels CT
Puerperal thrombophlebitis of the ovarian veins – diagnosis using CT
RÖFO 1984 Jun, Vol. 140 (6), P. 665–8

2368. Jacobs J E, Markowitz S K
CT diagnosis of uterine lipoma
Am J Roentgenol 1988 Jun, Vol. 150 (6), P. 1335–6

2369. Jansen O, Gmelin E
Die Darstellung der Extrauteringravidität in der Computertomographie
Imaging of extrauterine pregnancy in computed tomography
RÖFO 1987 Dec, Vol. 147 (6), P. 681–2

2370. Jaques P F, Staab E, Richey W, Photopulos G, Swanton M
CT-assisted pelvic and abdominal aspiration biopsies in gynecological malignancy
Radiology 1978 Sep, Vol. 128 (3), P. 651–5

2371. Jaramillo D, Allan N K, Raval B
Computed tomography of vaginitis emphysematosa
J Comput Assist Tomogr 1986 May-Jun, Vol. 10 (3), P. 521–3

2372. Johnson R J, Blackledge G, Eddleston B, Crowther D
Abdomino-pelvic computed tomography in the management of ovarian carcinoma
Radiology 1983 Feb, Vol. 146 (2), P. 447–52

2373. Kiefer H, Berle P, Harding P
Computertomographische Diagnose einer Endometritis puerperalis durch gasbildende Bak-
terien
Computer tomographic diagnosis of puerperal endometritis caused by gas-forming bacteria
RÖFO 1982 Oct, Vol. 137 (4), P. 476–8

2374. Kilcheski T S, Arger P H, Mulhern C B Jr, Coleman B G, Kressel H Y, Mikuta J I
Role of computed tomography in the presurgical evaluation of carcinoma of the cervix
J Comput Assist Tomogr 1981 Jun, Vol. 5 (3), P. 378–83

2375. Kim S H, Choi B I, Lee H P, Kang S B, Choi Y M, Han M C, Kim C W
Uterine cervical carcinoma: comparison of CT and MR findings
Radiology 1990 Apr, Vol. 175 (1), P. 45–51

2376. Kopernik G, Barmeir E, Leiberman J R, Hirsch M
Intrauterine balloon catheter in the CT evaluation of pelvic masses
J Comput Assist Tomogr 1983 Oct, Vol. 7 (5), P. 928–30

2377. Koster O, Braun P, Lackner K, Leyendecker G
Computertomographie und Klinik beim Karzinom des Collum uteri
Computed tomography and the clinical picture of carcinoma of the uterine cervix
RÖFO 1984 Feb, Vol. 140 (2), P. 136–44

2378. Kronthal A J, Fishman E K, Sanders R C, Epstein J I, Kuhlman J E, Brendler C B
Uterine perforation simulating urachal carcinoma: CT diagnosis
Am J Roentgenol 1990 Apr, Vol. 154 (4), P. 741–3

2379. Kuhlman J E, Fishman E K
CT evaluation of enterovaginal and vesicovaginal fistulas
J Comput Assist Tomogr 1990 May-Jun, Vol. 14 (3), P. 390–4

2380. Lee L L, McGahan J P
Combined use of ultrasound and computed tomography in evaluation of intraabdominal
pregnancy and fetal demise
J Comput Assist Tomogr 1984 Aug, Vol. 8 (4), P. 770–1

2381. Lentini J F, Love M B, Ritchie W G, Sedlacek T V
Computed tomography in retroconversion of hepatic metastases from immature ovarian tera-
toma
J Comput Assist Tomogr 1986 Nov-Dec, Vol. 10 (6), P. 1060–2

2382. Magarik D E, Dunne M G, Weksberg A P
CT appearance of intrauterine pregnancy
J Comput Assist Tomogr 1984 Jun, Vol. 8 (3), P. 469–72

2383. Matsumoto F, Yoshioka H, Hamada T, Ishida O, Noda K
Struma ovarii: CT and MR findings
J Comput Assist Tomogr 1990 Mar-Apr, Vol. 14 (2), P. 310–2

2384. Megibow A J, Hulnick D H, Bosniak M A, Balthazar E J
Ovarian metastases: computed tomographic appearances
Radiology 1985 Jul, Vol. 156 (1), P. 161–4

2385. Megibow A J, Bosniak M A, Ho A G, Beller U, Hulnick D H, Beckman E M
Accuracy of CT in detection of persistent or recurrent ovarian carcinoma: correlation with second-
look laparotomy
Radiology 1988 Feb, Vol. 166 (2), P. 341–5

2386. Mitchell D G, Mintz M C, Spritzer C E, Gussman D, Arger P H, Coleman B G, Axel L, Kressel
H Y
Adnexal masses: MR imaging observations at 1.5 T, with US and CT correlation
Radiology 1987 Feb, Vol. 162 (2), P. 319–24

2387. Newbold R, Safrit H, Cooper C
Surgical lateral ovarian transposition: CT appearance
Am J Roentgenol 1990 Jan, Vol. 154 (1), P. 119–20

2388. Nokes S R, Martinez C R, Arrington J A, Dauito R
Significance of vaginal air on computed tomography
J Comput Assist Tomogr 1986 Nov-Dec, Vol. 10 (6), P. 997–9

2389. Outwater E, Gerzof S G
Pedunculated leiomyosarcoma of the vaginal cuff after total hysterectomy: CT features
J Comput Assist Tomogr 1989 Oct, Vol. 13 (6), P. 1095–6

2390. Pandolfo I, Blandino A, Gaeta M, Racchiusa S, Freni O
Calcified peritoneal metastases from papillary cystadenocarcinoma of the ovary: CT features
J Comput Assist Tomogr 1986 May-Jun, Vol. 10 (3), P. 545–6

2391. Pistoia F, Markowitz S K, Sussman S K
Contrast material in posterior vaginal fornix mimicking bladder rupture: CT features
J Comput Assist Tomogr 1989 Jan-Feb, Vol. 13 (1), P. 153–5

2392. Raber G, Potzschke B
Wert der Computertomographie zur Parametrienbeurteilung bei Zervixkarzinomen
Value of computerized tomography for the assessment of the parametrium in cervical cancer
RÖFO 1985 Nov, Vol. 143 (5), P. 544–9

2393. Radin D R, Ray M J, Harrison E, Petruzzo R, Mayekawa D
CT demonstration of ovarian varices
J Comput Assist Tomogr 1986 Mar- Apr, Vol. 10 (2), P. 361–2

2394. Richardson M L, Kinard R E, Watters D H
Location of intrauterine devices: evaluation by computed tomography
Radiology 1982 Mar, Vol. 142 (3), P. 690

2395. Rieth K G, Comite F, Shawker T H, Cutler G B Jr
Pituitary and ovarian abnormalities demonstrated by CT and ultrasound in children with features
of the McCune-Albright syndrome
Radiology 1984 Nov, Vol. 153 (2), P. 389–93

2396. Rohde U, Steinbrich W, Friedmann G
Computertomographie der Ovarialtumoren – Fortschritte in der Diagnostik
Computed tomography of ovarian tumours-progress in diagnosis
Radiologe 1982 Apr, Vol. 22 (4), P. 146–53

2397. Rubens D, Thornbury J R, Angel C, Stoler M H, Weiss S L, Lerner R M, Beecham J
Stage IB cervical carcinoma: comparison of clinical, MR, and pathologic staging
Am J Roentgenol 1988 Jan, Vol. 150 (1), P. 135–8

2398. Salomon C G, Patel S K
Computed tomography of chronic nonpuerperal uterine inversion
J Comput Assist Tomogr 1990 Nov- Dec, Vol. 14 (6), P. 1024–6

2399. Sanders C, Rubin E
Malignant gestational trophoblastic disease: CT findings
Am J Roentgenol 1987 Jan, Vol. 148 (1), P. 165–8

2400. Savader S J, Otero R R, Savader B L
Puerperal ovarian vein thrombosis: evaluation with CT, US, and MR imaging
Radiology 1988 Jun, Vol. 167 (3), P. 637–9

2401. Sawyer R W, Vick C W, Walsh J W, McClure P H
Computed tomography of benign ovarian masses
J Comput Assist Tomogr 1985 Jul-Aug, Vol. 9 (4), P. 784–9

2402. Shamam O M, Bennett W F, Teteris N J, Finer R M
Primary fallopian tube adenocarcinoma presenting as a hydrosalpinx: CT appearance
J Comput Assist Tomogr 1988 Jul-Aug, Vol. 12 (4), P. 674–5

2403. Sheth S, Fishman E K, Buck J L, Hamper U M, Sanders R C
The variable sonographic appearances of ovarian teratomas: correlation with CT
Am J Roentgenol 1988 Aug, Vol. 151 (2), P. 331–4

2404. Silverman P M, Osborne M, Dunnick N R, Bandy L C
CT prior to second-look operation in ovarian cancer
Am J Roentgenol 1988 Apr, Vol. 150 (4), P. 829–32

2405. Skaane P, Klott K J
Fat – fluid level in in a cystic ovarian teratoma
J Comput Assist Tomogr 1981 Aug, Vol. 5 (4), P. 577–9

2406. Skaane P, Huebener K H
Computed tomography of cystic ovarian teratomas with gravity- dependent layering
J Comput Assist Tomogr 1983 Oct, Vol. 7 (5), P. 837–41

2407. Steinbrich W, Rohde U, Friedmann G
Wert der Computertomographie für die Diagnostik der Uterustumoren und ihrer Rezidive
Importance of computed tomography for the diagnosis of tumors of the uterus and recurrent
lesions
Radiologe 1982 Apr, Vol. 22 (4), P. 154–61

2408. Tada S, Tsukioka M, Ishii C, Tanaka H, Mizunuma K
Computed tomographic features of uterine myoma
J Comput Assist Tomogr 1981 Dec, Vol. 5 (6), P. 866–9

2409. Togashi K, Nishimura K, Nakano Y, Itoh H, Torizuka K, Ozasa H, Watanabe T
Cystic pedunculated leiomyomas of the uterus with unusual CT manifestations
J Comput Assist Tomogr 1986 Jul- Aug, Vol. 10 (4), P. 642–4

2410. Togashi K, Nishimura K, Itoh K, Nakano Y, Torizuka K, Satoh S, Ohshima M
Computed tomography of hydrosalpinx following tubal ligation
J Comput Assist Tomogr 1986 Jan-Feb, Vol. 10 (1), P. 78–80

2411. Togashi K, Noma S, Ozasa H
CT and MR demonstration of nabothian cysts mimicking a cystic adnexal mass
J Comput Assist Tomogr 1987 Nov-Dec, Vol. 11 (6), P. 1091–2

2412. Triller J, Goldhirsch A
Computertomographie, primäre Laparotomie und second-look-Operation bei Ovarialkarzinom

Computed tomography, primary laparotomy and second look surgery in ovarian carcinoma
RÖFO 1984 Mar, Vol. 140 (3), P. 294–303

2413. Tschakert H, Giesen V
Wertigkeit der Sonographie und Computertomographie bei Tumoren im kleinen Becken der Frau. Prospektive vergleichende Untersuchung bei 132 operierten pelvinen Raumforderungen
Value of sonography and computerized tomography in pelvic tumors in the female. Prospective comparative study of 132 surgically treated pelvic space-occupying lesions
Radiologe 1988 Mar, Vol. 28 (3), P. 125–31

2414. Twickler D M, Setiawan A T, Harrell R S, Brown C E
CT appearance of the pelvis after cesarean section
Am J Roentgenol 1991 Mar, Vol. 156 (3), P. 523–6

2415. Tyrrel R T, Murphy F B, Bernardino M E
Tubo-ovarian abscesses: CT-guided percutaneous drainage
Radiology 1990 Apr, Vol. 175 (1), P. 87–9

2416. van Heesewijk H P, Smit F W, Heitbrink M A, Kok F P
Herniation of an ovarian cyst through the inguinal canal: diagnosis with CT letter
Am J Roentgenol 1990 Jan, Vol. 154 (1), P. 202–3

2417. Vick C W, Walsh J W, Wheelock J B, Brewer W H
CT of the normal and abnormal parametria in cervical cancer
Am J Roentgenol 1984 Sep, Vol. 143 (3), P. 597–603

2418. Walsh J W, Rosenfield A T, Jaffe C C, Schwartz P E, Simeone J, Dembner A G, Taylor K J
Prospective comparison of ultrasound and computed tomography in the evaluation of gynecologic pelvic masses
Am J Roentgenol 1978 Dec, Vol. 131 (6), P. 955–60

2419. Walsh J W, Amendola M A, Konerding K F, Tisnado J, Hazra T A
Computed tomographic detection of pelvic and inguinal lymph- node metastases from primary and recurrent pelvic malignant disease
Radiology 1980 Oct, Vol. 137 (1 Pt 1), P. 157–66

2420. Walsh J W, Amendola M A, Hall D J, Tisnado J, Goplerud D R
Recurrent carcinoma of the cervix: CT diagnosis
Am J Roentgenol 1981 Jan, Vol. 136 (1), P. 117–22

2421. Walsh J W, Goplerud D R
Prospective comparison between clinical and CT staging in primary cervical carcinoma
Am J Roentgenol 1981 Nov, Vol. 137 (5), P. 997–1003

2422. Walsh J W, Goplerud D R
Computed tomography of primary, persistent, and recurrent endometrial malignancy
Am J Roentgenol 1982 Dec, Vol. 139 (6), P. 1149–54

2423. Woerner H, Kramann B, Brill G
Diagnose postpartaler Komplikationen mittels CT und MRT
Diagnosis of postpartum complications using CT and MRT
RÖFO 1989 Aug, Vol. 151 (2), P. 158–62

2424. Zapf S, Halbsguth A, Schweden F, Klose K, Lochner B, Beck T, Friese K, Kreienberg R
Magnetresonanztomographie in der Diagnostik des Kollumkarzinoms. Computertomographische und histologische Korrelation
Magnetic resonance tomography in the diagnosis of cervix cancer. Computed tomographic and histological correlations
RÖFO 1988 Jan, Vol. 148 (1), P. 34–7

The Retroperitoneal Cavity

2425. Baert A L, Marchal G, Staelens B, Coenen Y
C. T. evaluation of renal space occupying lesions
RÖFO 1977 Apr, Vol. 126 (4), P. 285–91

2426. Baron R L, McClennan B L, Lee J K, Lawson T L
Computed tomography of transitional-cell carcinoma of the renal pelvis and ureter
Radiology 1982 Jul, Vol. 144 (1), P. 125–30

2427. Beers G J, Carter J P, Leiter B, Shapiro J H
CT detection of retroperitoneal gas associated with gas in intervertebral disks
J Comput Assist Tomogr 1984 Apr, Vol. 8 (2), P. 232–6

2428. Beyer D, Lorenz R, Mödder U, Steinbrich W
Diagnostik des extranodalen Befalls bei Non-Hodgkin-Lymphom im Abdominal- und Retroperitonealraum mit Sonographie und Computertomographie
Diagnosis of extranodal involvement of non- Hodgkin's lymphoma in the abdominal and retroperitoneal space using sonography and computed tomography
Radiologe 1985 May, Vol. 25 (5), P. 206–12

2429. Birnbaum B A, Friedman J P, Lubat E, Megibow A J, Bosniak M A
Extrarenal genitourinary tuberculosis: CT appearance of calcified pipe-stem ureter and seminal vesicle abscess
J Comput Assist Tomogr 1990 Jul-Aug, Vol. 14 (4), P. 653–5

2430. Bjorgvinsson E, Friedman A C
Notching of the ureter: CT demonstration of periureteral collaterals
J Comput Assist Tomogr 1984 Dec, Vol. 8 (6), P. 1215–6

2431. Braverman R M, Lebowitz R L
Occult ectopic ureter in girls with urinary incontinence: diagnosis by using CT
Am J Roentgenol 1991 Feb, Vol. 156 (2), P. 365–6

2432. Brick S H, Friedman A C, Pollack H M, Fishman E K, Radecki P D, Siegelbaum M H, Mitchell D G, Lev Toaff A S, Caroline D F
Urachal carcinoma: CT findings
Radiology 1988 Nov, Vol. 169 (2), P. 377–81

2433. Brun B, Laursen K, Sorensen I N, Lorentzen J E, Kristensen J K
CT in retroperitoneal fibrosis
Am J Roentgenol 1981 Sep, Vol. 137 (3), P. 535–8

2434. Callen P W, Marks W M, Filly R A
Computed tomography and ultrasonography in the evaluation of the retroperitoneum in patients with malignant ascites
J Comput Assist Tomogr 1979 Oct, Vol. 3 (5), P. 581–4

2435. Choi B I, Chi J G, Kim S H, Chang K H, Han M C
MR imaging of retroperitoneal teratoma: correlation with CT and pathology
J Comput Assist Tomogr 1989 Nov-Dec, Vol. 13 (6), P. 1083–6

2436. Cohan R H, Baker M E, Cooper C, Moore J O, Saeed M, Dunnick N R
Computed tomography of primary retroperitoneal malignancies
J Comput Assist Tomogr 1988 Sep-Oct, Vol. 12 (5), P. 804–10

2437. Dannenmaier B, von Schweinitz D
Computertomographie der retroperitonealen Lymphangiomyomatose
Computed tomography of retroperitoneal lymphangiomyomatosis
RÖFO 1988 Jan, Vol. 148 (1), P. 86–8

2438. Davidson A J, Hartman D S
Lymphangioma of the retroperitoneum: CT and sonographic characteristic
Radiology 1990 May, Vol. 175 (2), P. 507–10

2439. Degesys G E, Dunnick N R, Silverman P M, Cohan R H, Illescas F F, Castagno A
Retroperitoneal fibrosis: use of CT in distinguishing among possible causes
Am J Roentgenol 1986 Jan, Vol. 146 (1), P. 57–60

2440. Dodds W J, Foley W D, Lawson T L, Stewart E T, Taylor A
Anatomy and imaging of the lesser peritoneal sac
Am J Roentgenol 1985 Mar, Vol. 144 (3), P. 567–75

2441. Dodds W J, Darweesh R M, Lawson T L, Stewart E T, Foley W D, Kishk S M, Hollwarth M
The retroperitoneal spaces revisited
Am J Roentgenol 1986 Dec, Vol. 147 (6), P. 1155–61

2442. Dunnick N R, Javadpour N
Value of CT and lymphography: distinguishing retroperitoneal metastases from nonseminomatous testicular tumors
Am J Roentgenol 1981 Jun, Vol. 136 (6), P. 1093–9

2443. Ellis J H, Bies J R, Kopecky K K, Klatte E C, Rowland R G, Donohue J P
Comparison of NMR and CT imaging in the evaluation of metastatic retroperitoneal lymphadenopathy from testicular carcinoma
J Comput Assist Tomogr 1984 Aug, Vol. 8 (4), P. 709–19

2444. Feldberg M A, van Waes P F
Computed tomography of pseudocysts in retroperitoneal fibrosis
J Comput Assist Tomogr 1987 May-Jun, Vol. 11 (3), P. 485–7

2445. Fischedick A R, Muller R P, Kramps H, Cramer B
Computertomographie retroperitonealer Traumen
Computer tomography of retroperitoneal trauma
RÖFO 1982 Jan, Vol. 136 (1), P. 56–9

2446. Gaeta M, Volta S, Minutoli A, Bartiromo G, Pandolfo I
Fournier gangrene caused by a perforated retroperitoneal appendix: CT demonstration
Am J Roentgenol 1991 Feb, Vol. 156 (2), P. 341–2

2447. Glazer G M, Goldberg H I, Moss A A, Axel L
Computed tomographic detection of retroperitoneal adenopathy
Radiology 1982 Apr, Vol. 143 (1), P. 147–9

2448. Glynn T P Jr, Kreipke D L, Irons J M
Amyloidosis: diffuse involvement of the retroperitoneum
Radiology 1989 Mar, Vol. 170 (3 Pt 1), P. 726

2449. Greenstein S, Fishman E K, Kaufman S L, Kadir S, Siegelman S S
Castleman disease of the retroperitoneum: CT demonstration
J Comput Assist Tomogr 1986 May-Jun, Vol. 10 (3), P. 547–8

2450. Hagen B, Vowinckel M
Computertomographische Dokumentation retroperitonealer Hämatome nach translumbaler Aortographie
Computed tomographic demonstration of retroperitoneal haematoma following translumbar aortography
RÖFO 1980 Nov, Vol. 133 (5), P. 496–501

2451. Hayes W S, Davidson A J, Grimley P M, Hartman D S
Extraadrenal retroperitoneal paraganglioma: clinical, pathologic, and CT findings
Am J Roentgenol 1990 Dec, Vol. 155 (6), P. 1247–50

2452. Hopper K D, Sherman J L, Ghaed N
Aortic rupture into retroperitoneum
Am J Roentgenol 1985, Vol.145, P.435–7

2453. Hulnick D H, Chatson G P, Megibow A J, Bosniak M A, Ruoff M
Retroperitoneal fibrosis presenting as colonic dysfunction: CT diagnosis
J Comput Assist Tomogr 1988 Jan-Feb, Vol. 12 (1), P. 159–61

2454. Illescas F F, Baker M E, McCann R, Cohan R H, Silverman P M, Dunnick N R
CT evaluation of retroperitoneal hemorrhage associated with femoral arteriography
Am J Roentgenol 1986 Jun, Vol. 146 (6), P. 1289–92

2455. Inaraja L, Franquet T, Caballero P, Encabo B, Humbert P
CT findings in circumscribed upper abdominal idiopathic retroperitoneal fibrosis
J Comput Assist Tomogr 1986 Nov-Dec, Vol. 10 (6), P. 1063–4

2456. Joseph N, Vogelzang R L, Hidvegi D, Neiman H L
Computed tomography of retroperitoneal castleman disease plasma cell type with sonographic and angiographic correlation
J Comput Assist Tomogr 1985 May-Jun, Vol. 9 (3), P. 570–2

2457. Lane R H, Stephens D H, Reiman H M
Primary retroperitoneal neoplasms: CT findings in 90 cases with clinical and pathologic correlation
Am J Roentgenol 1989 Jan, Vol. 152 (1), P. 83–9

2458. Lien H H, Kolbenstvedt A, Talle K, Fossa S D, Klepp O, Ous S
Comparison of computed tomography, lymphography, and phlebography in 200 consecutive patients with regard to retroperitoneal metastases from testicular tumor
Radiology 1983 Jan, Vol. 146 (1), P. 129–32

2459. Luning M, Bock A, Wolff H, Staffa G
Retroperitonealabszeß: Komplikation nach CT-gestützter Feinnadelbiopsie
Retroperitoneal abscess: a complication following CT-guided fine needle biopsy
RÖFO 1989 Apr, Vol. 150 (4), P. 485–6

2460. Marchal G, Coenen Y, Wilms G, Baert A L
The accuracy of tc-scan in the diagnosis of retroperitoneal metastases of malignant testicular tumours
RÖFO 1978 Jun, Vol. 128 (6), P. 746–53

2461. Mendez G Jr, Isikoff M B, Hill M C
Retroperitoneal processes involving the psoas demonstrated by computed tomography
J Comput Assist Tomogr 1980 Feb, Vol. 4 (1), P. 78–82

2462. Meranze S, Coleman B, Arger P, Mintz M, Markowitz L
Retroperitoneal manifestations of sarcoidosis on computed tomography
J Comput Assist Tomogr 1985 Jan-Feb, Vol. 9 (1), P. 50-2

2463. Metzger H, Welker H, Dannert J
Die retroperitoneale Darmduplikatur in US und CT. Ein Beitrag zur Differentialdiagnose
Retroperitoneal intestinal duplication in US and CT. A contribution to its differential diagnosis
RÖFO 1987 Dec, Vol. 147 (6), P. 683–5

2464. Mulligan S A, Holley H C, Koehler R E, Koslin D B, Rubin E, Berland L L, Kenney P J
CT and MR imaging in the evaluation of retroperitoneal fibrosis
J Comput Assist Tomogr 1989 Mar-Apr, Vol. 13 (2), P. 277–81

2465. Munechika H, Honda M, Kushihashi T, Koizumi K, Gokan T
Computed tomography of retroperitoneal cystic lymphangiomas
J Comput Assist Tomogr 1987 Jan-Feb, Vol. 11 (1), P. 116–9

2466. Rauws E A, Mallens W M, Bieger R
CT scanning for the follow-up of corticosteroid treatment of primary retroperitoneal fibrosis
J Comput Assist Tomogr 1983 Feb, Vol. 7 (1), P. 113–6

2467. Stephens D H, Sheedy P F, Hattery R R, Williamson B Jr
Diagnosis and evaluation of retroperitoneal tumors by computed tomography
Am J Roentgenol 1977 Sep, Vol. 129 (3), P. 395–402

2468. Takebayashi S, Ono Y, Sakai F, Tamura S, Unayama S
Computed tomography of amyloidosis involving retroperitoneal lymph nodes mimicking lymphoma
J Comput Assist Tomogr 1984 Oct, Vol. 8 (5), P. 1025–7

2469. Van Besien R, Fishman E K, Kuhlman J E, Almarez R
Breast prosthesis simulating retroperitoneal mass: CT appearance
J Comput Assist Tomogr 1988 Sep-Oct, Vol. 12 (5), P. 901–2

2470. Weinstein B J, Lenkey J L, Williams S
Ultrasound and CT demonstration of a benign cystic teratoma arising from the retroperitoneum
Am J Roentgenol 1979 Nov, Vol. 133 (5), P. 936–8

Muscle Tissue

2471. Amendola M A, Glazer G M, Agha F P, Francis I R, Weatherbee L, Martel W
Myositis ossificans circumscripta: computed tomographic diagnosis
Radiology 1983 Dec, Vol. 149 (3), P. 775–9

2472. Ashida C, Zerhouni E A, Fishman E K
CT demonstration of prominent right hilar soft tissue collections
J Comput Assist Tomogr 1987 Jan-Feb, Vol. 11 (1), P. 57–9

2473. Augustiny N, Goebel N, Jager K, Brunner U, von Schulthess G K
Zystische Adventitiadegeneration der A. poplitea: Kernspintomographie und Computertomographie
Cystic adventitial degeneration of the popliteal artery: nuclear magnetic resonance tomography and computerized tomography
RÖFO 1988 Apr, Vol. 148 (4), P. 452–3

2474. Berger P E, Kuhn J P
Computed tomography of tumors of the musculoskeletal system in children. Clinical applications
Radiology 1978 Apr, Vol. 127 (1), P. 171–5

2475. Biondetti P R, Vannier M W, Gilula L A, Knapp R
Wrist: coronal and transaxial CT scanning
Radiology 1987 Apr, Vol. 163 (1), P. 149–51

2476. Bodne D, Quinn S F, Cochran C F
Imaging foreign glass and wooden bodies of the extremities with CT and MR
J Comput Assist Tomogr 1988 Jul-Aug, Vol. 12 (4), P. 608–11

2477. Bulcke J A, Herpels V
Diagnostic value of CT scanning in neuromuscular diseases
Radiologe 1983 Nov, Vol. 23 (11), P. 523–8

2478. Cohen B A, Lanzieri C F, Mendelson D S, Sacher M, Hermann G, Train J S, Rabinowitz J G
CT evaluation of the greater sciatic foramen in patients with sciatica
AJNR 1986 Mar-Apr, Vol. 7 (2), P. 337–42

2479. deSantos L A, Goldstein H M, Murray J A, Wallace S
Computed tomography in the evaluation of musculoskeletal neoplasms
Radiology 1978 Jul, Vol. 128 (1), P. 89–94

2480. Deutsch A L, Hyde J, Miller S M, Diamond C G, Schanche A F
Cystic adventitial degeneration of the popliteal artery: CT demonstration and directed percutaneous therapy
Am J Roentgenol 1985 Jul, Vol. 145 (1), P. 117–8

2481. Dihlmann W, Bandick J
Computertomographie (CT) der Schulterweichteile. Teil 2: Rotatorenmanschette
Computed tomography CT of shoulder soft tissues. 2. The rotator cuff
RÖFO 1987 Aug, Vol. 147 (2), P. 147–51

2482. Dihlmann W, Bandick J
Computertomographie (CT) der Schulterweichteile. Teil 1: Synovialisreaktionen
Computed tomography of the soft tissues of the shoulder. 1. Synovial reactions
RÖFO 1987 Jul, Vol. 147 (1), P. 1–5

2483. Dihlmann W, Bandick J
Computertomographie der Schulterweichteile. Teil 3: Periarthropathia calcificans humeroscapularis
Computed tomography of the soft tissues of the shoulder. 3. Periarthropathia calcificans humeroscapularis
RÖFO 1988 Jan, Vol. 148 (1), P. 58–61

2484. Dihlmann W, Peters A, Tillmann B
Bursa iliopectinea – morphologisch-computertomographische Studie
The bursa iliopectinea – a morphologic-computed tomographic study
RÖFO 1989 Mar, Vol. 150 (3), P. 274–9

2485. Domingues R C, Mikulis D, Swearingen B, Tompkins R, Rosen B R
Subcutaneous sacrococcygeal myxopapillary ependymoma: CT and MR findings
AJNR 1991 Jan-Feb, Vol. 12 (1), P. 171–2

2486. Faro S H, Racette C D, Lally J F, Wills J S, Mansoory A
Traumatic lumbar hernia: CT diagnosis
Am J Roentgenol 1990 Apr, Vol. 154 (4), P. 757–9

2487. Feldberg M A, Koehler P R, van Waes P F
Psoas compartment disease studied by computed tomography. Analysis of 50 cases and subject review
Radiology 1983 Aug, Vol. 148 (2), P. 505–12

2488. Fisher D R, Hinke M L
Musculoskeletal case of the day
Am J Roentgenol 1986 May, Vol. 146 (5), P. 1087–93

2489. Fishman E K, Magid D, Ney D R, Drebin R A, Kuhlman J E
Three-dimensional imaging and display of musculoskeletal anatomy
J Comput Assist Tomogr 1988 May-Jun, Vol. 12 (3), P. 465–7

2490. Fourth International Workshop on Bone and Soft Tissue Densitometry Using Computed Tomography. Fontevraud, France, May 29-June 1, 1984
J Comput Assist Tomogr 1985 May-Jun, Vol. 9 (3), P. 602–41

2491. Giyanani V L, Grozinger K T, Gerlock A J Jr, Mirfakhraee M, Husbands H S
Calf hematoma mimicking thrombophlebitis: sonographic and computed tomographic appearance
Radiology 1985 Mar, Vol. 154 (3), P. 779–81

2492. Glickstein M F, Haggar A M, Coleman B G
Vascular and soft tissue calcification in systemic oxalosis: CT diagnosis
J Comput Assist Tomogr 1986 Jul-Aug, Vol. 10 (4), P. 691–3

2493. Gordon L F, Arger P H, Dalinka M K, Coleman B G
Computed tomography in soft tissue calcification layering
J Comput Assist Tomogr 1984 Feb, Vol. 8 (1), P. 71–3

2494. Gorich J, Seifert P
Das intramuskuläre Myxom. Sonographischer und computertomographischer Befund
Intramuscular myxoma. Sonographic and computerized tomography findings
RÖFO 1987 Sep, Vol. 147 (3), P. 354–5

2495. Hagino H, Eda I, Takashima S, Takeshita K, Sugitani A
Computed tomography in patients with Ehlers-Danlos syndrome
Neuroradiology 1985, Vol. 27 (5), P. 443–5

2496. Hall F M, Docken W P, Curtis H W
Calcific tendinitis of the longus coli: diagnosis by CT
Am J Roentgenol 1986 Oct, Vol. 147 (4), P. 742–3

2497. Haller J, Resnick D, Greenway G, Chevrot A, Murray W, Haghighi P, Sartoris D J, Chen C K
Juxtaacetabular ganglionic or synovial cysts: CT and MR features
J Comput Assist Tomogr 1989 Nov-Dec, Vol. 13 (6), P. 976–83

2498. Hermann G, Rose J S
Computed tomography in bone and soft tissue pathology of the extremities
J Comput Assist Tomogr 1979 Feb, Vol. 3 (1), P. 58–66

2499. Heuck A F, Steiger P, Stoller D W, Gluer C C, Genant H K
Quantification of knee joint fluid volume by MR imaging and CT using three-dimensional data processing J Comput Assist Tomogr 1989 Mar-Apr, Vol. 13 (2), P. 287–93

2500. Hudson T M, Springfield D S, Schiebler M
Popliteus muscle as a barrier to tumor spread: computed tomography and angiography
J Comput Assist Tomogr 1984 Jun, Vol. 8 (3), P. 498–501

2501. Jafri S Z, Bree R L, Glazer G M, Francis I R, Schwab R E
Computed tomography and ultrasound findings in Klippel-Trenaunay syndrome
J Comput Assist Tomogr 1983 Jun, Vol. 7 (3), P. 457–60

2502. Jiddane M, Gastaut J L, Pellissier J F, Pouget J, Serratrice G, Salamon G
CT of primary muscle diseases
AJNR 1983 May-Jun, Vol. 4 (3), P. 773–6

2503. John V, Nau H E, Nahser H C, Reinhardt V, Venjakob K
CT of carpal tunnel syndrome
AJNR 1983 May-Jun, Vol. 4 (3), P. 770–2

2504. Keyser C K, Gilula L A, Hardy D C, Adler S, Vannier M
Soft-tissue abnormalities of the foot and ankle: CT diagnosis
Am J Roentgenol 1988 Apr, Vol. 150 (4), P. 845–50

2505. Lohr E, Serdarevic M, Beck A, Wendt F C
CT-Diagnostik eines mykotischen Aneurysmas der Arteria femoralis nach Typhus-Infektion
CT diagnosis of a mycotic aneurysm of the femoral artery following typhoid infection
Radiologe 1986 Mar, Vol. 26 (3), P. 159–61

2506. Magid D, Fishman E K, Wharam M D Jr, Siegelman S S
Musculoskeletal desmoid tumors: CT assessment during therapy
J Comput Assist Tomogr 1988 Mar-Apr, Vol. 12 (2), P. 222–6

2507. Moncada R, Cardella R, Demos T C, Churchill R J, Cardoso M, Love L, Reynes C J
Evaluation of superior vena cava syndrome by axial CT and CT phlebography
Am J Roentgenol 1984 Oct, Vol. 143 (4), P. 731–6

2508. Morano J U, Russell W F
Nerve root enlargement in Charcot-Marie-Tooth disease: CT appearance
Radiology 1986 Dec, Vol. 161 (3), P. 784

2509. Muller N, Morris D C, Nichols D M
Popliteal artery entrapment demonstrated by CT
Radiology 1984 Apr, Vol. 151 (1), P. 157–8

2510. Newmark H 3d, Clifford O
CT of acute cervical tendinitis
AJNR 1987 May-Jun, Vol. 8 (3), P. 575–6

2511. O Doherty D S, Schellinger D, Raptopoulos V
Computed tomographic patterns of pseudohypertrophic muscular dystrophy: preliminary results
J Comput Assist Tomogr 1977 Oct, Vol. 1 (4), P. 482–6

2512. Osborn A G, Koehler P R
Computed tomography of the paraspinal musculature: normal and pathologic anatomy
Am J Roentgenol 1982 Jan, Vol. 138 (1), P. 93–8

2513. Osborn R E, DeWitt J D
Giant cauda equina schwannoma: CT appearance
AJNR 1985 Sep-Oct, Vol. 6 (5), P. 835–6

2514. Pate D, Resnick D, Andre M, Sartoris D J, Kursunoglu S, Bielecki D, Dev P, Vassiliadis A
Perspective: three-dimensional imaging of the musculoskeletal system
Am J Roentgenol 1986 Sep, Vol. 147 (3), P. 545–51

2515. Patel R B, Barton P, Salimi Z, Molitor J
Computed tomography of complicated psoas abscess with intraabscess contrast medium injection
J Comput Assist Tomogr 1983 Oct, Vol. 7 (5), P. 911–3

2516. Patten R M, Shuman W P, Teefey S
Subcutaneous metastases from malignant melanoma: prevalence and findings on CT
Am J Roentgenol 1989 May, Vol. 152 (5), P. 1009–12

2517. Pawar S V, Kay C J
Soft-tissue CT changes in pelvic venous thrombosis
Am J Roentgenol 1984 Sep, Vol. 143 (3), P. 605–7

2518. Pech P, Haughton V
A correlative CT and anatomic study of the sciatic nerve
Am J Roentgenol 1985 May, Vol. 144 (5), P. 1037–41

2519. Petasnick J P, Turner D A, Charters J R, Gitelis S, Zacharias C E
Soft-tissue masses of the locomotor system: comparison of MR imaging with CT
Radiology 1986 Jul, Vol. 160 (1), P. 125–33

2520. Pritchard R S, Shah H R, Nelson C L, FitzRandolph R L
MR and CT appearance of iliopsoas bursal distention secondary to diseased hips
J Comput Assist Tomogr 1990 Sep-Oct, Vol. 14 (5), P. 797–800

2521. Pullan B R, Fawcitt R A, Isherwood I
Tissue characterization by an analysis of the distribution of attenuation values in computed tomography scans: a preliminary report
J Comput Assist Tomogr 1978 Jan, Vol. 2 (1), P. 49–54

2522. Ralls P W, Boswell W, Henderson R, Rogers W, Boger D, Halls J
CT of inflammatory disease of the psoas muscle
Am J Roentgenol 1980 Apr, Vol. 134 (4), P. 767–70

2523. Ralls P W, Barakos J A, Kaptein E M, Friedman P E, Fouladian G, Boswell W D, Halls J, Massry S G
Renal biopsy-related hemorrhage: frequency and comparison of CT and sonography
J Comput Assist Tomogr 1987 Nov-Dec, Vol. 11 (6), P. 1031–4

2524. Rapoport S, Blair D N, McCarthy S M, Desser T S, Hammers L W, Sostman H D
Brachial plexus: correlation of MR imaging with CT and pathologic findings
Radiology 1988 Apr, Vol. 167 (1), P. 161–5

2525. Rickards D, Isherwood I, Hutchinson R, Gibbs A, Cumming W J
Computed tomography in dystrophia myotonica
Neuroradiology 1982, Vol. 24 (1), P. 27–31

2526. Rodiek S O, Kuther G
Technik computertomographischer Skelettmuskeluntersuchungen bei neuromuskulären Erkrankungen
Technic for computed tomographic study of skeletal muscles in neuromuscular diseases
RÖFO 1985 Jul, Vol. 143 (1), P. 24–8

2527. Rodiek S O, Kuther G
Computertomographie der Skelettmuskulatur bei neuromuskulären Erkrankungen
Computed tomography of the skeletal muscles in neuromuscular diseases
RÖFO 1985 Jun, Vol. 142 (6), P. 663–9

2528. Rosenberg Z S, Feldman F, Singson R D
Peroneal tendon injuries: CT analysis
Radiology 1986 Dec, Vol. 161 (3), P. 743–8

2529. Rosenberg Z S, Cheung Y, Jahss M H, Noto A M, Norman A, Leeds N E
Rupture of posterior tibial tendon: CT and MR imaging with surgical correlation
Radiology 1988 Oct, Vol. 169 (1), P. 229–35

2530. Rosenberg Z S, Jahss M H, Noto A M, Shereff M J, Cheung Y, Frey C C, Norman A
Rupture of the posterior tibial tendon: CT and surgical findings
Radiology 1988 May, Vol. 167 (2), P. 489–93

2531. Rotte K H, Kleinau H, Kriedemann E, Perlick E, Schmidt Peter P
Das maligne fibröse Histiozytom (MFH) der Weichteile. Möglichkeiten und Grenzen der Computertomographie
Malignant fibrous histiocytoma of soft tissue. Possibilities and limitations of computed tomography
RÖFO 1988 May, Vol. 148 (5), P. 520–3

2532. Rubenstein W A, Gray G, Auh Y H, Honig C L, Thorbjarnarson B, Williams J J, Haimes A B, Zirinsky K, Kazam E
CT of fibrous tissues and tumors with sonographic correlation
Am J Roentgenol 1986 Nov, Vol. 147 (5), P. 1067–74

2533. Sambrook P, Rickards D, Cumming W J
CT muscle scanning in the evaluation of patients with spinal muscular atrophy SMA
Neuroradiology 1988, Vol. 30 (6), P. 487–95

2534. Schwimmer M, Edelstein G, Heiken J P, Gilula L A
Synovial cysts of the knee: CT evaluation
Radiology 1985 Jan, Vol. 154 (1), P. 175–7

2535. Singer A M, Naimark A, Felson D, Shapiro J H
Comparison of overhead and cross-table lateral views for detection of knee- joint effusion
Am J Roentgenol 1985 May, Vol. 144 (5), P. 973–5

2536. Steiger P, Block J E, Friedlander A, Genant H K
Precise determination of paraspinous musculature by quantitative CT
J Comput Assist Tomogr 1988 Jul-Aug, Vol. 12 (4), P. 616–20

2537. Termote J L, Baert A, Crolla D, Palmers Y, Bulcke J A
Computed tomography of the normal and pathologic muscular system
Radiology 1980 Nov, Vol. 137 (2), P. 439–44

2538. Totty W G, Vannier M W
Complex musculoskeletal anatomy: analysis using three dimensional surface reconstruction
Radiology 1984 Jan, Vol. 150 (1), P. 173–7

2539. Towers M J, Downey D B, Poon P Y
Psoas muscle calcification and acute renal failure associated with nontraumatic rhabdomyolysis: CT features
J Comput Assist Tomogr 1990 Nov-Dec, Vol. 14 (6), P. 1027–9

2540. Tumeh S S, Butler G J, Maguire J H, Nagel J S
Pyogenic myositis: CT evaluation
J Comput Assist Tomogr 1988 Nov-Dec, Vol. 12 (6), P. 1002–5

2541. v d Vliet A M, Thijssen H O, Joosten E, Merx J L
CT in neuromuscular disorders: comparison of CT and histology
Neuroradiology 1988, Vol. 30 (5), P. 421–5

2542. Van Bockel S R, Mindelzun R E
Gas in the psoas muscle secondary to an intravertebral vacuum cleft: CT characteristics
J Comput Assist Tomogr 1987 Sep-Oct, Vol. 11 (5), P. 913–5

2543. von Rottkay P
CT signs of ischemic muscle necrosis
J Comput Assist Tomogr 1985 Jul-Aug, Vol. 9 (4), P. 833–4

2544. Wechsler R J, Schilling J F
CT of the gluteal region
Am J Roentgenol 1985 Jan, Vol. 144 (1), P. 185–90

2545. Wilbur A C, Spigos D G
Adventitial cyst of the popliteal artery: CT-guided percutaneous aspiration
J Comput Assist Tomogr 1986 Jan-Feb, Vol. 10 (1), P. 161–3

2546. Wilson J S, Korobkin M, Genant H K, Bovill E G Jr
Computed tomography of musculoskeletal disorders
Am J Roentgenol 1978 Jul, Vol. 131 (1), P. 55–61

2547. Yoshy C, Montana M
CT findings of metastatic breast carcinoma involving muscle
J Comput Assist Tomogr 1985 Sep-Oct, Vol. 9 (5), P. 967–8

Soft-Tissue Tumors and Bone Tumors

2548. Aisen A M, Martel W, Braunstein E M, McMillin K I, Phillips W A, Kling T F
MRI and CT evaluation of primary bone and soft-tissue tumors
Am J Roentgenol 1986 Apr, Vol. 146 (4), P. 749–56

2549. Ambrosetto P, Michelucci R, Forti A, Tassinari C A
CT findings in progressive supranuclear palsy
J Comput Assist Tomogr 1984 Jun, Vol. 8 (3), P. 406–9

2550. Ambrosetto P
CT in progressive supranuclear palsy
AJNR 1987 Sep-Oct, Vol. 8 (5), P. 849–51

2551. Arger P H, Mulhern C B Jr, Littman P S, Meadows A T, Coleman B G, Jarrett P T
Management of solid tumors in children: contribution of computed tomography
Am J Roentgenol 1981 Aug, Vol. 137 (2), P. 251–5

2552. Baleriaux Waha D, Terwinghe G, Jeanmart L
The value of computed tomography for the diagnosis of hourglass tumors of the spine
Neuroradiology 1977 Aug 25, Vol. 14 (1), P. 31–2

2553. Balthazar E J, Streiter M, Megibow A J
Anorectal giant condyloma acuminatum Buschke-Loewenstein tumor: CT and radiographic manifestations
Radiology 1984 Mar, Vol. 150 (3), P. 651–3

2554. Bernardino M E, Jing B S, Thomas J L, Lindell M M Jr, Zornoza J
The extremity soft-tissue lesion: a comparative study of ultrasound, computed tomography, and xeroradiography
Radiology 1981 Apr, Vol. 139 (1), P. 53–9

2555. Berthoty D, Haghighi P, Sartoris D J, Resnick D
Osseous invasion by soft-tissue sarcoma seen better on MR than on CT letter
Am J Roentgenol 1989 May, Vol. 152 (5), P. 1131

2556. Bloem J L, Taminiau A H, Eulderink F, Hermans J, Pauwels E K
Radiologic staging of primary bone sarcoma: MR imaging, scintigraphy, angiography, and CT correlated with pathologic examination
Radiology 1988 Dec, Vol. 169 (3), P. 805–10

2557. Boven F, De Boeck M, Potvliege R
Synovial plicae of the knee on computed tomography
Radiology 1983 Jun, Vol. 147 (3), P. 805–9

2558. Buck J, Heuck F H, Reichardt W, Ulbricht D
Die gutartigen Erkrankungen der Weichteile im Röntgen-Computer- Tomogram
Benign disorders of soft tissue on the roentgen computer tomogram
Radiologe 1983 Nov, Vol. 23 (11), P. 485–90

2559. Bunker S R
CT evaluation of soft-tissue hemorrhage letter
Am J Roentgenol 1986 Dec, Vol. 147 (6), P. 1331–2

2560. Castagno A A, Shuman W P, Kilcoyne R F, Haynor D R, Morris M E, Matsen F A
Complex fractures of the proximal humerus: role of CT in treatment
Radiology 1987 Dec, Vol. 165 (3), P. 759–62

2561. Cecchini A, Pezzotta S, Paoletti P, Rognone F
Dense dermoids in craniocervical region
J Comput Assist Tomogr 1983 Jun, Vol. 7 (3), P. 479–83

2562. Chao P W, Farman J, Kapelner S
CT features of presacral mass: an unusual focus of extramedullary hematopoiesis
J Comput Assist Tomogr 1986 Jul-Aug, Vol. 10 (4), P. 684–5

2563. Cohen M A, Mendelsohn D B
CT and MR imaging of myxofibroma of the jaws
J Comput Assist Tomogr 1990 Mar-Apr, Vol. 14 (2), P. 281–5

2564. Crone Munzebrock W, Baake S, Denkhaus H, Thoma G
Computertomographie bei Weichteiltumoren der Extremitäten
Computed tomography of soft tissue tumors of the extremities
RÖFO 1986 Jan, Vol. 144 (1), P. 83–8

2565. Crone Munzebrock W, Rehder U
Computertomographische Diagnose eines Knochenlipoms
Computed tomographic diagnosis of a bone lipoma
RÖFO 1986 Mar, Vol. 144 (3), P. 363–4

2566. deSantos L A, Bernardino M E, Murray J A
Computed tomography in the evaluation of osteosarcoma: experience with 25 cases
Am J Roentgenol 1979 Apr, Vol. 132 (4), P. 535–40

2567. Destouet J M, Gilula L A, Murphy W A
Computed tomography of long-bone osteosarcoma
Radiology 1979 May, Vol. 131 (2), P. 439–45

2568. DeVita V T, Hellman S, Rosenberg S A, (Eds.)
Cancer, principles and practice of oncology
1989, J.B.Lippincott Company, New York-St.Louis-San Francisco-London-Sidney-Tokyo

2569. Donoghue V, Daneman A, Mancer K, Krajbich I
CT features of reactive periostitis in the humerus: a lesion resembling myositis ossificans
J Comput Assist Tomogr 1985 Mar-Apr, Vol. 9 (2), P. 401–3

2570. Duda S, Bittner R, Laniado M, Lobeck H, Langer M
Bildgebende Diagnostik der aggressiven Fibromatosen und MRT- pathologische Korrelation
Imaging diagnosis of aggressive fibromatosis and the MRT- pathological correlation
RÖFO 1989 Jul, Vol. 151 (1), P. 57–62

2571. Dunnick N R, Seibert K, Cramer H R Jr
Cardiac metastasis from osteosarcoma
J Comput Assist Tomogr 1981 Apr, Vol. 5 (2), P. 253–5

2572. Egund N, Ekelund L, Sako M, Persson B
CT of soft-tissue tumors
Am J Roentgenol 1981 Oct, Vol. 137 (4), P. 725–9

2573. Enzinger F M, Weiss S W
Soft tissue tumors
1983 The C.V.Mosby Company, St.Louis Toronto London

2574. Farmlett E J, Magid D, Fishman E K
Osteoblastoma of the tibia: CT demonstration
J Comput Assist Tomogr 1986 Nov-Dec, Vol. 10 (6), P. 1068–70

2575. Forst R, Hausmann B
Zur Wertigkeit der spinalen Computertomographie in der Frühdiagnostik des Osteoidosteoms an der Wirbelsäule
Value of spinal computed tomography in the early diagnosis of spinal osteoid osteoma
RÖFO 1984 Jan, Vol. 140 (1), P. 100–2

2576. Friedrich M, Hoffmann E
Nichttraumatische Myositis ossificans circumscripta im CT
Nontraumatic myositis ossificans circumscripta in CT
RÖFO 1989 Feb, Vol. 150 (2), P. 225–7

2577. Gamba J L, Martinez S, Apple J, Harrelson J M, Nunley J A
Computed tomography of axial skeletal osteoid osteomas
Am J Roentgenol 1984 Apr, Vol. 142 (4), P. 769–72

2578. Gillespy T 3d, Manfrini M, Ruggieri P, Spanier S S, Pettersson H, Springfield D S
Staging of intraosseous extent of osteosarcoma: correlation of preoperative CT and MR imaging with pathologic macroslides
Radiology 1988 Jun, Vol. 167 (3), P. 765–7

2579. Ginaldi S, deSantos L A
Computed tomography in the evaluation of small round cell tumors of bone
Radiology 1980 Feb, Vol. 134 (2), P. 441–6

2580. Grabbe E, Heller M, Bocker W
Computertomographie bei Weichteilsarkomen
Computed tomography of soft tissue sarcomas
RÖFO 1979 Oct, Vol. 131 (4), P. 372–8

2581. Hadjis N S, Carr D H, Banks L, Pflug J J
The role of CT in the diagnosis of primary lymphedema of the lower limb
Am J Roentgenol 1985 Feb, Vol. 144 (2), P. 361–4

2582. Heelan R T, Watson R C, Smith J
Computed tomography of lower extremity tumors
Am J Roentgenol 1979 Jun, Vol. 132 (6), P. 933–7

2583. Heiken J P, Lee J K, Smathers R L, Totty W G, Murphy W A
CT of benign soft-tissue masses of the extremities
Am J Roentgenol 1984 Mar, Vol. 142 (3), P. 575–80

2584. Heller M, Oltmann K, Spielmann R P, Crone Munzebrock W
CT tumoröser Läsionen des knöchernen Beckens
CT of tumorous lesions of the osseous pelvis
RÖFO 1989 Apr, Vol. 150 (4), P. 383–9

2585. Heller M, Heyer D, Spielmann R P, Bucheler E
Computertomographische Differentialdiagnose primär pelviner Osteo-, Chondro- und Ewing-Sarkome
Computed tomographic differential diagnosis of primary pelvic osteo- , chondro- and Ewing's sarcomas
RÖFO 1990 Aug, Vol. 153 (2), P. 137–42

2586. Hermann G, Leviton M, Mendelson D, Norton K, Harris M, Weiner M, Lewis M
Osteosarcoma: relation between extent of marrow infiltration on CT and frequency of lung metastases
Am J Roentgenol 1987 Dec, Vol. 149 (6), P. 1203–6

2587. Heuchemer T, Bargon G, Wustner Hofmann M, Hofmann A
Beugesehnenlipom der tiefen Hohlhand – Sonographie versus Computertomographie
Lipoma of the flexor tendons of the palm: ultrasonography versus computed tomography
RÖFO 1990 Jul, Vol. 153 (1), P. 105–6

2588. Hollmann J, Valavanis A
Beitrag der Computertomographie zur radiologischen Abklärung eines Chondroms der zerviko-thorakalen Wirbelsäule
Contribution of computed tomography to the radiological clarification of a chondroma of the cervicothoracic spinal column
RÖFO 1983 Apr, Vol. 138 (4), P. 440–3

2589. Hudson T M, Springfield D S, Spanier S S, Enneking W F, Hamlin D J
Benign exostoses and exostotic chondrosarcomas: evaluation of cartilage thickness by CT
Radiology 1984 Sep, Vol. 152 (3), P. 595–9

2590. Hudson T M, Springfield D S, Benjamin M, Bertoni F, Present D A
Computed tomography of parosteal osteosarcoma
Am J Roentgenol 1985 May, Vol. 144 (5), P. 961–5

2591. Hudson T M, Bertoni F, Enneking W F
Computed tomography of a benign mesenchymoma of soft tissue
J Comput Assist Tomogr 1985 Jan-Feb, Vol. 9 (1), P. 205–8

2592. Iivanainen M, Hakola P, Erkinjuntti T, Sipponen J T, Ketonen L, Sulkava R, Sepponen R E
Cerebral MR and CT imaging in polycystic lipomembranous osteodysplasia with sclerosing leukoencephalopathy
J Comput Assist Tomogr 1984 Oct, Vol. 8 (5), P. 940–3

2593. Irnberger T
Die fibröse Knochendysplasie und das ossifizierende Knochenfibrom im orbitalen und periorbitalen Bereich unter besonderer Berücksichtigung der CT
Fibrous bone dysplasia and ossifying bone fibroma in the orbital and periorbital region with special reference to CT
RÖFO 1985 Nov, Vol. 143 (5), P. 569–74

2594. Irnberger T
Computertomographische Diagnose und Differentialdiagnose des juvenilen Angiofibroms und angiomatösen Polypen
Computed tomographic diagnosis and differential diagnosis of juvenile angiofibroma and angiomatous polyps
RÖFO 1985 Apr, Vol. 142 (4), P. 391–4

2595. Israels S J, Chan H S, Daneman A, Weitzman S S
Synovial sarcoma in childhood
Am J Roentgenol 1984 Apr, Vol. 142 (4), P. 803–6

2596. Jansen V O, Korner U, Reuter C, Arnholdt H
Angiographie und Computertomographie des Hibernoms
Angiography and computed tomography of a hibernoma
Am J Roentgenol 1988 Jan, Vol. 148 (1), P. 93–4

2597. Jeffrey R B, Callen P W, Federle M P
Computed tomography of psoas abscesses
J Comput Assist Tomogr 1980 Oct, Vol. 4 (5), P. 639–41

2598. Kaiser M C, Sperber M
Metastatic abscesses resulting from staphylococcal infection of the hand: CT appearance
RÖFO 1987 May, Vol. 146 (5), P. 603

2599. Kenney P J, Gilula L A, Murphy W A
The use of computed tomography to distinguish osteochondroma and chondrosarcoma
Radiology 1981 Apr, Vol. 139 (1), P. 129–37

2600. Ketyer S, Brownstein S, Cholankeril J
CT diagnosis of intraosseous lipoma of the calcaneus
J Comput Assist Tomogr 1983 Jun, Vol. 7 (3), P. 546–7

2601. Konig H, Kurtz B
Computertomographische Diagnostik der Liposarkome
Computed tomographic diagnosis of liposarcoma
RÖFO 1985 Mar, Vol. 142 (3), P. 260–3

2602. Kornreich L, Grunebaum M, Ziv N, Cohen Y
Osteogenic sarcoma of the calvarium in children: CT manifestations
Neuroradiology 1988, Vol. 30 (5), P. 439–41

2603. Koster O, Distelmaier W, Lackner K
Computertomographische Kontrolle konventionell röntgenologischer Befunde bei Raumforderungen des knöchernen Beckens
Computed tomographic control of the conventional X-ray findings in space-occupying lesions of the bony pelvis
RÖFO 1984 Aug, Vol. 141 (2), P. 148–54

2604. Krahe T, Nicolas V, Ring S, Warmuth Metz M, Koster O
Diagnostische Aussagefähigkeit von Röntgenübersichtsaufnahme und Computertomographie bei Knochentumoren der Wirbelsäule
Diagnostic evaluation of full X-ray pictures and computed tomography of bone tumors of the spine
RÖFO 1989 Jan, Vol. 150 (1), P. 13–9

2605. Kuckein D, Walter K, Kunlen H, Paal G
Beitrag der Computertomographie zur Diagnose und Lokalisation eines spinalen Agioms
Computer tomographic contribution to the diagnosis and localization of a spinal angioma
RÖFO 1979 Oct, Vol. 131 (4), P. 443–4

2606. Lanzieri C F, Solodnik P, Sacher M, Hermann G
Computed tomography of solitary spinal osteochondromas
J Comput Assist Tomogr 1985 Nov-Dec, Vol. 9 (6), P. 1042–4

2607. Levine E, Lee K R, Neff J R, Maklad N F, Robinson R G, Preston D F
Comparison of computed tomography and other imaging modalities in the evaluation of musculoskeletal tumors
Radiology 1979 May, Vol. 131 (2), P. 431–7

2608. Levinsohn E M, Bryan P J
Computed tomography in unilateral extremity swelling of unusual cause
J Comput Assist Tomogr 1979 Feb, Vol. 3 (1), P. 67–70

2609. Lindell M M Jr, Shirkhoda A, Raymond A K, Murray J A, Harle T S
Parosteal osteosarcoma: radiologic-pathologic correlation with emphasis on CT
Am J Roentgenol 1987 Feb, Vol. 148 (2), P. 323–8

2610. Lukens J A, McLeod R A, Sim F H
Computed tomographic evaluation of primary osseous malignant neoplasms
Am J Roentgenol 1982 Jul, Vol. 139 (1), P. 45–8

2611. Lynn M D, Braunstein E M, Wahl R L, Shapiro B, Gross M D, Rabbani R
Bone metastases in pheochromocytoma: comparative studies of efficacy of imaging
Radiology 1986 Sep, Vol. 160 (3), P. 701–6

2612. Mahboubi S
CT appearance of nidus in osteoid osteoma versus sequestration in osteomyelitis
J Comput Assist Tomogr 1986 May-Jun, Vol. 10 (3), P. 457–9

2613. Mail J T, Cohen M D, Mirkin L D, Provisor A J
Response of osteosarcoma to preoperative intravenous high-dose methotrexate chemotherapy: CT evaluation
Am J Roentgenol 1985 Jan, Vol. 144 (1), P. 89–93

2614. Majewski A, Freyschmidt J
Computertomographie bei Tumoren des Beckenskeletts
Computer-tomographic evaluation of tumors of the pelvis
RÖFO 1982 Jun, Vol. 136 (6), P. 635–40

2615. Marincek B, von Gumppenberg S, Triller J, Robotti G
Computertomographie bei chondrogenen Tumoren
Computed tomography of chondrogenic tumors
Radiologe 1984 May, Vol. 24 (5), P. 211–6

2616. Matsushima K, Shinohara Y, Yamamoto M, Tanigaki T, Ikeda A, Satoh O
Spinal extradural angiolipoma: MR and CT diagnosis
J Comput Assist Tomogr 1987 Nov-Dec, Vol. 11 (6), P. 1104–6

2617. Meyer J E, Lepke R A, Lindfors K K, Pagani J J, Hirschy J C, Hayman L A, Momose K J, McGinnis B
Chordomas: their CT appearance in the cervical, thoracic and lumbar spine
Radiology 1984 Dec, Vol. 153 (3), P. 693–6

2618. Morrison M C, Weiss K L, Moskos M M
CT and MR appearance of a primary intraosseous meningioma
J Comput Assist Tomogr 1988 Jan-Feb, Vol. 12 (1), P. 169–70

2619. Mueller P R, Ferrucci J T Jr, Wittenberg J, Simeone J F, Butch R J
Iliopsoas abscess: treatment by CT-guided percutaneous catheter drainage
Am J Roentgenol 1984 Feb, Vol. 142 (2), P. 359–62

2620. Omojola M F, Fox A J, Vinuela F V
Computed tomographic metrizamide myelography in the evaluation of thoracic spinal osteoblastoma
AJNR 1982 Nov-Dec, Vol. 3 (6), P. 670–3

2621. Oot R F, Parizel P M, Weber A L
Computed tomography of osteogenic sarcoma of nasal cavity and paranasal sinuses
J Comput Assist Tomogr 1986 May-Jun, Vol. 10 (3), P. 409–14

2622. Ortega W, Mahboubi S, Dalinka M K, Robinson T
Computed tomography of rib hemangiomas
J Comput Assist Tomogr 1986 Nov-Dec, Vol. 10 (6), P. 945–7

2623. Ottery F D, Carlson R A, Gould H, Weese J L
Retrorectal cyst-hamartomas: CT diagnosis
J Comput Assist Tomogr 1986 Mar-Apr, Vol. 10 (2), P. 260–3

2624. Paling M R
Plexiform neurofibroma of the pelvis in neurofibromatosis: CT findings
J Comput Assist Tomogr 1984 Jun, Vol. 8 (3), P. 476–8

2625. Pandolfo I, Gaeta M, Blandino A, La Spada F, Casablanca G, Caminiti R
Costal chondrosarcoma with pleural seeding: CT findings
J Comput Assist Tomogr 1985 Mar-Apr, Vol. 9 (2), P. 408–9

2626. Patten R M, Shuman W P, Teefey S
Metastases from malignant melanoma to the axial skeleton: a CT study of frequency and appearance
Am J Roentgenol 1990 Jul, Vol. 155 (1), P. 109–12

2627. Plonsky L, Virapongse C, Markowitz R I
Congenital orbital teratoma
J Comput Assist Tomogr 1983 Apr, Vol. 7 (2), P. 367–9

2628. Post M J, Seminer D S, Quencer R M
CT diagnosis of spinal epidural hematoma
AJNR 1982 Mar-Apr, Vol. 3 (2), P. 190–2

2629. Rauch R F, Silverman P M, Korobkin M, Dunnick N R, Moore A V, Wertman D, Martinez S
Computed tomography of benign angiomatous lesions of the extremities
J Comput Assist Tomogr 1984 Dec, Vol. 8 (6), P. 1143–6

2630. Romer T, Berger T, Berghaus A, Loeffler M
Juveniles ossifizierendes Fibrom des Gesichtsschädels. Computertomographie und Kernspintomographie
Juvenile ossifying fibroma of the facial skull. Computerized tomography and nuclear magnetic resonance tomography
Radiologe 1987 Oct, Vol. 27 (10), P. 479–82

2631. Rosenthal D I, Scott J A, Mankin H J, Wismer G L, Brady T J
Sacrococcygeal chordoma: magnetic resonance imaging and computed tomography
Am J Roentgenol 1985 Jul, Vol. 145 (1), P. 143–7

2632. Rotte K H, Kriedemann E, Geyer J, Kunde D, Melcher J, Perlick E, Schmidt Peter P
Zum Wert der Computertomographie für das Monitoring der präoperativen Chemotherapie des Osteosarkoms
The value of computed tomography in monitoring the preoperative chemotherapy of osteosarcoma
RÖFO 1989 Jan, Vol. 150 (1), P. 8–12

2633. Rubin E, Dunham W K, Stanley R J
Pancreatic metastases in bone sarcomas: CT demonstration
J Comput Assist Tomogr 1985 Sep- Oct, Vol. 9 (5), P. 886–8

2634. Schlesinger A E, Hernandez R J
Intracapsular osteoid osteoma of the proximal femur: findings on plain film and CT
Am J Roentgenol 1990 Jun, Vol. 154 (6), P. 1241–4

2635. Schmitt R, Kreiskother E, Lucas D, Lanz U
Fibrolipom des Nervus medianus. Bildgebung mittels CT und NMR
Fibrolipoma of the median nerve. Its imaging by CT and NMR
RÖFO 1987 Aug, Vol. 147 (2), P. 216–8

2636. Schmitt R, Lanz U, Feyerabend T
Schwannom des Nervus medianus – CT-Morphologie
Schwannoma of the median nerve – CT morphology
RÖFO 1988 Apr, Vol. 148 (4), P. 458–9

2637. Schmitt R, Warmuth Metz M, Lanz U, Lucas D, Feyerabend T, Schindler G
Computertomographie von Weichteiltumoren der Hand und des Unterarmes
Computed tomography of soft tissue tumors of the hand and the forearm
Radiologe 1990 Apr, Vol. 30 (4), P. 185–92

2638. Schultz S R, Bree R L, Schwab R E, Raiss G
CT detection of skeletal muscle metastases
J Comput Assist Tomogr 1986 Jan-Feb, Vol. 10 (1), P. 81–3

2639. Schwimer S R, Bassett L W, Mancuso A A, Mirra J M, Dawson E G
Giant cell tumor of the cervicothoracic spine
Am J Roentgenol 1981 Jan, Vol. 136 (1), P. 63–7

2640. Seeger J F, Burke D P, Knake J E, Gabrielsen T O
Computed tomographic and angiographic evaluation of hemangioblastomas
Radiology 1981 Jan, Vol. 138 (1), P. 65–73

2641. Shibuya H, Kurabayashi T, Iwaki H, Ohashi I, Yamada I, Suzuki S
CT findings in primary osteosarcoma of the jaw
RÖFO 1991 Feb, Vol. 154 (2), P. 139–42

2642. Steinbaum S, Liss A, Tafreshi M, Alexander L L
CT findings in metastatic adenocarcinoma of the skeletal muscles
J Comput Assist Tomogr 1983 Jun, Vol. 7 (3), P. 545–6

2643. Steinberg G G, Coumas J M, Breen T
Preoperative localization of osteoid osteoma: a new technique that uses CT
Am J Roentgenol 1990 Oct, Vol. 155 (4), P. 883–5

2644. Stojanovic J, Papa J, Cicin Sain T B
Das computertomographische und angiographische Bild eines Osteoidosteoms der Wirbel-
säule
Computer tomographic and angiographic pictures of an osteoid osteoma of the spine
RÖFO 1982 Aug, Vol. 137 (2), P. 226–9

2645. Stojanovic J, Papa J, Buljat G, Tetickovic E, Bradac G B
Ein Beitrag der Computertomographie und der spinalen Angiographie zur Diagnostik eines Wir-
belangioms
Computer tomography and spinal angiography in the diagnosis of spinal angioma
RÖFO 1985 Feb, Vol. 142 (2), P. 169–72

2646. Tehranzadeh J, Mnaymneh W, Ghavam C, Morillo G, Murphy B J
Comparison of CT and MR imaging in musculoskeletal neoplasms
J Comput Assist Tomogr 1989 May-Jun, Vol. 13 (3), P. 466–72

2647. Tehranzadeh J, Murphy B J, Mnaymneh W
Giant cell tumor of the proximal tibia: MR and CT appearance
J Comput Assist Tomogr 1989 Mar-Apr, Vol. 13 (2), P. 282–6

2648. Treu E B, de Slegte R G, Golding R P, Sperber M, van Zanten T E, Valk J
CT findings in paravertebral malignant sarcoma
J Comput Assist Tomogr 1986 May-Jun, Vol. 10 (3), P. 460–2

2649. Triebel H J, Heller M, Schumann R, Langkowski J H, Schafer H J, Weh H J
CT-Morphologie maligner Schwannome
CT morphology of malignant schwannoma
RÖFO 1988 Oct, Vol. 149 (4), P. 354–60

2650. Tschappeler H
Die Computertomographie bei primären Knochentumoren im Kindesalter
Computed tomography of primary bone tumors in children
Radiologe 1984 May, Vol. 24 (5), P. 217–21

2651. Wasenko J J, Rosenbloom S A
Temporomandibular joint chondrosarcoma: CT demonstration
J Comput Assist Tomogr 1990 Nov- Dec, Vol. 14 (6), P. 1002–3

2652. Webb W R, Jeffrey R B, Godwin J D
Thoracic computed tomography in superior sulcus tumors
J Comput Assist Tomogr 1981 Jun, Vol. 5 (3), P. 361–5

2653. Weekes R G, McLeod R A, Reiman H M, Pritchard D J
CT of soft-tissue neoplasms
Am J Roentgenol 1985 Feb, Vol. 144 (2), P. 355–60

2654. Weill A, del Carpio O Donovan R, Tampieri D, Melanson D, Ethier R
Spinal angiolipomas: CT and MR aspects
J Comput Assist Tomogr 1991 Jan-Feb, Vol. 15 (1), P. 83–5

2655. Weinberger G, Levinsohn E M
Computed tomography in the evaluation of sarcomatous tumors of the thigh
Am J Roentgenol 1978 Jan, Vol. 130 (1), P. 115–8

2656. Wojtowicz J, Karwowski A, Konkiewicz J, Lukaszewski B
Case report. Renal oncocytoma
J Comput Assist Tomogr 1979 Feb, Vol. 3 (1), P. 124–5

2657. Wolverson M K, Jagannadharao B, Sundaram M, Heiberg E, Grider R
Computed tomography in the diagnosis of gluteal abscess and other peripelvic fluid collec-
tions
J Comput Assist Tomogr 1981 Feb, Vol. 5 (1), P. 34–8

2658. Wood B P, Harwood Nash D C, Berger P, Goske M
Intradural spinal lipoma of the cervical cord
Am J Roentgenol 1985 Jul, Vol. 145 (1), P. 174–6

2659. Zeanah W R, Hudson T M, Springfield D S
Computed tomography of ossifying fibroma of the tibia
J Comput Assist Tomogr 1983 Aug, Vol. 7 (4), P. 688–91

2660. Zimmer W D, Berquist T H, McLeod R A, Sim F H, Pritchard D J, Shives T C, Wold L E,
May G R
Bone tumors: magnetic resonance imaging versus computed tomography
Radiology 1985 Jun, Vol. 155 (3), P. 709–18

Bones and Spine

2661. Abello R, Rovira M, Sanz M P, Gili J, Capdevila A, Escalada J, Peri J
MRI and CT of ankylosing spondylitis with vertebral scalloping
Neuroradiology 1988, Vol. 30 (3), P. 272–5

2662. Abrahams J J, Wood G W, Eames F A, Hicks R W
CT-guided needle aspiration biopsy of an intraspinal synovial cyst ganglion: case report and review
of the literature
AJNR 1988 Mar-Apr, Vol. 9 (2), P. 398–400

2663. Acheson M B, Livingston R R, Richardson M L, Stimac G K
High-resolution CT scanning in the evaluation of cervical spine fractures: comparison with plain
film examinations
Am J Roentgenol 1987 Jun, Vol. 148 (6), P. 1179–85

2664. Adams G W, Rauch R F, Kelvin F M, Silverman P M, Korobkin M
CT detection of typhlitis
J Comput Assist Tomogr 1985 Mar-Apr, Vol. 9 (2), P. 363–5

2665. Adams J E, Chen S Z, Adams P H, Isherwood I
Measurement of trabecular bone mineral by dual energy computed tomography
J Comput Assist Tomogr 1982 Jun, Vol. 6 (3), P. 601–7

2666. Adapon B D, Legada B D Jr, Lim E V, Silao J V Jr, Dalmacio Cruz A
CT-guided closed biopsy of the spine
J Comput Assist Tomogr 1981 Feb, Vol. 5 (1), P. 73–8

2667. Allen G J
Longitudinal stress fractures of the tibia: diagnosis with CT see comments
Radiology 1988 Jun, Vol. 167 (3), P. 799–801

2668. Altman N, Harwood Nash D C, Fitz C R, Chuang S H, Armstrong D
Evaluation of the infant spine by direct sagittal computed tomography
AJNR 1985 Jan-Feb, Vol. 6 (1), P. 65–9

2669. Alvarez O, Roque C T, Pampati M
Multilevel thoracic disk herniations: CT and MR studies
J Comput Assist Tomogr 1988 Jul- Aug, Vol. 12 (4), P. 649–52

2670. Anand A K, Lee B C
Plain and metrizamide CT of lumbar disk disease: comparison with myelography
AJNR 1982 Sep-Oct, Vol. 3 (5), P. 567–71

2671. Anda S, Dale L G, Vassal J
Intradural disc herniation with vacuum phenomenon: CT diagnosis
Neuroradiology 1987, Vol. 29 (4), P. 407

2672. Anda S, Stovring J, Ro M
CT of extraforaminal disc herniation with associated vacuum phenomenon
Neuroradiology 1988, Vol. 30 (1), P. 76–7

2673. Anda S, Terjesen T, Kvistad K A, Svenningsen S
Acetabular angles and femoral anteversion in dysplastic hips in adults: CT investigation
J Comput Assist Tomogr 1991 Jan-Feb, Vol. 15 (1), P. 115–20

2674. Aoki S, Machida T, Sasaki Y, Yoshikawa K, Iio M, Sasaki T, Takakura K
Enterogenous cyst of cervical spine: clinical and radiological aspects including CT and MRI
Neuroradiology 1987, Vol. 29 (3), P. 291–3

2675. Arredondo F, Haughton V M, Hemmy D C, Zelaya B, Williams A L
The computed tomographic appearance of the spinal cord in diastematomyelia
Radiology 1980 Sep, Vol. 136 (3), P. 685–8

2676. Artmann H, Salbeck R, Grau H
Technik und Ergebnisse der spinalen Computertomographie bei der Diagnose der zervikalen
Bandscheibenerkrankung
Technic and results of spinal computed tomography in the diagnosis of cervical disk disease
RÖFO 1985 Aug, Vol. 143 (2), P. 157–9

2677. Aubin M L, Vignaud J, Jardin C, Bar D
Computed tomography in 75 clinical cases of syringomyelia
AJNR 1981 May-Jun, Vol. 2 (3), P. 199–204

2678. Awwad E E, Sundaram M, Bucholz R D
Post-traumatic spinal synovial cyst with spondylolysis: CT features
J Comput Assist Tomogr 1989 Mar-Apr, Vol. 13 (2), P. 334–7

2679. Baker M E, Weinerth J L, Andriani R T, Cohan R H, Dunnick N R
Lumbar hernia: diagnosis by CT
Am J Roentgenol 1987 Mar, Vol. 148 (3), P. 565–7

2680. Baleriaux D, Noterman J, Ticket L
Recognition of cervical soft disk herniation by contrast-enhanced CT
AJNR 1983 May-Jun, Vol. 4 (3), P. 607–8

2681. Baleriaux Waha D, Osteaux M, Terwinghe G, de Meeus A, Jeanmart L
The management of anterior sacral meningocele with computed tomography
Neuroradiology 1977 Aug 25, Vol. 14 (1), P. 45–6

2682. Banks L M, Stevenson J C
Modified method of spinal computed tomography for trabecular bone mineral measurements
J Comput Assist Tomogr 1986 May-Jun, Vol. 10 (3), P. 463–7

2683. Banzer D, Schneider U, Wegener O H, Pleul O
Quantitative Mineralsalzbestimmung im Wirbelkörper mittels Computertomographie
RÖFO (1979) Vol. 130, P.77

2684. Beck B, Schindera F, Niederstadt T
Computertomographischer Befund bei Hämangiolipomatose des Skeletts
Computed tomographic findings in hemangiolipomatosis of the bones
RÖFO 1989 Dec, Vol. 151 (6), P. 749–51

2685. Becker H
Dreidimensionale kraniale und spinale Computertomographie
3-dimensional cranial and spinal computed tomography
Radiologe 1988 May, Vol. 28 (5), P. 239–42

2686. Beers G J, Carter A P, McNary W F
Vertical foramina in the lumbosacral region: CT appearance
Am J Roentgenol 1984 Nov, Vol. 143 (5), P. 1027–9

2687. Beltran J, Noto A M, Chakeres D W, Christoforidis A J Tumors of the osseous spine: staging with
MR imaging versus CT
Radiology 1987 Feb, Vol. 162 (2), P. 565–9

2688. Beres J, Pech P, Berns T F, Daniels D L, Williams A L, Haughton V M
Spinal epidural lymphomas: CT features in seven patients
AJNR 1986 Mar-Apr, Vol. 7 (2), P. 327–8

2689. Berns T F, Daniels D L, Williams A L, Haughton V M
Mesencephalic anatomy: demonstration by computed tomography
AJNR 1981 Jan-Feb, Vol. 2 (1), P. 65–7

2690. Bertolino G C, Cusmano F, Pichezzi P, Contini C, De Donatis M, Piazza P, Isgro E, Bruschi G,
Bassi P
Computed tomography of intradural cervical lipoma
Neuroradiology 1985, Vol. 27 (2), P. 184

2691. Bhasin S, Sartoris D J, Fellingham L, Zlatkin M B, Andre M, Resnick D
Three-dimensional quantitative CT of the proximal femur: relationship to vertebral trabecular bone density in postmenopausal women
Radiology 1988 Apr, Vol. 167 (1), P. 145–9

2692. Biggemann M, Hilweg D, Brinckmann P
Experimentelle Untersuchungen zur quantitativen computertomographischen Vorhersage der Kompressionsfestigkeit thorakolumbaler Wirbelkörper
Experimental research on the quantitative computed tomographic prediction of the compressive strength of the thoracolumbar vertebrae
RÖFO 1989 Sep, Vol. 151 (3), P. 322–5

2693. Biskjaer N L, Halaburt H
Traumatic lumbosacral nerve root avulsion demonstrated via computerised tomography
RÖFO 1986 Nov, Vol. 145 (5), P. 610–2

2694. Blews D E, Wang H, Kumar A J, Robb P A, Phillips P C, Bryan R N
Intradural spinal metastases in pediatric patients with primary intracranial neoplasms: Gd-DTPA enhanced MR vs CT myelography
J Comput Assist Tomogr 1990 Sep-Oct, Vol. 14 (5), P. 730–5

2695. Blumberg M L
CT of iliac unicameral bone cysts
Am J Roentgenol 1981 Jun, Vol. 136 (6), P. 1231–2

2696. Boccardo M, Macchia L, Carlotti G, Andrioli G
The value of enhanced "dynamic" computed tomography in localizing a spinal juxtamedullary meningioma. Enhanced dynamic CT in localizing a spinal meningioma
Neuroradiology 1987, Vol. 29 (3), P. 313

2697. Boechat M I
Spinal deformities and pseudofractures
Am J Roentgenol 1987 Jan, Vol. 148 (1), P. 97–8

2698. Boger D C
Traction device to improve CT imaging of lower cervical spine
AJNR 1986 Jul-Aug, Vol. 7 (4), P. 719–21

2699. Bonafe A, Ethier R, Melanccon D, Belanger G, Peters T
High resolution computed tomography in cervical syringomyelia
J Comput Assist Tomogr 1980 Feb, Vol. 4 (1), P. 42–7

2700. Bongartz G, Muller Miny H, Reiser M
Computertomographische Darstellung von Schultergelenkverletzungen
Computerized tomography imaging of shoulder joint injuries
Radiologe 1988 Feb, Vol. 28 (2), P. 73–8

2701. Borlaza G S, Seigel R, Kuhns L R, Good A E, Rapp R, Martel W
Computed tomography in the evaluation of sacroiliac arthritis
Radiology 1981 May, Vol. 139 (2), P. 437–40

2702. Bosnjakovic S, Reiser U, Bach D
Computertomographische und konventionelle radiologische Untersuchungen bei Knochener-krankungen
CT and conventional radiography in the evaluation of bony lesions
Radiologe 1981 Jan, Vol. 21 (1), P. 19–27

2703. Bostel F, Hauger W
CT-Kavographie: Diagnostik iliokavaler Thrombosen mit pedaler Kontrastmittelapplikation
CT cavography: diagnosis of iliocaval thrombosis by administration of contrast medium into the foot
RÖFO 1988 Oct, Vol. 149 (4), P. 423–6

2704. Bradley W G Jr, Waluch V, Yadley R A, Wycoff R R
Comparison of CT and MR in 400 patients with suspected disease of the brain and cervical spinal cord
Radiology 1984 Sep, Vol. 152 (3), P. 695–702

2705. Braitinger S, Heller H, Petsch R, Kunkel B, Dornemann H W, Stass P
Kernspintomographie der operierten Lendenwirbelsäule. Bildvergleich MR versus CT bei Band-scheibenrezidiven
Magnetic resonance tomography of the postoperative lumbar spine. A comparison of the MR versus CT images in recurrent intervertebral disk prolapse
RÖFO 1987 Aug, Vol. 147 (2), P. 185–91

2706. Braitinger S, Weigert F, Held P, Obletter N, Breit A
CT und MRT von Wirbelhämangiomen
CT and MRT of vertebral hemangiomas
RÖFO 1989 Oct, Vol. 151 (4), P. 399–407

2707. Brant Zawadzki M, Miller E M, Federle M P
CT in the evaluation of spine trauma
Am J Roentgenol 1981 Feb, Vol. 136 (2), P. 369–75

2708. Braun I F, Lin J P, Benjamin M V, Kricheff I I
Computed tomography of the asymptomatic postsurgical lumbar spine: analysis of the physiologic scar
Am J Roentgenol 1984 Jan, Vol. 142 (1), P. 149–52

2709. Braun I F, Lin J P, George A E, Kricheff I I, Hoffman J C Jr
Pitfalls in the computed tomographic evaluation of the lumbar spine in disc disease
Neuroradiology 1984, Vol. 26 (1), P. 15–20

2710. Braun I F, Hoffman J C Jr, Davis P C, Landman J A, Tindall G T
Contrast enhancement in CT differentiation between recurrent disk herniation and postoperative scar: prospective study
Am J Roentgenol 1985 Oct, Vol. 145 (4), P. 785–90

2711. Bressler E L, Marn C S, Gore R M, Hendrix R W
Evaluation of ectopic bone by CT
Am J Roentgenol 1987 May, Vol. 148 (5), P. 931–5

2712. Brody A S, Ball W S, Towbin R B
Computed arthrotomography as an adjunct to pediatric arthrography
Radiology 1989 Jan, Vol. 170 (1 Pt 1), P. 99–102

2713. Brown B M, Brant Zawadzki M, Cann C E
Dynamic CT scanning of spinal column trauma
Am J Roentgenol 1982 Dec, Vol. 139 (6), P. 1177–81

2714. Bundschuh C V, Stein L, Slusser J H, Schinco F P, Ladaga L E, Dillon J D
Distinguishing between scar and recurrent herniated disk in postoperative patients: value of contrast-enhanced CT and MR imaging
AJNR 1990 Sep-Oct, Vol. 11 (5), P. 949–58

2715. Burguet J L, Sick H, Dirheimer Y, Wackenheim A
CT of the main ligaments of the cervico-occipital hinge
Neuroradiology 1985, Vol. 27 (2), P. 112–8

2716. Burk D L Jr, Mears D C, Kennedy W H, Cooperstein L A, Herbert D L
Three-dimensional computed tomography of acetabular fractures
Radiology 1985 Apr, Vol. 155 (1), P. 183–6

2717. Burke D R, Brant Zawadzki M
CT of pyogenic spine infection
Neuroradiology 1985, Vol. 27 (2), P. 131–7

2718. Burmester E, Mendoza A S, Gmelin E
Computertomographie des Ellbogengelenkes
Computerized tomography of the elbow joint
RÖFO 1985 Dec, Vol. 143 (6), P. 671–6

2719. Burnstein M I, Pozniak M A
Computed tomography with stress maneuver to demonstrate sternoclavicular joint dislocation
J Comput Assist Tomogr 1990 Jan-Feb, Vol. 14 (1), P. 159–60

2720. Bush C H, Gillespy T 3d, Dell P C
High-resolution CT of the wrist: initial experience with scaphoid disorders and surgical fusions
Am J Roentgenol 1987 Oct, Vol. 149 (4), P. 757–60

2721. Carmody R F, Rickles D J, Johnson S F
Giant cell tumor of the sphenoid bone
J Comput Assist Tomogr 1983 Apr, Vol. 7 (2), P. 370–3

2722. Carrera G F, Haughton V M, Syvertsen A, Williams A L
Computed tomography of the lumbar facet joints
Radiology 1980 Jan, Vol. 134 (1), P. 145–8

2723. Carrera G F, Foley W D, Kozin F, Ryan L, Lawson T L
CT of sacroiliitis
Am J Roentgenol 1981 Jan, Vol. 136 (1), P. 41–6

2724. Carrera G F, Williams A L, Haughton V M
Computed tomography in sciatica
Radiology 1980 Nov, Vol. 137 (2), P. 433–7

2725. Carroll R, Miketic L M
Ewing sarcoma of the temporal bone: CT appearance
J Comput Assist Tomogr 1987 Mar-Apr, Vol. 11 (2), P. 362–3

2726. Casselman J W, Smet M H, Van Damme B, Lemahieu S F
Primary cervical neuroblastoma: CT and MR findings
J Comput Assist Tomogr 1988 Jul-Aug, Vol. 12 (4), P. 684–6

2727. Castor W R, Miller J D, Russell A S, Chiu P L, Grace M, Hanson J
Computed tomography of the craniocervical junction in rheumatoid arthritis
J Comput Assist Tomogr 1983 Feb, Vol. 7 (1), P. 31–6

2728. Chafetz N, Cann C E, Morris J M, Steinbach L S, Goldberg H I, Ax L
Pseudarthrosis following lumbar fusion: detection by direct coronal CT scanning
Radiology 1987 Mar, Vol. 162 (3), P. 803–5

2729. Chan F L, Ho E K, Chau E M
Spinal pseudarthrosis complicating ankylosing spondylitis: comparison of CT and conventional tomography
Am J Roentgenol 1988 Mar, Vol. 150 (3), P. 611–4

2730. Chang K H, Han M H, Choi Y W, Kim I O, Han M C, Kim C W
Tuberculous arachnoiditis of the spine: findings on myelography, CT, and MR imaging
AJNR 1989 Nov-Dec, Vol. 10 (6), P. 1255–62

2731. Chimon J L, Cantos E L
CT recognition of spinal epidural air after pelvic trauma
J Comput Assist Tomogr 1990 Sep-Oct, Vol. 14 (5), P. 795–6

2732. Chiras J, Bories J, Leger J M, Gaston A, Launay M
CT scan of dural arteriovenous fistulas
Neuroradiology 1982, Vol. 23 (4), P. 185–94

2733. Claussen C, Banniza von Bazan U, Jaschke W, Schilling V
Die Bedeutung der Computertomographie in der Diagnostik kongenitaler spinaler Mißbildungen, insbesondere der Diastematomyelie
The value of computer tomography in the diagnosis of congenital spinal malformations particularly diastematomyelia
RÖFO 1980 Nov, Vol. 133 (5), P. 520–7

2734. Cobb S R, Shohat M, Mehringer C M, Lachman R
CT of the temporal bone in achondroplasia
AJNR 1988 Nov-Dec, Vol. 9 (6), P. 1195–9

2735. Conrad M R, Pitkethly D T
Bilateral synovial cysts creating spinal stenosis: CT diagnosis
J Comput Assist Tomogr 1987 Jan-Feb, Vol. 11 (1), P. 196–7

2736. Coscina W F, Mintz M C, Rascoe R R, Coleman B G, Arger P H
CT characteristics of cervical mucocele mimicking a cystic adnexal mass
J Comput Assist Tomogr 1986 Mar-Apr, Vol. 10 (2), P. 352–3

2737. Coughlan J D
Extrusion of bone graft after lumbar fusion: CT appearance
J Comput Assist Tomogr 1986 May-Jun, Vol. 10 (3), P. 399–400

2738. Coughlin W F, McMurdo S K
CT diagnosis of spondylolysis of the axis vertebra letter
Am J Roentgenol 1989 Jul, Vol. 153 (1), P. 195–6

2739. Cramer B M, Kramps H A, Laumann U, Fischedick A R
CT- Diagnostik bei habitueller Schulterluxation
CT diagnosis of recurrent subluxation of the shoulder
RÖFO 1982 Apr, Vol. 136 (4), P. 440–3

2740. Crolla D, Hens L, Wilms G, Van den Bergh R, Baert A L
Metrizamide enhanced CT in hydrosyringomyelia
Neuroradiology 1980, Vol. 19 (1), P. 39–41

2741. Crone Munzebrock W, Spielmann R P, Meenen N M
Beziehungen zwischen dem computertomographisch bestimmten Mineralgehalt und dem Frak-turverhalten von gesunden und metastatischen Wirbelkörpern
The relation of computed tomography-determined mineral content and the fracture behavior of healthy and metastatic vertebral bodies
RÖFO 1989 Sep, Vol. 151 (3), P. 326–30

2742. Cunningham M J, Curtin H D, Butkiewicz B L
Histiocytosis X of the temporal bone: CT findings
J Comput Assist Tomogr 1988 Jan-Feb, Vol. 12 (1), P. 70–4

2743. Curtin H D
Radiologic approach to paragangliomas of the temporal bone
Radiology 1984 Mar, Vol. 150 (3), P. 837–8

2744. Curtin H D, Jensen J E, Barnes L Jr, May M
"Ossifying" hemangiomas of the temporal bone: evaluation with CT
Radiology 1987 Sep, Vol. 164 (3), P. 831–5

2745. Daffner R H, Kirks D R, Gehweiler J A Jr, Heaston D K
Computed tomography of fibrous dysplasia
Am J Roentgenol 1982 Nov, Vol. 139 (5), P. 943–8

2746. Dake M D, Jacobs R P, Margolin F R
Computed tomography of posterior lumbar apophyseal ring fractures
J Comput Assist Tomogr 1985 Jul-Aug, Vol. 9 (4), P. 730–2

2747. Dalley R W, Robertson W D, Nugent R A
Computed tomography of calvarial and petrous bone sarcoidosis
J Comput Assist Tomogr 1987 Sep-Oct, Vol. 11 (5), P. 884–6

2748. Daniels D L, Grogan J P, Johansen J G, Meyer G A, Williams A L, Haughton V M
Cervical radiculopathy: computed tomography and myelography compared
Radiology 1984 Apr, Vol. 151 (1), P. 109–13

2749. De Santis M, Crisi G, Folchi Vici F
Late contrast enhancement in the CT diagnosis of herniated lumbar disk
Neuroradiology 1984, Vol. 26 (4), P. 303–7

2750. Destouet J M, Gilula L A, Murphy W A, Sagel S S
Computed tomography of the sternoclavicular joint and sternum
Radiology 1981 Jan, Vol. 138 (1), P. 123–8

2751. Deutsch A L, Resnick D, Campbell G
Computed tomography and bone scintigraphy in the evaluation of tarsal coalition
Radiology 1982 Jul, Vol. 144 (1), P. 137–40

2752. Deutsch A L, Resnick D, Mink J H, Berman J L, Cone R O, Resnik C S, Danzig L, Guerra
J Jr
Computed and conventional arthrotomography of the glenohumeral joint: normal anatomy and
clinical experience
Radiology 1984 Dec, Vol. 153 (3), P. 603–9

2753. Di Chiro G, Rieth K G, Oldfield E H, Tievsky A L, Doppman J L, Davis D O
Digital subtraction angiography and dynamic computed tomography in the evaluation of arte-
riovenous malformations and hemangioblastomas of the spinal cord
J Comput Assist Tomogr 1982 Aug, Vol. 6 (4), P. 655–70

2754. Diankov L, Velitschkov L, Petkov D, Nedelkov G, Pampoulov L
Die Wertigkeit der Computertomographie zur Diagnostik der diabetischen Osteoarthropathie
The value of computerized tomography for the diagnosis of diabetic osteoarthropathy
Radiologe 1983 Dec, Vol. 23 (12), P. 560–6

2755. Dihlmann W
Koxale Computertomographie (KCT)
Computed tomography of the hip joint
RÖFO 1981 Sep, Vol. 135 (3), P. 333–42

2756. Dihlmann W, Nebel G
Computed tomography of the hip joint capsule
J Comput Assist Tomogr 1983 Apr, Vol. 7 (2), P. 278–85

2757. Dihlmann W, Heller M
Asterisk-Zeichen und adulte ischämische Femurkopfnekrose
The asterisk sign and adult ischemic femur head necrosis
RÖFO 1985 Apr, Vol. 142 (4), P. 430–5

2758. Dihlmann W
Lumbaler Reprolaps oder Narbengewebe? Versuch der Differenzierung mittels computertomo-
graphischem Bicolor- Modus
Lumbar reprolapse or scar tissue? An attempt at differentiation via a computer tomographic
bicolor mode
RÖFO 1987 Mar, Vol. 146 (3), P. 330–4

2759. Dihlmann W
Hochauflösende Computertomographie bei der Femurkopfnekrose. Stellungnahme zu dem Bei-
trag in: Fortschr. Röntgenstr. 148 (1988) 285–288
High-resolution computed tomography of femur head necrosis.
RÖFO 1988 Nov, Vol. 149 (5), P. 539–40

2760. Dock W, Grabenwoger F, Schratter M, Farres M T, Kwasny O
Diagnostik von Beckenfrakturen: Beckenübersichtsaufnahmen versus CT
Diagnosis of pelvic fractures: synoptic views of the pelvis versus CT
RÖFO 1989 Mar, Vol. 150 (3), P. 280–3

2761. Donaldson I, Gibson R
Spinal cord atrophy associated with arachnoiditis as demonstrated by computed tomography
Neuroradiology 1982, Vol. 24 (2), P. 101–5

2762. Donoghue V, Chuang S H, Chilton S J, Fitz C R, Harwood Nash D C
Intraspinal epidermoid cysts
J Comput Assist Tomogr 1984 Feb, Vol. 8 (1), P. 143–4

2763. Donoghue V, Daneman A, Krajbich I, Smith C R
CT appearance of sacroiliac joint trauma in children
J Comput Assist Tomogr 1985 Mar-Apr, Vol. 9 (2), P. 352–6

2764. Doppman J L, Marx S, Spiegel A, Brown E, Downs R, Brennan M F, Aurbach G
Differential diagnosis of brown tumor vs. cystic osteitis by arteriography and computed tomo-
graphy
Radiology 1979 May, Vol. 131 (2), P. 339–40

2765. Doppman J L, Sharon M, Gorden P
Metatarsal penciling in acromegaly: a proposed mechanism based on CT findings
J Comput Assist Tomogr 1988 Jul-Aug, Vol. 12 (4), P. 708–9

2766. Dorne H L, Lander P H
CT recognition of anomalies of the posterior arch of the atlas vertebra: differentiation from
fracture
AJNR 1986 Jan-Feb, Vol. 7 (1), P. 176–7

2767. Drebin R A, Magid D, Robertson D D, Fishman E K
Fidelity of three-dimensional CT imaging for detecting fracture gaps
J Comput Assist Tomogr 1989 May-Jun, Vol. 13 (3), P. 487–9

2768. Dublin A B, Phillips H E
Computed tomography of disseminated coccidiodomycosis
Radiology 1980 May, Vol. 135 (2), P. 361–8

2769. Dublin A B, McGahan J P, Reid M H
The value of computed tomographic metrizamide myelography in the neuroradiological evalua-
tion of the spine
Radiology 1983 Jan, Vol. 146 (1), P. 79–86

2770. Durand E P, Ruegsegger P
Cancellous bone structure: analysis of high-resolution CT images with the run-length method
J Comput Assist Tomogr 1991 Jan-Feb, Vol. 15 (1), P. 133–9

2771. Dvorak J, Hayek J
Diagnostik der Instabilität der oberen Halswirbelsäule mittels funktioneller Computertomo-
graphie
Diagnosis of instability of the upper cervical spine by functional computed tomography
RÖFO 1986 Nov, Vol. 145 (5), P. 582–5

2772. Dvorak J, Penning L, Hayek J, Panjabi M M, Grob D, Zehnder R
Functional diagnostics of the cervical spine using computer tomography
Neuroradiology 1988, Vol. 30 (2), P. 132–7

2773. Edelstein G, Levitt R G, Slaker D P, Murphy W A
CT observation of rib abnormalities: spectrum of findings
J Comput Assist Tomogr 1985 Jan-Feb, Vol. 9 (1), P. 65–72

2774. Efremidis S C, Dan S J, Cohen B A, Mitty H A, Rabinowitz J G
Displaced paraspinal line: role of CT and lymphography
Am J Roentgenol 1981 Mar, Vol. 136 (3), P. 505–9

2775. Elster A D, Jensen K M
Vacuum phenomenon within the cervical spinal canal: CT demonstration of a herniated disc
J Comput Assist Tomogr 1984 Jun, Vol. 8 (3), P. 533–5

2776. Elster A D, Jensen K M
Computed tomography of spondylolisthesis: patterns of associated pathology
J Comput Assist Tomogr 1985 Sep-Oct, Vol. 9 (5), P. 867–74

2777. Enzmann D R, Murphy Irwin K, Silverberg G D, Djang W T, Golden J B
Spinal cord tumor imaging with CT and sonography
AJNR 1985 Jan-Feb, Vol. 6 (1), P. 95–7

2778. Eubanks B A, Cann C E, Brant Zawadzki M
CT measurement of the diameter of spinal and other bony canals: effects of section angle and
thickness
Radiology 1985 Oct, Vol. 157 (1), P. 243–6

2779. Feldman F, Singson R D, Rosenberg Z S, Berdon W E, Amodio J, Abramson S J
Distal tibial triplane fractures: diagnosis with CT
Radiology 1987 Aug, Vol. 164 (2), P. 429–35

2780. Felsenberg D
Quantitative Knochenmineralgehaltsbestimmung mit der Zwei-Spektren- Computertomo-
graphie
Quantitative determination of bone mineral content by double- spectrum computer tomo-
graphy
Radiologe 1988 Apr, Vol. 28 (4), P. 166–72

2781. Felsenberg D, Kalender W A, Banzer D, Schmilinsky G, Heyse M, Fischer E, Schneider U
Quantitative computertomographische Knochenmineralgehaltsbestimmung
Quantitative computerized tomographic determination of bone mineral content
RÖFO 1988 Apr, Vol. 148 (4), P. 431–6

2782. Firooznia H, Benjamin V, Kricheff I I, Rafii M, Golimbu C
CT of lumbar spine disk herniation: correlation with surgical findings
Am J Roentgenol 1984 Mar, Vol. 142 (3), P. 587–92

2783. Firooznia H, Golimbu C, Rafii M, Schwartz M S
Rate of spinal trabecular bone loss in normal perimenopausal women: CT measurement
Radiology 1986 Dec, Vol. 161 (3), P. 735–8

2784. Firooznia H, Rafii M, Golimbu C, Schwartz M S, Ort P
Trabecular mineral content of the spine in women with hip fracture: CT measurement
Radiology 1986 Jun, Vol. 159 (3), P. 737- 40

2785. Fishman E K, Zinreich S J, Kumar A J, Rosenbaum A E, Siegelman S S
Sacral abnormalities in Marfan syndrome
J Comput Assist Tomogr 1983 Oct, Vol. 7 (5), P. 851–6

2786. Fishman E K, Magid D, Robertson D D, Brooker A F, Weiss P, Siegelman S S
Metallic hip implants: CT with multiplanar reconstruction
Radiology 1986 Sep, Vol. 160 (3), P. 675–81

2787. Fishman E K, Drebin B, Magid D, Scott W W Jr, Ney D R, Brooker A F Jr, Riley L H Jr, St Ville
J A, Zerhouni E A, Siegelman S S
Volumetric rendering techniques: applications for three-dimensional imaging of the hip
Radiology 1987 Jun, Vol. 163 (3), P. 737–8

2788. Frager D H, Elkin C M, Kansler F, Mendelsohn S L, Leeds N E
Extraspinal abnormalities identified on lumbar spine CT
Neuroradiology 1986, Vol. 28 (1), P. 58–60

2789. Frahm R, Drescher E
Radiologische Diagnostik nach komplizierter distaler Radiusfraktur unter besonderer Berück-
sichtigung der Computertomographie
Radiologic diagnosis following compound fracture of the distal radius with special reference to
computed tomography
RÖFO 1988 Mar, Vol. 148 (3), P. 295–300

2790. Frahm R, Saul O, Drescher E
CT-Diagnostik bei Fehlstellungen nach distaler Radiusfraktur
CT diagnosis of malalignment following distal radius fracture
Radiologe 1989 Feb, Vol. 29 (2), P. 68–72

2791. Frahm R, Lowka K, Wimmer B
Computed tomography of the wrist
Computertomographie des Handgelenkes
Radiologe 1990 Aug, Vol. 30 (8), P. 366–72

2792. Frahm R, Wimmer B
Suche nach freien Gelenkkörpern im Ellbogengelenk – Konventionelle oder CT-Arthro-
graphie?
The search for joint loose bodies in the elbow joint – conventional or CT arthrography?
Radiologe 1990 Mar, Vol. 30 (3), P. 113–5

2793. Franklin P D, Dunlop R W, Whitelaw G, Jacques E Jr, Blickman J G, Shapiro J H
Computed tomography of the normal and traumatized elbow
J Comput Assist Tomogr 1988 Sep-Oct, Vol. 12 (5), P. 817–23

2794. Friedburg H, Hendrich V, Wimmer B, Riede U N
Computertomographie bei komplexen Sprunggelenksfrakturen
Computed tomography in complex fractures of the ankle joint
Radiologe 1983 Sep, Vol. 23 (9), P. 421–5

2795. Friedman L, Yong Hing K, Johnston G H
Forty degree angled coronal CT scanning of scaphoid fractures through plaster and fiberglass
casts
J Comput Assist Tomogr 1989 Nov-Dec, Vol. 13 (6), P. 1101–4

2796. Fries J W, Abodeely D A, Vijungco J G, Yeager V L, Gaffey W R
Computed tomography of herniated and extruded nucleus pulposus
J Comput Assist Tomogr 1982 Oct, Vol. 6 (5), P. 874–87

2797. Frocrain L, Duvauferrier R, Husson J L, Noel J, Ramee A, Pawlotsky Y
Recurrent postoperative sciatica: evaluation with MR imaging and enhanced CT
Radiology 1989 Feb, Vol. 170 (2), P. 531–3

2798. Fuchs W A
Computertomographie in der orthopädischen Radiologie
Computed tomography in orthopedic radiology
Radiologe 1984 May, Vol. 24 (5), P. 201–4

2799. Gacetta D J, Yandow D R
Computed tomography of spontaneous osteoporotic sacral fractures
J Comput Assist Tomogr 1984 Dec, Vol. 8 (6), P. 1190–1

2800. Gado M, Patel J, Hodges F J
Lateral disk herniation into the lumbar intervertebral foramen: differential diagnosis
AJNR 1983 May-Jun, Vol. 4 (3), P. 598–600

2801. Gagnerie F, Taillan B, Bruneton J N, Bonnard J M, Denis F, Commandre F, Euller Ziegler L,
Ziegler G
Three cases of pigmented villonodular synovitis of the knee. Ultrasound and computed tomo-
graphic findings
RÖFO 1986 Aug, Vol. 145 (2), P. 227–8

2802. Gambari P I, Giuliani G, Poppi M, Pozzati E
Ganglionic cysts of the peroneal nerve at the knee: CT and surgical correlation
J Comput Assist Tomogr 1990 Sep-Oct, Vol. 14 (5), P. 801–3

2803. Ganti S R, Silver A J, Diefenbach P, Hilal S K, Mawad M E, Sane P
Computed tomography of primitive neuroectodermal tumors
AJNR 1983 May-Jun, Vol. 4 (3), P. 819–21

2804. Gellad F E, Levine A M, Joslyn J N, Edwards C C, Bosse M
Pure thoracolumbar facet dislocation: clinical features and CT appearance
Radiology 1986 Nov, Vol. 161 (2), P. 505–8

2805. Genez B M, Willis J J, Lowrey C E, Lauerman W C, Woodruff W, Diaz M J, Higgs J B
CT findings of degenerative arthritis of the atlantoodontoid joint
Am J Roentgenol 1990 Feb, Vol. 154 (2), P. 315–8

2806. Gentry L R, Turski P A, Strother C M, Javid M J, Sackett J F
Chymopapain chemonucleolysis: CT changes after treatment
Am J Roentgenol 1985 Aug, Vol. 145 (2), P. 361–9

2807. Giles D J, Thomas R J, Osborn A G, Clayton P D, Miller M H, Bahr A L, Frederick P R, O Connor G D, Ostler D
Lumbar spine: pretest predictability of CT findings
Radiology 1984 Mar, Vol. 150 (3), P. 719–22

2808. Gluer C C, Genant H K
Impact of marrow fat on accuracy of quantitative CT
J Comput Assist Tomogr 1989 Nov-Dec, Vol. 13 (6), P. 1023–35

2809. Goiney R C, Connell D G, Nichols D M
CT evaluation of tarsometatarsal fracture-dislocation injuries
Am J Roentgenol 1985 May, Vol. 144 (5), P. 985–90

2810. Golimbu C, Firooznia H, Rafii M
CT of osteomyelitis of the spine
Am J Roentgenol 1984 Jan, Vol. 142 (1), P. 159–63

2811. Goodsitt M M, Kilcoyne R F, Gutcheck R A, Richardson M L, Rosenthal D I
Effect of collagen on bone mineral analysis with CT
Radiology 1988 Jun, Vol. 167 (3), P. 787–91

2812. Gould E S, Abdelwahab I F
Role of diskography after negative postmyelography CT scans letter
AJNR 1989 Jul-Aug, Vol. 10 (4), P. 848

2813. Gould R, Rosenfield A T, Friedlaender G E
Loose body within the glenohumeral joint in recurrent anterior dislocation: CT demonstration
J Comput Assist Tomogr 1985 Mar-Apr, Vol. 9 (2), P. 404–6

2814. Gouliamos A, Carvounis E, Kalovidouris A, Vlahos L, Pontifex G, Papavassiliou C, Deligeorgi Politi H
Computed tomography in the evaluation of spinal aneurysmal bone cyst
Radiologe 1986 Nov, Vol. 26 (11), P. 528–30

2815. Goupille P, Giraudet Le Quintrec J S, Job Deslandre C, Menkes C J
Longitudinal stress fractures of the tibia: diagnosis with CT letter; comment
Radiology 1989 May, Vol. 171 (2), P. 583

2816. Graves V B, Keene J S, Strother C M, Bennett L N, Hackelthorn J C, Houston L
CT of bilateral lumbosacral facet dislocation
AJNR 1988 Jul-Aug, Vol. 9 (4), P. 809

2817. Grehn S
Hochauflösende Computertomographie bei der Femurkopfnekrose
High-resolution computed tomography of femur head necrosis
RÖFO 1988 Mar, Vol. 148 (3), P. 285–8

2818. Grenier N, Vital J M, Greselle J F, Richard O, Houang B, Pinol Daubisse H, Senegas J, Caille J M
CT-diskography in the evaluation of the postoperative lumbar spine. Preliminary results
Neuroradiology 1988, Vol. 30 (3), P. 232–8

2819. Grogan J P, Daniels D L, Williams A L, Rauschning W, Haughton V M
The normal conus medullaris: CT criteria for recognition
Radiology 1984 Jun, Vol. 151 (3), P. 661–4

2820. Grosman H, Gray R, St Louis E L
CT of long-standing ankylosing spondylitis with cauda equina syndrome
AJNR 1983 Sep- Oct, Vol. 4 (5), P. 1077–80

2821. Guinto F C Jr, Hashim H, Stumer M
CT demonstration of disk regression after conservative therapy
AJNR 1984 Sep-Oct, Vol. 5 (5), P. 632–3

2822. Gulati A N, Weinstein Z R
Gas in the spinal canal in association with the lumbosacral vacuum phenomenon: CT findings
Neuroradiology 1980 Dec, Vol. 20 (4), P. 191–2

2823. Gulati A N, Weinstein R, Studdard E
CT scan of the spine for herniated discs
Neuroradiology 1981, Vol. 22 (2), P. 57–60

2824. Guyer B H, Levinsohn E M, Fredrickson B E, Bailey G L, Formikell M
Computed tomography of calcaneal fractures: anatomy, pathology, dosimetry, and clinical relevance
Am J Roentgenol 1985 Nov, Vol. 145 (5), P. 911–9

2825. Haberbeck Modesto M A, Servadei F, Greitz T, Steiner L
Computed tomography for anterior sacral and intracorporal meningoceles
Neuroradiology 1981, Vol. 21 (3), P. 155–8

2826. Habibian A, Stauffer A, Resnick D, Reicher M A, Rafii M, Kellerhouse L, Zlatkin M B, Newman C, Sartoris D J
Comparison of conventional and computed arthrotomography with MR imaging in the evaluation of the shoulder
J Comput Assist Tomogr 1989 Nov-Dec, Vol. 13 (6), P. 968–75

2827. Hall F M, Sussman S K
Coning of spinal CT images in low back pain letter
Am J Roentgenol 1985 Jun, Vol. 144 (6), P. 1320

2828. Hall F M
CT in atlantoaxial rotatory fixation letter
Am J Roentgenol 1988 Apr, Vol. 150 (4), P. 947–8

2829. Hammer B, Bohm Jurkovic H, zur Nedden D, Valencak E, Moshenipour I
Der Wert der frühen postoperativen CT-Untersuchung nach lumbaler Bandscheibenoperation
The value of early postoperative CT study after lumbar intervertebral disk surgery
RÖFO 1986 Nov, Vol. 145 (5), P. 586–90

2830. Han S S, Love M B, Simeone F A
Diagnosis and treatment of a lumbar extradural arteriovenous malformation
AJNR 1987 Nov-Dec, Vol. 8 (6), P. 1129–30

2831. Handel S, Grossman R, Sarwar M
Case report: computed tomography in the diagnosis of spinal cord astrocytoma
J Comput Assist Tomogr 1978 Apr, Vol. 2 (2), P. 226–8

2832. Hannesschlager G, Riedelberger W, Neumuller H, Schwarzl G
Computertomographie der Rotatorenmanschette – Vergleich mit anderen bildgebenden Verfahren
Computed tomography of the rotator cuff – a comparison with other imaging technics
RÖFO 1989 Jun, Vol. 150 (6), P. 643–9

2833. Hansen S T Jr
CT for pelvic fractures
Am J Roentgenol 1982 Mar, Vol. 138 (3), P. 592–3

2834. Harbin W P
Metastatic disease and the nonspecific bone scan: value of spinal computed tomography
Radiology 1982 Oct, Vol. 145 (1), P. 105–7

2835. Hardy D C, Murphy W A, Gilula L A
Computed tomography in planning percutaneous bone biopsy
Radiology 1980 Feb, Vol. 134 (2), P. 447–50

2836. Hardy D C, Totty W G, Funk K C
CT-directed rib biopsy
J Comput Assist Tomogr 1987 Nov-Dec, Vol. 11 (6), P. 994–7

2837. Harley J D, Mack L A, Winquist R A
CT of acetabular fractures: comparison with conventional radiography
Am J Roentgenol 1982 Mar, Vol. 138 (3), P. 413–7

2838. Hasso A N, McKinney J M, Killeen J, Hinshaw D B Jr, Thompson J R
Computed tomography of children and adolescents with suspected spinal stenosis
J Comput Assist Tomogr 1987 Jul-Aug, Vol. 11 (4), P. 609–11

2839. Haughton V M, Eldevik O P, Magnaes B, Amundsen P
A prospective comparison of computed tomography and myelography in the diagnosis of herniated lumbar disks
Radiology 1982 Jan, Vol. 142 (1), P. 103–10

2840. Heger L, Wulff K, Seddiqi M S
Computed tomography of calcaneal fractures
Am J Roentgenol 1985 Jul, Vol. 145 (1), P. 131–7

2841. Heger L, Wulff K
Computed tomography of the calcaneus: normal anatomy
Am J Roentgenol 1985 Jul, Vol. 145 (1), P. 123–9

2842. Heinz E R, Yeates A, Burger P, Drayer B P, Osborne D, Hill R
Opacification of epidural venous plexus and dura in evaluation of cervical nerve roots: CT technique
AJNR 1984 Sep- Oct, Vol. 5 (5), P. 621–4

2843. Heller M, Kotter D, Wenzel E
Computertomographische Diagnostik des traumatisierten Beckens
Computer-tomographic diagnosis of the traumatised pelvis
RÖFO 1980 Apr, Vol. 132 (4), P. 386–91

2844. Heller M, Dihlmann W
Computertomographie der Paget- Koxopathie
Computed tomography of Paget's disease of the hip
RÖFO 1983 Apr, Vol. 138 (4), P. 427–34

2845. Heller M, Wenk M, Jend H H
Vergleichende Untersuchungen zur Darstellung artifizieller Knochenläsionen – konventionelle Tomographie und Computertomographie
Comparative studies on imaging artificial bone lesions -conventional tomography and computed tomography
RÖFO 1984 Jun, Vol. 140 (6), P. 631–8

2846. Helms C A, Cann C E, Brunelle F O, Gilula L A, Chafetz N, Genant H K
Detection of bone-marrow metastases using quantitative computed tomography
Radiology 1981 Sep, Vol. 140 (3), P. 745–50

2847. Helms C A, Dorwart R H, Gray M
The CT appearance of conjoined nerve roots and differentiation from a herniated nucleus pulposus
Radiology 1982 Sep, Vol. 144 (4), P. 803–7

2848. Helms C A, McCarthy S
CT scanograms for measuring leg length discrepancy
Radiology 1984 Jun, Vol. 151 (3), P. 802

2849. Helzel M V, Betz H, Gladziwa U, Frey M
Sonographische Spinalkanal-Weitenbestimmung. Vergleich zur Computertomographie, Myelographie und konventionellen Röntgenuntersuchung der Lendenwirbelsäule
Sonographic determination of spinal canal width. Comparison of computed tomography, myelography and conventional roentgen study of the lumbar spine
Radiologe 1985 Jun, Vol. 25 (6), P. 277–83

2850. Helzel M V, Schindler G, Gay B
Sonographische Messung des Gelenkknorpels über den Femurkondylen. Vergleich zur Arthrographie und Pneumarthrocomputertomographie
Sonographic measurement of the articular cartilage over the femoral condyles. A comparison with arthrography and computed tomographic pneumoarthrography
RÖFO 1987 Jul, Vol. 147 (1), P. 10–4

2851. Henkes H, Schorner W, Jochens R, Lang P, Ruf B, Heise W, Trautmann M, Felix R
Zerebrale und meningeale Manifestation des AIDS: Sensitivität von CT und T2-gewichteter MRT (129 Patienten)
Cerebral and meningeal manifestations of AIDS: sensitivity of CT and T2-weighted MRT 129 patients
RÖFO 1990 Sep, Vol. 153 (3), P. 303–12

2852. Herman G T, Coin C G
The use of three-dimensional computer display in the study of disk disease
J Comput Assist Tomogr 1980 Aug, Vol. 4 (4), P. 564–7

2853. Hermanus N, de Becker D, Baleriaux D, Hauzeur J P
The use of CT scanning for the study of posterior lumbar intervertebral articulations
Neuroradiology 1983, Vol. 24 (3), P. 159–61

2854. Hernandez R J, Tachdjian M O, Poznanski A K, Dias L S
CT determination of femoral torsion
Am J Roentgenol 1981 Jul, Vol. 137 (1), P. 97–101

2855. Hernandez R J, Tachdjian M O, Dias L S
Hip CT in congenital dislocation: appearance of tight iliopsoas tendon and pulvinar hypertrophy
Am J Roentgenol 1982 Aug, Vol. 139 (2), P. 335–7

2856. Hernandez R J
Concentric reduction of the dislocated hip. Computed-tomographic evaluation
Radiology 1984 Jan, Vol. 150 (1), P. 266–8

2857. Herter M, Steudel H, Steudel A
Histologische Sicherung eines monoostotischen Paget im Os sacrum durch CT-gesteuerte Knochenstanzung
Histological confirmation of monostotic Paget's disease in the sacrum by CT-guided bone puncture biopsy
RÖFO 1986 Nov, Vol. 145 (5), P. 608–10

2858. Heuchemer T, Bargon G, Bauer G, Mutschler W
Vorteile in Diagnose und Einteilung der intraartikulären Kalkaneusfraktur durch die Computer-
tomographie
Advantages in the diagnosis and classification of intra-articular fractures of the calcaneus using
computed tomography
RÖFO 1988 Jul, Vol. 149 (1), P. 8–14

2859. Heuck F, Weiske R
Informationswert der Röntgen-Computer-Tomographie für den Nachweis und die Kontrolle der
Spondylitis
Information value of x-ray computed tomography for the detection and control of spondylitis
Radiologe 1985 Jul, Vol. 25 (7), P. 307–17

2860. Heuck F, Schneider R
Nachweis maskierter Frakturen des Beckenskelettes mit der Röntgen- Computer-Tomo-
graphie
Detection of occult fractures of the pelvic bones by roentgen computed tomography
Radiologe 1985 Mar, Vol. 25 (3), P. 114–20

2861. Hindman B W, Schreiber R R, Wiss D A, Ghilarducci M J, Avolio R E
Supracondylar fractures of the humerus: prediction of the cubitus varus deformity with CT
Radiology 1988 Aug, Vol. 168 (2), P. 513–5

2862. Hindman B W, Kulik W J, Lee G, Avolio R E
Occult fractures of the carpals and metacarpals: demonstration by CT
Am J Roentgenol 1989 Sep, Vol. 153 (3), P. 529–32

2863. Hirschy J C, Leue W M, Berninger W H, Hamilton R H, Abbott G F
CT of the lumbosacral spine: importance of tomographic planes parallel to vertebral end
plate
Am J Roentgenol 1981 Jan, Vol. 136 (1), P. 47–52

2864. Hofmann W, Grobovschek M, Rahim H
Spinale Computertomographie lumbosakral/lumbosakrale Funktionsmyelographie. Dosime-
trischer Vergleich – Vergleich der Indikation
Lumbosacral computed tomography and lumbosacral functional myelography. Dosimetric com-
parison and comparison of indications
RÖFO 1986 Oct, Vol. 145 (4), P. 392–6

2865. Holbert J M, Lewis E
CT evaluation of the pelvis after hemipelvectomy
Am J Roentgenol 1985 Dec, Vol. 145 (6), P. 1233–9

2866. Hopf C, Schaub T
Eine computertomographische Analyse zur Wirbelrotation vor und nach der operativen Korrektur
der idiopathischen Skoliose
A computed tomographic analysis of vertebral rotation before and after surgical correction of
idiopathic scoliosis
RÖFO 1989 Oct, Vol. 151 (4), P. 408–13

2867. Hudson T M
Fluid levels in aneurysmal bone cysts: a CT feature
Am J Roentgenol 1984 May, Vol. 142 (5), P. 1001–4

2868. Hudson TM, Vandergriend RA, Springfield DS, Hawkins IF Jr, Spanier SS, Enneking WF, Hamlin D
J
Aggressive fibromatosis: evaluation by computed tomography and angiography
Radiology 1984 Feb, Vol. 150 (2), P. 495–501

2869. Imhof H, Hajek P, Kumpan W, Schratter M, Wagner M
CT in der Akutdiagnostik von Wirbelsäulendiagnostik
Computerized tomography in the acute diagnosis of spinal injuries
Radiologe 1986 May, Vol. 26 (5), P. 242–7

2870. Inoue N, Motomura S, Murai Y, Tsukamoto Y, Nakata H, Ito K, Ijichi M
Computed tomography in calcification of ligamenta flava of the cervical spine
J Comput Assist Tomogr 1983 Aug, Vol. 7 (4), P. 704–6

2871. Ishida Y, Suzuki K, Ohmori K
Dynamics of the spinal cord: an analysis of functional myelography by CT scan
Neuroradiology 1988, Vol. 30 (6), P. 538–44

2872. Jahnke R W
Low density in the posterior portion of the lumbar disk: a new CT finding in disk herniations
J Comput Assist Tomogr 1983 Apr, Vol. 7 (2), P. 313–5

2873. James H E, Oliff M
Computed tomography in spinal dysraphism
J Comput Assist Tomogr 1977 Oct, Vol. 1 (4), P. 391–7

2874. Janson R, Kuhr J, Lackner K, Brecht G
CT-Diagnostik der chronischen Osteomyelitis
CT diagnosis of chronic osteomyelitis
RÖFO 1981 May, Vol. 134 (5), P. 517–22

2875. Jend H H, Heller M, Schontag H, Schoettle H
Eine computertomographische Methode zur Bestimmung der Tibiatorsion
A computer tomographic method for the determination of tibial torsion
RÖFO 1980 Jul, Vol. 133 (1), P. 22–5

2876. Jend H H, Helmke K, Heller M, Kuhne D
Die Computertomographie bei Fehlbildungen, entzündlichen und degenerativen Veränderungen der
Wirbelsäule
Computer tomography in malformations, inflammatory and degenerative changes in the spine
RÖFO 1982 Nov, Vol. 137 (5), P. 523–9

2877. Jensen P S, Orphanoudakis S C, Rauschkolb E N, Baron R, Lang R, Rasmussen H
Assessment of bone mass in the radius by computed tomography
Am J Roentgenol 1980 Feb, Vol. 134 (2), P. 285–92

2878. Johansen J G
Tissue inhomogeneity within lumbar costotransverse foramen
Neuroradiology 1987, Vol. 29 (4), P. 406

2879. Johansen J G, Stenwig J T
Paraspinal schwannoma with cystic appearance on CT
Neuroradiology 1987, Vol. 29 (3), P. 314

2880. Johansen J G
Demonstration of anterior intervertebral disc herniation by CT
Neuroradiology 1987, Vol. 29 (2), P. 214

2881. Jungreis C A, Cohen W A
Spinal cord compression induced by steroid therapy: CT findings
J Comput Assist Tomogr 1987 Mar- Apr, Vol. 11 (2), P. 245–7

2882. Kaftori J K, Kleinhaus U, Naveh Y
Progressive diaphyseal dysplasia Camurati-Engelmann: radiographic follow-up and CT find-
ings
Radiology 1987 Sep, Vol. 164 (3), P. 777–82

2883. Kaiser M C, Pettersson H, Harwood Nash D C, Fitz C R, Armstrong E
Direct coronal CT of the spine in infants and children
AJNR 1981 Sep-Oct, Vol. 2 (5), P. 465–6

2884. Kaiser M C, Capesius P, Ohanna F, Roilgen A
Computed tomography of acute spinal epidural hematoma associated with cervical root avul-
sion
J Comput Assist Tomogr 1984 Apr, Vol. 8 (2), P. 322–3

2885. Kaiser M C, Sandt G, Roilgen A, Capesius P, Poos D, Ohanna F
Intradural disk herniation with CT appearance of gas collection
AJNR 1985 Jan-Feb, Vol. 6 (1), P. 117–8

2886. Kaiser M C, Capesius P, Veiga Pires J A, Bruch J M
Recognition of gas-containing disc herniation on lateral CT- scoutview
Neuroradiology 1987, Vol. 29 (1), P. 98

2887. Kaiser M C, Capesius P, Roilgen A, Sandt G, Poos D, Gratia G
Epidural venous stasis in spinal stenosis. CT appearance
Neuroradiology 1984, Vol. 26 (6), P. 435–8

2888. Kalender W A, Klotz E, Suess C
Vertebral bone mineral analysis: an integrated approach with CT
Radiology 1987 Aug, Vol. 164 (2), P. 419–23

2889. Kalender W A, Brestowsky H, Felsenberg D
Bone mineral measurement: automated determination of midvertebral CT section
Radiology 1988 Jul, Vol. 168 (1), P. 219–21

2890. Kalender W A
Neue Entwicklungen in der Knochendichtemessung mit quantitativer Computertomographie
(QCT)
New developments in bone density measurement by quantitative computer tomography
Radiologe 1988 Apr, Vol. 28 (4), P. 173–8

2891. Kalender W A, Felsenberg D, Louis O, Lopez P, Osteaux M, Fraga J
Reference values for trabecular and cortical vertebral bone density in single and dual-energy
quantitative computed tomography
Europ.J.Radiol.1989, Vol. 9, P. 75–80

2892. Kan S, Fox A J, Vinuela F, Barnett H J, Peerless S J
Delayed CT metrizamide enhancement of syringomyelia secondary to tumor
AJNR 1983 Jan-Feb, Vol. 4 (1), P. 73–8

2893. Kapila A, Lines M
Neuropathic spinal arthropathy: CT and MR findings
J Comput Assist Tomogr 1987 Jul-Aug, Vol. 11 (4), P. 736–9

2894. Karnaze M G, Gado M H, Sartor K J, Hodges F J
Comparison of MR and CT myelography in imaging the cervical and thoracic spine
Am J Roentgenol 1988 Feb, Vol. 150 (2), P. 397–403

2895. Kattapuram S V, Phillips W C, Boyd R
CT in pyogenic osteomyelitis of the spine
Am J Roentgenol 1983 Jun, Vol. 140 (6), P. 1199–201

2896. Kattapuram S V, Rosenthal D I
Percutaneous biopsy of the cervical spine using CT guidance
Am J Roentgenol 1987 Sep, Vol. 149 (3), P. 539–41

2897. Kerr R, Resnick D, Pineda C
CT analysis of proximal femoral trabecular pattern simulating skeletal pathology
J Comput Assist Tomogr 1988 Mar-Apr, Vol. 12 (2), P. 227–30

2898. Ketonen L, Gyldensted C
Lumbar disc disease evaluated by myelography and postmyelography spinal computed tomo-
graphy
Neuroradiology 1986, Vol. 28 (2), P. 144–9

2899. Kieft G J, Bloem J L, Rozing P M, Obermann W R
MR imaging of recurrent anterior dislocation of the shoulder: comparison with CT arthro-
graphy
Am J Roentgenol 1988 May, Vol. 150 (5), P. 1083–7

2900. Kilcoyne R F, Mack L A, King H A, Ratcliffe S S, Loop J W
Thoracolumbar spine injuries associated with vertical plunges: reappraisal with computed tomo-
graphy
Radiology 1983 Jan, Vol. 146 (1), P. 137–40

2901. Kish K K, Wilner H I
Spondylolysis of C2: CT and plain film findings
J Comput Assist Tomogr 1983 Jun, Vol. 7 (3), P. 517–8

2902. Klein J, Sumner T E, Volberg F M, Orbon R J
Combined CT-arthrography in recurrent traumatic hip dislocation
Am J Roentgenol 1982 May, Vol. 138 (5), P. 963–4

2903. Knudsen L L, Voldby B, Stagaard M
Computed tomographic myelography in spinal subdural empyema
Neuroradiology 1987, Vol. 29 (1), P. 99

2904. Kock C
Sagittale Weiten des zervikalen Wirbelkanales im Computertomogramm
Sagittal widths of the cervical spinal canal in the computerized tomogram
Radiologe 1986 May, Vol. 26 (5), P. 239–41

2905. Kolin J, Kolar J
Posterior lumbar apophyseal ring fracture simulating a mass lesion in computed tomograms
RÖFO 1989 Jul, Vol. 151 (1), P. 114–5

2906. Konig H, Majer M, Konermann M, Sell S
Möglichkeiten der hochauflösenden Nativ-Computertomographie für die Meniskusdiagnostik
Potentials of high-resolution native computed tomography in meniscal diagnosis
RÖFO 1989 Jan, Vol. 150 (1), P. 39–43

2907. Kopecky K K, Gilmor R L, Scott J A, Edwards M K
Pitfalls of computed tomography in diagnosis of discitis
Neuroradiology 1985, Vol. 27 (1), P. 57–66

2908. Kowalski H M, Cohen W A, Cooper P, Wisoff J H
Pitfalls in the CT diagnosis of atlantoaxial rotary subluxation
Am J Roentgenol 1987 Sep, Vol. 149 (3), P. 595–600

2909. Krause P, Hedtler W
Morphometrischer Ansatz zur Beurteilung des Fersenbeines im Computertomogramm
Morphometric approach to the assessment of the heel bone in the computed tomogram
RÖFO 1990 Mar, Vol. 152 (3), P. 303–6

2910. Kreitner K F, Lehmann M, Zapf S, Wenda K, Schild H H
Möglichkeiten der CT-Arthrographie in der Diagnostik von Schulterinstabilitäten
CT arthrography in the diagnosis of shoulder instability
RÖFO 1990 Nov, Vol. 153 (5), P. 510–5

2911. Krol G, Khomeini R, Deck M F
CT of the spine
Neuroradiology 1978, Vol. 16, P. 362–3

2912. Krol G, Sundaresan N, Deck M
Computed tomography of axial chordomas
J Comput Assist Tomogr 1983 Apr, Vol. 7 (2), P. 286–9

2913. Krol G, Sze G, Malkin M, Walker R
MR of cranial and spinal meningeal carcinomatosis: comparison with CT and myelography
Am J Roentgenol 1988 Sep, Vol. 151 (3), P. 583–8

2914. Krone A, Klawki P, Oldenkott P
Zervikale Myelographie mit assistierender Computertomographie. Indikation, Durchführung und Ergebnisse
Cervical myelography with supplemental computer tomography. Indications, execution and results
RÖFO 1982 Nov, Vol. 137 (5), P. 530–4

2915. Kuckein D, Walter K, Paal G
Computertomographischer Nachweis einer intraspinalen Arachnoidalzyste
Computerized tomography of an intraspinal arachnoid cyst
RÖFO 1981 Mar, Vol. 134 (3), P. 323–4

2916. Kuhlman J E, Fishman E K, Magid D, Scott W W Jr, Brooker A F, Siegelman S S
Fracture nonunion: CT assessment with multiplanar reconstruction
Radiology 1988 May, Vol. 167 (2), P. 483–8

2917. Kuhn J P, Berger P E
Computed tomographic diagnosis of osteomyelitis
Radiology 1979 Feb, Vol. 130 (2), P. 503–6

2918. Kumar R, Roper P R, Guinto F C Jr
Subcutaneous ossification of the legs in chronic venous stasis
J Comput Assist Tomogr 1983 Apr, Vol. 7 (2), P. 377–8

2919. Kurokawa H, Miura S, Goto T
Ecchordosis physaliphora arising from the cervical vertebra, the CT and MRI appearance
Neuroradiology 1988, Vol. 30 (1), P. 81–3

2920. Laasonen E M, Lahdenranta U
Lipomembranous polycystic osteodysplasia with progressive dementia
J Comput Assist Tomogr 1981 Aug, Vol. 5 (4), P. 580–2

2921. Laasonen E M, Kankaanpaa U, Paukku P, Sandelin J, Servo A, Slatis P
Computed tomographic myelography CTM in atlanto-axial rheumatoid arthritis
Neuroradiology 1985, Vol. 27 (2), P. 119–22

2922. LaBerge J M, Brant Zawadzki M
Evaluation of Pott's disease with computed tomography
Neuroradiology 1984, Vol. 26 (6), P. 429–34

2923. Lackner K, Schroeder S, Koster O
Quantitative Auswertung, Indikationen und Wertigkeit der Computertomographie der Lendenwirbelsäule
Quantitative evaluation, indications and value of computer tomography of the lumbar spine
RÖFO 1982 Sep, Vol. 137 (3), P. 309–15

2924. Lackner K, Schroeder S, Koster O
Computertomographische Beurteilung der freien Fettplastik nach Laminektomie
Computer tomographic evaluation of free fatty tissue grafts following laminectomy
RÖFO 1982 Jun, Vol. 136 (6), P. 744–5

2925. Lafferty C M, Sartoris D J, Tyson R, Resnick D, Kursunoglu S, Pate D, Sutherland D
Acetabular alterations in untreated congenital dysplasia of the hip: computed tomography with multiplanar re-formation and three- dimensional analysis
J Comput Assist Tomogr 1986 Jan-Feb, Vol. 10 (1), P. 84–91

2926. Lambiase R, Sartoris D J, Fellingham L, Andre M, Resnick D
Vertebral mineral status: assessment with single- versus multi- section CT
Radiology 1987 Jul, Vol. 164 (1), P. 221–6

2927. Landman J A, Hoffman J C Jr, Braun I F, Barrow D L
Value of computed tomographic myelography in the recognition of cervical herniated disk
AJNR 1984 Jul-Aug, Vol. 5 (4), P. 391–4

2928. Lang P, Genant H K, Steiger P, Chafetz N, Morris J M
Dreidimensionale Computertomographie und multiplanare CT- Reformationen bei lumbalen Spondylodesen
3-dimensional computed tomography and multiplanar CT-reformations in lumbar spondylodesis
RÖFO 1988 May, Vol. 148 (5), P. 524–9

2929. Lang P, Steiger P, Genant H K, Chafetz N, Lindquist T, Skinner S, Moore S
Three-dimensional CT and MR imaging in congenital dislocation of the hip: clinical and technical considerations
J Comput Assist Tomogr 1988 May-Jun, Vol. 12 (3), P. 459–64

2930. Lange T A, Alter A J Jr
Evaluation of complex acetabular fractures by computed tomography
J Comput Assist Tomogr 1980 Dec, Vol. 4 (6), P. 849–52

2931. Langston J W, Gavant M L
"Incomplete ring" sign: a simple method for CT detection of spondylolysis
J Comput Assist Tomogr 1985 Jul-Aug, Vol. 9 (4), P. 728–9

2932. Lanzieri C F, Hilal S K
Computed tomography of the sacral plexus and sciatic nerve in the greater sciatic foramen
Am J Roentgenol 1984 Jul, Vol. 143 (1), P. 165–8

2933. Lanzieri C F, Sacher M, Solodnik P, Moser F
CT myelography of spontaneous spinal epidural hematoma
J Comput Assist Tomogr 1985 Mar-Apr, Vol. 9 (2), P. 393–4

2934. Lapointe J S, Graeb D A, Nugent R A, Robertson W D
Value of intravenous contrast enhancement in the CT evaluation of intraspinal tumors
Am J Roentgenol 1986 Jan, Vol. 146 (1), P. 103–7

2935. Larde D, Mathieu D, Frija J, Gaston A, Vasile N
Spinal vacuum phenomenon: CT diagnosis and significance
J Comput Assist Tomogr 1982 Aug, Vol. 6 (4), P. 671–6

2936. Larde D, Mathieu D, Frija J, Gaston A, Vasile N
Vertebral osteomyelitis: disk hypodensity on CT
Am J Roentgenol 1982 Nov, Vol. 139 (5), P. 963–7

2937. Laros G S, Leo J S
Role of diskography after negative postmyelography CT scans letter
AJNR 1988 Nov-Dec, Vol. 9 (6), P. 1244

2938. Latack J T, Gabrielsen T O, Knake J E, Gebarski S S, Dorovini Zis K
Computed tomography of spinal cord necrosis from multiple sclerosis
AJNR 1984 Jul-Aug, Vol. 5 (4), P. 485–7

2939. Lauten G J, Wehunt W D
Computed tomography in absent cervical pedicle
AJNR 1980 Mar-Apr, Vol. 1 (2), P. 201–3

2940. Laval Jeantet A M, Roger B, Bouysee S, Bergot C, Mazess R B
Influence of vertebral fat content on quantitative CT density
Radiology 1986 May, Vol. 159 (2), P. 463–6

2941. Lawson T L, Foley W D, Carrera G F, Berland L L
The sacroiliac joints: anatomic, plain roentgenographic, and computed tomographic analysis
J Comput Assist Tomogr 1982 Apr, Vol. 6 (2), P. 307–14

2942. Le Minor J M, Rosset P, Favard L, Burdin P
Fracture of the anterior arch of the atlas associated with a congenital cleft of the posterior arch. Demonstration by CT
Neuroradiology 1988, Vol. 30 (5), P. 444–6

2943. Lecklitner M L, Potter J L, Growcock G
Computed tomography in acquired absence of thoracic pedicle
J Comput Assist Tomogr 1985 Mar-Apr, Vol. 9 (2), P. 395–7

2944. Lee B C, Kazam E, Newman A D
Computed tomography of the spine and spinal cord
Radiology 1978 Jul, Vol. 128 (1), P. 95–102

2945. Lee J K, McClennan B L, Stanley R J, Sagel S S
Utility of computed tomography in the localization of the undescended testis
Radiology 1980 Apr, Vol. 135 (1), P. 121–5

2946. Lee K R, Cox G G, Neff J R, Arnett G R, Murphey M D
Cystic masses of the knee: arthrographic and CT evaluation
Am J Roentgenol 1987 Feb, Vol. 148 (2), P. 329–34

2947. Lee Y Y, Van Tassel P, Nauert C, Raymond A K, Edeiken J
Craniofacial osteosarcomas: plain film, CT, and MR findings in 46 cases
Am J Roentgenol 1988 Jun, Vol. 150 (6), P. 1397–402

2948. Lee Y Y, Van Tassel P
Craniofacial chondrosarcomas: imaging findings in 15 untreated cases
AJNR 1989 Jan-Feb, Vol. 10 (1), P. 165–70

2949. Leehey P, Naseem M, Every P, Russell E, Sarwar M
Vertebral hemangioma with compression myelopathy: metrizamide CT demonstration
J Comput Assist Tomogr 1985 Sep-Oct, Vol. 9 (5), P. 985–6

2950. Leemans J, Deboeck M, Claes H, Boven F, Potvliege R
Computed tomography of ununited neurocentral synchondrosis in the cervical spine
J Comput Assist Tomogr 1984 Jun, Vol. 8 (3), P. 540–3

2951. Lefkowitz D M, Quencer R M
Vacuum facet phenomenon: a computed tomographic sign of degenerative spondylolisthesis
Radiology 1982 Aug, Vol. 144 (3), P. 562

2952. Lehner K, Reiser M, Hawe W, Smasal V
Die Defekte der Patellarückfläche im CT-Arthrogramm. Nachweis und Differentialdiagnose
Posterior defects of the patella on CT arthrograms. Detection and differential diagnosis
RÖFO 1986 Jan, Vol. 144 (1), P. 95–9

2953. Leonardi M, Biasizzo E, Fabris G, Penco T, Bertolissi D
CT evaluation of the lumbosacral spine
AJNR 1983 May-Jun, Vol. 4 (3), P. 846–7

2954. Levitan L H, Wiens C W
Chronic lumbar extradural hematoma: CT findings
Radiology 1983 Sep, Vol. 148 (3), P. 707–8

2955. Lewis C A, Castillo M, Hudgins P A
Cervical prevertebral fat stripe: a normal variant simulating prevertebral hemorrhage
Am J Roentgenol 1990 Sep, Vol. 155 (3), P. 559–60

2956. Li Y P, Srikantaswamy S, Zweig G, Chiu S, Guico R
Computed tomography of cervical epidermoid cysts
J Comput Assist Tomogr 1989 Jan-Feb, Vol. 13 (1), P. 164–6

2957. Lin Greenberg A, Cholankeril J
Vertebral arch destruction in tuberculosis: CT features
J Comput Assist Tomogr 1990 Mar-Apr, Vol. 14 (2), P. 300–2

2958. Lingg G, Hering L
Computertomographie der Chondropathia patellae. Experimentelle und klinische Ergebnisse
Computed tomography of patellar chondropathy. Experimental and clinical results
RÖFO 1983 Dec, Vol. 139 (6), P. 663–8

2959. Lochner B, Grumme T, Claussen C
Computertomographische Diagnostik einer Pseudomeningozele nach lumbaler Bandscheibenoperation
Computer tomographic diagnosis of pseudomeningocele after lumbar intervertebral disk operations
RÖFO 1982 Aug, Vol. 137 (2), P. 224–4

2960. Lusins J O, Danielski E J Jr
Lumbar arteriovenous malformation presenting as an acute disc syndrome: CT findings
J Comput Assist Tomogr 1984 Oct, Vol. 8 (5), P. 1028–9

2961. Mack L A, Harley J D, Winquist R A
CT of acetabular fractures: analysis of fracture patterns
Am J Roentgenol 1982 Mar, Vol. 138 (3), P. 407–12

2962. Mack L A, Duesdieker G A, Harley J D, Bach A W, Winquist R A
CT of acetabular fractures: postoperative appearances Am J Roentgenol 1983 Nov, Vol. 141 (5), P. 891–4

2963. Mafee M F, Folk E R, Langer B G, Miller M T, Lagouros P, Mittleman D
Computed tomography in the evaluation of Brown syndrome of the superior oblique tendon sheath
Radiology 1985 Mar, Vol. 154 (3), P. 691–5

2964. Magid D, Fishman E K, Brooker A F Jr, Mandelbaum B R, Siegelman S S
Multiplanar computed tomography of acetabular fractures
J Comput Assist Tomogr 1986 Sep-Oct, Vol. 10 (5), P. 778–83

2965. Magid D, Michelson J D, Ney D R, Fishman E K
Adult ankle fractures: comparison of plain films and interactive two- and three-dimensional CT scans
Am J Roentgenol 1990 May, Vol. 154 (5), P. 1017–23

2966. Magid D, Fishman E K, Ney D R
Sacral foramina: view at CT
Radiology 1991 Feb, Vol. 178 (2), P. 573–4

2967. Mahboubi S, Horstmann H
Femoral torsion: CT measurement
Radiology 1986 Sep, Vol. 160 (3), P. 843–4

2968. Mahoney M C, Shipley R T, Corcoran H L, Dickson B A
CT demonstration of calcification in carcinoma of the lung
Am J Roentgenol 1990 Feb, Vol. 154 (2), P. 255–8

2969. Manaster B J, Osborn A G
CT patterns of facet fracture dislocations in the thoracolumbar region
Am J Roentgenol 1987 Feb, Vol. 148 (2), P. 335–40

2970. Manco L G, Lozman J, Coleman N D, Kavanaugh J H, Bilfield B S, Dougherty J
Noninvasive evaluation of knee meniscal tears: preliminary comparison of MR imaging and CT
Radiology 1987 Jun, Vol. 163 (3), P. 727–30

2971. Manco L G, Berlow M E, Czajka J, Alfred R
Bucket-handle tears of the meniscus: appearance at CT
Radiology 1988 Sep, Vol. 168 (3), P. 709–12

2972. Mann F A, Gilula L A
Direct sagittal CT of the foot letter
Am J Roentgenol 1989 Oct, Vol. 153 (4), P. 886

2973. Maravilla K R, Lesh P, Weinreb J C, Selby D K, Mooney V
Magnetic resonance imaging of the lumbar spine with CT correlation
AJNR 1985 Mar-Apr, Vol. 6 (2), P. 237–45

2974. Marin M L, Austin J H, Markowitz A M
Elastofibroma dorsi: CT demonstration
J Comput Assist Tomogr 1987 Jul-Aug, Vol. 11 (4), P. 675–7

2975. Marincek B, Porcellini B, Robotti G
Computertomographische Klassifikation von Acetabulumfrakturen
Computed tomographic classification of acetabular fractures
Radiologe 1984 May, Vol. 24 (5), P. 205–10

2976. Martinez S, Korobkin M, Fondren F B, Goldner J L
A device for computed tomography of the patellofemoral joint
Am J Roentgenol 1983 Feb, Vol. 140 (2), P. 400–1

2977. Matozzi F, Moreau J J, Jiddane M, Beranger M, Ito T, Nazarian S, Gambarelli J, Michotey P, Raybaud C, Salamon G
Correlative anatomic and CT study of the lumbar lateral recess
AJNR 1983 May-Jun, Vol. 4 (3), P. 650–2

2978. Mawad M E, Hilal S K, Fetell M R, Silver A J, Ganti S R, Sane P
Patterns of spinal cord atrophy by metrizamide CT
AJNR 1983 May-Jun, Vol. 4 (3), P. 611–3

2979. Mayr B, Siuda S, Will A, Frenzl G, Habermeier P
Pneumarthro-Computertomographie in der Diagnostik von rezidivierenden Luxationen und Instabilitäten der Schulter
Pneumarthro-computed tomography in the diagnosis of recurring luxations and instabilities of the shoulder
RÖFO 1991 Jan, Vol. 154 (1), P. 81–6

2980. McGahan J P, Graves D S, Palmer P E, Stadalnik R C, Dublin A B
Classic and contemporary imaging of coccidioidomycosis
Am J Roentgenol 1981 Feb, Vol. 136 (2), P. 393–404

2981. McNiesh L M, Callaghan J J
CT arthrography of the shoulder: variations of the glenoid labrum
Am J Roentgenol 1987 Nov, Vol. 149 (5), P. 963–6

2982. Mehta R C, Wilson M A, Perlman S B
False-negative bone scan in extensive metastatic disease: CT and MR findings
J Comput Assist Tomogr 1989 Jul-Aug, Vol. 13 (4), P. 717–9

2983. Mercader J, Munoz Gomez J, Cardenal C
Intraspinal synovial cyst: diagnosis by CT. Follow-up and spontaneous remission
Neuroradiology 1985, Vol. 27 (4), P. 346–8

2984. Merine D, Wang H, Kumar A J, Zinreich S J, Rosenbaum A E
CT myelography and MR imaging of acute transverse myelitis
J Comput Assist Tomogr 1987 Jul-Aug, Vol. 11 (4), P. 606–8

2985. Merine D, Fishman E K, Magid D
CT detection of sacral osteomyelitis associated with pelvic abscesses
J Comput Assist Tomogr 1988 Jan-Feb, Vol. 12 (1), P. 118–21

2986. Merine D, Fishman E K
Hemangioendothelioma of bone: CT findings
J Comput Assist Tomogr 1989 Nov-Dec, Vol. 13 (6), P. 1098–100

2987. Mesgarzadeh M, Revesz G, Bonakdarpour A
Femoral neck torsion angle measurement by computed tomography
J Comput Assist Tomogr 1987 Sep-Oct, Vol. 11 (5), P. 799–803

2988. Meyer J D, Latchaw R E, Roppolo H M, Ghoshhajra K, Deeb Z L
Computed tomography and myelography of the postoperative lumbar spine
AJNR 1982 May-Jun, Vol. 3 (3), P. 223–8

2989. Miller J D, Grace M G, Lampard R
Computed tomography of the upper cervical spine in Down syndrome
J Comput Assist Tomogr 1986 Jul-Aug, Vol. 10 (4), P. 589–92

2990. Mitchell D G, Kressel H Y, Arger P H, Dalinka M, Spritzer C E, Steinberg M E
Avascular necrosis of the femoral head: morphologic assessment by MR imaging, with CT correlation
Radiology 1986 Dec, Vol. 161 (3), P. 739–42

2991. Miyasaka K, Isu T, Iwasaki Y, Abe S, Takei H, Tsuru M
High resolution computed tomography in the diagnosis of cervical disc disease
Neuroradiology 1983, Vol. 24 (5), P. 253–7

2992. Montag M, Doren M, Meyer Galander H M, Montag T, Peters P E
Computertomographisch bestimmter Mineralgehalt in der LWS-Spongiosa. Normwerte für gesunde perimenopausale Frauen und Vergleich dieser Werte mit der mechanischen Wirbelsäulenbelastung
Mineral content of the spongiosa of the lumbar spine determined by computer tomography. Normal values for healthy perimenopausal women and their relation to mechanical stress of the vertebral column
Radiologe 1988 Apr, Vol. 28 (4), P. 161–5

2993. Montag M, Roos N, Peters P E
Wirbelkörperläsionen als Störfaktor bei der quantitativen Computertomographie der Lendenwirbelsäule. Eine Analyse von 1166 standardisiert durchgeführten Messungen
Vertebral body lesions as an interference factor in quantitative computed tomography of the lumbar spine. An analysis of 1116 standardized performed measurements
RÖFO 1989 Sep, Vol. 151 (3), P. 317–21

2994. Montana M A, Richardson M L, Kilcoyne R F, Harley J D, Shuman W P, Mack L A
CT of sacral injury
Radiology 1986 Nov, Vol. 161 (2), P. 499–503

2995. Mostrom U, Ytterbergh C
Reliability of attenuation measurements in CT of the lumbar spine: evaluation with an anthropomorphic phantom
J Comput Assist Tomogr 1988 May-Jun, Vol. 12 (3), P. 474–81

2996. Muller H A, Sachsenheimer W, van Kaick G
Die Wertigkeit der CT bei der präoperativen Diagnostik von Bandscheibenvorfällen
The value of CT in the pre-operative diagnosis of disc prolapse
RÖFO 1981 Nov, Vol. 135 (5), P. 535–40

2997. Muraki A S, Mancuso A A, Harnsberger H R
Metastatic cervical adenopathy from tumors of unknown origin: the role of CT
Radiology 1984 Sep, Vol. 152 (3), P. 749–53

2998. Nagashima C, Yamaguchi T, Tsuji R
Arteriovenous malformation of the spinal cord: computed tomography with intraarterial enhancement
J Comput Assist Tomogr 1981 Aug, Vol. 5 (4), P. 586–7

2999. Naidich T P, King D G, Moran C J, Sagel S S
Computed tomography of the lumbar thecal sac
J Comput Assist Tomogr 1980 Feb, Vol. 4 (1), P. 37–41

3000. Naidich T P, Harwood Nash D C
Diastematomyelia: hemicord and meningeal sheaths; single and double arachnoid and dural tubes
AJNR 1983 May-Jun, Vol. 4 (3), P. 633–6

3001. Nakada T, Kwee I L, Palmaz J C
Computed tomography of spinal cord atrophy
Neuroradiology 1982, Vol. 24 (2), P. 97–9

3002. Nakagawa H, Huang Y P, Malis L I, Wolf B S
Computed tomography of intraspinal and paraspinal neoplasms
J Comput Assist Tomogr 1977 Oct, Vol. 1 (4), P. 377–90

3003. Nakagawa H, Okumura T, Sugiyama T, Iwata K
Discrepancy between metrizamide CT and myelography in diagnosis of cervical disk protrusions
AJNR 1983 May-Jun, Vol. 4 (3), P. 604–6

3004. Nebel G, Lingg G, Reid W
Diagnostische Möglichkeiten mit der Computertomographie bei Koxopathien. Paget-Koxopathie, Femurkopfnekrose, Koxarthrose, Koxarthritis
Diagnostic possibilities of computer tomography in hip joint diseases. Paget's disease, femur head necrosis, coxarthrosis, coxarthritis
RÖFO 1982 Oct, Vol. 137 (4), P. 363–71

3005. Nepper Rasmussen J
CT of dens axis fractures
Neuroradiology 1989, Vol. 31 (1), P. 104–6

3006. Nesbit D, Levine E, Neff J R
Direct longitudinal computed tomography of the forearm
J Comput Assist Tomogr 1981 Feb, Vol. 5 (1), P. 144–6

3007. Nickoloff E L, Feldman F, Atherton J V
Bone mineral assessment: new dual-energy CT approach
Radiology 1988 Jul, Vol. 168 (1), P. 223–8

3008. Nijboer E W, Penning L
Hypertrophic anterior tubercles of C5 and C6 on CT
Neuroradiology 1987, Vol. 29 (1), P. 78–80

3009. Nijensohn E, Russell E J, Milan M, Brown T
Calcified synovial cyst of the cervical spine: CT and MR evaluation
J Comput Assist Tomogr 1990 May-Jun, Vol. 14 (3), P. 473–6

3010. Novetsky G J, Berlin L, Epstein A J, Lobo N, Miller S H
The extraforaminal herniated disc: detection by computed tomography
AJNR 1982 Nov-Dec, Vol. 3 (6), P. 653–5

3011. Nutz V, von Uexkull Guldenband
Computertomographische Untersuchungen der Frakturheilung
Computed tomographic studies of fracture healing
RÖFO 1988 Oct, Vol. 149 (4), P. 396–401

3012. Nyberg D A, Jeffrey R B, Brant Zawadzki M, Federle M, Dillon W
Computed tomography of cervical infections
J Comput Assist Tomogr 1985 Mar-Apr, Vol. 9 (2), P. 288–96

3013. O Callaghan J P, Ullrich C G, Yuan H A, Kieffer S A
CT of facet distraction in flexion injuries of the thoracolumbar spine: the "naked" facet
Am J Roentgenol 1980 Mar, Vol. 134 (3), P. 563–8

3014. Oesterreich F U, Heller M, Triebel H J, Kruse H P
Morphologie der Osteodystrophia deformans Paget im Computertomogramm
Morphology of Paget's osteodystrophia deformans in the computed tomogram
RÖFO 1988 Dec, Vol. 149 (6), P. 603–8

3015. Orrison W W, Lilleas F G
CT demonstration of gas in a herniated nucleus pulposus
J Comput Assist Tomogr 1982 Aug, Vol. 6 (4), P. 807–8

3016. Orrison W W, Johansen J G, Eldevik O P, Haughton V M
Optimal computed-tomographic techniques for cervical spine imaging
Radiology 1982 Jul, Vol. 144 (1), P. 180–2

3017. Ortore P G, Bonatti G P, Gostner P
Ungewöhnliches computertomographisches Bild einer Kolloidzyste des 3. Ventrikels
Unusual computed tomographic picture of a colloid cyst of the 3d ventricle
RÖFO 1984 Nov, Vol. 141 (5), P. 588–9

3018. Osborn A G, Hood R S, Sherry R G, Smoker W R, Harnsberger H R
CT/MR spectrum of far lateral and anterior lumbosacral disk herniations
AJNR 1988 Jul-Aug, Vol. 9 (4), P. 775–8

3019. Osborne D, Triolo P, Dubois P, Drayer B, Heinz E
Assessment of craniocervical junction and atlantoaxial relation using metrizamide-enhanced CT in flexion and extension
AJNR 1983 May-Jun, Vol. 4 (3), P. 843–5

3020. Pan G, Shirkhoda A
Pelvic exenteration: role of CT in follow-up
Radiology 1987 Sep, Vol. 164 (3), P. 665–70

3021. Passariello R, Trecco F, De Paulis F, Bonanni G, Masciocchi C, Zobel B B
Computed tomography of the knee joint: technique of study and normal anatomy
J Comput Assist Tomogr 1983 Dec, Vol. 7 (6), P. 1035–42

3022. Passariello R, Trecco F, de Paulis F, Masciocchi C, Bonanni G, Zobel B B
Meniscal lesions of the knee joint: diagnosis
Radiology 1985 Oct, Vol. 157 (1), P. 29–34

3023. Passariello R, Trecco F, De Paulis F, Masciocchi C, Bonanni G, Beomonte Zobel B
CT demonstration of capsuloligamentous lesions of the knee joint
J Comput Assist Tomogr 1986 May-Jun, Vol. 10 (3), P. 450–6

3024. Pastakia B, Herdt J R
Radiolucent "zones" in parietal bones seen on computed tomography: a normal anatomic variant
J Comput Assist Tomogr 1984 Feb, Vol. 8 (1), P. 108–9

3025. Pech P, Kilgore D P, Pojunas K W, Haughton V M
Cervical spinal fractures: CT detection
Radiology 1985 Oct, Vol. 157 (1), P. 117–20

3026. Pennes D R, Jonsson K, Buckwalter K A
Direct coronal CT of the scaphoid bone
Radiology 1989 Jun, Vol. 171 (3), P. 870–1

3027. Pennes D R, Jonsson K, Buckwalter K, Braunstein E, Blasier R, Wojtys E
Computed arthrotomography of the shoulder: comparison of examinations made with internal and external rotation of the humerus
Am J Roentgenol 1989 Nov, Vol. 153 (5), P. 1017–9

3028. Pennes D R
Shoulder joint: arthrographic CT appearance letter
Radiology 1990 Jun, Vol. 175 (3), P. 878–9

3029. Pennisi A K, Davis D O, Wiesel S, Moskovitz P
CT appearance of Candida diskitis
J Comput Assist Tomogr 1985 Nov- Dec, Vol. 9 (6), P. 1050–4

3030. Pettersson H, Harwood Nash D C, Fitz C R, Chuang H S, Armstrong E
Conventional metrizamide myelography MM and computed tomographic metrizamide myelography
CTMM in scoliosis. A comparative study
Radiology 1982 Jan, Vol. 142 (1), P. 111–4

3031. Pfadenhauer K, Ebeling U, Bergleiter R, Stoeter P
Zuverlässigkeit der Computertomographie bei der Diagnostik von Rezidivbeschwerden nach
lumbalen Bandscheibenoperationen
The reliability of computer tomography in the diagnosis of recurrent symptoms after lumbar disc
operations
RÖFO 1983 Aug, Vol. 139 (2), P. 127–31

3032. Plumley T F, Kilcoyne R F, Mack L A
Computed tomography in evaluation of gunshot wounds of the spine
J Comput Assist Tomogr 1983 Apr, Vol. 7 (2), P. 310–2

3033. Pressman B D, Mink J H, Turner R M, Rothman B J
Low-dose metrizamide spinal computed tomography in outpatients
J Comput Assist Tomogr 1986 Sep-Oct, Vol. 10 (5), P. 817–21

3034. Psarras H, Faraj J, Gouliamos A, Kalovidouris A, Vlahos L, Papavassiliou C
Tuberculosis of the spine. CT demonstration of paravertebral abscess
Radiologe 1985 Jul, Vol. 25 (7), P. 339–41

3035. Pullicino P, Kendall B E
Computed tomography of "cystic" intramedullary lesions
Neuroradiology 1982, Vol. 23 (3), P. 117–21

3036. Quinn S F, Murray W, Watkins T, Kloss J
CT for determining the results of treatment of fractures of the wrist
Am J Roentgenol 1987 Jul, Vol. 149 (1), P. 109–11

3037. Quint D J
CT of bilateral cervical spondylolysis letter
Am J Roentgenol 1991 Jan, Vol. 156 (1), P. 200–1

3038. Quiroga O, Matozzi F, Beranger M, Nazarian S, Gambarelli J, Salamon G
Normal CT anatomy of the spine. Anatomo-radiological correlations
Neuroradiology 1982, Vol. 24 (1), P. 1–6

3039. Rafii M, Firooznia H, Golimbu C, Bonamo J
Computed tomography of tibial plateau fractures
Am J Roentgenol 1984 Jun, Vol. 142 (6), P. 1181–6

3040. Rafii M, Firooznia H, Golimbu C, McCauley D I
Hematogenous osteomyelitis with fat-fluid level shown by CT
Radiology 1984 Nov, Vol. 153 (2), P. 493–4

3041. Rafii M, Firooznia H, Golimbu C, Minkoff J, Bonamo J
CT arthrography of capsular structures of the shoulder
Am J Roentgenol 1986 Feb, Vol. 146 (2), P. 361–7

3042. Rafii M, Firooznia H, Bonamo J J, Minkoff J, Golimbu C
Athlete shoulder injuries: CT arthrographic findings
Radiology 1987 Feb, Vol. 162 (2), P. 559–64

3043. Rafii M, Firooznia H, Golimbu C, Horner N
Radiation induced fractures of sacrum: CT diagnosis
J Comput Assist Tomogr 1988 Mar-Apr, Vol. 12 (2), P. 231–5

3044. Raininko R
The value of CT after total block on myelography. Experience with 25 patients
RÖFO 1983 Jan, Vol. 138 (1), P. 61–5

3045. Ram P C, Martinez S, Korobkin M, Breiman R S, Gallis H R, Harrelson J M
CT detection of intraosseous gas: a new sign of osteomyelitis
Am J Roentgenol 1981 Oct, Vol. 137 (4), P. 721–3

3046. Ramirez H Jr, Blatt E S, Cable H F, McComb B L, Zornoza J, Hibri N S
Intraosseous pneumatocysts of the ilium. Findings on radiographs and CT scans
Radiology 1984 Feb, Vol. 150 (2), P. 503–5

3047. Ramirez H Jr, Navarro J E, Bennett W F
"Cupid's bow" contour of the lumbar vertebral endplates detected by computed tomography
J Comput Assist Tomogr 1984 Feb, Vol. 8 (1), P. 121–4

3048. Ramos A, Quintana F, Diez C, Leno C, Berciano J
CT findings in spinocerebellar degeneration
AJNR 1987 Jul-Aug, Vol. 8 (4), P. 635–40

3049. Randall B C, Muraki A S, Osborn R E, Brown F
Epidural lipomatosis with lumbar radiculopathy: CT appearance
J Comput Assist Tomogr 1986 Nov-Dec, Vol. 10 (6), P. 1039–41

3050. Raskin S P
Demonstration of nerve roots on unenhanced computed tomographic scans
J Comput Assist Tomogr 1981 Apr, Vol. 5 (2), P. 281–4

3051. Raskin S P, Keating J W
Recognition of lumbar disk disease: comparison of myelography and computed tomography
Am J Roentgenol 1982 Aug, Vol. 139 (2), P. 349–55

3052. Rauschning W, Bergstrom K, Pech P
Correlative craniospinal anatomy studies by computed tomography and cryomicrotomy
J Comput Assist Tomogr 1983 Feb, Vol. 7 (1), P. 9–13

3053. Reddy S C, Vijayamohan G, Rao G R
Delayed CT myelography in spinal intramedullary metastasis
J Comput Assist Tomogr 1984 Dec, Vol. 8 (6), P. 1182–5

3054. Reede D L, Bergeron R T
Cervical tuberculous adenitis: CT manifestations
Radiology 1985 Mar, Vol. 154 (3), P. 701–4

3055. Reiser M, Rupp N, Karpf P M, Feuerbach S, Paar O
Erfahrungen mit der CT-Arthrographie der Kreuzbänder des Kniegelenkes. Bericht über 512
Untersuchungen
Experience with CT- arthrography of the cruciate ligaments of the knee. Report on 512 exami-
nations
RÖFO 1982 Oct, Vol. 137 (4), P. 372–9

3056. Reiser M, Rupp N
Computertomographie bei Sportverletzungen
Computer tomography of sports injuries
Radiologe 1984 Jan, Vol. 24 (1), P. 40–5

3057. Reiser M, Rupp N, Aigner R, Rimar E, Hipp E, Sommer B
Die Gelenke des Rückfußes im Computertomogramm. Untersuchungen am Amputationspräparat
und klinische Ergebnisse
The joints in the posterior part of the foot in the computed tomogram. Studies on amputation
preparations and clinical observations

RÖFO 1984 Jun, Vol. 140 (6), P. 638–45

3058. Reiser U, Heuck F, Lichtenau L
Untersuchungen der Mineraltopographie am menschlichen Wirbelkörper mit der Röntgen-Com-
puter-Tomographie
Investigations of the mineral topography in human vertebral bodies. A comparison of results derived
from bone- ashing, photodensitometry and attenuation coefficients by CT
Radiologe 1980 Nov, Vol. 20 (11), P. 554–7

3059. Reiser V M, Rupp N, Lehner K, Paar O, Gradinger R, Karpf P M
Die Darstellung der Achillessehne im Computertomogramm. Normalbefunde und pathologische
Veränderungen
Imaging of the Achilles tendon on the computed tomogram. Normal findings and pathological
changes
RÖFO 1985 Aug, Vol. 143 (2), P. 173–7

3060. Reuther G, Mutschler W
Wertigkeit von CT und MRT in der Diagnostik knorpelbildender Tumoren
The value of CT and MRT in the diagnosis of cartilage-forming tumors
RÖFO 1989 Dec, Vol. 151 (6), P. 647–52

3061. Revak C S
Mineral content of cortical bone measured by computed tomography
J Comput Assist Tomogr 1980 Jun, Vol. 4 (3), P. 342–50

3062. Richardson P, Young J W, Porter D
CT detection of cortical fracture of the femoral head associated with posterior hip dislocation
Am J Roentgenol 1990 Jul, Vol. 155 (1), P. 93–4

3063. Rieber A, Brambs H J, Friedl P
CT beim Echinokokkus der LWS und den paravertebralen Strukturen
CT in echinococcosis of the lumbar spine and paravertebral structures
RÖFO 1989 Sep, Vol. 151 (3), P. 379–80

3064. Rieden K, Adolph J, Flentje M, Mende U, Lellig U, zum Winkel K
Indikation und Wertigkeit von Computertomographie und konventioneller Skelettdiagnostik bei
Verdacht auf Knochenmetastasen
Indications for and value of computed tomography and conventional skeletal diagnosis in suspected
bone metastases
RÖFO 1988 May, Vol. 148 (5), P. 505–15

3065. Risius B, Modic M T, Hardy R W Jr, Duchesneau P M, Weinstein M A
Sector computed tomographic spine scanning in the diagnosis of lumbar nerve root entrap-
ment
Radiology 1982 Apr, Vol. 143 (1), P. 109–14

3066. Rodiek S O
Computertomographische Untersuchungen bei zervikaler spinaler Stenose
Computed tomographic studies in cervical spinal stenosis
RÖFO 1983 Oct, Vol. 139 (4), P. 383–8

3067. Roger D J, Richli W R
A CT table attachment for parasagittal scanning of the axilla
Am J Roentgenol 1987 Sep, Vol. 149 (3), P. 555–6

3068. Rosenberg Z S, Feldman F, Singson R D, Price G J
Peroneal tendon injury associated with calcaneal fractures: CT findings
Am J Roentgenol 1987 Jul, Vol. 149 (1), P. 125–9

3069. Rosenbloom S, Cohen W A, Marshall C, Kricheff I I
Imaging factors influencing spine and cord measurements by CT: a phantom study
AJNR 1983 May-Jun, Vol. 4 (3), P. 646–9

3070. Rosenthal D I, Stauffer A E, Davis K R, Ganott M, Taveras J M
Evaluation of multiplanar reconstruction in CT recognition of lumbar disk disease
Am J Roentgenol 1984 Jul, Vol. 143 (1), P. 169–76

3071. Rosenthal D I, Mayo Smith W, Goodsitt M M, Doppelt S, Mankin H J
Bone and bone marrow changes in Gaucher disease: evaluation with quantitative CT
Radiology 1989 Jan, Vol. 170 (1 Pt 1), P. 143–6

3072. Rossier A B, Foo D, Naheedy M H, Wang A M, Rumbaugh C L, Levine H
Radiography of posttraumatic syringomyelia
AJNR 1983 May- Jun, Vol. 4 (3), P. 637–40

3073. Rothman S L, Dobben G D, Rhodes M L, Glenn W V Jr, Azzawi Y M
Computed tomography of the spine: curved coronal reformations from serial images
Radiology 1984 Jan, Vol. 150 (1), P. 185–90

3074. Rovira M, Romero F, Ibarra B, Torrent O
Prolapsed lumbar disk: value of CT in diagnosis
AJNR 1983 May-Jun, Vol. 4 (3), P. 593–4

3075. Ruegsegger P, Anliker M, Dambacher M
Quantification of trabecular bone with low dose computed tomography
J Comput Assist Tomogr 1981 Jun, Vol. 5 (3), P. 384–90

3076. Ruggiero R, Capece W, Del Vecchio E, Palmieri A, Ambrosio A, Calabro A
High resolution CT spinal scanning with Acta 0200 FS
Neuroradiology 1981, Vol. 22 (1), P. 23–5

3077. Ruscalleda J, Rovira A, Guardia E, de Juan M
Short review of CT in the study of some intraspinal diseases
Neuroradiology 1984, Vol. 26 (4), P. 421–7

3078. Russell E J, D Angelo C M, Zimmerman R D, Czervionke L F, Huckman M S
Cervical disk herniation: CT demonstration after contrast enhancement
Radiology 1984 Sep, Vol. 152 (3), P. 703–12

3079. Ryan R W, Lally J F, Kozic Z
Asymptomatic calcified herniated thoracic disks: CT recognition
AJNR 1988 Mar-Apr, Vol. 9 (2), P. 363–6

3080. Salamon O, Freilich M D
Calcified hemangioma of the spinal canal: unusual CT and MR presentation
AJNR 1988 Jul-Aug, Vol. 9 (4), P. 799–802

3081. Sarno R C, Carter B L, Bankoff M S, Semine M C
Computed tomography in tarsal coalition
J Comput Assist Tomogr 1984 Dec, Vol. 8 (6), P. 1155–60

3082. Sartor K
Computertomographie bei spinalen Tumoren
Computer tomography for spinal tumours
RÖFO 1980 Apr, Vol. 132 (4), P. 391–8

3083. Sartor K
Computertomographie bei Verletzungen der Halswirbelsäule und der oberen Brustwirbelsäule
Computed tomography after injuries of the cervical and upper thoracic spine
RÖFO 1980 Feb, Vol. 132 (2), P. 132–8

3084. Sartor K
Spinale Compoutertomographie. Neue Perspektiven in der Diagnostik der Wirbelsäule und des
Rückenmarks
Spinal computed tomography. New perspectives in the diagnosis of the spine and spinal cord
Radiologe 1980 Oct, Vol. 20 (10), P. 485–93

3085. Sartoris D J, Kursunoglu S, Pineda C, Kerr R, Pate D, Resnick D
Detection of intra-articular osteochondral bodies in the knee using computed arthrotomography
Radiology 1985 May, Vol. 155 (2), P. 447–50

3086. Sartoris D J, Andre M, Resnik C S, Resnick D, Resnick C corrected to Resnik C S
Trabecular bone density in the proximal femur: quantitative CT assessment. Work in progress
published erratum appears in Radiology 1986 Dec; 1613:855
Radiology 1986 Sep, Vol. 160 (3), P. 707–12

3087. Sauser D D, Billimoria P E, Rouse G A, Mudge K
CT evaluation of hip trauma
Am J Roentgenol 1980 Aug, Vol. 135 (2), P. 269–74

3088. Schick R M, Humphrey C C, Wang A M, Brooks M L, Rumbaugh C L
CT guided lateral C1-C2 puncture
J Comput Assist Tomogr 1988 Jul-Aug, Vol. 12 (4), P. 715–6

3089. Schild H, Muller H A, Menke W
Computertomographie nach Tibiamarknagelung
Computer tomography after medullary nailing of the tibia
RÖFO 1982 Nov, Vol. 137 (5), P. 554–60

3090. Schild H, Muller H A, Menke W
Die Tibiakopffraktur – eine CT-Indikation?
Fractures of the head of the tibia – an indication for CT?
RÖFO 1983 Aug, Vol. 139 (2), P. 135–42

3091. Schipper J, Kardaun J W, Braakman R, van Dongen K J, Blaauw G
Lumbar disk herniation: diagnosis with CT or myelography
Radiology 1987 Oct, Vol. 165 (1), P. 227–31

3092. Schmitt R, Schindler G, Gay B, Brendel H, Riemenschneider J
Computertomographische Diagnostik bei Azetabulumfrakturen
Computerized tomography diagnosis of acetabulum fractures
RÖFO 1987 Jun, Vol. 146 (6), P. 628–35

3093. Schmitt W G, Mahmalat M O, Beyer H K
Die Meßgenauigkeit der computertomographischen Densitometrie in der Nachbarschaft des Beckenskeletts
Accuracy of computed tomographic densitometry in the neighborhood of the pelvic bones
RÖFO 1987 Jan, Vol. 146 (1), P. 34–8

3094. Schneider P, Borner W
Vergleichende Messung des Knochenmineralgehalts mit DPA und DPX – Erste klinische Erfahrungen
Comparative measurement of bone mineral content using DPA and DPX – initial clinical experiences
letter
RÖFO 1991 Jan, Vol. 154 (1), P. 123–5

3095. Schoter I, Wappenschmidt J
Die intraspinale Raumforderung im computerassistierten Myelogramm (CAM)
Computer assisted myelography in the investigation of intraspinal space-occupying lesions
RÖFO 1980 Nov, Vol. 133 (5), P. 527–30

3096. Schratter M
CT-gezielte, perkutane Biopsie in der Orthopädie. Indikationen – Planung – Technik – eigene Erfahrungen, unter besonderer Berücksichtigung des Achsenskeletts
CT-guided percutaneous biopsy in orthopedics. Indications – planning – technic – personal experiences, with special reference to the spine
Radiologe 1990 May, Vol. 30 (5), P. 201–13

3097. Schrijvers A, Sauerwein W, Lohr E
Wertigkeit der Computertomographie bei der Diagnostik von Tumoren und entzündlichen Prozessen des knöchernen Beckens
Value of computer tomography in the diagnosis of tumors and inflammatory changes in the pelvis
Radiologe 1983 Nov, Vol. 23 (11), P. 512–7

3098. Schubiger O, Valavanis A
CT differentiation between recurrent disc herniation and postoperative scar formation: the value of contrast enhancement
Neuroradiology 1982, Vol. 22 (5), P. 251–4

3099. Schubiger O, Valavanis A
Postoperative lumbar CT: technique, results, and indications
AJNR 1983 May-Jun, Vol. 4 (3), P. 595–7

3100. Schubiger O, Valavanis A, Hollmann J
Computed tomography of the intervertebral foramen
Neuroradiology 1984, Vol. 26 (6), P. 439–44

3101. Schuler M, Naegele M, Lienemann A, Munch O, Siuda S, Hahn D, Lissner J
Die Wertigkeit der hochauflösenden CT und der Kernspintomographie im Vergleich zu den Standardverfahren bei der Diagnostik von Meniskusläsionen
Value of high-resolution CT and nuclear magnetic resonance tomography compared to the standard procedures in the diagnosis of meniscal lesions
RÖFO 1987 Apr, Vol. 146 (4), P. 391–7

3102. Schumacher M, Fischer R, Thoden U
CT- Verlaufsuntersuchungen bei konservativ behandelten lumbalen Bandscheibenvorfällen
CT follow-up studies of conservatively treated lumbar intervertebral disk herniation
Radiologe 1990 Oct, Vol. 30 (10), P. 492–6

3103. Schweitzer M E, Felsberg G, Bardfeld P
CT of hyoid osteomyelitis letter
Am J Roentgenol 1989 Aug, Vol. 153 (2), P. 432–3

3104. Scotti G, Harwood Nash D C, Hoffman H J
Congenital thoracic dermal sinus: diagnosis by computer assisted metrizamide myelography
J Comput Assist Tomogr 1980 Oct, Vol. 4 (5), P. 675–7

3105. Scotti G, Harwood Nash D C
Computed tomography of rhabdomyosarcomas of the skull base in children
J Comput Assist Tomogr 1982 Feb, Vol. 6 (1), P. 33–9

3106. Scotti G, Scialfa G, Pieralli S, Boccardi E, Valsecchi F, Tonon C
Myelopathy and radiculopathy due to cervical spondylosis: myelographic-CT correlations
AJNR 1983 May-Jun, Vol. 4 (3), P. 601–3

3107. Seltzer S E, Weissman B N, Braunstein E M, Adams D F, Thomas W H
Computed tomography of the hindfoot
J Comput Assist Tomogr 1984 Jun, Vol. 8 (3), P. 488–97

3108. Seltzer S E
Value of computed tomography in planning medical and surgical treatment of chronic osteomyelitis
J Comput Assist Tomogr 1984 Jun, Vol. 8 (3), P. 482–7

3109. Shen W C, Yang C F
Herniated lumbar disk shown by dynamic computed tomography
J Comput Assist Tomogr 1988 Jul-Aug, Vol. 12 (4), P. 713–4

3110. Shirkhoda A, Johnston R E, Staab E V, McCartney W H
Technical note. Optimal computed tomography technique for bone evaluation
J Comput Assist Tomogr 1979 Feb, Vol. 3 (1), P. 134–9

3111. Shirkhoda A, Jaffe N, Wallace S, Ayala A, Lindell M M, Zornoza J
Computed tomography of osteosarcoma after intraarterial chemotherapy
Am J Roentgenol 1985 Jan, Vol. 144 (1), P. 95–9

3112. Sievers K W, Werner W R, Loehr E
CT-Nachweis einer spinalen Fistel nach Tumorresektion
CT detection of a spinal fistula following tumor resection
RÖFO 1989 Mar, Vol. 150 (3), P. 360

3113. Singson R D, Feldman F, Rosenberg Z S
Elbow joint: assessment with double-contrast CT arthrography
Radiology 1986 Jul, Vol. 160 (1), P. 167–73

3114. Singson R D, Feldman F, Bigliani L
CT arthrographic patterns in recurrent glenohumeral instability
Am J Roentgenol 1987 Oct, Vol. 149 (4), P. 749–53

3115. Singson R D, Feldman F, Bigliani L U, Rosenberg Z S
Recurrent shoulder dislocation after surgical repair: double- contrast CT arthrography. Work in progress
Radiology 1987 Aug, Vol. 164 (2), P. 425–8

3116. Singson R D, Feldman F, Slipman C W, Gonzalez E, Rosenberg Z S, Kiernan H
Postamputation neuromas and other symptomatic stump abnormalities: detection with CT
Radiology 1987 Mar, Vol. 162 (3), P. 743–5

3117. Sinnott R G, Citrin C M
Computed tomography of intrathecal thorotrast
Neuroradiology 1981 Jan, Vol. 20 (5), P. 257–9

3118. Sisler W J
CT of the wrist: what is abnormal? letter
Am J Roentgenol 1990 May, Vol. 154 (5), P. 1127

3119. Sklar E, Quencer R M, Green B A, Montalvo B M, Post M J
Acquired spinal subarachnoid cysts: evaluation with MR, CT myelography, and intraoperative sonography
Am J Roentgenol 1989 Nov, Vol. 153 (5), P. 1057–64

3120. Smith D K, Berquist T H, An K N, Robb R A, Chao E Y
Validation of three-dimensional reconstructions of knee anatomy: CT vs MR imaging
J Comput Assist Tomogr 1989 Mar-Apr, Vol. 13 (2), P. 294–301

3121. Smith D K, Gilula L A, Totty W G
Subtalar arthrosis: evaluation with CT
Am J Roentgenol 1990 Mar, Vol. 154 (3), P. 559–62

3122. Sobel D F, Barkovich A J, Munderloh S H
Metrizamide myelography and postmyelographic computed tomography: comparative adequacy in the cervical spine
AJNR 1984 Jul-Aug, Vol. 5 (4), P. 385–90

3123. Solomon M A, Gilula L A, Oloff L M, Oloff J
CT scanning of the foot and ankle: 2. Clinical applications and review of the literature
Am J Roentgenol 1986 Jun, Vol. 146 (6), P. 1204–14

3124. Solomon M A, Gilula L A, Oloff L M, Oloff J, Compton T
CT scanning of the foot and ankle: 1. Normal anatomy
Am J Roentgenol 1986 Jun, Vol. 146 (6), P. 1192–203

3125. Som P M, Hermann G, Sacher M, Stollman A L, Moscatello A L, Biller H F
Paget disease of the calvaria and facial bones with an osteosarcoma of the maxilla: CT and MR findings
J Comput Assist Tomogr 1987 Sep-Oct, Vol. 11 (5), P. 887–90

3126. Somer K, Meurman K O
Computed tomography of stress fractures
J Comput Assist Tomogr 1982 Feb, Vol. 6 (1), P. 109–15

3127. Sotiropoulos S, Chafetz N I, Lang P, Winkler M, Morris J M, Weinstein P R, Genant H K
Differentiation between postoperative scar and recurrent disk herniation: prospective comparison of MR, CT, and contrast-enhanced CT
AJNR 1989 May-Jun, Vol. 10 (3), P. 639–43

3128. Soulen R L, Fishman E K, Pyeritz R E, Zerhouni E A, Pessar M L
Marfan syndrome: evaluation with MR imaging versus CT
Radiology 1987 Dec, Vol. 165 (3), P. 697–701

3129. Soye I, Levine E, Batnitzky S, Price H I
Computed tomography of sacral and presacral lesions
Neuroradiology 1982, Vol. 24 (2), P. 71–6

3130. Space T C, Louis D S, Francis I, Braunstein E M
CT findings in distal radioulnar dislocation
J Comput Assist Tomogr 1986 Jul-Aug, Vol. 10 (4), P. 689–90

3131. Spencer R R, Jahnke R W, Hardy T L
Dissection of gas into an intraspinal synovial cyst from contiguous vacuum facet
J Comput Assist Tomogr 1983 Oct, Vol. 7 (5), P. 886–8

3132. Stanley J H, Schabel S I, Frey G D, Hungerford G D
Quantitative analysis of the cervical spinal canal by computed tomography
Neuroradiology 1986, Vol. 28 (2), P. 139–43

3133. Stark P
Invasion of the sternum by lymphoma – role of CT
Radiologe 1984 Mar, Vol. 24 (3), P. 130–2

3134. Steiger P, Block J E, Steiger S, Heuck A F, Friedlander A, Ettinger B, Harris S T, Gluer C C, Genant H K
Spinal bone mineral density measured with quantitative CT: effect of region of interest, vertebral level, and technique
Radiology 1990 May, Vol. 175 (2), P. 537–43

3135. Stein R A, Pearce K I, Nosil J, Strecker T C
Toward quantitative characterization of the caudate nucleus through CT image enhancement
J Comput Assist Tomogr 1985 Jul-Aug, Vol. 9 (4), P. 708–14

3136. Steiner H, Lammer J, Schreyer H, Papaefthymiou G, Schneider G H
Computertomographische und myelographische Befunde nach lumbalen Bandscheibenoperationen
Computerized tomography and myelography findings following lumbar intervertebral disk surgery
RÖFO 1987 Jun, Vol. 146 (6), P. 697–704

3137. Stober T, Wussow W, Schimrigk K
Bicaudate diameter – the most specific and simple CT parameter in the diagnosis of Huntington's disease
Neuroradiology 1984, Vol. 26 (1), P. 25–8

3138. Stoeter P, Bergleiter R, Schumacher M
Diagnostische Bedeutung der spinalen Computertomographie unter besonderer Berücksichtigung einer achsengerechten Schichteinstellung

The diagnostic significance of spinal computer tomography with special reference to perpendicular projection
RÖFO 1981 Feb, Vol. 134 (2), P. 123-7

3139. Stoeter P, Schneider I, Bergleiter R, Ebeling U
Diagnostischer Wert der computertomographischen Untersuchung der Lumbosakralregion bei Patienten mit Lumboischialgien
Diagnostic importance of CT examination of the lumbosacral region of patients with lumbo-sciatica
RÖFO 1982 May, Vol. 136 (5), P. 515-24

3140. Stollman A, Pinto R, Benjamin V, Kricheff I
Radiologic imaging of symptomatic ligamentum flavum thickening with and without ossification
AJNR 1987 Nov-Dec, Vol. 8 (6), P. 991-4

3141. Strohecker J, Grobovschek M
CT- und Myelographiebefund bei der Neurofibromatose von Recklinghausen
CT and myelographic findings in Recklinghausen's neurofibromatosis
RÖFO 1984 Nov, Vol. 141 (5), P. 590-1

3142. Sutker B, Balthazar E J, Fazzini E
Presacral myelolipoma: CT findings
J Comput Assist Tomogr 1985 Nov-Dec, Vol. 9 (6), P. 1128-30

3143. Tadmor R, Cacayorin E D, Kieffer S A
Advantages of supplementary CT in myelography of intraspinal masses
AJNR 1983 May-Jun, Vol. 4 (3), P. 618-21

3144. Tan W S, Spigos D G, Khine N, Capek V
Computed air myelography of the lumbosacral spine
AJNR 1983 May-Jun, Vol. 4 (3), P. 609-10

3145. Tan W S, Wilbur A C, Spigos D G
Postmyelographic CT evaluation of multiple blocks due to metastases
J Comput Assist Tomogr 1985 Sep-Oct, Vol. 9 (5), P. 979-81

3146. Tantana S, Pilla T J, Luisiri A
Computed tomography of acute spinal subdural hematoma
J Comput Assist Tomogr 1986 Sep- Oct, Vol. 10 (5), P. 891-2

3147. Tash R R, Weitzner I Jr
Acute intervertebral gas following vertebral fracture: CT demonstration
J Comput Assist Tomogr 1986 Jul-Aug, Vol. 10 (4), P. 707-8

3148. Taylor A J, Haughton V M, Doust B D
CT imaging of the thoracic spinal cord without intrathecal contrast medium
J Comput Assist Tomogr 1980 Apr, Vol. 4 (2), P. 223-4

3149. Taylor G A, Eggli K D
Lap-belt injuries of the lumbar spine in children: a pitfall in CT diagnosis published erratum appears in AJR 1988 Sep; 1513 :preceding 641
Am J Roentgenol 1988 Jun, Vol. 150 (6), P. 1355-8

3150. Tehranzadeh J, Gabriele O F
The prone position for CT of the lumbar spine
Radiology 1984 Sep, Vol. 152 (3), P. 817-8

3151. Tehranzadeh J, Vanarthos W, Pais M J
Osteochondral impaction of the femoral head associated with hip dislocation: CT study in 35 patients
Am J Roentgenol 1990 Nov, Vol. 155 (5), P. 1049-52

3152. Teplick J G, Teplick S K, Goodman L, Haskin M E
Pitfalls and unusual findings in computed tomography of the lumbar spine
J Comput Assist Tomogr 1982 Oct, Vol. 6 (5), P. 888-93

3153. Teplick J G, Haskin M E
Review. Computed tomography of the postoperative lumbar spine
Am J Roentgenol 1983 Nov, Vol. 141 (5), P. 865-84

3154. Teplick J G, Peyster R G, Teplick S K, Goodman L R, Haskin M E
CT Identification of postlaminectomy pseudomeningocele
Am J Roentgenol 1983 Jun, Vol. 140 (6), P. 1203-6

3155. Teplick J G, Haskin M E
Intravenous contrast-enhanced CT of the postoperative lumbar spine: improved identification of recurrent disk herniation, scar, arachnoiditis, and diskitis
Am J Roentgenol 1984 Oct, Vol. 143 (4), P. 845-55

3156. Teplick J G, Laffey P A, Berman A, Haskin M E
Diagnosis and evaluation of spondylolisthesis and/or spondylolysis on axial CT
AJNR 1986 May-Jun, Vol. 7 (3), P. 479-91

3157. Teruel Agustin J J, Gomez Martinench E, Castanyer Corretger F, Cando Salcines L, Davalos Errando A
Computed tomography of a post traumatic spinal arachnoid cyst
Neuroradiology 1989, Vol. 31 (4), P. 354-5

3158. Thiede G, Schadel A
CT-Diagnostik der ventralen Spaltbildung des 1. HWK
CT diagnosis of the ventral slit formation of the lst cervical vertebrae
RÖFO 1982 May, Vol. 136 (5), P. 613-4

3159. Thompson J R, Christiansen E, Sauser D, Hasso A N, Hinshaw D B Jr
Dislocation of the temporomandibular joint meniscus: contrast arthrography vs. computed tomography
Am J Roentgenol 1985 Jan, Vol. 144 (1), P. 171-4

3160. Toombs B D, Rayschkolb E N, Gibbs B J
CT of acetabular fractures: software and image display letter
Am J Roentgenol 1982 Aug, Vol. 139 (2), P. 416-7

3161. Torricelli P, Spina V, Martinelli C
CT diagnosis of lumbosacral conjoined nerve roots. Findings in 19 cases published erratum appears in Neuroradiology 1987; 296:584
Neuroradiology 1987, Vol. 29 (4), P. 374-9

3162. Tosch U, Hertel P, Lais E, Witt H
Zweidimensionale (2-D) CT-Arthrotomographie zur postoperativen Kontrolle einer neuen vorderen Kreuzbandplastik
2-dimensional CT arthrotomography in the postoperative follow-up of a new anterior cruciate ligament plasty
Radiologe 1989 Nov, Vol. 29 (11), P. 546-9

3163. Treisch J, Claussen C
Computertomographische Diagnostik von Wirbelsäulenverletzungen
Computer tomographic diagnosis of spinal injuries
RÖFO 1983 May, Vol. 138 (5), P. 588-91

3164. Tsuji H, Takazakura E, Terada Y, Makino H, Yasuda A, Oiko Y
CT demonstration of spinal epidural emphysema complicating bronchial asthma and violent coughing
J Comput Assist Tomogr 1989 Jan-Feb, Vol. 13 (1), P. 38-9

3165. Tully R J, Pickens J, Oro J, Levine C
Hereditary multiple exostoses and cervical cord compression: CT and MR studies
J Comput Assist Tomogr 1989 Mar-Apr, Vol. 13 (2), P. 330-3

3166. Ullrich C G, Binet E F, Sanecki M G, Kieffer S A
Quantitative assessment of the lumbar spinal canal by computed tomography
Radiology 1980 Jan, Vol. 134 (1), P. 137-43

3167. Vadala G, Dore R, Garbagna P
Unusual osseous changes in lumbar herniated disks: CT features
J Comput Assist Tomogr 1985 Nov-Dec, Vol. 9 (6), P. 1045-9

3168. van Kuijk C
Vertebral bone density in children: effect of puberty
Radiology 1989 Mar, Vol. 170 (3 Pt 1), P. 895-6

3169. van Schaik J J, Verbiest H, van Schaik F D
Morphometry of lower lumbar vertebrae as seen on CT scans: newly recognized characteristics
Am J Roentgenol 1985 Aug, Vol. 145 (2), P. 327-35

3170. Vas W G, Wolverson M K, Sundaram M, Heiberg E, Pilla T, Shields J B, Crepps L
The role of computed tomography in pelvic fractures
J Comput Assist Tomogr 1982 Aug, Vol. 6 (4), P. 796-801

3171. Veiga Pires J A, Kaiser M C
Direct coronal slices on CT scanning of the spine. Technical note
Neuroradiology 1982, Vol. 22 (4), P. 203-5

3172. Verstraete K L, Martens F, Smeets P, Vandekerckhove T, Meire D, Parizel P M, Van de Velde E, Calliauw L
Traumatic lumbosacral nerve root meningoceles. The value of myelography, CT and MRI in the assessment of nerve root continuity
Neuroradiology 1989, Vol. 31 (5), P. 425-9

3173. Vogelzang R L, Hendrix R W, Neiman H L
Computed tomography of tuberculous osteomyelitis of the pubis
J Comput Assist Tomogr 1983 Oct, Vol. 7 (5), P. 914-5

3174. Vogler J B, Brown W H, Helms C A, Genant H K
The normal sacroiliac joint: a CT study of asymptomatic patients
Radiology 1984 May, Vol. 151 (2), P. 433-7

3175. Volle E, Kern A, Stoltenburg G, Claussen C
CT reconstruction technique in lumbar intraneuroforaminal disc herniation
Neuroradiology 1988, Vol. 30 (2), P. 138-44

3176. Vollrath T, Eberle C, Grauer W
Computertomographie intraartikulärer Kalkaneusfrakturen
Computed tomography of intra- articular calcaneal fractures
RÖFO 1987 Apr, Vol. 146 (4), P. 400-3

3177. Wagner Manslau C, Rupp N, Paar O, Rodammer G
Die Computertomographie der Menisci
Computed tomography of the menisci
RÖFO 1988 Oct, Vol. 149 (4), P. 392-5

3178. Walker M D, Bennett W F
Iliac bone marrow harvesting: CT appearance
J Comput Assist Tomogr 1985 Nov-Dec, Vol. 9 (6), P. 1148-9

3179. Wang A M, Lewis M L, Rumbaugh C L, Zamani A A, O Reilly G V
Spinal cord or nerve root compression in patients with malignant disease: CT evaluation
J Comput Assist Tomogr 1984 Jun, Vol. 8 (3), P. 420-8

3180. Wang A M, Lipson S J, Haykal H A, Weinberg D S, Zamani A A, Rumbaugh C L
Computed tomography of aneurysmal bone cyst of the L1 vertebral body
J Comput Assist Tomogr 1984 Dec, Vol. 8 (6), P. 1186-9

3181. Wang A M, Joachim C L, Shillito J Jr, Morris J H, Zamani A A, Rumbaugh C L
Cervical chordoma presenting with intervertebral foramen enlargement mimicking neurofibroma: CT findings
J Comput Assist Tomogr 1984 Jun, Vol. 8 (3), P. 529-32

3182. Warmuth Metz M, Schmitt R, Schindler G, Gay B
Die Computertomographie in der traumatologischen Diagnostik des hinteren Beckenrings
Computed tomography in the diagnosis of injuries of the posterior pelvic girdle
RÖFO 1988 Mar, Vol. 148 (3), P. 289-94

3183. Warmuth Metz M, Krauss J, Becker T, Hofmann E
Der lumbosakrale Nervenwurzelabriß. Diagnostik mit Computertomographie (CT), Magnetresonanztomographie (MRT) und Myelographie
Lumbosacral nerve root avulsion. Diagnosis using computed tomography, magnetic resonance tomography and myelography
RÖFO 1990 Apr, Vol. 152 (4), P. 374-7

3184. Weinreb J C, Arger P H, Grossman R, Samuel L
CT metrizamide myelography in multiple bilateral intrathoracic meningoceles
J Comput Assist Tomogr 1984 Apr, Vol. 8 (2), P. 324-6

3185. Weisberg L A
Non-neoplastic gliotic cerebellar cysts: clinical and computed tomographic correlations
Neuroradiology 1982, Vol. 24 (1), P. 53-7

3186. Weiss T, Treisch J, Claussen C, Banzer D
Irrtumsmöglichkeiten und Schwierigkeiten in der computertomographischen Diagnostik lumbaler Bandscheibenvorfälle
Possibility of error and difficulties in the computerized tomographic diagnosis of lumbar intervertebral disk prolapse
RÖFO 1983 Jan, Vol. 138 (1), P. 54-60

3187. Weiss T, Treisch J, Kazner E, Claussen C, Schorner W, Fiegler W
Intravenöse Kontrastmittelgabe bei der Computertomographie (CT) der operierten Lendenwirbelsäule
Intravenous administration of contrast medium during computed tomography CT of the operated lumbar spine
RÖFO 1984 Jul, Vol. 141 (1), P. 30-4

3188. Weiss T, Treisch J, Kohler D, Claussen C
Spondylolysis und -listhesis. Eine computertomographische Differentialdiagnose der lumbalen Diskopathie
Spondylolysis and -listhesis. A computed tomographic differential diagnosis of lumbar discopathy
RÖFO 1985 Jul, Vol. 143 (1), P. 68-73

3189. Whelan M A, Hilal S K, Gold R P, Luken M G, Michelson W J
Computed tomography of the sacrum: 2. Pathology
Am J Roentgenol 1982 Dec, Vol. 139 (6), P. 1191-5

3190. Whelan M A, Gold R P
Computed tomography of the sacrum: 1. Normal Anatomy
Am J Roentgenol 1982 Dec, Vol. 139 (6), P. 1183-90

3191. Whelan M A, Naidich D P, Post J D, Chase N E
Computed tomography of spinal tuberculosis
J Comput Assist Tomogr 1983 Feb, Vol. 7 (1), P. 25-30

3192. Whelan M A, Schonfeld S, Post J D, Svigals P, Meisler W, Weingarten K, Kricheff I I
Computed tomography of nontuberculous spinal infection
J Comput Assist Tomogr 1985 Mar-Apr, Vol. 9 (2), P. 280–7

3193. Wiesen E J, Crass J R, Bellon E M, Ashmead G G, Cohen A M
Improvement in CT pelvimetry
Radiology 1991 Jan, Vol. 178 (1), P. 259–62

3194. Williams A L, Haughton V M, Syvertsen A
Computed tomography in the diagnosis of herniated nucleus pulposus
Radiology 1980 Apr, Vol. 135 (1), P. 95–9

3195. Williams A L, Haughton V M, Daniels D L, Thornton R S
CT recognition of lateral lumbar disk herniation
Am J Roentgenol 1982 Aug, Vol. 139 (2), P. 345–7

3196. Williams A L, Haughton V M, Daniels D L, Grogan J P
Differential CT diagnosis of extruded nucleus pulposus
Radiology 1983 Jul, Vol. 148 (1), P. 141–8

3197. Wilmink J T, Korte J H, Penning L
Dimensions of the spinal canal in individual symptomatic and non-symptomatic for sciatica: a CT study
Neuroradiology 1988, Vol. 30 (6), P. 547–50

3198. Wilmink J T
CT morphology of intrathecal lumbosacral nerve-root compression
AJNR 1989 Mar-Apr, Vol. 10 (2), P. 233–48

3199. Wilson A J, Totty W G, Murphy W A, Hardy D C
Shoulder joint: arthrographic CT and long-term follow-up, with surgical correlation
Radiology 1989 Nov, Vol. 173 (2), P. 329–33

3200. Wimmer B, Friedburg H, Hennig J, Kauffmann G W
Möglichkeiten der diagnostischen Bildgebung durch Kernspintomographie. Veränderungen an Wirbeln, Bändern und Bandscheiben im Vergleich mit der Computertomographie
Diagnostic imaging potentialities of nuclear resonance tomography. Changes in vertebrae, ligaments and intervertebral disks in comparison with computed tomography
Radiologe 1986 Mar, Vol. 26 (3), P. 137–43

3201. Wimmer B
Computertomographie bei Wirbelsäulentrauma
Computed tomography of spinal injuries
Radiologe 1989 Sep, Vol. 29 (9), P. 441–6

3202. Wing V W, Jeffrey R B Jr, Federle M P, Helms C A, Trafton P
Chronic osteomyelitis examined by CT
Radiology 1985 Jan, Vol. 154 (1), P. 171–4

3203. Wirth R L, Zatz L M, Parker B R
CT detection of a Jefferson fracture in a child
Am J Roentgenol 1987 Nov, Vol. 149 (5), P. 1001–2

3204. Yagan R
CT diagnosis of limbus vertebra
J Comput Assist Tomogr 1984 Feb, Vol. 8 (1), P. 149–51

3205. Yang P J, Seeger J F, Dzioba R B, Carmody R F, Burt T B, Komar N N, Smith J R
High-dose i.v. contrast in CT scanning of the postoperative lumbar spine
AJNR 1986 Jul-Aug, Vol. 7 (4), P. 703-7

3206. Yeh H C, Rabinowitz J G
Ultrasonography of the extremities and pelvic girdle and correlation with computed tomography
Radiology 1982 May, Vol. 143 (2), P. 519–25

3207. Yoshimura T, Takeo G, Souda M, Ohe H, Ohe N
CT demonstration of spinal epidural emphysema after strenuous exercise
J Comput Assist Tomogr 1990 Mar-Apr, Vol. 14 (2), P. 303–4

3208. Yousem D, Magid D, Fishman E K, Kuhajda F, Siegelman S S
Computed tomography of stress fractures
J Comput Assist Tomogr 1986 Jan-Feb, Vol. 10 (1), P. 92–5

3209. Yu Y L, du Boulay G H, Stevens J M, Kendall B E
Morphology and measurements of the cervical spinal cord in computer-assisted myelography
Neuroradiology 1985, Vol. 27 (5), P. 399–402

3210. Zatz L M
Pseudocyst of spinal cord on metrizamide ct letter
AJNR 1984 Jul-Aug, Vol. 5 (4), P. 489–90

3211. Zee C S, Segall H D, Ahmadi J, Tsai F Y, Apuzzo M
CT myelography in spinal cysticercosis
J Comput Assist Tomogr 1986 Mar-Apr, Vol. 10 (2), P. 195–8

3212. Ziegler V M, Mendoza A S, Borgis K J, Weiss H D, Kuhnel W
CT des oberen Sprunggelenkes. Anatomie – Pathologie
CT of the upper ankle joint. Anatomy – pathology
RÖFO 1989 May, Vol. 150 (5), P. 588–91

3213. Zilkha A, Irwin G A, Fagelman D
Computed tomography of spinal epidural hematoma
AJNR 1983 Sep-Oct, Vol. 4 (5), P. 1073–6

3214. Zinreich S J, Wang H, Updike M L, Kumar A J, Ahn H S, North R B, Rosenbaum A E
CT myelography for outpatients. An inpatient/outpatient pilot study to assess methodology
Radiology 1985 Nov, Vol. 157 (2), P. 387–90

3215. Zlatkin M B, Bjorkengren A G, Gylys Morin V, Resnick D, Sartoris D J
Cross-sectional imaging of the capsular mechanism of the glenohumeral joint
Am J Roentgenol 1988 Jan, Vol. 150 (1), P. 151–8

3216. Zucker Pinchoff B, Hermann G, Srinivasan R
Computed tomography of the carpal tunnel: a radioanatomical study
J Comput Assist Tomogr 1981 Aug, Vol. 5 (4), P. 525–8

3217. Zwaan M, Borgis K J, Weiss H D, Burmester E
CT-Diagnostik des Ellbogengelenkes
CT diagnosis of the elbow joint
Radiologe 1990 Mar, Vol. 30 (3), P. 106–12

Further Literature

3218. Abbitt P L, Armstrong P
Percutaneous catheter drainage of necrotic tumors: CT demonstration
J Comput Assist Tomogr 1989 May- Jun, Vol. 13 (3), P. 437–9

3219. Abdelwahab I F, Gould E S
The role of diskography after negative postmyelography CT scans: retrospective review
AJNR 1988 Jan-Feb, Vol. 9 (1), P. 187–90

3220. Abel M
Prämedikation und Risiken bei Computertomographien im Neugeborenen- und Säuglingsalter
Premedication and risks in computed tomography of newborn and infant children
Radiologe 1985 Dec, Vol. 25 (12), P. 599–601

3221. Adam P, Bec P, Mathis A, Alberge Y
Morning glory syndrome: CT findings
J Comput Assist Tomogr 1984 Feb, Vol. 8 (1), P. 134–6

3222. Agnoli A L, Tzavaras N, Reisig L
Computertomographische Befunde bei Alkoholismus
Computer tomographic findings in alcoholism
RÖFO 1980 May, Vol. 132 (5), P. 565–72

3223. Akine Y, Hosoba M, Berardo P A
Clinical merit of simulation images generated from CT
Radiology 1982 Nov, Vol. 145 (2), P. 528–31

3224. Alemdaroglu A
Os supra-petrosum of Meckel: CT appearance
J Comput Assist Tomogr 1986 Jan-Feb, Vol. 10 (1), P. 164–5

3225. Allard J C, Tilak S, Carter A P
CT and MR of MELAS syndrome
AJNR 1988 Nov-Dec, Vol. 9 (6), P. 1234–8

3226. Allen H A, Scatarige J C, Kim M H
Actinomycosis: CT findings in six patients
Am J Roentgenol 1987 Dec, Vol. 149 (6), P. 1255–8

3227. Allgayer B, Reiser M, Feuerbach S
CT-Diagnostik einer Phlebothrombose bei einer Baker-Zyste
CT diagnosis of phlebothrombosis in Baker's cyst
RÖFO 1984 Nov, Vol. 141 (5), P. 593–4

3228. Allgayer B, Reiser M, Kramann B
Typische computertomographische Befunde bei der Neurofibromatose
Typical computed tomographic findings in neurofibromatosis
RÖFO 1984 Jun, Vol. 140 (6), P. 669–72

3229. Allibone G, Porter S C, Becker S N
Lipid granulomatosis causing lymph node enlargement: CT appearance
Am J Roentgenol 1982 Apr, Vol. 138 (4), P. 744–5

3230. Alpern M B, Thorsen M K, Kellman G M, Pojunas K, Lawson T L
CT appearance of hemangiopericytoma
J Comput Assist Tomogr 1986 Mar-Apr, Vol. 10 (2), P. 264–7

3231. Altman N R
MR and CT characteristics of gangliocytoma: a rare cause of epilepsy in children
AJNR 1988 Sep, Vol. 9 (5), P. 917–21

3232. Altman N R, Altman D H, Wolfe S A, Morrison G
Three- dimensional CT reformation in children
Am J Roentgenol 1986 Jun, Vol. 146 (6), P. 1261–7

3233. Altman N, Fitz C R, Chuang S, Harwood Nash D, Cotter C, Armstrong D
Radiologic characteristics of primitive neuroectodermal tumors in children
AJNR 1985 Jan-Feb, Vol. 6 (1), P. 15–8

3234. Ambrosetto P
CT changes in dementing diseases letter
AJNR 1987 Jul-Aug, Vol. 8 (4), P. 734–5

3235. Ambrosetto P
MR imaging, CT scan, and clinical examination in multiple sclerosis letter
AJNR 1986 Nov-Dec, Vol. 7 (6), P. 1101–2

3236. Ambrosetto P
CT scan in progressive supranuclear palsy letter
AJNR 1986 May-Jun, Vol. 7 (3), P. 529

3237. Anderson R E, Radmehr A, Osborn A G, Wing S D
Impact of a "fast" scanner on image quality in pediatric computed tomography
Radiology 1980 Jan, Vol. 134 (1), P. 251–2

3238. Anderson R E, Thomas D G, du Boulay G H
Radiological aspects of CT-guided stereotactic neurosurgical procedures
Neuroradiology 1983, Vol. 24 (3), P. 163–6

3239. Andreou J, George A E, Wise A, de Leon M, Kricheff I I, Ransohoff J, Foo S H
CT prognostic criteria of survival after malignant glioma surgery
AJNR 1983 May-Jun, Vol. 4 (3), P. 488–90

3240. Arasaki K, Kwee I L, Nakada T
Limbic lymphoma
Neuroradiology 1987, Vol. 29 (4), P. 389–92

3241. Armington W G, Osborn A G, Cubberley D A, Harnsberger H R, Boyer R, Naidich T P, Sherry R G
Supratentorial ependymoma: CT appearance
Radiology 1985 Nov, Vol. 157 (2), P. 367–72

3242. Armstrong E A, Harwood Nash D C, Hoffman H, Fitz C R, Chuang S, Pettersson H
Benign suprasellar cysts: the CT approach
AJNR 1983 Mar-Apr, Vol. 4 (2), P. 163–6

3243. Armstrong E A, Harwood Nash D C, Ritz C R, Chuang S H, Pettersson H, Martin D J
CT of neuroblastomas and ganglioneuromas in children
Am J Roentgenol 1982 Sep, Vol. 139 (3), P. 571–6

3244. Aronson D, Kier R
CT pelvimetry: the foveae are not an accurate landmark for the level of the ischial spines
Am J Roentgenol 1991 Mar, Vol. 156 (3), P. 527–30

3245. Ashley D G, Zee C S, Chandrasoma P T, Segall H D
Lhermitte-Duclos disease: CT and MR findings
J Comput Assist Tomogr 1990 Nov-Dec, Vol. 14 (6), P. 984–7

3246. Ascencio Ferreira V, Bancovsky I, Diament A J, Gherpelli J L, Moreira F A
Computed tomography in ataxia- telangiectasia
J Comput Assist Tomogr 1981 Oct, Vol. 5 (5), P. 660–1

3247. Aubourg P, Diebler C
Adrenoleukodystrophy-its diverse CT appearances and an evolutive or phenotypic variant: the leukodystrophy without adrenal insufficiency
Neuroradiology 1982, Vol. 24 (1), P. 33–42

3248. Auh Y H, Rosen A, Rubenstein W A, Engel I A, Whalen J P, Kazam E
CT of the papillary process of the caudate lobe of the liver
Am J Roentgenol 1984 Mar, Vol. 142 (3), P. 535–8

3249. Auh Y H, Rubenstein W A, Schneider M, Reckler J M, Whalen J P, Kazam E
Extraperitoneal paravesical spaces: CT delineation with US correlation
Radiology 1986 May, Vol. 159 (2), P. 319–28

3250. Austin R M, Bankoff M S, Carter B L
Gas collections in the spinal cord on computed tomography
J Comput Assist Tomogr 1981 Aug, Vol. 5 (4), P. 522–4

3251. Avrahami E, Yust Y, Cohn D F
Falx myeloid metaplasia in myelofibrosis. A CT demonstration
Neuroradiology 1981, Vol. 21 (3), P. 165–6

3252. Awwad E E, DiIorio G, Martin D S, Smith K R
Fat deposition adjacent to chronic subdural hematoma: CT demonstration
J Comput Assist Tomogr 1990 Jul-Aug, Vol. 14 (4), P. 665–7

3253. Azar Kia B, Naheedy M H, Fine M
Spinal subarachnoid clot detected by CT letter
AJNR 1986 Jan-Feb, Vol. 7 (1), P. 178–9

3254. Badami J P, Norman D, Barbaro N M, Cann C E, Weinstein P R, Sobel D F
Metrizamide CT myelography in cervical myelopathy and radiculopathy: correlation with conventional myelography and surgical findings
Am J Roentgenol 1985 Apr, Vol. 144 (4), P. 675–80

3255. Badcock P C
The role of computed tomography in the planning of radiotherapy fields
Radiology 1983 Apr, Vol. 147 (1), P. 241–4

3256. Bajcsy R, Lieberson R, Reivich M
A computerized system for the elastic matching of deformed radiographic images to idealized atlas images
J Comput Assist Tomogr 1983 Aug, Vol. 7 (4), P. 618–25

3257. Balfe D M, Chezmar J, Koehler R E, Lichtenstein J E, Nelson R
Abdominal-gastrointestinal radiology
Radiology 1991 Mar, Vol. 178 (3), P. 911–3

3258. Banna M
Computed tomographic arteriography of microadenoma
J Comput Assist Tomogr 1980 Oct, Vol. 4 (5), P. 690–2

3259. Banzer D, Risch W D, Wegener O H
Eine neue Methode zur Messung des Rotationswinkels der Wirbelskoliose
A new method for measuring rotation of a vertebral scoliosis
RÖFO 1980 Apr, Vol. 132 (4), P. 403–5

3260. Barack B M
Persistence of the cardinal veins and thrombosis: CT demonstration
J Comput Assist Tomogr 1986 Mar-Apr, Vol. 10 (2), P. 327–8

3261. Barnes P A, Bernardino M E, Thomas J L
Flow phenomenon mimicking thrombus: a possible pitfall of the pedal infusion technique
J Comput Assist Tomogr 1982 Apr, Vol. 6 (2), P. 304–6

3262. Baron B, Goldberg A L, Rothfus W E, Sherman R L
CT features of sarcoid infiltration of a lumbosacral nerve root
J Comput Assist Tomogr 1989 Mar-Apr, Vol. 13 (2), P. 364–5

3263. Baron R L, Kuyper S J, Lee S P, Rohrmann C A Jr, Shuman W P, Nelson J A
In vitro dissolution of gallstones with MTBE: correlation with characteristics at CT and MR imaging
Radiology 1989 Oct, Vol. 173 (1), P. 117–21

3264. Baum P A, Matsumoto A H, Teitelbaum G P, Zuurbier R A, Barth K H
Anatomic relationship between the common femoral artery and vein: CT evaluation and clinical significance
Radiology 1989 Dec, Vol. 173 (3), P. 775–7

3265. Becker H, Vogelsang H, Schwarzrock R
Vergleichende MR- und CT-Untersuchungen bei ausgewählten neuroradiologischen Fragestellungen
Comparative MR and CT research in selected neuroradiological problems
RÖFO 1985 Jan, Vol. 142 (1), P. 23–30

3266. Beers G J, Carter A P, Leiter B E, Tilak S P, Shah R R
Interobserver discrepancies in distance measurements from lumbar spine CT scans
Am J Roentgenol 1985 Feb, Vol. 144 (2), P. 395–8

3267. Beggs I
The radiology of hydatid disease
Am J Roentgenol 1985 Sep, Vol. 145 (3), P. 639–48

3268. Bellamy E A, Husband J E, Blaquiere R M, Law M R
Bleomycin-related lung damage: CT evidence
Radiology 1985 Jul, Vol. 156 (1), P. 155–8

3269. Bellamy E A, Meller S, Westbury G, Husband J E
CT demonstration of calcified subcutaneous masses following parenteral pentamidine isethionate injection
J Comput Assist Tomogr 1985 Jan-Feb, Vol. 9 (1), P. 210–1

3270. Bellamy E A, Perez D J, Husband J E
CT demonstration of a spinal subarachnoid haematoma following lumbar puncture
J Comput Assist Tomogr 1984 Aug, Vol. 8 (4), P. 791–2

3271. Beltran J, Gray L A, Bools J C, Zuelzer W, Weis L D, Unverferth L J
Rotator cuff lesions of the shoulder: evaluation by direct sagittal CT arthrography
Radiology 1986 Jul, Vol. 160 (1), P. 161–5

3272. Berbaum K S, Franken E A, Honda H, McGuire C, Weis R R, Barloon T
Evaluation of a PACS workstation for assessment of body CT studies
J Comput Assist Tomogr 1990 Sep-Oct, Vol. 14 (5), P. 853–8

3273. Bergstrand G, Oxenstierna G, Flyckt L, Larsson S A, Sedvall G
Radionuclide cisternography and computed tomography in 30 healthy volunteers
Neuroradiology 1986, Vol. 28 (2), P. 154–60

3274. Bergstrom K, Nyberg G, Pech P, Rauschning W, Ytterbergh C
Multiplanar spinal anatomy: comparison of CT and cryomicrotomy in postmortem specimens
AJNR 1983 May-Jun, Vol. 4 (3), P. 590–2

3275. Berkmen Y M, Auh Y H, Davis S D, Kazam E
Anatomy of the minor fissure: evaluation with thin-section CT
Radiology 1989 Mar, Vol. 170 (3 Pt 1), P. 647–51

3276. Bernardino M E
Percutaneous biopsy
Am J Roentgenol 1984 Jan, Vol. 142 (1), P. 41–5

3277. Bernardino M E, Chuang V P, Wallace S, Thomas J L, Soo C S 50
Therapeutically infarcted tumors: ct findings
Am J Roentgenol 1981 Mar, Vol. 136 (3), P. 527–30

3278. Berninger W, Redington R, Leue W, Axel L, Norman D, Brundage B, Carlsson E, Herfkens R, Lipton M
Technical aspects and clinical applications of CT/X, a dynamic CT scanner
J Comput Assist Tomogr 1981 Apr, Vol. 5 (2), P. 206–15

3279. Bettmann M A
Venous air embolism on contrast-enhanced CT: chimera or Trojan horse? editorial
Radiology 1988 May, Vol. 167 (2), P. 571–2

3280. Beyer Enke S A, Gorich J, Gamroth A
Axiale Myopie- computertomographischer und kernspintomographischer Befund
Axial myopia-computed tomography and magnetic resonance tomography findings
Radiologe 1987 Aug, Vol. 27 (8), P. 375–6

3281. Beyer Enke S A, Gorich J, van Kaick G
Größen- und Dichtebestimmung mit der Dünnschicht-CT in Abhängigkeit von Strukturdurchmesser und Umgebungskontrast
Size and density determination by thin-layer CT in relation to structural diameter and the contrast of the surrounding tissue
RÖFO 1989 Jul, Vol. 151 (1), P. 93–6

3282. Bianco F, Floris R
Computed tomography abnormalities in hanging
Neuroradiology 1987, Vol. 29 (3), P. 297–8

3283. Biondetti P R, Vigo M, Fiore D, De Faveri D, Ravasini R, Benedetti L
CT appearance of generalized von Recklinghausen neurofibromatosis
J Comput Assist Tomogr 1983 Oct, Vol. 7 (5), P. 866–9

3284. Bird C R, McMahan J R, Gilles F H, Senac M O, Apthorp J S
Strangulation in child abuse: CT diagnosis
Radiology 1987 May, Vol. 163 (2), P. 373–5

3285. Bisceglia M, Donaldson J S
Calcification of the ligamentum arteriosum in children: a normal finding on CT
Am J Roentgenol 1991 Feb, Vol. 156 (2), P. 351–2

3286. Black W C, Burke J W, Feldman P S, Johnson C M, Swanson S
CT appearance of cervical lipoblastoma
J Comput Assist Tomogr 1986 Jul-Aug, Vol. 10 (4), P. 696–8

3287. Blom R J
Pleomorphic xanthoastrocytoma: CT appearance
J Comput Assist Tomogr 1988 Mar-Apr, Vol. 12 (2), P. 351–2

3288. Boechat M I, Ortega J, Hoffman A D, Cleveland R H, Kangarloo H, Gilsanz V
Computed tomography in stage III neuroblastoma
Am J Roentgenol 1985 Dec, Vol. 145 (6), P. 1283–7

3289. Bolen J W Jr, Lipper M H, Caccamo D
Intraventricular central neurocytoma: CT and MR findings
J Comput Assist Tomogr 1989 May-Jun, Vol. 13 (3), P. 495–7

3290. Bolender N F, Cromwell L D, Graves V, Margolis M T, Kerber C W, Wendling L
Interval appearance of glioblastomas not evident in previous CT examinations
J Comput Assist Tomogr 1983 Aug, Vol. 7 (4), P. 599–603

3291. Bonafe A, Manelfe C, Espagno J, Guiraud B, Rascol A
Evaluation of syringomyelia with metrizamide computed tomographic myelography
J Comput Assist Tomogr 1980 Dec, Vol. 4 (6), P. 797–802

3292. Bonafe A, Manelfe C, Scotto B, Pradere M Y, Rascol A
Role of computed tomography in vertebrobasilar ischemia
Neuroradiology 1985, Vol. 27 (6), P. 484–93

3293. Bonatti G P, Huber R, Gostner P, Simeoni J
Lyme- Krankheit: computertomographisches und MR-tomographisches Bild
Lyme disease: the computed tomographic and MR tomographic images
RÖFO 1987 Jul, Vol. 147 (1), P. 97–8

3294. Bonneville J F, Cattin F, Racle A, Bouchareb M, Boulard D, Potelon P, Tang Y S
Dynamic CT of the laterosellar extradural venous spaces
AJNR 1989 May-Jun, Vol. 10 (3), P. 535–42

3295. Bories J, Derhy S, Chiras J
CT in hemispheric ischaemic attacks
Neuroradiology 1985, Vol. 27 (6), P. 468–83

3296. Bourjat P, Cartier J, Woerther J P
Thyroglossal duct cyst in hyoid bone: CT confirmation
J Comput Assist Tomogr 1988 Sep- Oct, Vol. 12 (5), P. 871–3

3297. Brant Zawadzki M, Jeffrey R B Jr
CT with image reformation for noninvasive screening of the carotid bifurcation: early experience
AJNR 1982 Jul-Aug, Vol. 3 (4), P. 395–400

3298. Brasch R C, Cann C E
Computed tomographic scanning in children: II. An updated comparison of radiation dose and resolving power of commercial scanners
Am J Roentgenol 1982 Jan, Vol. 138 (1), P. 127–33

3299. Braun I F, Chambers E, Leeds N E, Zimmerman R D
The value of unenhanced scans in differentiating lesions producing ring enhancement
AJNR 1982 Nov-Dec, Vol. 3 (6), P. 643–7

3300. Braun J, Guilburd J N, Borovich B, Goldsher D, Mendelson H, Kerner H
Occipital aneurysmal bone cyst: CT features
J Comput Assist Tomogr 1987 Sep-Oct, Vol. 11 (5), P. 880–3

3301. Braunwald E, Isselbacher K J, Petersdorf R G, Wilson J D, Martin J B, Fauci A S, (Eds)
Harrison's principles of internal medicine
1987 11 thed., McGraw-Hill Book Company, New York St Louis San Francisco Hamburg Paris Sidney Tokyo Toronto

3302. Brazeau Lamontagne L, Charlin B, Levesque R Y, Lussier A
Cricoarytenoiditis: CT assessment in rheumatoid arthritis
Radiology 1986 Feb, Vol. 158 (2), P. 463–6

3303. Brecht G, Janson R, Schilling G
Das Aneurysma dissecans im Computertomogramm
Computerized tomography of a dissecting aneurysm
RÖFO 1980 Mar, Vol. 132 (3), P. 343–5

3304. Brecht G, Lackner K, Janson R, Thurn P
Die Computertomographie in der Notfalldiagnostik
Computer tomography in emergency diagnosis
RÖFO 1980 Mar, Vol. 132 (3), P. 272–81

3305. Bressler E L, Weinberg P E, Zaret C R
Silicone encircling bands for retinal detachment: CT appearance
J Comput Assist Tomogr 1984 Oct, Vol. 8 (5), P. 960–2

3306. Brinkman S D, Sarwar M, Levin H S, Morris H H
Quantitative indexes of computed tomography in dementia and normal aging
Radiology 1981 Jan, Vol. 138 (1), P. 89–92

3307. Brodey P A, Randel S, Lane B, Fisch A E
Computed tomography of axial myopia
J Comput Assist Tomogr 1983 Jun, Vol. 7 (3), P. 484–5

3308. Brody A S, Kuhn J P, Seidel F G, Brodsky L S
Airway evaluation in children with use of ultrafast CT: pitfalls and recommendations
Radiology 1991 Jan, Vol. 178 (1), P. 181–4

3309. Brody W R, Cassel D M, Sommer F G, Lehmann L A, Macovski A, Alvarez R E, Pelc N J, Riederer S J, Hall A L
Dual-energy projection radiography: initial clinical experience
Am J Roentgenol 1981 Aug, Vol. 137 (2), P. 201–5

3310. Brooks B S, el Gammal T
Metrizamide CT ventriculography in the evaluation of a pseudoballooned fourth ventricle
AJNR 1984 Nov-Dec, Vol. 5 (6), P. 825–7

3311. Brooks B S, El Gammal T
Case report. An additional case of adrenoleukodystrophy with both type I and type II CT features
J Comput Assist Tomogr 1982 Apr, Vol. 6 (2), P. 385–8

3312. Brooks B S, El Gammal T, Hungerford G D, Acker J, Trevor R P, Russell W
Radiologic evaluation of neurosarcoidosis: role of computed tomography
AJNR 1982 Sep-Oct, Vol. 3 (5), P. 513–21

3313. Brown B M, Stark E H, Dion G, Ono H
Computed tomography and chymopapain chemonucleolysis: preliminary findings
Am J Roentgenol 1985 Apr, Vol. 144 (4), P. 667–70

3314. Brown J J, Hesselink J R, Rothrock J F
MR and CT of lacunar infarcts
Am J Roentgenol 1988 Aug, Vol. 151 (2), P. 367–72*

3315. Brown R A, Roberts T, Osborn A G
Simplified CT-guided stereotaxic biopsy
AJNR 1981 Mar-Apr, Vol. 2 (2), P. 181–4

3316. Brown T R, Quinn S F, D Agostino A N
Deposition of calcium pyrophosphate dihydrate crystals in the ligamentum flavum: evaluation with MR imaging and CTRadiology 1991 Mar, Vol. 178 (3), P. 871–3

3317. Brugieres P, Gaston A, Heran F, Voisin M C, Marsault C
Percutaneous biopsies of the thoracic spine under CT guidance: transcostovertebral approach
J Comput Assist Tomogr 1990 May-Jun, Vol. 14 (3), P. 446–8

3318. Bruhl K, Kramer G, Bornemann A
Computertomographische Verlaufsdokumentation und Magnetresonanztomographie
Radiologe 1988 Nov, Vol. 28 (11), P. 514–6

3319. Bruneton J N, Falewee M N, Franccois E, Cambon P, Philip C, Riess J G, Balu Maestro C, Rogopoulos A
Liver, spleen, and vessels: preliminary clinical results of CT with perfluorooctylbromide
Radiology 1989 Jan, Vol. 170 (1 Pt 1), P. 179–83

3320. Bryan R N, Miller R H, Ferreyro R I, Sessions R B
Computed tomography of the major salivary glands
Am J Roentgenol 1982 Sep, Vol. 139 (3), P. 547–54

3321. Buff B L Jr, Schick R M, Norregaard T
Meningeal metastasis of leiomyosarcoma mimicking meningioma: CT and MR findings
J Comput Assist Tomogr 1991 Jan-Feb, Vol. 15 (1), P. 166–7

3322. Burbank F
Imaging-directed percutaneous biopsies with a biopsy gun letter
Radiology 1990 Jul, Vol. 176 (1), P. 286–7

3323. Burgess A E, Colborne B, Zoffmann E
Vertebral trabecular bone: comparison of single and dual-energy CT measurements with chemical analysis
J Comput Assist Tomogr 1987 May-Jun, Vol. 11 (3), P. 506–15

3324. Bursztyn E M, Lee B C, Bauman J
CT of acquired immunodeficiency syndrome
AJNR 1984 Nov-Dec, Vol. 5 (6), P. 711–4

3325. Burton E M, Ball W S Jr, Crone K, Dolan L M
Hamartoma of the tuber cinereum: a comparison of MR and CT findings in four cases
AJNR 1989 May-Jun, Vol. 10 (3), P. 497–501

3326. Burton E M, Keith J W, Linden B E, Lazar R H
CSF fistula in a patient with Mondini deformity: demonstration by CT cisternography
AJNR 1990 Jan-Feb, Vol. 11 (1), P. 205–7

3327. Busch G
Ungewöhnlicher computertomographischer Befund nach Shuntoperation bei Hydrocephalus internus permagnus
Unusual computed tomographic findings following shunting of hydrocephalus internus permagnus
RÖFO 1986 Apr, Vol. 144 (4), P. 470–3

3328. Buy J N, Moss A A, Singler R C
CT guided celiac plexus and splanchnic nerve neurolysis
J Comput Assist Tomogr 1982 Apr, Vol. 6 (2), P. 315–9

3329. Byrd S E, Winter J, Takahashi M, Joyce P
Symptomatic Rathke's cleft cyst demonstrated on computed tomography
J Comput Assist Tomogr 1980 Jun, Vol. 4 (3), P. 411–4

3330. Calvy T M, Segall H D, Gilles F H, Bird C R, Zee C S, Ahmadi J, Biddle R
CT anatomy of the craniovertebral junction in infants and children
AJNR 1987 May-Jun, Vol. 8 (3), P. 489–94

3331. Cann C E
Quantitative CT for determination of bone mineral density: a review
Radiology 1988 Feb, Vol. 166 (2), P. 509–22

3332. Cann C E
Low-dose CT scanning for quantitative spinal mineral analysis
Radiology 1981 Sep, Vol. 140 (3), P. 813–5

3333. Cann C E, Genant H K
Precise measurement of vertebral mineral content using computed tomography
J Comput Assist Tomogr 1980 Aug, Vol. 4 (4), P. 493–500

3334. Carter B L, Karmody C S, Blickman J R, Panders A K
Computed tomography and sialography: 2. Pathology
J Comput Assist Tomogr 1981 Feb, Vol. 5 (1), P. 46–53

3335. Carter B L, Karmody C S, Blickman J R, Panders A K
Computed tomography and sialography: 1. Normal anatomy
J Comput Assist Tomogr 1981 Feb, Vol. 5 (1), P. 42–5

3336. Cassel D M, Young S W, Brody W R, Hall A L
Cancer imaging by scanned projection radiography
J Comput Assist Tomogr 1981 Aug, Vol. 5 (4), P. 557–62

3337. Casselman J W, Mancuso A A
Major salivary gland masses: comparison of MR imaging and CT
Radiology 1987 Oct, Vol. 165 (1), P. 183–9

3338. Cassleman E S, Hasso A N, Ashwal S, Schneider S
Computed tomography of tuberculous meningitis in infants and children
J Comput Assist Tomogr 1980 Apr, Vol. 4 (2), P. 211–6

3339. Castillo M, Davis P C, Ross W K, Hoffman J C Jr
Meningioma of the chiasm and optic nerves: CT and MR findings
J Comput Assist Tomogr 1989 Jul-Aug, Vol. 13 (4), P. 679–81

3340. Castillo M, Hudgins P A, Hoffman J C Jr
Lockjaw secondary to skull base osteochondroma: CT findings
J Comput Assist Tomogr 1989 Mar-Apr, Vol. 13 (2), P. 338–9

3341. Caughran M, White T J, Gerald B, Gardner G
Computed tomography of jugulotympanic paragangliomas
J Comput Assist Tomogr 1980 Apr, Vol. 4 (2), P. 194–8

3342. Cazenave F L, Glass Royal M C, Teitelbaum G P, Zuurbier R, Zeman R K, Silverman P M
CT analysis of a safe approach for translumbar access to the aorta and inferior vena cava
Am J Roentgenol 1991 Feb, Vol. 156 (2), P. 395–6

3343. Chakeres D W, Bryan R N
Acute subarachnoid hemorrhage: in vitro comparison of magnetic resonance and computed tomography
AJNR 1986 Mar-Apr, Vol. 7 (2), P. 223–8

3344. Chakeres D W, Weider D J
Computed tomography of the ossicles
Neuroradiology 1985, Vol. 27 (2), P. 99–107

3345. Chamberlain M C, Press G A, Hesselink J R
MR imaging and CT in three cases of Sturge-Weber syndrome: prospective comparison
AJNR 1989 May-Jun, Vol. 10 (3), P. 491–6

3346. Chambers E F, Manelfe C, Cellerier P
Metrizamide CT cisternography and perioptic subarachnoid space imaging
J Comput Assist Tomogr 1981 Dec, Vol. 5 (6), P. 875–80

3347. Chang C H, Nesbit D E, Fisher D R, Fritz S L, Dwyer S J, Templeton A W, Lin F, Jewell W R
Computed tomographic mammography using a conventional body scanner
Am J Roentgenol 1982 Mar, Vol. 138 (3), P. 553–8

3348. Chang W
Slice characteristics of the Imatron Cine-CT scanner
J Comput Assist Tomogr 1987 May-Jun, Vol. 11 (3), P. 554–7

3349. Chi J G, Yoo H W, Chang K H, Kim C W, Moon H R, Ko K W
Leigh's subacute necrotizing encephalomyelopathy: possible diagnosis by CT scan
Neuroradiology 1981, Vol. 22 (3), P. 141–4

3350. Chintapalli K, Unger J M, Shaffer K, Millen S J
Otosclerosis: comparison of complex-motjon tomography and computed tomography
AJNR 1985 Jan-Feb, Vol. 6 (1), P. 85–9

3351. Chirathivat S, Post M J
CT demonstration of dural metastases in neuroblastoma
J Comput Assist Tomogr 1980 Jun, Vol. 4 (3), P. 316–9

3352. Cho P S, Huang H K, Tillisch J, Kangarloo H
Clinical evaluation of a radiologic picture archiving and communication system for a coronary care unit
Am J Roentgenol 1988 Oct, Vol. 151 (4), P. 823–7

3353. Choi B I, Kim S H, Yu E S, Chung H S, Han M C, Kim C W
Retained surgical sponge: diagnosis with CT and sonography
Am J Roentgenol 1988 May, Vol. 150 (5), P. 1047–50

3354. Cholankeril J V, Ravipati M, Khedekar S, Janeira L F, Villacin A
Unusually large sialocele: CT characteristics
J Comput Assist Tomogr 1989 Mar-Apr, Vol. 13 (2), P. 367–8

3355. Chow P P, Horgan J G, Taylor K J
Neonatal periventricular leukomalacia: real-time sonographic diagnosis with CT correlation
Am J Roentgenol 1985 Jul, Vol. 145 (1), P. 155–60

3356. Chui M C, Bird B L, Rogers J
Extracranial and extraspinal nerve sheath tumors: computed tomographic evaluation
Neuroradiology 1988, Vol. 30 (1), P. 47–53

3357. Claussen C, Lochner B
Dynamische Computertomographie
Springer-Verlag, Berlin Heidelberg New York Tokyo

3358. Claussen C, Lochner B, Kohler D, Banzer D
Dynamische Computertomographie bei Gesichtsschädeltumoren
Dynamic computer tomographic for tumours of the facial skeleton
RÖFO 1982 Feb, Vol. 136 (2), P. 144–50

3359. Clavier E, Thiebot J, Delangre T, Hannequin D, Samson M, Benozio M
Marchiafava-Bignami disease. A case studied by CT and MR imaging
Neuroradiology 1986, Vol. 28 (4), P. 376

3360. Cohen C R, Duchesneau P M, Weinstein M A
Calcification of the basal ganglia as visualized by computed tomography
Radiology 1980 Jan, Vol. 134 (1), P. 97–9

3361. Cohen L M, Hill M C, Siegel R S, Lande I M
CT manifestations of Richter syndrome
J Comput Assist Tomogr 1987 Nov-Dec, Vol. 11 (6), P. 1007–8

3362. Cohen M D
Pediatric sedation editorial; comment
Radiology 1990 Jun, Vol. 175 (3), P. 611–2

3363. Cohen W A, Pinto R S, Kricheff I I
Dynamic CT scanning for visualization of the parasellar carotid arteries
Am J Roentgenol 1982 May, Vol. 138 (5), P. 905–9

3364. Coin C G, Coin J T
Computed tomography of cervical disk disease: technical considerations with representative case reports
J Comput Assist Tomogr 1981 Apr, Vol. 5 (2), P. 275–80

3365. Coleman B G, Arger P H, Dalinka M K, Obringer A C, Raney B R, Meadows A T
CT of sarcomatous degeneration in neurofibromatosis
Am J Roentgenol 1983 Feb, Vol. 140 (2), P. 383–7

3366. Colosimo C Jr, Fileni A, Moschini M, Guerrini P
CT findings in eclampsia
Neuroradiology 1985, Vol. 27 (4), P. 313–7

3367. Conti J, Deck M D, Rottenberg D A
An inexpensive video patient repositioning system for use with transmission and emission computed tomographs
J Comput Assist Tomogr 1982 Apr, Vol. 6 (2), P. 417–21

3368. Controversy: Mis-use of contrast detail curves
Am J Roentgenol 1980 Dec, Vol. 135 (6), P. 1310–5 3369. Cordes M, Christe W, Henkes H, Delavier U, Eichstadt H, Schorner W, Langer R, Felix R
Focal epilepsies: HM-PAO SPECT compared with CT, MR, and EEG
J Comput Assist Tomogr 1990 May-Jun, Vol. 14 (3), P. 402–9

3370. Coscina W F, Arger P H, Herlinger H, Levine M S, Coleman B G, Mintz M C
CT diagnosis of villous adenoma
J Comput Assist Tomogr 1986 Sep-Oct, Vol. 10 (5), P. 764–6

3371. Cox H E, Bennett W F
Computed tomography of absent cervical pedicle
J Comput Assist Tomogr 1984 Jun, Vol. 8 (3), P. 537–9

3372. Cunat J S, Haaga J R, Rhodes R, Bekeny J, El Yousef S
Periaortic fluid aspiration for recognition of infected graft: preliminary report
Am J Roentgenol 1982 Aug, Vol. 139 (2), P. 251–3

3373. Curtin H D, Wolfe P, May M
Malignant external otitis: CT evaluation
Radiology 1982 Nov, Vol. 145 (2), P. 383–8

3374. Dake M D, Dillon W P, Dorwart R H
CT of extraarachnoid metrizamide instillation
Am J Roentgenol 1986 Sep, Vol. 147 (3), P. 583–6

3375. Dal Pozzo G, Mascalchi M, Fonda C, Cadelo M, Ronchi O, Inzitari D
Lower cranial nerve palsy due to dissection of the internal carotid artery: CT and MR imaging
J Comput Assist Tomogr 1989 Nov-Dec, Vol. 13 (6), P. 989–95

3376. Damsma H, Mali W P, Zonneveld F W
CT diagnosis of an aberrant internal carotid artery in the middle ear
J Comput Assist Tomogr 1984 Apr, Vol. 8 (2), P. 317–9

3377. Daneman A, Mancer K, Sonley M
CT appearance of thickened nerves in neurofibromatosis
Am J Roentgenol 1983 Nov, Vol. 141 (5), P. 899–900

3378. Daniels D L, Haughton V M, Williams A L, Berns T F
The flocculus in computed tomography
AJNR 1981 May-Jun, Vol. 2 (3), P. 227–9

3379. Daniels D L, Haughton V M, Williams A L, Gager W E, Berns T F
Computed tomography of the optic chiasm
Radiology 1980 Oct, Vol. 137 (1 Pt 1), P. 123–7

3380. Daniels D L, Williams A L, Haughton V M
Computed tomography of the medulla
Radiology 1982 Oct, Vol. 145 (1), P. 63–9

3381. Daniels D L, Williams A L, Syvertsen A, Gager W E, Harris G J
CT recognition of optic nerve sheath meningioma: abnormal sheath visualization
AJNR 1982 Mar-Apr, Vol. 3 (2), P. 181–3

3382. Darwish H, Haslam R H, Johns R
Enlarged CSF spaces in infants with subdural hematoma letter
Radiology 1983 Apr, Vol. 147 (1), P. 286

3383. Davis J M, Davis K R, Hesselink J R, Greene R
Malignant glomus jugulare tumor: a case with two unusual radiographic features
J Comput Assist Tomogr 1980 Jun, Vol. 4 (3), P. 415–7

3384. Davis J R, Zito J L, Hesselink J R, Taveras J M, Kjellberg R N
Metrizamide sagittal tomography: adjunct to CT cisternography of the sellar region
Am J Roentgenol 1980 Jun, Vol. 134 (6), P. 1205–08

3385. de Leon M J, George A E, Ferris S H, Rosenbloom S, Christman D R, Gentes C I, Reisberg B, Kricheff I I, Wolf A P
Regional correlation of PET and CT in senile dementia of the Alzheimer type
AJNR 1983 May-Jun, Vol. 4 (3), P. 553–6

3386. de Leon M J, George A E, Reisberg B, Ferris S H, Kluger A, Stylopoulos L A, Miller J D, La Regina M E, Chen C, Cohen J
Alzheimer's disease: longitudinal CT studies of ventricular change
Am J Roentgenol 1989 Jun, Vol. 152 (6), P. 1257–62

3387. Delavelle J, Lalanne B, Megret M
Man-in-the barrel syndrome: first CT images
Neuroradiology 1987, Vol. 29 (5), P. 501

3388. Delavelle J, Megret M
CT sagittal reconstruction of posterior fossa tumors
Neuroradiology 1980, Vol. 19 (2), P. 81–8

3389. Destian S, Heier L A, Zimmerman R D, Morgello S, Deck M D
Differentiation between meningeal fibrosis and chronic subdural hematoma after ventricular shunting: value of enhanced CT and MR scans
AJNR 1989 Sep-Oct, Vol. 10 (5), P. 1021–6

3390. Di Chiro G, Eiben R M, Manz H J, Jacobs I B, Schellinger D
A new CT pattern in adrenoleukodystrophy
Radiology 1980 Dec, Vol. 137 (3), P. 687–92

3391. Dietemann J L, Bonneville J F, Cattin F, Poulignot D
Computed tomography of the sellar spine
Neuroradiology 1983, Vol. 24 (3), P. 173–4

3392. Dietemann J L, Heldt N, Burguet J L, Medjek L, Maitrot D, Wackenheim A
CT findings in malignant meningiomas
Neuroradiology 1982, Vol. 23 (4), P. 207–9

3393. Dietemann J L, Portha C, Cattin F, Mollet E, Bonneville J F
CT follow-up of microprolactinoma during bromocriptine-induced pregnancy
Neuroradiology 1983, Vol. 25 (3), P. 133–8

3394. Dietemann J L, Sick H, Wolfram Gabel R, Cruz da Silva R, Koritke J G, Wackenheim A
Anatomy and computed tomography of the normal lumbosacral plexus
Neuroradiology 1987, Vol. 29 (1), P. 58–68

3395. Dihlmann W, Nebel G, Lingg G
Das Dorsum sellae als Indikator der Stammskelettosteoporose. Ergebnisse der computertomographischen Densitometrie
The dorsum sellae as an indicator of axial skeletal osteoporosis. The results of computer tomographic densitometry
RÖFO 1983 Nov, Vol. 139 (5), P. 531–4

3396. Dillon W, Brant Zawadzki M, Sherry R G
Transient computed tomographic abnormalities after focal seizures
AJNR 1984 Jan-Feb, Vol. 5 (1), P. 107–9

3397. Distelmaier P, Kaiser R, Palleske H
Computertomographische Ventrikulographie
Computer tomographic ventriculography
RÖFO 1982 Apr, Vol. 136 (4), P. 421–7

3398. Dold U, Sack H
Praktische Tumortherapie
3. Auflage, 1985 Georg Thieme, Stuttgart New York

3399. Dolinskas C A, Simeone F A
CT characteristics of intraventricular oligodendrogliomas
AJNR 1987 Nov-Dec, Vol. 8 (6), P. 1077–82

3400. Donaldson J S, Luck S R, Vogelzang R
Preoperative CT and MR imaging of ischiopagus twins
J Comput Assist Tomogr 1990 Jul-Aug, Vol. 14 (4), P. 643–6

3401. Dietemann J S, Poznanski A K, Nieves A
CT of children's feet: an immobilization technique
Am J Roentgenol 1987 Jan, Vol. 148 (1), P. 169–70

3402. Doubleday L C, Bernardino M E
CT findings in the perirectal area following radiation therapy
J Comput Assist Tomogr 1980 Oct, Vol. 4 (5), P. 634–8

3403. Downey E F Jr, Buck D R, Ray J W
Arachnoiditis simulating acoustic neuroma on air-CT cisternography
AJNR 1981 Sep-Oct, Vol. 2 (5), P. 470–1

3404. Drayer B P
Functional applications of CT of the central nervous system
AJNR 1981 Nov-Dec, Vol. 2 (6), P. 495–510

3405. du Boulay G H, Ruiz J S, Rose F C, Stevens J M, Zilkha K J
CT changes associated with migraine
AJNR 1983 May-Jun, Vol. 4 (3), P. 472–3

3406. Dubois P J, Beardsley T, Klintworth G, Sydnor C, Cook W, Osborne D, Heinz E R, Drayer B P
Computed tomography of sarcoidosis of the optic nerve
Neuroradiology 1983, Vol. 24 (3), P. 179–82

3407. Dubois P J, Nashold B S, Perry J, Burger P, Bowyer K, Heinz E R, Drayer B P, Bigner S, Higgins A C
CT-guided stereotaxis using a modified conventional stereotaxic frame
AJNR 1982 Jul-Aug, Vol. 3 (3), P. 345–51

3408. Duchazeaubeneix J C, Faivre J C, Garreta D, Guilleminet B, Rouger M, Saudinos J, Palmieri P, Raybaud C, Salamon G, Charpak G, Melchart G, Perrin Y, Santiard J C, Sauli F
Nuclear scattering radiography
J Comput Assist Tomogr 1980 Dec, Vol. 4 (6), P. 803–18

3409. Earnest F 4th, McCullough E C, Frank D A
Fact or artifact: an analysis of artifact in high-resolution computed tomographic scanning of the sella
Radiology 1981 Jul, Vol. 140 (1), P. 109–13

3410. Edelstein W A, Bottomley P A, Hart H R, Smith L S
Signal, noise, and contrast in nuclear magnetic resonance NMR imaging
J Comput Assist Tomogr 1983 Jun, Vol. 7 (3), P. 391–401

3411. Edwards M K, Gilmor R L, Franco J M
Computed tomography of chiasmal optic neuritis
AJNR 1983 May-Jun, Vol. 4 (3), P. 816–8

3412. Eftekhari F, Bernardino M E, Headley D L, Corry P M
Technical note. Use of CT in the placement of heat monitoring thermocouples for hyperthermia therapy
J Comput Assist Tomogr 1981 Dec, Vol. 5 (6), P. 933–6

3413. Ege G N
Computed tomographic demonstration of internal mammary lymph node metastasis in patients with locally recurrent breast carcinoma letter
Radiology 1982 Jan, Vol. 142 (1), P. 253–4

3414. Egger J, Kendall B E
Computed tomography in mitochondrial cytopathy
Neuroradiology 1981, Vol. 22 (2), P. 73–8

3415. Eldevik O P, Dugstad G, Orrison W W, Haughton V M
The effect of clinical bias on the interpretation of myelography and spinal computed tomography
Radiology 1982 Oct, Vol. 145 (1), P. 85–9

3416. Ellert J, Kreel L
The role of computed tomography in the initial staging and subsequent management of the lymphomas
J Comput Assist Tomogr 1980 Jun, Vol. 4 (3), P. 368–91

3417. Elster A D, Stark P
Episternal ossicles: a normal CT variant
RÖFO 1985 Aug, Vol. 143 (2), P. 246–7

3418. Enlow R A, Hodak J A, Pullen K W, Bedworth D D, Moor W C, Reahard T M, Milligan V A
The effect of the computed tomographic scanner on utilization and charges for alternative diagnostic procedures
Radiology 1980 Aug, Vol. 136 (2), P. 413–7

3419. Enzmann D R, Brant Zawadzki M, Britt R H
CT of central nervous system infections in immunocompromised patients
Am J Roentgenol 1980 Aug, Vol. 135 (2), P. 263–7

3420. Enzmann D R, Wheat R, Marshall W H, Bird R, Murphy Irwin K, Karbon K, Hanbery J, Silverberg G D, Britt R H, Shuer L
Tumors of the central nervous system studied by computed tomography and ultrasound
Radiology 1985 Feb, Vol. 154 (2), P. 393–9

3421. Esfahani F, Dolan K D
Air CT cisternography in the diagnosis of vascular loop causing vestibular nerve dysfunction
AJNR 1989 Sep-Oct, Vol. 10 (5), P. 1045–9

3422. Evens R G
Economic implications of a new technology installation: a CT model
Am J Roentgenol 1981 Apr, Vol. 136 (4), P. 673–7

3423. Evens R G, Mettler F A
National CT use and radiation exposure: United States
Am J Roentgenol 1985 May, Vol. 144 (5), P. 1077–81

3424. Fagelman D, Lawrence L P, Black K S, Javors B R
Inferior vena cava pseudothrombus in computed tomography using a contrast medium power injector: a potential pitfall
J Comput Assist Tomogr 1987 Nov-Dec, Vol. 11 (6), P. 1042–3

3425. Farrelly C, Daneman A, Chan H S, Martin D J
Occult neuroblastoma presenting with opsomyoclonus: utility of computed tomography
Am J Roentgenol 1984 Apr, Vol. 142 (4), P. 807–10

3426. Fearon T, Vucich J
Pediatric patient exposures from CT examinations: GE CT/T 9800 scanner
Am J Roentgenol 1985 Apr, Vol. 144 (4), P. 805–9

3427. Fearon T, Vucich J
Normalized pediatric organ-absorbed doses from CT examinations
Am J Roentgenol 1987 Jan, Vol. 148 (1), P. 171–4

3428. Federle M P, Moss A A, Margolin F R
Role of computed tomography in patients with "sciatica"
J Comput Assist Tomogr 1980 Jun, Vol. 4 (3), P. 335–41

3429. Feinstein R S, Gatewood O M, Fishman E K, Goldman S M, Siegelman S S
Computed tomography of adult neuroblastoma
J Comput Assist Tomogr 1984 Aug, Vol. 8 (4), P. 720–6

3430. Felsenberg D, Kalender W A, Trinkwalter W, Wolf K J
CT- Untersuchungen mit reduzierter Strahlendosis
CT examinations using a reduced radiation dosage
RÖFO 1990 Nov, Vol. 153 (5), P. 516–21

3431. Fenzl G, Heywang S H, Vogl T, Obermuller J, Einhaupl K, Clados D, Steinhoff H
Die Kernspintomographie der Wirbelsäule und des Rückenmarks im Vergleich zu Computertomographie und Myelographie

Nuclear magnetic resonance tomography of the spine and spinal cord compared with computed tomography and myelography
RÖFO 1986 Jun, Vol. 144 (6), P. 636–43

3432. Fernandez G G, Coblentz C L, Cooper C, Sallee D S
Hickman nodule: a mimic of metastatic disease
Radiology 1989 May, Vol. 171 (2), P. 401–2

3433. Fernbach S K, Naidich T P, McLone D G, Leestma J E
Computed tomography of primary intrathecal Wilms tumor with diastematomyelia
J Comput Assist Tomogr 1984 Jun, Vol. 8 (3), P. 523–8

3434. Feuerstein I M, Margulis A R
Semierect computed tomography of the abdomen using the Imatron ultrafast CT scanner
J Comput Assist Tomogr 1987 Nov-Dec, Vol. 11 (6), P. 1107–8

3435. Feuerstein I M, Zeman R K, Jaffe M H, Clark L R, David C L
Perirenal cobwebs: the expanding CT differential diagnosis
J Comput Assist Tomogr 1984 Dec, Vol. 8 (6), P. 1128–30

3436. Fiegler W
Der Canalis basilaris medianus im Röntgenbild und Computertomogramm
The canalis basilaris medianus on the x-ray and computed tomogram
RÖFO 1980 Oct, Vol. 133 (4), P. 416–9

3437. Fiegler W, Claussen C, Hedde J P
Vergleich Computertomographie, automatisierter Multisektorscanner (Octoson), konventioneller Ultraschall bei Pankreaserkrankungen
Comparison of computed tomography, automated multisector scanner Octoson and conventional ultrasound in pancreatic diseases
RÖFO 1984 Jan, Vol. 140 (1), P. 50–3

3438. Fileni A, Colosimo C Jr, Mirk P, De Gaetano A M, Di Rocco C
Dandy-Walker syndrome: diagnosis in utero by means of ultrasound and CT correlations
Neuroradiology 1983, Vol. 24 (4), P. 233–5

3439. Fine M, Barron J T, Gordon D L, Horowitz S W
Sellar enlargement due to ectatic carotid arteries: CT and MR demonstration
J Comput Assist Tomogr 1990 May-Jun, Vol. 14 (3), P. 488

3440. Fineberg H V, Wittenberg J, Ferrucci J T Jr, Mueller P R, Simeone J F, Goldman J
The clinical value of body computed tomography over time and technologic change
Am J Roentgenol 1983 Nov, Vol. 141 (5), P. 1067–72

3441. Finelli P F
Bilateral hemorrhagic infarction of the pallidum
J Comput Assist Tomogr 1984 Feb, Vol. 8 (1), P. 125–7

3442. Fink I J, Danziger A, Dillon W P, Brant Zawadzki M, Rechthand E
Atypical CT findings in bacterial meningoencephalitis
Neuroradiology 1984, Vol. 26 (1), P. 51–4

3443. Fink I J, Garra B S, Zabell A, Doppman J L
Computed tomography with metrizamide myelography to define the extent of spinal canal block due to tumor
J Comput Assist Tomogr 1984 Dec, Vol. 8 (6), P. 1072–5

3444. Fisher D M
Sedation of pediatric patients: an anesthesiologist's perspective comment
Radiology 1990 Jun, Vol. 175 (3), P. 613–5

3445. Fishman E K, Pakter R L, Gayler B W, Wheeler P S, Siegelman S S
Jugular venous thrombosis: diagnosis by computed tomography
J Comput Assist Tomogr 1984 Oct, Vol. 8 (5), P. 963–8

3446. Fitzgerald S W, Donaldson J S, Poznanski A K
Pediatric thoracic aorta: normal measurements determined with CT
Radiology 1987 Dec, Vol. 165 (3), P. 667–9

3447. Fletcher G, Haughton V M, Ho K C, Yu S W
Age-related changes in the cervical facet joints: studies with cryomicrotomy, MR, and CT
Am J Roentgenol 1990 Apr, Vol. 154 (4), P. 817–20

3448. Flodmark O, Becker L E, Harwood Nash D C, Fitzhardinge P M, Fitz C R, Chuang S H
Correlation between computed tomography and autopsy in premature and full-term neonates that have suffered perinatal asphyxia
Radiology 1980 Oct, Vol. 137 (1 Pt 1), P. 93–103

3449. Foley W D
Diagnosis with CT at an electronic workstation editorial; comment
Radiology 1991 Mar, Vol. 178 (3), P. 631–2

3450. Foley W D, Lawson T L, Berland L L, Chintapalli K, Berninger W H, Reddington R W
Reformatted coronal display of upper abdominal computed tomography: comparison with ultrasonography
J Comput Assist Tomogr 1981 Aug, Vol. 5 (4), P. 496–502

3451. Ford K, Sarwar M
Computed tomography of dural sinus thrombosis
AJNR 1981 Nov-Dec, Vol. 2 (6), P. 539–43

3452. Fram E K, Godwin J D, Putman C E
Three-dimensional display of the heart, aorta, lungs, and airway using CT
Am J Roentgenol 1982 Dec, Vol. 139 (6), P. 1171–6

3453. Fraser R G, Pare' J A
Diagnoses of diseases of the chest
1979, W.B.Saunders Company, Philadelphia London Toronto

3454. Frederick P R
Licensing agreements and resale of CT equipment editorial
Am J Roentgenol 1980 Mar, Vol. 134 (3), P. 617

3455. Freyschmidt J, Ostertag H
Knochentumoren
1988 Springer Verlag , Berlin Heidelberg New York London Paris Tokyo

3456. Frija J, Yana C, Laval Jeantet M
Anatomy of the minor fissure: evaluation with thin-section CT letter
Radiology 1989 Nov, Vol. 173 (2), P. 571–2

3457. Fuchs W A (ed.)
Advances in CT
1990 Springer Verlag , Berlin Heidelberg New York London Paris Tokyo Hong Kong

3458. Fujioka M, Ohyama N, Honda T, Tsujiuchi J, Suzuki M, Hashimoto S, Ikeda S
Holography of 3D surface reconstructed CT images
J Comput Assist Tomogr 1988 Jan-Feb, Vol. 12 (1), P. 175–8

3459. Futrell N N, Osborn A G, Cheson B D
Pineal region tumors: computed tomographic-pathologic spectrum
Am J Roentgenol 1981 Nov, Vol. 137 (5), P. 951–6

3460. Gaeta M, Pandolfo I, Russi E, Blandino A, Volta S, Racchiusa S
Pelvic carcinomatous neuropathy: CT findings and implications for radiation treatment planning
J Comput Assist Tomogr 1988 Sep-Oct, Vol. 12 (5), P. 811–6

3461. Galanski M, Dickob M, Wittkowski W
CT-Zisternographie der basalen Zisternen. Eine röntgenanatomische Studie
CT- cisternography of the basal cisterns. A roentgen anatomic study
RÖFO 1986 Aug, Vol. 145 (2), P. 149–57

3462. Gale M E
Bochdalek hernia: prevalence and CT characteristics
Radiology 1985 Aug, Vol. 156 (2), P. 449–52

3463. Gale M E, Pugatch R D
Sagittal and coronal CT reconstruction for demonstration of subcarinal adenopathy
J Comput Assist Tomogr 1982 Apr, Vol. 6 (2), P. 249–53

3464. Galvin J R, Rooholamini S A, Stanford W
Obstructive sleep apnea: diagnosis with ultrafast CT
Radiology 1989 Jun, Vol. 171 (3), P. 775–8

3465. Gardner T W, Zaparackas Z G, Naidich T P
Congenital optic nerve colobomas: CT demonstration
J Comput Assist Tomogr 1984 Feb, Vol. 8 (1), P. 95–102

3466. Gatenby R A, Coia L R, Richter M P, Katz H, Moldofsky P J, Engstrom P, Brown D Q, Brookland R, Broder G J
Oxygen tension in human tumors: in vivo mapping using CT-guided probes
Radiology 1985 Jul, Vol. 156 (1), P. 211–4

3467. Gatenby R A, Hartz W H, Engstrom P F, Rosenblum J S, Hammond N D, Kessler H B, Moldofsky P J, Clair M R, Unger E, Broder G J
CT-guided laser therapy in resistant human tumors: phase I clinical trials
Radiology 1987 Apr, Vol. 163 (1), P. 172- 5

3468. Gebarski K S, Glazer G M, Gebarski S S
Brachial plexus: anatomic, radiologic, and pathologic correlation using computed tomography
J Comput Assist Tomogr 1982 Dec, Vol. 6 (6), P. 1058–63

3469. Gebarski S S, Gebarski K S, Gabrielsen T O, Knake J E, Latack J T, Yang P J
Gas as a mass: a symptomatic spinal canalicular collection
J Comput Assist Tomogr 1984 Feb, Vol. 8 (1), P. 145–6

3470. Gebarski S S, Knake J E
Prominent internal occipital protuberance misdiagnosed as fourth ventricular mass
J Comput Assist Tomogr 1984 Aug, Vol. 8 (4), P. 780–2

3471. Gebarski S S, Maynard F W, Gabrielsen T O, Knake J E, Latack J T, Hoff J T
Posttraumatic progressive myelopathy. Clinical and radiologic correlation employing MR imaging, delayed CT metrizamide myelography, and intraoperative sonography
Radiology 1985 Nov, Vol. 157 (2), P. 379–85

3472. Gellad F, Rao K C, Joseph P M, Vigorito R D
Morphology and dimensions of the thoracic cord by computer-assisted metrizamide myelography
AJNR 1983 May-Jun, Vol. 4 (3), P. 614–7

3473. George A E, de Leon M J, Ferris S H, Kricheff I I
Parenchymal CT correlates of senile dementia Alzheimer disease: loss of gray-white matter discriminability
AJNR 1981 May-Jun, Vol. 2 (3), P. 205–13

3474. George A E, de Leon M J, Stylopoulos L A, Miller J, Kluger A, Smith G, Miller D C
CT diagnostic features of Alzheimer disease: importance of the choroidal/hippocampal fissure complex
AJNR 1990 Jan-Feb, Vol. 11 (1), P. 101–7

3475. Gerber J D, Ney D R, Magid D, Fishman E K
Simulated femoral repositioning with three-dimensional CT
J Comput Assist Tomogr 1991 Jan-Feb, Vol. 15 (1), P. 121–5

3476. Gerlock A J Jr, Giyanani V L, Venable D D, Mirfakhraee M
Membranous obstruction of the inferior vena cava: an ultrasound, computed tomography, and inferior vena cavogram image correlation
J Comput Assist Tomogr 1984 Jun, Vol. 8 (3), P. 567–9

3477. Gerzof S G
Triangulation: indirect CT guidance for abscess drainage
Am J Roentgenol 1981 Nov, Vol. 137 (5), P. 1080–1

3478. Geyer C A, Sartor K J, Prensky A J, Abramson C L, Hodges F J, Gado M H
Leigh disease subacute necrotizing encephalomyelopathy: CT and MR in five cases
J Comput Assist Tomogr 1988 Jan-Feb, Vol. 12 (1), P. 40–4

3479. Gillespie J E, Adams J E, Isherwood I
Three-dimensional computed tomographic reformations of sellar and para-sellar lesions
Neuroradiology 1987, Vol. 29 (1), P. 30–5

3480. Ginsberg F, Peyster R G, Rose W S, Drapkin A J
Sixth nerve schwannoma: MR and CT demonstration
J Comput Assist Tomogr 1988 May-Jun, Vol. 12 (3), P. 482–4

3481. Giorgi C, Broggi G, Garibotto G, Passerini A, Cerchiari U, Abele M G, Koslow M
Three-dimensional neuroanatomic images in CT-guided stereotaxic neurosurgery
AJNR 1983 May-Jun, Vol. 4 (3), P. 719–21

3482. Glassberg R M, Sussman S K, Glickstein M F
CT anatomy of the internal mammary vessels: importance in planning percutaneous transthoracic procedures
Am J Roentgenol 1990 Aug, Vol. 155 (2), P. 397–400

3483. Glatt S L, Lantos G, Danziger A, Katzman R
Efficacy of CT in the diagnosis of vascular dementia
AJNR 1983 May-Jun, Vol. 4 (3), P. 703–5

3484. Gluck E, Radu E W, Mundt C, Gerhardt P
A computed tomographic prolective trohoc study of chronic schizophrenics
Neuroradiology 1980 Dec, Vol. 20 (4), P. 167–71

3485. Gmelin E, Rosenthal M, Schmeller W, Tichy P, Busch D
Computertomographie und Kernspintomographie des Unterschenkels bei chronischer Venen-insuffizienz
Computed tomography and magnetic resonance tomography of the lower leg in chronic venous insufficiency
RÖFO 1989 Jul, Vol. 151 (1), P. 50–6

3486. Goebel N, Brunner U, Bollinger A
CT-Aspekt der häufigsten Variante des Entrapmentsyndroms der Arteria poplitea
CT aspects of the most common variant of the popliteal artery entrapment syndrome
RÖFO 1985 Jun, Vol. 142 (6), P. 698–700

3487. Goitein M, Meyer J
The radiologist, computed tomography, and radiation therapy
Radiology 1982 Jun, Vol. 143 (3), P. 799–801

3488. Goldberg A L, Rosenbaum A E, Wang H, Kim W S, Lewis V L, Hanley D F
Computed tomography of dural sinus thrombosis
J Comput Assist Tomogr 1986 Jan-Feb, Vol. 10 (1), P. 16–20

3489. Goldmann A, Sautter C, Schumacher K A
Computertomographische Befunde bei Plesiomonas-shigelloides- Meningitis
Computed tomographic findings in Plesiomonas shigelloides meningitis
RÖFO 1990 Nov, Vol. 153 (5), P. 601–2

3490. Goldstein J D, Zeifer B, Chao C, Moser F G, Dickson D W, Hirschfeld A D, Davis L
CT appearance of primary CNS lymphoma in patients with acquired immunodeficiency syndrome
J Comput Assist Tomogr 1991 Jan-Feb, Vol. 15 (1), P. 39–44

3491. Golimbu C, Firooznia H, Rafii M, Engler G, Delman A
Computed tomography of thoracic and lumbar spine fractures that have been treated with Harrington instrumentation
Radiology 1984 Jun, Vol. 151 (3), P. 731–3

3492. Gomori J M, Grossman R I, Goldberg H I, Bilaniuk L T, Zimmerman R A
Wall of infundibular recess: a CT and MR study
J Comput Assist Tomogr 1985 Jul-Aug, Vol. 9 (4), P. 705–7

3493. Gomori J M, Leibovici V, Zlotogorski A, Wirguin I, Haham Zadeh S
Computed tomography in Sjogren-Larsson syndrome
Neuroradiology 1987, Vol. 29 (6), P. 557–9

3494. Goodman L R, Almassi G H, Troup P J, Gurney J W, Veseth Rogers J, Chapman P D, Wetherbee J N
Complications of automatic implantable cardioverter defibrillators: radiographic, CT, and echocardiographic evaluation
Radiology 1989 Feb, Vol. 170 (2), P. 447–52

3495. Gooskens R H, Veiga Pires J A, van Nieuwenhuizen O, Kaiser M C
CT of sebaceous nevus syndrome Jadassohn disease
AJNR 1983 Mar-Apr, Vol. 4 (2), P. 203–5

3496. Gore R M, Ghahremani G G, Joseph A E, Nemeck A A, Marn C S, Vogelzang R L
Acquired malposition of the colon and gallbladder in patients with cirrhosis: CT findings and clinical implications
Radiology 1989 Jun, Vol. 171 (3), P. 739–42

3497. Gorich J, Beyer Enke S A, Muller M, Guckel F, Probst G, van Kaick G
Die Wertigkeit der Computertomographie bei der Suche nach unbekanntem Primärtumor
The value of computed tomography in the search for an unknown primary tumor
RÖFO 1988 Sep, Vol. 149 (3), P. 277–9

3498. Grant E G, Borts F T, Schellinger D, McCullough D C, Sivasubramanian K N, Smith Y
Real-time ultrasonography of neonatal intraventricular hemorrhage and comparison with computed tomography
Radiology 1981 Jun, Vol. 139 (3), P. 687–91

3499. Gregl A, Fischer U, von Heyden D, Imschweiler E, Korber H J, Stichnoth F, Terwey B
Computertomographie und Kernspintomographie beim peripheren Lymphödem
Computed tomography and nuclear spin tomography in peripheral lymphedema
RÖFO 1985 Aug, Vol. 143 (2), P. 219–26

3500. Groen J J, Hekster R E
Computed tomography in Pick's disease: findings in a family affected in three consecutive generations
J Comput Assist Tomogr 1982 Oct, Vol. 6 (5), P. 907–11

3501. Groenhout C M, Gooskens R H, Veiga Pires J A, Ramos L, Willemse J, van Nieuwenhuizen O
Value of sagittal sonography and direct sagittal CT of the Dandy- Walker syndrome
AJNR 1984 Jul- Aug, Vol. 5 (4), P. 476–7

3502. Grönemeyer D H W, Seidel R M M (ed.)
Interventionelle Computertomographie
1989 Ueberreuter Wissenschaft, Wien Berlin

3503. Guyon J J, Brant Zawadzki M, Seiff S R
CT demonstration of optic canal fractures
Am J Roentgenol 1984 Nov, Vol. 143 (5), P. 1031–4

3504. Haaga J R, Kori S H, Eastwood D W, Borkowski G P
Improved technique for CT-guided celiac ganglia block
Am J Roentgenol 1984 Jun, Vol. 142 (6), P. 1201–4

3505. Hahn F J, Gurney J
CT signs of central descending transtentorial herniation letter
AJNR 1985 Sep-Oct, Vol. 6 (5), P. 844–5

3506. Hall A, Wagle V
CT enhancement after use of cocaine letter
AJNR 1990 Sep-Oct, Vol. 11 (5), P. 1083

3507. Hall F M
Workup of adenocarcinoma of unknown primary site letter
Radiology 1982 Oct, Vol. 145 (1), P. 233

3508. Hall F M, Joffe N
CT imaging of the anserine bursa
Am J Roentgenol 1988 May, Vol. 150 (5), P. 1107–8

3509. Hammer B
Experiences with intrathecally enhanced computed tomography
Neuroradiology 1980, Vol. 19 (5), P. 221–8

3510. Hammer B, Jellinger K
Computertomographische Diagnostik der Zystizerkose
Computer tomographic diagnosis of cysticercosis
RÖFO 1981 Sep, Vol. 135 (3), P. 365–7

3511. Hammerschlag S B, O Reilly G V, Naheedy M H
Computed tomography of the optic canals
AJNR 1981 Nov-Dec, Vol. 2 (6), P. 593–4

3512. Hanafee W N, Mancuso A, Winter J, Jenkins H, Bergstrom L
Edge enhancement computed tomography scanning in inflammatory lesions of the middle ear
Radiology 1980 Sep, Vol. 136 (3), P. 771–5

3513. Harder T, Dewes W, Solymosi L, Steudel A, Brassel F
MR- Tomographie, CT und Angiographie vaskulärer Malformationen des zentralen Nervensystems
MR tomography, CT and angiography of vascular malformations of the central nervous system
RÖFO 1989 Feb, Vol. 150 (2), P. 119–24

3514. Harnsberger H R, Mancuso A A, Muraki A S, Byrd S E, Dillon W P, Johnson L P, Hanafee W N
Branchial cleft anomalies and their mimics: computed tomographic evaluation
Radiology 1984 Sep, Vol. 152 (3), P. 739–48

3515. Harter L P, Moss A A, Goldberg H I, Gross B H
CT-guided fine-needle aspirations for diagnosis of benign and malignant disease
Am J Roentgenol 1983 Feb, Vol. 140 (2), P. 363–7

3516. Harvey G D, Mayer D P, Radecki P D
Simplified patient positioning to reduce beam hardening in CT of the lower neck
AJNR 1984 Nov-Dec, Vol. 5 (6), P. 796

3517. Hashimoto T, Mitomo M, Hirabuki N, Miura T, Kawai R, Nakamura H, Kawai H, Ono K, Kozuka T
Nerve root avulsion of birth palsy: comparison of myelography with CT myelography and somatosensory evoked potential
Radiology 1991 Mar, Vol. 178 (3), P. 841–5

3518. Hasuo K, Tamura S, Yasumori K, Uchino A, Goda S, Ishimoto S, Kamikaseda K, Wakuta Y, Kishi M, Masuda K
Computed tomography and angiography in MELAS mitochondrial myopathy, encephalopathy, lactic acidosis and stroke-like episodes; report of 3 cases
Neuroradiology 1987, Vol. 29 (4), P. 393–7

3519. Hatam A, Bergstrom M, Noren G
Effects of dexamethasone treatment on acoustic neuromas: evaluation by computed tomography
J Comput Assist Tomogr 1985 Sep-Oct, Vol. 9 (5), P. 857–60

3520. Hatfield K D, Segal S D, Tait K
Barium sulfate for abdominal computer assisted tomography
J Comput Assist Tomogr 1980 Aug, Vol. 4 (4), P. 570

3521. Haughton V M, Rimm A A, Sobocinski K A, Papke R A, Daniels D L, Williams A L, Lynch R, Levine R
A blinded clinical comparison of MR imaging and CT in neuroradiology
Radiology 1986 Sep, Vol. 160 (3), P. 751–5

3522. Haughton V M, Rosenbaum A E, Williams A L, Drayer B
Recognizing the empty sella by CT: the infundibulum sign
Am J Roentgenol 1981 Feb, Vol. 136 (2), P. 293–5

3523. Haughton V M, Williams A L
Computed tomography of the spine
1982 C.V.Mosby Company ,St Louis Toronto London

3524. Haughton V, Schmidt J, Syvertsen A, Khatri B, Ho K C, Wilson C
Detection of demyelinated plaques with xenon-enhanced computed tomography
Neuroradiology 1980 Dec, Vol. 20 (4), P. 181–3

3525. Hawkins I F Jr
Robotic intervention: why not? editorial
Am J Roentgenol 1984 Jun, Vol. 142 (6), P. 1292–3

3526. Hayashi T, Shyojima K, Honda E, Hashimoto T
Lipoma of corpus callosum associated with frontoethmoidal lipomeningocele: CT findings
J Comput Assist Tomogr 1984 Aug, Vol. 8 (4), P. 795–6

3527. Hayes E, Lavelle W
Sphenochoanal polyp: CT findings
J Comput Assist Tomogr 1989 Mar-Apr, Vol. 13 (2), P. 365–6

3528. Haykal H A, Wang A M, Zamani A A, Rumbaugh C L
Computed tomography of spontaneous acute cervical epidural hematoma
J Comput Assist Tomogr 1984 Apr, Vol. 8 (2), P. 229–31

3529. Hayman L A, Evans R A, Bastion F O, Hinck V C
Delayed high dose contrast CT: identifying patients at risk of massive hemorrhagic infarction
Am J Roentgenol 1981 Jun, Vol. 136 (6), P. 1151–9

3530. Haynor D R, Borning A W, Griffin B A, Jacky J P, Kalet I J, Shuman W P
Radiotherapy planning: direct tumor location on simulation and port films using CT. Part I. Principles
Radiology 1986 Feb, Vol. 158 (2), P. 537–40

3531. Heelan R T, Demas B E, Caravelli J F, Martini N, Bains M S, McCormack P M, Burt M, Panicek D M, Mitzner A
Superior sulcus tumors: CT and MR imaging
Radiology 1989 Mar, Vol. 170 (3 Pt 1), P. 637–41

3532. Heelan R T, Hilaris B S, Anderson L L, Nori D, Martini N, Watson R C, Caravelli J F, Linares L A
Lung tumors: percutaneous implantation of I-125 sources with CT treatment planning
Radiology 1987 Sep, Vol. 164 (3), P. 735–40

3533. Heiberg E, Wolverson M K, Sundaram M, Shields J B
CT findings in leukemia
Am J Roentgenol 1984 Dec, Vol. 143 (6), P. 1317–23

3534. Heinz E R, Dubois P J, Drayer B P, Hill R
A preliminary investigation of the role of dynamic computed tomography in renovascular hypertension
J Comput Assist Tomogr 1980 Feb, Vol. 4 (1), P. 63–6

3535. Heinz E R, Heinz T R, Radtke R, Darwin R, Drayer B P, Fram E, Djang W T
Efficacy of MR vs CT in epilepsy
Am J Roentgenol 1989 Feb, Vol. 152 (2), P. 347–52

3536. Heinz E R, Ward A, Drayer B P, Dubois P J
Distinction between obstructive and atrophic dilatation of ventricles in children
J Comput Assist Tomogr 1980 Jun, Vol. 4 (3), P. 320–5

3537. Heiss E, Huk W
Das computertomographische Bild des subduralen Empyems
The computer tomographic appearances of subdural empyemas
RÖFO 1981 May, Vol. 134 (5), P. 500–2

3538. Heller M, Guthoff R, Hagemann J, Jend H H
CT of malignant choroidal melanoma – morphology and perfusion characteristics
Neuroradiology 1982, Vol. 23 (1), P. 23–30

3539. Heller M, Jend H J, (Hrg)
Computertomographie in der Traumatologie
Georg Thieme, Stuttgart New York

3540. Helmberger T, Schmitt R, Wuttke V
CT-Diagnose einer diffusen Episkleritis
CT diagnosis of a diffuse episcleritis
RÖFO 1989 Dec, Vol. 151 (6), P. 752–3

3541. Helmer M, Gritzmann N, Schlegl A
Computertomographische Diagnostik eines Aneurysmas einer "Arteria lusoria"
Computed tomographic diagnosis of an aneurysm of an arteria lusoria
RÖFO 1987 Jul, Vol. 147 (1), P. 99–100

3542. Helms C A, Munk P L, Witt W S, Davis G W, Morris J, Onik G
Retrorenal colon: implications for percutaneous diskectomy
Radiology 1989 Jun, Vol. 171 (3), P. 864–5

3543. Hemmingsson A, Jung B, Ytterbergh C
Ellipsoidal body phantom for evaluation of CT scanners
J Comput Assist Tomogr 1983 Jun, Vol. 7 (3), P. 503–8

3544. Hendrickx P, Dohring W
Computertomographischer Nachweis chemotherapie-induzierter Thymusveranderungen bei Patienten mit metastasierten Hodentumoren
Computed tomographic detection of chemotherapy-induced thymus changes in patients with metastatic testicular tumors
RÖFO 1989 Mar, Vol. 150 (3), P. 268–73

3545. Henriksen L H, Trebo S
Post-traumatic coronoid process impingement on zygomatic arch: CT demonstration
J Comput Assist Tomogr 1988 Jul-Aug, Vol. 12 (4), P. 712–3

3546. Heran F, Defer G, Brugieres P, Brenot F, Gaston A, Degos J D
Cortical blindness during chemotherapy: clinical, CT, and MR correlations
J Comput Assist Tomogr 1990 Mar-Apr, Vol. 14 (2), P. 262–6

3547. Herbert D L, Gur D, Shabason L, Good W F, Rinaldo J E, Snyder J V, Borovetz H S, Mancici M C
Mapping of human local pulmonary ventilation by xenon enhanced computed tomography
J Comput Assist Tomogr 1982 Dec, Vol. 6 (6), P. 1088–93

3548. Herman G T, Lewitt R M
Evaluation of a preprocessing algorithm for truncated CT projections
J Comput Assist Tomogr 1981 Feb, Vol. 5 (1), P. 127–35

3549. Hertzanu Y, Hirsch M, Peiser J, Avinoach I
Computed tomography of elephantiasis neuromatosa
J Comput Assist Tomogr 1989 Jan-Feb, Vol. 13 (1), P. 156–8

3550. Herzog S, Mafee M
Synovial chondromatosis of the TMJ: MR and CT findings
AJNR 1990 Jul-Aug, Vol. 11 (4), P. 742–5

3551. Hidalgo H, Korobkin M, Breiman R S, Heaston D K, Moore A V, Ram P C
CT demonstration of subcutaneous venous collaterals J Comput Assist Tomogr 1982 Jun, Vol. 6 (3), P. 514–8

3552. Hill S C, Hoeg J M, Dwyer A J, Vucich J J, Doppman J L
CT findings in acid lipase deficiency: wolman disease and cholesteryl ester storage disease
J Comput Assist Tomogr 1983 Oct, Vol. 7 (5), P. 815–8

3553. Hinshaw D B Jr, Fahmy J L, Peckham N, Thompson J R, Hasso A N, Holshouser B, Paprocki T
The bright choroid plexus on MR: CT and pathologic correlation
AJNR 1988 May-Jun, Vol. 9 (3), P. 483–6

3554. Hiraoka M, Akuta K, Nishimura Y, Nagata Y, Jo S, Takahashi M, Abe M
Tumor response to thermoradiation therapy: use of CT in evaluation
Radiology 1987 Jul, Vol. 164 (1), P. 259–62

3555. Holland B A, Perrett L V, Mills C M
Meningovascular syphilis: CT and MR findings
Radiology 1986 Feb, Vol. 158 (2), P. 439–42

3556. Holland I M, Kendall B E
Computed tomography in Alexander's disease
Neuroradiology 1980, Vol. 20 (2), P. 103–6

3557. Holtas S, Monajati A, Utz R
Computed tomography of malignant lymphoma involving the skull
J Comput Assist Tomogr 1985 Jul-Aug, Vol. 9 (4), P. 725–7

3558. Hong Magno E T, Muraki A S, Huttenlocher P R
Atypical CT scans in adrenoleukodystrophy
J Comput Assist Tomogr 1987 Mar-Apr, Vol. 11 (2), P. 333–6

3559. Hopper K D, Diehl L F, Lesar M, Barnes M, Granger E, Baumann J
Hodgkin disease: clinical utility of CT in initial staging and treatment
Radiology 1988 Oct, Vol. 169 (1), P. 17–22

3560. Hopper K D, Sherman J L, Luethke J M, Ghaed N
The retrorenal colon in the supine and prone patient
Radiology 1987 Feb, Vol. 162 (2), P. 443–6

3561. Hopper K D, Yakes W F
The posterior intercostal approach for percutaneous renal procedures: risk of puncturing the lung, spleen, and liver as determined by CT
Am J Roentgenol 1990 Jan, Vol. 154 (1), P. 115–7

3562. Hornig K
Ausgedehnte osteolytische Kalottendestruktionen bei primarem Mammakarzinom
Extensive osteolytic calotte destructions in primary breast cancer
Radiologe 1988 Mar, Vol. 28 (3), P. 132–3

3563. Houston L W, Hinke M L
Neuroradiology case of the day
Am J Roentgenol 1986 May, Vol. 146 (5), P. 1094–7

3564. Hubener K H, Pahl W M
Computertomographische Untersuchungen an altägyptischen Mumien
Computer tomographic investigation of ancient Egyptian mummies
RÖFO 1981 Aug, Vol. 135 (2), P. 213–9

3565. Huggins T J, Lesar M L, Friedman A C, Pyatt R S, Thane T T
CT appearance of persistent left superior vena cava
J Comput Assist Tomogr 1982 Apr, Vol. 6 (2), P. 294–7

3566. Hughes G M
National survey of computed tomography unit capacity
Radiology 1980 Jun, Vol. 135 (3), P. 699–703

3567. Huk W, Baer U
A new targeting device for stereotaxic procedures within the CT scanner
Neuroradiology 1980, Vol. 19 (1), P. 13–7

3568. Huk W, Heindel W, Deimling M, Stetter E
Nuclear magnetic resonance NMR tomography of the central nervous system: comparison of two imaging sequences
J Comput Assist Tomogr 1983 Jun, Vol. 7 (3), P. 468–75

3569. Hunter T B
The value of a worksheet in body-CT examinations letter
Am J Roentgenol 1987 May, Vol. 148 (5), P. 1060

3570. Hunter T B, Paplanus S H, Chernin M M, Coulthard S W
Dermoid cyst of the floor of the mouth: CT appearance
Am J Roentgenol 1983 Dec, Vol. 141 (6), P. 1239–40

3571. Hurst R W, Erickson S, Cail W S, Newman S A, Levine P A, Burke J, Cantrell R W
Computed tomographic features of esthesioneuroblastoma
Neuroradiology 1989, Vol. 31 (3), P. 253–7

3572. Hurst R W, Kerns S R, McIlhenny J, Park T S, Cail W S
Neonatal dural venous sinus thrombosis associated with central venous catheterization: CT and MR studies
J Comput Assist Tomogr 1989 May-Jun, Vol. 13 (3), P. 504–7

3573. Ieshima A, Eda I, Matsui A, Yoshino K, Takashima S, Takeshita K
Computed tomography in Krabbe's disease: comparison with neuropathology
Neuroradiology 1983, Vol. 25 (5), P. 323–7

3574. Ieshima A, Kisa T, Yoshino K, Takashima S, Takeshita K
A morphometric CT study of Down's syndrome showing small posterior fossa and calcification of basal ganglia
Neuroradiology 1984, Vol. 26 (6), P. 493–8

3575. Igidbashian V, Mahboubi S, Zimmerman R A
CT and MR findings in Aicardi syndrome
J Comput Assist Tomogr 1987 Mar-Apr, Vol. 11 (2), P. 357–8

3576. Im J G, Gamsu G, Gordon D, Stein M G, Webb W R, Cann C E, Niklason L T
CT densitometry of pulmonary nodules in a frozen human thorax
Am J Roentgenol 1988 Jan, Vol. 150 (1), P. 61–6

3577. Imai A, Meyer J S, Kobari M, Ichijo M, Shinohara T, Oravez W T
LCBF values decline while L lambda values increase during normal human aging measured by stable xenon-enhanced computed tomography
Neuroradiology 1988, Vol. 30 (6), P. 463–72

3578. Imamura K, Fujii M
Empirical beam hardening correction in the measurement of vertebral bone mineral content by computed tomography
Radiology 1981 Jan, Vol. 138 (1), P. 223–6

3579. Inoue Y, Fukuda T, Takashima K, Ochi H, Onoyama Y, Kusuda S, Matsuoka O, Murata R
Adrenoleukodystrophy: new CT findings
AJNR 1983 Jul-Aug, Vol. 4 (4), P. 951–4

3580. Inoue Y, Saiwai S, Miyamoto T, Ban S, Yamamoto T, Takemoto K, Taniguchi S, Sato S, Namba K, Ogata M
Postcontrast computed tomography in subarachnoid hemorrhage from ruptured aneurysms
J Comput Assist Tomogr 1981 Jun, Vol. 5 (3), P. 341–4

3581. International symposium and course on computed tomography and other computer assisted imaging techniques. New Orleans, Louisiana. April 12–16, 1982. Abstracts
J Comput Assist Tomogr 1982 Dec, Vol. 6 (6), P. 1220–5

3582. International symposium and course on computed tomography. Las Vegas, Nevada April 7–11, 1980. Abstracts
J Comput Assist Tomogr 1980 Oct, Vol. 4 (5), P. 700–17

3583. Irnberger T
Die hochauflösende Computertomographie bei primären und sekundären Läsionen des Optikus-scheidenkomplexes
High-resolution computed tomography in primary and secondary lesions of the optic nerve sheath complex
RÖFO 1985 Aug, Vol. 143 (2), P. 151–7

3584. Irnberger T
Computertomographische Diagnose eines kongenitalen Optikuskoloboms
Computed tomographic diagnosis of a congenital optic nerve coloboma
RÖFO 1985 Jul, Vol. 143 (1), P. 112–3

3585. Irnberger T
Zur Diagnose und Differentialdiagnose der Drüsenpapille unter besonderer Berücksichtigung der Computertomographie
Diagnosis and differential diagnosis of drusen of the optic papilla with special reference to computed tomography
RÖFO 1984 Aug, Vol. 141 (2), P. 136–9

3586. Jack C R Jr, O Neill B P, Banks P M, Reese D F
Central nervous system lymphoma: histologic types and CT appearance
Radiology 1988 Apr, Vol. 167 (1), P. 211–5

3587. Jacobs C J, Harnsberger H R, Lufkin R B, Osborn A G, Smoker W R, Parkin J L
Vagal neuropathy: evaluation with CT and MR imaging
Radiology 1987 Jul, Vol. 164 (1), P. 97–102

3588. Jacoby C G
Need for precision in experimental design letter
Am J Roentgenol 1986 Jan, Vol. 146 (1), P. 174–5

3589. Janon E A
Gadolinium-DPTA: a radiographic contrast agent letter
Am J Roentgenol 1989 Jun, Vol. 152 (6), P. 1348

3590. Jaques P F, Parker L A, Mauro M A
Fulminant systemic necrotizing arteritis: CT findings
J Comput Assist Tomogr 1988 Jan-Feb, Vol. 12 (1), P. 104–8

3591. Jeffrey R B Jr, Federle M P
The collapsed inferior vena cava: CT evidence of hypovolemia
Am J Roentgenol 1988 Feb, Vol. 150 (2), P. 431–2

3592. Jend H H
Die computertomographische Antetorsionswinkelbestimmung. Voraussetzungen und Möglichkeiten
Computed tomographic determination of the anteversion angle. Premises and possibilities
RÖFO 1986 Apr, Vol. 144 (4), P. 447–52

3593. Jewel K L
Sensitivity of MRI vs. CT for neuroimaging letter
Am J Roentgenol 1985 Jun, Vol. 144 (6), P. 1319–20

3594. Jinkins J R
Optic hydrops: isolated nerve sheath dilation demonstrated by CT
AJNR 1987 Sep-Oct, Vol. 8 (5), P. 867–70

3595. Jinkins J R
Dynamic CT of tuberculous meningeal reactions
Neuroradiology 1987, Vol. 29 (4), P. 343–7

3596. Jinkins J R
CT findings in complete premature craniosynostosis
Neuroradiology 1987, Vol. 29 (2), P. 216

3597. Jinkins J R, Bashir R, Al Kawi M Z, Siquiera E
The parenchymal CT myelogram: in vivo imaging of the gray matter of the spinal cord
AJNR 1987 Nov-Dec, Vol. 8 (6), P. 979–82

3598. Johansen J G, Hemminghytt S, Haughton V M
CT Appearance of the retroisthmic cleft
AJNR 1984 Nov-Dec, Vol. 5 (6), P. 835–6

3599. Johansen J G, McCarty D J, Haughton V M
Retrosomatic clefts: computed tomographic appearance
Radiology 1983 Aug, Vol. 148 (2), P. 447–8

3600. Johnson D W, Voorhees R L, Lufkin R B, Hanafee W, Canalis R
Cholesteatomas of the temporal bone: role of computed tomography
Radiology 1983 Sep, Vol. 148 (3), P. 733–7

3601. Johnson J E, Yang P J, Seeger J F, Iacono R P
Vertical fracture of the odontoid: CT diagnosis
J Comput Assist Tomogr 1986 Mar-Apr, Vol. 10 (2), P. 311–2

3602. Johnson K K, Russ P D, Bair J H, Friefeld G D
Diagnosis of synthetic vascular graft infection: comparison of CT and gallium scans
Am J Roentgenol 1990 Feb, Vol. 154 (2), P. 405–9

3603. Junker J A, Totty W G, Stanley R J, McClennan B L
Computed-tomographic confirmation of femoral vein distension with the Valsalva maneuver
Radiology 1983 Apr, Vol. 147 (1), P. 275

3604. Kaiser M C, Capesius P, Veiga Pires J A, Sandt G
A sign of lumbar disk herniation recognizable on lateral CT generated digital radiograms
J Comput Assist Tomogr 1984 Dec, Vol. 8 (6), P. 1066–71

3605. Kaiser M C, Pettersson H, Harwood Nash D C, Fitz C R, Chuang S
CT for trauma to the base of the skull and spine in children
Neuroradiology 1981, Vol. 22 (1), P. 27–31

3606. Kaiser M C, Veiga Pires J A, Descamps P, Brihaye C
CT in the diagnostic work-up of hypogenetic lung syndrome HLS in homozygotic twins
RÖFO 1986 Apr, Vol. 144 (4), P. 476–8

3607. Kalovidouris A, Gouliamos A, Demou L, Vassilopoulos P, Vlachos L, Papavassiliou K
Postsurgical evaluation of hydatid disease with CT: diagnostic pitfalls
J Comput Assist Tomogr 1984 Dec, Vol. 8 (6), P. 1114–9

3608. Kam J, Patel S, Ward R E
Computed tomography of aortic and aortoiliofemoral grafts
J Comput Assist Tomogr 1982 Apr, Vol. 6 (2), P. 298–303

3609. Kapila A, Chakeres D W
Clivus fracture: CT demonstration
J Comput Assist Tomogr 1985 Nov-Dec, Vol. 9 (6), P. 1142–4

3610. Kapila A, Gupta K L, Garcia J H
CT and MR of lymphomatoid granulomatosis of the CNS: report of four cases and review of the literature
AJNR 1988 Nov-Dec, Vol. 9 (6), P. 1139–43

3611. Kappelle L J, Ramos L M, van Gijn J
The role of computed tomography in patients with lacunar stroke in the carotid territory
Neuroradiology 1989, Vol. 31 (4), P. 316–9

3612. Karasawa H, Tomita S, Suzuki S
Chronic subdural hematomas. Time-density curve and iodine concentration in enhanced CT
Neuroradiology 1987, Vol. 29 (1), P. 36–9

3613. Kart B H, Reddy S C, Rao G R, Poveda H
Choroid plexus metastasis: CT appearance
J Comput Assist Tomogr 1986 May-Jun, Vol. 10 (3), P. 537–40

3614. Kaufman H H, Singer J M, Sadhu V K, Handel S F, Cohen G
Isodense acute subdural hematoma
J Comput Assist Tomogr 1980 Aug, Vol. 4 (4), P. 557–9

3615. Kaufman J L, Fereshetian A, Chang B, Shah D M, Leather R P
Septicemia presenting with endoaneurysmal gas: CT demonstration
Am J Roentgenol 1988 Aug, Vol. 151 (2), P. 287–8

3616. Kaufman R A, Stalker H P
Hypovolemic shock in children letter
Radiology 1988 Feb, Vol. 166 (2), P. 579–80

3617. Kazui S, Kuriyama Y, Naritomi H, Sawada T, Ogawa M, Maruyama M
Estimation of vertebral arterial asymmetry by computed tomography
Neuroradiology 1989, Vol. 31 (3), P. 237–9

3618. Kearfott K J, Rottenberg D A, Knowles R J
A new headholder for PET, CT, and NMR imaging
J Comput Assist Tomogr 1984 Dec, Vol. 8 (6), P. 1217–20

3619. Kelekis L, Kelekis D, Mameletzis K, Kelemouridis B, Artopoulos J
Thoracopagus twins studied with computed tomography
J Comput Assist Tomogr 1980 Jun, Vol. 4 (3), P. 405–6

3620. Kelly D R, Grant E G, Zeman R K, Choyke P L, Bolan J C, Warsof S L
In utero diagnosis of congenital diaphragmatic hernia by CT amniography
J Comput Assist Tomogr 1986 May-Jun, Vol. 10 (3), P. 500–2

3621. Kendall B, Reider Grosswasser I, Valentine A
Diagnosis of masses presenting within the ventricles on computed tomography
Neuroradiology 1983, Vol. 25 (1), P. 11–22

3622. Kennard D R, Spigos D G, Tan W S
Cervical aortic arch: CT correlation with conventional radiologic studies
Am J Roentgenol 1983 Aug, Vol. 141 (2), P. 295–7

3623. Ketonen L, Oksanen V, Kuuliala I, Somer H
Hypodense white matter lesions in computed tomography of neurosarcoidosis
J Comput Assist Tomogr 1986 Mar-Apr, Vol. 10 (2), P. 181–3

3624. Keyes J W Jr, Singer D, Satterlee W, Kalff V, Harkness B A
Liver-spleen studies with the rotating gamma camera. II: Utility of tomography
Radiology 1984 Nov, Vol. 153 (2), P. 537–41

3625. Khouri M R, Mintz M C, Coleman B G
Aneurysmal dilatation of a patent umbilical vein masquerading as a pancreatic pseudocyst: CT characteristics
J Comput Assist Tomogr 1988 Jul- Aug, Vol. 12 (4), P. 662–3

3626. Kido D K, LeMay M, Levinson A W, Benson W E
Computed tomographic localization of the precentral gyrus
Radiology 1980 May, Vol. 135 (2), P. 373–7

3627. Kim K S, Rogers L F, Goldblatt D
CT features of hyperostosing meningioma en plaque
Am J Roentgenol 1987 Nov, Vol. 149 (5), P. 1017–23

3628. Kinard R E, Orrison W W, Brogdon B G
The value of a worksheet in reporting body-CT examinations
Am J Roentgenol 1986 Oct, Vol. 147 (4), P. 848–9

3629. Kingsley D P, Harwood Nash D C
Parameters of infiltration in posterior fossa tumours of childhood using a high resolution CT scanner
Neuroradiology 1984, Vol. 26 (5), P. 347–50

3630. Kingsley D P, Harwood Nash D C
Radiological features of the neuroectodermal tumours of childhood
Neuroradiology 1984, Vol. 26 (6), P. 463–7

3631. Kingsley D P, Kendall B E
CT of the adverse effects of therapeutic radiation of the central nervous system
AJNR 1981 Sep- Oct, Vol. 2 (5), P. 453–60

3632. Kirzner H, Oh Y K, Lee S H
Intraspinal air: a CT finding of epidural abscess
Am J Roentgenol 1988 Dec, Vol. 151 (6), P. 1217–8

3633. Kizer K W
The role of computed tomography in the management of dysbaric diving accidents
Radiology 1981 Sep, Vol. 140 (3), P. 705–7

3634. Kjaer M, Boris P, Hansen L G
Abnormal CT scan in a patient with Gilles de la Tourette syndrome
Neuroradiology 1986, Vol. 28 (4), P. 362–3

3635. Kjos B O, Brant Zawadzki M, Young R G
Early CT findings of global central nervous system hypoperfusion
Am J Roentgenol 1983 Dec, Vol. 141 (6), P. 1227–32

3636. Klein B, McGahan J P
Thorn synovitis: CT diagnosis
J Comput Assist Tomogr 1985 Nov-Dec, Vol. 9 (6), P. 1135–6

3637. Klein M A, Kelly J K, Jacobs I G
Diffuse pneumocephalus from Clostridium perfringens meningitis: CT findings
AJNR 1989 Mar-Apr, Vol. 10 (2), P. 447

3638. Knaus W A, Wagner D P, Davis D O
CT for headache: cost/benefit for subarachnoid hemorrhage
Am J Roentgenol 1981 Mar, Vol. 136 (3), P. 537–42

3639. Knopp E A, Chynn K Y
Spontaneous expulsive choroidal hemorrhage: CT findings
AJNR 1990 Nov-Dec, Vol. 11 (6), P. 1208–9

3640. Kobari M, Meyer J S, Ichijo M, Oravez W T
Leukoaraiosis: correlation of MR and CT findings with blood flow, atrophy, and cognition
AJNR 1990 Mar-Apr, Vol. 11 (2), P. 273–81

3641. Kobayashi T, Negoro M, Awaya S
Cavernous sinus subarachnoid diverticulum and sixth nerve palsy
Neuroradiology 1987, Vol. 29 (3), P. 306–7

3642. Koehler P R, Anderson R E
Computed angiotomography
Radiology 1980 Dec, Vol. 137 (3), P. 843–5

3643. Kogutt M S, Jones J P, Perkins D D
Low-dose digital computed radiography in pediatric chest imaging
Am J Roentgenol 1988 Oct, Vol. 151 (4), P. 775–9

3644. Kohlmeyer K, Lehmkuhl G, Poutska F
Computed tomography of anorexia nervosa
AJNR 1983 May-Jun, Vol. 4 (3), P. 437–8

3645. Kokubo T, Itai Y, Ohtomo K, Yoshikawa K, Iio M, Atomi Y
Retained surgical sponges: CT and US appearance
Radiology 1987 Nov, Vol. 165 (2), P. 415–8

3646. Komaiko M S, Lee M E, Birnberg F A
The contrast enhanced paravascular neoplasm: a potential CT pitfall
J Comput Assist Tomogr 1980 Aug, Vol. 4 (4), P. 516–20

3647. Konig R, Brendlein F
Computertomographischer Nachweis von eisenspeichernden Lymphknoten bei transfusionsbedürftigen Anämien
Computer tomographic detection of iron-storing lymph nodes in transfusion requiring anemias
RÖFO 1982 Sep, Vol. 137 (3), P. 350–2

3648. Kopans D B, Meyer J E
Computed tomography guided localization of clinically occult breast carcinoma-the "N" skin guide
Radiology 1982 Oct, Vol. 145 (1), P. 211–2

3649. Kopp W, Schneider G H, Kaulfersch W, Fritsch G, Schmidberger H
Computertomographische und klinische Verlaufsuntersuchungen bei intraventrikulärer Hämorrhagie
Computed tomographic and clinical follow-up studies in intraventricular hemorrhage
RÖFO 1985 Feb, Vol. 142 (2), P. 154–8

3650. Koslin D B, Kenney P J, Stanley R J, Van Dyke J A
Aortocaval fistula: CT appearance with angiographic correlation
J Comput Assist Tomogr 1987 Mar-Apr, Vol. 11 (2), P. 348–50

3651. Koster O, Lackner K, Simons H, Joka T
Computertomographische Untersuchungen von Gefäßprothesen und Venentransplantaten
Computer tomographic studies of vascular prostheses and vein transplants
RÖFO 1982 Nov, Vol. 137 (5), P. 548–54

3652. Krantz P, Holtas S
Postmortem computed tomography in a diving fatality
J Comput Assist Tomogr 1983 Feb, Vol. 7 (1), P. 132–4

3653. Krassanakis K, Sourtsis E, Karvounis P
Unusual appearance of an acoustic neuroma on computed tomography
Neuroradiology 1981 Feb, Vol. 21 (1), P. 51–3

3654. Kratz H W, Bartel H
Pseudothrombose der Vena cava inferior
Radiologe 1987 Jan, Vol. 27 (1), P. 43–4

3655. Krause D, Drape J L,Maitrot D, Woerly B, Tongio J
CT and MRI of disk herniations
1991 Springer Verlag , Berlin Heidelberg New York London Paris Tokyo Hong Kong Barcelona

3656. Kreel L, Bydder G
Use of a portable syringe pump for glucagon administration in abdominal computed tomography
Radiology 1980 Aug, Vol. 136 (2), P. 507–8

3657. Kressel E
Bildgebende Systeme für die medizinische Diagnostik
1988 Siemens Aktiengesellschaft Berlin München

3658. Kressel H Y, McLean G K, Troupin R H
Correlative imaging conference: Hospital of the University of PennsylvaniaAm J Roentgenol 1980 Dec, Vol. 135 (6), P. 1305–9

3659. Kretzschmar K, Gutjahr P, Kutzner J
CT studies before and after CNS treatment for acute lymphoblastic leukemia and malignant non-hodgkin's lymphoma in childhood
Neuroradiology 1980 Dec, Vol. 20 (4), P. 173–80

3660. Kricheff I I, Pinto R S, Bergeron R T, Cohen N
Air-CT cisternography and canaliography for small acoustic neuromas
AJNR 1980 Jan-Feb, Vol. 1 (1), P. 57–63

3661. Kricun R, Kricun M E
Computed tomography of the spine
1987 Aspen Publishers, Rockville Maryland

3662. Kubota K, Itoh M, Yamada K, Endo S, Matsuzawa T
Some devices for computed tomography radiotherapy treatment planning
J Comput Assist Tomogr 1980 Oct, Vol. 4 (5), P. 697–9

3663. Kucharczyk W, Peck W W, Kelly W M, Norman D, Newton T H
Rathke cleft cysts: CT, MR imaging, and pathologic features
Radiology 1987 Nov, Vol. 165 (2), P. 491–5

3664. Kuhn M J, Clark H B, Morales A, Shekar P C
Group III Mobius syndrome: CT and MR findings
AJNR 1990 Sep-Oct, Vol. 11 (5), P. 903–4

3665. Kuhns L R, Marks B, Brown R A
Delineation of masses identified on axial computed tomography
Radiology 1982 Feb, Vol. 142 (2), P. 536

3666. Kumar A J, Rosenbaum A E, Naidu S, Wener L, Citrin C M, Lindenberg R, Kim W S, Zinreich S J, Molliver M E, Mayberg H S, et al
Adrenoleukodystrophy: correlating MR imaging with CT
Radiology 1987 Nov, Vol. 165 (2), P. 497–504

3667. Kushner M J, Luken M G
Posterior fossa epidural hematoma. A report of three cases diagnosed with computed tomography
Neuroradiology 1983, Vol. 24 (3), P. 169–71

3668. Kwan E, Drace J, Enzmann D
Specific CT findings in Krabbe disease
Am J Roentgenol 1984 Sep, Vol. 143 (3), P. 665–70

3669. Laffey P A, Peyster R G, Nathan R, Haskin M E, McGinley J A
Computed tomography and aging: results in a normal elderly population
Neuroradiology 1984, Vol. 26 (4), P. 273–8

3670. Laissy J P, Milon P, Freger P, Hattab N, Creissard P, Thiebot J
Cervical epidural hematomas: CT diagnosis in two cases that resolved spontaneously
AJNR 1990 Mar-Apr, Vol. 11 (2), P. 394–6

3671. LaMasters D L, Watanabe T J, Chambers E F, Norman D, Newton T H
Multiplanar metrizamide-enhanced CT imaging of the foramen magnum
AJNR 1982 Sep-Oct, Vol. 3 (5), P. 485–94

3672. Lang C
Is direct CT caudatometry superior to indirect parameters in confirming Huntington's disease?
Neuroradiology 1985, Vol. 27 (2), P. 161–3

3673. Lanzieri C F, Sabato U, Sacher M
Third ventricular lymphoma: CT findings
J Comput Assist Tomogr 1984 Aug, Vol. 8 (4), P. 645–7

3674. Larsson E M, Holtas S
False diagnosis of acoustic neuroma due to subdural injection during gas CT cisternogram
J Comput Assist Tomogr 1986 Nov-Dec, Vol. 10 (6), P. 1025–6

3675. Laster D W, Penry J K, Moody D M, Ball M R, Witcofski R L, Riela A R
Chronic seizure disorders: contribution of MR imaging when CT is normal
AJNR 1985 Mar-Apr, Vol. 6 (2), P. 177–80

3676. Latchaw R E, Lunsford L D, Kennedy W H
Reformatted imaging to define the intercommissural line for CT-guided stereotaxic functional neurosurgery
AJNR 1985 May-Jun, Vol. 6 (3), P. 429–33

3677. Lee B C, Deck M D
Sellar and juxtasellar lesion detection with MR
Radiology 1985 Oct, Vol. 157 (1), P. 143–7

3678. Lee B C, Kneeland B, Knowles R J, Cahill P T
Quantification of gray/white matter in neonates and adults
AJNR 1983 May-Jun, Vol. 4 (3), P. 692–5

3679. Lee J K T, Sagel S S, Stanley R J (ed.)
Computed body tomography
2nd ed. 1989 Raven Press, New York

3680. Lee K F
Ischemic chiasma syndrome
AJNR 1983 May-Jun, Vol. 4 (3), P. 777–80

3681. Lee K R, Dwyer S J, Anderson W H, Betz D, Faszold S, Preston D F, Robinson R G, Templeton A W
Continuous image recording using gray-tone, dry-process silver paper
Radiology 1981 May, Vol. 139 (2), P. 493–6

3682. Lee K R, Mansfield C M, Dwyer S J, Cox H L, Levine E, Templeton A W
CT for intracavitary radiotherapy planning
Am J Roentgenol 1980 Oct, Vol. 135 (4), P. 809–13

3683. Lee K R, Tines S C, Yoon J W
CT findings of suprapatellar synovial cysts
J Comput Assist Tomogr 1984 Apr, Vol. 8 (2), P. 296–9

3684. Lee Y Y, Glass J P, van Eys J, Wallace S
Medulloblastoma in infants and children: computed tomographic follow-up after treatment
Radiology 1985 Mar, Vol. 154 (3), P. 677–82

3685. Lee Y Y, Van Tassel P, Bruner J M, Moser R P, Share J C
Juvenile pilocytic astrocytomas: CT and MR characteristics
Am J Roentgenol 1989 Jun, Vol. 152 (6), P. 1263–70

3686. LeMay M
CT changes in dementing diseases: a review
Am J Roentgenol 1986 Nov, Vol. 147 (5), P. 963–75

3687. LeMay M, Stafford J L, Sandor T, Albert M, Haykal H, Zamani A
Statistical assessment of perceptual CT scan ratings in patients with Alzheimer type dementia
J Comput Assist Tomogr 1986 Sep-Oct, Vol. 10 (5), P. 802–9

3688. Levin S, Robinson R O, Aicardi J, Hoare R D
Computed tomography appearances in the linear sebaceous naevus syndrome
Neuroradiology 1984, Vol. 26 (6), P. 469–72

3689. Lewin P K
First stereoscopic images from CT reconstructions of mummies letter
Am J Roentgenol 1988 Dec, Vol. 151 (6), P. 1249

3690. Lewis L K, Hinshaw D B Jr, Will A D, Hasso A N, Thompson J R
CT and angiographic correlation of severe neurological disease in toxemia of pregnancy
Neuroradiology 1988, Vol. 30 (1), P. 59–64

3691. Lien H H, von Krogh J
Varicosity of the left renal ascending lumbar communicant vein: a pitfall in CT diagnosis
Radiology 1984 Aug, Vol. 152 (2), P. 484

3692. Lilja A, Bergstrom K, Spannare B, Olsson Y
Reliability of computed tomography in assessing histopathological features of malignant supratentorial gliomas
J Comput Assist Tomogr 1981 Oct, Vol. 5 (5), P. 625–36

3693. Lindfors K K, Meyer J E, Busse P M, Kopans D B, Munzenrider J E, Sawicka J M
CT evaluation of local and regional breast cancer recurrence
Am J Roentgenol 1985 Oct, Vol. 145 (4), P. 833–7

3694. Lingg G, Hering L
Computertomographie und pathogenes Potential der Plica parapatellaris medialis
Computed tomography and the pathogenic potential of the medial parapatellar fold
RÖFO 1984 May, Vol. 140 (5), P. 561–6

3695. Lipinski J K, McCreath G, Matheson M
Computed tomography of fetal specimens
J Comput Assist Tomogr 1980 Aug, Vol. 4 (4), P. 568–9

3696. Lisson G, Leupold D, Bechinger D, Wallesch C
CT findings in a case of deficiency of 3-hydroxy-3-methylglutaryl-Co A-lyase
Neuroradiology 1981, Vol. 22 (2), P. 99–101

3697. Lo W W, Solti Bohman L G
High-resolution CT of the jugular foramen: anatomy and vascular variants and anomalies
Radiology 1984 Mar, Vol. 150 (3), P. 743–7

3698. Loffler E, Sauer O, Baier K
CT in der Strahlentherapie. Stellenwert bei der rechnerunterstützten 3D-Bestrahlungsplanung der Mamma
CT in radiotherapy. Its value in computer-supported 3D- irradiation planning for the breast
RÖFO 1985 Dec, Vol. 143 (6), P. 685–91

3699. Lovrencic M, Schmutzer L
CT measurement of the normal ventricular system in premature infants
AJNR 1983 May-Jun, Vol. 4 (3), P. 683–4

3700. Ludwig B, Kishikawa T, Wende S, Rochel M, Gehler J
Cranial computed tomography in disorders of complex carbohydrate metabolism and related storage diseases
AJNR 1983 May-Jun, Vol. 4 (3), P. 431–3

3701. Lutgemeier J, Brandtner M, Neumann D
Dreidimensionale Bestrahlungsplanung am Computertomographen
Three dimensional radiation planning using computer tomography
RÖFO 1981 Sep, Vol. 135 (3), P. 343–6

3702. Macpherson P, Teasdale E
CT demonstration of a 5th ventricle-a finding to KO boxers?
Neuroradiology 1988, Vol. 30 (6), P. 506–10

3703. Mafee M F, Lachenauer C S, Kumar A, Arnold P M, Buckingham R A, Valvassori G E
CT and MR imaging of intralabyrinthine schwannoma: report of two cases and review of the literature
Radiology 1990 Feb, Vol. 174 (2), P. 395–400

3704. Mafee M F, Singleton E L, Valvassori G E, Espinosa G A, Kumar A, Aimi K
Acute otomastoiditis and its complications: role of CT
Radiology 1985 May, Vol. 155 (2), P. 391–7

3705. Maier W
Computertomographische Diagnostik des doppelten Aortenbogens beim Neugeborenen
Computed tomographic diagnosis of double aortic arch in the newborn infant
RÖFO 1988 Aug, Vol. 149 (2), P. 223–4

3706. Manelfe C, Clanet M, Gigaud M, Bonafe A, Guiraud B, Rascol A
Internal capsule: normal anatomy and ischemic changes demonstrated by computed tomography
AJNR 1981 Mar-Apr, Vol. 2 (2), P. 149–55

3707. Mann F A, Hildebolt C F
Inappropriate use of a chi 2 test in modality comparison study of related samples letter
Radiology 1991 Feb, Vol. 178 (2), P. 582–3

3708. Mann H, Kozic Z, Boulos M I
CT of lightning injury
AJNR 1983 Jul-Aug, Vol. 4 (4), P. 976–7

3709. Mann H, Kozic Z, Medinilla O R
Computed tomography of lambdoid calvarial defect in neurofibromatosis. A case report
Neuroradiology 1983, Vol. 25 (3), P. 175–6

3710. Marc J A, Khan A, Pillari G, Rosenthal A, Baron M G
Positive contrast ventriculography combined with computed tomography: technique and applications
J Comput Assist Tomogr 1980 Oct, Vol. 4 (5), P. 608–13

3711. Margulis A R
Whitehouse lecture. Radiologic imaging: changing costs, greater benefits
Am J Roentgenol 1981 Apr, Vol. 136 (4), P. 657–65

3712. Martelli A, Scotti G, Harwood Nash D C, Fitz C R, Chuang S H
Aneurysms of the vein of Galen in children: CT and angiographic correlations
Neuroradiology 1980, Vol. 20 (3), P. 123–33

3713. Martin N, Debroucker T, Mompoint D, Akoun J, Cambier J, Nahum H
Sarcoidosis of the pineal region: CT and MR studies
J Comput Assist Tomogr 1989 Jan-Feb, Vol. 13 (1), P. 110–2

3714. Marx M, D Auria S H
Three-dimensional CT reconstructions of an ancient human Egyptian mummy
Am J Roentgenol 1988 Jan, Vol. 150 (1), P. 147–9

3715. Masdeu J C
Infarct versus neoplasm on CT: four helpful signs
AJNR 1983 May-Jun, Vol. 4 (3), P. 522–4

3716. Masdeu J C, Dobben G D, Azar Kia B
Dandy-Walker syndrome studied by computed tomography and pneumoencephalography
Radiology 1983 Apr, Vol. 147 (1), P. 109–14

3717. Mason T O, Rose B S, Goodman J H
Gas bubbles in polymethylmethacrylate cranioplasty simulating abscesses: CT appearance
AJNR 1986 Sep-Oct, Vol. 7 (5), P. 829–31

3718. Masuzawa T, Kumagai M, Sato F
Computed tomographic evolution of post-traumatic subdural hygroma in young adults
Neuroradiology 1984, Vol. 26 (3), P. 245–8

3719. Mathias K, Lambers U, Hoffmann J
Cardiac arrhythmias. Amiodarone liver
Herzrhythmusstorungen. Amiodaronleber
Radiologe 1990 Nov, Vol. 30 (11), P. 553–4

3720. Mayo Smith W, Hayes C W, Biller B M, Klibanski A, Rosenthal H, Rosenthal D I
Body fat distribution measured with CT: correlations in healthy subjects, patients with anorexia nervosa, and patients with Cushing syndrome
Radiology 1989 Feb, Vol. 170 (2), P. 515–8

3721. Mayo Smith W, Rosenthal D I, Goodsitt M M, Klibanski A
Intravertebral fat measurement with quantitative CT in patients with Cushing disease and anorexia nervosa
Radiology 1989 Mar, Vol. 170 (3 Pt 1), P. 835–8

3722. McAdams H P, Geyer C A, Done S L, Deigh D, Mitchell M, Ghaed V N
CT and MR imaging of Canavan disease
AJNR 1990 Mar-Apr, Vol. 11 (2), P. 397–9

3723. McAlister W H, Siegel M J
Pediatric radiology case of the day. Diffuse infiltrating lipomatosis
Am J Roentgenol 1989 Jun, Vol. 152 (6), P. 1331–2

3724. McAllister M D, O Leary D H
CT myelography of subarachnoid leukemic infiltration of the lumbar thecal sac and lumbar nerve roots
AJNR 1987 May-Jun, Vol. 8 (3), P. 568–9

3725. McClellan R L, Eisenberg R L, Giyanani V L
Routine CT screening of psychiatry inpatients
Radiology 1988 Oct, Vol. 169 (1), P. 99–100

3726. McCormack J, Peyster R G, Brodner R A, Cooper V R
CT visualization of ruptured berry aneurysm within hematoma: the flip-flop sign
J Comput Assist Tomogr 1986 Jan-Feb, Vol. 10 (1), P. 28–31

3727. McCort J J
Caring for the major trauma victim: the role for radiology
Radiology 1987 Apr, Vol. 163 (1), P. 1–9

3728. McGinnis B D, Brady T J, New P F, Buonanno F S, Pykett I L, DeLaPaz R L, Kistler J P, Taveras J M
Nuclear magnetic resonance NMR imaging of tumors in the posterior fossa
J Comput Assist Tomogr 1983 Aug, Vol. 7 (4), P. 575–84

3729. McLoughlin M J
CT and percutaneous fine-needle aspiration biopsy in tropical myositis
Am J Roentgenol 1980 Jan, Vol. 134 (1), P. 167–8

3730. McNeil B J, Hanley J A, Funkenstein H H, Wallman J
Paired receiver operating characteristic curves and the effect of history on radiographic interpretation. CT of the head as a case study
Radiology 1983 Oct, Vol. 149 (1), P. 75–7

3731. Meese W, Kluge W, Grumme T, Hopfenmuller W
CT evaluation of the CSF spaces of healthy persons
Neuroradiology 1980 Apr, Vol. 19 (3), P. 131–6

3732. Mehler M F, Rabinowich L
Inflammatory myelinoclastic diffuse sclerosis Schilder's disease: neuroradiologic findings
AJNR 1989 Jan-Feb, Vol. 10 (1), P. 176–80

3733. Mendelson D S, Som P M, Crane R, Cohen B A, Spiera H
Relapsing polychondritis studied by computed tomography
Radiology 1985 Nov, Vol. 157 (2), P. 489–90

3734. Merine D S, Fishman E K, Jones B, Nussbaum A R, Simmons T
Right lower quadrant pain in the immunocompromised patient: CT findings in 10 cases
Am J Roentgenol 1987 Dec, Vol. 149 (6), P. 1177–9

3735. Meyer J E, Oot R F, Lindfors K K
CT appearance of clival chordomas
J Comput Assist Tomogr 1986 Jan-Feb, Vol. 10 (1), P. 34- 8

3736. Meyers M A (ed.)
Computed tomography of the gastrointestinal tract
1986 Springer-Verlag, New York Berlin Heidelberg Tokyo

3737. Mezzacappa P M, Price A P, Haller J O, Kassner E G, Hansbrough F
MR and CT demonstration of levator sling in congenital anorectal anomalies
J Comput Assist Tomogr 1987 Mar- Apr, Vol. 11 (2), P. 273–5

3738. Micklos T J, Proto A V
CT demonstration of the coronary sinus
J Comput Assist Tomogr 1985 Jan-Feb, Vol. 9 (1), P. 60–4

3739. Middleton W D, Smith D F, Foley W D
CT detection of aortocaval fistula
J Comput Assist Tomogr 1987 Mar-Apr, Vol. 11 (2), P. 344–7

3740. Miller C L, Wechsler R J
CT evaluation of Kimray- Greenfield filter complications
Am J Roentgenol 1986 Jul, Vol. 147 (1), P. 45–50

3741. Miner D G, Cohan R H, Davis W K, Braun S D
CT-guided percutaneous aspiration of septic thrombosis of the inferior vena cava
Am J Roentgenol 1987 Jun, Vol. 148 (6), P. 1213–4

3742. Mirich D R, McArdle C B, Kulkarni M V
Benign pleomorphic adenomas of the salivary glands: surface coil MR imaging versus CT
J Comput Assist Tomogr 1987 Jul-Aug, Vol. 11 (4), P. 620–3

3743. Mitnick J S, Pinto R S
Computed tomography in the diagnosis of eosinophilic granuloma
J Comput Assist Tomogr 1980 Dec, Vol. 4 (6), P. 791–3

3744. Mitnick J S, Pinto R S, Lin J P, Rose H, Lieberman A
CT of thrombosed arteriovenous malformations in children
Radiology 1984 Feb, Vol. 150 (2), P. 385–9

3745. Modic M T, Weinstein M A, Rothner A D, Erenberg G, Duchesneau P M, Kaufman B
Calcification of the choroid plexus visualized by computed tomography
Radiology 1980 May, Vol. 135 (2), P. 369–72

3746. Montagno E D, Romer T
Computertomographische Stereotaxie (CTS): Entwicklung eines neuen Systems
Computed tomographic stereotaxy: development of a new system
RÖFO 1986 Oct, Vol. 145 (4), P. 396–401

3747. Moon K L Jr, Federle M P, Abrams D I, Volberding P, Lewis B J
Kaposi sarcoma and lymphadenopathy syndrome: limitations of abdominal CT in acquired immunodeficiency syndrome
Radiology 1984 Feb, Vol. 150 (2), P. 479–83

3748. Moore W E, Ganti S R, Mawad M E, Hilal S K
CT and angiography of primary extradural juxtasellar tumors
Am J Roentgenol 1985 Sep, Vol. 145 (3), P. 491–6

3749. Moran C J, Naidich T P, Marchoski J A
CT-guided needle placement in the central nervous system: results in 146 consecutive patients
Am J Roentgenol 1984 Oct, Vol. 143 (4), P. 861–8

3750. Mori H, Fukuda T, Isomoto I, Maeda H, Hayashi K
CT diagnosis of catheter-induced septic thrombus of vena cava
J Comput Assist Tomogr 1990 Mar-Apr, Vol. 14 (2), P. 236–8

3751. Mori K, Handa H, Itoh M, Okuno T
Benign subdural effusion in infants
J Comput Assist Tomogr 1980 Aug, Vol. 4 (4), P. 466–71

3752. Morris R E, Hasso A N, Thompson J R, Hinshaw D B Jr, Vu L H
Traumatic dural tears: CT diagnosis using metrizamide
Radiology 1984 Aug, Vol. 152 (2), P. 443–6

3753. Moseley I
Long term effects of the introduction of non invasive investigations in neuroradiology. Part 2: Effects on management of individual patients
Neuroradiology 1988, Vol. 30 (3), P. 193–200

3754. Moseley I F
Long term effects of the introduction of noninvasive investigations in neuroradiology. Part 1: Overall trends
Neuroradiology 1988, Vol. 30 (3), P. 187–92

3755. Mostrom U, Bergstrom K, Pech P, Ytterbergh C
Deep-frozen biologic phantom for performance evaluation of CT scanners
J Comput Assist Tomogr 1986 Nov-Dec, Vol. 10 (6), P. 1016–24

3756. Mostrom U, Ytterbergh C
Artifacts in computed tomography of the posterior fossa: a comparative phantom study
J Comput Assist Tomogr 1986 Jul-Aug, Vol. 10 (4), P. 560–6

3757. Muller J W, van Waes P F, Koehler P R
Computed tomography of breast lesions: comparison with x-ray mammography
J Comput Assist Tomogr 1983 Aug, Vol. 7 (4), P. 650–4

3758. Munk P L, Helms C A
Coronoid process hyperplasia: CT studies
Radiology 1989 Jun, Vol. 171 (3), P. 783–4

3759. Munk P L, Robertson W D, Durity F A
Middle fossa arachnoid cyst and subdural hematoma: CT studies
J Comput Assist Tomogr 1988 Nov-Dec, Vol. 12 (6), P. 1073–5

3760. Murphy W A
How does magnetic resonance compare with computed tomography?
Radiology 1984 Jul, Vol. 152 (1), P. 235–6

3761. Murray K, Nixon G W
Epiphyseal growth plate: evaluation with modified coronal CT
Radiology 1988 Jan, Vol. 166 (1 Pt 1), P. 263–5

3762. Nabawi P, Dobben G D, Mafee M, Espinosa G A
Diagnosis of lipoma of the corpus callosum by CT in five cases
Neuroradiology 1981, Vol. 21 (3), P. 159–62

3763. Nagata Y, Nishidai T, Abe M, Hiraoka M, Takahashi M, Fujiwara K, Okajima K
Laser projection system for radiotherapy and CT-guided biopsy
J Comput Assist Tomogr 1990 Nov-Dec, Vol. 14 (6), P. 1046–8

3764. Naheedy M H, Kido D K, O Reilly G V
Computed tomographic evaluation of subdural and epidural metastases
J Comput Assist Tomogr 1980 Jun, Vol. 4 (3), P. 311–5

3765. Nahser H C, Grote W, Lohr E, Gerhard L
Multiple meningiomas. Clinical and computer tomographic observations
Neuroradiology 1981, Vol. 21 (5), P. 259–63

3766. Nahser H C, Hanssler L, Nau H E, Lohr E
Computertomographische Befunde in der Diagnostik und Verlaufskontrolle von germinalen Matrixblutungen bei Neugeborenen
Diagnosis and follow-up studies by computed tomography in hemorrhage of germinal matrix of newborns
Radiologe 1981 Nov, Vol. 21 (11), P. 516–20

3767. Naidich D P, Zerhouni E A, Siegelman S S
Computed tomography and magnetic resonance of the thorax
2nd ed. 1991 Raven Press , New York

3768. Naidich T P, Tomita T, Pech P, Haughton V
Direct coronal computed tomography for presurgical evaluation of posterior fossa tumors
J Comput Assist Tomogr 1985 Nov-Dec, Vol. 9 (6), P. 1065- 72

3769. Naidich T P, Yu R H, King D G, Wholahan J D
Superimposition reformatted CT for preoperative lesion localization and surgical planning
J Comput Assist Tomogr 1980 Oct, Vol. 4 (5), P. 693–6

3770. Naim ur Rahman
Chronic subdural hematoma: correlation of computerized tomography with colour
Neuroradiology 1987, Vol. 29 (1), P. 40–2

3771. Nakasu S, Yoshida M, Nakajima M, Handa J
Cystic cavernous angioma in an infant: CT features
J Comput Assist Tomogr 1991 Jan- Feb, Vol. 15 (1), P. 163–5

3772. Nakstad P, Sortland O, Hovind K
The evaluation of ventriculography as a supplement to computed tomography
Neuroradiology 1982, Vol. 23 (2), P. 85–8

3773. Nanni D, Lotz P R
Hemorrhagic nerve sheath tumors plexiform neurofibromas of the scalp: CT findings
J Comput Assist Tomogr 1985 Mar-Apr, Vol. 9 (2), P. 272–4

3774. Nardis P F, Teramo M, Giunta S, Bellelli A
Unusual cholesteatoma shell: CT findings
J Comput Assist Tomogr 1988 Nov- Dec, Vol. 12 (6), P. 1084–5

3775. Neave V C, Wycoff R R
Computed tomography of cystic nerve root sleeve dilatation
J Comput Assist Tomogr 1983 Oct, Vol. 7 (5), P. 881–5

3776. Nelson J, Grebbell F S
The value of computed tomography in patients with mucopolysaccharidosis
Neuroradiology 1987, Vol. 29 (6), P. 544–9

3777. Neufang K F, Modder U, Friedmann G
Nicht-invasive Diagnostik der Karotis-Sinus-cavernosus-Fisteln durch die Computertomographie
Non-invasive diagnosis of carotid artery- cavernous sinus fistulas using computed tomography
RÖFO 1983 Dec, Vol. 139 (6), P. 639–43

3778. New P F, Hesselink J R, O Carroll C P, Kleinman G M
Malignant meningiomas: CT and histologic criteria, including a new CT sign
AJNR 1982 May-Jun, Vol. 3 (3), P. 267–76

3779. Newman G E, Warner M A, Heaston D K
Diagnosis of lithokelyphos by computed tomography
J Comput Assist Tomogr 1983 Feb, Vol. 7 (1), P. 166–8

3780. Nicolas V, Krahe T, Lackner K, Ruther W, Siedek S
Computertomographische Untersuchungen zur Vitalität des freien Fettlappens im Laminektomiebereich
Computed tomographic research on the viability of a free fat pedicle flap in the area of a laminectomy
RÖFO 1987 May, Vol. 146 (5), P. 565–9

3781. Nishitani H, Umezu Y, Ogawa K, Yuzuriha H, Tanaka H, Matsuura K
Dual-energy projection radiography using condenser x-ray generator and digital radiography apparatus
Radiology 1986 Nov, Vol. 161 (2), P. 533–5

3782. Noldge G, Reinke M
Nose injury Nasentrauma
Radiologe 1984 Sep, Vol. 24 (9), P. 447–8

3783. Noorbehesht B, Fabrikant J I, Enzmann D R
Size determination of supratentorial arteriovenous malformations by MR, CT and angio
Neuroradiology 1987, Vol. 29 (6), P. 512–8

3784. Norton K I, Shugar J M, Som P M, Bernard P J, Murphy R J
Sternocleidomastoid tumor of infancy: CT manifestations
J Comput Assist Tomogr 1991 Jan-Feb, Vol. 15 (1), P. 158–9

3785. Nov A A, Cromwell L D
Computed tomography of neuraxis aspergillosis
J Comput Assist Tomogr 1984 Jun, Vol. 8 (3), P. 413–5

3786. Nussel F, Huber P
High resolution computed tomography of superior sagittal sinus-thrombosis and -abnormalities
Neuroradiology 1989, Vol. 31 (4), P. 307–11

3787. O Mara E M, Pennes D R, Argenta L C
Combination gel- inflatable mammary prosthesis: appearance at CT
Radiology 1989 Jan, Vol. 170 (1 Pt 1), P. 78

3788. O Tuama L A, Laster D W
Oculocerebrorenal syndrome: case report with CT and MR correlates
AJNR 1987 May-Jun, Vol. 8 (3), P. 555-7

3789. Oldendorf W H
Some possible applications of computerized tomography in pathology
J Comput Assist Tomogr 1980 Apr, Vol. 4 (2), P. 141-4

3790. Olier J, Gallego J, Digon E
Computerized tomography in primary hyperammonemia
Neuroradiology 1989, Vol. 31 (4), P. 356-7

3791. Olm M, Blesa R, Ribera G, Cardenal C
Lipoma of the corpus callosum: CT and MR for diagnosis letter
Am J Roentgenol 1988 Sep, Vol. 151 (3), P. 613-4

3792. Onik G, Costello P, Cosman E, Wells T Jr, Goldberg H, Moss A, Kane R, Clouse M E, Hoddick W, Moore S, et al
CT body stereotaxis: an aid for CT-guided biopsies
Am J Roentgenol 1986 Jan, Vol. 146 (1), P. 163-8

3793. Onik G, Goodman P C
CT of Castleman disease
Am J Roentgenol 1983 Apr, Vol. 140 (4), P. 691-2

3794. Oot R F, Melville G E, New P F, Austin Seymour M, Munzenrider J, Pile Spellman J, Spagnoli M, Shoukimas G M, Momose K J, Carroll R, et al
The role of MR and CT in evaluating clival chordomas and chondrosarcomas
Am J Roentgenol 1988 Sep, Vol. 151 (3), P. 567-75

3795. Orcutt J, Ragsdale B D, Curtis D J, Levine M I
Misleading CT in parosteal osteosarcoma
Am J Roentgenol 1981 Jun, Vol. 136 (6), P. 1233-5

3796. Ormson M J, Kispert D B, Sharbrough F W, Houser O W, Earnest F 4th, Scheithauer B W, Laws E R Jr
Cryptic structural lesions in refractory partial epilepsy: MR imaging and CT studies
Radiology 1986 Jul, Vol. 160 (1), P. 215-9

3797. Osborn A G, Anderson R E, Wing S D
The false falx sign
Radiology 1980 Feb, Vol. 134 (2), P. 421-5

3798. Osborn A G, Harnsberger H R, Smoker W R, Boyer R S
Multiple sclerosis in adolescents: CT and MR findings
Am J Roentgenol 1990 Aug, Vol. 155 (2), P. 385-90

3799. Osborne D R, Foulks G N
Computed tomographic analysis of deformity and dimensional changes in the eyeball
Radiology 1984 Dec, Vol. 153 (3), P. 669-74

3800. Otto J, Henderson R, Dandekar M
MR and CT findings in infected ventricular aneurysm repair
J Comput Assist Tomogr 1987 Nov-Dec, Vol. 11 (6), P. 1069-70

3801. Packer R J, Bilaniuk L T, Zimmerman R A
CT parenchymal abnormalities in bacterial meningitis: clinical significance
J Comput Assist Tomogr 1982 Dec, Vol. 6 (6), P. 1064-8

3802. Pagani J J
Significance in statistical analysis of data letter
Am J Roentgenol 1982 Jan, Vol. 138 (1), P. 180-1

3803. Pagani J J, Bernardino M E
Incidence and significance of serendipitous CT findings in the oncologic patient
J Comput Assist Tomogr 1982 Apr, Vol. 6 (2), P. 268-75

3804. Paling M R, Hyams D M
Computed tomography in malignant fibrous histiocytoma
J Comput Assist Tomogr 1982 Aug, Vol. 6 (4), P. 785-8

3805. Papavasiliou C, Andreou J, Stringaris K, Vlahos L, Pontifex G
The CT findings of extramedullary hematopoiesis
Radiologe 1982 Feb, Vol. 22 (2), P. 86-7

3806. Parienty R A, Pradel J, Lepreux J F, Nicodeme C, Dologa M
Computed tomography of sponges retained after laparotomy
J Comput Assist Tomogr 1981 Apr, Vol. 5 (2), P. 187-9

3807. Parisi M, Mehdizadeh H M, Hunter I V, Finch I J
Evaluation of craniosynostosis with three-dimensional CT imaging
J Comput Assist Tomogr 1989 Nov-Dec, Vol. 13 (6), P. 1006-12

3808. Partain C L, James A E, Watson J T, Price R R, Coulam C M, Rollo F D
Nuclear magnetic resonance and computed tomography: comparison of normal human body images
Radiology 1980 Sep, Vol. 136 (3), P. 767-70

3809. Patel D V, Neuman M J, Hier D B
Reversibility of CT and MR findings in neuro-Behcet disease
J Comput Assist Tomogr 1989 Jul-Aug, Vol. 13 (4), P. 669-73

3810. Pedersen H, Gjerris F, Klinken L
Malignancy criteria in computed tomography of primary supratentorial tumors in infancy and childhood
Neuroradiology 1989, Vol. 31 (1), P. 24-8

3811. Pedersen H, Gjerris F, Klinken L
Computed tomography of benign supratentorial astrocytomas of infancy and childhood
Neuroradiology 1981 Mar, Vol. 21 (2), P. 87-91

3812. Perani D, Colombo N, Scotti G, Tonon C
Rapid size reduction of giant prolactinoma following medical treatment
J Comput Assist Tomogr 1984 Feb, Vol. 8 (1), P. 131-3

3813. Perry R D, Parker G D, Hallinan J M
CT and MR imaging of fourth ventricular meningiomas
J Comput Assist Tomogr 1990 Mar- Apr, Vol. 14 (2), P. 276-80

3814. Peters E, Bublitz G, Grapp B, Grupe G, Herrmann B
Computertomographische Untersuchung mittelalterlicher Särge
Computerized tomographic study of medieval coffins
RÖFO 1986 Jul, Vol. 145 (1), P. 97-9

3815. Peters P E, Beyer K
Querdurchmesser normaler Lymphknoten in verschiedenen anatomischen Regionen und ihre Bedeutung für die computertomographische Diagnostik
Radiologe 1985 May, Vol. 25 (5), P. 193-8

3816. Peters T M, Clark J A, Olivier A, Marchand E P, Mawko G, Dieumegarde M, Muresan L V, Ethier R
Integrated stereotaxic imaging with CT, MR imaging, and digital subtraction angiography
Radiology 1986 Dec, Vol. 161 (3), P. 821-6

3817. Petersen O F, Espersen J O
How to distinguish between bleeding and coagulated extradural hematomas on the plain CT scanning
Neuroradiology 1984, Vol. 26 (4), P. 285-92

3818. Petersen O F, Espersen J O
Extradural hematomas: measurement of size by volume summation on CT scanning
Neuroradiology 1984, Vol. 26 (5), P. 363-7

3819. Petras A F, Sobel D F, Mani J R, Lucas P R
CT myelography in cervical nerve root avulsion
J Comput Assist Tomogr 1985 Mar- Apr, Vol. 9 (2), P. 275-9

3820. Pettersson H, Harwood Nash D C, Fitz C R, Chuang S, Armstrong E
The CT appearance of avulsion of the posterior vertebral apophysis. A case report
Neuroradiology 1981, Vol. 21 (3), P. 145-7

3821. Peyster R G, Augsburger J J, Shields J A, Satchell T V, Markoe A M, Clarke K, Haskin M E
Choroidal melanoma: comparison of CT, fundoscopy, and US
Radiology 1985 Sep, Vol. 156 (3), P. 675-80

3822. Peyster R G, Ginsberg F, Hoover E D
Computed tomography of familial pineoblastoma
J Comput Assist Tomogr 1986 Jan-Feb, Vol. 10 (1), P. 32-3

3823. Peyster R G, Hoover E D, Hershey B L, Haskin M E
High- resolution CT of lesions of the optic nerve
Am J Roentgenol 1983 May, Vol. 140 (5), P. 869-74

3824. Pfeiffer K
Computertomographie und Speicheldrüsendiagnostik
Computed tomography and diagnosis of salivary gland diseases
Radiologe 1987 Jun, Vol. 27 (6), P. 262-8

3825. Pinto J A, Pereira J R, Guimaraes A, Veiga Pires J A
The value of CT-scanning in supratentorial haemangioblastomas
Neuroradiology 1987, Vol. 29 (6), P. 573-5

3826. Pinto R S, Kricheff I I, Bergeron R T, Cohen N
Small acoustic neuromas: detection by high resolution gas CT cisternography
Am J Roentgenol 1982 Jul, Vol. 139 (1), P. 129-32

3827. Podlas H B, Gritzman M C, Thomaides S, Roos H
CT of CNS lesions in lymphomatoid granulomatosis: case report
AJNR 1988 May- Jun, Vol. 9 (3), P. 592-4

3828. Pomeranz S J, Hawkins H H, Towbin R, Lisberg W N, Clark R A
Granulocytic sarcoma chloroma: CT manifestations
Radiology 1985 Apr, Vol. 155 (1), P. 167-70

3829. Pond G D, Castellino R A, Horning S, Hoppe R T
Non- Hodgkin lymphoma: influence of lymphography, CT, and bone marrow biopsy on staging and management
Radiology 1989 Jan, Vol. 170 (1 Pt 1), P. 159-64

3830. Poser C M
Neuroimaging and the lesion of multiple sclerosis: an addendum letter
AJNR 1987 Nov-Dec, Vol. 8 (6), P. 1146

3831. Post M J, Mendez D R, Kline L B, Acker J D, Glaser J S
Metastatic disease to the cavernous sinus: clinical syndrome and CT diagnosis
J Comput Assist Tomogr 1985 Jan-Feb, Vol. 9 (1), P. 115-20

3832. Post M J, Tate L G, Quencer R M, Hensley G T, Berger J R, Sheremata W A, Maul G
CT, MR, and pathology in HIV encephalitis and meningitis
Am J Roentgenol 1988 Aug, Vol. 151 (2), P. 373-80

3833. Prasad S C, Pilepich M V, Perez C A
Contribution of CT to quantitative radiation therapy planning
Am J Roentgenol 1981 Jan, Vol. 136 (1), P. 123-8

3834. Price D B, Nardi P, Teitcher J
Venous air embolization as a complication of pressure injection of contrast media: CT findings
J Comput Assist Tomogr 1987 Mar-Apr, Vol. 11 (2), P. 294- 5

3835. Proto A V, Ball J B Jr
Computed tomography of the major and minor fissures
Am J Roentgenol 1983 Mar, Vol. 140 (3), P. 439-48

3836. Pullicino P, Kendall B E
Contrast enhancement in ischaemic lesions. I. Relationship to prognosis
Neuroradiology 1980 Mar, Vol. 19 (5), P. 235-9

3837. Quinn S F, Murtagh F R, Chatfield R, Kori S H
CT-guided nerve root block and ablation
Am J Roentgenol 1988 Dec, Vol. 151 (6), P. 1213-6

3838. Quint L E, Gross B H, Glazer G M, Braunstein E M, White S J
CT evaluation of chondroblastoma
J Comput Assist Tomogr 1984 Oct, Vol. 8 (5), P. 907-10

3839. Radin D R, Allgood M R, Johnson M B, Pentecost M
CT diagnosis of superior mesenteric arteriovenous fistula
J Comput Assist Tomogr 1989 Jul-Aug, Vol. 13 (4), P. 721-3

3840. Rahatzad M, Adamson D A, Henderson S
Computed tomography and ultrasound of retained placenta from abdominal pregnancy
J Comput Assist Tomogr 1983 Aug, Vol. 7 (4), P. 730-1

3841. Ramirez H Jr, Bennett W F, Peters V
CT diagnosis of hernia through iliac bone-graft donor site
J Comput Assist Tomogr 1985 Mar-Apr, Vol. 9 (2), P. 411-2

3842. Ramirez H, Blatt E S, Hibri N S
Computed tomographic identification of calcified optic nerve drusen
Radiology 1983 Jul, Vol. 148 (1), P. 137-9

3843. Ramsey R G, Geremia G K
CNS complications of AIDS: CT and MR findings
Am J Roentgenol 1988 Sep, Vol. 151 (3), P. 449-54

3844. Ramsey R G, Penn R D
Computed tomography of a false postoperative meningocele
AJNR 1984 May-Jun, Vol. 5 (3), P. 326-8

3845. Randell C P, Collins A G, Young I R, Haywood R, Thomas D J, McDonnell M J, Orr J S, Bydder G M, Steiner R E
Nuclear magnetic resonance imaging of posterior fossa tumors
Am J Roentgenol 1983 Sep, Vol. 141 (3), P. 489-96

3846. Rao C V, Kishore P R, Bartlett J, Brennan T G
Computed tomography in the postoperative patient
Neuroradiology 1980, Vol. 19 (5), P. 257-63

3847. Reed D, Robertson W D, Graeb D A, Lapointe J S, Nugent R A, Woodhurst W B
Acute subdural hematomas: atypical CT findings
AJNR 1986 May-Jun, Vol. 7 (3), P. 417-21

3848. Regenbogen V S, Zinreich S J, Kim K S, Kuhajda F P, Applebaum B I, Price J C, Rosenbaum A E
Hyperostotic esthesioneuroblastoma: CT and MR findings
J Comput Assist Tomogr 1988 Jan-Feb, Vol. 12 (1), P. 52–6

3849. Reid M H, Dublin A B
QUAC: a modest proposal for optimal use of CT scanning equipment a parody
Am J Roentgenol 1984 Apr, Vol. 142 (4), P. 845–6

3850. Remley K B, Coit W E, Harnsberger H R, Smoker W R, Jacobs J M, McIff E B
Pulsatile tinnitus and the vascular tympanic membrane: CT, MR, and angiographic findings
Radiology 1990 Feb, Vol. 174 (2), P. 383–9

3851. Ren H, Kuhlman J E, Hruban R H, Fishman E K, Wheeler P S, Hutchins G M
CT-pathology correlation of amiodarone lung
J Comput Assist Tomogr 1990 Sep-Oct, Vol. 14 (5), P. 760–5

3852. Retrum E R, Schmidlin T M, Taylor W K, Pepe R G
CT myelography of extradural pigmented villonodular synovitis
AJNR 1987 Jul-Aug, Vol. 8 (4), P. 727–9

3853. Reuther G, Wernecke K, Peters P E
Localization technic for percutaneous punctures under CT control Lokalisationstechnik für perkutane Punktionen unter CT-Kontrolle
Radiologe 1990 May, Vol. 30 (5), P. 217–20

3854. Reyes G D
A guidance device for CT-guided procedures
Radiology 1990 Sep, Vol. 176 (3), P. 863–4

3855. Rice C A, Anderson T M, Sepahdari S
Computed tomography and ultrasonography of carcinoma in duplication cysts
J Comput Assist Tomogr 1986 Mar-Apr, Vol. 10 (2), P. 233–5

3856. Richardson M L, Kinard R E, Gray M B
CT of generalized gray matter infarction due to hypoglycemia
AJNR 1981 Jul-Aug, Vol. 2 (4), P. 366–7

3857. Richter E, Feyerabend T
Normal lymph node topography
1991 Springer Verlag , Berlin Heidelberg New York London Paris Tokyo Hong Kong Barcelona

3858. Robb W L
Future advances and directions in imaging research
Am J Roentgenol 1988 Jan, Vol. 150 (1), P. 39–42

3859. Robbins A H, Pugatch R D, Gerzof S G, Faling L J, Johnson W C, Spira R, Gale D R
Further observations on the medical efficacy of computed tomography of the chest and abdomen
Radiology 1980 Dec, Vol. 137 (3), P. 719–25

3860. Roberts L Jr, Dunnick N R, Thompson W M, Foster W L Jr, Halvorsen R A, Gibbons R G, Feldman J M
Primary aldosteronism due to bilateral nodular hyperplasia: CT demonstration
J Comput Assist Tomogr 1985 Nov-Dec, Vol. 9 (6), P. 1125–7

3861. Robertson D D, Walker P S, Granholm J W, Nelson P C, Weiss P J, Fishman E K, Magid D
Design of custom hip stem prostheses using three-dimensional CT modeling
J Comput Assist Tomogr 1987 Sep-Oct, Vol. 11 (5), P. 804–9

3862. Robertson H J, Hatten H P Jr, Keating J W
False-positive CT gas cisternogram
AJNR 1983 May-Jun, Vol. 4 (3), P. 474–7

3863. Robinson D A, Steiner R E, Young I R
The MR contribution after CT demonstration of supratentorial mass effect without additional localising features
J Comput Assist Tomogr 1988 Mar- Apr, Vol. 12 (2), P. 275–9

3864. Rodacki M A, Detoni X A, Teixeira W R, Boer V H, Oliveira G G
CT features of cellulosae and racemosus neurocysticercosis
J Comput Assist Tomogr 1989 Nov-Dec, Vol. 13 (6), P. 1013–6

3865. Rodacki M A, Teixeira W R, Boer V H, Caropreso J, Oliveira G G
Intradural, extramedullary high cervical neurenteric cyst
Neuroradiology 1987, Vol. 29 (6), P. 588

3866. Rodiek S
Exogen-toxische bilaterale Stammganliennekrosen im Computertomogramm
Exogenous-toxic bilateral basal ganglia necroses in computer tomography
RÖFO 1982 Sep, Vol. 137 (3), P. 316–21

3867. Rodiek S O, Rupp N, von Einsiedel H G
MR- und CT-Muster der Neurozystizerkose
MR and CT patterns of neurocysticercosis
RÖFO 1987 May, Vol. 146 (5), P. 570–7

3868. Roex L, Casselman J, Lemahieu S F, Baert A L
CT- appearance of cervical actinomycosis. Case report
RÖFO 1987 Mar, Vol. 146 (3), P. 357–8

3869. Rohloff R, Hitzler H, Arndt W, Frey K W
Experimentelle Untersuchungen zur Genauigkeit der Mineralsalzgehaltsbestimmung spongioser Knochen mit Hilfe der quantitativen CT (Einenergiemessung)
Experimental studies on the accuracy of mineral content assessment in spongiosa bone using quantitative CT single energy measurement
RÖFO 1985 Dec, Vol. 143 (6), P. 692–7

3870. Romano A J, Shoemaker E I, Gado M
Neuroradiology case of the day. Choroid plexus papilloma, third ventricle
Am J Roentgenol 1989 Jun, Vol. 152 (6), P. 1333–5

3871. Romano A J, Shoemaker E I, Gado M, Hodges F J
Neuroradiology case of the day. Plasmacytoma of the skull vault
Am J Roentgenol 1989 Jun, Vol. 152 (6), P. 1335–7

3872. Rommel T, Hamer J
Development of ganglioglioma in computed tomography
Neuroradiology 1983, Vol. 24 (4), P. 237–9

3873. Rosa U, Wade K C
CT findings in hemitruncus
J Comput Assist Tomogr 1987 Jul-Aug, Vol. 11 (4), P. 698–700

3874. Rosenthal D I, Hayes C W, Rosen B, Mayo Smith W, Goodsitt M M
Fatty replacement of spinal bone marrow due to radiation: demonstration by dual energy quantitative CT and MR imaging
J Comput Assist Tomogr 1989 May-Jun, Vol. 13 (3), P. 463–5

3875. Rossi P, Cozzi F, Iannaccone G
CT for assessing feasibility of separation of thoracopagus twins
J Comput Assist Tomogr 1981 Aug, Vol. 5 (4), P. 574–6

3876. Rostock R A, Fishman E K, Zinreich E S, Lee D J
Computed tomography in radiation therapy treatment planning of hepatic metastases
J Comput Assist Tomogr 1985 Jul-Aug, Vol. 9 (4), P. 755–9

3877. Rothfus W E, Curtin H D, Slamovits T L, Kennerdell J S
Optic nerve/sheath enlargement. A differential approach based on high-resolution CT morphology
Radiology 1984 Feb, Vol. 150 (2), P. 409–15

3878. Rothfus W E, Goldberg A L, Tabas J H, Deeb Z L
Callosomarginal infarction secondary to transfalcial herniation
AJNR 1987 Nov-Dec, Vol. 8 (6), P. 1073–6

3879. Rothfus W E, Hirsch W L, Latchaw R E, Starzl T E
Neuroradiologic aspects of pediatric orthotopic liver transplantation
AJNR 1988 Mar-Apr, Vol. 9 (2), P. 303–6

3880. Rovira M, Romero F, Torrent O, Ibarra B
Study of tuberculous meningitis by CT
Neuroradiology 1980 Apr, Vol. 19 (3), P. 137–41

3881. Rubin J, Curtin H D, Yu V L, Kamerer D B
Malignant external otitis: utility of CT in diagnosis and follow- up
Radiology 1990 Feb, Vol. 174 (2), P. 391–4

3882. Ruscalleda J, Guardia E, dos Santos F M, Carvajal A
Dynamic study of arachnoid cysts with metrizamide
Neuroradiology 1980 Dec, Vol. 20 (4), P. 185–9

3883. Ruskin J A, Haughton V M
CT findings in adult Reye syndrome
AJNR 1985 May-Jun, Vol. 6 (3), P. 446–7

3884. Russell E J, Naidich T P
The enhancing septal/alveal wedge: a septal sign of intraaxial mass
Neuroradiology 1982, Vol. 23 (1), P. 33–40

3885. Sabattini L
Evaluation and measurement of the normal ventricular and subarachnoid spaces by CT
Neuroradiology 1982, Vol. 23 (1), P. 1–5

3886. Sacher M, Som P M, Shugar J M, Leeds N E
Kissing intrasellar carotid arteries in acromegaly: CT demonstration
J Comput Assist Tomogr 1986 Nov-Dec, Vol. 10 (6), P. 1033–5

3887. Sadatoh N, Hatabu H, Takahashi M, Imanaka K, Sano A
Oxygen-assisted breath-holding in computed tomography
J Comput Assist Tomogr 1987 Jul-Aug, Vol. 11 (4), P. 742–4

3888. Sadhu V K, Handel S F, Pinto R S, Glass T F
Neuroradiologic diagnosis of subdural empyema and CT limitations
AJNR 1980 Jan-Feb, Vol. 1 (1), P. 39–44

3889. Salazar J E, Duke R A, Ellis J V
Second branchial cleft cyst: unusual location and a new CT diagnostic sign
Am J Roentgenol 1985 Nov, Vol. 145 (5), P. 965–6

3890. Samuel E
Plain radiographs and CT scans in the diagnosis of sinus disease letter
Am J Roentgenol 1990 Aug, Vol. 155 (2), P. 425

3891. Sandhu A, Kendall B
Computed tomography in management of medulloblastomas
Neuroradiology 1987, Vol. 29 (5), P. 444–52

3892. Sandor T, Albert M, Stafford J, Harpley S
Use of computerized CT analysis to discriminate between Alzheimer patients and normal control subjects
AJNR 1988 Nov-Dec, Vol. 9 (6), P. 1181–7

3893. Sano N, Nagao H, Morimoto T, Takahashi M, Habara S, Aoi T, Matsuda H, Kamoshita S
Infantile sudanophilic leukodystrophy: computed tomography demonstration
Neuroradiology 1986, Vol. 28 (2), P. 170–2

3894. Sargent S K, Young W, Crow P, Simpson W
CT amniography: value in detecting a monoamniotic pair in a triplet pregnancy
Am J Roentgenol 1991 Mar, Vol. 156 (3), P. 559–60

3895. Sartoris D J, Resnick D, Guerra J Jr
Vertebral venous channels: CT appearance and differential considerations
Radiology 1985 Jun, Vol. 155 (3), P. 745–9

3896. Sarwar M, Ford K
Rapid development of basal ganglia calcification
AJNR 1981 Jan-Feb, Vol. 2 (1), P. 103–4

3897. Sarwar M, Virapongse C, Bhimani S, Freilich M
Interhemispheric fissure sign of dysgenesis of the corpus callosum
J Comput Assist Tomogr 1984 Aug, Vol. 8 (4), P. 637–44

3898. Sato M, Tanaka S, Kohama A
"Top of the basilar" syndrome: clinico-radiological evaluation
Neuroradiology 1987, Vol. 29 (4), P. 354–9

3899. Sauerwein W, Towfigh H
Fistelbildung nach Periduralanästhesie. Sichere Diagnose einer seltenen Katheterkomplikation mittels Computertomographie
Fistula formation after peridural anesthesia. A reliable diagnosis of a rare catheter complication by computed tomography
RÖFO 1985 Jan, Vol. 142 (1), P. 109–11

3900. Scatarige J C, Fishman E K, Zinreich E S, Brem R F, Almaraz R
Internal mammary lymphadenopathy in breast carcinoma: CT appraisal of anatomic distribution
Radiology 1988 Apr, Vol. 167 (1), P. 89–91

3901. Scatliff J H, Williams A L, Krigman M R, Whaley R A
CT recognition of subcortical hematomas
AJNR 1981 Jan-Feb, Vol. 2 (1), P. 49–53

3902. Schauwecker D S, Burt R W, Richmond B D
Comparison of CVA imaging with 99mTc phosphates, 99mTc pertechnetate, and computed tomography
Neuroradiology 1981, Vol. 21 (4), P. 199–205

3903. Schellinger D, Grant E G, Richardson J D
Cystic periventricular leukomalacia: sonographic and CT findings
AJNR 1984 Jul-Aug, Vol. 5 (4), P. 439–45

3904. Schellinger D, McCullough D C, Pederson R T
Computed tomography in the hydrocephalic patient after shunting
Radiology 1980 Dec, Vol. 137 (3), P. 693–704

3905. Schepp S, Reiser M, Ingianni G, Holscher M
Diagnostik der Neurofibromatose durch Kernspintomographie
Diagnosis of neurofibromatosis by nuclear resonance tomography
RÖFO 1986 Apr, Vol. 144 (4), P. 473–6

3906. Schild H H, Schweden F E
Computertomographie in der Urologie
1989 Georg Thieme ,Stuttgart New York

3907. Schild H, Geier G, Schaub T
Jugulovenöser Reflux im CT
Jugular vein reflux in the CT x-ray
RÖFO 1984 May, Vol. 140 (5), P. 615-6

3908. Schild H, Gronniger J, Gunther R, Thelen M, Schwab R
Transabdominelle CT-gesteuerte Sympathektomie
Transabdominal CT- guided sympathectomy
RÖFO 1984 Nov, Vol. 141 (5), P. 504-8

3909. Schild H, Gunther R, Hoffmann J, Goedecke R
CT-gesteuerte Blockade des Plexus coeliacus mit ventralem Zugang
CT-guided celiac plexus block with ventral approach
RÖFO 1983 Aug, Vol. 139 (2), P. 202-5

3910. Schils J, Hermanus N, Flament Durant J, Van Gansbeke D, Baleriaux D
Cerebral schistosomiasis
AJNR 1985 Sep-Oct, Vol. 6 (5), P. 840-1

3911. Schipper H I, Seidel D
Computed tomography in late-onset metachromatic leucodystrophy
Neuroradiology 1984, Vol. 26 (1), P. 39-44

3912. Schlenska G K, Walter G F
Serial computed tomography findings in Creutzfeldt-Jakob disease
Neuroradiology 1989, Vol. 31 (4), P. 303-6

3913. Schlolaut K H, Lackner K, von Uexkull Guldenband V, Nicolas V, Vogel J
Ergebnisse und Komplikationen perkutaner CT- gesteuerter Punktionen mit einer großlumigen Punktionsnadel
Results and complications of CT-guided puncture biopsies with a wide-lumen puncture needle
RÖFO 1987 Jul, Vol. 147 (1), P. 25-32

3914. Schmitt R, Wuttke V, Buchner U, Preger R
Diagnostik posttraumatischer Neurome mittels Sonographie und CT
The diagnosis of posttraumatic neuroma via sonography and CT
RÖFO 1990 Feb, Vol. 152 (2), P. 180-4

3915. Schmitt W G, Hubener K H
Computertomographische Densitometrie formalinfixierter und gefrorener menschlicher Gewebe
Computer tomographic densitometry of formalin-fixed and frozen human tissue
RÖFO 1980 Nov, Vol. 133 (5), P. 531-4

3916. Schmitz L, Jeffrey R B, Palubinskas A J, Moss A A
CT demonstration of septic thrombosis of the inferior vena cava
J Comput Assist Tomogr 1981 Apr, Vol. 5 (2), P. 259-61

3917. Schorner W, Meencke H J, Sander B, Henkes H, Felix R
Psychomotorische Epilepsie-Vergleich von CT und MR bei 100 Patienten
Psychomotor epilepsy-a comparison of CT and MR in 100 patients
RÖFO 1989 Aug, Vol. 151 (2), P. 202-9

3918. Schreiman J S, Gisvold J J, Greenleaf J F, Bahn R C
Ultrasound transmission computed tomography of the breast
Radiology 1984 Feb, Vol. 150 (2), P. 523-30

3919. Schreiman J S, McLeod R A, Kyle R A, Beabout J W
Multiple myeloma: evaluation by CT
Radiology 1985 Feb, Vol. 154 (2), P. 483-6

3920. Schroeder B A, Samaraweera R N, Starshak R J, Oechler H W
Intraparenchymal meningioma in a child: CT and MR findings
J Comput Assist Tomogr 1987 Jan-Feb, Vol. 11 (1), P. 192-3

3921. Schroeder B A, Wells R G, Starshak R J, Sty J R
Clivus chordoma in a child with tuberous sclerosis: CT and MR demonstration
J Comput Assist Tomogr 1987 Jan-Feb, Vol. 11 (1), P. 195-6

3922. Schroth G, Thron A, Voigt K
Raumforderungen der hinteren Schädelgrube. Ein Vergleich von Magnetresonanztomographie und Computertomographie
Posterior fossa masses. Comparison of magnetic resonance tomography and computed tomography
RÖFO 1984 Dec, Vol. 141 (6), P. 635-41

3923. Schuknecht B, Muller J, Nadjmi M
Maligne Melanome der Meningen-MR- und CT-Diagnostik
Malignant melanoma of the meninges- MR and CT diagnosis
RÖFO 1990 Jan, Vol. 152 (1), P. 80-6

3924. Schultz S M, Twickler D M, Wheeler D E, Hogan T D
Ameloblastoma associated with basal cell nevus Gorlin syndrome: CT findings
J Comput Assist Tomogr 1987 Sep-Oct, Vol. 11 (5), P. 901-4

3925. Schwaighofer B W, Sobel D F, Klein M V, Zyroff J, Hesselink J R
Mucocele of the anterior clinoid process: CT and MR findings
J Comput Assist Tomogr 1989 May-Jun, Vol. 13 (3), P. 501-3

3926. Schwartz A, Aulich A, Hammer B
CT-Verlaufsbeobachtungen bei Neurocysticerkose unter Praziquanteltherapie
CT follow-up of neurocysticercosis treated with praziquantel
Radiologe 1987 May, Vol. 27 (5), P. 237-42

3927. Schwartz J M, Holliday R A, Breda S D
CT diagnosis of pyriform sinus perforation
J Comput Assist Tomogr 1988 Sep-Oct, Vol. 12 (5), P. 869-70

3928. Sciuk J, Peters P E
CT-Untersuchungen im höheren Lebensalter
Radiologe 1989 Dec, Vol. 29 (12), P. 592-5

3929. Scotti G, Musgrave M A, Fitz C R, Harwood Nash D C
The isolated fourth ventricle in children: CT and clinical review of 16 cases
Am J Roentgenol 1980 Dec, Vol. 135 (6), P. 1233-8

3930. Scotti G, Musgrave M A, Harwood Nash D C, Fitz C R, Chuang S H
Diastematomyelia in children: metrizamide and CT metrizamide myelography
Am J Roentgenol 1980 Dec, Vol. 135 (6), P. 1225-32

3931. Second International Workshop on Bone and Soft Tissue Densitometry Using Computed Tomography. Zuoz, Switzerland, April 13-16, 1981. Abstracts
J Comput Assist Tomogr 1982 Feb, Vol. 6 (1), P. 197-220

3932. Seemann W R, Ernst H U, Wimmer B
Computertomographische Befunde bei der pigmentierten villonodulären Synovitis
Computertomographic findings in pigmented villonodular synovitis
RÖFO 1983 Dec, Vol. 139 (6), P. 606-7

3933. Seerup A, Svendsen F, Iversen G, Schmidt E B
Tuberous sclerosis. CT findings versus clinical state
RÖFO 1987 Aug, Vol. 147 (2), P. 196-7

3934. Segal A J, Spataro R F
Computed tomography of adult polycystic disease
J Comput Assist Tomogr 1982 Aug, Vol. 6 (4), P. 777-80

3935. Seidenwurm D, Novotny E Jr, Marshall W, Enzmann D
MR and CT in cytoplasmically inherited striatal degeneration
AJNR 1986 Jul-Aug, Vol. 7 (4), P. 629-32

3936. Seigel R S, Sell J, Magnus D E
CT appearance of traumatic dislocated lens
AJNR 1988 Mar-Apr, Vol. 9 (2), P. 390

3937. Servo A, Porras M, Jaaskelainen J, Paetau A, Haltia M
Computed tomography and angiography do not reliably discriminate malignant meningiomas from benign ones
Neuroradiology 1990, Vol. 32 (2), P. 94-7

3938. Servo A, Porras M, Jaaskinen J
Diagnosis of ependymal intraventricular cysts of the third ventricle by computed tomography
Neuroradiology 1983, Vol. 24 (3), P. 155-7

3939. Sevel D, Krausz H, Ponder T, Centeno R
Value of computed tomography for the diagnosis of a ruptured eye
J Comput Assist Tomogr 1983 Oct, Vol. 7 (5), P. 870-5

3940. Shackelford G D, Siegel M J
CT appearance of cystic adenomatoid malformations
J Comput Assist Tomogr 1989 Jul-Aug, Vol. 13 (4), P. 612-6

3941. Shaffer K A
Comparison of computed tomography and complex motion tomography in the evaluation of cholesteatoma
Am J Roentgenol 1984 Aug, Vol. 143 (2), P. 397-400

3942. Shapeero L G, Young S W
Mycosis fungoides: manifestations on computed tomography
Radiology 1983 Jul, Vol. 148 (1), P. 202

3943. Shapir J, Coblentz C, Malanson D, Ethier R, Robitaille Y
New CT finding in aggressive meningioma
AJNR 1985 Jan-Feb, Vol. 6 (1), P. 101-2

3944. Sharif H S, Clark D C, Aabed M Y, Aideyan O A, Mattsson T A, Haddad M C, Ohman S O, Joshi R K, Hasan H A, Haleem A
Mycetoma: comparison of MR imaging with CT
Radiology 1991 Mar, Vol. 178 (3), P. 865-70

3945. Sheldon J J, Siddharthan R, Tobias J, Sheremata W A, Soila K, Viamonte M Jr
MR imaging of multiple sclerosis: comparison with clinical and CT examinations in 74 patients
Am J Roentgenol 1985 Nov, Vol. 145 (5), P. 957-64

3946. Shenouda N F, Hyams B B, Rosenbloom M B
Evaluation of Spigelian hernia by CT
J Comput Assist Tomogr 1990 Sep-Oct, Vol. 14 (5), P. 777-8

3947. Sherman J L, Citrin C, Johns T, Black J
Erdheim-Chester disease: computed tomography in two cases
AJNR 1985 May-Jun, Vol. 6 (3), P. 444-5

3948. Sherman J L, McLean I W, Brallier D R
Coats' disease: CT- pathologic correlation in two cases
Radiology 1983 Jan, Vol. 146 (1), P. 77-8

3949. Shin M S, Berland L L, Ho K J
Postoperative malignant seroma: CT demonstration of its formation mechanism
J Comput Assist Tomogr 1984 Oct, Vol. 8 (5), P. 1001-4

3950. Shoemaker E I, Romano A J, Gado M
Neuroradiology case of the day. Moyamoya disease
Am J Roentgenol 1989 Jun, Vol. 152 (6), P. 1337-8

3951. Shoemaker E I, Romano A J, Gado M Hodges F J
Neuroradiology case of the day. Chordoma of the clivus
Am J Roentgenol 1989 Jun, Vol. 152 (6), P. 1333

3952. Shuman W P, Griffin B R, Yoshy C S, Listerud J A, Mack L A, Rowberg A H, Moss A A
The impact of CT CORRELATE ScoutView images on radiation therapy planning
Am J Roentgenol 1985 Sep, Vol. 145 (3), P. 633-8

3953. Shuman W P, Griffin B W, Luk K H, Mack L A, Hanson J A
CT and radiation therapy planning: impact of LOCATE ScoutView images
Am J Roentgenol 1982 Nov, Vol. 139 (5), P. 985-9

3954. Shuman W P, Kilcoyne R F, Matsen F A, Rogers J V, Mack L A
Double-contrast computed tomography of the glenoid labrum
Am J Roentgenol 1983 Sep, Vol. 141 (3), P. 581-4

3955. Sibala J L, Chang C H, Lin F, Thomas J H
CT of angiolipoma of the breast
Am J Roentgenol 1980 Apr, Vol. 134 (4), P. 840-1

3956. Siegel H A, Seltzer S E, Miller S
Prenatal computed tomography: are there indications?
J Comput Assist Tomogr 1984 Oct, Vol. 8 (5), P. 871-6

3957. Silver A J, Pederson M E Jr, Ganti S R, Hilal S K, Michelson W J
CT of subarachnoid hemorrhage due to ruptured aneurysm
AJNR 1981 Jan-Feb, Vol. 2 (1), P. 13-22

3958. Simmons J D, Norman D, Newton T H
Preoperative demonstration of postinflammatory syringomyelia
AJNR 1983 May-Jun, Vol. 4 (3), P. 625-8

3959. Skirkhoda A, Whaley R A, Boone S C, Scatliff J H, Schnapf D
Varied CT appearance of aneurysms of the vein of Galen in infancy
Neuroradiology 1981, Vol. 21 (5), P. 265-70

3960. Slanina J, Sigmund G, Hinkelbein W, Wenz W, Wannenmacher M
Die pulmonale Strahlenreaktion nach Mantelfeldbestrahlung. Vergleich der Verlaufsstadien im konventionellen Rontgenbild und im Computertomogram
Pulmonary reaction to radiation following mantle-field irradiation. Comparison of follow-up by conventional x-ray and by computed tomography
Radiologe 1988 Jan, Vol. 28 (1), P. 20-8

3961. Smith D, Bloch S, Al Rashid R A
Basal ganglia calcification on CT scanning in children with acute lymphocytic leukemia
Neuroradiology 1980, Vol. 20 (2), P. 91-3

3962. Smith J R, Hadgis C, Van Hasselt A, Metreweli C
CT of Kimura disease
AJNR 1989 Sep-Oct, Vol. 10 (5 Suppl), P. S34-6

3963. Smith V, Parker D L, Stanley J H, Phillips T L, Boyd D P, Kan P T
Development of a computed tomographic scanner for radiation therapy treatment planning
Radiology 1980 Aug, Vol. 136 (2), P. 489-93

3964. Smoker W R, Corbett J J, Gentry L R, Keyes W D, Price M J, McKusker S
High-resolution computed tomography of the basilar artery: 2. Vertebrobasilar dolichoectasia: clinical-pathologic correlation and review
AJNR 1986 Jan-Feb, Vol. 7 (1), P. 61-72

3965. Smoker W R, Price M J, Keyes W D, Corbett J J, Gentry L R
High-resolution computed tomography of the basilar artery: 1. Normal size and position
AJNR 1986 Jan-Feb, Vol. 7 (1), P. 55–60

3966. Society for pediatric radiology: abstracts from 1983 meeting
Am J Roentgenol 1983 Oct, Vol. 141 (4), P. 846–553967. Solti Bohman L G, Magaram D L, Lo W W,
Wade C T, Witten R M, Shimizu F H, McMonigle E M, Rao A K
Gas-CT cisternography for detection of small acoustic nerve tumors
Radiology 1984 Feb, Vol. 150 (2), P. 403–7

3968. Som P M, Biller H F
The combined CT-sialogram
Radiology 1980 May, Vol. 135 (2), P. 387–90

3969. Som P M, Reede D L, Bergeron R T, Parisier S C, Shugar J M, Cohen N L
Computed tomography of glomus tympanicum tumors
J Comput Assist Tomogr 1983 Feb, Vol. 7 (1), P. 14–7

3970. Som P M, Shugar J M
Antral mucoceles: a new look
J Comput Assist Tomogr 1980 Aug, Vol. 4 (4), P. 484–8

3971. Som P M, Shugar J M
The CT classification of ethmoid mucoceles
J Comput Assist Tomogr 1980 Apr, Vol. 4 (2), P. 199–203

3972. Sonnenblick E B, Buchness M R, Austin J H
CT demonstration of steatocystoma multiplex
J Comput Assist Tomogr 1986 Mar-Apr, Vol. 10 (2), P. 357–9

3973. Spallone A, Tanfani G, Vassilouthis J, Dazzi M
Benign extramedullary foramen magnum tumors: diagnosis by computed tomography
J Comput Assist Tomogr 1980 Apr, Vol. 4 (2), P. 225–9

3974. Spiegel S M, Vinuela F, Fox A J, Pelz D M
CT of multiple sclerosis: reassessment of delayed scanning with high doses of contrast material
Am J Roentgenol 1985 Sep, Vol. 145 (3), P. 497–500

3975. Spiessl B, Beahrs O H, Hermanek P, Hutter R V P, Scheibe O, Sobin L H , Wagner G
TNM Atlas
3rd ed., 1990 Springer Verlag , Berlin Heidelberg New York London Paris Tokyo Hong Kong
Barcelona

3976. Sprecher S, Steinberg R, Serchuk L
Foot-in-mouth disease no April fools' joke letter
Am J Roentgenol 1990 Sep, Vol. 155 (3), P. 651

3977. Stanford W, Galvin J
Cine CT in obstructive sleep apnea letter
Am J Roentgenol 1988 Feb, Vol. 150 (2), P. 468

3978. Stark D D, Brasch R C, Moss A A, deLorimier A A, Albin A R, London D A, Gooding
C A
Recurrent neuroblastoma: the role of CT and alternative imaging tests
Radiology 1983 Jul, Vol. 148 (1), P. 107–12

3979. Stark D D, Moss A A, Brasch R C, deLorimier A A, Albin A R, London D A, Gooding
C A
Neuroblastoma: diagnostic imaging and staging
Radiology 1983 Jul, Vol. 148 (1), P. 101–5

3980. Stark P, Aguilar E A Jr, Robbins K T
Diagnostik der obstruktiven Schlafapnoe (Pickwickian Syndrome). Wertigkeit der Computerto-
mographie
Diagnosis of obstructive sleep apnea Pickwickian syndrome. Value of computed tomography
RÖFO 1984 Jan, Vol. 140 (1), P. 46–7

3981. Stark P, Wareham G, Hildebrandt Stark H E
CT-Diagnose des zystischen Hygroms
CT diagnosis of cystic hygroma
Radiologe 1989 Feb, Vol. 29 (2), P. 82–4

3982. Statz A, Boltshauser E, Schinzel A, Spiess H
Computed tomography in Pelizaeus-Merzbacher disease
Neuroradiology 1981, Vol. 22 (2), P. 103–5

3983. Stein M G, Gamsu G, de Geer G, Golden J A, Crumley R L, Webb W R
Cine CT in obstructive sleep apnea
Am J Roentgenol 1987 Jun, Vol. 148 (6), P. 1069–74

3984. Stephenson T F, Lincoln A J, Mehnert P J, Paul G J
Comparison of X-ray film and photographic paper in recording CT images
J Comput Assist Tomogr 1984 Dec, Vol. 8 (6), P. 1161–3

3985. Stevens J M, Kendall B E, Love S
Radiological features of subependymoma with emphasis on computed tomography
Neuroradiology 1984, Vol. 26 (3), P. 223–8

3986. Stevens J M, Ruiz J S, Kendall B E
Observations on peritumoral oedema in meningioma. Part II: Mechanisms of oedema produc-
tion
Neuroradiology 1983, Vol. 25 (3), P. 125–31

3987. Stimac G K, Mills R P, Dailey R A, Shults W T, Kalina R E
CT of acquired hyperopia with choroidal folds
AJNR 1987 Nov-Dec, Vol. 8 (6), P. 1107–11

3988. Stimac G K, Solomon M A, Newton T H
CT and MR of angiomatous malformations of the choroid plexus in patients with Sturge-Weber
disease
AJNR 1986 Jul-Aug, Vol. 7 (4), P. 623–7

3989. Strain J D, Campbell J B, Harvey L A, Foley L C
IV Nembutal: safe sedation for children undergoing CT
Am J Roentgenol 1988 Nov, Vol. 151 (5), P. 975–9

3990. Strain J D, Harvey L A, Foley L C, Campbell J B
Intravenously administered pentobarbital sodium for sedation in pediatric CT
Radiology 1986 Oct, Vol. 161 (1), P. 105–8

3991. Suss R A, Resta S, Diehl J T
Persistent cortical enhancement in tuberculous meningitis
AJNR 1987 Jul-Aug, Vol. 8 (4), P. 716–20

3992. Swartz J D, Bazarnic M L, Naidich T P, Lowry L D, Doan H T
Aberrant internal carotid artery lying within the middle ear. High resolution CT diagnosis and
differential diagnosis
Neuroradiology 1985, Vol. 27 (4), P. 322–6

3993. Swartz J D, Berger A S, Zwillenberg S, Granoff D W, Popky G L
Synthetic ossicular replacements: normal and abnormal CT appearance
Radiology 1987 Jun, Vol. 163 (3), P. 766–8

3994. Swartz J D, Berger A S, Zwillenberg S, Popky G L
Ossicular erosions in the dry ear: CT diagnosis
Radiology 1987 Jun, Vol. 163 (3), P. 763–5

3995. Swartz J D, Faerber E N
Congenital malformations of the external and middle ear: high-resolution CT findings of surgical
import
Am J Roentgenol 1985 Mar, Vol. 144 (3), P. 501–6

3996. Swartz J D, Faerber E N, Wolfson R J, Marlowe F I
Fenestral otosclerosis: significance of preoperative CT evaluation
Radiology 1984 Jun, Vol. 151 (3), P. 703–7

3997. Swartz J D, Mandell D M, Faerber E N, Popky G L, Ardito J M, Steinberg S B, Rojer C L
Labyrinthine ossification: etiologies and CT findings
Radiology 1985 Nov, Vol. 157 (2), P. 395–8

3998. Swartz J D, Russell K B, Basile B A, O Donnell P C, Popky G L
High-resolution computed tomographic appearance of the intrasellar contents in women of
childbearing age
Radiology 1983 Apr, Vol. 147 (1), P. 115–7

3999. Swartz J D, Wolfson R J, Marlowe F I, Popky G L
Postinflammatory ossicular fixation: CT analysis with surgical correlation
Radiology 1985 Mar, Vol. 154 (3), P. 697–700

4000. Swartz J D, Zwillenberg S, Berger A S
Acquired disruptions of the incudostapedial articulation: diagnosis with CT
Radiology 1989 Jun, Vol. 171 (3), P. 779–81

4001. Taccone A, Di Rocco M, Fondelli P, Cottafava F
Leigh disease: value of CT in presymptomatic patients and variability of the lesions with time
J Comput Assist Tomogr 1989 Mar-Apr, Vol. 13 (2), P. 207–10

4002. Takahashi M, Saito Y, Konno K
Intraventricular hemorrhage in childhood moyamoya disease
J Comput Assist Tomogr 1980 Feb, Vol. 4 (1), P. 117–20

4003. Takeuchi S, Kobayashi K, Tsuchida T, Imamura H, Tanaka R, Ito J
Computed tomography in moyamoya disease
J Comput Assist Tomogr 1982 Feb, Vol. 6 (1), P. 24–32

4004. Tan C T, Kuan B B
Cryptococcus meningitis, clinical-CT scan considerations
Neuroradiology 1987, Vol. 29 (1), P. 43–6

4005. Tapies Barba C, Alvarez Moro F J, Palmer Sancho J A, Comet Segu R, Ruiz Marcellan M C
Unusually low CT density in a peripheral neurofibroma
J Comput Assist Tomogr 1988 Nov-Dec, Vol. 12 (6), P. 1086–7

4006. Tatcher M, Elgrabli S, Kuten A, Kleinhaus U
An analog patient model derived from computed tomograms for three- dimensional radiotherapy
planning
Radiology 1980 Jul, Vol. 136 (1), P. 236–8

4007. Taveras J M
Nuclear magnetic resonance imaging editorial
AJNR 1982 Sep-Oct, Vol. 3 (5), P. 586–7

4008. Taylor A J, Haughton V M, Syvertsen A, Ho K C
Taylor- Haughton line revisited
AJNR 1980 Jan-Feb, Vol. 1 (1), P. 55–6

4009. Taylor G A, Glass P, Fitz C R, Miller M K
Neurologic status in infants treated with extracorporeal membrane oxygenation: correlation of
imaging findings with developmental outcome
Radiology 1987 Dec, Vol. 165 (3), P. 679–82

4010. Taylor R, Holgate R C
Carbon monoxide poisoning: asymmetric and unilateral changes on CT
AJNR 1988 Sep, Vol. 9 (5), P. 975–7

4011. Taylor S B, Quencer R M, Holzman B H, Naidich T P
Central nervous system anoxic-ischemic insult in children due to near- drowning
Radiology 1985 Sep, Vol. 156 (3), P. 641–6

4012. Terasaki K K, Zee C S
Evolution of central necrosis in a meningioma: CT and MR features
J Comput Assist Tomogr 1990 May- Jun, Vol. 14 (3), P. 464–6

4013. Terhorst L L
National survey of computed tomography unit capacity: an update. Special report
Radiology 1984 Oct, Vol. 153 (1), P. 207–10

4014. Thomas J L, Barnes P A, Bernardino M E, Hagemeister F B
Limited CT studies in monitoring treatment of lymphoma
Am J Roentgenol 1982 Mar, Vol. 138 (3), P. 537–9

4015. Thompson J R, Schneider S, Ashwal S, Holden B S, Hinshaw D B Jr, Hasso A N
The choice of sedation for computed tomography in children: a prospective evaluation
Radiology 1982 May, Vol. 143 (2), P. 475–9

4016. Titelbaum D S, Hayward J C, Zimmerman R A
Pachygyriclike changes: topographic appearance at MR imaging and CT and correlation with
neurologic status
Radiology 1989 Dec, Vol. 173 (3), P. 663–7

4017. Tobben P J, Zajko A B, Sumkin J H, Bowen A, Fuhrman C R, Skolnick M L, Bron K M, Esquivel C O,
Starzl T E
Pseudoaneurysms complicating organ transplantation: roles of CT, duplex sonography, and
angiography
Radiology 1988 Oct, Vol. 169 (1), P. 65–70

4018. Tokiguchi S, Kurashima A, Ito J, Takahashi H, Shimbo Y
Fat in the dural sinus-CT and anatomical correlations
Neuroradiology 1988, Vol. 30 (1), P. 78–80

4019. Tolly E, Ebner F, Oberbauer R W
Pränatale Diagnostik des Dandy-Walker-Syndroms durch Sonographie und Computertomo-
graphie
Prenatal diagnosis of the Dandy-Walker syndrome using sonography and computed tomo-
graphy
RÖFO 1984 Jul, Vol. 141 (1), P. 40–3

4020. Trattnig S, Schindler E, Ungersbock K, Schmidbauer M, Heimberger K, Hubsch P, Stiglbauer
R
Extra-CNS metastases of glioblastoma: CT and MR studies
J Comput Assist Tomogr 1990 Mar- Apr, Vol. 14 (2), P. 294–6

4021. Trattnig S, Stiglbauer R, Ungersbock K, Cech T, Schindler E, Imhof H
Magnetresonanztomographie beim "failed back surgery syndrome": Vergleich zur Computer-
tomographie
Magnetic resonance tomography of the failed back surgery syndrome: a comparison with computed
tomography
RÖFO 1990 Apr, Vol. 152 (4), P. 369–73

4022. Traupe H, Heiss W D, Hoeffken W, Zulch K J
Perfusion patterns in CT transit studies
Neuroradiology 1980, Vol. 19 (4), P. 181–91

4023. Trefler M, Haughton V M
Patient dose and image quality in computed tomography
Am J Roentgenol 1981 Jul, Vol. 137 (1), P. 25–7

4024. Tress B M, Davis S, Lavain J, Kaye A, Hopper J
Incremental dynamic computed tomography: practical method of imaging the carotid bifurcation
Am J Roentgenol 1986 Mar, Vol. 146 (3), P. 465–70

4025. Triebel H J, Menck J, Beese M, Rix J
Computertomographische und anatomische Untersuchungen zur Morphologie des kleinen Lappenspaltes
RÖFO 1991 Vol.155

4026. Trommer B L, Naidich T P, Dal Canto M C, McLone D G, Larsen M B
Noninvasive CT diagnosis of infantile Alexander disease: pathologic correlation
J Comput Assist Tomogr 1983 Jun, Vol. 7 (3), P. 509–16

4027. Tsai F Y, Teal J S, Heishima G B, Zee C S, Grinnell V S, Mehringer C M, Segall H D
Computed tomography in acute posterior fossa infarcts
AJNR 1982 Mar-Apr, Vol. 3 (2), P. 149–56

4028. Tsai F Y, Teal J S, Itabashi H H, Huprich J E, Hieshima G B, Segall H D
Computed tomography of posterior fossa trauma
J Comput Assist Tomogr 1980 Jun, Vol. 4 (3), P. 291–305

4029. Tschakert H, Grosse Hokamp H
Computertomographischer Nachweis eines beidseitigen Aderhautosteoms
Computed tomographic detection of a bilateral choroidal osteoma
RÖFO 1985 Jul, Vol. 143 (1), P. 113–5

4030. Turner R M, Gutman I, Hilal S K, Behrens M, Odel J
CT of drusen bodies and other calcific lesions of the optic nerve: case report and differential diagnosis
AJNR 1983 Mar-Apr, Vol. 4 (2), P. 175–8

4031. Valavanis A, Kubik S, Schubiger O
High-resolution CT of the normal and abnormal fallopian canal
AJNR 1983 May-Jun, Vol. 4 (3), P. 748–51

4032. van Gijn J, van Dongen K J
The time course of aneurysmal haemorrhage on computed tomograms
Neuroradiology 1982, Vol. 23 (3), P. 153–6

4033. Van Tassel P, Lee Y Y, Bruner J M
Synchronous and metachronous malignant gliomas: CT findings
AJNR 1988 Jul-Aug, Vol. 9 (4), P. 725–32

4034. Vannier M W, Hildebolt C F, Marsh J L, Pilgram T K, McAlister W H, Shackelford G D, Offutt C J, Knapp R H
Craniosynostosis: diagnostic value of three-dimensional CT reconstruction
Radiology 1989 Dec, Vol. 173 (3), P. 669–73

4035. Villforth J C
Medical radiation protection: a long view
Am J Roentgenol 1985 Dec, Vol. 145 (6), P. 1114–8

4036. Vinuela F V, Fox A J, Debrun G M, Feasby T E, Ebers G C
New perspectives in computed tomography of multiple sclerosis
Am J Roentgenol 1982 Jul, Vol. 139 (1), P. 123–7

4037. Virapongse C, Rothman S L, Sasaki C, Kier E L
The role of high resolution computed tomography in evaluating disease of the middle ear
J Comput Assist Tomogr 1982 Aug, Vol. 6 (4), P. 711–20

4038. Vogelzang R L, Limpert J D, Yao J S
Detection of prosthetic vascular complications: comparison of CT and angiography
Am J Roentgenol 1987 Apr, Vol. 148 (4), P. 819–23

4039. Vogl G, Schimek F, Ozdoba C, Steuhl P K, Voigt K, Nusslin F
Stereotactic retrobulbar anesthesia using CT
J Comput Assist Tomogr 1990 Sep-Oct, Vol. 14 (5), P. 859–61

4040. Vogl G, Schwer C, Jauch M, Wietholter H, Kindermann U, Muller Schauenburg W
A simple superimposition method for anatomical adjustments of CT and SPECT images
J Comput Assist Tomogr 1989 Sep-Oct, Vol. 13 (5), P. 929–31

4041. von Kummer R, Kober B
Mehrdeutiger CT-Befund bei einer fulminant verlaufenden Pneumokokkenmeningitis
Ambiguous CT finding in a fulminant pneumococcal meningitis
RÖFO 1983 Sep, Vol. 139 (3), P. 324–5

4042. Vonofakos D, Marcu H, Hacker H
CT diagnosis of basilar artery occlusion
AJNR 1983 May-Jun, Vol. 4 (3), P. 525–8

4043. Vouge M, Pasquini U, Salvolini U
CT findings of atypical forms of phakomatosis
Neuroradiology 1980, Vol. 20 (2), P. 99–101

4044. Vukanovic S, Hauser H, Wettstein P
CT localization of myonecrosis for surgical decompression
Am J Roentgenol 1980 Dec, Vol. 135 (6), P. 1298

4045. Waggenspack G A, Guinto F C Jr
MR and CT of masses of the anterosuperior third ventricle
Am J Roentgenol 1989 Mar, Vol. 152 (3), P. 609–14

4046. Waldron R L, Abbott D C, Vellody D
Computed tomography in preeclampsia-eclampsia syndrome
AJNR 1985 May-Jun, Vol. 6 (3), P. 442–3

4047. Walkey M M
And what is your sign? letter
Radiology 1991 Mar, Vol. 178 (3), P. 894

4048. Wang A M, Fischer E G, Ofori Kwakye S K, Rumbaugh C L, Lewis M L
Posterior fossa ependymal cyst and atlantoaxial subluxation in a patient with Down syndrome: CT findings
J Comput Assist Tomogr 1984 Aug, Vol. 8 (4), P. 783–7

4049. Wang A M, Lin J C, Rumbaugh C L
What is expected of CT in the evaluation of stroke?
Neuroradiology 1988, Vol. 30 (1), P. 54–8

4050. Wang A M, Morris J H, Hickey W F, Hammerschlag S B, O Reilly G V, Rumbaugh C L
Unusual CT patterns of multiple sclerosis
AJNR 1983 Jan-Feb, Vol. 4 (1), P. 47–50

4051. Wang A M, Skias D D, Rumbaugh C L, Schoene W C, Zamani A
Central nervous system changes after radiation therapy and/or chemotherapy: correlation of CT and autopsy findings
AJNR 1983 May-Jun, Vol. 4 (3), P. 466–71

4052. Ward M P, Glazer H S, Heiken J P, Spector J G
Traumatic perforation of the pyriform sinus: CT demonstration
J Comput Assist Tomogr 1985 Sep-Oct, Vol. 9 (5), P. 982–4

4053. Watanabe A S, Smoker W R
Computed tomography and angiographic findings in metastatic choriocarcinoma
J Comput Assist Tomogr 1989 Mar-Apr, Vol. 13 (2), P. 319–22

4054. Watanabe A T, Jeffrey R B Jr
CT diagnosis of traumatic rupture of the cisterna chyli
J Comput Assist Tomogr 1987 Jan-Feb, Vol. 11 (1), P. 175–6

4055. Weisberg L A, Stazio A, Elliott D, Shamsnia M
Putaminal hemorrhage: clinical-computed tomographic correlations
Neuroradiology 1990, Vol. 32 (3), P. 200–6

4056. Weissman J L, Tabor E K, Curtin H D
Sphenochoanal polyps: evaluation with CT and MR imaging
Radiology 1991 Jan, Vol. 178 (1), P. 145–8

4057. Welch K, Naheedy M H, Abroms I F, Strand R D
Computed tomography of Sturge-Weber syndrome in infants
J Comput Assist Tomogr 1980 Feb, Vol. 4 (1), P. 33–6

4058. Welch T J, Sheedy P F, Johnson C D, Johnson C M, Stephens D H
CT-guided biopsy: prospective analysis of 1,000 procedures
Radiology 1989 May, Vol. 171 (2), P. 493–6

4059. Welker H, Metzger H, Reich L
CT bei der Amyloidose der Zunge und des Mundbodens. Ein kasuistischer Beitrag zur Differentialdiagnose der Makroglossie
CT of tongue and mouth floor amyloidosis. A case contribution to the differential diagnosis of macroglossia
RÖFO 1986 Oct, Vol. 145 (4), P. 470–2

4060. Wells R G, Sty J R, Starshak R J
CT findings in noma
J Comput Assist Tomogr 1988 Jul-Aug, Vol. 12 (4), P. 711–2

4061. Wende K, Kishikawa T, Huwel N, Kazner E, Grumme T, Lanksch W
Do we need ventriculography in the era of computed tomography?
Neuroradiology 1982, Vol. 23 (2), P. 89–90

4062. Wende K, Kishikawa T, Huwel N, Kazner E, Grumme T, Lanksch W
Computer-Tomographie und / oder Ventrikulographie?
Computed tomography and/or ventriculography?
Radiologe 1982 Jan, Vol. 22 (1), P. 38–44

4063. Wester K, Kjartansson O, Bakke S J
CT guided stereotaxy based on scout view imaging
Neuroradiology 1987, Vol. 29 (3), P. 287–90

4064. Whelan M A, Myung K H, Bergeron R T
The innominate line
Neuroradiology 1984, Vol. 26 (2), P. 119–22

4065. Wichmann W, Schubiger O, Valavanis A, Kasdaglis K
Zur kernspintomographischen Diagnostik von Mikroadenomen der Hypophyse: Vergleich MRT, CT und OP
NMR tomographic diagnosis of microadenomas of the hypophysis: a comparison of MRT, CT and operation
RÖFO 1988 Sep, Vol. 149 (3), P. 239–44

4066. Willeit J, Schmutzhard E, Aichner F, Mayr U, Weber F, Gerstenbrand F
CT and MR imaging in neuro-Behcet disease
J Comput Assist Tomogr 1986 Mar-Apr, Vol. 10 (2), P. 313–5

4067. Willgeroth F, Breit A (ed.)
Weibliches Genitale-Mamma- Geburtshilfe
1989 Springer Verlag , Berlin Heidelberg New York London Paris Tokyo Hong Kong

4068. Wilms G, Van Roost W, Van Russelt J, Smits J
Biparietal thinning: correlation with CT findings
Radiologe 1983 Aug, Vol. 23 (8), P. 385–6

4069. Wilson D M, Enzmann D R, Hintz R L, Rosenfeld G
Computed tomographic findings in septo-optic dysplasia: discordance between clinical and radiological findings
Neuroradiology 1984, Vol. 26 (4), P. 279–83

4070. Wimmer B, Hofmann E, Jacob
Trauma of the spine
1990 Springer Verlag , Berlin Heidelberg New York London Paris Tokyo Hong Kong

4071. Winkler S, Turski P
Potential hazards of xenon inhalation editorial
AJNR 1985 Nov-Dec, Vol. 6 (6), P. 974–5

4072. Wittenberg J, Fineberg H V, Ferrucci J T Jr, Simeone J F, Mueller P R, van Sonnenberg E, Kirkpatrick R H
Clinical efficacy of computed body tomography, II
Am J Roentgenol 1980 Jun, Vol. 134 (6), P. 1111–20

4073. Wodarz R
Watershed infarctions and computed tomography. A topographical study in cases with stenosis or occlusion of the carotid artery
Neuroradiology 1980, Vol. 19 (5), P. 245–8

4074. Wodarz R, Ratzka M, Grosse D
Der Grenzzoneninfarkt als besondere Infarktkonstellation bei Karotisinsuffizienz. Eine computertomographisch-angiographische Korrelationsstudie
Watershed infarctions-a special type of infarction in cases with carotid artery stenosis or occlusion verified by CT and angiography
RÖFO 1981 Feb, Vol. 134 (2), P. 128–31

4075. Wong W S, Sherman N E, Moss A A
Malignant histiocytosis in a patient with sickle cell anemia: CT findings
J Comput Assist Tomogr 1983 Oct, Vol. 7 (5), P. 908–10

4076. Woo E, Chan F L, Yu Y L, Huang C Y, Mak E, Lee P K, So S Y
Bulbar palsy aggravated by metrizamide CT cisternography
Neuroradiology 1987, Vol. 29 (2), P. 219

4077. Woolfitt R A, Brantly P N, Neal R K
CT demonstration of a neurofibrosarcoma causing femoral neuropathy
J Comput Assist Tomogr 1982 Oct, Vol. 6 (5), P. 1013–4

4078. Wunschik F, Georgi M, Pastyr O
Stereotactic biopsy using computed tomography
J Comput Assist Tomogr 1984 Feb, Vol. 8 (1), P. 32–7

4079. Xu G L, Haughton V M, Carrera G F
Lumbar facet joint capsule: appearance at MR imaging and CT
Radiology 1990 Nov, Vol. 177 (2), P. 415–20

4080. Yamamoto M, Shinohara Y, Kamei T, Yoshii F
Diagnosis of internal carotid artery occlusion by dynamic computed tomography
J Comput Assist Tomogr 1981 Oct, Vol. 5 (5), P. 637–40

4081. Yamato M, Fuhrman C R
Computed tomography of fatty replacement in extramedullary hematopoiesis
J Comput Assist Tomogr 1987 May-Jun, Vol. 11 (3), P. 541–2

4082. Yamato M, Ido K, Izutsu M, Narimatsu Y, Hiramatsu K
CT and ultrasound findings of surgically retained sponges and towels
J Comput Assist Tomogr 1987 Nov-Dec, Vol. 11 (6), P. 1003–6

4083. Yang P J, Seeger J F, Carmody R F, Fleischer A S
Chondroma of falx: CT findings
J Comput Assist Tomogr 1986 Nov- Dec, Vol. 10 (6), P. 1075–6

4084. Yang W C, Rudansky M C, Stiller J, Shanzer S
Value of metrizamide CT in the demonstration of spinal arachnoid cysts
AJNR 1983 Sep-Oct, Vol. 4 (5), P. 1115–8

4085. Yock D H Jr, Larson D A
Computed tomography of hemorrhage from anterior communicating artery aneurysms, with angiographic correlation
Radiology 1980 Feb, Vol. 134 (2), P. 399–407

4086. Yonas H, Grundy B, Gur D, Shabason L, Wolfson S K Jr, Cook E E
Side effects of xenon inhalation
J Comput Assist Tomogr 1981 Aug, Vol. 5 (4), P. 591–2

4087. Young J W, Burgess A R
Use of CT in acute trauma victims letter
Radiology 1988 Mar, Vol. 166 (3), P. 903

4088. Young S C, Grossman R I, Goldberg H I, Spagnoli M V, Hackney D B, Zimmerman R A, Bilaniuk L T
MR of vascular encasement in parasellar masses: comparison with angiography and CT
AJNR 1988 Jan-Feb, Vol. 9 (1), P. 35–8

4089. Young S W, Noon M A, Nassi M, Castellino R A
Dynamic computed tomography body scanning
J Comput Assist Tomogr 1980 Apr, Vol. 4 (2), P. 168–73

4090. Yousem D, Scott W Jr, Fishman E K, Watson A J, Traill T, Gimenez L
Saphenous vein graft aneurysms demonstrated by computed tomography
J Comput Assist Tomogr 1986 May-Jun, Vol. 10 (3), P. 526–8

4091. Yu W S, Sagerman R H, Chung C T, King G A, Dalal P S, Bassano D A, Ames T E
Anatomical relationships in intracavitary irradiation demonstrated by computed tomography
Radiology 1982 May, Vol. 143 (2), P. 537–41

4092. Zanella F E, Kirchhof B, Modder U
Drüsenverkalkungen des Sehnervkopfes in der CT
Calcification of optic disk drusen on CT
RÖFO 1984 Dec, Vol. 141 (6), P. 647–8

4093. Zanella F E, Modder U, Benz Bohm G, Thun F
Die Neurofibromatose im Kindesalter. Computertomographische Befunde im Schädel- und Hals-bereich
Neurofibromatosis in childhood. Computed tomographic findings in the skull and neck areas
RÖFO 1984 Nov, Vol. 141 (5), P. 498–504

4094. Zee C S, Segall H D, Miller C, Ahmadi J, McComb J G, Han J S, Park S H
Less common CT features of medulloblastoma
Radiology 1982 Jul, Vol. 144 (1), P. 97–102

4095. Zerhouni E A, Barth K H, Siegelman S S
Demonstration of venous thrombosis by computed tomography
Am J Roentgenol 1980 Apr, Vol. 134 (4), P. 753–8

4096. Zhu X P, Checkley D R, Hickey D S, Isherwood I
Accuracy of area measurements made from MR images compared with computed tomography
J Comput Assist Tomogr 1986 Jan-Feb, Vol. 10 (1), P. 96–102

4097. Zilkha A, Daiz A S
Computed tomography in the diagnosis of superior sagittal sinus thrombosis
J Comput Assist Tomogr 1980 Feb, Vol. 4 (1), P. 124–6

4098. Zimmerman R A, Bilaniuk L T
Age-related incidence of pineal calcification detected by computed tomography
Radiology 1982 Mar, Vol. 142 (3), P. 659–62

4099. Zimmerman R A, Bilaniuk L T
Computed tomography of acute intratumoral hemorrhage
Radiology 1980 May, Vol. 135 (2), P. 355–9

4100. Zimmerman R A, Bilaniuk L T, Packer R J, Goldberg H I, Grossman R I
Computed tomographic-arteriographic correlates in acute basal ganglionic infarction of child-hood
Neuroradiology 1983, Vol. 24 (5), P. 241–8

4101. Zimmerman R D, Leeds N E, Danziger A
Subdural empyema: CT findings
Radiology 1984 Feb, Vol. 150 (2), P. 417–22

4102. Zimmerman R D, Russell E J, Leeds N E
Axial CT recognition of anteroposterior displacement of fourth ventricle
AJNR 1980 Jan-Feb, Vol. 1 (1), P. 65–70

4103. Zimmerman R D, Russell E J, Yurberg E, Leeds N E
Falx and interhemispheric fissure on axial CT: II. Recognition and differentiation of interhemispheric subarachnoid and subdural hemorrhage
AJNR 1982 Nov-Dec, Vol. 3 (6), P. 635–42

4104. Zimmerman R D, Yurberg E, Russell E J, Leeds N E
Falx and interhemispheric fissure on axial CT: I. Normal anatomy
Am J Roentgenol 1982 May, Vol. 138 (5), P. 899–904

4105. Zinreich S J, Long D M, Davis R, Quinn C B, McAfee P C, Wang H
Three-dimensional CT imaging in postsurgical "failed back" syndrome
J Comput Assist Tomogr 1990 Jul-Aug, Vol. 14 (4), P. 574–80

4106. Zonneveld F W, de Groot J A, Damsma H, van Waes P F, Huizing E H
Die Anwendbarkeit der hochauflösenden CT zur Darstellung des Aquaeductus vestibuli (Meniere) und der Otospongiosis des Labyrinths
Feasibility of high resolution CT in the demonstration of the vestibular aqueduct Meniere and otospongiosis of the labyrinth
Radiologe 1984 Nov, Vol. 24 (11), P. 508–15

Keyword Index

Acetabulum, fracture of
2716, 2798, 2833, 2837, 2843, 2860, 2930, 2961, 2962, 2964, 2975, 3087, 3092, 3151, 3160, 3170

Adrenal gland
–, atrophy of
2177, 3311
–, hemorrhage in
2214, 2233, 2238
–, hyperplasia and hyperfunction of
2178, 2185, 2235, 2881, 3860
–, metastases to
984, 1230, 2195, 2206, 2232, 2311, 2611, 3351
–, neoplasms of
1708, 2171, 2178, 2181, 2182, 2185, 2187, 2188, 2190, 2192, 2200, 2203, 2207, 2211, 2217, 2219

Aneurysm
–, abdominal
198, 301, 303, 307, 434, 444, 447, 475, 482, 485, 491, 841, 1676, 1721, 1742, 1775, 1831, 1856, 2439, 3303, 3650
–, aortic
198, 233, 255, 276, 278, 279, 289, 298, 301, 303, 353, 442, 447, 474, 491, 546, 660, 761, 790, 3303

Angiomyolipoma
1979, 1983, 2003, 2023, 2035, 2059, 2109, 2119, 2124, 2150, 2154

Aorta, thoracic
169, 195, 198, 233, 238, 244, 255, 267, 270, 276, 278, 279, 289, 298, 300, 301, 303, 304, 307, 326, 329, 353, 402, 428, 442, 447, 455, 474, 491, 508, 546, 660, 761, 790, 3303, 3446, 3622, 3705

Appendicitis
1187, 1495, 1500, 1692, 1737, 1763, 1916, 2446

Asbestos-related diseases
577, 578, 584, 585, 652, 653, 720, 767, 768, 769, 779, 853, 871, 897, 1846

Ascites
113, 280, 830, 1175, 1210, 1311, 1672, 1681, 1701, 1715, 1716, 1745, 1754, 1765, 1797, 1813, 1874, 1900, 1915, 1918, 1976, 2434, 3434

Azygos vein
227, 272, 279, 296, 305, 344, 400, 401, 426, 432, 456, 619, 759, 788, 1862, 1903, 3260

Biliary tract, tumor of
917, 991, 995, 1051, 1067, 1131, 1233, 1247, 1258, 1273, 1275, 1276, 1284, 1301, 1323, 1335

Biloma
1311

Biopsy, CT-guided
128, 252, 310, 316, 322, 632, 752, 814, 815, 862, 893, 940, 967, 996, 1050, 1097, 1100, 1135, 1136, 1225, 1242, 1385, 1461, 1716, 1966, 2244, 2323, 2392, 2523, 2525, 2630, 2835, 2877, 2896, 3238, 3315, 3389, 3406, 3459, 3556, 3827, 3829, 3919, 3972, 4026, 4078

Bolus injection *see* Contrast media

Bone tumor, benign chondrogenic
424, 797, 879, 2588, 2589, 2599, 2606, 2615, 2650, 2897, 3060, 3340, 3563, 3838, 4083

Bronchiectasis
452, 618, 633, 654, 657, 686, 712, 727, 753, 812, 820, 827, 859, 869, 894, 911

Bronchogenic carcinoma
114, 217, 232, 264, 274, 309, 385, 388, 411, 457, 458, 465, 489, 607, 621, 651, 661, 667, 668, 681, 683, 688, 693, 700, 702, 734, 736, 740, 741, 763, 772, 779, 795, 796, 824, 829, 842, 848, 849, 852, 857, 860, 879, 906, 910, 923, 924, 932, 938, 941, 1746, 1885, 3701, 3859

Bronchogenic cyst
579

Bronchopneumonia, pneumonia
225, 359, 392, 712, 716, 783, 819, 830, 906, 923, 955

Carcinoid
462, 590, 638, 682, 735, 755, 782, 826, 859, 889, 923, 984, 1243, 1300, 1482, 1507, 1529, 1542, 1624, 1633, 1693, 4089

Carcinoma
–, bronchoalveolar
718, 721, 747, 802, 907, 938, 4047
–, colorectal
13, 134, 154, 182, 571, 959, 1019, 1031, 1062, 1103, 1104, 1146, 1147, 1151, 1157, 1206, 1209, 1230, 1494, 1497, 1515, 1535, 1540, 1543, 1560, 1562, 1563, 1577, 1588, 1603, 1604, 1610, 1622, 1638, 1647, 1717, 1732, 1747, 1825, 1830, 1905, 2348, 2384, 2501, 3020, 3876
–, fibrolamellar
1234
–, hepatocellular
990, 1009, 1045, 1057, 1065, 1066, 1080, 1083, 1115, 1126, 1137, 1145, 1152, 1176, 1234, 1249, 1251, 1252, 1894

Cardiac chambers
43, 489, 490, 492, 500, 502, 503, 521, 522, 527, 536, 538, 544, 551, 559, 565, 568, 570, 573, 2119, 2571, 3463, 3800, 3834

Caroli's disease
1010, 1016, 1017, 1321

Cervix neoplasm
13, 1650, 1747, 1828, 1855, 1883, 1884, 2262, 2360, 2361, 2363, 2369, 2374, 2375, 2377, 2379, 2387, 2392, 2397, 2407, 2417, 2419, 2420, 2421, 2424, 3779, 4091

Cholangiocarcinoma
1233, 1273, 1275, 1276, 1323

Cholangitis
963, 1274, 1280, 1302, 1329, 1331, 1338

Cholecystitis
998, 1039, 1260, 1262, 1268, 1270, 1271, 1278, 1280, 1281, 1289, 1293, 1294, 1297, 1298, 1303, 1304, 1305, 1308, 1313, 1315, 1316, 1322, 1324, 1325, 1327, 1332, 1334, 1337, 1339, 1342, 1344, 1348, 1349, 1916, 3496

Choledochal cyst
1285

Cholelithiasis
1079, 1150, 1260, 1264, 1265, 1268, 1270, 1271, 1274, 1281, 1282, 1288, 1294, 1295, 1297, 1298, 1304, 1308, 1315, 1320, 1325, 1331, 1332, 1335, 1342, 1344, 1345, 1348, 1725, 3263

Cholestasis *see* Obstruction, biliary

Chondrosarcoma
2585, 2589, 2610, 2614, 2615, 2625, 2651, 2948, 3060, 3084, 3097, 3794

Colitis, ulcerative
1535, 1541, 1550, 1574, 1576, 1627, 1643, 1702, 2664

Computed tomography, technology
9, 11, 23, 24, 31, 51, 54, 76, 78, 79, 84, 98, 99, 108, 121, 122, 160, 179, 514, 672, 792, 936, 977, 1167, 1393, 1917, 2405, 2521, 2535, 2538, 3073, 3076, 3138, 3148, 3160, 3186, 3223, 3363, 3368, 3372, 3408, 3422, 3440, 3548, 3564, 3681, 3711, 3763, 3885, 3954

Contrast media
–, barium sulfate
160, 168, 223, 235, 236, 1471, 1493, 1497, 1515, 1517, 1528, 1535, 1538, 1573, 1576, 1579, 1597, 1599, 1619, 1660, 1664, 1686, 1764, 1788, 2374, 3370, 3520, 3875
–, bolus injection
17, 136, 138, 139, 147, 169, 214, 620, 988, 1029, 1030, 1068, 1132, 1183, 1459, 1980

Coxitis
2484, 2755, 2756, 3004

Crohn's disease
1535, 1537, 1538, 1546, 1550, 1569, 1576, 1581, 1585, 1619, 1625, 1639, 1643, 1664, 1666, 1707, 1811, 1919, 2278

CT-Myelography
144, 190, 451, 1691, 2616, 2620, 2624, 2668, 2670, 2674, 2675, 2690, 2693, 2694, 2699, 2724, 2730, 2748, 2761, 2769, 2796, 2800, 2812, 2819, 2823, 2839, 2849, 2864, 2881, 2885, 2894, 2898, 2903, 2912, 2913, 2914, 2915, 2921, 2927, 2933, 2934, 2937, 2938, 2959, 2980, 2984, 2988, 2991, 2996, 3000, 3001, 3003, 3030, 3044, 3051, 3053, 3070, 3072, 3074, 3077, 3082, 3091, 3095, 3104, 3106, 3119, 3122, 3136, 3139, 3140, 3141, 3143, 3144, 3145, 3154, 3157, 3161, 3179, 3181, 3183, 3184, 3195, 3196, 3207, 3209, 3211, 3214, 3219, 3243, 3262, 3291, 3326, 3364, 3371, 3374, 3403, 3415, 3420, 3431, 3433, 3443, 3471, 3472, 3509, 3517, 3597, 3753, 3754, 3805, 3819, 3852, 3865, 3914, 3930, 3958, 4076, 4084

CT-Portography (CT during arterial portography)
1023, 1059, 1111, 1144, 1145, 1146, 1152, 1180, 1182, 1205, 1237

Densitometry
21, 66, 143, 339, 423, 663, 673, 879, 927, 1068, 1264, 1344, 2406, 2511, 2691, 2784, 2940, 2958, 3058, 3071, 3086, 3093, 3538, 3564, 3576, 3614, 3915, 3931

Dermoid cyst
343, 477, 549, 1734, 1842, 2346, 2354, 2403, 2405, 2406, 2470, 2561, 3084, 3570

Diastematomyelia
2675, 2733, 3000, 3433, 3930

Disc, intervertebral
2671, 2672, 2709, 2775, 2880, 2886, 2898, 2960, 2991, 2996, 3031, 3098, 3175

Dissection, aortic
233, 241, 255, 276, 278, 279, 286, 289, 290, 298, 301, 303, 323, 353, 357, 410, 419, 430, 431, 442, 445, 474, 475, 482, 491, 494, 546, 635, 660, 761, 790, 1698, 1742, 1775, 1876, 3303, 3375

Diverticulitis
1462, 1493, 1497, 1517, 1528, 1535, 1547, 1553, 1557, 1558, 1565, 1566, 1573, 1579, 1597, 1644, 1651, 1659, 1729, 1825, 2295, 2296, 3641

Drainage, CT-guided
90, 113, 116, 128, 347, 351, 412, 440, 579, 895, 918, 979, 1002, 1046, 1312, 1345, 1379, 1430, 1476, 1500, 1760, 1763, 1817, 1871, 1891, 1966, 1975, 2002, 2030, 2086, 2123, 2415, 2480, 2619, 3218, 3477, 3913

Ductus thyreoglossus
–, cysts of
3296

Echinococcosis
997, 1000, 1008, 1015, 1039, 1040, 1090, 1110, 1191, 1196, 1217, 1219, 1829, 2263, 3267, 3607

Esophagus
–, cysts of
320, 463
–, diverticula of
362
–, fistula of
197, 236, 374
–, neoplasms of
208, 235, 236, 293, 294, 317, 338, 342, 367, 370, 373, 375, 380, 425, 443, 445, 458, 468, 470, 702, 1501, 1593, 1657, 1658, 2638, 3463, 3701
–, varices of
224, 229, 293, 305, 547, 968, 1075, 1148, 1177, 1492, 1862, 1939

Fibrosis, retroperitoneal
1721, 2325, 2433, 2439, 2444, 2448, 2453, 2455, 2464, 2466, 2532

Focal nodular hyperplasia (FNH)
1018, 1074, 1090, 1098, 1110, 1129, 1215, 1231, 3860

Gallbladder, tumor of
995, 1281, 1290, 1296, 1298, 1300, 1306, 1318, 1324, 1334, 1335, 1341, 1344, 1346, 1350, 1825, 1830

Giant cell tumor
39, 2479, 2500, 2610, 2639, 2647, 2721, 3057, 3084

Goiter
203, 210, 273, 275, 408, 422, 810

Heart (general)
863, 49, 67, 535, 528, 498, 501, 524, 3452, 43, 515, 571, 523, 562, 507, 557, 490, 554, 530, 561, 3049, 558, 495, 543, 572, 542, 522
–, aneurysm of
43, 493, 506, 568, 3800
–, coronary diseases of
43, 169, 231, 336, 339, 340, 341, 379, 387, 484, 505, 510, 514, 522, 525, 528, 535, 537, 539, 541, 542, 543, 553, 569, 1148, 1184, 3352, 3738, 4090
–, (congenital) defects of
270, 500, 508, 531, 544
–, enlargement of
493, 501, 509, 531, 828, 1063, 1169, 1745, 1765, 3434, 3463
–, neoplasms of
16, 43, 221, 478, 492, 496, 497, 504, 513, 519, 521, 527, 536, 545, 548, 553, 561, 565, 573, 575, 612, 2119, 2311, 2571

Hemochromatosis
503, 968, 1125, 1160, 1201

Hepatic vein thrombosis
1027, 1055, 1143, 1165, 1194, 1208, 1240, 1248

Hepatitis
1088, 1238, 1331

Histiocytosis X
617, 807

Hydronephrosis
1217, 1721, 1829, 1986, 2000, 2002, 2010, 2011, 2021, 2096, 2115, 2142, 2144, 2161, 2257, 2258, 2259, 2286, 2425, 2466, 3020

Iliopsoas muscle
2461, 2487, 2515, 2520, 2522, 2539, 2542, 2597, 2619, 2855

Ischemia, mesenteric
1113, 1491, 1516, 1518, 1574, 1774

Islet cell tumor
984, 1362, 1363, 1370, 1376, 1381, 1387, 1388, 1394, 1406, 1423, 1458, 1468, 3859

Kidney
–, abscess in
2034, 2044, 2062, 2073, 2111, 2138, 2139, 2145, 2223, 2429
–, adenoma of
2217
–, calculi of
1987, 2043, 2105, 2127, 2142, 2149, 2160
–, cysts of
1887, 1980, 1996, 1997, 2004, 2008, 2009, 2010, 2022, 2052, 2054, 2061, 2062, 2070, 2071, 2074, 2075, 2077, 2082, 2085, 2088, 2089, 2090, 2094, 2095, 2115, 2126, 2134, 2136, 2143, 2147, 2148, 2165, 2166, 2259, 2425, 3658
–, infarction of
2026, 2027, 2034, 2041, 2096, 2152, 2158, 2168, 3534
–, lypmhoma of
1732, 1977, 1992, 1995, 2040, 2055, 2065, 2120, 2156
–, polycystic disease of
2071, 2072, 2087
–, renal cell carcinoma
1989, 1993, 2016, 2037, 2058, 2063, 2067, 2084, 2098, 2107, 2117, 2118, 2129, 2132, 2137, 2154, 2155, 2163, 2426
–, thrombosis of renal vein
1750, 1939, 1998, 2028, 2037, 2080, 2140, 2157, 2158
–, transitional cell carcinoma
1988, 1989, 2261, 2426
–, trauma to
1375, 1503, 1719, 1735, 1771, 1856, 1980, 1984, 2014, 2015, 2022, 2025, 2038, 2049, 2062, 2080, 2092, 2096, 2105, 2115, 2131, 2146, 2159, 2202, 2238, 2355, 2445, 2523
–, tuberculosis of
2013, 2019, 2031, 2198, 2429

Leiomyoma, uterine
2363, 2407, 2408, 2409
Lipomatosis
–, pancreatis
1433
–, renal
2046, 2090, 2142
Liver
–, abscess in
979, 1002, 1044, 1050, 1053, 1091, 1138, 1164, 1203
–, adenoma of
980, 1277
–, circulation of
1041, 1054, 1063, 1076, 1081, 1155, 1158, 1177, 1209
–, cirrhosis of
968, 1109, 1117, 1221, 1236
–, cysts in
994, 995, 998, 1038, 1060, 1099, 1110, 1132, 1217, 1218, 1221, 1289, 1324
–, fatty infiltration of
24, 956, 960, 968, 969, 995, 1020, 1049, 1097, 1121, 1185, 1192, 1197, 1201, 1250
–, hemangioma in
965, 973, 992, 1015, 1029, 1032, 1048, 1078, 1082, 1084, 1090, 1093, 1153, 1193, 1195, 1787, 2501
–, lymphoma of
1064, 1225, 3416
–, metastases to
996, 1007, 1057, 1058, 1121, 1124, 1146, 1149, 1154, 1157, 1209, 1254, 2381
–, trauma to
1043, 1053, 1119, 1130, 1159, 1161, 1164, 1192, 1210, 1212, 1218, 1310, 1503, 1735, 1859, 1932, 2014, 2355

–, tumor (general) of
220, 689, 917, 962, 973, 977, 981, 983, 990, 991, 1009, 1013, 1018, 1027, 1028, 1030, 1031, 1045, 1048, 1051, 1057, 1059, 1065, 1066, 1067, 1069, 1070, 1081, 1084, 1086, 1089, 1103, 1110, 1115, 1126, 1131, 1132, 1137, 1144, 1145, 1151, 1152, 1154, 1163, 1167, 1168, 1171, 1174, 1176, 1179, 1213, 1227, 1243, 1247, 1249, 1251, 1252, 1258, 1344, 1543, 1708, 1844, 1885, 1894, 1970, 2101, 2195, 3416
Lung
–, abscess in
702, 902, 918, 1739
–, benign tumor of
682, 702, 755, 782, 923
–, collapse of
378, 397, 473, 628, 637, 640, 655, 664, 682, 735, 753, 778, 779, 798, 827, 828, 829, 844, 846, 866, 931
–, emphysema of
1289, 1348, 1523, 1613, 2284, 2371, 2427, 2542, 3164, 3207
–, idiopathic fibrosis of
77, 207, 578, 602, 603, 604, 605, 623, 663, 674, 712, 754, 768, 779, 780, 781, 789, 814, 815, 838, 878, 882, 901, 925
–, infarction of
214, 225, 595, 597, 639, 670, 697, 713, 725, 905
–, lymphangiomatosis of
690, 752, 862, 887, 912, 1923, 2437
–, lymphangitic carcinomatosis of
602, 754
–, nodule, pulmonary
21, 44, 61, 129, 661, 672, 702, 715, 751, 813, 852, 858, 875, 888, 891, 892, 900, 937, 3576
–, sarcoidosis of
348, 592, 602, 604, 605, 616, 663, 695, 768, 780, 789, 816, 817, 838, 913
–, sequestration of
472, 596, 730, 805, 840, 847, 916
–, trauma to
922
Lymph node, metastases
1624, 1747, 1820, 1821, 1863, 1885, 2067, 2301, 2326, 2439, 2442, 2443, 2447, 2458
Lymphadenopathy
1004, 1862, 1888, 2039, 2439, 2447, 2461, 2468, 3012
Lymphoma, malignant (general)
205, 316, 445, 450, 453, 458, 460, 504, 571, 625, 664, 680, 690, 758, 889, 941, 948, 952, 975, 981, 1064, 1116, 1188, 1256, 1469, 1487, 1504, 1512, 1521, 1529, 1532, 1555, 1575, 1587, 1595, 1599, 1604, 1620, 1625, 1639, 1691, 1732, 1762, 1783, 1804, 1816, 1820, 1821, 1825, 1840, 1887, 1905, 1922, 1936, 1942, 1948, 1956, 1964, 1992, 2040, 2055, 2098, 2120, 2128, 2204, 2247, 2277, 2428, 2439, 2468, 2488, 2579, 2610, 2638, 2688, 2773, 2774, 2997, 3133, 3196, 3206, 3324, 3416, 3435, 3490, 3557, 3659, 3673, 3831, 3843, 4014, 4089
–, gastrointestinal
1532, 1599, 1604, 1607, 1620, 1625, 1762, 1808, 2428
–, giant follicular
1992
–, histiocytic
1211, 1992, 2097, 3240, 3361, 3557, 4014
–, lymphocytic
1225, 1687, 3586
–, retroperitoneal
1504, 1732, 1762, 1783, 1816, 1820, 1821, 1840, 1887, 1905, 2428, 2439, 2468

Mediastinitis
199, 216, 218, 282, 368, 461, 702, 2507
Mediastinum
–, cystic masses of
249, 257, 266, 273, 275, 318, 350, 358, 369, 395, 409,

421, 423, 460, 462, 477, 548, 579, 746, 766, 770, 839, 1734
–, neurogenic neoplasms of
213, 314, 445, 460, 571, 888, 941, 3184, 3283, 3288, 3425, 3429
–, trauma to
273, 329, 366, 384
Meningocele
273, 2681, 2785, 2825, 2876, 2959, 3153, 3154, 3172, 3184, 3517, 3526, 3844
Mesenteric cysts
1412, 1622, 1751, 1818, 1886
Mesothelioma
327, 407, 464, 575, 586, 612, 684, 732, 769, 776, 1862, 3949
Muscle
–, abscess of
308, 1546, 1811, 2461, 2515, 2558, 2597, 2619, 3034, 3206
–, atrophy of
2477, 2508, 2527, 2537
–, dystrophy of
2511, 2525
–, hematoma of
308, 1835, 1917, 2461, 2491, 2558, 3206, 3533
–, inflammatory diseases of
2461, 2487, 2522, 2540, 2541, 2608, 3729
Myelolipoma
2170, 2186, 2194, 2213, 2220, 2237
Myositis ossificans
2471, 2488, 2569, 2576, 2583

Nephritis
–, acute bacterial, local
1073, 1916, 2006, 2030, 2036, 2044, 2045, 2116, 2127, 2138, 2139, 2145, 3435
–, xanthogranulomatous
2030, 2127, 2145
Nephroma, multilocular cystic
2100
Neuroblastoma
3351, 3978
Non-Hodgkin's lymphoma
257, 465, 622, 762, 1064, 1514, 1797, 1822, 1836, 1978, 1992, 1995, 2040, 2065, 2066, 2156, 2204, 2248, 2382, 2436, 3189, 3586, 3829

Obstruction, biliary
998, 1040, 1261, 1262, 1266, 1268, 1291, 1324, 1333, 1334, 1338, 1340, 1342, 1440, 1461
Oncocytoma
1994, 2003, 2005, 2064, 2069, 2125, 2656
Osteoarthritis of hip *see* Coxitis
Osteoma
2488, 2574, 2575, 2577, 2593, 2612, 2620, 2634, 2643, 2644, 2650, 2659, 4029, 4030
Osteosarcoma
627, 687, 692, 2162, 2500, 2548, 2564, 2566, 2567, 2571, 2578, 2582, 2585, 2586, 2590, 2599, 2602, 2609, 2610, 2613, 2614, 2621, 2632, 2633, 2641, 2650, 2702, 2867, 2947, 3111, 3125, 3795
Ovary
–, cysts of
1751, 1884, 2357, 2369, 2386, 2387, 2396, 2401, 2416
–, neoplasms of
114, 436, 1126, 1697, 1713, 1745, 1747, 1855, 1884, 1885, 1905, 1922, 2007, 2253, 2339, 2341, 2344, 2345, 2346, 2348, 2354, 2357, 2363, 2364, 2366, 2372, 2381, 2383, 2384, 2385, 2386, 2387, 2390, 2396, 2401, 2403, 2404, 2405, 2406, 2409, 2412, 2418, 2638, 3218

Pancreas
–, abscess in
1355, 1357, 1377, 1379, 1404, 1412, 1421, 1475, 1509, 1513, 1651, 1695, 1724, 1840, 1871, 1887
–, adenoma of
1374, 1409, 1414, 1452
–, carcinoma of
1324, 1353, 1366, 1369, 1370, 1390, 1397, 1398, 1400, 1406, 1407, 1411, 1416, 1417, 1418, 1426, 1429, 1454, 1479, 1922, 3450
–, cystadenocarcinoma of
714, 1409, 1414, 1439
–, cysts in
128, 358, 1298, 1359, 1368, 1380, 1382, 1383, 1391, 1396, 1406, 1416, 1421, 1422, 1427, 1428, 1438, 1446, 1464, 1473, 1477, 1625, 1640, 1786, 1843, 1887, 3625
–, lymphoma of
1469, 1620, 1625, 1825, 1840, 1887, 1905, 1922, 3435
–, neoplasms of
13, 714, 984, 1042, 1112, 1126, 1162, 1186, 1230, 1262, 1291, 1299, 1324, 1331, 1346, 1352, 1353, 1354, 1362, 1363, 1366, 1367, 1368, 1369, 1370, 1372, 1373, 1374, 1376, 1380, 1381, 1385, 1387, 1388, 1390, 1394, 1395, 1397, 1398, 1399, 1400, 1401, 1405, 1406, 1407, 1409, 1411, 1414, 1416, 1417, 1418, 1419, 1420, 1423, 1425, 1426, 1427, 1428, 1429, 1431, 1439, 1440, 1442, 1450, 1451, 1452, 1454, 1458, 1460, 1461, 1465, 1467, 1468, 1469, 1470, 1473, 1474, 1478, 1479, 1825, 1840, 1885, 1887, 1905, 1922, 1930, 1952, 2455, 2633, 2649, 3437, 3859
–, trauma to
1413
Pancreatitis (general)
114, 1262, 1298, 1311, 1324, 1331, 1355, 1356, 1357, 1364, 1365, 1367, 1372, 1373, 1377, 1380, 1383, 1390, 1392, 1399, 1404, 1405, 1406, 1407, 1412, 1415, 1417, 1419, 1420, 1421, 1424, 1425, 1428, 1429, 1431, 1432, 1433, 1434, 1435, 1441, 1456, 1465, 1466, 1469, 1471, 1473, 1474, 1475, 1476, 1509, 1580, 1695, 1697, 1745, 1823, 1887, 1959, 2086, 2355, 3435, 3437, 3450
–, acute
1355, 1356, 1357, 1392, 1404, 1415, 1421, 1424, 1433, 1434, 1435, 1441, 1466, 1471
–, chronic
1372, 1380, 1390, 1417, 1432, 1959
Pararenal and perirenal space, diseases of
1856, 1935, 2007, 2033, 2044, 2056, 2086, 2128, 2157, 3435
Parathyroid glands
252, 253
–, neoplasms of
252, 253, 702
Pelvic fractures
2355, 2760, 2843, 2860, 3092, 3170
Pericarditis, constrictive
502, 562
Pericardium (general)
467, 478, 486, 494, 499, 504, 513, 519, 521, 534, 547, 548, 549, 554, 555, 556, 560, 561, 567, 612
–, effusion of
460, 509, 511, 516, 519, 521, 523, 529, 532, 533, 539, 546, 553, 562, 564, 567, 674, 1063, 3494
–, neoplasms of
467, 478, 519
Peritoneal cavity (general)
1395, 1672, 1793, 2078, 3249
–, abscesses in see Peritonitis
–, hemorrhage in
1503, 1719, 1768, 1827, 1849
–, neoplasms (primary and metastatic) of
29, 970, 1284, 1395, 1504, 1624, 1690, 1697, 1761, 1767,

1784, 1788, 1792, 1797, 1812, 1815, 1816, 1819, 1842, 1846, 1886, 1900, 1904, 1905, 1918, 2340, 2345, 2390, 2412, 3803, 3828

Peritonitis
1622, 1633, 1667, 1768, 1799, 1827

Pheochromocytoma
1539, 2206, 2209, 2212, 2221, 2226, 2228, 2234, 2236, 2611

Plasmocytoma
1142, 1522, 2181, 3871, 3874

Pleura (general)
295, 351, 407, 441, 448, 597, 605, 629, 656, 720, 785, 798, 816, 831, 866, 871, 902, 3275
–, effusion of
586, 888, 429, 395, 1365, 381, 713, 637, 448, 477, 1976, 330, 760, 288, 757, 776, 1210, 830, 458, 635, 473, 396, 674, 282, 1748, 608, 846, 397
–, empyema of
330, 448, 458, 473, 608, 635, 757, 769

Pneumonia
225, 359, 392, 716, 783, 819, 830, 906, 923, 955

Portal vein, thrombosis of
1027, 1069, 1070, 1081, 1123, 1140, 1143, 1163, 1194, 1205, 1240, 1241, 1627, 1674, 1851, 1894

Prostate gland
–, abscess in
2303, 2327, 2330
–, cysts in
2324
–, hypertrophy of
2316, 2296, 2317, 2327
–, neoplasms of
45, 1347, 1874, 2241, 2247, 2298, 2302, 2305, 2306, 2307, 2309, 2315, 2316, 2319, 2327, 2331, 2332, 2419

Pseudocyst, pancreatic
114, 128, 1379, 1382, 1391, 1406, 1421, 1422, 1438, 1469, 1473, 1477, 1592, 1640, 1651, 1695, 1751, 1843, 1959, 2445, 3437, 3450, 3625

Pseudomyxoma peritonei
1781, 1814, 1832, 1877

Pulmonary artery
16, 214, 228, 231, 238, 239, 245, 272, 292, 332, 348, 349, 360, 372, 389, 453, 454, 522, 524, 552, 648, 664, 665, 670, 671, 696, 697, 717, 721, 725, 760, 765, 791, 844, 929, 935, 2472, 3834, 3873

Retroperitoneal neoplasms
29, 112, 478, 641, 690, 1353, 1469, 1638, 1708, 1732, 1733, 1808, 1821, 2130, 2209, 2213, 2226, 2313, 2325, 2326, 2428, 2434, 2435, 2436, 2437, 2438, 2439, 2442, 2451, 2457, 2458, 2460, 2461, 2463, 2465, 2467, 2468, 2469, 2470, 2615, 2649, 2788, 3230, 3803

Retroperitoneal space (general)
1004, 1148, 1551, 1782, 1852, 1888, 2039, 2056, 2078, 2086, 2133, 2288, 2427, 2441, 2463, 3560

Sacroiliitis
2701, 2723, 2763, 2941, 2966

Seminal vesicles
2309, 2312, 2318, 2319, 2321, 2328, 2337, 2429

Silicosis
600, 602, 768

Small intestine
–, tumor (general) of
1400, 1498, 1499, 1507, 1508, 1522, 1532, 1603, 1604, 1607, 1633, 1665, 1792, 1807, 1808, 1815, 2428, 3855
–, benign tumors
1607, 1808

Soft tissue tumors
–, (origin. from) adipose tissue (except lipoma)
345, 369, 445, 1298, 1318, 1398, 1714, 1886, 2046, 2090, 2142, 2478, 2544, 2601, 2684, 3049, 3723
–, (origin. from) autonomic ganglions
472, 941, 1670, 2104, 2130, 2726, 3231, 3243, 3245, 3288, 3289, 3351, 3425, 3429, 3630, 3872, 3978, 3979
–, (origin. from) blood vessels
427, 565, 689, 917, 981, 1108, 1204, 1226, 1239, 1691, 1950, 2457, 2519, 2564, 2610, 2637, 2640, 2702, 2753, 2986, 3230, 3825
–, (origin. from) fibrous tissue
43, 211, 468, 1401, 1677, 1710, 1907, 2129, 2344, 2396, 2457, 2469, 2506, 2531, 2532, 2544, 2564, 2570, 2572, 2593, 2610, 2637, 2659, 2868, 2946, 2974, 3804, 4089
–, (origin. from) lymph vessels
259, 273, 390, 438, 690, 752, 754, 818, 862, 887, 912, 1451, 1700, 1923, 1965, 2437, 2438, 2465, 2488, 3981
–, (origin. from) mesothelial tissue
327, 407, 464, 575, 586, 612, 684, 732, 769, 776, 897, 1846, 1862, 1905, 1918, 3949
–, (origin. from) muscle tissue
497, 521, 628, 648, 797, 1186, 1243, 1369, 1487, 1529, 1532, 1584, 1593, 1607, 1631, 1645, 1690, 1697, 1784, 1808, 1857, 1886, 1892, 1920, 2129, 2245, 2298, 2346, 2363, 2389, 2407, 2408, 2409, 2457, 2467, 2544, 2564, 2583, 2655, 3105, 3321
–, (origin. from) paraganglionic structures
408, 797, 2226, 2451, 2457, 2743, 3341, 3383, 3850, 3969
–, (origin. from) peripheral nerves
314, 571, 2457, 2513, 2519, 2624, 2636, 2649, 2655, 2879, 3002, 3084, 3116, 3181, 3196, 3356, 3365, 3480, 3703, 3748, 3773, 3914, 4005
–, (origin. from) pluripotential mesenchyme
1886, 2591
–, (origin. from) synovial tissue
2555, 2595, 2637, 2648, 2655
–, lipoma
23, 317, 398, 476, 496, 800, 888, 899, 944, 947, 1021, 1086, 1096, 1251, 1526, 1532, 1562, 1603, 1647, 1665, 1710, 1717, 1733, 1740, 1843, 1847, 1899, 1979, 1983, 2003, 2023, 2035, 2059, 2062, 2102, 2109, 2119, 2124, 2149, 2150, 2154, 2194, 2213, 2220, 2237, 2368, 2457, 2519, 2564, 2565, 2572, 2583, 2587, 2596, 2600, 2616, 2635, 2637, 2654, 2658, 2668, 2690, 3002, 3077, 3142, 3526, 3762, 3791, 3955, 4005, 4018

Spinal stenosis
2735, 2776, 2782, 2798, 2807, 2838, 2849, 2876, 2887, 2904, 2905, 2921, 2923, 3044, 3049, 3066, 3122, 3145, 3197, 3198, 3266, 3316, 3431

Spine
–, degenerative diseases of
74, 2698, 2748, 2876, 2887, 2894, 2923, 2953, 2978, 2991, 3066, 3106, 3122, 3132, 3139
–, injury to
42, 2678, 2707, 2713, 2798, 2804, 2869, 2994, 3032, 3066, 3084, 3088, 3132, 3163, 3200, 3201, 3471, 3605, 3752
–, meningeal neoplasms of
2696, 2913, 3002, 3077, 3082, 3084, 3671, 3973
–, spinal cord neoplasms
2552, 2605, 2658, 2690, 2694, 2704, 2753, 2777, 2819, 2831, 2892, 2894, 2913, 2934, 3035, 3044, 3053, 3077, 3084, 3095, 3141, 3243, 3265, 3420, 3431, 3443, 3671, 3724

Spleen
–, cysts in
994, 1218, 1948, 1964
–, infarction of
1924, 1925, 1930, 1947, 1973
–, neoplasms of
758, 1116, 1156, 1230, 1787, 1942, 1948, 1950, 1956, 1960, 1964, 1965, 2311, 3319, 3416, 4053

758, 1116, 1156, 1230, 1787, 1942, 1948, 1950, 1956, 1960, 1964, 1965, 2311, 3319, 3416, 4053

–, thrombosis of splenic vein
1240, 1674, 1851, 1930, 1939

–, trauma to
1218, 1503, 1509, 1735, 1840, 1866, 1917, 1927, 1931, 1937, 1961, 1972, 1973, 2014, 2355, 3533

Spondylitis, Spondylodiscitis
42, 2715, 2717, 2859, 2907, 2923, 2936, 3139, 3186, 3200, 3317

Spondylolysis
2678, 2738, 2901, 2931, 2991, 3037, 3156, 3188

Stomach
–, inflammation of
1523, 1545, 1564, 1568, 1571, 1586, 1613, 1631, 1663, 1745

–, neoplasms of
133, 687, 797, 1243, 1486, 1487, 1509, 1512, 1521, 1527, 1542, 1554, 1555, 1586, 1587, 1593, 1595, 1599, 1604, 1612, 1616, 1618, 1624, 1626, 1631, 1645, 1647, 1655, 1657, 1658, 1663, 1697, 1825, 1922, 2311, 2348, 2384, 2428

Syringomyelia
451, 2677, 2699, 2740, 2831, 2876, 2892, 3035, 3072, 3077, 3084, 3132, 3291, 3431, 3471, 3597, 3671, 3958

Teratoma
251, 384, 423, 450, 460, 548, 771, 1873

Thorac wall, diseases of
373, 459, 720, 777, 841, 942, 944, 946, 950, 2577, 2615, 2622, 2625, 2650, 2773, 2836, 3191, 3317, 3900, 4020

Thymus gland (general)
201, 202, 226, 237, 247, 254, 272, 284, 299, 302, 331, 334, 409, 462, 3416

–, hyperplasia of
281, 284, 409, 462, 3544

–, neoplasms of
201, 247, 261, 284, 302, 313, 318, 331, 334, 384, 409, 445, 450, 462, 476, 478, 536, 680, 702, 766, 941, 1482, 3793, 4006

Thyroid gland
182, 210, 272, 352, 422, 2209

–, neoplasms of
114, 971, 1149, 3646

Trachea
26, 206, 212, 215, 234, 262, 316, 332, 354, 355, 363, 367, 392, 393, 406, 415, 424, 446, 461, 615, 719, 737, 1714, 3308, 3452

Transplant, renal
1732, 2051, 2091, 2123, 2153, 2233, 4017

Urachal cyst
1843, 2268, 2270, 2273, 2281, 2292, 2295, 2378, 2432

Urinary bladder
–, diseases of
2096, 2240, 2244, 2251, 2271, 2278, 2296

–, tumor of
150, 1309, 1347, 1650, 1830, 1836, 1843, 1874, 1885, 2128, 2195, 2241, 2245, 2246, 2247, 2253, 2254, 2255, 2256, 2260, 2262, 2268, 2273, 2275, 2276, 2281, 2282, 2285, 2287, 2290, 2291, 2292, 2297, 2298, 2377, 2378, 2419, 2432, 2501

Uterine neoplasm
228, 1922, 2083, 2340, 2350, 2362, 2363, 2364, 2365, 2368, 2399, 2407, 2408, 2409, 2418, 2422, 2478, 3682, 4053

Vena cava inferior, diseases of
227, 233, 285, 333, 344, 456, 502, 550, 619, 1036, 1039, 1133, 1143, 1171, 1248, 1736, 1742, 1857, 1892, 1897, 1920, 1922, 1979, 2063, 2108, 2119, 2135, 2163, 2257, 2288, 2293, 2311, 2442, 3248, 3342, 3591, 3650, 3739

–, thrombosis of
118, 483, 489, 1165, 1240, 1708, 1851, 1896, 2703, 3260, 3261, 3424, 3476, 3654, 3741, 3750, 3916

Vena cava superior, diseases of
231, 250, 256, 272, 279, 305, 333, 456, 522, 527, 598, 1076, 1746, 2507, 3565, 3738, 3750

Vertebra, tumor/tumorlike lesions
42, 396, 1862, 2316, 2474, 2565, 2566, 2575, 2577, 2588, 2604, 2606, 2615, 2616, 2617, 2620, 2639, 2644, 2645, 2650, 2654, 2668, 2687, 2688, 2690, 2696, 2706, 2741, 2799, 2814, 2834, 2859, 2879, 2905, 2911, 2912, 2919, 2923, 2949, 2982, 3002, 3082, 3084, 3096, 3100, 3143, 3145, 3180, 3181, 3189, 3196, 3200, 3274, 3317, 3428, 3431, 3568, 3874, 3905, 3973

Wilms tumor
1985, 2020, 2102, 2104, 2113, 3433

Xenon, contrast media
3524, 3547, 3577, 4071, 4086

Author Index

Aabed M Y: 3944
Aakhus T: 1421
Aarimaa M: 1420
Aasen A O: 1645
Abbitt P L: 3218
Abbott D C: 4046
Abbott G F: 2863
Abbott J: 500
Abboud R: 817
Abdelwahab I F: 2812, 3219
Abe M: 3554, 3763
Abe S: 2991
Abel M: 3220
Abele M G: 3481
Abello R: 2661
Abeln E L: 1977
Aberle D R: 416, 577, 578, 779
Abodeely D A: 2796
Abols I B: 1679
Abraham J L: 523
Abrahams J J: 2662
Abrams D I: 1762, 3747
Abrams H L: 959, 1402, 1428, 1855, 2169, 2203
Abramson C L: 3478
Abramson S J: 2779
Abroms I F: 4057
Achatzy R: 574
Acheson M B: 2663
Acker J: 3312
Acker J D: 3831
Acritidis N C: 194
Adachi Y: 1665
Adam A: 579
Adam E J: 477, 1614
Adam J L: 107
Adam P: 3221
Adams A J: 1005
Adams D F: 106, 959, 1402, 1855, 2169, 3107
Adams G W: 2664
Adams J E: 2665, 3479
Adams M D: 182
Adams P H: 2665
Adamson D A: 3840
Adamson R H: 180
Adapon B D: 2666
Adbullah A K: 727
Adisoejoso B: 2238
Adkins M C: 956
Adler J: 957
Adler O: 192
Adler O B: 224, 580
Adler S: 2504
Adolph J: 1019, 1104, 2209, 3064
Adolph J M: 1482
Adson M A: 1093
Aeikens B: 2033
Aggarwal S: 581
Agha F P: 472, 2471
Agnoli A L: 3222
Agostini S: 1483
Aguilar E A Jr: 3980
Ahlgren J D: 1254
Ahmadi P: 958, 3211, 3330, 4094
Ahn H S: 3214
Aicardi J: 3688
Aichner F: 1, 4066
Aideyan O A: 3944
Aiello M R: 482
Aigner R: 3057
Aihara H: 657
Aikawa H: 1164, 1165, 2219
Aimi K: 3704
Aisen A M: 666, 1411, 2240, 2241, 2548
Aisner J: 327, 467, 806
Aizenstein R: 483
Aizpuru R N: 1661

Akashi H: 1818
Akine Y: 3223
Akira M: 582, 583, 584, 585
Akoun J: 3713
Akuta K: 3554
Akwari O: 2265
Akwari O E: 5
Al Ansari A G: 1012
Al Kawi M Z: 3597
Al Rashid R A: 3961
Alberge Y: 3221
Albert M: 3687, 3892
Albig M: 2366
Albin A R: 3978, 3979
Albin J: 1863
Albrecht A: 1034, 1377
Albrechtsson U: 484
Alderson P O: 551, 959, 1402, 1855
Alegret X: 1953
Alemdaroglu A: 3224
Alerci M: 639, 1711
Alexander E: 586
Alexander L L: 2642
Alexander T J: 1463
Alexiadis I: 1726
Alfidi R J: 232, 1135, 1297
Alfred R: 2971
Aliferopoulos D: 2235
Alker G: 55
Allan N K: 2371
Allard J C: 3225
Allen G J: 2667
Allen H A: 2038, 3226
Allen K S: 1484
Allgayer B: 2355, 3227, 3228
Allgood M R: 3839
Allhoff E: 2275
Allibone G: 3229
Allolio B: 2211
Almaraz R: 3900
Almarez R: 2469
Almassi G H: 3494
Almog C: 898
Alonso J P: 1127
Alpern M B: 849, 960, 984, 1307, 1707, 2132, 3230
Alspaugh J P: 961
Alter A J: 1740
Alter A J Jr: 2930
Alterman D D: 1516, 1517, 1667, 1797
Altman D H: 3232
Altman N: 2668, 3233
Altman N R: 587, 3231, 3232
Alvarez C P: 1548
Alvarez J L: 1039
Alvarez Moro F J: 4005
Alvarez O: 2669
Alvarez R: 75
Alvarez R E: 76, 3309
Amamoto Y: 2147
Amato M: 1668
Amberg J R: 1702
Ambrosetto P: 2549, 2550, 3234, 3235, 3236
Ambrosio A: 3076
Amendola B E: 962, 2339
Amendola M A: 962, 1410, 1883, 2028, 2050, 2204, 2234, 2241, 2339, 2419, 2420, 2471
Ament A E: 963
Ames T E: 4091
Amis E S: 2001
Amis E S Jr: 2283
Ammann R: 1008
Amodio J: 2779
Amundsen P: 2839
An K N: 3120

Anacker H: 1403
Anand A K: 2670
Anda S: 193, 2671, 2672, 2673
Andersen P E Jr: 485
Anderson D J: 274, 685
Anderson J C: 1748
Anderson L L: 3532
Anderson P: 111
Anderson R E: 1828, 3237, 3238, 3642, 3797
Anderson R U: 2045
Anderson S D: 391
Anderson T M: 3855
Anderson W: 2117
Anderson W H: 3681
Andersson I: 2152
Andoh K: 964
Andonopoulos A P: 194
Andre M: 2514, 2691, 2926, 3086
Andreou J: 519, 3239, 3805
Andriani R T: 2679
Andriole J G: 1351
Andrioli J: 2696
Ang J G: 588
Angel C: 2397
Angelelli G: 133, 134, 1485
Angelini F: 1698
Angtuaco T L: 1860
Anliker M: 3075
Antman K H: 684
Anton P: 2149
Antonucci F: 1674
Antoun N: 624
Aoi T: 3893
Aoki S: 2674
Appell R G: 356
Apple J: 2577
Applebaum B I: 3848
Applegate G R: 1669
Aprahamian C: 1024, 1944
Apter S: 2168, 2242
Apthorp J S: 3284
Apuzzo M: 3211
Araki T: 1078, 1079, 1080, 1082, 1089, 1300, 1301, 1407, 1409, 1670, 1978, 2160
Araki Y: 1066
Arams R S: 837
Aranda C P: 832
Arasaki K: 3240
Arata J A Jr: 1662
Archer B R: 119
Ardito J M: 3997
Arenson A M: 1979
Arevalos E: 960
Argenta L C: 3787
Arger P: 2296, 2462
Arger P H: 19, 358, 628, 802, 1347, 1996, 1997, 2105, 2315, 2352, 2374, 2386, 2493, 2551, 2736, 2990, 3184, 3365, 3370
Arisawa J: 404, 716
Arlart I P: 291
Armas R R: 1955
Armington W G: 3241
Armstrong D: 2668, 3233
Armstrong E: 2883, 3030, 3820
Armstrong E A: 3242, 3243
Armstrong P: 211, 610, 611, 3218
Arndt R D: 1352
Arndt W: 3869
Arnett G R: 2946
Arnholdt H: 2596
Arnold G: 1792
Arnold P M: 3703
Aronberg D J: 195, 196, 272, 461, 486, 589, 667, 668, 952, 1671

Aronchick J: 258
Aronchick J M: 373, 590
Aronchik J M: 643
Aronson D: 366, 3244
Arranda C: 835
Arredondo F: 2675
Arrington J A: 2388
Artmann H: 2676
Artopoulos J: 3619
Asakura K: 964
Asamoto H: 821
Asato T: 1071
Ascher N L: 1119
Ashida C: 965, 2472
Ashida H: 1076, 1177
Ashizawa A: 2219
Ashley D G: 3245
Ashmead G G: 3193
Ashton P R: 2197
Ashwal S: 3338, 4015
Asling C W: 1556
Aspelin P: 2253
Aspestrand F: 197
Assencio Ferreira V J: 3246
Assinger S: 177
Astinet F: 1257, 1258, 1923
Atherton J V: 3007
Atlas S W: 198
Atomi Y: 1079, 1082, 1408, 1409, 3645
Atwell D T: 1740
Aubin A: 2764
Aubourg P: 3247
Aufderheide J F: 154
Augsburger J J: 3821
Augustin N: 1255
Augustiny N: 2473
Auh Y: 703
Auh Y H: 208, 256, 966, 1210, 1672, 1852, 1921, 1922, 2056, 2166, 2167, 2312, 2532, 3248, 3249, 3275
Aulich A: 3926
Aurbach G: 2764
Aurbach G D: 253
Austin H M: 608
Austin J H: 365, 591, 592, 2974, 3972
Austin R: 2143
Austin R M: 3250
Austin Seymour M: 3794
Avallone A: 2309
Avila N A: 2042
Avinoach I: 3549
Avolio R E: 2861, 2862
Avrahami E: 3251
Awaya S: 3641
Awwad E E: 595, 2678, 3252
Ax L: 2728
Axel L: 2, 258, 967, 1167, 1201, 1942, 2386, 2447, 3278
Ayala A: 3111
Ayer G: 1895
Ayuso M C: 593, 1128
Azar Kia B: 3253, 3716
Azon A: 1128
Azzawi Y M: 3073

Baake S: 2564
Babaian E: 2192
Babcock D S: 1771
Baber C E: 594
Bach A W: 2962
Bach D: 2702
Badcock P C: 3255
Bader M: 1767
Bae W K: 765
Baehner R: 627

Baer U: 3567
Baert A: 1459, 1460, 1800, 2238, 2537
Baert A L: 97, 219, 968, 998, 1132, 1486, 1596, 1685, 1703, 1910, 1980, 2425, 2460, 2740, 3868
Baeten C G: 1582
Bahn R C: 3918
Bahr A L: 433, 2807
Bahr R: 1219
Bahren W: 940
Baier K: 3698
Bailey G L: 2824
Baim R S: 487
Bains M S: 701, 3531
Bair J H: 3602
Bajcsy R: 3256
Baker B K: 595
Baker E L: 596, 1546
Baker H L Jr: 94
Baker L P: 1905
Baker M E: 344, 397, 494, 969, 970, 1353, 1573, 1642, 1694, 1995, 2205, 2298, 2436, 2454, 2679
Baker R R: 478
Baker S: 1319
Bakke S J: 4063
Balachandran S: 1860
Balakrishnan J: 597
Balcar I: 1924
Baleriaux D: 2680, 2853, 3910
Baleriaux Waha D: 2552, 2681
Balfe D M: 367, 1059, 1228, 1261, 1284, 1400, 1457, 1487, 1488, 1569, 1639, 1838, 2016, 2131, 2340, 3257
Baliga K: 549
Balikian J P: 448
Ball D S: 1673
Ball J B Jr: 3835
Ball M R: 3675
Ball T J: 1384
Ball W S: 3, 2712
Ball W S Jr: 3325
Balthazar E J: 308, 1354, 1355, 1356, 1357, 1489, 1490, 1491, 1492, 1493, 1494, 1495, 1496, 1497, 1498, 1565, 1566, 1604, 1605, 1606, 1607, 1652, 1759, 1925, 2142, 2384, 2553, 3142
Balu Maestro C: 3319
Ban S: 3580
Bancovsky I: 3246
Banderali A: 2176, 2220
Bandick J: 2481, 2482, 2483
Bando B: 1333
Bandy L C: 2404
Bangert Burroughs K: 1280
Bank E R: 1499
Bankoff M S: 598, 971, 1188, 3081, 3250
Banks L: 2581
Banks L M: 1273, 2682
Banks P M: 3586
Banna M: 3258
Banner M: 1997
Banner M P: 1347, 1996, 2105
Bannerjee A K: 1514
Banniza von Bazan U: 2733
Banyoczki G: 1674
Banzer D: 139, 2683, 2781, 3186, 3259, 3358
Bar D: 2677
Bar Ziv J: 1401
Barack B M: 3260
Barakos J A: 1260, 1500, 2523
Barat J L: 983

Barbier J Y: 68
Barbier P: 1501, 1973
Barbier P A: 1133
Barbot D J: 373
Bardfeld P: 3103
Barefield K P: 1175
Bargon G: 1896, 2587, 2858
Baris S: 1705
Barkin J: 1404, 1416, 1466
Barkin J S: 1383
Barkmeier J D: 963
Barkovich A J: 3122
Barloon T: 3272
Barloon T J: 809, 1064, 2046
Barmeir E: 2376
Barnes G T: 12, 44
Barnes L Jr: 2744
Barnes M: 3559
Barnes P A: 154, 773, 972, 1121, 3261, 4014
Barnett H J: 2892
Barnett P H: 973
Barnett S M: 199
Barnhart G R: 524
Baron B: 3262
Baron M G: 3710
Baron R: 2877
Baron R L: 200, 201, 202, 1122, 1261, 1262, 1263, 1264, 1265, 1331, 1338, 1881, 2085, 2426, 3263
Barone C M: 1354
Barr I: 289
Barrett M R: 1680
Barron J T: 3439
Barrow D L: 2927
Bartel H: 3654
Barth K H: 3264, 4095
Barth V: 1473, 1981
Bartiromo G: 2446
Bartlett J: 3846
Barton P: 1220, 2515
Bartscher K H: 96
Barzen G: 2341
Bashi S A: 727
Bashir R: 3597
Bashist B: 203, 551, 884, 974, 2040
Basile B A: 3998
Bass I: 792
Bassano D A: 872, 4091
Bassett L W: 2639
Bassi P: 2690
Bassiony H: 1012, 1718
Bastion F O: 3529
Bates H R: 1009
Batnitzky S: 3129
Battikha J G: 1399
Bauer G: 2858
Baum E S: 2017
Baum M L: 2243
Baum P A: 3264
Baum R D: 2243
Bauman J: 3324
Bauman J S: 1490
Baumann J: 3559
Baumgartner B R: 1199, 1890, 2141, 2173
Baumgartner W A: 712
Bautz W: 599, 1591
Bayer N: 1691
Bayless T M: 1537, 1575, 1576, 1585, 1619, 2278
Bazarnic M L: 3992
Bazot M: 217, 2346
Beabout J W: 3919
Beachley M C: 2234
Beardsley T: 3406
Bec P: 3221
Becher H: 561
Bechinger D: 3696
Bechtold R E: 204, 975, 1515
Beck A: 2505
Beck B: 2684
Beck C L: 947
Beck J W: 5
Beck S: 228
Beck T: 2424

Becker C D: 1133, 1266, 1339, 1501
Becker H: 607, 1778, 2685, 3265
Becker L E: 3448
Becker R: 2035
Becker R D: 762, 2271
Becker R L: 958
Becker S: 2237
Becker S N: 3229
Becker T: 3183
Becker W: 1675, 2019
Beckman E M: 2385
Beckman I: 1796, 1859
Bednarek D R: 55
Bedworth D D: 3418
Beecham J: 2397
Beecham J B: 2365
Beeckman P: 853
Beers G J: 1505, 2427, 2686, 3266
Beese M: 4025
Began N: 1397
Beggs I: 3267
Begin R: 600
Behan M: 2170
Behr J: 729
Behrens M: 4030
Bein M E: 261
Bekeny J: 3372
Belanger G: 2699
Bell D Y: 604, 605
Bellah R D: 2342
Bellamy E A: 2311, 3268, 3269, 3270
Belldegrun A: 2203
Bellelli A: 3774
Beller U: 2385
Bellin M F: 264
Belloir C: 761, 2023
Bellon E M: 1782, 1976, 3193
Belton R L: 976
Beltran J: 2286, 2687, 3271
Belzberg H: 330
Benator R M: 60
Bender C E: 1323
Benedetti L: 1894, 3283
Beneventano T C: 1538
Benjamin M: 2590
Benjamin M V: 2708
Benjamin S B: 1481
Benjamin V: 2782, 3140
Bennett L L: 601
Bennett L N: 2816
Bennett W F: 251, 2402, 3047, 3178, 3371, 3841
Bennum R R: 205
Benozio M: 3359
Benson M: 1502
Benson W E: 3626
Benton W K: 2309
Benz Bohm G: 4093
Beomonte Zobel B: 3023
Beranbaum E R: 831, 1605
Beranger M: 2977, 3038
Berard H: 1239
Berardo P A: 3223
Berbaum K S: 3272
Berciano J: 3048
Berdon W E: 2779
Beres J: 2688
Berg E: 2092
Bergan J J: 198
Berger A S: 3993, 3994, 4000
Berger J R: 3832
Berger N: 145
Berger P: 2658
Berger P E: 206, 1503, 2474, 2917
Berger T: 2630
Bergeron D: 600
Bergeron R T: 3054, 3660, 3826, 3969, 4064
Berghaus A: 2630
Bergin C: 207
Bergin C J: 602, 603, 604, 605, 606, 812
Bergleiter R: 3031, 3138, 3139
Bergot C: 2940
Bergstrand G: 3273

Bergstrom K: 3052, 3274, 3692, 3755
Bergstrom L: 3512
Bergstrom M: 3519
Berkman W A: 961, 979, 1148
Berkmen Y M: 208, 633, 701, 703, 3275
Berland L L: 229, 390, 430, 889, 977, 1022, 1023, 1063, 1107, 1267, 1268, 1862, 1926, 1939, 2171, 2464, 2941, 3450, 3949
Berle P: 2373
Berlin L: 1449, 2094, 3010
Berliner L: 2172
Berlow M E: 2971
Berman A: 3156
Berman D: 1290
Berman J L: 2752
Bernard P J: 3784
Bernardino M: 1358
Bernberg F A: 923, 3646
Bernardino M E: 154, 347, 434, 773, 961, 972, 978, 979, 1121, 1148, 1175, 1180, 1181, 1182, 1183, 1199, 1200, 1236, 1237, 1340, 1374, 1504, 1620, 1688, 1889, 2141, 2173, 2174, 2325, 2329, 2360, 2415, 2554, 2566, 3261, 3277, 3402, 3412, 3803, 4014
Bernardy M O: 2343
Berne A S: 1825
Berninger W: 967, 1166, 3278
Berninger W H: 493, 2863, 3450
Berns T F: 2688, 2689, 3378, 3379
Beron G: 692
Berquist T H: 2660, 3120
Berry D F: 1505
Berry G J: 606
Berry M: 581
Berson B D: 325
Berthoty D: 2555
Bertolino G C: 2690
Bertolissi D: 2953
Bertoni F: 2590, 2591
Bescos J M: 1940
Bettmann M A: 3279
Betz D: 3681
Betz H: 2849
Beuscart R: 865
Beute G H: 363, 848, 849, 950
Beyer D: 1311, 1599, 1948, 2275, 2428
Beyer Enke I A: 518
Beyer Enke S: 661, 681
Beyer Enke S A: 209, 284, 607, 682, 683, 941, 1739, 1746, 3280, 3281, 3497
Beyer H K: 2155, 3093
Beyer J: 1394
Beyer K: 3815
Bezahler G H: 2271
Bhalla M: 942
Bharathi M V: 1781
Bhasin S: 2691
Bhatt G M: 608
Bhimani S: 3897
Bianchi G: 549
Bianco F: 3282
Biasizzo E: 153, 2953
Biddle R: 3330
Bidwell J K: 2244
Bieber J: 1104
Bieger R: 2466
Bielecki D: 2514
Biempica L: 1162
Bierman S M: 2344
Biersack H J: 3286
Bies J R: 2443
Bigelow R H: 161
Biggemann M: 2692
Biggers W P: 1637
Bigliani L: 3114
Bigliani L U: 3115
Bigner S: 3407
Bigongiari L R: 1595
Bigot J M: 824
Bihl H: 2209
Bilaniuk L T: 3492, 3801, 4088, 4098, 4099, 4100

Bilbey J H: 488
Bilfield B S: 2970
Billah K: 2284
Biller B M: 3720
Biller H F: 2137, 3125, 3968
Billimoria P E: 1004, 1506, 3087
Bilotta W: 1893
Binder J P: 1363
Binder R E: 210
Binet E F: 3166
Bini R M: 389
Biondetti P R: 260, 609, 646, 980, 1714, 2475, 3283
Biondetti P R Jr: 1894
Birbas A: 1834
Bird B L: 3356
Bird C R: 3284, 3330
Bird R: 3420
Birnbaum B A: 1794, 2429
Birnbaum S: 1737
Birnberg F A: 923, 3646
Bisceglia M: 3285
Biskjaer N L: 2693
Bissonette M B: 1308
Bittner R: 943, 2570
Bjorgvinsson E: 2430
Bjorkengren A G: 3215
Blaauw G: 3091
Black E B: 1380
Black J: 3947
Black K S: 3424
Black W C: 211, 610, 611
Blackledge G: 2372
Blaha H: 879
Blair D N: 2524
Blair R H: 1676
Blanco E: 1769
Bland P H: 2299
Blandino A: 1621, 1830, 2390, 2625, 3460
Blandino G: 1191
Blane C E: 962
Blane C E: 1564
Blanck C E: 1564
Bluth R: 1913
Bobba V S: 890
Boccardi E: 3106
Boccardo M: 2696
Bock A: 2459
Bocker F: 125
Bocker W: 2580
Boctor M: 600
Bodne D: 2476
Bodne D J: 1202
Boechat M I: 981, 2697, 3288
Boer V H: 3864, 3865
Boerner N: 1215
Boetes C: 418
Boger D: 2522
Boger D C: 2698
Bogman M J: 1970
Bohan L: 2103
Bohlman M E: 1905
Bohm Jurkovic H: 2829
Bohm N: 1289
Bohndorf K: 612, 740
Boijsen E: 1982
Boitz F: 2082
Bokemeier R B: 1045
Bolan J C: 3620
Bolen J W: 1540
Bolen J W Jr: 3289
Bolender N F: 3290
Boller M: 930
Bollinger A: 3486

Bollmann J: 2196
Bolte H D: 502
Boltshauser E: 3982
Bolwell B J: 1351
Bombi J A: 593
Bona E: 1973
Bonafe A: 2699, 3291, 3292, 3706
Bonakdarpour A: 2987
Bonamo J: 3039, 3041
Bonamo J F: 3042
Bonanni G: 3021, 3022, 3023
Bonati P: 1321
Bonatti G P: 1507, 3017, 3293
Bonfiglio P: 764
Bongartz G: 2700
Bonnard J M: 2801
Bonneville J F: 3294, 3391, 3393
Bookstein F L: 371, 687
Bools J C: 3271
Boone S C: 3959
Borgis K J: 3212, 3217
Bories J: 2732, 3295
Boris P: 3634
Borkowski G: 1192
Borkowski G P: 468, 613, 1992, 2188, 3504
Borlaza G: 751, 1114
Borlaza G S: 1359, 1633, 2701
Bornemann A: 3318
Borner N: 1216
Borner W: 3094
Borning A W: 3530
Borovetz H S: 3547
Borovich B: 3300
Borre D: 880
Borts F T: 489, 3498
Bos C J: 1352
Bosniak M A: 160, 308, 1160, 1461, 1565, 1603, 1604, 1606, 1607, 1958, 1983, 2048, 2109, 2118, 2142, 2172, 2217, 2230, 2243, 2324, 2384, 2385, 2429, 2453
Bosnjakovic S: 2702
Bosse M: 2804
Bostel F: 356, 1677, 2703
Boswell W: 2522
Boswell W D: 810, 861, 2227, 2523
Boswell W D Jr: 1260, 2228
Botet J F: 1211
Bottger E: 1927
Bottles K: 212, 1762, 1824
Botto H: 2023
Bottomley P A: 3410
Botvinick E: 505
Botvinick E H: 512
Bouchard A: 490, 543
Bouchareb M: 3294
Boukadoum M: 129, 1269
Boulard D: 3294
Boulos M I: 3708
Bourgouin P M: 213
Bourjat P: 3296
Bouysee S: 2940
Boven F: 2557, 2950
Bovill E G Jr: 2546
Bowen A: 4017
Bowich B: 1508
Bowerman R A: 1248
Bowman L M: 1867
Bowyer K: 3407
Boyd A D: 832
Boyd C M: 1860
Boyd D P: 542, 3963
Boyd R: 2895
Boyer R: 3241
Boyer R S: 3798
Braakman R: 3091
Brachlow M: 1360, 1678
Bracken R B: 2329
Bradac G B: 2645
Bradaczek M: 1257
Bradley W G Jr: 2704
Brady T J: 2631, 3728
Brady T M: 472, 2027
Braedel H U: 1984, 2006, 2304

Braga C: 2350
Braitinger S: 2705, 2706
Brakel K: 1270
Brallier D R: 3948
Bramble J M: 4
Brambs H J: 1361, 3063
Brandt H: 385
Brandt J: 982
Brandt T D: 1044, 2119
Brandtner M: 3701
Brant W E: 1651, 2245
Brant Zawadzki M: 614, 2707, 2713, 2717, 2778, 2922, 3012, 3297, 3396, 3419, 3442, 3503, 3635
Brant Zawadzki M N: 2353
Brantly P N: 2194, 4077
Brasch R C: 615, 781, 1679, 1985, 3298, 3978, 3979
Brassel F: 3513
Brassow F: 2249
Braun G: 1425
Braun I F: 2708, 2709, 2710, 2927, 3299
Braun J: 3300
Braun P: 2377
Braun S D: 16, 326, 3741
Brauner M W: 616, 617
Braunstein E: 3027
Braunstein E M: 2548, 2611, 3107, 3130, 3838
Braunstein S: 1653
Braunsteiner H: 339
Braunwald E: 3301
Braver J H: 555
Braverman R M: 892, 2431
Bravo E L: 2188
Brazeau Lamontagne L: 3302
Breatnach E: 214, 1986, 1987
Breatnach E S: 618, 1362, 1988
Brecht G: 491, 531, 758, 767, 2874, 3303, 3304
Breckenridge J W: 619
Breda S D: 3927
Bree R L: 1502, 1989, 2204, 2319, 2501, 2638
Breen T: 2643
Breiman R S: 5, 278, 514, 527, 642, 672, 1366, 3045, 3551
Breit A: 2706
Brem R F: 3900
Brenbridge A N: 400, 2106
Brendel A J: 983
Brendel H: 3092
Brendlein F: 3647
Brendler C: 1547
Brendler C B: 2378
Brennan J: 361
Brennan M F: 252, 253, 2764
Brennan R E: 1959
Brennan R P: 1990
Brennan T G: 3846
Brenot F: 3546
Bressel M: 2285
Bressler E L: 198, 620, 984, 2711, 3305
Brestowsky H: 2889
Brett C M: 449
Brewer W H: 2038, 2417
Brewster D C: 1831
Breyer D: 825
Brick S H: 985, 986, 2432
Brihaye C: 3606
Brill G: 2423
Brinckmann P: 2692
Brink J A: 1271
Brinkman S D: 3306
Brion J P: 621
Brisson L J: 6
Britt A R: 622
Britt R H: 3419, 3420
Brock J G: 560
Brockmann W P: 1042, 1521, 2249
Brodell G K: 1844
Broder G J: 662, 3466, 3467
Brodey P A: 1272, 3307
Brodner R A: 3726
Brodsky L S: 3308

Brody A S: 7, 1928, 2712, 3308
Brody W R: 495, 3309, 3336
Brogdon B G: 3628
Broggi G: 3481
Brolsch C: 1131
Bron K M: 4017
Bronskill M J: 857
Brooker A F: 2786, 2916
Brooker A F Jr: 2787, 2964
Brookland R: 3466
Brooks B S: 3310, 3311, 3312
Brooks M L: 3088
Brooks R A: 8
Brooks R D: 9
Brost F: 473
Brotman S: 1053, 1684
Brown B M: 215, 216, 1509, 2713, 3313
Brown C E: 2414
Brown D L: 1680
Brown D Q: 3466
Brown E: 2764
Brown F: 3049
Brown J J: 3314
Brown J M: 1941
Brown R A: 3315, 3665
Brown T: 3009
Brown T R: 2015, 3316
Brown W H: 3174
Brownlie K: 2175
Brownstein S: 2600
Bru C: 1128
Bruch J M: 2886
Brugieres P: 3317, 3546
Bruhl K: 3318
Brun B: 2433
Bruna J: 1991
Brundage B: 505, 3278
Brundage B H: 277
Brunelle F O: 2846
Bruner J M: 3685, 4033
Brunet W G: 1929
Bruneton J N: 2801, 3319
Brunner U: 2473, 3486
Brunt E M: 1059
Bruschi G: 2690
Bryan P J: 36, 232, 1135, 2246, 2608
Bryan R N: 2694, 3320, 3343
Bryk D: 269
Bublitz G: 3814
Bucheler E: 38, 125, 913, 2285, 2585
Buchner U: 3914
Buchness M R: 3972
Bucholz R D: 2678
Buck D R: 3403
Buck J: 42, 492, 1298, 1363, 1981, 2200, 2558
Buck J L: 2403
Buckingham R A: 3703
Bucklein W: 1722
Buckner B C: 2232
Buckwalter K: 3027
Buckwalter K A: 3026
Buda A J: 513
Budorick N E: 249
Bueschen A J: 1987
Buff B L Jr: 3321
Buijs P H: 116
Bulas D I: 1510, 1867
Bulcke J A: 2477, 2537
Buljat G: 2645
Bulzacchi A: 1698
Bunce L A: 1638
Bundschuh C V: 2714
Bunker S R: 2559
Buonanno F S: 3728
Burbank F: 3322
Burch D: 111
Burch P A: 745
Burdin P: 2942
Burgener F A: 136, 987, 988, 1559, 2247, 2256, 2365
Burger P: 2842, 3407
Burgess A E: 10, 3323
Burgess A R: 4087
Burghuber O C: 882
Burguet J L: 2715, 3392

Burigo E: 1698
Burk D L Jr: 2716
Burke D P: 2640
Burke D R: 1234, 2717
Burke J: 3571
Burke J W: 1364
Burke M: 898
Burkhalter J L: 2300
Burks D D: 1634
Burmester E: 1391, 2051, 2718, 3217
Burnam R E: 947
Burney B T: 2301
Burnstein M I: 2719
Burrell M I: 1484, 1643, 1644
Burstein S: 1757
Bursztyn E M: 3324
Burt M: 3531
Burt R W: 3902
Burt T B: 3205
Burton E M: 3325, 3326
Burton G M: 2197
Busch D: 3485
Busch G: 3327
Buschi A J: 400, 805, 2106
Buschman D L: 807
Bush C H: 2720
Busse P M: 3693
Butch R J: 1230, 1476, 1511, 2619
Butkiewicz B L: 2742
Butler G J: 2540
Butler H E: 2246
Butler S: 623
Buurman R: 1425
Buxton R C: 944
Buy J N: 217, 629, 1512, 1544, 2345, 2346, 3328
Bydder G: 3656
Bydder G M: 1365, 1681, 3845
Byrd S E: 3329, 3514
Byrne W J: 1499

Caballero P: 2455
Cable H F: 3046
Cacak R K: 148
Cacayorin E D: 3143
Caccamo D: 3289
Caccavale R: 1355
Caceres J: 788
Cachera J P: 442, 790
Cadelo M: 3375
Cahalane M: 239
Cahill P T: 3678
Cail W S: 3571, 3572
Caille J M: 2818
Cain J B: 565
Calabro A: 3076
Calabro F: 260, 646
Calavreszos A: 612
Califf R M: 514, 515
Callaghan J J: 2981
Callen P W: 989, 1366, 1367, 1513, 1682, 1745, 1804, 2434, 2597
Calliauw L: 3172
Calonge E: 786
Calvo T M: 3330
Cambier J: 3713
Cambier L: 2268
Cambon P: 3319
Cameron J C: 1576
Cameron J L: 1462, 1553, 1631, 2349
Caminiti R: 2625
Campbell G: 2751
Campbell J B: 3989, 3990
Campbell W L: 1094, 1875
Canalis R: 3600
Candardjis G: 1217, 2295
Cando Salcines L: 3157
Canellos G: 1820, 1821
Cangir A: 254
Cann C: 21
Cann C E: 66, 673, 1166, 1743, 2353, 2713, 2728, 2778, 2846, 3298, 3331, 3332, 3333, 3576
Cantin A: 600
Cantos E L: 2731

Cantrell R W: 3571
Capdevila A: 2661
Capece W: 3076
Capek M: 1836
Capek P: 70
Capek V: 825, 3144
Capesius P: 312, 2884, 2885, 2886, 2887, 3604
Capra R E: 7
Capron F: 217
Caputi Jambrenghi O: 1485
Caravelli J F: 701, 3531, 3532
Carberry D: 591
Carbonneau R J: 448
Cardella R: 2507
Cardenal C: 2983, 3791
Cardoso M: 2507
Carette M F: 824
Cariati M: 2287
Carlotti G: 2696
Carlson R A: 2623
Carlsson E: 493, 3278
Carlucci M: 1372
Carmody R F: 2721, 3205, 4083
Caroline D F: 652, 1120, 1579, 1673, 2261, 2432
Caropreso J: 3865
Carpenter H A: 1414
Carpenter J T Jr: 1986
Carr D H: 1273, 2581
Carrasquillo J A: 1158
Carrera G F: 2722, 2723, 2724, 2941, 4079
Carrol C L: 218
Carroll R: 2725, 3794
Carson P L: 2299
Carson R: 64
Carter A P: 2427, 2686, 3225, 3266
Carter B L: 598, 886, 948, 1221, 2292, 3081, 3250, 3334, 3335
Cartier J: 3296
Carvajal A: 3882
Carvalho P: 1514
Carvounis E: 2814
Casabianca J: 2625
Casanova R: 1324, 1325, 1723
Casarella W J: 979, 1148
Caskey C I: 945
Casola G: 440, 441, 918
Cassel D: 75
Cassel D M: 3309, 3336
Casselman J: 3868
Casselman J W: 219, 2726, 3337
Casselman E S: 3338
Castagno A: 2439
Castagno A A: 2560
Castanyer Corretger F: 3157
Castellino R A: 189, 207, 215, 220, 221, 222, 604, 606, 625, 1003, 1186, 1683, 1687, 1888, 3829, 4089
Castilla M T: 1805
Castillo M: 2955, 3339, 3340
Castor W R: 2727
Castro J M: 1453
Castronovo F P Jr: 11
Castrucci M: 1372
Catala F: 786
Cates J D: 990, 1024
Catsikis B D: 1684
Cattau E L: 1481
Cattin F: 3294, 3391, 3393
Caughran M: 3341
Cavouras D: 2032
Cayea P D: 223
Cazenave F L: 3342
Ceballos R: 389
Cecchini A: 2561
Cech T: 4021
Cellerier P: 3346
Cengiz K: 1705
Centeno R: 3939
Cerchiari U: 3481
Certo A: 1191
Ceulemans R: 1596
Ceuterick L: 1685
Chafetz N: 2728, 2846, 2928, 2929

Chafetz N I: 3127
Chahinian A P: 1918
Chait S: 224
Chakeres D W: 1769, 1770, 2687, 3343, 3344, 3609
Chakraborty D P: 12
Chalif M: 347
Chamberlain C C: 872
Chamberlain D W: 650, 862
Chamberlain M C: 3345
Chambers E: 3299
Chambers E F: 3346, 3671
Champion P: 817
Chan F L: 1274, 1686, 2729, 4076
Chan H S: 2595, 3425
Chandler W F: 417
Chandrasoma P T: 3245
Chang A E: 1157, 1158, 1206
Chang B: 3615
Chang C H: 3347, 3955
Chang C M: 4076
Chang F C: 1091
Chang K H: 718, 2435, 2730, 3349
Chang R: 1157, 2180
Chang W: 3348
Chanin D S: 37
Chao C: 3490
Chao E Y: 3120
Chao P: 1285
Chao P W: 2562
Chapman P D: 3494
Charache S: 1798
Charboneau J W: 13, 1388, 1414, 1450
Charlin B: 3302
Charnsangavej C: 1326
Charpak G: 3408
Charters J R: 2519
Chase N E: 3191
Chatani M: 1065
Chatfield R: 3837
Chatson G P: 2453
Chatterji D C: 180, 182
Chatterji D G: 1156
Chau E M: 2729
Checkley D R: 624, 4096
Chen C: 3386
Chen C K: 2497
Chen C T: 71
Chen G T: 71
Chen H H: 2248
Chen J T: 698
Chen M: 2224
Chen S Z: 624, 2665
Chen Y M: 1515
Chenevert T L: 2226, 2299
Cheng J: 1687
Cherian M J: 1718
Chernin M M: 1702, 3570
Cherryman G R: 2260
Chesler D A: 18
Cheson B D: 3459
Cheung Y: 2529, 2530
Chevrot A: 2497
Chezmar J: 3257
Chezmar J L: 1180, 1181, 1182, 1183, 1688, 2141
Chi J G: 1690, 2435, 3349
Chilcote W A: 1992
Childs T L: 2111
Chiles C: 494, 570, 604, 605, 818, 887
Chilton S J: 2762
Chimon J L: 2731
Chintapalli K: 14, 225, 1689, 3350, 3450
Chintapalli K N: 977
Chinwuba C E: 1567
Chiodini P G: 2231
Chiras J: 2732, 3295
Chirathivat S: 3351
Chirico G: 1191, 1830
Chiu L C: 1844
Chiu P L: 2727
Chiu S: 2956
Cho C: 221
Cho C S: 625
Cho K C: 1516, 1517, 1667, 1759, 1797, 2348

Cho P S: 3352
Choe K O: 626
Choi B I: 718, 991, 992, 1275, 1276, 1277, 1368, 1690, 2076, 2375, 2435, 3353
Choi Y M: 2375
Choi Y W: 2730
Cholankeril J: 2600, 2957
Cholankeril J V: 728, 3354
Choplin R H: 204
Chopp M: 15
Choto S: 1146
Choussat A: 541
Choutoh S: 423
Chow P P: 1758, 3355
Choyke P L: 226, 1198, 2081, 2223, 3620
Christ G: 122
Christe W: 3369
Christen B: 590
Christensen R: 441
Christiansen E: 3159
Christman D R: 3385
Christoforidis A J: 2687
Chrousos G P: 638, 2178, 2179, 2180
Chuang H S: 3030
Chuang S: 3233, 3242, 3605, 3820
Chuang S H: 2668, 2762, 3243, 3448, 3512, 3930
Chuang V P: 1036, 1121, 2325, 3277
Chui M: 1691
Chui M C: 3356
Chun G: 1533
Chun G H: 1697
Chung C T: 4091
Chung D H: 1286
Chung H S: 3353
Chung J W: 719
Churchill B M: 2117
Churchill R: 332
Churchill R J: 227, 333, 994, 1793, 2507
Chynn K Y: 3639
Cicin Sain T B: 2644
Cicio G R: 2220
Cienfuegos J A: 1039
Cimanowski N: 2082
Ciolina A: 1833
Cipriano P R: 495
Cirimelli K M: 228
Citrin C: 3947
Citrin C M: 3117, 3666
Citron M: 870
Clados D: 3431
Claes H: 2950
Clair M R: 3467
Clanet M: 3706
Clark D C: 3944
Clark D L: 544, 557, 558
Clark H B: 3664
Clark J A: 3816
Clark K E: 229
Clark L R: 1198, 1253, 1254, 2081, 2163, 3435
Clark M: 212
Clark R A: 586, 1076, 1202, 1317, 1518, 3828
Clark W M: 2008
Clarke K: 3821
Clarke P D: 1692
Clary G: 889
Claussen C: 137, 562, 776, 1015, 1369, 1993, 2733, 2959, 3163, 3175, 3186, 3187, 3188, 3357, 3358, 3437
Claussen C D: 138, 139
Clavier E: 3359
Claypool H R: 2012
Clayton P D: 2807
Clement J P: 1483
Clements J L Jr: 1199
Clements L A: 1253
Clemett A: 1442
Cleveland R H: 3288
Clifford O: 2510
Clorius J: 607
Clouse M E: 1153, 3792

Co C S: 1278
Cobb R J: 230
Cobb S R: 2734
Cobet H: 231, 2082
Coblentz C: 3943
Coblentz C L: 424, 604, 605, 3432
Coburn T P: 163
Cochran C F: 2476
Cochran S T: 2143, 2158
Cockett A T: 2256
Cockey B M: 1693
Cockshott W P: 2270
Coenen Y: 2425, 2460
Cohan R H: 16, 344, 970, 1353, 1655, 1694, 1994, 1995, 2145, 2328, 2436, 2439, 2454, 2679, 3741
Cohen A J: 1669, 1755, 2274
Cohen A M: 232, 3193
Cohen B A: 476, 801, 1930, 1955, 2218, 2478, 2774, 3733
Cohen C R: 3360
Cohen D J: 1370
Cohen E P: 2148
Cohen G: 3614
Cohen H A: 2353
Cohen J: 3386
Cohen J M: 1695
Cohen L M: 1120, 3361
Cohen M: 627
Cohen M A: 2563
Cohen M D: 237, 2613, 3362
Cohen M I: 233, 234
Cohen N: 3660, 3826
Cohen N L: 3969
Cohen W A: 2881, 2908, 3069, 3363
Cohen W N: 482
Cohen Y: 2602
Cohn D F: 3251
Coia L R: 3466
Coin C G: 2852, 3364
Coin J T: 3364
Coit W E: 3850
Colborne B: 3323
Cole B A: 306
Cole P J: 820
Coleman B: 2296, 2462
Coleman B G: 19, 358, 373, 628, 802, 1347, 1996, 1997, 2105, 2315, 2352, 2374, 2386, 2492, 2493, 2551, 2736, 3365, 3370, 3625
Coleman C C: 1998
Coleman N D: 2970
Coleman P: 2330
Coleman R E: 605
Collen M J: 1423
Colletti P M: 228, 810, 1203, 1204, 1260, 2228
Colley D P: 586
Collins A G: 3845
Collins D L: 1786
Collins R: 1285
Colodny A: 1756
Colognato A: 609
Colombo N: 3812
Colosimo C Jr: 242, 3366, 3438
Colvin R S: 405
Comet Segu R: 4005
Comite F: 2395
Commandre F: 2801
Compton T: 3124
Conces D J Jr: 235, 496, 911
Condom E: 1128
Cone R O: 2752
Confer D J: 2327
Conley C R: 1562
Connell D G: 488, 928, 2809
Connor R: 1696
Connors J: 298
Conoley P M: 1342
Conrad M R: 17, 1931, 1932, 2735
Conti J: 3367
Contini C: 2690
Cook E E: 4086
Cook W: 3406

Cooke J C: 820
Coolbaugh B L: 1455
Cools L: 1933
Coombs R J: 1096
Cooper C: 570, 629, 1642, 1697, 2387, 2436, 3432
Cooper C J: 344
Cooper M D: 71
Cooper M M: 1355
Cooper P: 2908
Cooper P H: 211
Cooper V R: 3726
Cooperberg P L: 1304, 2320
Cooperman A M: 1297
Cooperman A V: 1396
Cooperstein L A: 2716
Copeland J: 2223
Coppa G F: 2118
Coray T: 1343, 1474
Corbett J J: 3964, 3965
Corbetti F: 1698
Corcoran H L: 524, 2968
Cordes M: 1934, 2302, 2341, 3369
Cordes U: 1394, 2189
Cork R D: 1183
Cormier P J: 1999
Cornalba G: 497, 1711
Cornblath M: 1005, 1006
Cornwell J: 236
Corrales M: 140
Correia J A: 18
Corry P M: 3412
Cory D A: 237
Coscina W F: 19, 2736, 3370
Cosman E: 3792
Cosman E R: 86
Costello P: 86, 205, 630, 1126, 1153, 1305, 1306, 3792
Cottafava F: 4001
Cotter C: 3233
Couanet D: 993
Coughlan J D: 2737
Coughlin W F: 2738
Coulam C M: 1765, 3808
Coulthard S W: 3570
Coumas J M: 2643
Cox G G: 2946
Cox H E: 3371
Cox H L: 3371
Cozzi F: 3875
Craig J R: 1204
Cramer B: 2445
Cramer B C: 2000
Cramer B M: 144, 2739
Cramer H R Jr: 2571
Cramer M: 238
Crampton A R: 233
Crane R: 3733
Cranston P E: 1519
Crass J R: 128, 1119, 1520, 1541, 1785, 3193
Crass R A: 1379, 1413
Craven R M: 2290
Crawford W O Jr: 922
Creissard P: 3670
Crepps J T: 1961
Crepps L: 3170
Crepps L F: 1917
Creviston S: 232
Crisi G: 2749
Crist D W: 1462
Crivello M S: 239
Crofford M J: 147
Crolla D: 2537, 2740
Cromwell L D: 240, 3290, 3785
Cronan J J: 1768, 1974, 2001, 2163
Crone K: 3325
Crone Munzebrock W: 1279, 1521, 2249, 2564, 2565, 2584, 2741
Crooks L E: 1168, 1709
Crotte E: 2297
Crowther D: 2372
Crumley R L: 3983
Cruz Da Silva R: 3394
Cruz V: 2224
Csobaly S: 710

Cuasay N S: 944
Cubberley D A: 3241
Cubillo E: 1699
Cucco J: 1700
Cuevas A: 1723
Culham J A: 498
Cumming W J: 2525, 2533
Cunat J S: 1053, 3372
Cunningham D G: 994
Cunningham M J: 2742
Curcio C M: 1522
Currie D C: 820
Curry N: 2143
Curry N S: 2002, 2003
Curtin H D: 2742, 2743, 2744, 3373, 3877, 3881, 4056
Curtis A M: 631
Curtis D J: 3795
Curtis H W: 2496
Cusmano F: 2690
Cusumano G: 1208
Cutillo D P: 995, 1700
Cutler G B: 2178
Cutler G B Jr: 638, 2179, 2180, 2395
Cutz E: 1371
Cyran J: 502
Czajka J: 2971
Czarnecki R: 1915
Czervionke L F: 3078

D Agostino A N: 3316
D Agostino H B: 918
D Andrea F: 639
D Angelo C M: 3078
D Auria S H: 3714
D Cruz I: 2119
D Orsi C J: 168, 1846
Dacey R G: 111
Daepp M: 921
Daffner R H: 20, 1796, 2080, 2745
Dahlene D H Jr: 1701
Dailey R A: 3987
Daiz A S: 4097
Dake M D: 2746, 3374
Dal Canto M C: 4026
Dal Pozzo G: 3375
Dalal P S: 4091
Dale L G: 2671
Dalinka M: 2990
Dalinka M K: 2493, 2622, 3365
Dallabonzana D: 2231
Dallant P: 66
Dalley R W: 2747
Dalman H R: 477
Dalton S C: 1107
Daly B D: 598, 632
Dambacher M: 3075
Damgaard Pedersen K: 2212
Dammann H G: 1392
Damsma H: 3376, 4106
Dan S J: 2774
Dandekar N: 3800
Daneman A: 1371, 2569, 2595, 2763, 3377, 3425
Daniel T M: 211, 611
Daniels D L: 1753, 2225, 2688, 2689, 2748, 2819, 3195, 3196, 3378, 3379, 3380, 3381, 3521
Danielski E J Jr: 2960
Danielson K: 1702
Danielson K S: 996
Dannenmaier B: 2437
Dannert J: 2463
Danza F M: 241, 242, 2176
Danzig L: 2752
Danziger A: 3442, 3483, 4101
Darling J D: 1935
Darling R C: 1831
Darweesh R M: 2441
Darwin R: 3535
Darwish H: 3382
Dash M: 1859
Dauito R: 2388
Dautenhahn L W: 1936
Davalos Errando A: 3157
Daves M L: 499
David C L: 1007, 3435

Davidoff A: 168, 1455, 1772
Davidson A J: 2036, 2438, 2451
Davis C A: 34
Davis C J Jr: 2036
Davis D O: 2753, 3029, 3638
Davis G W: 3542
Davis J M: 2004, 3383
Davis J R: 3384
Davis K R: 18, 3070, 3383
Davis L: 3490
Davis M: 267
Davis M A: 168, 1455
Davis M C: 2349
Davis P C: 2710, 3339
Davis P L: 1168, 1469, 1875
Davis R: 4105
Davis S: 1924, 4024
Davis S D: 633, 634, 703, 3275
Davis T M Jr: 394
Davis W K: 2350, 3741
Dawson E G: 2639
Day D L: 243, 244, 1119, 1785
Daykin E L: 245
Daza R C: 2334
Dazzi M: 3973
De Agostini A: 639, 1711
De Baets M: 1909
De Becker D: 2853
De Boeck M: 246, 2557
De Carvalho C R: 807
De Cremoux H: 616
De Diego Choliz J: 997
De Donatis M: 2690
De Faveri D: 1894, 3283
De Fracquen P: 621
De Francesco F: 1621
De Gaetano A M: 3438
De Geer G: 21, 247, 953, 954, 3983
De Groot J A: 4106
De Juan M: 3077
De La Torre S: 1325
De Lange E E: 1523
De Leon M: 3239
De Leon M J: 3385, 3386, 3473, 3474
De Maeyer P: 968
De Martini W J: 1366
De Mayer P: 1980
De Meeus A: 2681
De Paulis F: 3021, 3022, 3023
De Pauw B E: 1970
De Ronde T: 1659
De Santis M: 2749
De Schepper A: 1196
De Slegte R G: 2648
De Smedt E: 246
De Somer F: 968, 1980
De Verbizier J: 2181
Dean P B: 319, 543, 1167
Deboeck M: 2950
Debroucker T: 3713
Debrun G M: 4036
Deck M: 74, 2912
Deck M F: 92, 3367, 3389, 3677
Deck M F: 2911
Decker T: 1129
Decroix Y: 2345
Decurtins M: 1134
Dedrick C G: 388, 393, 406
Dee P: 357
Deeb Z L: 2988, 3878
Deering T F: 631
Defer G: 3546
Degenhart A T: 1
Degesys G E: 1994, 2439
Degos J D: 3546
Degreef J M: 865
Deider S: 353
Deigh D: 3722
Deimling M: 3568
Deininger H K: 385, 1543, 1677
Del Carpio O Donovan R: 2654
Del Vecchio E: 3076
Delaney J P: 1541
Delaney V B: 2141
Delangre T: 3359
Delany D J: 791
Delapaz R L: 3728
Delavelle J: 3387, 3388

Delavier U: 3369
Deligeorgi Politi H: 2814
Dell P C: 2720
Delman A: 3491
Delmaschio A: 1372
Delorimier A A: 3978, 3979
Delorme S: 1801
Delphendahl A: 811
Demaerel P: 998, 1703
Demas B: 86
Demas B E: 1561, 1704, 3531
Dembner A G: 1373, 2418
Demetris A J: 1094
Demirci A: 1705
Demos T C: 248, 249, 332, 333, 549, 2005, 2078, 2507
Demou L: 3607
Denath F M: 1706
Denis F: 2801
Denkhaus H: 2564
Dennis M A: 1280, 2303
Depauw L: 621
Derchi L E: 1321, 2176, 2220
Derhy S: 3295
Deridder P H: 1463
Derouet H: 2006, 2304
Dery R: 490, 500, 501
Desai K K: 851
Desai M B: 1832
Desantos L A: 1374, 2479, 2566, 2579
Desbleds M T: 824
Descamps P: 3606
Deschamps J P: 1000
Deschler T W: 118
Deshmukh S: 1319
Desmarais R: 637
Desser T S: 2524
Destian S: 3389
Destouet J M: 2567, 2750
Detoni X A: 3864
Deutch B M: 2187
Deutch S J: 1707
Deutsch A L: 439, 2480, 2751, 2752
Dev P: 2514
Deveney C W: 1468
Devita V T: 2568
Dewes W: 3513
Dewey C: 1129
Dewilde D: 1486
Dewitt J D: 2513
Dey C: 1524
Di Chiro G: 8, 2753, 3390
Di Giulio C: 639
Di Rocco C: 3438
Di Rocco M: 4001
Diament A J: 3246
Diamond C G: 2480
Diankov L: 2754
Dias L S: 2854, 2855
Diaz M J: 2805
Dibianca F A: 9
Dibie C: 1139
Dick L: 999
Dickey J E: 250
Dickob M: 3461
Dickson B A: 2968
Dickson D W: 3490
Didier D: 1000, 1708
Diebler C: 3247
Diefenbach P: 2803
Diehl J T: 3991
Diehl L F: 306, 3559
Dietemann J L: 3391, 3392, 3393, 3394
Diethelm E: 490
Diethelm L: 501
Dieumegarde M: 3816
Diez C: 3048
Digon E: 3790
Dihlmann W: 22, 2481, 2482, 2483, 2484, 2755, 2756, 2757, 2758, 2759, 2844, 3395
Diiorio G: 3252
Dilley R B: 444
Dillon J D: 2714
Dillon W: 3012, 3396
Dillon W P: 3374, 3442, 3514
Dingler W: 385

Dinkel E: 462, 635
Dion G: 3313
Dipietro M A: 2299
Dirheimer Y: 2715
Distelmaier P: 3397
Distelmaier W: 1108, 2603
Divano L: 1933
Divine M: 1142
Dixon A K: 660, 1001, 1869, 1908
Dixon G D: 1002
Djang W T: 1003, 2777, 3535
Do Y S: 991
Doan H T: 3992
Dobben G D: 3073, 3716, 3762
Dobranowski J: 251
Dock W: 1043, 2760
Docken W P: 2496
Dodd G D: 1169
Dodds W J: 1130, 1375, 2440, 2441
Dodo Y: 1618
Doerr J: 2284
Dohring W: 23, 24, 33, 286, 636, 1555, 1984, 2033, 3544
Doi H: 1069
Doi K: 25
Doi O: 755
Dolan K D: 3421
Dolan L M: 3325
Dolinskas C A: 2351, 3399
Dologa M: 3806
Domingues R C: 2485
Don C: 637
Donaldson I: 2761
Donaldson J S: 1004, 1525, 1999, 2017, 3285, 3400, 3401, 3446
Done S L: 717, 3722
Donnal J F: 422
Donoghue V: 2569, 2762, 2763
Donohue J P: 2443
Donohue R E: 2303
Donovan A T: 1526
Doolas A M: 1171, 1172
Dooms G C: 1709, 1710, 2309
Doost Hoseini A: 75
Doppelt S: 3071
Doppman J L: 180, 182, 252, 253, 502, 503, 638, 742, 777, 804, 1005, 1006, 1009, 1125, 1154, 1155, 1156, 1157, 1206, 1308, 1381, 1423, 1835, 2060, 2177, 2178, 2179, 2180, 2182, 2753, 2764, 2765, 3443, 3552
Dorcier F: 541
Dore R: 497, 639, 1711, 3167
Doren M: 2992
Dorfman G S: 1768, 2001
Doringer E: 1527, 1528
Dorkin H L: 1221
Dorne H L: 2766
Dornemann H W: 2705
Dornhorst A: 2193
Dorovini Zis K: 2938
Dorwart R H: 2847, 3374
Dos Santos F M: 3882
Doshi V: 2338
Dosoretz D E: 1610
Doubleday L C: 3402
Doucet M: 2346
Dougan H: 1700
Dougherty J: 2970
Doust B D: 1267, 3148
Downey D B: 2539
Downey E F Jr: 1734, 3403
Downs R: 2764
Doyle T B: 1052
Doyle T C: 640
Drace J: 3668
Drach G W: 2043
Drake J: 2268
Drapkin A J: 3480
Drayer B: 3019, 3522
Drayer B P: 2842, 3404, 3406, 3407, 3534, 3535, 3536
Drebin B: 2787
Drebin R A: 30, 2489, 2767
Drescher E: 32, 2789, 2790
Dretler S P: 2283
Drewes G: 144

Drexler G: 91
Dritschilo A: 1254
Drosos A A: 194
Drouillard J: 541, 983
Drouineau J: 2181
Druy E M: 1712
Du Boulay G: 1902
Du Boulay G H: 141, 190, 3209, 3238, 3405
Duber C: 572, 576, 1281, 1584, 2125
Dublin A B: 2768, 2769, 2980, 3849
Dubois P: 3019
Dubois P J: 3406, 3407, 3534, 3536
Dubrow R A: 1007, 1713
Ducassou D: 983
Ducellier R: 1452, 1622, 2101
Duchazeaubeneix J C: 3408
Duchesneau P M: 3065, 3360, 3745
Ducret R P: 956
Duda S: 2570
Dudiak K M: 1529
Duesdieker G A: 2962
Duewell S: 1008
Dugstad G: 3415
Duke R A: 1680, 3889
Dumler J S: 711
Duncan Meyer J: 668
Dunham C M: 376
Dunham W K: 2633
Dunlap H J: 857
Dunlop R W: 2793
Dunn D L: 1430
Dunn M G: 1282, 2244, 2382
Dunne M G: 1282, 2244, 2382
Dunnick N R: 16, 326, 334, 344, 641, 842, 1009, 1345, 1353, 1458, 1750, 1850, 1851, 1865, 1994, 1995, 2007, 2008, 2009, 2060, 2083, 2182, 2183, 2205, 2214, 2259, 2328, 2404, 2436, 2439, 2442, 2454, 2571, 2629, 2679, 3860
Durand E P: 2770
Durham J R: 1702
Durity F A: 3759
Durizch M L: 775
Duszlak E: 1305
Dutcher J P: 327
Duvauferrier R: 2797
Duvoisin B: 1524, 1530, 2250
Dvorak J: 2771, 2772
Dwyer A: 1006
Dwyer A J: 638, 1005, 1206, 2178, 3552
Dwyer S J: 3347, 3681, 3682
Dyer R B: 2162
Dzioba R B: 3205

Eames F A: 2662
Earll J M: 2177
Earnest F 4th: 3409, 3796
Eastwood D W: 3504
Ebeling U: 3031, 3139
Eberle C: 3176
Ebers G C: 4036
Ebersberger J: 57
Ebner F: 4019
Eckhauser F: 1359
Eckmann A: 1216
Ecoiffier J: 2346
Eda I: 2495, 3573
Edeiken J: 2947
Edelstein G: 946, 2534, 2773
Edelstein W A: 3410
Edmonds P R: 873
Edwards C C: 2804
Edwards F M: 61
Edwards M K: 2907, 3411
Eelkema E A: 1376
Eenhoorn P C: 116
Effmann E L: 316, 446, 642
Efremidis S C: 801, 2774
Eftekhari F: 254, 3412
Egan T J: 255
Ege G: 856
Ege G N: 3413

Egger J: 3414
Eggleston J C: 782
Eggli K D: 3149
Eghrari M: 2184
Egund N: 2572
Ehlenz P: 767
Ehrlich C P: 504
Ehrlich S M: 1628
Ehrman K O: 2010
Eiben R M: 3390
Eichberger D: 661
Eichelberger M R: 399, 986, 1510, 1867, 1878, 1880
Eichler H: 2222
Eichstadt H: 3369
Eickhoff U: 982
Einhaupl K: 3431
Eisenberg B: 697
Eisenberg D: 1283
Eisenberg R L: 3725
Eisenberger F: 1981
Eisenhardt H J: 1311
Eising E G: 1010
Eisner R L: 9
Ekberg O: 1640
Ekelund L: 2572
Ekstrom J E: 1122
El Gammal T: 3310, 3311, 3312
El Magdy W: 1012
El Yousef S: 3372
El Yousef S J: 680, 1135
Elbrechtz F: 1377
Eldevik O P: 2839, 3016, 3415
Elgeti H: 1312
Elgrabli S: 4006
Elizondo G: 1033
Elkin C M: 2788
Ell S R: 26
Ellert J: 3416
Elliott D: 4055
Ellis D A: 2208
Ellis J: 2025
Ellis J V: 622, 909, 1378, 1602, 2264, 2443
Ellis J V: 3889
Ellis K: 203
Ellwood R A: 2050
Elman A: 1956
Elouaer Blanc L: 1142
Elster A D: 27, 2775, 2776, 3417
Emami B: 274, 667, 948
Emerich B: 1014
Emory T H: 2305
Encabo B: 2455
Endo S: 3662
Engel I A: 256, 966, 3248
Engel K: 1593
Engelmann U: 2124, 2125
Engels J T: 1284
Engelstad B L: 505, 2011
Engler G: 3491
English J T: 257
Engstrom P: 3466
Engstrom P F: 3467
Enlow R A: 3418
Enneking W F: 2589, 2591, 2868
Enomoto K: 452
Ensminger W D: 984
Enzi G: 1714
Enzinger F M: 2573
Enzmann D: 3668, 3935
Enzmann D R: 2777, 3419, 3420, 3783, 4069
Epstein A J: 1449, 2094, 3010
Epstein B M: 1715, 2251
Epstein D: 590
Epstein D M: 258, 373, 643, 802, 2352
Epstein J I: 2378
Epstein N E: 267
Erbel R: 572, 576
Erenberg G: 3745
Eresue J: 983
Erickson S: 3571
Erickson S J: 432, 1130, 1364, 1375, 2148
Erkinjuntti T: 2592
Ernst H U: 3932
Erwin B C: 1199, 1200, 2173

Escalada J: 2661
Escarous A: 506, 534
Esfahani F: 3421
Espagno J: 3291
Esparza J: 1940
Espersen J O: 3817, 3818
Espinosa G A: 3704, 3762
Esposito W J: 324
Esquivel C O: 4017
Esser P D: 551
Et Al: 129, 217, 309, 638, 701, 716, 857, 937, 1057, 1083, 1146, 1173, 1215, 1246, 1249, 1254, 1372, 2180, 2282, 3666, 3792, 3794
Ethier R: 2654, 2699, 3816, 3943
Etievent J P: 1708
Ettenger N A: 480, 833, 835
Ettinger B: 3134
Eubanks B A: 2778
Eulderink F: 2556
Euler A: 692
Euller Ziegler L: 2801
Evans K G: 411, 814, 883
Evans R A: 149, 3529
Evans S J: 1639
Evans W K: 856
Evens R G: 3422
Every P: 2949
Ewald L: 15
Ewen K: 507
Eybel C E: 569
Eyler W R: 289

Fabian T M: 1004, 1506
Fabrikant J I: 3783
Fabris G: 153, 2953
Faer M J: 947
Faerber E N: 3995, 3996, 3997
Fagan C J: 267
Fagelman D: 463, 800, 1285, 1370, 1531, 1937, 3213, 3424
Fagniez P L: 1138
Fahl M H: 877
Fahmy A: 2239
Fahmy J S: 3553
Fahr L M: 149
Fahrendorf G: 1011
Faivre J C: 3408
Fajardo L L: 2012
Fajman W J: 1101
Fakhri A: 1716
Falappa P: 241
Faling L J: 210, 369, 372, 555, 632, 3859
Falke T H: 575, 726, 2185
Falkoff G E: 2013
Fallat M E: 1878
Fallone B G: 1224
Fan S T: 1274
Farah J: 2050
Farah M C: 1532
Faraj J: 3034
Faravelli A: 1372
Farber B: 2068
Farha P: 773
Farman J: 1285, 2562
Farmer D: 542
Farmer D W: 335, 490, 508, 543
Farmlett E: 1018
Farmlett E J: 1717, 2574
Faro S H: 2486
Farrelly C: 3425
Farres M T: 1043, 2760
Fasciano M G: 995
Faszold S: 3681
Fataar S: 1012, 1718, 1858
Fauci A S: 3301
Favard L: 2942
Fawcitt R A: 2021, 2521
Fazzini E: 3142
Fazzio F: 1327
Fearon T: 3426, 3427
Feasby T E: 4036
Federle M: 1442, 3012
Federle M P: 102, 218, 276, 412, 449, 455, 456, 902, 1013, 1091, 1115, 1161, 1302, 1303, 1379,

1412, 1413, 1417, 1438, 1469, 1475, 1500, 1509, 1533, 1544, 1549, 1571, 1572, 1697, 1719, 1720, 1762, 1763, 1797, 1824, 1826, 1849, 1913, 1938, 1945, 1950, 1964, 2014, 2015, 2044, 2115, 2158, 2252, 2262, 2353, 2597, 2707, 3202, 3428, 3591, 3747
Feig S: 981
Fein A B: 2016
Feinberg S B: 1731
Feiner H D: 1160
Feinstein K A: 2017
Feinstein R S: 1522, 3429
Feiring A J: 558
Fekete F: 443
Feld R: 856, 857
Feldberg M A: 116, 1660, 1721, 2354, 2444, 2487
Feldman F: 2528, 2779, 3007, 3068, 3113, 3114, 3115, 3116
Feldman J M: 1458, 3860
Felix R: 137, 138, 509, 943, 1015, 1051, 1257, 1258, 1727, 2341, 2366, 2851, 3369, 3917
Fellingham L: 2691, 2926
Felmlee J P: 28
Felsberg G: 3103
Felsenberg D: 2780, 2781, 2889, 2891, 3430
Felson B: 644
Felson D: 2535
Fender B: 557
Fenzl G: 3431
Fereshetian A: 3615
Fernandez G G: 3432
Fernandez M: 1358
Fernandez Sanchez J: 1722
Fernbach S K: 2017, 3433
Ferner R: 1528
Ferrane J: 761
Ferreiros J: 1723
Ferreyro R I: 3320
Ferris D T: 1828
Ferris E J: 2232
Ferris R A: 1286
Ferris S H: 3385, 3386, 3473
Ferrucci J T: 895, 1033, 1271, 1380, 1470
Ferrucci J T Jr: 440, 1054, 1230, 1476, 1511, 1816, 1817, 1831, 1891, 2619, 2644, 3440, 4072
Fertig S: 1272
Fetell M R: 2978
Fettig O: 96
Feuerbach S: 29, 1014, 1403, 1724, 2355, 3055, 3227
Feuerstein I M: 578, 638, 1725, 3434, 3435
Fevery J: 998
Feyerabend T: 2636, 2637
Fezoulidis I: 259, 1726
Fichte H: 729
Fiedler H: 1815
Fiegler W: 1015, 1727, 1777, 1993, 3187, 3436, 3437
Fiel S B: 652, 653
Field D R: 7
Figueredo A: 919
Fileni A: 3366, 3438
Filippa D A: 1211
Filly R A: 989, 1013, 1055, 1320, 1679, 1682, 1745, 2434
Filson R G: 1882
Finberg H J: 684, 959, 1402, 1811, 1855, 2169
Finch I J: 187, 3807
Findling J W: 638
Fine M: 3253, 3439
Fineberg H V: 3440, 4072
Finelli P F: 3441
Finer R M: 2402
Finizio J P: 2030
Fink D W: 2186
Fink I: 645
Fink I J: 1381, 3442, 3443
Fink M P: 1967
Finkbeiner W E: 925
Finley R: 556

Fiore D: 260, 609, 646, 980, 1714, 3283
Fiorooznia H: 2782, 2783, 2784, 2810, 3039, 3040, 3041, 3042, 3043, 3491
Fisch A E: 1272, 3307
Fischedick A R: 1011, 1016, 1017, 1296, 1382, 2018, 2024, 2445, 2739
Fischer A P: 1431
Fischer C: 2155
Fischer E: 2781
Fischer E G: 4048
Fischer H J: 1675, 2019
Fischer H W: 142
Fischer P: 507, 1109
Fischer R: 2092, 3102
Fischer U: 3499
Fish G: 2003
Fishbach R: 2211
Fisher D M: 3444
Fisher D R: 2488, 3347
Fisher J K: 1534, 1535, 1536, 1728
Fisher M S: 652
Fisher R I: 180
Fishman A: 1383
Fishman E K: 30, 83, 101, 166, 320, 546, 597, 647, 695, 712, 744, 745, 746, 747, 748, 749, 782, 866, 867, 892, 945, 965, 1018, 1149, 1151, 1213, 1214, 1247, 1307, 1314, 1462, 1537, 1547, 1553, 1574, 1575, 1576, 1585, 1608, 1609, 1619, 1631, 1649, 1666, 1693, 1696, 1716, 1717, 1729, 1766, 1798, 1879, 1949, 1960, 2020, 2030, 2031, 2087, 2138, 2139, 2187, 2278, 2323, 2349, 2356, 2361, 2378, 2379, 2403, 2432, 2449, 2469, 2472, 2489, 2506, 2574, 2767, 2785, 2786, 2787, 2916, 2964, 2965, 2966, 2985, 2986, 3128, 3208, 3429, 3445, 3475, 3734, 3851, 3861, 3876, 3900, 4090
Fishman E K,: 750, 868
Fitz C R: 2668, 2762, 2883, 3030, 3233, 3242, 3448, 3605, 3712, 3820, 3929, 3930, 4009
Fitzgerald P M: 648
Fitzgerald S W: 3446
Fitzhardinge P M: 3448
Fitzrandolph R L: 2520
Fiumara F: 1451
Flament Durant J: 3910
Flanigan R C: 2343
Fleischer A S: 4083
Fleischer D F: 1481
Flentje M: 683, 1019, 1104, 1746, 3064
Fletcher G: 3447
Fletcher T B: 1730
Flickinger F W: 1935
Flint A: 688
Flisak M E: 248
Flodmark O: 3448
Flory J G: 1020
Flournoy D J: 1020
Flueckinger F: 649
Flyckt L: 3273
Flye M W: 1059
Fobbe F: 1021
Folchi Vici F: 2749
Foley L C: 3989, 3990
Foley W D: 31, 229, 238, 430, 960, 977, 990, 1022, 1023, 1024, 1025, 1026, 1130, 1267, 1287, 1315, 1341, 1689, 1939, 2148, 2440, 2441, 2723, 2941, 3449, 3450, 3739
Folk E R: 2963
Fon G T: 261
Fonda C: 3375
Fondelli P: 4001
Fondren F B: 2976
Foo D: 3072
Foo S H: 3239
Foo S S: 650
Forbes W S: 2021

Ford K: 3451, 3896
Fork F T: 1288
Forman B H: 895
Formikell M: 2824
Forrest J V: 296
Forst R: 2575
Forti A: 2549
Fortune J B: 1837
Fossa S: 2291
Fossa S D: 2458
Foster M A: 1331
Foster W Jr: 1658
Foster W L: 1050
Foster W L Jr: 294, 651, 1458, 1477, 1657, 2009, 3860
Fotter R: 1778
Fougner R: 193
Fouladian G: 2523
Foulks G N: 3799
Fournier D: 2250
Fox A J: 2620, 2892, 3974, 4036
Fraga J: 2891
Frager D: 2272
Frager D H: 1538, 2788
Frahm R: 32, 2789, 2790, 2791, 2792
Fram E K: 316, 446, 672, 673, 3452
Franccois E: 3319
Francis I: 3130
Francis I R: 371, 383, 513, 521, 620, 622, 664, 666, 700, 855, 926, 984, 1307, 1336, 1478, 1532, 1539, 1952, 2027, 2028, 2204, 2226, 2241, 2264, 2471, 2501
Franco J M: 3411
Frank D A: 3409
Frank J A: 226, 1206
Franken E A: 3272
Franken E A Jr: 262, 263, 1064
Franken T: 2222
Franklin P D: 2793
Franquet Casas T: 997
Franquet T: 1940, 2455
Fraser R G: 44, 3453
Fratello A: 133
Frederick P R: 433, 2807, 3454
Fredrickson B E: 2824
Freedy R M: 2306
Freeny P C: 1027, 1028, 1029, 1030, 1031, 1032, 1331, 1338, 1384, 1385, 1540
Freger P: 3670
Freidmann G: 2211
Freilich M: 3897
Freilich M D: 3080
French W M: 1684
Freni O: 2390
Freni O F: 1829
Frenkel T L: 1247
Frennby B: 2253
Frenzl G: 2979
Fretz C: 1218, 2022
Fretz C J: 1033
Freund U: 1401
Frey C C: 2530
Frey E E: 262, 263, 510
Frey G D: 3132
Frey K W: 3869
Frey M: 2849
Freyschmidt J: 2614
Friberg J: 621
Frick M P: 1119, 1386, 1520, 1541, 1731, 1732
Fricke M: 1387
Fried A M: 188, 2114
Friedburg H: 1056, 1289, 2794, 3200
Friedl P: 3063
Friedlaender G E: 2813
Friedland J T: 1383
Friedlander A: 2536, 3134
Friedman A C: 652, 653, 762, 873, 1120, 1579, 1673, 1733, 1734, 1900, 1920, 2064, 2087, 2112, 2261, 2272, 2430, 2432, 3565
Friedman J P: 2429

Friedman L: 2795
Friedman M A: 1166, 1167
Friedman P E: 2523
Friedman P J: 440, 441, 654, 655, 760
Friedman W: 2341
Friedmann G: 43, 741, 1311, 1441, 1589, 1590, 1735, 1874, 1948, 2221, 2396, 2407, 3777
Friedrich J M: 381, 1896
Friedrich M: 1034, 1051, 2576
Friefeld G D: 1853, 3602
Fries J W: 2796
Friese K: 2424
Frija J: 824
Frija J: 37, 264, 656, 761, 2023, 2935, 2936, 3456
Fritsch G: 3649
Fritschy P: 1035
Fritz H: 32
Fritz S L: 3347
Frocrain L: 2797
Frohlich H: 33
Frommhold H: 1425
Fromowitz F B: 762, 2064, 2271
Fruauff A: 1542
Fuchs H D: 1390
Fuchs W A: 143, 436, 445, 1398, 2196, 2331, 2332, 2798
Fuessl H S: 1839
Fugazzola C: 1041
Fuhrman C R: 4017, 4081
Fujii H: 2147
Fujii M: 553, 1075, 3578
Fujikawa J: 2257
Fujikawa M: 1075
Fujino Y: 2282
Fujioka M: 3458
Fujisawa I: 82, 1057
Fujisawa M: 1333
Fujita M: 755, 2281, 2282
Fujiwara K: 3763
Fukakusa S: 1736
Fukaya T: 1876
Fukuda T: 1164, 1165, 2357, 3579, 3750
Fukushima K: 657
Fukushima Y: 2146
Fukuya T: 1665
Fuks J Z: 467
Fund G: 2024
Fung C Y: 2326
Funk K C: 2836
Funkenstein H H: 3730
Funt S: 835
Furui S: 1078, 1079, 1080, 1082, 1083, 1300, 1301, 1409
Furukawa T: 1736
Furuse M: 657
Furuta M: 821
Fusco A: 241
Futagawa S: 1164, 2147
Futrell N N: 3459
Futyu Y: 1072, 1073

Gaa J: 1543
Gabriele O F: 3150
Gabrielsen T O: 417, 2640, 2938, 3469, 3471
Gacetta D J: 2799
Gademann G: 736
Gado M: 2800, 3870, 3871, 3950
Gado M H: 2894, 3478
Gado M Hodges F J: 3951
Gaeta M: 1051, 1813, 1830, 2390, 2446, 2625, 3460
Gaffey W R: 2796
Gager R M: 3379, 3381
Gagnerie F: 2801
Gaines J A: 2043
Galanski M: 144, 3461
Gale D R: 100, 511, 3859
Gale M E: 511, 632, 658, 659, 859, 886, 1223, 1737, 1738, 2358, 3462, 3463
Galiber A K: 1388
Gallagher J H: 79
Gallagher S: 660
Gallego J: 3790
Gallis H R: 3045

Gallmann W H: 2145
Galvin J: 3977
Galvin J R: 26, 809, 3464
Gamba J L: 265, 2577
Gambarelli J: 2977, 3038
Gambari P I: 2802
Gamroth A: 266, 661, 681, 1103, 1389, 1739, 3280
Gamstatter G: 380
Gamsu G: 21, 247, 335, 415, 416, 453, 454, 455, 456, 457, 458, 577, 578, 605, 645, 670, 720, 779, 780, 792, 813, 876, 923, 924, 925, 3576, 3983
Gamsu G G: 673
Ganott M: 3070
Ganti S R: 566, 2803, 2978, 3748, 3957
Garagiola D M: 2359
Garay S M: 713, 832, 833
Garbagna P: 3167
Garcia A T: 1548
Garcia J H: 3610
Gardeur D: 145
Gardner G: 3341
Gardner J D: 1423
Gardner T W: 3465
Garibotto G: 3481
Garnick M B: 2326
Garra J: 1253
Garra B S: 1254, 1465, 1481, 3443
Garreta D: 3408
Garrett J: 490
Garrett J S: 500, 512
Garrett P R: 146
Garvey J: 734
Garvin A J: 2003
Gasano V A: 536
Gaskin L: 1371
Gasparaitis A: 1545
Gastaut J L: 2502
Gaston A: 2732, 2935, 2936, 3317, 3546
Gatenby R A: 662, 3466, 3467
Gatewood O M: 1547, 2030, 2054, 2138, 2193, 2361, 3429
Gatsonis C: 926
Gaupp R J: 267
Gavant M L: 929, 2025, 2931
Gay B: 2850, 3092, 3182
Gay S B: 733
Gayet B: 443
Gayler B W: 647, 3445
Gayou D E: 117
Gearhart J P: 2159
Gebarski K: 664
Gebarski K S: 3468, 3469
Gebarski S S: 417, 2938, 3468, 3469, 3470, 3471
Gebauer A: 879
Geboes K: 1685
Gedgaudas E: 1386
Gedgaudas Mcclees K: 1199, 1236, 1732, 2173
Geffen A: 2279
Gefter W: 258
Gefter W B: 373, 590, 643, 685, 802
Gehler J: 3700
Gehweiler J A Jr: 2745
Geier G: 3907
Geisinger M A: 2188
Geiss A C: 1531
Gelfand D W: 1515
Gelfand M J: 1771
Gellad F: 3472
Gellad F E: 2804
Geller S: 1924
Geller S C: 335
Genant H K: 34, 2499, 2536, 2546, 2808, 2846, 2928, 2929, 3127, 3134, 3174, 3333
Gendal E S: 325
Genereux G P: 268
Genez B M: 2805
Genkins S: 108
Gens D R: 1159, 1957
Gentes C I: 3385

Gentry L R: 1740, 1941, 2806, 3964, 3965
Geoffray A: 1741
George A E: 2709, 3239, 3385, 3386, 3473, 3474
Georgi M: 2189, 2190, 4078
Georgi P: 464, 1482
Gerald B: 3341
Gerard P S: 269, 1290
Gerber J D: 3475
Gerber R: 1312
Geremia G K: 3843
Gerhard L: 3765
Gerhardt P: 29, 3484
Gerlock A J Jr: 2157, 2491, 3476
Gersten K C: 734
Gerstenbrand F: 4066
Gerza C B: 1020
Gerzof S G: 100, 1737, 1738, 2389, 3477, 3859
Geyer C A: 3478, 3722
Geyer J: 2632
Ghaed N: 382, 2452, 3560
Ghaed V N: 545, 3722
Ghahremani G G: 236, 3496
Ghavam C: 2646
Gherpelli J L: 3246
Ghilarducci M J: 2861
Ghoshhajra K: 2988
Ghossain M A: 217, 2345, 2346
Gianola F J: 1155
Giargiana F A: 1960
Gibbons R G: 1458, 3860
Gibbs A: 2525
Gibbs B J: 3160
Gibbs D A: 1902
Gibbs F A: 1828
Gibson D: 1793
Gibson L: 2359
Gibson R: 2761
Gibson R N: 1291
Giesen V: 2413
Gigaud M: 3706
Gilabert R: 593
Gilbert B K: 98
Gilbert P M: 1757
Giles D J: 2807
Gili J: 2661
Gill J R: 2182
Gill J R Jr: 2177
Gilles F H: 3284, 3330
Gillespie J E: 3479
Gillespy T 3d: 2578, 2720
Gilman M J: 663
Gilmor R L: 2907, 3411
Gilsanz V: 981, 1525, 3288
Gilula L A: 2475, 2504, 2534, 2567, 2599, 2750, 2835, 2846, 2972, 3121, 3123, 3124
Gimenez L: 4090
Ginaldi S: 1036, 1256, 1742, 2360, 2579
Gingrich R D: 809
Ginsberg F: 3480, 3822
Ginsberg R J: 857
Giorgi C: 3481
Girard P: 824
Giraudet Le Quintrec J S: 2815
Girton M: 180, 182, 1006, 1308
Girton M E: 1005
Gisvold J J: 3918
Gitelis S: 2519
Gittes R F: 2203
Giuliani G: 2802
Giunta A: 1829
Giunta S: 3774
Given Wilson R: 1614
Giyanani V L: 1037, 2491, 3476, 3725
Gjerris F: 3810, 3811
Gladziwa U: 2849
Glanz S: 270, 1285
Glaser J S: 3831
Glasier C M: 1864
Glass J P: 3684
Glass P: 4009
Glass Royal M C: 3342
Glass T A: 975
Glass T F: 3888
Glassberg R M: 3482

Glatt S L: 3483
Glazer G: 453, 454
Glazer G M: 165, 271, 288, 370, 371, 513, 521, 620, 622, 664, 665, 666, 687, 688, 700, 855, 860, 926, 951, 962, 984, 1167, 1248, 1330, 1336, 1410, 1411, 1539, 1544, 1942, 1952, 2026, 2027, 2028, 2204, 2226, 2240, 2241, 2362, 2363, 2447, 2471, 2501, 3468, 3838
Glazer H S: 195, 196, 272, 273, 274, 275, 396, 409, 486, 667, 668, 771, 772, 952, 1058, 1624, 2016, 2040, 2191, 4052
Glenn W V Jr: 3073
Glenny R: 5
Gleysteen J J: 1939
Glick A G: 427
Glick S N: 1545
Glickman M G: 2116
Glickstein M F: 2492, 3482
Glover G H: 9
Gluck E: 3484
Gluer C C: 34, 2499, 2808, 3134
Glynn T P Jr: 2448
Gmeinwieser J: 39
Gmelin E: 1390, 1391, 2051, 2192, 2369, 2718, 3485
Gnann H: 1591
Gobien B S: 669
Gobien R P: 669, 2002
Goda S: 3518
Godwin J D: 276, 277, 278, 279, 280, 426, 514, 515, 670, 671, 672, 673, 674, 675, 717, 807, 843, 894, 911, 2652, 3452
Goebel N: 1563, 1674, 2473, 3486
Goedecke R: 3909
Goei R: 1582
Goerich J: 607
Goff S: 1702
Goff W B: 1795, 2254
Gohel V: 358
Goiney R C: 2809
Goitein M: 3487
Gokan T: 2465
Golbey S H: 269
Gold B: 1542
Gold B M: 2348
Gold K: 2272
Gold P: 904
Gold R P: 203, 2029, 2040, 3189, 3190
Goldberg A L: 676, 3262, 3488, 3878
Goldberg H: 1442, 3792
Goldberg H I: 86, 792, 1038, 1055, 1081, 1167, 1168, 1201, 1278, 1406, 1417, 1468, 1469, 1544, 1546, 1556, 1719, 1743, 1807, 1942, 2044, 2195, 2363, 2447, 2728, 3492, 3515, 4088, 4100
Goldberg M E: 1541, 1785
Goldberg N: 366
Goldberg R E: 281
Goldberg R P: 504, 1292, 2144
Goldblatt D: 3627
Golden J: 780
Golden J A: 335, 3983
Golden J B: 2777
Goldhirsch A: 436, 2412
Goldin M D: 569
Golding R H: 1304
Golding R P: 1892, 2648
Goldman J: 3440
Goldman M: 1538, 1733
Goldman M J: 2064
Goldman S M: 1526, 1547, 2020, 2030, 2031, 2036, 2054, 2087, 2138, 2139, 2187, 2193, 2361, 3429
Goldmann A: 3489
Goldner J L: 2976
Goldsher D: 1776, 3300
Goldstein D P: 1756
Goldstein H M: 2479
Goldstein J D: 3490

Goldstein L: 516
Goldstein L D: 329
Goldstein M S: 677
Goldstein R B: 1293
Goldstein S: 289
Golimbu C: 942, 2782, 2783, 2784, 2810, 3039, 3040, 3041, 3042, 3043, 3491
Golkow R S: 678
Gomez Leon N: 1723
Gomez M T: 2179
Gomez Martinench E: 3157
Gomori J M: 3492, 3493
Gonzalez A: 1190
Gonzalez Crussi F: 1999
Gonzalez E: 3116
Gonzalez J G: 1548
Gonzalez L R: 1039
Gonzalez R R: 1548
Good A E: 2701
Good W F: 1875, 3547
Gooding C A: 615, 1679, 3978, 3979
Gooding G A: 1943
Goodman A: 1040, 1514
Goodman J H: 3717
Goodman M: 429, 3152
Goodman L R: 31, 225, 282, 283, 431, 678, 679, 738, 1944, 3154, 3494
Goodman P: 1744
Goodman P C: 412, 902, 1549, 1945, 2252, 3793
Goodsitt M M: 2811, 3071, 3721, 3874
Gooskens R H: 517, 3495, 3501
Gootenberg J E: 226
Goplerud D R: 2339, 2420, 2421, 2422
Goralnik C H: 680
Gorden P: 1381, 1423, 2765
Gordon A: 476
Gordon D: 3576
Gordon D H: 270
Gordon D L: 3439
Gordon L F: 2493
Gordon P: 1126
Gordon P M: 2064
Gordon R: 1496, 1497
Gordon R B: 1493, 1495, 1775, 1794
Gore R M: 118, 198, 233, 234, 596, 1240, 1546, 1550, 1745, 2307, 2711, 3496
Gorich J: 209, 266, 284, 518, 661, 681, 682, 683, 941, 1739, 1746, 2494, 3280, 3281, 3497
Gorman B: 1388
Goske M: 2658
Gossmann A: 29
Gossner W: 29
Gostner P: 1041, 3017, 3293
Gothi R: 1877
Goto T: 2919
Gottlieb R: 1795
Gould E S: 2812, 3219
Gould H: 2623
Gould H R: 1617, 1740
Gould R: 792, 2813
Gould R G: 501, 615, 1985
Gould R J: 1171, 1172
Gouliamos A: 285, 519, 2263, 2814, 3034, 3607
Gouliamos A D: 948
Goupille P: 2815
Gourtsoyiannis N: 2032
Gouverne M L: 784
Govoni A F: 634
Grabbe E: 38, 1042, 1392, 1551, 1552, 1747, 2580
Grabenwoger F: 1043, 2760
Grably D: 1138
Grace M: 2727
Grace M G: 2989
Gradinger R: 3059
Graeb D A: 520, 2934, 3847
Graen J: 286
Grage T: 1785
Graham R T: 1979
Graham S: 1846

Graham S D Jr: 2173
Graif M: 2140
Grandgeorge S: 262
Granger E: 3559
Granholm J W: 3861
Graninger W: 882
Granoff D W: 3993
Grant C S: 1388
Grant D C: 684
Grant E G: 1465, 3498, 3620, 3903
Grant J P: 2265
Grant T: 1044
Grantham J J: 2070, 2071, 2072, 2075
Grapp B: 3814
Gratia G: 2887
Grau H: 2676
Grauer W: 3176
Grauthoff H: 1425
Graves D S: 2980
Graves V: 3290
Graves V B: 2816
Gray G: 2532
Gray J E: 28
Gray L A: 3271
Gray M: 2847
Gray M B: 3856
Gray R: 2820
Gray R K: 1352
Gray R R: 1814
Greathouse J L: 2070
Grebbell F S: 3776
Grecos G P: 1212
Green B A: 3119
Greenberg B M: 1294, 1393
Greenberg H M: 1929
Greenberg I M: 1393
Greenberg J N: 226
Greenberg M: 1294, 1393
Greenberg R W: 336
Greene A J: 1635
Greene K M: 2194
Greene R: 287, 685, 878, 903, 3383
Greenleaf J F: 3918
Greenspan R H: 631
Greenstein S: 1553, 2449
Greenway G: 2497
Gregl A: 3499
Grehn S: 705, 2201, 2817
Greif W L: 659
Greiner K G: 2255
Greiner R: 914
Greitz T: 2825
Grendell J H: 1475
Grenier N: 2818
Grenier P: 616, 617, 686, 824, 1137, 1139, 1140, 1150
Greselle J F: 2818
Greve L H: 932
Gribbin C J: 837
Grider R: 2657
Griffin B A: 3530
Griffin B R: 3952
Griffin B W: 3953
Griffin D J: 288
Griffin G K: 846
Griffiths B: 1938
Griffiths B G: 1849
Grilias D: 1834
Grillo F: 2176
Grillo H C: 406
Grimaud J C: 1483
Grimes G: 180, 182, 1156
Grimes M M: 591
Grimley P M: 2451
Gritzman M C: 3827
Gritzmann N: 259, 1220, 3541
Grizzard M: 163
Grob D: 2772
Grobovschek M: 2864, 3141
Groen J J: 3500
Groenhout C M: 3501
Groenninger J: 1215
Grogan J P: 1753, 2748, 2819, 3196
Gronniger J: 3908

Grosfeld J: 627
Grosman H: 1814, 2820
Gross B H: 271, 288, 383, 407, 408, 513, 521, 620, 666, 687, 688, 700, 855, 951, 1055, 1330, 1539, 2028, 2195, 2240, 2277, 2322, 2362, 2363, 3515, 3838
Gross M D: 2611
Gross S C: 35, 289, 1446
Grosse D: 4074
Grosse Hokamp H: 4029
Grosser G: 462, 1554
Grossman H B: 2241
Grossman R: 2831, 3184
Grossman R A: 1997
Grossman R I: 3492, 4088, 4100
Grote R: 286, 1045, 1555, 2033
Grote W: 3765
Groves B M: 499
Growcock G: 2943
Grozinger K T: 2491
Grube E: 531, 561, 3286
Gruessner R: 1430
Grumbach K: 1295
Grumme T: 2959, 3731, 4061, 4062
Grundy B: 4086
Grunebaum M: 2602
Grupe G: 3814
Gruson B: 1623
Guardia E: 3077, 3882
Guckel F: 1746, 3497
Guerra J J: 2347
Guerra J J Jr: 2752, 3895
Guerrini P: 3366
Guhl L: 689, 690, 691
Guice K S: 1771
Guico J: 2956
Guigui B: 1141
Guilburd J N: 3300
Guilford W B: 1806
Guillaumin E: 1556
Guillerminet B: 3408
Guimaraes A: 3825
Guinto F C Jr: 147, 2821, 2918, 4045
Guion C J: 1880
Guiraud B: 3291, 3706
Gulati A N: 2822, 2823
Gullotta U: 1724, 2355
Gunderson L L: 1610
Gunther R: 1584, 3908, 3909
Gunther R W: 1394
Gupta K L: 3610
Gur D: 1875, 3547, 4086
Gurney J: 1748, 3494, 3505
Gurney J W: 31, 3494
Gurret J P: 2198
Gurtler K F: 692
Gussman D: 2386
Gustafson K D: 1395
Gustafson T: 1124
Gutcheck R A: 2811
Guthaner D F: 364, 387, 475, 522
Guthoff R: 3538
Gutierrez F R: 410
Gutjahr P: 3659
Gutman I: 4030
Guyer B H: 2824
Guyon J J: 3503
Gyldensted C: 2898
Gylys Morin V: 3215

Haaga J R: 36, 79, 232, 250, 281, 470, 680, 963, 1046, 1135, 1192, 1297, 1351, 1396, 1397, 1597, 1844, 1971, 2034, 2127, 2149, 3372, 3504
Haasner E: 2302
Habara S: 3893
Haberbeck Modesto M A: 2825
Haberle H J: 1896
Habermeier P: 2979
Habibian A: 2826
Hachiya J: 1085
Hackelthorn J C: 2816
Hacker H: 4042
Hackney D: 523
Hackney D B: 4088
Haddad M C: 3944

Haddock J A: 1614
Hadgis C: 3962
Hadjis N S: 1273, 2581
Haertel M: 143, 290, 920, 935, 1047, 1218, 1296, 1360, 1398, 1678, 1857, 2022, 2196, 2364
Hagemann J: 3538
Hagemeister F B: 4014
Hagen B: 2450
Hager T: 1632
Hagerstrand I: 1124
Haggar A M: 2492
Haghighi P: 2497, 2555
Hagino H: 2495
Haham Zadeh S: 3493
Hahn C: 291
Hahn D: 3101
Hahn F J: 3505
Hahn P F: 895, 1470
Haimes A B: 2532
Hain E: 612
Hajek P: 259, 693, 2869
Hakola M: 2592
Halaburt H: 2693
Halbsguth A: 292, 576, 2424
Halden W J: 293
Haleem A: 3944
Hales E D: 2308
Haliasos N: 285
Hall A: 3506
Hall A L: 3309, 3336
Hall D A: 1380
Hall D J: 2339, 2420
Hall E: 75
Hall F M: 72, 694, 1048, 1557, 1558, 2496, 2827, 2828, 3507, 3508
Hall T: 903, 981
Haller J: 704, 2497
Haller J O: 3737
Hallinan A J: 3813
Halls J: 1842, 2522, 2523
Halls J M: 810, 861, 1203, 1204, 1260, 2227, 2228
Halm H: 574
Halpert R D: 1601
Halter F: 1474
Haltia M: 3937
Halvorsen R: 2183
Halvorsen R A: 1049, 1050, 1458, 1477, 1657, 1658, 1694, 1749, 3860
Halvorsen R A Jr: 128, 294, 571, 956, 970, 1430, 1655, 2197
Hamada T: 2383
Hamer J: 3872
Hamilton D W: 1598
Hamilton P: 1630
Hamilton R H: 2863
Hamilton S R: 1576
Hamlin D J: 136, 319, 987, 988, 1559, 2247, 2256, 2365, 2589, 2868
Hamm B: 1021, 1051, 2366
Hammar S P: 807
Hammer B: 2829, 3509, 3510, 3926
Hammerman A M: 295, 1052
Hammers L: 1227
Hammers L W: 2524
Hammerschlag S B: 3511, 4050
Hammond N D: 3467
Hamper P: 2059
Hamper U M: 695, 2403
Han C H: 321
Han J K: 721, 1690
Han J S: 4094
Han M C: 310, 321, 718, 719, 721, 722, 765, 991, 992, 1275, 1276, 1277, 1368, 2076, 2375, 2435, 2730, 3353
Han M H: 991, 992, 2730
Han S K: 719
Han S S: 2830
Han S Y: 1362
Hanafee W: 3600
Hanafee W N: 3512, 3514
Hanbery J: 3420
Handa H: 3751
Handa J: 3771

Handel D B: 1750
Handel S: 2831
Handel S F: 3614, 3888
Hanefeld F: 2110
Haney P J: 327, 1053, 1751
Hanley D F: 3488
Hanley J A: 3730
Hanna R: 1012
Hannequin D: 3359
Hannesschlager G: 2832
Hansbrough F: 3737
Hansen F C: 166
Hansen G C: 2035
Hansen L G: 3634
Hansen M F: 1364
Hansen S T Jr: 2833
Hanson J: 2727
Hanson J A: 3953
Hanson R D: 1752
Hanssler L: 3766
Hanto D W: 1732
Hara K: 1344
Harada J: 474
Harada K: 425
Harada S: 838
Haraguchi Y: 1665
Haramati N: 2272
Harbin W P: 1054, 1816, 2834
Harbury O L: 2099
Harder T: 303, 315, 491, 696, 1111, 1112, 1587, 3513
Harding P: 2373
Hardy D C: 2504, 2835, 2836, 3199
Hardy K A: 781
Hardy R W Jr: 3065
Hardy T L: 3131
Harell G: 522
Harell G S: 567
Harker C: 918
Harkness B A: 3624
Harle T S: 1235, 2609
Harley J D: 2837, 2961, 2962, 2994
Harley W D: 974
Harms D: 1629
Harnsberger H R: 293, 2997, 3018, 3241, 3514, 3587, 3798, 3850
Harpley S: 3892
Harrell R S: 1730, 2414
Harrelson J M: 2577, 3045
Harries Jones E P: 1040
Harris A E: 647
Harris G J: 3381
Harris L P: 98
Harris M: 2586
Harris N L: 1956
Harris R D: 1684
Harris S T: 3134
Harrison D A: 245
Harrison E: 2393
Harrison P B: 520
Harrison W L: 1748
Hart H R: 3410
Hartenberg M A: 60
Harter L P: 645, 1055, 2195, 3515
Hartman B: 1842
Hartman B J: 2167
Hartman D S: 1733, 1734, 1920, 2020, 2030, 2031, 2036, 2187, 2438, 2451
Hartman G W: 2165
Hartmann K: 1727
Hartshorne M F: 697
Hartson M: 15
Hartz W H: 3467
Harvey G D: 3516
Harvey L A: 3989, 3990
Harwood Nash D: 3233
Harwood Nash D C: 173, 2658, 2668, 2762, 2883, 3000, 3030, 3104, 3105, 3242, 3243, 3448, 3605, 3629, 3630, 3712, 3820, 3929, 3930
Harzendorf E: 2082
Hasan H A: 3944
Hasegawa B H: 148
Hasegawa H: 1233
Hashim H: 147, 2821

Hashimoto H: 2357
Hashimoto K: 2046
Hashimoto S: 3458
Hashimoto T: 1818, 3517, 3526
Haslam M E: 429, 678, 738, 3152, 3153, 3154, 3155, 3156, 3669, 3821, 3823
Haslam R H: 3382
Hassler H: 1266
Hasso A N: 2838, 3159, 3338, 3553, 3690, 3752, 4015
Hasuo K: 1249, 3518
Hata Y: 2037
Hatabu H: 2293, 3887
Hatakeyama M: 844
Hatam A: 3519
Hatfield K D: 3520
Hattab N: 3670
Hatten H P Jr: 3862
Hattery R R: 996, 1093, 1395, 1840, 2165, 2236, 2467
Hattori N: 2257
Haubner W: 1632
Hauenstein K: 1911
Hauenstein K H: 1056, 1245
Hauer R: 562
Hauger W: 377, 2703
Haughton V: 2518, 3524, 3768
Haughton V M: 1753, 2225, 2675, 2688, 2689, 2722, 2724, 2748, 2819, 2839, 3016, 3025, 3148, 3194, 3195, 3196, 3378, 3379, 3380, 3415, 3447, 3521, 3522, 3598, 3599, 3883, 4008, 4023, 4079
Hauser H: 525, 1399, 1625, 2198, 4044
Hausmann B: 2575
Haussinger K: 794, 795, 796
Hauuy M P: 824
Hauzeur J P: 2853
Haveson S B: 1352
Havrilla T R: 79, 1297
Hawe W: 2952
Hawkes D J: 2310
Hawkins H H: 3828
Hawkins I F Jr: 2868, 3525
Hawkins W G: 1247
Hayabuchi N: 346
Hayashi K: 1163, 1164, 1165, 1318, 3750
Hayashi N: 1057
Hayashi S: 1074
Hayashi T: 3526
Hayek J: 2771, 2772
Hayes C: 239
Hayes C W: 3720, 3874
Hayes E: 3527
Hayes R: 1989
Hayes W S: 2451
Haykal H: 3687
Haykal H A: 3180, 3528
Hayman L A: 149, 161, 2617, 3529
Haynes J W: 2038, 2039
Haynor D R: 2560, 3530
Hays D: 168
Hayward I: 296
Hayward J C: 4016
Haywood R: 3845
Hazra T A: 2419
Headley D L: 3412
Healy M E: 2258
Heaston D: 2183
Heaston D K: 5, 265, 326, 334, 698, 842, 1750, 2197, 2265, 2745, 3551, 3779
Heater K: 699
Heavey L R: 700
Hebbar G: 1718
Hebel R: 57
Hecht H L: 974
Hecht S T: 1875
Hedde J P: 3437
Hedlund L W: 594, 642
Hedtler W: 2909
Heelan R T: 701, 926, 937, 2582, 3531, 3532
Heger L: 2840, 2841

Heiberg E: 112, 297, 298, 299, 300, 301, 1917, 2199, 2336, 2657, 3170, 3533
Heier L A: 3389
Heiken J P: 401, 1058, 1059, 1228, 1334, 1400, 2016, 2040, 2534, 2583, 4052
Heimberger K: 4020
Heindel W: 3568
Heintz A: 1653
Heinz E: 3019
Heinz E R: 2842, 3406, 3407, 3534, 3535, 3536
Heinz T R: 3535
Heise W: 2851
Heishima G B: 4027
Heiss J: 3537
Heiss W D: 4022
Hekali P: 2041
Hekster R E: 3500
Held P: 2706
Heldt N: 3392
Helenon O: 37
Heller H: 2705
Heller M: 38, 380, 692, 869, 913, 1392, 2580, 2584, 2585, 2649, 2757, 2843, 2844, 2845, 2875, 2876, 3014, 3538, 3539
Hellman S: 2568
Hellsten S F: 150
Hellwig H: 502
Helmberger T: 3540
Helmer M: 3541
Helmke K: 2876
Helms C A: 2846, 2847, 2848, 3174, 3202, 3542, 3758
Helzel M V: 2332, 2849, 2850
Hemingway A P: 1273
Hemminghytt S: 1753, 3598
Hemmingsson A: 39, 3543
Hemmy D C: 2675
Hendee W R: 148
Henderson R: 2522, 3800
Henderson S: 3840
Hendrich V: 2794
Hendricks P J: 1560
Hendrickx P: 1131, 3544
Hendriks M J: 2354
Hendrix R W: 2711, 3173
Henkelman R M: 77, 857
Henkes H: 2851, 3369, 3917
Hennig J: 1056, 3200
Hennig R C: 533
Henriksen L H: 3545
Henry D A: 524
Hens L: 2740
Henschke C I: 701, 703
Hensley G T: 3832
Heran F: 3317, 3546
Herbert D E: 775
Herbert D L: 2716, 3547
Herbst C A: 1638
Herdt J R: 742, 3024
Herfkens R: 505, 3278
Herfkens R J: 277
Herfkens R L: 276
Hering L: 2958, 3694
Herlinger H: 3370
Herlong F H: 965, 1214
Herman G T: 40, 41, 2852, 3548
Herman P G: 384, 823
Herman R J: 255
Herman S J: 650, 862
Herman T E: 1060, 1946
Hermann G: 2478, 2498, 2586, 2606, 3125, 3216
Hermann H J: 1103
Hermans J: 2556
Hermans P: 1486
Hermanus N: 2853, 3910
Hermreck A S: 1595
Hernandez Mora M: 1039
Hernandez R J: 1499, 2634, 2854, 2855, 2856
Herold C: 882
Herold C J: 704
Heron C W: 302, 469, 2260

Herpels V: 2477
Herrmann B: 3814
Herschorn S: 1979
Hershey B L: 3823
Hertel P: 3162
Herter M: 303, 2857
Hertz M: 2090, 2168, 2242
Hertz M A: 1937
Hertzanu Y: 1401, 3549
Hertzler G: 1358
Herzog S: 3550
Hessel S J: 106, 959, 1402, 1448, 1855, 2169
Hesselink J R: 3314, 3345, 3383, 3384, 3778, 3925
Hesselman C W: 129
Heuchemer T: 2587, 2858
Heuck A: 1403
Heuck A F: 2499, 3134
Heuck F: 42, 492, 689, 863, 1298, 2200, 2859, 2860, 3058
Heuck F H: 2558
Heuser L: 43, 525, 526, 1425
Hewer W: 705
Heydemann J: 2334
Heyer D: 2585
Heyse M: 2781
Heywang S H: 794, 3431
Hibri N S: 3046, 3842
Hickey D S: 4096
Hickey N M: 44
Hickey W F: 4050
Hicks R W: 2662
Hidalgo R: 471, 527, 2259, 3551
Hidvegi D: 2456
Hidvegi R S: 706
Hieckel H G: 707
Hier D B: 3809
Hieshima G B: 4028
Higashihara T: 404, 582, 583, 584, 585
Higgins A C: 3407
Higgins C B: 500, 508, 512, 523, 528, 529, 542, 543, 1709, 1710
Higgins W L: 304
Higgs J B: 2805
Highman L M: 1396
Hightower D R: 1500
Hilal S K: 53, 566, 2803, 2932, 2978, 3189, 3748, 3957, 4030
Hilaris B S: 3532
Hildebolt C F: 3707, 4034
Hildebrandt Stark H E: 3981
Hildell J: 2096, 2151, 2152, 2153
Hildell J G: 150
Hill A L: 2305
Hill M C: 985, 1404, 1440, 1466, 1568, 2461, 3361
Hill R: 2842, 3534
Hill R C: 651
Hill S C: 2042, 3552
Hillesheimer W: 1912
Hillman B J: 2012, 2043
Hilton S: 830, 1461, 1759, 1925
Hilweg D: 2692
Himmelfarb E: 1634
Himmelstein E: 678
Hinchcliffe W A: 212
Hinck V C: 149, 3529
Hindman B W: 2861, 2862
Hinke M L: 438, 1843, 2488, 3563
Hinkelbein W: 45, 3960
Hino K: 1246
Hinshaw D B Jr: 2838, 3159, 3553, 3690, 3752, 4015
Hintz R L: 4069
Hipp E: 3057
Hirabuki N: 3517
Hiramatsu K: 4082
Hirano T: 379
Hirao K: 1164
Hiraoka M: 3554, 3763
Hiraoka T: 82
Hirata K: 1074
Hirayama T: 553
Hirji M: 924
Hirji M K: 533
Hirning T: 1389
Hirohashi S: 1099

Hirose J: 305, 1146
Hirose N: 355
Hirota K: 1069
Hirsch M: 1754, 2376, 3549
Hirsch W L: 3879
Hirschfeld A D: 3490
Hirschy J C: 2617, 2863
Hitomi S: 354
Hitzler H: 3869
Hiyama Y: 1179
Hjelmquist B: 1640
Hjermstad B M: 1508, 1764
Ho A G: 2385
Ho E K: 2729
Ho K C: 3447, 3524, 4008
Ho K J: 389, 390, 391, 392, 564, 565, 888, 3949
Ho M: 441
Hoare R D: 3688
Hoch W H: 2290
Hodak J A: 3418
Hodapp N: 45
Hoddick W: 2044, 3792
Hoddick W I: 86
Hoddick W K: 1561
Hodges F J: 2800, 2894, 3478, 3871
Hodgman C G: 1562
Hodler J: 530, 1061
Hodson J: 2116
Hoeffken W: 4022
Hoeg J M: 2042, 3552
Hoel M J: 1183
Hoer P W: 292
Hoevels J: 1062
Hoey G B: 182
Hofbauer J: 2190
Hofer B: 1895
Hofer G A: 1755
Hoff J T: 3471
Hoffer F: 226
Hoffer F A: 1756
Hoffman A D: 3288
Hoffman E P: 2045
Hoffman H: 3242
Hoffman H J: 3104
Hoffman J: 1162, 1346
Hoffman J C Jr: 2709, 2710, 2927, 3339, 3340
Hoffman R B: 2035
Hoffman Tretin J C: 1516, 2330
Hoffmann E: 2576
Hoffmann J: 3719, 3909
Hoffmann T: 572
Hoffstein V: 874
Hofmann A: 2587
Hofmann E: 3183
Hofmann W: 2864
Hogan T D: 3924
Hohenberger P: 1019
Hohne K H: 125
Holbert B L: 708
Holbert J M: 708, 2865
Holden B S: 4015
Holden R W: 909
Holgate R C: 4010
Holland B A: 3555
Holland I M: 3556
Holle J P: 767
Holley H C: 1063, 2464
Holliday R A: 3927
Hollmann J: 2588, 3100
Hollmann J P: 1563
Hollwarth M: 2441
Holscher M: 3905
Holshouser B: 3553
Holtas S: 3557, 3652, 3674
Holzkamp J: 550
Holzman B H: 4011
Honda E: 3526
Honda H: 1064, 2046, 3272
Honda M: 2465
Honda T: 3458
Hong Magno E T: 3558
Honickman S J: 35
Honig C L: 2532
Honig E G: 663
Hood R S: 3018
Hoogewoud H M: 2108
Hoover E D: 3822, 3823

Hopf C: 2866
Hopfenmuller W: 3731
Hopkins R M: 182
Hoppe E: 2215
Hoppe R T: 220, 221, 3829
Hoppe Seyler P: 1361
Hopper J: 4024
Hopper K D: 306, 382, 1635, 2452, 3559, 3560, 3561
Hordvik M: 176
Horejs D: 1757
Horgan J G: 1758, 3355
Hori S: 2282
Horii S: 1983
Horii S C: 2142
Horikawa Y: 50
Horner N: 3043
Horner S: 74
Hornig K: 3562
Horning S: 3829
Horowitz L: 1603
Horowitz S W: 3439
Horst M: 2276, 2316
Horstmann H: 2967
Horton W A: 1786
Horvath F: 709, 710
Horvath K: 1835
Hosoba M: 3223
Hosoki T: 1065, 1066, 1405
Houang B: 2818
Hounsfield G N: 46, 47
Houser O W: 3796
Houston L: 2816
Houston L W: 3563
Houttuin E: 2335, 2336
Hovind K: 3772
Howard J: 1212
Howie J L: 268
Hricak H: 1709, 1710, 2309
Hruban R H: 30, 711, 712, 866, 867, 3851
Hruban R H,: 868
Hruby W: 177, 307, 1067
Huang C Y: 4076
Huang H K: 3352
Huang K M: 563
Huang R M: 713
Huang Y P: 3002
Hubener K H: 48, 49, 450, 599, 1068, 1219, 2201, 3564, 3915
Huber D J: 2367
Huber P: 3786
Huber R: 795, 3293
Huber R M: 794, 796
Hubsch P: 2123, 4020
Hubsch T: 342
Huckman M S: 3078
Hudgins P A: 2955, 3340
Hudson A: 1691
Hudson T M: 2500, 2589, 2590, 2591, 2659, 2867, 2868
Huebener K H: 881, 2202, 2406
Huggins T J: 3565
Hughes G M: 3566
Hughes J J: 714, 1564, 2047
Hugol D: 2346
Huizing E H: 4106
Huk W: 3537, 3567, 3568
Hulnick D: 1491, 1493, 1494, 1495, 1496
Hulnick D H: 308, 828, 829, 830, 1565, 1566, 1605, 1607, 1688, 1759, 1983, 2048, 2230, 2324, 2384, 2385, 2453
Humbert P: 2455
Hummelsheim P: 2155
Humphrey C C: 3088
Humphrey R L: 1522
Hundgen R: 104
Hungerford G D: 3132, 3312
Hunter J C: 3807
Hunter R E: 2344
Hunter T B: 1752, 2012, 2095, 3569, 3570
Huntrakoon M: 2069, 2074
Hupke R: 97
Huprich J E: 4028
Hurd R N: 297
Hurst R W: 3571, 3572
Hurwitz E F: 1048

Hurwitz L: 1283
Husband J E: 302, 469, 771, 1624, 2260, 2310, 2311, 3268, 3269, 3270
Husbands H S: 2491
Husberg B: 2096
Hussain S: 2203
Husselmann H: 612
Husson J L: 2797
Huston J 3d: 715
Hutchins D: 1649
Hutchins G M: 711, 712, 866, 867, 868, 3851
Hutchinson R: 2525
Hutchinson R J: 2299
Huttenlocher P R: 3558
Hutton S: 1386
Huwel N: 4061, 4062
Hyams B B: 3946
Hyams D M: 3804
Hyde J: 2480

Iacono R P: 3601
Iannaccone G: 3875
Ibarra B: 3074, 3880
Ibukuro K: 1252
Ichijo M: 3577, 3640
Ida M: 1144, 1145, 1146, 1251, 1333
Ideguchi S: 1246
Ideker R E: 515
Ido K: 4082
Iechima S: 2219
Ieshima A: 3573, 3574
Igdbashian V: 3575
Ignatoff J M: 2248
Ihde D C: 641, 1009
Ihori M: 1736
Iio M: 1082, 1301, 1439, 1670, 2674, 3645
Iivanainen M: 2592
Ijichi M: 2870
Ikeda A: 2616
Ikeda H: 716
Ikeda M: 50, 723
Ikeda S: 3458
Ikeuchi M: 2357
Ikeya S: 1233
Ikezoe J: 309, 404, 425, 582, 583, 585, 716, 717
Iko B O: 1567
Illanas M: 1039
Illescas F F: 1655, 2439, 2454
Ilves R: 1310
Im J G: 310, 321, 718, 719, 720, 721, 722, 765, 876, 925, 3576
Imaeda T: 1069
Imai A: 3577
Imamura H: 4003
Imamura K: 3578
Imanaka K: 2293, 3887
Imbert M C: 2100
Imhof H: 259, 693, 2869, 4021
Imschweiler E: 3499
Inada Y: 553
Inamoto K: 1070, 1299
Inaraja L: 1805, 2455
Inatsuki S: 2161
Ind P W: 579
Ingianni G: 1724, 2355, 3905
Ingrisch H: 794, 795, 796
Inoue E: 2282
Inoue K: 1144, 1145
Inoue N: 2870
Inoue Y: 1252, 2357, 3579, 3580
Inscoe S: 181
Inzitari D: 3375
Irnberger T: 2593, 2594, 3583, 3584, 3585
Irngartinger G: 464
Irons J M: 2448
Irwin G A: 245, 1542, 3213
Isaza M: 716
Isgro E: 2690
Isherwood I: 624, 2021, 2521, 2525, 2665, 3479, 4096
Ishida O: 2383
Ishida Y: 1102, 2871
Ishigaki T: 50, 723
Ishii C: 2408

Ishii S: 331
Ishikawa I: 1071, 1072, 1073, 2049
Ishikawa N: 1074
Ishikawa T: 553, 1074, 1075, 1076, 1077
Ishikawa Y: 1177, 1299
Ishimoto S: 3518
Isikoff M B: 1383, 1404, 1416, 1466, 2461
Isomoto I: 1165, 3750
Israels S J: 2595
Isselbacher K J: 3301
Isu T: 2991
Itabashi H H: 4028
Itai Y: 1078, 1079, 1080, 1081, 1082, 1083, 1084, 1085, 1086, 1087, 1088, 1089, 1300, 1301, 1406, 1407, 1408, 1409, 1439, 1670, 3645
Itatani H: 2154
Ito J: 4003, 4018
Ito K: 2870
Ito M: 2147
Ito T: 2977
Itoh H: 82, 423, 821, 822, 1144, 1145, 2154, 2409
Itoh K: 82, 1057, 1105, 2410
Itoh M: 3662, 3751
Itoh T: 821
Itoh Y: 723
Ivancev K: 155
Iversen G: 3933
Iwai S: 723
Iwaki H: 2641
Iwao M: 1163
Iwasaki S: 844
Iwasaki Y: 2991
Iwata K: 1178, 3003
Iyer G N: 1195
Izumi T: 822
Izutsu M: 4082

Jaaskelainen J: 3937
Jaaskinen J: 3938
Jack C R Jr: 3586
Jackson H: 1856
Jackson R M: 392
Jacky J P: 3530
Jacob F: 2255
Jacobs C J: 3587
Jacobs D: 2309
Jacobs I B: 3390
Jacobs I G: 3637
Jacobs J E: 2368
Jacobs J M: 1568, 3850
Jacobs R: 1306
Jacobs R P: 2746
Jacobson D R: 31
Jacoby C G: 3588
Jacques E Jr: 2793
Jaffe J: 2261
Jaffe M H: 1198, 1253, 1410, 1465, 1481, 2081, 2163, 3435
Jaffe N: 3111
Jafri S Z: 1411, 1532, 2050, 2204, 2362, 2501
Jagannadharao B: 297, 1916, 2335, 2657
Jager K: 2473
Jahnke R W: 2872, 3131
Jahss M H: 2529, 2530
Jain C: 1832
Jain S: 1877
James A E: 3808
James A E Jr: 2185
James E M: 1323, 1388
James H E: 2873
James S: 1569
Jamshidi S: 676
Janeira L F: 3354
Janicki P C: 548
Janon E A: 3589
Janowitz P: 1332
Jansen O: 2051, 2369
Jansen V O: 2596
Jansen W: 526
Janson R: 531, 758, 1090, 2874, 3303, 3304

Jantzen R: 73
Janus C L: 325
Jaques P: 1760
Jaques P F: 1962, 2370, 3590
Jaramillo D: 1570, 2371
Jardin C: 2677
Jardin M: 311, 724
Jaretzki A 3d: 365
Jarrell B E: 1242
Jarrett P T: 2551
Jaschke W: 725, 1927, 2052, 2189, 2733
Jasper M P: 1781
Jaspers M J: 726
Jauch M: 4040
Javadpour N: 2007, 2182, 2442
Javid M J: 2806
Javors B: 1285
Javors B R: 3424
Jeanmart L: 1933, 2552, 2681
Jeffrey R B: 449, 532, 1293, 1302, 1379, 1412, 1509, 1533, 1571, 1572, 1697, 1824, 1913, 1950, 2014, 2044, 2115, 2262, 2309, 2597, 2652, 3012, 3916
Jeffrey R B Jr: 218, 614, 1091, 1092, 1123, 1303, 1413, 1475, 1500, 1556, 1600, 1719, 1720, 1761, 1762, 1763, 1797, 1827, 1938, 2053, 3202, 3297, 3591, 4054
Jellinger K: 3510
Jend H H: 2845, 2875, 2876, 3538, 3592
Jend H J: 3539
Jenkins H: 3512
Jenkins M: 1304
Jensen J E: 2744
Jensen K M: 27, 2775, 2776
Jensen P S: 2877
Jensen R T: 1423
Jenss H: 1219
Jeong H J: 626
Jewel K L: 3593
Jewell W R: 3347
Jiddane M: 2502, 2977
Jing B S: 1504, 2360, 2554
Jinkins J R: 3594, 3595, 3597, 3788
Jinnouchi Y: 2093
Jitsukawa K: 1736
Jo S: 3554
Joachim C L: 3181
Job Deslandre C: 2815
Jochelson M S: 2326
Jochens R: 2851
Joffe N: 3508
Johansen J G: 2748, 2878, 2879, 2880, 3016, 3598, 3599
Joharjy I A: 727
John V: 2503
Johns C J: 695
Johns R: 3382
Johns T: 3947
Johns T T: 1635
Johnson A R: 1764
Johnson C D: 1323, 1414, 1415, 1529, 1573, 1648, 2205, 4058
Johnson C M: 1093, 4058
Johnson D W: 3600
Johnson G A: 51, 672
Johnson H A: 598
Johnson J B Jr: 1680
Johnson J E: 3601
Johnson J F: 1773
Johnson K K: 3602
Johnson K W: 1998
Johnson L P: 3514
Johnson M A: 533
Johnson M B: 1260, 3839
Johnson M L: 1282
Johnson P: 677
Johnson R J: 2372
Johnson S F: 2721
Johnson W C: 1737, 1738, 3859
Johnston Early A: 641
Johnston G H: 2795
Johnston R E: 3110
Johnston W W: 2197
Joka T: 3651

Jolesz F: 451
Jolles H: 26, 1765
Jolles P R: 564
Jones B: 547, 1522, 1537, 1547, 1553, 1574, 1575, 1576, 1608, 1609, 1619, 1631, 1666, 1693, 1696, 1716, 1717, 1729, 1766, 2278, 3734
Jones E: 1327
Jones E C: 1183
Jones J P: 3643
Jones K R: 52, 103
Jones M A: 1749
Jonsson K: 3026, 3027
Joosten E: 2541
Jordan R L: 1883
Joseph A E: 3496
Joseph G: 547
Joseph N: 2456
Joseph P M: 53, 54, 3472
Joseph R C: 2347
Joseph R R: 1446
Joshi R K: 3944
Joshi R R: 728
Joslyn J N: 2804
Joyce P: 3329
Joyce P F: 1916
Joyce P W: 1352
Judmaier G: 1095
Juettner-Smolle F: 649
Jung B: 39, 3543
Jung Legg Y: 632
Jung S Y: 765
Junginger T: 740, 1216
Jungreis C A: 2881
Junker J A: 3603

Kaczmarek R G: 55
Kaczmarek R V: 55
Kadir S: 1018, 1345, 2449
Kadowaki K: 309, 716, 2282
Kadoya M: 1144, 1145, 1146
Kaftori J K: 1776, 2882
Kahn T: 1767
Kaiser D: 943
Kaiser J A: 455, 456, 1719, 1951, 2014, 2252
Kaiser L R: 274, 295
Kaiser M C: 56, 312, 517, 2598, 2883, 2884, 2885, 2886, 2887, 3171, 3495, 3604, 3605, 3606
Kaiser R: 2206, 3397
Kakimoto S: 2147
Kakuda K: 1251
Kalavritinos M: 1726
Kalender W A: 49, 57, 58, 139, 729, 921, 2781, 2888, 2889, 2890, 2891, 3430
Kalet I J: 3530
Kalff V: 3624
Kalina R E: 3987
Kalkhoff R K: 1753
Kalovidouris A: 519, 2263, 2814, 3034, 3607
Kalser M: 1404
Kam J: 1337, 3608
Kamei T: 4080
Kamerer D B: 3881
Kameyama T: 1146
Kamikaseda K: 3518
Kamimura R: 1145
Kaminsky R I: 1856
Kamoi I: 1592
Kamoshita S: 3893
Kampmann H: 1577
Kan P T: 3963
Kan S: 2892
Kanai K: 1178
Kanaoka M: 821
Kanayama H: 452
Kane N M: 1768, 2264
Kane R: 3792
Kane R A: 86, 1305, 1306
Kane V G: 1578
Kanehann L B: 1579
Kaneko M: 1876
Kang H S: 310
Kang S B: 2375
Kangarloo H: 981, 3288, 3352

Kangasniemi P: 167
Kankaanpaa U: 2921
Kansler F: 2788
Kanter R A: 210
Kanzow G: 913
Kapelner S: 2562
Kapila A: 1769, 1770, 2893, 3609, 3610
Kaplan H S: 220
Kaplan I L: 313
Kaplan J O: 1416
Kaplan M M: 1188
Kaplan S B: 1094
Kappeler M: 1343, 1474
Kappelle L J: 3611
Kaptein E M: 2523
Karadanas A H: 194
Karagiannis E: 470
Karagoz F: 1705
Karantanas A H: 314, 730
Karasawa E: 1417
Karasawa H: 3612
Karasick S R: 151
Karavias D: 1834
Karbon K: 3420
Kardaun J W: 3091
Karellas A: 168, 1455
Karl R C: 1202
Karmody C S: 3334, 3335
Karnaze G C: 1395, 1580
Karnaze M G: 2894
Karnel F: 259, 1220, 2123
Karp J E: 745
Karpatkin M: 1160
Karpf P M: 3055, 3059
Karstaedt N: 204, 975, 1479, 1487, 2207
Karsteadt N: 1515
Karstens J H: 2055
Kart B H: 3613
Karvounis P: 3653
Karwowski A: 2656
Kasdaglis K: 4065
Kashima H K: 647
Kassner E G: 3737
Katayama K: 1250
Katayama M: 1232
Kathrein H: 1095
Kato K: 452
Kato Y: 2037
Katsiotis P: 194
Katsumata Y: 964
Kattapuram S V: 2895, 2896
Katz D: 2000
Katz H: 3466
Katz J: 1306
Katz M: 656
Katzman R: 3483
Kauczor H U: 1801
Kauffmann G W: 3200
Kaufman B: 3745
Kaufman H H: 3614
Kaufman J L: 3615
Kaufman L: 1168
Kaufman R A: 59, 731, 1229, 1771, 3616
Kaufman S L: 1237, 2449
Kaufmann H J: 2110
Kaulfersch W: 3649
Kaurich J D: 1096
Kavanaugh J H: 2970
Kavuru M: 749
Kawaguchi M: 1612
Kawahira K: 355, 1249, 2093
Kawai H: 3517
Kawai R: 3517
Kawamoto E H: 1479
Kawamura I: 423, 1251
Kawanami T: 1249
Kawashima A: 732, 1097
Kay C J: 2517
Kay H: 283
Kay H R: 282
Kaye A: 4024
Kayser K: 681, 682
Kazam E: 256, 703, 966, 1210, 1672, 1852, 1921, 1922, 2056, 2166, 2167, 2170, 2312, 2532, 2944, 3248, 3249, 3275
Kazner E: 137, 3187, 4061, 4062

Kazui S: 3617
Keane T: 783
Kearfott K J: 3618
Keating J W: 3051, 3862
Keefe B: 1560
Keene J S: 2816
Keesey J C: 261
Keeter S: 60
Keilbach H: 562
Keita K: 442, 790
Keith J W: 3326
Kelcz F: 53
Kelekis D: 3619
Kelekis L: 3619
Kelemouridis B: 3619
Keller E: 380
Keller J M: 61
Keller W: 2190
Kellerhouse L: 2826
Kellermeyer R W: 1397
Kellman G M: 1024, 3230
Kellum C D: 1364
Kelly D R: 3620
Kelly J: 1772
Kelly J K: 3637
Kelly K M: 2143
Kelly R B: 1773
Kelly W M: 3663
Kelvin F M: 1642, 1774, 1851, 1865, 2133, 2265, 2664
Kempf P: 1584
Kempmann G: 725
Kendall B: 3621, 3891
Kendall B E: 152, 1902, 3035, 3209, 3414, 3556, 3631, 3836, 3985, 3986
Kennard D R: 3622
Kennedy W H: 2716, 3676
Kennerdell J S: 3877
Kenney P J: 2171, 2208, 2266, 2267, 2464, 2599, 3650
Kenny J M: 1214
Kerber C W: 3290
Kern A: 3175
Kerner H: 3300
Kerns S R: 733, 3572
Kerr I H: 820
Kerr R: 2897, 3085
Kerremans R: 1685
Kersjes W: 315
Kessler A: 2140
Kessler H B: 3467
Ketonen L: 2592, 2898, 3623
Ketyer S: 2600
Keyes J W Jr: 3624
Keyes W D: 26, 3964, 3965
Keyser C K: 2504
Khaffaji S: 1012
Khaja F: 289
Khalifa A: 1718
Khan A: 734, 823, 3710
Khan F A: 734
Kharasch M: 18
Khatri B: 3524
Khedekar S: 3354
Khine N: 3144
Khine N M: 944
Khomeini R: 2911
Khorsandian C: 2304
Khouri M R: 3625
Khouri N F: 348, 349, 695, 747, 827, 828, 829, 891, 892
Khoury P T: 402
Kido D K: 3626, 3764
Kido M: 838
Kiefer H: 2373
Kieffer S A: 3013, 3143, 3166
Kieft G J: 2899
Kier E L: 1848, 4037
Kier R: 1098, 3244
Kiernan H: 3116
Kihm W D: 725
Kilcheski T S: 2374
Kilcoyne R F: 2560, 2811, 2900, 2994, 3032, 3954
Kilgore D P: 3025
Killebrew E J: 490, 543
Killeen J: 2838
Kim B S: 2273
Kim C: 1532

Kim C W: 310, 321, 718, 719, 721, 765, 992, 1276, 1277, 1368, 2076, 2375, 2730, 3349, 3353
Kim C Y: 1275
Kim D: 239
Kim H J: 991
Kim I O: 2076, 2730
Kim K S: 3627, 3848
Kim K W: 1368
Kim M H: 3226
Kim M J: 1784
Kim S H: 992, 1275, 1276, 1277, 2375, 2435, 3353
Kim S Y: 1418
Kim W H: 1275
Kim W S: 321, 2054, 3488, 3666
Kim Y C: 2031
Kim Y H: 765
Kim Y I: 1275, 1277, 1368
Kimmig B: 1103, 2209
Kimmig B N: 1482
Kimoto T: 350, 838, 1447
Kimura A: 1099
Kimura N: 1447
Kimura S: 346
Kinard R E: 2394, 3628, 3856
Kindermann U: 4040
King B F: 1113
King D G: 2999, 3769
King D L: 2040
King G A: 4091
King H A: 2900
King T: 633
Kingsley D P: 3629, 3630, 3631
Kinlaw W B: 619
Kinsey J H: 98
Kirby D F: 1550
Kirchhof B: 4092
Kirchhoff P G: 537
Kirchner R: 1289
Kirklin J K: 565
Kirkpatrick R H: 1380, 1816, 4072
Kirks D R: 316, 2745
Kirsch J D: 534
Kirschner L P: 1286
Kirschner P A: 476, 801
Kirzner H: 3632
Kisa T: 3574
Kish K K: 2901
Kishi M: 3518
Kishikawa T: 3700, 4061, 4062
Kishk S M: 2441
Kishore P R: 3846
Kispert D B: 3796
Kisslo J R: 527
Kistler J P: 3728
Kita N: 582, 583, 584, 585
Kitada H: 1072
Kitagawa K: 1145
Kitagawa M: 934
Kitagawa S: 1665
Kitamura I: 844
Kitamura S: 844
Kitano M: 331
Kitani F: 582
Kitchens H H: 2273
Kitoh F: 964
Kittredge R D: 1775
Kivisaari L: 1419, 1420, 2041
Kiwak M G: 511
Kizer K W: 3633
Kjaer M: 3634
Kjartansson O: 4063
Kjellberg R N: 3384
Kjos B O: 3635
Klapdor R: 1042
Klappenbach R S: 2223
Klatte E C: 910, 2301, 2443
Klauber G: 2292
Klawki P: 2914
Klech H: 693
Kleckow M: 464
Klein A: 2902
Klein B: 3636
Klein J S: 360
Klein M A: 3637
Klein M L: 1643
Klein M V: 3925

Kleinau H: 2531
Kleinhaus U: 1581, 1776, 2882, 4006
Kleinman G M: 3778
Klepp O: 2458
Klibanski A: 3720, 3721
Kline L B: 3831
Kling G A: 2297
Kling T F: 2548
Klingensmith W C: 535
Klingmuller V: 2122
Klinken L: 3810, 3811
Klintworth G: 3406
Klooster N J: 1582
Klose K: 473, 2424
Klose K C: 568, 1100, 1583, 2055, 2255
Klose K J: 1394, 1584, 2124
Kloss J: 3036
Klott K: 1219
Klott K J: 48, 2405
Klotter H J: 1394
Klotz E: 58, 2888
Kluge W: 3731
Kluger A: 3386, 3474
Knake J E: 2640, 2938, 3469, 3470, 3471
Knapp E: 339, 340, 341
Knapp R: 2475
Knapp R H: 4034
Knappschneider U: 96
Knaus W A: 3638
Kneeland B: 3678
Kneeland J B: 966, 1852, 1921, 1922, 2056, 2312
Kniffert T: 1777
Knipper H: 1993
Knopf D R: 1101
Knopp E A: 3639
Knowles C: 748, 1585
Knowles R J: 3618, 3678
Knudsen L L: 2903
Knuth A: 1216
Ko K W: 3349
Kobari M: 3577, 3640
Kobayashi A: 1102
Kobayashi K: 425, 4003
Kobayashi N: 1057
Kobayashi S: 85
Kobayashi T: 839, 3641
Kobayashi Y: 2154
Kober B: 109, 1019, 1103, 1104, 4041
Kock C: 2904
Kodama K: 755
Koehler P R: 1660, 1828, 2487, 2512, 3642, 3757
Koehler R E: 367, 1261, 1262, 1329, 1487, 1488, 1701, 1783, 2464, 3257
Koenigsberg M: 1346, 1467
Koeppe P: 927
Kogutt M S: 62, 3643
Kohama A: 3898
Kohler D: 1777, 3188, 3358
Kohlmeyer K: 3644
Kohno A: 573
Kohno H: 1179
Kohno S: 2257
Koischwitz D: 317, 1110, 1903, 2062
Koizumi K: 2465
Kojima K: 1105, 1178
Kojoh K: 1246
Kok F P: 2416
Kokubo T: 1084, 1085, 1086, 1088, 1089, 1105, 1408, 3645
Kolar J: 2905
Kolbenstvedt A: 1421, 1868, 2057, 2091, 2458
Kolin J: 2905
Kolmannskog F: 1421, 2091
Komaiko M S: 3646
Komaki S: 1586
Komar N N: 3205
Kondoh S: 1105
Konerding K F: 2234, 2419
Konermann M: 2906
Koneru B: 1947
Kong Y: 514

Konig H: 756, 1422, 2601, 2906
Konig R: 318, 735, 736, 906, 3647
Konishi H: 1145, 1146
Konkiewicz J: 2656
Konno K: 4002
Kopans D B: 1610, 3648, 3693
Kopernik G: 2376
Kopp W: 753, 1778, 3649
Koppenhofer H: 1106
Korber H J: 3499
Korec S M: 1254
Kori S H: 3504, 3837
Koritke J G: 3394
Kormano M: 737, 1419
Kormano M J: 319
Korner U: 2596
Kornreich L: 2602
Korobkin M: 5, 51, 108, 265, 326, 334, 471, 514, 527, 536, 567, 672, 698, 842, 1049, 1050, 1226, 1307, 1366, 1442, 1478, 1657, 1658, 1682, 1750, 1774, 1850, 1851, 1865, 1966, 1994, 2008, 2009, 2083, 2133, 2183, 2210, 2214, 2259, 2265, 2268, 2298, 2322, 2546, 2629, 2664, 2976, 3045, 3551
Korte J H: 3197
Koschel G: 612
Koslin D B: 1063, 1107, 2171, 2464, 3650
Koslow M: 3481
Kosowicz J: 2229
Kossol J M: 2269
Koster K: 684
Koster O: 880, 949, 1108, 1109, 1110, 1111, 1587, 1593, 2377, 2603, 2604, 2923, 2924, 3651
Kostrubiak I: 329, 330
Kostrubiak I S: 516
Kotake T: 2281
Kothari K: 2058
Kotner L M Jr: 1052
Kott M M: 903
Kotter D: 2843
Kotterer O: 385
Kowal L E: 738
Kowalski H M: 2908
Kowalski J B: 35
Koyano K: 1876
Kozakewich H: 1756
Kozic Z: 3079, 3708, 3709
Kozin F: 2723
Kozuka T: 309, 425, 582, 583, 584, 585, 3517
Kraft R: 1884, 1885
Krahe T: 303, 1112, 2604, 3780
Krajbich I: 2569, 2763
Kramann B: 1349, 2423, 3228
Kramer E L: 1588
Kramer G: 3318
Kramer J: 704
Kramer S S: 1879, 2159
Kramps H: 2445
Kramps H A: 2739
Krantz P: 3652
Krappel W: 559
Krassanakis K: 3653
Kratz H W: 2059, 3654
Kraus A P Jr: 1680
Krause P: 2909
Krauss J: 3183
Krausz M: 3939
Kreel L: 1365, 1681, 2175, 2333, 3416, 3656
Kreienberg R: 2424
Kreipke D L: 739, 2448
Kreiskother E: 2635
Kreitner K F: 1215, 2910
Krellenstein D J: 325
Kremer B: 1279
Krempa J: 1883
Kressel H: 258
Kressel H Y: 2210, 2374, 2386, 2990, 3658
Krestin G P: 740, 741, 1589, 1590, 1792, 2211
Kretzschmar K: 3659

Kricheff I: 3140
Kricheff I I: 2708, 2709, 2782, 3069, 3192, 3239, 3363, 3385, 3473, 3660, 3826
Kriedemann E: 2531, 2632
Kriegshauser J S: 1113
Krigman M R: 3901
Kristensen J K: 2433
Kriz R J: 123
Krohn B P: 2070
Krol G: 2911, 2912, 2913
Krolikowski F J: 1846
Krone A: 2914
Kronthal A J: 2378
Krudy A G: 252, 253, 742, 1308, 1381, 1423, 2060
Kruglik G D: 743
Kruis F J: 116
Kruse H P: 3014
Kryscio R J: 2114
Kuan B B: 4004
Kubale R: 933
Kubik S: 4031
Kubo K: 4031
Kubota K: 3662
Kucharczyk W: 3663
Kuckein D: 2605, 2915
Kudo S: 1249
Kuhajda F: 1716, 3208
Kuhajda F P: 747, 2323, 3848
Kuhlman J E: 83, 166, 320, 712, 744, 745, 746, 747, 748, 749, 866, 867, 1151, 1585, 2278, 2378, 2379, 2469, 2489, 2916, 3851
Kuhlman J E,: 750, 868
Kuhn F: 473
Kuhn F P: 1255, 1394
Kuhn G: 621
Kuhn J P: 206, 1503, 1928, 2474, 2917, 3308
Kuhn M J: 3664
Kuhne D: 2876
Kuhnel W: 3212
Kuhns L R: 206, 751, 785, 1114, 1359, 1472, 1633, 2701, 3665
Kuhr J: 2874
Kuklinski M E: 342
Kulik W J: 2862
Kulkarni M V: 1634, 2185, 3742
Kullmann G: 2313
Kullnig P: 649, 752, 753, 754, 816, 818, 1778
Kumagai J: 3718
Kumar A: 581, 3703, 3704
Kumar A J: 2694, 2785, 2984, 3214, 3666
Kumar K: 1877
Kumar M: 2284
Kumar R: 2918
Kumpan W: 693, 1779, 2869
Kunde D: 2632
Kunieda E: 657
Kunin M: 63, 2061
Kunkel B: 2705
Kunlen H: 2605
Kunstlinger F: 1115
Kuper K: 1591
Kuppers S: 1801
Kurabayashi T: 2641
Kurashima A: 4018
Kurauchi S: 1612
Kuriyama K: 755, 2281, 2282
Kuriyama Y: 3617
Kuroda A: 1079, 1408
Kuroda M: 2281
Kuroda Y: 2293
Kurokawa H: 2919
Kurosaki M: 1102
Kursawe R: 1424
Kursh E D: 2246
Kursunoglu S: 2514, 2925, 3085
Kurtz A: 1184, 1959, 2272
Kurtz A B: 1242
Kurtz B: 599, 756, 757, 1116, 1117, 2601
Kurtz D: 1835
Kushihashi T: 2465

Kushner M J: 3667
Kusuda S: 3579
Kuten A: 4006
Kuther G: 2526, 2527
Kutin N: 1160
Kutzner J: 3659
Kuuliala I: 3623
Kuwabara Y: 1592
Kuwahara O: 309
Kuyper S J: 3263
Kvale P: 363
Kvicala V: 1118
Kvistad K A: 2673
Kwan E: 3668
Kwasny O: 2760
Kwee I L: 3001, 3240
Kwok Liu J P: 2270
Kyle R A: 3919

La France N D: 2159
La Regina M E: 3386
La Spada F: 2625
Laasonen E M: 2920, 2921
Laberge J M: 2922
Lacey S R: 1636
Lachenauer C S: 3703
Lachman R: 2734
Lackner K: 507, 509, 525, 531, 537, 538, 539, 561, 758, 767, 949, 1090, 1109, 1110, 1112, 1425, 1593, 1903, 2062, 2377, 2603, 2874, 2923, 2924, 3286, 3304, 3651, 3780, 3913
Ladaga L E: 2714
Ladd W A: 850
Ladeb M F: 1141
Lafferty C M: 2925
Laffey P A: 3156, 3669
Lagouros P: 2963
Lahdenranta U: 2920
Laing F C: 1293, 1302, 1303, 1412, 1475, 1500, 1572, 1762, 2044
Lais E: 3162
Laissy J P: 3670
Lakshminarayanan A V: 12
Lalanne B: 3387
Lallemand D: 824
Lally J F: 2486, 3079
Lam A H: 2104
Lam S C: 939
Lamasters D L: 3671
Lambers U: 3719
Lambiase R: 2926
Lameris J S: 1270
Lammer J: 3136
Lamont B M: 1837
Lamorgese B: 1780
Lampard R: 2989
Landay M J: 759
Lande I M: 985, 3361
Lander P H: 2766
Landman J A: 2710, 2927
Landwehr P: 3286
Lane C: 3307
Lane R H: 2457
Lang C: 3672
Lang E K: 2063
Lang E V: 760
Lang P: 2851, 2928, 2929, 3127
Lang R: 2877
Langdon T: 1024
Lange K: 64
Lange P H: 2305
Lange T A: 2930
Langenbruch K: 2024
Langer B G: 2963
Langer M: 1257, 1258, 1777, 1923, 2341, 2570
Langer R: 1257, 1258, 3369
Langkowski J H: 2649
Langle F: 2123
Langston J W: 2931
Laniado M: 137, 2570
Lanksch W: 4061, 4062
Lantieri R: 1003
Lantos C: 3483
Lantz E J: 1562
Lanz U: 2635, 2636, 2637

Lanzieri C F: 403, 2478, 2606, 2932, 2933, 3673
Lapin S A: 810, 1260, 2228
Lapointe J S: 520, 2934, 3847
Lappas J C: 235
Larde D: 761, 1136, 1137, 1138, 1239, 2023, 2935, 2936
Largiader F: 1134
Laros G S: 2937
Larossa D: 2352
Larsen C R: 1654
Larsen M B: 4026
Larson D A: 4085
Larsson E M: 3674
Larsson S J: 3273
Larsson S G: 1594
Larusso N F: 996
Lasker R D: 252
Lassegue A: 1000
Lassen M N: 65
Laster D W: 3675
Latack J T: 417, 2938, 3469, 3471
Latchaw R E: 2988, 3676, 3879
Lattimer J: 2289
Lau D H: 182
Lauerman W C: 2805
Laumann O: 2739
Launay M: 2732
Laurens R G Jr: 663
Laurent J: 541
Laursen K: 2212, 2433
Lausen M: 1348
Lauten G J: 2939
Lautin E M: 762, 1733, 2064, 2271, 2272
Lautrou J: 145
Lavain J: 4024
Laval Jeantet A M: 66, 2940
Laval Jeantet M: 37, 264, 656, 3456
Lavaroni A: 153
Lavelle W: 3527
Law M R: 3268
Lawate P S: 1781
Lawler G A: 640
Lawrence E R: 3424
Laws E R Jr: 3796
Lawson D W: 351
Lawson T L: 229, 238, 430, 960, 977, 990, 1022, 1023, 1024, 1130, 1268, 1287, 1315, 1341, 1375, 1939, 2426, 2440, 2441, 2723, 2941, 3230, 3450
Lawton J S: 2145
Layer G: 763
Lazar R H: 3326
Le Minor J M: 2942
Leather R P: 3615
Leavitt D D: 1828
Lebeau B: 217
Lebowitz R L: 2431
Leccia F: 983
Lecklitner M L: 2943
Lecumberri F J: 1940
Lecumberri Olaverri F J: 997
Leder R A: 1353, 1995
Lee B C: 2670, 2944, 3324, 3677, 3678
Lee B H: 765
Lee D H: 1277
Lee D J: 3876
Lee G: 2862
Lee H: 1782
Lee H C: 67
Lee H P: 2375
Lee J D: 721, 1418
Lee J H: 1276
Lee J J: 832
Lee J K: 68, 201, 202, 401, 772, 952, 1058, 1059, 1228, 1238, 1261, 1262, 1284, 1307, 1309, 1334, 1429, 1488, 1569, 1783, 2016, 2086, 2107, 2314, 2340, 2426, 2583, 2945
Lee J S: 2076
Lee J T: 1784
Lee J Y: 764, 2171
Lee K F: 3680
Lee K R: 1595, 2067, 2068, 2607, 2946, 3681, 3682, 3683

Lee K S: 321, 721, 765
Lee L L: 2380
Lee M E: 3646
Lee M O: 354
Lee P K: 4076
Lee S H: 35, 991, 2273, 3632
Lee S P: 1264, 3263
Lee T G: 1828
Lee W J: 1690
Lee Y S: 582
Lee Y Y: 2947, 2948, 3684, 3685, 4033
Leeds N E: 2529, 2788, 3299, 3886, 4101, 4102, 4103, 4104
Leehey P: 2949
Leekam R N: 1310
Leemans J: 2950
Leestma J E: 3433
Leetzow M L: 28
Lefcoe M S: 893
Lefkovitz Z: 269
Lefkowitz D M: 2951
Lefleur R S: 1354, 1489, 1492
Legada B D Jr: 2666
Leger J M: 2732
Lehar S C: 1947
Lehmann L A: 3309
Lehmann J: 2910
Lehmkuhl G: 3644
Lehner E: 2952, 3059
Lehr J L: 69, 70
Leiberman J R: 2376
Leibman A J: 766, 1162
Leibovici L: 3493
Leichner P K: 1247
Leipner N: 303, 767, 768, 880, 1108
Leiter B: 2427
Leiter B E: 3266
Leitman B S: 828, 829, 942
Lelbach W K: 1108
Lellig U: 3064
Lellouche D: 442
Lemahieu S F: 2726, 3868
Lemaitre L: 311
Lemay M: 2953, 3686, 3687
Lemmens H A: 932
Lenkel S C: 487
Lenkey J L: 2470
Leno C: 3048
Lenoir S: 616, 617
Lentini J F: 2381
Lenz M: 940
Leo F P: 129, 891, 892, 936
Leo J S: 2937
Leonardi M: 153, 2953
Leong H J: 1784
Leong L L: 1274
Lepke R A: 161, 1426, 2617
Lepreux J F: 1623, 3806
Lequire M H: 850
Lerner H J: 1661
Lerner R M: 2397
Lesar M: 3559
Lesar M L: 3565
Lesar M S: 601
Lesh P: 2973
Letourneau J G: 128, 1119, 1430, 1785
Leue W: 3278
Leue W M: 2863
Leung A N: 769
Leung C H: 67
Leupold D: 3696
Lev Toaff A S: 652, 1120, 1579, 2261, 2432
Leveen H H: 1241
Levesque R Y: 3302
Levin D C: 1427, 1428
Levin D N: 71
Levin H S: 3306
Levin S: 3688
Levine A M: 2804
Levine C: 770, 2065, 2066, 3165
Levine E: 1595, 1786, 1787, 2066, 2067, 2068, 2069, 2070, 2071, 2072, 2073, 2074, 2075, 2135, 2216, 2607, 3006, 3129, 3682
Levine H: 3072

Levine M I: 3795
Levine M L: 72
Levine M S: 1295, 1545, 2315, 3370
Levine P A: 3571
Levine R: 1925, 3521
Levinsohn E M: 2608, 2655, 2824
Levinson A W: 3626
Levitan L H: 2954
Leviton M: 2586
Levitt R: 1668
Levitt R G: 200, 201, 410, 668, 685, 771, 772, 946, 1262, 1309, 1429, 1624, 1671, 1788, 2011, 2191, 2207, 2773
Lewin J R: 1789, 1790
Lewin P K: 3689
Lewis B J: 3747
Lewis C A: 2955
Lewis E: 154, 773, 1121, 2129, 2865
Lewis J W Jr: 849, 950
Lewis L K: 3690
Lewis M: 2586
Lewis M L: 3179, 4048
Lewis T D: 524
Lewis V L: 3488
Lewitt R M: 3548
Leyendecker G: 2377
Leyman P: 1596
Li D K: 1791, 1823
Li Y P: 2956
Libshitz H I: 161, 322, 359, 708, 732, 774, 852, 1007
Lichtenau L: 3058
Lichtenstein J E: 3257
Lichtman D: 1795
Lichtman J B: 2136
Liddell R M: 1122
Lieberman A: 3744
Lieberman J M: 1597
Liebermann D: 917
Lieberson R: 3256
Liebman R: 2213
Lien H H: 2057, 2313, 2458, 3691
Lienemann A: 3101
Lierse W: 1551
Lilja A: 3692
Lilleas F G: 3015
Lillington G: 793
Lim E V: 2666
Lim G M: 1123
Lim J H: 1277, 1418
Lim T H: 2076
Limpert J D: 4038
Lin A S: 439
Lin F: 3347, 3955
Lin G: 1124, 1982
Lin Greenberg A: 2957
Lin J C: 4049
Lin J P: 2708, 2709, 3744
Linares L A: 3532
Lincoln A J: 3984
Lind J A Jr: 2079
Lindecken K D: 1109
Lindell M M: 3111
Lindell M M Jr: 2554, 2609
Lindemann S R: 878
Linden B E: 3326
Lindenberg R: 3666
Linder M: 2190
Lindfors K K: 803, 2617, 3693, 3735
Lindgren R D: 1941
Lindner P: 1904
Lindquist T: 2929
Lines M: 2893
Ling A: 638
Ling D: 265, 1058, 2016, 2214
Lingeman R E: 739
Lingg G: 2092, 2958, 3004, 3395, 3694
Linggood R M: 803
Linke G: 23, 24, 138, 636
Lipinski J K: 1040, 3695
Lipper M H: 3289
Lipson S J: 3180
Lipton M: 505, 3278
Lipton M J: 276, 277, 455, 456,

490, 493, 500, 501, 508, 512, 542, 543, 615
Lipuma J P: 36, 232, 1135, 2149, 2246
Lis L E: 2274
Lisberg W N: 3828
Liss A: 2642
Lissner J: 502, 503, 794, 879, 1870, 3101
Lisson G: 3696
Listerud J A: 3952
Litt A W: 480
Littleton J T: 775
Littman P S: 2551
Litwiller T: 80
Livingston R R: 111, 2663
Livingstone A S: 1416
Llauger J: 788, 1953
Llewellyn H J: 878
Lloyd K: 1988
Lloyd R: 1873
Lo J: 1598
Lo W W: 3697, 3967
Lobeck H: 2570
Lobo N: 2094, 3010
Lochner B: 138, 776, 1369, 2424, 2959, 3357, 3358
Lochner R: 576
Loddenkemper R: 776, 943
Loeffler M: 2630
Loehr E: 3112
Loffler E: 3698
Lohlein D: 1555
Lohr E: 2505, 3097, 3765, 3766
Lohr H: 73
Loisance D: 790
London D A: 3978, 3979
London S S: 1367, 1417, 1964, 2026, 2158
Long D M: 4105
Long J A Jr: 777, 1125, 2007, 2177
Long R W: 951
Long W D: 1742
Longley D G: 1430
Longmaid H E: 1126
Longo J M: 1127
Longo M: 1191, 1451
Loop J W: 240, 2900
Lopez P: 2891
Lopez Rasines G J: 1127
Lorcher U: 778
Lorentzen J E: 485, 2433
Lorenz R: 1311, 1599, 1792, 1815, 1948, 2275, 2428
Lorenz W J: 736
Loriaux D L: 2178, 2179
Lorigan J G: 1007
Lorman J G: 2114
Lorphelin J M: 1143, 1150
Lotan D: 2140
Lotz P R: 3773
Loudenslager D M: 1247
Loughlin T: 2178
Louis D S: 3130
Louis O: 2891
Louvet J P: 1436
Love L: 227, 333, 1793, 2077, 2078, 2079, 2232, 2507
Love M B: 2381, 2830
Love S: 3985
Lovrencic M: 3699
Low R N: 1600
Lowe J E: 570
Lower R R: 524
Lowka K: 2791
Lowrey C E: 2805
Lowry L D: 3992
Lozada C: 549
Lozman J: 2970
Lubat E: 713, 1794, 2429
Lubbers D J: 1444
Lubbers M J: 1975
Lubbers P R: 1795
Lubrano J M: 1452, 1622, 2101
Luburich P: 1128
Lucas D: 2635, 2637
Lucas P R: 3819
Luck S R: 3400
Luckener H G: 465

Luckner H: 177
Ludwig B: 3700
Ludwigsen B: 1993
Luethke J M: 3560
Luetmer P H: 1431, 1432
Luetzeler J: 180
Lufkin R B: 1594, 3587, 3600
Luhrs M: 2613
Luisiri A: 3146
Luk K H: 3953
Lukas P: 1898
Lukaszewski B: 2656
Luken M G: 3189, 3667
Lukens J A: 2610
Lullig H: 811
Lundell C: 861, 2227
Lunderquist A: 155, 1124
Luning M: 707, 1129, 1170, 1424, 2215, 2459
Lunsford L D: 3676
Luoma A A: 488
Lupetin A R: 261, 1796, 1859, 2080
Lupo L: 1485
Lusins J O: 2960
Luska G: 1312
Lussier A: 3302
Lutgemeier J: 2276, 2316, 3701
Lutz R J: 1158
Lutzeler A: 758
Lynch D: 925
Lynch D A: 779, 780, 781
Lynch J C: 306
Lynch J H: 2163, 2223
Lynch M A: 1797
Lynch R: 3521
Lynn M D: 2611

Maas R: 2285
Macarini L: 133, 134, 1485
Maccarty R L: 1323
Macchia G: 2696
Macdonald I L: 487
Macgregor J M: 280
Machida K: 323
Machida T: 1086, 2037, 2674
Macintyre N R: 605
Macintyre W: 36
Mack L A: 240, 2837, 2900, 2961, 2962, 2994, 3032, 3952, 3953, 3954
Macmillan R M: 544, 557, 558
Macovski A: 75, 76, 3309
Macpherson P: 3702
Macrander S J: 1130
Macsweeney J E: 579
Maddison F E: 229
Maddrey W C: 1242
Madgar I: 2168
Madrazo B L: 362, 363, 848, 950, 1601
Madsen K: 195
Maeda H: 1163, 1164, 1165, 1612, 2219, 3750
Maeda T: 1165
Maeshima S: 2282
Mafee M: 3550, 3762
Mafee M F: 2963, 3703, 3704
Magaram D L: 3967
Magarik D E: 2382
Magid D: 30, 83, 101, 782, 1729, 1798, 1949, 2349, 2489, 2506, 2574, 2767, 2786, 2787, 2916, 2964, 2965, 2966, 2985, 3208, 3475, 3861
Magill H L: 1799, 2102
Magilner A D: 151
Magin E: 2189
Magnaes B: 2839
Magnus D E: 3936
Magnuson J E: 1433
Magnussen H: 767, 869, 913
Magrath I T: 2060
Magruder Habib K: 294
Maguire G Q: 1588
Maguire J H: 2540
Mah K: 783
Mahboubi S: 2612, 2622, 2967, 3575
Mahmalat M O: 3093

Mahoney L T: 510
Mahoney M C: 2968
Mahoney P D: 1773
Mahony B: 1950
Mahony B S: 397
Mai A: 1424
Maier W: 156, 1434, 1435, 3705
Mail J T: 2613
Maile C W: 1119, 1520, 1541
Mainwaring B L: 2080
Maitrot D: 3392
Majer M: 2906
Majesky I F: 783
Majewski A: 1131, 2614
Majurin M L: 167
Makela P: 1420
Makino H: 3164
Makita K: 1084, 1085, 1086
Maklad N F: 2607
Makuuchi M: 1099, 1233
Malanson D: 3943
Malat J: 1227
Malave S R: 255
Malbec L: 217, 2345
Mali W P: 116, 3376
Malis L I: 3002
Malkin J: 2913
Mall J C: 1719, 1951, 2014, 2252
Mallens W M: 2466
Malone A J Jr: 2005
Maltby J D: 784
Malvar T C: 1443
Mameletzis K: 3619
Man S W: 1274
Manaster B J: 2969
Mancer K: 2569, 3377
Mancici M C: 3547
Manco Johnson M L: 1280
Manco L G: 2970, 2971
Mancuso A: 3512
Mancuso A A: 261, 293, 2639, 2997, 3337, 3514
Mandelbaum B R: 2964
Mandell D M: 3997
Mandell V S: 1806, 1962
Mandon V: 2224
Manelfe C: 1436, 3291, 3292, 3346, 3706
Manfrini M: 2578
Mangano F A: 2081
Mangkuwerdojo S: 2238
Mani J R: 1366, 3819
Mani R K: 1877
Mankin H J: 2631, 3071
Mann F A: 2972, 3707
Mann H: 3708, 3709
Mann J H: 1715
Mansfeld L: 2082
Mansfield C M: 3682
Mansoory A: 2486
Mantello M T: 324
Mantravadi R: 825
Manz H J: 3390
Maranhao V: 544
Maravilla K R: 74, 1695, 2973
Marc J A: 3710
Marcelis S: 853
Marchal G: 97, 968, 998, 1486, 1596, 1685, 1800, 1980, 2238, 2425, 2460
Marchal G J: 1132
Marchal W: 1459
Marchand E P: 3816
Marchoski J A: 3749
Marciniak H: 2082
Marcos J: 1039
Marcu H: 4042
Marcus F S: 989, 1166
Margolin F R: 2746, 3428
Margolis M T: 3290
Margulis A R: 337, 338, 1168, 1546, 1615, 1656, 3434, 3711
Marin Grez M: 1801
Marin M L: 2974
Marincek B: 437, 1008, 1133, 1134, 1802, 1884, 1885, 2615, 2975
Mark A S: 1803
Markisz J A: 1672
Markivee C: 1893

Markoe A M: 3821
Markowitz A M: 2974
Markowitz L: 2462
Markowitz R I: 2627
Markowitz S K: 1965, 2368, 2391
Marks B: 3665
Marks B W: 785
Marks G: 1628
Marks W: 1115
Marks W M: 1028, 1029, 1030, 1031, 1384, 1385, 1540, 1804, 2434
Marlowe F I: 3996, 3999
Marmor J B: 88
Marn C S: 1123, 1550, 1602, 1952, 2711, 3496
Marsan B: 333
Marsan R E: 227
Marsault C: 3317
Marsh J L: 4034
Marshall C: 3221
Marshall C H: 837
Marshall F F: 2054
Marshall W: 75, 3935
Marshall W H: 127, 3420
Marshall W H Jr: 76
Martel W: 2471, 2548, 2701
Martelli A: 3712
Marti Bonmati L: 786
Martens F: 3172
Martin C: 787
Martin D J: 1371, 3243, 3425
Martin D S: 3252
Martin E C: 2170
Martin F: 1041
Martin J: 787, 1805
Martin J B: 3301
Martin L F: 251
Martin N: 2023, 3713
Martin R: 1453
Martin R E: 1374
Martinelli C: 3161
Martinez C R: 937, 2388
Martinez S: 2577, 2629, 2976, 3045
Martini N: 701, 3531, 3532
Martino C R: 1135
Maruyama M: 1407, 3617
Marx M: 3714
Marx S: 2764
Marx S J: 252, 253
Marzoli G P: 1041
Mascalchi M: 3375
Masciocchi C: 3021, 3022, 3023
Masdeu J C: 3715, 3716
Masler J A: 467
Mason T O: 3717
Massry S G: 2523
Mast G J: 2006
Mastrodomenico L: 2083
Masuda F: 2037
Masuda K: 1665, 3518
Masuzaki S: 1072
Masuzawa T: 3718
Mata J: 1953
Mata J M: 786, 788, 1805
Mata M I: 1723
Matalon T A: 183, 569, 1171, 1172
Mather D: 919
Matherne G P: 510
Matheson M: 3695
Mathias K: 3719
Mathieson J R: 789, 817
Mathieu D: 442, 790, 1136, 1137, 1138, 1139, 1140, 1141, 1142, 1143, 1239, 1954, 2935, 2936
Mathis A: 3221
Mathis J M: 191
Matozzi F: 2977, 3038
Matsen F A: 2560, 3954
Matsuda H: 3893
Matsuda M: 755
Matsui A: 3573
Matsui O: 305, 1102, 1144, 1145, 1146, 1147, 1250, 1251
Matsumoto A H: 791, 3264
Matsumoto M: 2383
Matsumura K: 379
Matsunaga N: 2147

Matsuo T: 1318
Matsuoka O: 3579
Matsuoka Y: 1163
Matsushima K: 2616
Matsuura H: 1073, 2049
Matsuura K: 355, 1592, 2093, 3781
Matsuzawa T: 3662
Mattrey R: 523
Mattrey R F: 157, 158, 439, 529
Mattsson T A: 3944
Mauceri R A: 872
Maul G: 3832
Maurer D E: 434
Maurice F: 686
Mauro M: 1760
Mauro M A: 999, 1488, 1806, 1962, 2084, 2107, 3590
Maus T P: 1562
Mawad M E: 2803, 2978, 3748
Mawko G: 3816
Mawson J B: 817
May G R: 2660
May M: 2744, 3373
Mayberg H S: 3666
Mayekawa D: 2393
Mayer D P: 1673, 2085, 3516
Mayer J: 1010
Maynard F W: 3471
Mayo J: 416
Mayo J R: 77, 789, 792, 793
Mayo Smith W: 3071, 3720, 3721, 3874
Mayr A C: 2341
Mayr B: 794, 795, 796, 1870, 2979
Mayr U: 1, 4066
Mazess R B: 2940
Mazzoleni F: 1714
Mc Clennan B L: 2016
Mc Connell J R: 1860
Mc Cormack P M: 3531
Mc Donnell M J: 3845
Mcadams H P: 545, 3722
Mcafee P C: 4105
Mcalister W H: 3723, 4034
Mcallister M D: 3724
Mcaninch J W: 2014, 2015, 2252
Mcardle C: 2143
Mcardle C B: 3742
Mcarthur K: 1423
Mccain A H: 1148
Mccann R: 2454
Mccarron J P: 2312
Mccarthy M J: 1508
Mccarthy S: 159, 1437, 2350, 2848
Mccarthy S M: 1803, 1807, 2524
Mccartney W H: 1638, 3110
Mccarty D J: 3599
Mccaughan B C: 701
Mccauley D I: 348, 480, 713, 826, 827, 828, 829, 832, 833, 837, 942, 3040
Mccauslin M A: 306
Mcclellan R L: 3725
Mcclennan B L: 68, 1309, 2011, 2029, 2084, 2086, 2107, 2150, 2191, 2314, 2340, 2426, 2945, 3603
Mcclure P H: 2401
Mccomb B L: 3046
Mccomb J G: 4094
Mcconnell B J: 1197
Mccormack J: 3726
Mccormack P M: 701
Mccormick J F: 2064
Mccormick T L: 1633
Mccort J J: 3727
Mccowin M J: 1438
Mccracken S: 288
Mccray P: 262
Mccrea E S: 467
Mccreath G: 3695
Mccullough D C: 3498, 3904
Mccullough E C: 78, 94, 3409
Mcdaniel E C: 191
Mcdonnell C H: 1149
Mcelvein R B: 618

Mcgahan J P: 797, 2380, 2769, 2980, 3636
Mcginley J A: 3669
Mcginnis B: 2617
Mcginnis B D: 3728
Mcguire C: 3272
Mcguire C W: 2046
Mchugh K: 798
Mciff E B: 3850
Mcilhenny J: 3572
Mcintyre W J: 79
Mckinney J M: 2838
Mcknight R C: 410
Mckusick M A: 1231
Mckusker S: 3964
Mclaughlin A P: 2004
Mclean G K: 3658
Mclean I W: 3948
Mclendon R E: 651
Mcleod A J: 1808
Mcleod R A: 1580, 1899, 2610, 2653, 2660, 3919
Mclone D G: 3433, 4026
Mcloud T: 685
Mcloud T C: 213, 336, 388, 393, 406, 631, 799, 803, 912
Mcloughlin M J: 2184, 3729
Mcloughlin M L: 856
Mcmahan J R: 3284
Mcmanus R P: 365
Mcmillan J H: 2216
Mcmillin K: 1313
Mcmillin K I: 2277, 2548
Mcmonigle E M: 3967
Mcmurdo S K: 2738
Mcnary W F: 2686
Mcneil B J: 926, 959, 1402, 1855, 2169, 3730
Mcniesh L M: 2981
Mcvary K T: 2248
Mcvay L: 1465
Mcvay L V: 1481
Meadows A T: 2551, 3365
Meaney T F: 79
Mears D C: 2716
Meary E: 217
Medinilla O R: 3709
Medjek L: 3392
Meencke H J: 3917
Meenen N M: 2741
Meese W: 3731
Megibow A: 1489, 1497, 1925, 2172
Megibow A J: 160, 308, 830, 831, 1160, 1355, 1357, 1461, 1490, 1491, 1492, 1493, 1494, 1495, 1565, 1566, 1588, 1603, 1604, 1605, 1606, 1607, 1688, 1759, 1794, 1809, 1958, 1983, 2109, 2142, 2217, 2230, 2324, 2384, 2385, 2429, 2453, 2553
Megret M: 3387, 3388
Mehdizadeh H M: 3807
Mehler M F: 3732
Mehnert P J: 3984
Mehringer C M: 2734, 4027
Mehta A: 1977
Mehta R C: 2982
Meier P: 1061
Meier W L: 405
Meilstrup J W: 306
Meire D: 3172
Meisler W: 3192
Melanccon D: 2699
Melange M: 1659
Melanson D: 2654
Melchart G: 3408
Melcher J: 2632
Meller S: 3269
Mellone R: 1372
Melnick G S: 1810
Melrose B L: 977
Melson G L: 1261, 1783, 2107, 2150, 2207
Melville G E: 3794
Melzer G: 649, 752
Memeo V: 1485
Menck J: 4025
Mende U: 1103, 3064
Mendelsohn D B: 2563

Mendelsohn S L: 800, 2788
Mendelson D: 2586
Mendelson D S: 230, 325, 801, 1930, 1955, 2478, 3733
Mendelson H: 3300
Mendez D R: 3831
Mendez G Jr: 2461
Mendoza A S: 2718, 3212
Menke W: 3089, 3090
Menkes C J: 2815
Menu Y: 443, 686, 1143, 1150
Meranze S: 2462
Meranze S G: 1234
Mercader J: 2983
Merine D: 1151, 1152, 1314, 1608, 1609, 2278, 2984, 2985, 2986
Merine D S: 3734
Merkle N: 518
Merle M: 518
Mero J H: 1286
Merrick S H: 336
Merx J L: 2541
Mesgarzadeh M: 2987
Meshkov S L: 146, 1811
Metreweli C: 3962
Mettler D: 1133
Mettler F A Jr: 3, 1636
Metz C E: 1033
Metz V: 1043
Metzger H: 1117, 2463, 4059
Metzger H O: 49
Metzger J: 145
Metzger R A: 802
Meurman K O: 3126
Mewissen M W: 432
Meyer G A: 2748
Meyer Galander H M: 2992
Meyer H J: 1555
Meyer J: 576, 3487
Meyer J D: 2988
Meyer J E: 803, 1610, 1956, 2617, 3648, 3693, 3735
Meyer J S: 3577, 3640
Meyer Pannwitt U: 1279
Meyer W H: 2249
Meyers M A: 1611, 1793
Meyers P C: 1037
Meyers W C: 1458, 1655
Meziane M: 1314
Meziane M A: 546, 597, 711, 2087
Meziane M M: 747
Mezwa D G: 1532
Mezzacappa P M: 3737
Michalis A: 519
Michelson J D: 2965
Michelson W J: 3189, 3957
Michelucci R: 2549
Michielsen P: 1910
Michotey P: 2977
Micklos T J: 1662, 3738
Middleton W D: 1024, 1315, 3739
Mieza M: 2279
Miguet J P: 1000
Mihara K: 2363
Miketic L M: 2725
Miki T: 2281
Mikulis D: 2485
Mikulis D J: 1153
Mikuta J I: 2374
Milan M: 3009
Mildenberger P: 1216
Miles S G: 80
Millard J C: 145
Millen S J: 3350
Miller B L: 1169
Miller C: 4094
Miller C A: 958
Miller C L: 1242, 3740
Miller D: 1006
Miller D C: 3474
Miller D L: 253, 804, 1154, 1155, 1156, 1157, 1158, 1206, 1812, 2178, 2179, 2180
Miller E M: 2707
Miller F J Jr: 1662
Miller G A Jr: 326
Miller J: 3474

Miller J D: 2727, 2989, 3386
Miller J W: 1316
Miller K D Jr: 2306
Miller L R: 2136
Miller M H: 433, 2807
Miller M K: 4009
Miller M T: 2963
Miller P A: 805
Miller P R: 2039
Miller R H: 3320
Miller R R: 411, 769, 814, 815, 816, 819, 883, 893, 901, 938
Miller S: 3956
Miller S A: 1990
Miller S H: 2094, 3010
Miller S M: 2480
Miller S W: 287, 336
Miller W: 258, 590
Miller W T: 373, 643
Milligan V A: 3418
Mills C M: 3555
Mills R P: 3987
Mills S R: 1125
Millward S F: 547
Milon P: 3670
Minagi H: 614, 1938
Minami M: 1088, 1089, 1439
Minami R: 82
Mindell H J: 2088, 2089
Mindelzun R E: 2045, 2542
Miner D G: 3741
Mink J H: 2752, 3033
Minkoff J: 3041, 3042
Minor G R: 805
Mintz M: 2296, 2462
Mintz M C: 19, 1996, 2352, 2386, 2736, 3370, 3625
Minutoli A: 1813, 2446
Miraldi F: 36
Mirfakhraee M: 147, 2491, 3476
Mirich D R: 1814, 3742
Mirk P: 3438
Mirkin L D: 2613
Mirra J M: 2639
Mirvis S: 327
Mirvis S E: 328, 329, 330, 376, 516, 806, 1159, 1316, 1957, 1961
Mitani T: 755
Mitchell D G: 1440, 2386, 2432, 2990
Mitchell M: 3722
Mitchell S E: 586, 1317, 2159
Mitnick J S: 1160, 1958, 2217, 3743, 3744
Mitomo M: 3517
Mitsuoka A: 331
Mittal B B: 890
Mittelstaedt C A: 1464, 1962
Mittleman D: 2963
Mitty H A: 1930, 2218, 2280, 2774
Mitzkat H J: 1387
Mitzner A: 3531
Miura K: 1176, 1177
Miura S: 1333, 2919
Miura T: 1070, 1176, 1177, 3517
Miyake H: 1165, 1318, 1612, 2219
Miyamoto T: 2357, 3580
Miyasaka K: 2991
Miyata S: 934, 1251
Miyazaki N: 838
Miyazawa N: 808
Mizumoto S: 1818
Mizunuma K: 2408
Mizutani M: 2293
Mnaymneh W: 2646, 2647
Mockbee B: 2012
Modder U: 740, 1425, 1441, 1599, 1735, 1815, 1948, 2221, 2275, 2428, 3777, 4092, 4093
Modic M T: 548, 3065, 3745
Moeller G: 775
Moes N: 340
Moffat R E: 1595
Moguillansky S J: 549
Molde A: 2096, 2153
Moldofsky P J: 662, 3466, 3467
Molina P L: 274, 275

Molitor B: 2062
Molitor J: 2515
Mollet E: 3393
Molliver M E: 3666
Momose K J: 2617, 3794
Mompoint D: 443, 616, 617, 3713
Monajati A: 3557
Moncada R: 227, 332, 333, 549, 1793, 2507
Monden Y: 404
Montag J P: 2210
Montagno E D: 3746
Montag M: 1010, 2992, 2993
Montag T: 2992
Montagne J P: 2210
Montalvo B M: 3119
Montana M: 2547
Montana M A: 2994
Monteferrante M: 1613
Montemayor K A: 1889, 1890
Montes M: 1940
Moody A R: 1614
Moody D M: 3675
Moody M: 806
Moon H R: 3349
Moon K L Jr: 1161, 3747
Mooney N: 2973
Moor W C: 3418
Moore A D: 807
Moore A V: 5, 334, 514, 515, 1966, 2183, 2629, 3551
Moore A V Jr: 326, 1850
Moore E H: 213, 335, 336, 912
Moore J O: 2436
Moore M M: 81
Moore S: 2929, 3792
Moore T: 3748
Moore T S: 2106
Morag B: 2090
Morales E: 3664
Moran C J: 2999, 3749
Moran J F: 668
Morano J U: 2300, 2508
Moreau J J: 2977
Morehouse H: 1162, 1346
Morehouse H T: 766, 1319, 1517, 2330
Moreira F A: 3246
Morgan J A: 574
Morgan R H: 936
Morgello S: 3389
Mori H: 1163, 1164, 1165, 1318, 3750
Mori K: 808, 1057, 3751
Mori M: 809
Mori S: 1065, 1066
Mori Y: 1736
Moriarty P E: 324
Morillo G: 2646
Morimoto S: 309, 404, 425, 582, 583, 585, 716
Morimoto T: 3893
Morin R L: 78
Morinaga K: 584, 585
Moritz E: 693
Moriuchi A: 2219
Moriyama N: 1173
Morris D C: 2509
Morris H H: 3306
Morris J: 3542
Morris J A Jr: 1913
Morris J H: 3181, 4050
Morris J M: 2728, 2928, 3127
Morris M E: 2560
Morris R E: 3752
Morris U L: 810
Morrison G: 3232
Morrison H: 2056
Morrison H S: 2167
Morrison M C: 2618
Morrison S C: 963, 2034
Moscatello A L: 3125
Moschini M: 3366
Moseley I: 3753
Moseley I F: 3754
Moser F: 2933
Moser F G: 3490
Moser R P: 3685
Moshenipour I: 2829
Moskos M M: 2618

Moskovitz P: 3029
Moss A: 3792
Moss A A: 86, 107, 159, 337, 338, 596, 629, 967, 1013, 1038, 1081, 1115, 1166, 1167, 1168, 1201, 1302, 1320, 1367, 1406, 1417, 1437, 1442, 1468, 1469, 1512, 1544, 1546, 1561, 1615, 1650, 1656, 1704, 1719, 1743, 1803, 1804, 1807, 1942, 1964, 2158, 2195, 2210, 2258, 2307, 2345, 2346, 2350, 2363, 2447, 3328, 3428, 3515, 3916, 3952, 3978, 3979, 4075
Moss G D: 1443
Mostbeck G: 704, 2123
Mostowfi K: 2334
Mostrom U: 2995, 3755, 3756
Motomura S: 2870
Mouelhi M M: 617
Moulton J S: 1169, 1444
Moutsopoulos H M: 194
Moyers J H: 1183
Mrose H E: 878
Muchmore H G: 2239
Mudge K: 3087
Muecke E C: 2170
Mueller C F: 847
Mueller P R: 440, 895, 1470, 1476, 1511, 1816, 1817, 1831, 1891, 2619, 3440, 4072
Muhlbacher F: 1220
Muhlberger V: 339, 340, 341
Muhler A: 1170
Muhling T: 342
Muhm J R: 715, 937
Mukai J K: 1171, 1172
Mukai K: 1233
Mukhopadhyay S: 581
Mulhern C B Jr: 358, 662, 802, 2105, 2315, 2374, 2551
Muller C: 1934
Muller H A: 811, 2996, 3089, 3090
Muller H H: 127
Muller J: 1281, 3923
Muller J W: 3757
Muller M: 284, 3497
Muller Miny H: 2700
Muller N: 416, 2509
Muller N L: 77, 131, 343, 345, 411, 488, 602, 603, 675, 769, 789, 793, 807, 812, 813, 814, 815, 816, 817, 818, 819, 883, 893, 901, 912, 928, 938, 939, 1445
Muller R P: 1017, 1382, 2024, 2445
Muller Rensing R: 2024
Muller S: 707
Muller Schauenburg W: 4040
Mulligan S A: 2464
Mullin D: 1616
Mulvaney J A: 148
Munch O: 3101
Munda R: 1444
Munderloh S H: 3122
Mundt C: 3484
Mundth E D: 282
Munechika H: 344, 2465
Munk P L: 345, 1445, 3542, 3758, 3759
Munoz Gomez J: 2983
Munoz S J: 1242
Munro N C: 820
Munzenrider J: 3794
Munzenrider J E: 3693
Murai Y: 2870
Murakami J: 346, 1480
Murakami M: 1171, 1172
Murakami Y: 1409
Muraki A S: 2997, 3049, 3514, 3558
Muramatsu Y: 1173, 1233
Murata K: 821, 822, 823
Murata R: 3579
Murayama S: 717, 1097, 1174
Muresan L V: 3816
Murphey M D: 2946
Murphy B J: 2646, 2647

Murphy F B: 347, 1175, 2141, 2415
Murphy Irwin K: 2777, 3420
Murphy R J: 3784
Murphy W A: 772, 946, 2567, 2583, 2599, 2750, 2773, 2835, 3199, 3760
Murray D R: 1182
Murray J A: 2479, 2566, 2609
Murray K: 3761
Murray W: 2497, 3036
Murry R C: 74
Murtagh F R: 3837
Musante F: 1321, 2220
Musgrave M A: 3929, 3930
Musset D: 686, 824
Muta T: 1318
Mutschler W: 2858, 3060
Muzzio P C: 980
Myers J: 391
Myers J L: 889
Myung K H: 4064

Nabawi P: 825, 3762
Nachbur B: 437, 1802
Nacianceno S E: 1446
Nadel S N: 396, 409, 1353
Nadjmi M: 3923
Naegele M: 3101
Nagae T: 2293
Nagai H: 1408
Nagao H: 3893
Nagashima C: 2998
Nagashima T: 964
Nagata Y: 2257, 3554, 3763
Nagatomo H: 2219
Nagayama Y: 354
Nagel J S: 2540
Nagel K: 1216
Nagorney D M: 1323
Nahakara K: 404
Naheedy M H: 3072, 3253, 3511, 3764, 4057
Nahser H C: 2503, 3765, 3766
Nahum H: 443, 686, 1150, 3713
Naidich D: 1489, 1925
Naidich D P: 308, 348, 349, 480, 713, 807, 826, 827, 828, 829, 830, 831, 832, 833, 834, 835, 836, 837, 937, 942, 1355, 1492, 1494, 1565, 1604, 1607, 1652, 1759, 2217, 3191
Naidich T P: 2999, 3000, 3241, 3433, 3465, 3749, 3768, 3769, 3884, 3992, 4011, 4026
Naidu S: 3666
Naim Ur Rahman: 3770
Naimark A: 2535
Nakada T: 3001, 3240
Nakagawa H: 3002, 3003
Nakagawa S: 1074
Nakahara K: 309
Nakajima M: 3771
Nakajima Y: 1179, 1232
Nakamoto S K: 440
Nakamura H: 1818, 3517
Nakanishi K: 716
Nakano N: 309
Nakano T: 379
Nakano Y: 82, 1057, 1618, 2409, 2410
Nakao N: 1176, 1177
Nakashima A: 1165
Nakasu S: 3771
Nakata H: 350, 838, 839, 1174, 1447, 2870
Nakata K: 1178
Nakaya S: 1333
Nakayama C: 350
Nakayama T: 350, 838, 839, 1179, 1447
Nakazima H: 2357
Nakstad P: 2091, 3772
Nalesnik W J: 2335
Namba K: 3580
Nanni D: 3773
Narayan R: 2309
Nardi G L: 1476
Nardi P: 3834
Nardi P M: 1322, 1819

Nardis P F: 3774
Narimatsu Y: 4082
Narita N: 844
Naritomi H: 3617
Narumi Y: 755, 2281, 2282
Naseem M: 2949
Nash G: 448
Nashold B S: 3407
Nassi M: 495, 4089
Nath P H: 618
Nathan R: 3669
Nau H E: 2503, 3766
Naucnauck C J: 1853
Nauert C: 2947nauert C: 2947
Nauta R J: 1254
Navarro J E: 3047
Naveh Y: 2882
Nazarian S: 2977, 3038
Neal R K: 4077
Nealey P: 2112
Neave V C: 3775
Nebel G: 550, 1629, 2092, 2756, 3004, 3395
Nedelkov G: 2754
Needleman L: 1242
Neff C C: 351, 440, 441, 1476
Neff J R: 1787, 2607, 2946, 3006
Neglia W: 762
Negoro M: 3641
Neidl E: 2302
Neiman H L: 118, 183, 233, 255, 1550, 2456, 3173
Nejatheim M: 352
Nelems B: 411, 488, 883
Nelson C L: 2520
Nelson H S Jr: 1617
Nelson J: 3776
Nelson J A: 3263
Nelson P C: 3861
Nelson R: 3257
Nelson R C: 1180, 1181, 1182, 1183, 1688, 2141
Nemcek A A Jr: 890
Nemeck A A: 3496
Nemeth L: 709
Nepper Rasmussen J: 3005
Nesbit D: 3006
Nesbit D E: 3347
Nesbit G M: 1323
Neufang K F: 353, 526, 2211, 3777
Neuman M J: 3809
Neumann C: 220
Neumann C H: 1448, 1820, 1821
Neumann D: 3701
Neumann D R: 1822
Neumann G: 2221
Neumayer K: 840
Neumuller H: 2832
Nevelsteen A: 1703
Nevsimalova S: 1118
New P F: 3728, 3778, 3794
Newbold J M: 129
Newbold R: 2387
Newhouse J H: 1211, 2283, 2289, 2321
Newman A D: 2944
Newman C: 2826
Newman G E: 16, 3779
Newman L M: 459
Newman S A: 3571
Newmark H 3d: 2510
Newton T H: 3663, 3671, 3958, 3988
Ney C: 2284
Ney D R: 30, 83, 2489, 2787, 2965, 2966, 3475
Neylan J: 1358
Ng K K: 841
Ng S H: 841
Ngan H: 1686
Nichols D M: 812, 1823, 2509, 2809
Nicholson E: 698
Nickoloff E L: 551, 3007
Nicodeme C: 3806
Nicolas V: 315, 2222, 2285, 2604, 3780, 3913
Nicosia S V: 1202

Niederstadt T: 2684
Nielsen M E Jr: 842
Nieman L: 2178, 2179, 2180
Nieman L K: 638
Nienhuis A W: 777, 2177
Nienhus A W: 1125
Niethammer J G: 1617
Nieuwenhuizen Kruseman A C: 2185
Nieves A: 3401
Nijboer E W: 3008
Nijensohn E: 3009
Nijs H G: 1270
Nikesch W: 84
Niklason L T: 44, 3576
Nilsson U: 915
Nino Murcia M: 1184, 1959
Nishida Y: 1250
Nishidai T: 3763
Nishihara H: 1480
Nishimura K: 82, 822, 1618, 2409, 2410
Nishimura Y: 3554
Nishitani H: 355, 1249, 1592, 2093, 3781
Nishiyama Y: 452
Nishizawa S: 2293
Nixon G W: 3761
Nobe T: 350
Noda K: 2383
Noel J: 2797
Nokes S R: 2388
Noldge G: 3782
Noma S: 354, 821, 2411
Nomura F: 1185
Noon M A: 1186, 4089
Noorbehesht B: 3783
Norcus G: 1684
Noren G: 3519
Nori D: 3532
Norlindh S T: 150
Norman A: 2529, 2530
Norman D: 3278, 3663, 3671, 3958
Norregaard T: 3321
North R B: 3214
Norton J A: 253, 1381, 1423, 2179, 2180
Norton K: 2586
Norton K I: 2137, 3784
Norton L: 2137
Norton P: 1772
Noseworthy J: 1771
Nosil J: 3135
Nostrant C H: 1410
Nostrant T T: 1602
Noterman J: 2680
Noto A M: 2286, 2529, 2530, 2687
Noujaim S: 1532
Nov A A: 3785
Novetsky G J: 1449, 2094, 3010
Novotny E Jr: 3935
Noz M E: 1588
Nugent R A: 520, 2747, 2934, 3847
Numaguchi Y: 1592
Nunley J A: 2577
Nussbaum A: 1960, 2095
Nussbaum A R: 3734
Nussel F: 2873
Nusslin F: 4039
Nutz V: 3011
Nyberg D A: 212, 1762, 1824, 3012
Nyberg G: 3274
Nyman U: 1288, 1640, 2096, 2151, 2152, 2153, 2253
Nyman U R: 150

O Brien P C: 2165
O Brien W M: 2223
O Callaghan J P: 552, 3013
O Carroll C P: 3778
O Connell D M: 680
O Connor G D: 2807
O Doherty D S: 2511
O Donnell P C: 3998
O Donovan P B: 613, 2188
O Leary D H: 3724

Niederstadt T: 2684
O Leary J F: 1386
O Leary T: 1963
O Leary T J: 1156
O Mara E M: 3787
O Neill B P: 3586
O Reilly G V: 3179, 3511, 3764, 4050
Obara T: 1074
Oberbauer R W: 4019
Obermann W R: 2899
Obermuller J: 3431
Obletter N: 2706
Obringer A C: 3365
Ochi H: 3579
Ochi K: 2161
Ochiai T: 1185
Oddson T A: 594
Odel J: 4030
Oechler H W: 3920
Oei T K: 932, 1187
Oeser H: 927
Oesterreich F U: 3014
Oestmann J: 685
Offutt C J: 4034
Ofori Kwakye S K: 4048
Ogata M: 3580
Ogawa K: 3781
Ogawa M: 3617
Oh Y K: 3632
Ohanna F: 2884, 2885
Ohara T: 657
Ohashi I: 2641
Ohba T: 2093
Ohe H: 3207
Ohe N: 3207
Ohhashi K: 1409
Ohishi H: 844, 1344
Ohman S O: 3944
Ohmori K: 2871
Ohmoto K: 1246
Ohnishi K: 1179, 1185
Ohshima M: 2410
Ohshima T: 1318
Ohto M: 1442
Ohtomo K: 1082, 1084, 1085, 1086, 1088, 1089, 1105, 1301, 1408, 1409, 1439, 3645
Ohumi T: 1246
Ohyama N: 3458
Ohyama Y: 1075
Oiko Y: 3164
Okada K: 354
Okada Y: 1084, 1086
Okajima K: 3763
Okrent D H: 248
Oksanen V: 3623
Okuda K: 1179, 1185
Okuda Y: 379
Okudera H: 85
Okumura T: 1333, 3003
Okuno T: 3751
Okuyama A: 808
Olanow W: 334
Olazabal A: 1805
Oldendorf W H: 3789
Oldenkott P: 2914
Oldfield E: 2178
Oldfield E H: 2753
Oldham K T: 1771
Olier J: 3790
Oliff M: 2873
Oliphant M: 1825
Oliva L: 2287
Oliveira G G: 3864, 3865
Olivier A: 3816
Ollier P: 443
Olliff J F: 2260
Ollinger G: 238
Olm M: 3791
Olmsted W W: 1508
Oloff J: 3123, 3124
Oloff L M: 3123, 3124
Olson D L: 225, 2148
Olson M: 2097
Olson M C: 2079
Olson R: 1358
Olson W B: 1734
Olsson Y: 3692
Oltmann K: 2584

Omojola M F: 2620
Onik G: 86, 3542, 3792, 3793
Onishi T: 2037
Onitsuka H: 355, 1249, 1665, 2093
Ono H: 3313
Ono K: 3517
Ono M: 1249, 2093
Ono Y: 2468
Onouchi Z: 1071, 1072, 1073, 2049
Onoyama Y: 3579
Ontyd J: 559
Oon C L: 87
Oonishi M: 2357
Oot R F: 2621, 3735, 3794
Oppenheimer D A: 88, 89
Oppermann H C: 356
Opulencia J F: 1491
Oravez W T: 3577, 3640
Orbon R J: 2902
Orcutt J: 3795
Order S: 1151
Order S E: 1247
Ordonez N: 2325
Orel S G: 1619
Orellano L: 303, 315, 537, 561
Ormson M J: 1450, 3796
Oro J: 3165
Orphanoudakis S C: 2877
Orr J S: 3845
Orringer M B: 271, 370, 371, 513, 666, 688, 700, 855, 860, 951
Orrison W W: 3015, 3016, 3415, 3628
Ort P: 2784
Ortega E: 1190
Ortega J: 981, 3288
Ortega W: 2622
Ortore P G: 1507, 3017
Orwig D: 1826
Orwig D S: 1827
Osatavanichvong K: 179
Osborn A G: 1828, 2512, 2807, 2969, 3018, 3237, 3241, 3315, 3459, 3587, 3797, 3798
Osborn R E: 2513, 3049
Osborne D: 843, 2842, 3019, 3406
Osborne D R: 674, 3799
Osborne M: 2404
Oshima S: 822
Oshita A K: 215
Oshiumi Y: 1480
Osik A: 80
Ossoff R H: 234
Osteaux M: 1933, 2681, 2891
Osteaux M J: 853
Ostertag H: 933
Ostiz Zubieta S: 997
Ostler D: 2807
Ostrow D: 901
Ostrow D N: 812, 814, 815, 817
Otero R R: 2400
Otsuji H: 844
Ott D J: 1515
Ottery F D: 2623
Otto R: 3800
Oudkerk M: 357
Ouimette M: 1502
Ous S: 2291, 2458
Outwater E: 1188, 2389
Ovenfors C O: 670
Overbosch E: 357
Overlack P: 768
Ow E P: 549
Owen J W: 367
Owens D B: 1397
Owens F J: 1396
Owens G R: 358
Oxenstierna G: 3273
Oyama Y: 553
Oyen R: 1910
Ozasa H: 2409, 2411
Ozdoba C: 4039

Paal G: 2605, 2915
Paar O: 3055, 3059, 3177
Packer R J: 3801, 4100

Paetau A: 3937
Pagani J J: 161, 359, 845, 1189, 1426, 1620, 2098, 2143, 2617, 3802, 3803
Page D L: 427
Pagola M A: 1127
Pagola Serrano M A: 1190
Pahira J J: 2081
Pahl W M: 3564
Pai S C: 841
Pais M J: 3151
Pajari R: 2041
Pakter R L: 1960, 3445
Palacio A: 787
Palazzo L: 443
Palestrant A M: 90
Paling M R: 554, 846, 2624, 3804
Palleske H: 3397
Palmaz J C: 3001
Palmer J: 788
Palmer P E: 2980
Palmer Sancho J A: 4005
Palmer T E: 238
Palmers Y: 2537
Palmieri A: 162, 3076
Palmieri P: 3408
Palmtag H: 2052
Palubinskas A J: 2262, 3916
Pampati M: 2669
Pampoulov L: 2754
Pan G: 3020
Panaccione J L: 324
Panders A K: 3334, 3335
Pandolfo I: 1191, 1451, 1621, 1829, 1830, 2390, 2446, 2625, 3460
Panella J S: 2248
Panicek D M: 2266, 3531
Paniel B J: 2345
Panjabi M M: 2772
Pannarale O: 1485
Pantelidis N: 2032
Panzer W: 91
Paoletti P: 2561
Papa J: 2644, 2645
Papaefthymiou G: 3136
Papanicolaou N: 1831, 2099, 2337
Papavasiliou C: 519, 3805
Papavassiliou C: 2263, 2814, 3034
Papavassiliou K: 3607
Papke R A: 3521
Paplanus S H: 3570
Pappas D: 1961
Paprocki T: 3553
Paquet K J: 1090
Pardes J C: 966
Pardes J G: 1192
Pare' J A: 3453
Parienty R: 1193, 1194
Parienty R A: 1452, 1622, 1623, 2100, 2101, 2317, 3806
Parikh V P: 1195, 1832
Parisi M: 187, 3807
Parisier S C: 3969
Parizel P: 1196
Parizel P M: 2621, 3172
Park C K: 360
Park J H: 310, 718, 722, 992, 1275
Park J M: 721
Park S H: 958, 4094
Park T S: 3572
Parker B R: 3203
Parker D L: 3963
Parker G D: 3813
Parker L A: 791, 999, 1962, 3590
Parkin J L: 3587
Parolini D: 1372
Partain C L: 2185, 3808
Parvey H R: 1121
Parvey L S: 163, 2102
Pasmantier M W: 2166
Pasquini U: 164, 4043
Pass H I: 638, 2180
Passariello R: 164, 1460, 1833, 3021, 3022, 3023
Passas V: 1834
Passerini A: 3481

Pastakia B: 1835, 1963, 3024
Pastyr O: 4078
Pate D: 2514, 2925, 3085
Patel D V: 3809
Patel J: 2800
Patel P S: 2318
Patel R: 2150
Patel R B: 2515
Patel S: 361, 1197, 1337, 2111, 3608
Patel S K: 2269, 2398
Patel V: 2251
Paterson H S: 1598
Patino J V: 1548
Patten R M: 2516, 2626
Patterson E A: 1789
Patton A S: 351
Paukku P: 2921
Paul D J: 847
Paul G J: 3984
Paulus D D: 1374
Paushter D M: 1198, 1253, 1977
Pauwels E K: 2556
Pavone P: 1459, 1460
Pawar S V: 2517
Pawlotsky Y: 2797
Pazmino P: 2103
Pearce K I: 3135
Pearlberg J L: 362, 363, 848, 849, 950, 1601, 2132
Pearlstein A E: 1822, 1990
Peartree R J: 2058
Pech P: 2518, 2688, 3025, 3052, 3274, 3755, 3768
Peck W W: 523, 3663
Peckham M J: 2310
Peckham N: 3553
Peclet M H: 1866
Pedersen H: 3810, 3811
Pedersen M L: 850
Pederson M E Jr: 3957
Pederson R T: 3904
Pedrosa C S: 1324, 1325, 1548, 1723
Peerless S J: 2892
Peiken S R: 1959
Peiser J: 3549
Pekanan P: 179, 419
Pelc N J: 3309
Pelizzari C A: 71
Pellegrini C A: 1437
Pellissier J F: 2502
Pelz D M: 3974
Pena F: 1039
Penco T: 153, 2953
Pendergrass T W: 2156
Penn R D: 3844
Pennes D R: 951, 3026, 3027, 3028, 3787
Penninckx F: 1703
Penning L: 2772, 3008, 3197
Pennisi A K: 3029
Penry J K: 3675
Pentea S: 2263
Pentecost M: 3839
Pentlow K S: 92
Pepe R G: 3852
Pera A: 1836
Perani D: 3812
Pereira J R: 3825
Peretz G S: 2104
Perez C A: 3833
Perez D J: 3270
Peri J: 2661
Perkerson R B Jr: 1199
Perkins D D: 3643
Perlick E: 2531, 2632
Perlman S B: 2982
Perlman S J: 960
Perlmutter G S: 146
Perman W H: 551
Perret R: 238
Perrett L V: 3555
Perrin Y: 3408
Perry J: 3407
Perry R D: 3813
Persigehl M: 1583
Persson B: 2572
Pessar M: 1151
Pessar M L: 3128

Petasnick J P: 1171, 1172, 2519
Peters A: 2484
Peters E: 3814
Peters J C: 851, 1837
Peters M E: 438
Peters P E: 465, 1017, 1243, 2018, 2992, 2993, 3815, 3853, 3928
Peters T: 2699
Peters T M: 3816
Peters V: 3841
Petersdorf R G: 3301
Petersen D: 1901
Petersen O F: 3817, 3818
Peterson I M: 364
Peterson J E: 1181, 1183
Peterson M W: 365
Peterson R R: 196, 202, 486, 1488, 2086
Petit J: 787
Petkov D: 2754
Petras A F: 3819
Petruzzo R: 2393
Petsch R: 2705
Pettersson H: 2578, 2883, 3030, 3242, 3243, 3605, 3820
Petti M: 312
Peuchot M: 852
Peyster R G: 3154, 3480, 3669, 3726, 3821, 3822, 3823
Pezzella A T: 448
Pezzotta S: 2561
Pezzulli F A: 366
Pfadenhauer K: 3031
Pfeiffer K: 3824
Pfeiler M: 863
Pfister R C: 2099, 2283, 2337
Pflug J J: 2581
Pfretzschner C: 139
Philip C: 3319
Phillips H E: 2768
Phillips J J: 63
Phillips P C: 2694
Phillips T L: 3963
Phillips V M: 1199, 1200, 2173
Phillips W A: 2548
Phillips W C: 2895
Photopulos G: 2370
Piazza P: 2690
Picard J D: 1452, 2100, 2101
Picciotto M: 1621
Pichezzi P: 2690
Pichler W: 1043
Pickens J: 3165
Picouto J P: 1039
Picus D: 367, 1059, 1400, 1488, 1569, 1624, 1838
Piechowiak H: 1839
Piekarski J: 1201, 1964
Pieralli S: 2231, 3106
Piggott B: 1760
Pilai K: 1397
Pilate I: 853
Pile Spellman E A: 878
Pile Spellman J: 3794
Pilepich M V: 3833
Pilgram T K: 4034
Pilla T: 112, 3170
Pilla T J: 3146
Pillari G: 2224, 2288, 3710
Pineda C: 2897, 3085
Pinol Daubisse H: 2818
Pinstein M L: 854
Pinto J A: 3825
Pinto R: 3140
Pinto R S: 3363, 3660, 3743, 3744, 3826, 3888
Piomelli S: 1160
Pissiotis C: 2263
Pistoia F: 1965, 2391
Pitha J V: 2239
Pitkethly D T: 2735
Pitts L H: 614
Pizer S M: 93
Pizzo P A: 1963
Plaine L: 2243
Platt J F: 165, 855, 2319
Plauth M: 1117
Plemmons M: 979
Pleul O: 2683

Plojoux O: 1625
Plonsky L: 2627
Plumley T F: 3032
Podlas H B: 3827
Podrasky A E: 902
Poehls C: 2082
Poirson F: 217
Poitout P: 2346
Pojunas K: 3230
Pojunas K W: 2225, 3025
Polansky S M: 1837
Polga J P: 1676
Polger M: 166
Pollack H M: 1347, 1996, 1997, 2085, 2105, 2315, 2432
Pollack M: 1326
Pollack M S: 368
Pollard S G: 1869
Pollock W J: 714
Polsky M S: 1984
Polzleitner D: 882
Pombo F: 1453
Pomeranz S J: 3828
Pond G D: 3829
Ponder T: 3939
Ponette E: 968, 1596, 1800
Pongratz M: 753
Pontifex G: 285, 519, 2235, 2263, 2814, 3805
Poon P Y: 783, 856, 857, 2539
Poos D: 2885, 2887
Pope T L Jr: 400, 2106
Popky G L: 3993, 3994, 3997, 3998, 3999
Poppi M: 2802
Porcellini B: 1501, 2975
Porras M: 3937, 3938
Porst H: 2285
Porteous P H: 2251
Porter D: 3062
Porter S C: 3229
Portha C: 3393
Poser C M: 3830
Poskitt K J: 2320
Posniak H: 2078, 2097
Posniak H V: 249
Post J D: 3191, 3192
Post M J: 587, 2628, 3119, 3351, 3831, 3832
Postlethwait R W: 294, 1657
Potelon P: 3294
Potter B M: 986, 1880
Potter J L: 1020, 2943
Potter R: 465
Potvliege R: 246, 2557, 2950
Potzschke B: 2392
Pouget J: 2502
Poulignot D: 3391
Poutska F: 3644
Poveda H: 3613
Pozderac R: 1359
Poznanski A K: 2854, 3401, 3446
Pozniak M A: 2719
Pozzati E: 2802
Pradel J: 1452, 1622, 2100, 2101, 2317, 3806
Pradere M Y: 3292
Prasad S C: 3833
Prassopoulos P: 2032
Preger R: 3914
Premkumar A: 2289, 2321
Prensky A J: 3478
Presbrey T: 2237
Present D A: 2590
Press G A: 952, 1228, 2107, 3345
Pressman B D: 3033
Preston D F: 2607, 3681
Pretorius D: 1280
Price A P: 3737
Price D: 1803
Price D B: 3834
Price G J: 3068
Price H I: 3129
Price J C: 28, 3848
Price M J: 3964, 3965
Price R B: 961, 979
Price R R: 3808
Prien E L: 2283
Princenthal R A: 1643
Pringot J: 1143

Pritchard D J: 2653, 2660
Pritchard R S: 2520
Probst G: 284, 607, 661, 3497
Probst P: 437, 935, 2108, 2196
Proto A V: 378, 588, 858, 937, 3738, 3835
Provisor A J: 2613
Prudent J: 217
Psarras H: 3034
Pugatch R D: 100, 210, 369, 372, 555, 632, 859, 885, 3463, 3859
Pullan B R: 2521
Pullen K W: 3418
Pullicino P: 152, 3035, 3836
Pupols A: 1626
Purser R K: 587
Putman C E: 471, 594, 605, 631, 672, 698, 3452
Pyatt R: 2103
Pyatt R S: 1734, 3565
Pyeritz R E: 3128
Pykett I L: 3728

Quencer R M: 2628, 2951, 3119, 3832, 4011
Quinlan D M: 2159
Quinn C: 4105
Quinn M: 810
Quinn M J: 1840
Quinn S F: 1202, 1327, 2476, 3036, 3316, 3837
Quint D J: 3037
Quint L E: 271, 370, 371, 666, 855, 860, 2226, 2838
Quintana F: 3048
Quiroga O: 3038
Quiroz F: 1341
Quiroz F A: 1130, 1287

Raasch B N: 872
Rabbani R: 2611
Raber G: 2392
Rabinowich L: 3732
Rabinowitz J G: 1663, 1664, 1919, 2478, 2774, 3206
Racchiusa S: 1829, 1830, 2390, 3460
Racette C D: 2486
Racle A: 1708, 3294
Radecki P D: 652, 653, 1120, 1579, 1673, 1900, 2261, 2432, 3516
Radin D R: 861, 1203, 1204, 1227, 1260, 1328, 1454, 1644, 1841, 1842, 2227, 2228, 2393, 3839
Radmehr A: 3237
Radtke R: 3535
Radu E W: 3484
Rafii M: 2782, 2783, 2784, 2810, 2826, 3039, 3040, 3041, 3042, 3043, 3491
Raghavendra B N: 1958, 1983, 2109, 2324
Ragosin R J: 2286
Ragsdale B D: 3795
Rahatzad M: 3840
Rahatzad M T: 1362
Rahim H: 2864
Rahmouni A D: 945
Rahn N H: 1329
Raininko R: 167, 3044
Raiss G: 2638
Raju J S: 1446
Ralls P W: 810, 861, 1123, 1203, 1204, 1260, 1842, 2227, 2228, 2522, 2523
Ram P C: 5, 334, 471, 1049, 1226, 2259, 3045, 3551
Ramee A: 2797
Ramirez H: 3842
Ramirez H Jr: 3046, 3047, 3841
Ramos A: 3048
Ramos L: 3501
Ramos L M: 3611
Ramos L R: 116
Ramsewak W: 547
Ramsey R G: 3843, 3844
Ramzy I: 1020
Randall B C: 3049

Randel S: 3307
Randel S B: 1985
Randell C P: 3845
Raney B R: 3365
Rankin R N: 556
Rankin S: 372
Rankin S C: 100
Ranner G: 753
Ransohoff J: 3239
Ranson J H: 1355, 1357
Rantakokko V: 1419
Rao A K: 3967
Rao B K: 1843, 1844
Rao C V: 3846
Rao G R: 3053, 3613
Rao K C: 3472
Rao V M: 459
Rapaccini G L: 2176
Rapoport S: 2524
Rapp R: 2701
Rappaport D C: 862
Raptopoulos V: 168, 1455, 1772, 1845, 1846, 1967, 2511
Rascoe R R: 2736
Rascol A: 3291, 3292, 3706
Raskin S P: 3050, 3051
Rasmussen H: 2877
Rasmussen J F: 80
Ratcliffe S S: 2900
Ratzka M: 4074
Rau W: 1110
Rauch R F: 1774, 1966, 2629, 2664
Raudkivi U: 79
Rausch H P: 2110
Rauschkolb E N: 1197, 1235, 1337, 1471, 2111, 2877
Rauschning W: 2819, 3052, 3274
Rauws E A: 2466
Raval B: 556, 1456, 1570, 1744, 2371
Ravasini R: 609, 3283
Ravin C E: 631, 642, 698
Ravipati M: 3354
Ray C S: 577, 578, 779, 876
Ray J W: 3403
Ray M J: 2393
Raybaud C: 2977, 3408
Raymond A K: 2609, 2947
Rayor R: 1533
Rayschkolb E N: 3160
Rea F: 260
Reading C C: 13, 1113, 1388
Reahard T M: 3418
Reale F: 1846
Rebner M: 408, 1330, 2322
Recht M P: 373
Rechthand E: 3442
Reckler J M: 3249
Reddington R W: 3450
Reddy S C: 374, 3053, 3613
Redington R: 3278
Redington R W: 493
Redman H C: 1730
Redmond P E: 1603
Reed D: 3847
Reed K: 395
Reed M D: 2112
Reede D L: 2137, 3054, 3969
Rees M R: 544, 557, 558
Reese D F: 94, 3586
Regenbogen V S: 3848
Reggiani L: 2287
Rego J: 1302
Regulla D: 91
Reh T E: 1627
Rehder U: 2565
Rehpenning W: 73
Reich L: 4059
Reich N E: 79, 1297
Reichardt W: 2558
Reicher M A: 2826
Reid A: 764
Reid M H: 95, 2769, 3849
Reid W: 3004
Reider Grosswasser I: 3621
Reif L J: 960
Reilly L M: 1600
Reiman H M: 2457, 2653
Reiman T A: 2113

Reiman T H: 1457
Reinbold W D: 635
Reinertson J S: 1837
Reinhardt V: 2503
Reinig J W: 375, 1205, 1206
Reinke D B: 2305
Reinke M: 3782
Reisberg B: 3385, 3386
Reiser M: 1014, 1390, 1403, 1724, 1767, 1898, 2355, 2700, 2952, 3055, 3056, 3057, 3227, 3228, 3905
Reiser U: 42, 863, 2200, 2702, 3058
Reiser U J: 34, 169
Reiser V M: 3059
Reisig L: 3222
Reisner K: 96
Reiter J D: 1531
Reither M: 2122
Reitz B A: 712
Reivich M: 3256
Remberger K: 899
Remley K B: 3850
Remy J: 311, 724, 864, 865
Remy Jardin M: 864, 865
Ren H: 712, 866, 867, 868, 3851
Rene E: 1142
Renner P: 1377
Rennie C S: 1791
Resnick C S: 3086
Resnick D: 2497, 2514, 2555, 2691, 2751, 2752, 2826, 2897, 2925, 2926, 3085, 3086, 3215, 3895
Resnick M I: 2246
Resnik C S: 2752, 3086
Resnik M D: 1676
Resser K J: 1166
Resta S: 3991
Retrum E R: 3852
Retterbush D W: 1914
Reuter C: 2596
Reuter K: 1846
Reuter K L: 2344
Reuter M: 869
Reuther G: 1847, 3060, 3853
Revak C S: 3061
Revesz G: 2987
Revzani L: 699
Reyes G D: 3854
Reynes C: 332, 333
Reynes C J: 227, 994, 1793, 2507
Rhodes M L: 3073
Rhodes R: 3372
Rhodes R A: 2114
Rhyner P: 2115
Riaz M A: 1916, 2335
Ribera G: 3791
Rice C A: 3855
Rice R P: 1573, 1749, 1774
Richard O: 2818
Richardson J D: 3903
Richardson M L: 2394, 2663, 2811, 2994, 3856
Richardson P: 376, 3062
Richey W: 2370
Richie J P: 2203, 2326
Richli W R: 3067
Richmond B D: 910, 3902
Richmond T: 1848
Richter J O: 1644, 1758
Richter K: 231
Richter M P: 3466
Rickards D: 2525, 2533
Rickles D J: 2721
Rideout D F: 783, 857
Riebel T: 692
Rieber A: 3063
Riede U N: 2794
Riedelberger W: 2832
Rieden K: 1104, 3064
Riederer S J: 3309
Riedmiller H: 2121, 2124
Riela A R: 3675
Riemenschneider J: 3092
Riemer M: 125
Rienmuller R: 502, 503, 559, 729
Rieser R: 377
Riess J G: 3319

Rieth K G: 2395, 2753
Rifkin M D: 1628
Rigauts H: 97
Rigsby C M: 1227, 2013, 2116
Riley L H Jr: 2787
Rimm A A: 960, 3521
Rinaldo J E: 3547
Ring S: 2604
Ringertz H: 508
Ringertz H G: 543, 615
Risch W D: 3259
Risius B: 3065
Risius B F: 2188
Ritchie W G: 2381
Ritman E L: 98
Ritz C R: 3243
Riviezzo G C: 2220
Rix J: 4025
Rizk G K: 877
Rizzo M J: 1849
Ro M: 2672
Road J: 793
Rob P: 2051
Robb P A: 2694
Robb R A: 98, 3120
Robb W L: 99, 3858
Robbins A H: 100, 369, 555, 1737, 1738, 3859
Robbins G L: 2208
Robbins K T: 3980
Robbins S: 434
Robert N J: 1054, 1820, 1821
Roberts C M: 870
Roberts G S: 1272
Roberts J: 2252
Roberts L: 1658
Roberts L Jr: 294, 651, 1458, 3860
Roberts T: 3315
Robertson D D: 101, 2767, 2786, 3861
Robertson H J: 3862
Robertson J: 102
Robertson W D: 520, 2747, 2934, 3759, 3847
Robinson D A: 3863
Robinson D L: 1357
Robinson P J: 52, 103
Robinson R G: 2607, 3681
Robinson R O: 3688
Robinson T: 2622
Robitaille Y: 3943
Robotti G: 1886, 2615, 2975
Robotti G C: 935
Robsen C J: 2117
Robson D: 905
Rochel M: 3700
Rochemaure J: 217
Rochester D: 233, 2248
Rockoff S D: 871
Rocmans: 621
Rodacki M A: 3864, 3865
Rodammer G: 3177
Rodan B A: 698
Rodiek S: 3866
Rodiek S O: 2526, 2527, 3066, 3867
Rodl W: 1629
Rodriguez A: 328, 329
Rodriguez R: 1324
Roels F: 246
Roesler P J Jr: 1207
Roex L: 1486, 3868
Rofsky N M: 2118
Roger B: 66, 2940
Roger D J: 3067
Rogers C I: 560, 1241
Rogers J: 3356
Rogers J V: 3954
Rogers J V Jr: 405
Rogers L F: 3627
Rogers R E: 2359
Rogers W: 2522
Roggli V: 887
Rognone F: 2561
Rogopoulos A: 3319
Rohatgi P K: 489
Rohde U: 1904, 2396, 2407
Rohloff R: 3869
Rohmer P: 1000

Rohrmann C A: 1338
Rohrmann C A Jr: 1264, 1331, 3263
Roilgen A: 2884, 2885, 2887
Rojer C L: 3997
Rollo F D: 3808
Rolston D D: 1781
Romani S: 609
Romano A J: 3870, 3871, 3950, 3951
Romano P: 703
Romanzi F: 2287
Romer T: 1051, 2366, 2630, 3746
Romero F: 3074, 3880
Rommel T: 3872
Rona G: 1936
Ronchi O: 3375
Rooholamini S A: 3464
Roos H: 3827
Roos N: 2993
Roper C L: 274, 367, 772
Roper P R: 2918
Roppolo H M: 2988
Roque C T: 2669
Ros P R: 1508, 1764
Rosa U: 3873
Rosato E F: 373
Rose B S: 1854, 3717
Rose F C: 3405
Rose H: 3744
Rose J S: 801, 2498
Rose R M: 630
Rose W S: 3480
Rosen A: 108, 720, 1850, 1851, 3248
Rosen B: 3874
Rosen B R: 2485
Rosen I E: 2184
Rosenbaum A E: 2785, 2984, 3214, 3488, 3522, 3666, 3848
Rosenbaum D M: 2156
Rosenbaum R C: 1154
Rosenberg E R: 2259
Rosenberg S A: 220, 2568
Rosenberg Z S: 2528, 2529, 2530, 2779, 3068, 3113, 3115, 3116
Rosenberger A: 192, 224, 580
Rosenberger J: 1441
Rosenblatt M: 762
Rosenbloom M B: 3946
Rosenbloom S: 3069, 3385
Rosenbloom S A: 2651
Rosenblum J S: 3467
Rosenblum L J: 872
Rosenbusch G: 418
Rosenfeld G: 4069
Rosenfield A T: 1098, 1227, 1758, 1972, 2013, 2116, 2163, 2418, 2813
Rosenshein N B: 2356, 2361
Rosenstein F: 2227
Rosenthal A: 3710
Rosenthal D: 1820, 1821
Rosenthal D I: 2631, 2811, 2896, 3070, 3071, 3720, 3721, 3874
Rosenthal H: 1045, 3720
Rosenthal M: 3485
Rosenthal M S: 1875
Rosenthal R: 1389
Rosenwein M F: 2353
Rosler H: 1016
Ross A S: 1937
Ross C R: 831
Ross G J: 873
Ross W K: 3339
Rosser S B: 2308
Rosset P: 2942
Rossi P: 164, 1208, 1459, 1460, 3875
Rossier A B: 3072
Rost R C Jr: 378
Rostock R A: 3876
Roth J: 1209
Rothberg M: 1958
Rothenberg D M: 2119
Rothfus W E: 3262, 3877, 3878, 3879
Rothman B J: 3033
Rothman S: 1848

Rothman S L: 3073, 4037
Rothner A D: 3745
Rothrock J F: 3314
Rotstein J M: 2279
Rotte K H: 2531, 2632
Rottenberg D A: 92, 3367, 3618
Rottenberg R R: 2029
Rotter M: 29
Rouger M: 3408
Roukema J G: 185, 186
Rouse G A: 3087
Roush G: 1319
Rousseau M: 790, 1141
Roux V J: 1567
Rovighi L: 1833
Rovira A: 3077
Rovira M: 2661, 3074, 3880
Rowberg A A: 110
Rowberg A H: 3952
Rowedder A: 1279
Rowland R G: 2443
Roy S 3d: 1799
Royal H D: 1048
Royal S A: 1201
Roysland P: 193
Rozing P M: 2899
Rubens D: 2397
Rubens J R: 878
Rubenstein W A: 256, 966, 1210,
    1672, 1852, 1921, 1922, 2056,
    2166, 2167, 2312, 2532, 3248,
    3249
Rubesin S E: 1576, 1619
Rubin B E: 1712, 2120
Rubin E: 2399, 2464, 2633
Rubin J: 25, 1861, 3881
Rubin J M: 699, 1294, 1393, 1713
Rubinstein I: 874
Rubinstein Z J: 1335, 2090, 2242
Ruchman R B: 1322, 1819
Ruchti C: 1133
Ruckert K: 1394
Rudansky M C: 4084
Rudin S: 55
Rudwan M: 1718
Rudwan M A: 1012
Ruegsegger P: 2770, 3075
Ruf B: 2851
Ruf G: 1289, 1554
Ruggieri P: 2578
Ruggieri P M: 1330
Ruggiero R: 3076
Ruhl G: 2155
Ruijs J H: 418
Ruijs S H: 116
Ruiz J: 2322
Ruiz J S: 3405, 3986
Ruiz Marcellan M C: 4005
Ruiz Perales F: 786
Rumancik W M: 1461, 1688
Rumbaugh C L: 451, 3072, 3088,
    3179, 3180, 3181, 3528, 4048,
    4049, 4050, 4051
Rumberger J A: 558
Rumpf K D: 1312
Rundle R: 61
Ruoff M: 2453
Rupp N: 1014, 3055, 3056, 3057,
    3059, 3177, 3867
Ruscalleda J: 3077, 3882
Rush M: 677
Ruskin J A: 3883
Russ P D: 1853, 3602
Russell A S: 2727
Russell E: 2949
Russell E J: 170, 3009, 3078,
    3884, 4102, 4103, 4104
Russell K B: 3998
Russell W: 3312
Russell W F: 2508
Russell W J: 346, 1097
Russi E: 3460
Rustige J: 568
Ruther W: 3780
Rutt B K: 34
Ruzicka F F: 1626
Ryan J: 1211
Ryan J A: 1385, 1540
Ryan K G: 2290
Ryan L: 2723

Ryan R W: 3079
Rynties M: 1307
Rzehak L: 1984
Rzymski K: 1915, 2229

Sabato U: 3673
Sabattini L: 3885
Sabbagh E: 44
Sacher M: 403, 2478, 2606, 2933,
    3125, 3673, 3886
Sachs M: 930
Sachsenheimer W: 2996
Sackett J F: 2806
Sacks G A: 1634
Sadatoh N: 2293, 3887
Sadhu V K: 3614, 3888
Saeed M: 571, 1655, 2145, 2436
Saeger H D: 1062
Safi F: 1209
Safrit H: 1760, 2387
Saga T: 2257
Sagawa F: 1232
Sage M R: 171, 1598
Sagel S S: 195, 196, 200, 201,
    202, 272, 273, 274, 275, 296,
    384, 395, 396, 431, 461, 486,
    589, 667, 668, 875, 916, 937,
    952, 955, 1309, 1329, 1429,
    1487, 1671, 1783, 1788, 1864,
    2011, 2130, 2191, 2207, 2314,
    2750, 2945, 2999
Sager E M: 2291
Sagerman R H: 4091
Sagoh Y: 82
Saiki S: 2281, 2282
Saini S: 895, 1470, 1511
Saito I: 1246
Saito K: 657
Saito S: 1592
Saito T: 1072, 1073
Saito Y: 1071, 1072, 1073, 4002
Saitoh R: 573
Saitou Y: 808
Saiwai S: 2357, 3580
Sakaguchi S: 1876
Sakai F: 876, 2468
Sakamoto M: 1099
Sako M: 2572
Sakowicz B A: 183
Saks B J: 7
Saksouk F A: 877, 1213, 2356
Sakuma H: 379
Sakuma S: 50, 723
Sakuyama K: 1075
Salamon G: 2502, 2977, 3038,
    3408
Salamon O: 3080
Salazar J: 854
Salazar J E: 2025, 3889
Salbeck R: 2676
Salducci J: 1483
Salerno M D: 1854
Salimi Z: 2515
Sallee D S: 3432
Salomon C G: 2398
Salomonowitz E: 1386, 1732
Salvador A: 593
Salvi L: 1621
Salvolini U: 164, 4043
Samaraweera R N: 3920
Sambrook P: 2533
Sample W F: 2035, 2327
Samson L: 600
Samson M: 3359
Samuel E: 3890
Samuel L: 3184
Samuels B I: 664
Samuels T: 1630
San Dretto M A: 430
San Galli F: 983
Sanchez F W: 1205
Sandbaek G: 1647
Sandelin J: 2921
Sander B: 943, 3917
Sanders C: 2399
Sanders J H: 255
Sanders L M: 1211
Sanders R: 959, 1402, 2169
Sanders R C: 1631, 1855, 2378,
    2403

Sandhu A: 3891
Sandilos P: 519
Sandler C M: 1197, 1235, 1337,
    1342, 1856, 2111
Sandler M A: 362, 363, 848, 849,
    950, 1601, 1707, 2132
Sandler M P: 2185
Sandor T: 3687, 3892
Sandt G: 2885, 2887, 3604
Sane P: 2803, 2978
Sanecki M G: 3166
Sanger J J: 1588
Sano A: 2293, 3887
Sano N: 3893
Santiago E M: 1454
Santiard J C: 3408
Sanz M P: 2661
Saperstein M L: 1936
Sargent S K: 3894
Sarno R C: 2292, 3081
Sarr M G: 1415
Sartor K: 3082, 3083, 3084
Sartor K J: 2894, 3478
Sartori F: 609, 646
Sartoris D J: 2497, 2514, 2555,
    2691, 2826, 2925, 2926, 3085,
    3086, 3215, 3895
Sarwar M: 1848, 2831, 2949,
    3306, 3451, 3896, 3897
Sasagawa M: 808
Sasai K: 2293
Sasaki C: 4037
Sasaki T: 2674
Sasaki Y: 2674
Sashin D: 1875
Satchell T V: 3821
Sato F: 3718
Sato H: 1333
Sato M: 3898
Sato S: 3580
Sato T: 2281, 2282
Sato Y: 262, 263, 510, 839
Satoh O: 2641
Satoh S: 2410
Satterlee W: 3624
Satyanath S: 1012, 1718
Saudinos J: 3408
Sauer O: 3698
Sauerwein W: 3097, 3899
Saul O: 2790
Saul S H: 1234
Sauli F: 3408
Sauser D: 3159
Sauser D D: 3087
Sautter C: 3489
Savader B L: 2400
Savader S J: 2400
Savarese D M: 1725
Savart P: 2100
Savit R M: 2294
Savolaine E R: 1212
Sawada T: 3617
Sawicka J M: 3693
Sawin C T: 210
Sawyer R W: 2401
Saxena K M: 1998
Scanlan K A: 1843
Scarborough D: 971
Scardino P T: 2327
Scatamacchia S A: 1967
Scatarige J C: 744, 1213, 1214,
    1462, 1631, 1649, 2323, 2356,
    3226, 3900
Scatliff J H: 3901, 3959
Schaaf J: 811, 906, 907
Schaaf M: 253, 2180
Schabel S I: 375, 2002, 2003,
    3132
Schadel A: 3158
Schadlbauer E: 1726
Schaefer C: 685
Schaefer C M: 878
Schaefer P S: 545
Schaeffer A: 1954
Schafer H J: 2649
Schafer K: 982
Schaffstein J: 982
Schanche A F: 2480
Schaner E G: 2182
Scharp D W: 1400

Schaub T: 2866, 3907
Schauwecker D S: 3902
Scheibler M L: 1198
Scheid K F: 879
Scheithauer B W: 1395, 3796
Schellinger D: 2511, 3390, 3498,
    3903, 3904
Schepke P: 1632
Schepp S: 3905
Scherer K: 1349, 1425
Scherholz K: 758
Scherrer A: 1150
Scheurer C: 91
Scheurer U: 1343
Schick R M: 3088, 3321
Schiebler M: 2500
Schienman M M: 500
Schiffer M S: 172
Schild H: 380, 1215, 1216, 1653,
    2121, 2124, 2125, 3089, 3090,
    3907, 3908, 3909
Schild H H: 2910
Schildge J: 462
Schiller N B: 490, 501, 512
Schilling G: 3303
Schilling J F: 2544
Schilling V: 2733
Schils J: 3910
Schimek F: 4039
Schimke R N: 1786
Schimpf P P: 922
Schimrigk K: 3137
Schinco F P: 2714
Schindera F: 2684
Schindler E: 1984, 4020, 4021
Schindler G: 2637, 2850, 3092,
    3182
Schinella R: 713, 836
Schinella R A: 1497
Schinzel A: 3982
Schipper H I: 3911
Schipper J: 3091
Schlegl A: 3541
Schlenska G K: 3912
Schlesinger A E: 2634
Schlolaut K H: 561, 768, 880,
    3913
Schmachtenberg A: 104
Schmeller W: 3485
Schmid P: 1857
Schmidbauer M: 4020
Schmidberger H: 3649
Schmidlin T M: 3852
Schmidt E B: 3933
Schmidt E H: 1627
Schmidt J: 3524
Schmidt Peter P: 2531, 2632
Schmidt S: 2062
Schmied W: 1555
Schmilinsky G: 2781
Schmit P: 656
Schmitt R: 2635, 2636, 2637,
    3092, 3182, 3540, 3914
Schmitt W G: 105, 757, 3093,
    3915
Schmitt W G H: 881
Schmitteckert H: 209, 1739
Schmitz L: 3916
Schmitz Rixen T: 1792
Schmoll E: 1045
Schmutzer L: 3699
Schmutzhard E: 4066
Schnapf D: 3959
Schneekloth G: 1035, 1885
Schneider G H: 3136, 3649
Schneider H: 691
Schneider I: 3139
Schneider M: 3249
Schneider P: 252, 3094
Schneider P D: 804, 1155
Schneider R: 2860
Schneider S: 3338, 4015
Schneider U: 2683, 2781
Schnorr H: 2082
Schnur M J: 2040
Schnyder P: 337, 338, 1530,
    1615, 1656, 2295
Schnyder P A: 1217
Schoene W C: 4051
Schoenecker S A: 107

Schoettle H: 2875
Schonfeld S: 3192
Schontag H: 2875
Schopf R: 935, 1218
Schopke W: 2215
Schoppe W D: 106
Schorner W: 137, 139, 562, 943,
    1015, 2851, 3187, 3369, 3917
Schoter I: 3095
Schratter M: 693, 2760, 2869,
    3096
Schreiber R R: 2861
Schreiman J S: 3918, 3919
Schreiner C: 576
Schreyer H: 3136
Schrijvers A: 3097
Schroeder B A: 3920, 3921
Schroeder S: 2923, 2924
Schroth G: 3922
Schubiger O: 3098, 3099, 3100,
    4031, 4065
Schuknecht B: 3923
Schuler M: 3101
Schuller H: 768
Schulman A: 1858
Schulte S J: 1331, 1881
Schultz S M: 3924
Schultz S R: 1989, 2638
Schulz E E: 1506
Schulz R A: 53
Schulze K: 1219, 2201
Schulze W: 292
Schumacher K A: 381, 1332,
    1896, 3489
Schumacher M: 3102, 3138
Schumacher R: 2122
Schumann R: 2649
Schuppan U: 537
Schurawitzki H: 882, 1220, 1726,
    2123
Schutz B: 1361
Schutz H: 1015
Schwab R: 3908
Schwab R E: 1463, 1502, 1532,
    2319, 2501, 2638
Schwaighofer B W: 3925
Schwarting R: 1021
Schwartz A: 3926
Schwartz A M: 1221
Schwartz J M: 2230, 2324, 3927
Schwartz J R: 995
Schwartz K: 2218
Schwartz M S: 2783, 2784
Schwartz P E: 2418
Schwartz R: 2055, 2255
Schwarz G: 63
Schwarzinger I: 704
Schwarzl G: 2832
Schwarzrock R: 3265
Schweden F: 473, 1216, 1584,
    1653, 2124, 2125, 2424
Schweitzer M E: 3103
Schwer C: 4040
Schwimer S R: 2639
Schwimmer M: 2534
Schworm C P: 714
Scialfa G: 2231, 3106
Sciot C: 2345
Sciuk J: 3928
Scorpio R: 376
Scott I R: 883
Scott J A: 2631, 2907
Scott R L: 854
Scott V F: 1567
Scott W Jr: 4090
Scott W W Jr: 349, 478, 2787,
    2916
Scotti G: 173, 2231, 3104, 3105,
    3106, 3712, 3812, 3929, 3930
Scotto B: 3292
Scribano E: 1191, 1451, 1621
Sechtem U: 353
Seddiqi M S: 2840
Sedlacek T V: 2381
Sedvall G: 3273
Seeger J F: 2640, 3205, 3601,
    4083
Seemann W R: 3932
Seerup A: 3933
Sefczek R J: 1859

Segal A J: 2058, 2126, 3934
Segal S D: 3520
Segall H D: 958, 3211, 3245, 3330, 4027, 4028, 4094
Segui S: 1138
Sehgal E: 489
Seibel D G: 382
Seibert K: 2571
Seidel D: 3911
Seidel F G: 1928, 3308
Seidelmann F E: 1297
Seidenwurm D: 3935
Seidmon E J: 2261
Seifert P: 2494
Seiff S R: 3503
Seigel R: 1359, 2701
Seigel R S: 1633, 3936
Seigler H F: 698
Seissler W: 58, 729
Seitz K H: 492
Seki M: 1069
Seki T: 1333
Sekine I: 2147
Selby D K: 2973
Self J: 2272
Seline T H: 383
Sell J: 3936
Sell S: 2906
Seltzer S E: 223, 384, 684, 1126, 1811, 1924, 2203, 3107, 3108, 3956
Semerak M: 1927
Semine M C: 3081
Seminer D S: 2628
Senac M O: 3284
Senda M: 822
Senegas J: 2818
Sens M: 385
Seo J W: 721
Sepahdari S: 3855
Sepponen R E: 2592
Serchuk L: 3976
Serdarevic M: 2505
Sereerat P: 419
Serratrice G: 2502
Servadei F: 2825
Servo A: 2921, 3937, 3938
Sessions R B: 3320
Setiawan A T: 2414
Setiawan H: 1730
Sevel D: 3939
Sewell C W: 961, 2173
Sexton C C: 1222
Seymour E Q: 560
Shabason L: 3547, 4086
Shaer A H: 884
Shaff M: 2237
Shaff M I: 427, 1634, 2157, 2185
Shaffer H A Jr: 1523
Shaffer K: 885, 3350
Shaffer K A: 3941
Shah D M: 3615
Shah H R: 1860, 2232, 2520
Shah K K: 1463
Shah M: 2127
Shah R R: 3266
Shakudo M: 2357
Shamam O M: 2402
Shamsnia M: 4055
Shank B: 764
Shankar L: 1310
Shanzer S: 4084
Shapeero L G: 386, 387, 3942
Shapir J: 1861, 3943
Shapiro B: 513, 1539, 2226, 2611
Shapiro H A: 1442
Shapiro J H: 2427, 2535, 2793
Shapiro M: 481
Shapiro M P: 886, 1223
Sharbrough F W: 3796
Share J C: 3685
Sharif H S: 3944
Sharon M: 2765
Shatney C H: 1906
Shaw E: 1959
Shaw P: 1630, 1979
Shawker T H: 253, 1157, 1381, 1423, 1725, 1963, 2060, 2395

Shea P: 529
Shea W J: 1556
Shea W J Jr: 953, 954, 1278
Shearer D R: 81
Sheedy P F: 996, 1093, 1376, 1388, 1580, 1840, 2236, 2467, 4058
Shekar P C: 3664
Sheldon J J: 3945
Shen J H: 1033
Shen W C: 3109
Shenouda N F: 3946
Shepard J A: 336, 393, 406, 407, 912
Shepard J O: 213, 388
Shepp L A: 174
Sheps S G: 2236
Shereff M J: 2530
Sheremata W A: 3832, 3945
Sherman J: 1733
Sherman J L: 1635, 2452, 3560, 3947, 3948
Sherman N E: 4075
Sherman R L: 3262
Sherman S J: 2167
Sherrier R H: 887
Sherry R G: 3018, 3241, 3396
Sherwood T: 175
Sheth S: 2403
Sheward S E: 1636
Shibakiri I: 1736
Shibata A: 2146
Shibata T: 1057
Shibuya H: 2641
Shields J A: 3821
Shields J B: 112, 300, 301, 1916, 1917, 2336, 3170, 3533
Shigematsu N: 355
Shigeta A: 573
Shih T T: 563
Shillito J Jr: 3181
Shimbo Y: 4018
Shimizu F H: 3967
Shimizu H: 1333
Shimkin P: 1613
Shin M S: 389, 390, 391, 392, 564, 565, 888, 889, 1107, 1701, 1862, 3949
Shina D: 1397
Shinoda A: 1071, 1072
Shinohara T: 3577
Shinohara Y: 2616, 4080
Shiozaki H: 425
Shipley R T: 393, 2968
Shirazi K K: 2234
Shirey M P: 129
Shirkhoda A: 254, 993, 1224, 1225, 1326, 1464, 1616, 1637, 1638, 1741, 1808, 1836, 1863, 2128, 2129, 2609, 3020, 3110, 3111
Shives T C: 2660
Shoemaker E I: 3870, 3871, 3950, 3951
Shogen K: 425
Shohat M: 2734
Shor M J: 944
Shoukimas G M: 3794
Shreck E H: 2338
Shuer L: 3420
Shugar J M: 403, 2137, 3784, 3886, 3969, 3970, 3971
Shulman H S: 857
Shults W T: 3987
Shumaker E: 2297
Shuman L S: 774
Shuman W P: 107, 1122, 1264, 1331, 1338, 1881, 2516, 2560, 2626, 2994, 3263, 3530, 3952, 3953, 3954
Shyojima K: 3526
Sibala J L: 3955
Sick H: 2715, 3394
Sidbury J: 1005
Siddharthan R: 3945
Siddiky M A: 129, 1269
Sider L: 394, 890
Siedek S: 3780
Siegel H A: 3956
Siegel M J: 273, 275, 395, 396,

409, 1060, 1639, 1838, 1864, 1946, 2113, 2130, 2131, 3723
Siegel R S: 3361
Siegel S C: 2132
Siegelbaum M H: 2432
Siegelman S: 2278
Siegelman S S: 320, 348, 349, 478, 546, 597, 647, 695, 744, 745, 746, 747, 748, 749, 782, 826, 827, 828, 829, 830, 831, 891, 892, 936, 937, 959, 965, 973, 1018, 1213, 1214, 1247, 1402, 1462, 1522, 1537, 1547, 1553, 1574, 1575, 1608, 1619, 1631, 1693, 1696, 1716, 1717, 1729, 1766, 1798, 1855, 1879, 1949, 2020, 2030, 2031, 2054, 2087, 2169, 2187, 2193, 2323, 2349, 2356, 2361, 2449, 2506, 2785, 2786, 2787, 2916, 2964, 3208, 3429, 3445, 4095
Siegert A: 917
Sieghart S: 259
Sievers K W: 3112
Sigmund G: 940, 3960
Sigurjonsson S: 1288
Sigurjonsson S V: 1640
Silao J V Jr: 2666
Silprasert W: 896
Silva W E: 1967
Silver A J: 566, 2803, 2978, 3957
Silver S F: 893
Silverberg G D: 2777, 3420
Silverman P: 1573
Silverman P M: 108, 334, 397, 422, 494, 567, 571, 843, 894, 969, 970, 1050, 1226, 1253, 1254, 1465, 1481, 1641, 1642, 1655, 1694, 1697, 1750, 1774, 1850, 1851, 1865, 1966, 2009, 2083, 2133, 2214, 2298, 2328, 2404, 2439, 2454, 2629, 2664, 3342
Silverman S G: 895
Silverstein G S: 1578
Silverstein W: 1404, 1466
Sim F H: 2610, 2660
Simeone F A: 2351, 2830, 3399
Simeone J: 1033, 1373, 2418
Simeone J F: 440, 895, 1470, 1476, 1511, 1816, 1831, 2619, 3440, 4072
Simeoni J: 3293
Simmons J D: 3958
Simmons J L: 1633
Simmons J T: 1157
Simmons R L: 1520
Simmons T: 3734
Simon C: 1129
Simon H: 537
Simon R M: 1156
Simonetti G: 164, 1208, 1460, 1833
Simons H: 3651
Simonson J S: 501
Simpson W: 3894
Singcharoen T: 896
Singer A M: 2535
Singer D: 3624
Singer J M: 3614
Singer P: 109
Singh S P: 1781
Singjaroen T: 419
Singler R C: 3328
Singleton E L: 3704
Singson R D: 2528, 2779, 3068, 3113, 3114, 3115, 3116
Sinner W N: 398
Sinnott R G: 3117
Sinterhauf K: 2189
Sipponen J T: 2592
Siquiera E: 3597
Siram S M: 1567
Sironi S: 1372
Sischy B: 1559
Siskind B N: 1227, 1484, 1643, 1644
Sisler J: 793
Sisler W J: 3118
Sisson J C: 1539

Sitzmann J V: 1151
Siuda S: 2979, 3101
Sivasubramanian K N: 3498
Sivit C J: 399, 1866, 1867
Skaane P: 1645, 1646, 1647, 2405, 2406
Skalpe I O: 176
Skias D D: 4051
Skinner S: 2929
Skinner S R: 7
Skioldebrand C G: 276, 493
Skirkhoda A: 3959
Sklar E: 3119
Skolnick L: 2134
Skolnick M L: 1875, 4017
Skora T: 1100
Slaker D P: 946, 2773
Slamovits T L: 3877
Slanina J: 45, 3960
Slatis P: 2921
Slipman C W: 3116
Sloan G: 1737
Slusher S L: 2070, 2075
Slusser J H: 2714
Slutsky R A: 523
Slutsky V S: 1523
Small W C: 347
Smasal V: 2952
Smathers R L: 400, 401, 623, 1228, 1334, 2583
Smeets P: 3172
Smerud M J: 1648
Smet M H: 2726
Smevik B: 1868
Smit F W: 2416
Smith C: 1449
Smith C R: 2763
Smith D: 3961
Smith D F: 110, 238, 430, 1022, 1023, 1341, 1939, 3739
Smith D K: 3120, 3121
Smith E H: 168, 1455, 1846
Smith F P: 1254
Smith G: 3474
Smith G B: 1651
Smith J: 2582
Smith J A: 237
Smith J L: 1064, 1684
Smith J R: 3205, 3962
Smith K R: 3252
Smith L S: 3410
Smith P L: 579
Smith S J: 118
Smith T R: 402, 1467
Smith V: 3963
Smith W L: 262, 263, 510
Smith W P: 2135
Smith Y: 685
Smits J: 3498
Smits N J: 1975
Smoker W R: 3018, 3587, 3798, 3850, 3964, 3965, 4053
Smolarski N: 1452, 1622, 2101
Smolle Juttner F M: 752
Snider G L: 632
Sniderman K: 256
Snyder J V: 3547
So S: 4076
Sobel D F: 3122, 3819, 3925
Sobieszczyk S: 2229
Sobocinski K A: 3521
Socinski M A: 2326
Sodal G: 2091
Soffer O: 2136
Sohaey R: 447
Sohn H Y: 626
Sohotra P: 1900
Soila K: 3945
Soler R: 1453
Sollitto R A: 1600, 1710
Solodnik P: 2606, 2933
Solomon A: 897, 898, 1335, 2090
Solomon M A: 3123, 3124, 3988
Solomon N: 2233
Solti Bohman L G: 3697, 3967
Solymosi L: 3513
Som M L: 2137
Som P M: 403, 2137, 3125, 3733, 3784, 3886, 3968, 3969, 3970, 3971

Somer H: 3623
Somer K: 3126
Somers J M: 1869
Sommer B: 899, 1839, 1870, 3057
Sommer F G: 3309
Sommer H J: 1111
Somogyi J W: 552, 663
Sone S: 404
Sones P J: 1871
Sones P J Jr: 405, 961, 979, 1101, 1148
Song K S: 310
Song S H: 1446
Sonley M J: 3377
Sonnenblick E B: 3972
Soo C S: 1121, 2325, 3277
Sorensen I N: 2433
Sorensen K W: 664, 1336
Sortland O: 3772
Sostman H D: 2524
Sotiropoulos S: 3127
Soucek M: 921
Souda M: 3207
Soule E H: 1899
Soulen M C: 1649, 2138, 2139
Soulen R L: 3128
Sourtsis E: 3653
Soye I: 3129
Space T C: 3130
Spagnoli A: 3794
Spagnoli M V: 4088
Spallone A: 3973
Spanier S S: 2578, 2589, 2868
Spannare B: 3692
Spataro R F: 3934
Speck U: 184
Speckman J M: 278, 455, 456, 457, 672
Spector J G: 4052
Spellacy E: 1902
Spelta B: 2231
Spencer R R: 3131
Sperber M: 2598, 2648
Spiegel A: 2764
Spiegel A M: 253
Spiegel R: 2060
Spiegel S M: 3974
Spiegel T: 446
Spielmann R: 2285
Spielmann R P: 2584, 2585, 2741
Spiera H: 3733
Spies J B: 850
Spiess H: 3982
Spigos D G: 944, 2545, 3144, 3145, 3622
Spina V: 3161
Spira R: 100, 369, 3859
Spirn P W: 685
Spirt B A: 552, 900, 2208
Spitzer R M: 2058, 2126
Spitzer V M: 535
Spivey J F: 129, 936
Spizarny D L: 388, 406, 407, 408, 688
Sposato S: 1208
Sposito M: 1208
Sprawls P: 405
Sprayregen S: 2218
Sprecher S: 3976
Spring D B: 1650, 1872
Springfield D S: 2578, 2589, 2590, 2659, 2868
Spritzer C E: 2386, 2990
Sprung C L: 677
Srigley J: 1979
Srikantaswamy S: 2213, 2956
Srinivasan R: 3216
Srivisal S: 1627
St Amour T E: 409, 410
St Hilaire J: 1055
St Louis E L: 2184, 2820
St Ville J A: 2787
Staab E: 2370
Staab E V: 93, 1638, 3110
Stables D P: 2095
Stack C M: 1171, 1172
Stadalnik R C: 2980
Staelens K: 2425
Staffa G: 2459
Stafford J: 3892

Stafford J L: 3687
Stafford S A: 2337
Stagaard M: 2903
Stahl E: 484
Stalker H P: 1229, 3616
Standerskjold Nordenstam C G: 2041
Stanford W: 510, 809, 3464, 3977
Stanley J: 1897
Stanley J H: 375, 669, 3132, 3963
Stanley P: 981
Stanley R J: 68, 200, 214, 1063, 1107, 1261, 1262, 1268, 1307, 1309, 1329, 1362, 1429, 1487, 1671, 1701, 1783, 1788, 1914, 1986, 1987, 1988, 2011, 2084, 2171, 2207, 2267, 2314, 2633, 2945, 3603, 3650
Stanson A W: 1093
Staples C A: 411, 789, 815, 819, 901
Stapleton F B: 1799
Starinsky R: 2140
Stark D B: 1168
Stark D D: 412, 629, 902, 1033, 1230, 1468, 1469, 1470, 1511, 1807, 1978, 3978, 3979
Stark E H: 3313
Stark P: 413, 414, 685, 903, 904, 905, 1610, 3133, 3417, 3980, 3981
Starshak R J: 3920, 3921, 4060
Starzl T E: 3879, 4017
Stass P: 2705
Statz A: 3982
Staudacher C: 1372
Stauffer A: 2826
Stauffer A E: 1831, 3070
Stazio A: 4055
Steely J W: 1785
Steen G: 1270
Steffen R: 1257
Steiger J: 2499, 2536, 2928, 2929, 3134
Steiger S: 3134
Stein L: 2714
Stein M G: 415, 416, 792, 925, 3576, 3983
Stein R A: 3135
Steinbach L S: 2728
Steinbacher M: 906, 907
Steinbaum S: 1770, 2642
Steinberg A W: 1873
Steinberg D L: 908
Steinberg G G: 2643
Steinberg H: 734
Steinberg H V: 434, 1175, 2141
Steinberg M E: 2990
Steinberg R: 3976
Steinberg S B: 3997
Steinberg W M: 1568
Steinbrich W: 741, 1589, 1590, 1874, 2396, 2407, 2428
Steiner E: 895, 1470
Steiner H: 3136
Steiner L: 2825
Steiner R E: 3845, 3863
Steiner R M: 420, 678
Steinhardt M I: 857
Steinhoff H: 3431
Stellamor K: 177, 307, 1067
Stenberg P B: 150
Stenwig A E: 2291
Stenwig J T: 2879
Stephens D H: 996, 1093, 1231, 1307, 1376, 1414, 1415, 1431, 1432, 1433, 1450, 1529, 1580, 1648, 1840, 1899, 2236, 2457, 2467, 4058
Stephens R H: 2216
Stephenson L W: 628, 643
Stephenson T F: 3984
Steriotis J: 519
Stern D: 535, 898
Stetter E: 3568
Steudel A: 1111, 2857, 3513
Steudel M: 2857
Steuhl P K: 4039
Stevens J M: 3209, 3405, 3985, 3986

Stevenson J C: 2682
Stevenson W: 1947
Stewart E T: 31, 1341, 2440, 2441
Stichnoth F: 3499
Stiglbauer R: 882, 1220, 4020, 4021
Stiller J: 4084
Stimac G K: 111, 2663, 3987, 3988
Stiris M G: 1968, 1969
Stirnemann P: 437, 914
Stitik F P: 129, 348, 827, 891, 936, 937, 1269
Stober T: 3137
Stockham C D: 54
Stoeter P: 3031, 3138, 3139
Stojanovic J: 2644, 2645
Stoler M H: 2397
Stoller C: 1339
Stoller D W: 2499
Stollman A: 3140
Stollman A L: 3125
Stoltenberg P: 1386
Stoltenburg G: 3175
Stomper P C: 803, 1956, 2326
Stone D C: 129
Stone E E: 1651
Stork J: 178
Storkel S: 1281, 2125
Storme L: 1909
Stosiek M: 568
Stovring J: 193, 2672
Strain J D: 3989, 3990
Strand R D: 4057
Strashun A M: 352
Strasser S F: 569
Straub W H: 1875
Strauer B E: 502, 559
Straus D J: 1211
Strauss J E: 1652
Strax R: 1235, 1337, 1471
Strecker T C: 3135
Streiter M: 2553
Streiter M L: 1606
Strickland B: 820, 870
Stricof D D: 417
Stridbeck H: 155
Strife J L: 113
Strigaris K: 2235
Striggaris K: 285
Strijk S P: 418, 1970
Stringaris K: 3805
Strohecker J: 3141
Stroka D: 31
Strother C M: 2806, 2816
Strott C A: 2182
Strunk H: 1653
Struyven J: 621
Strzembosz A: 295
Stuck K J: 1472
Stuckmann G: 1674
Studdard E: 2823
Studlo J D: 248
Stulbarg M: 780
Stulbarg M S: 415
Stumer M: 2821
Sty J R: 3921, 4060
Styles R A: 1654
Stylopoulos L A: 3386, 3474
Subramanian R: 549
Subramanyam B R: 1354, 1958, 2142
Suchato C: 179, 419
Suehiro S: 1097
Suess C: 2888
Sugarbaker P: 180, 181, 1006
Sugarbaker P H: 1154, 1156, 1180, 1182, 1206, 1812
Sugarman L A: 2064
Sugihara M: 1102
Sugiki K: 1070
Sugita K: 85
Sugitani A: 2495
Sugiura H: 1250
Sugiyama T: 3003
Suh C H: 2076
Suh J H: 1784
Sukov R J: 2327
Sulkava R: 2592
Sullivan B M: 1020

Sullivan K L: 420, 421
Sullivan L D: 2320
Sumkin J: 1947, 2233
Sumkin J H: 1094, 4017
Sumner T E: 2902
Sundaram M: 112, 297, 298, 300, 301, 1893, 1916, 1917, 2335, 2336, 2657, 2678, 3170, 3533
Sundaresan N: 2912
Sunder Plassmann L: 795, 796, 1870
Susman N: 295, 298
Suss R A: 3991
Sussman J: 2143
Sussman S K: 422, 570, 571, 1655, 2144, 2145, 2328, 2391, 2827, 3482
Sutherland D: 2925
Sutherland D E: 1430
Sutker B: 3142
Sutton C S: 1971
Suy R: 1703
Suzuki E: 1299
Suzuki H: 350
Suzuki K: 2219, 2871
Suzuki M: 305, 423, 723, 1069, 1073, 1144, 1145, 1146, 2049, 3458
Suzuki S: 1232, 1252, 2641, 3612
Svendsen F: 3933
Svenningsen S: 2673
Svigals P: 3192
Swain M E: 424
Swanson S: 1523
Swanton M: 2370
Swartz J D: 3992, 3993, 3994, 3995, 3996, 3997, 3998, 3999, 4000
Swayne L C: 313, 995, 1700
Swearingen B: 2485
Swensen T: 1868
Swerdlow C D: 387
Swobodnik W: 1332
Sydnor C: 3406
Syvertsen A: 2722, 3194, 3381, 3524, 4008
Sze G: 2913
Szentpetery S: 524

Tabas J H: 3878
Tabor E K: 4056
Taccone A: 4001
Tachdjian M O: 2854, 2855
Tada S: 474, 2037, 2408
Tadmor R: 3164
Tafreshi M: 2642
Taillan B: 2801
Tait K: 3520
Takahashi H: 1177, 4018
Takahashi M: 1876, 2146, 3329, 3554, 3763, 3887, 3893, 4002
Takajasu K: 1173
Takakura K: 2674
Takanaka T: 1251
Takano M: 379
Takao R: 2147
Takashima E: 2357
Takashima S: 309, 425, 716, 2495, 3573, 3574, 3579
Takashima T: 305, 423, 934, 1102, 1144, 1145, 1146, 1250, 1251
Takasugi J E: 426, 675, 807
Takayama S: 1333
Takayanagi N: 1102
Takayasu K: 1099, 1152, 1233
Takayasu Y: 1176
Takazakura E: 3164
Takebayashi S: 2468
Takeda H: 1318
Takeda N: 379
Takehara Y: 1876
Takei H: 2991
Takeichi M: 452
Takemoto K: 3580
Takeo G: 3207
Takeshita K: 2495, 3573, 3574
Takeuchi M: 2161
Takeuchi N: 309, 425, 716
Takeuchi S: 4003

Takizawa K: 1232
Takizawa Y: 1074
Talbert A J: 9
Talle K: 2291, 2458
Tamakawa Y: 2146
Tamaki M: 1736
Tamaki N: 1057
Taminiau A H: 2556
Tampieri D: 2654
Tamura S: 1249, 2468, 3518
Tan C S: 944
Tan C T: 4004
Tan W S: 3144, 3145, 3622
Tanabe M: 2257
Tanada S: 1618
Tanagho E A: 2309
Tanaka H: 2408, 3781
Tanaka R: 4003
Tanaka S: 1299, 3898
Taneja K: 1877
Tanfani G: 3973
Tang Y S: 3294
Tanigaki T: 2616
Taniguchi S: 3580
Tanohata K: 964
Tantana S: 3146
Tapies Barba C: 4005
Tarr R J: 328
Tarr R W: 427
Tarver R D: 235, 496, 909, 910, 911, 2359
Tasaka A: 323, 1078, 1079, 1080, 1300, 1407
Tasaki T: 2147
Tash R R: 3147
Tashiro M: 2219
Tassinari C A: 2549
Tatcher M: 4006
Tate L G: 3832
Tateishi H: 1071, 1072
Tateishi R: 755
Tatsuta M: 755
Taveras J M: 18, 3070, 3384, 3728, 4007
Tavernier J: 541
Taylor A: 2440
Taylor A J: 31, 977, 1375, 2148, 3148, 4008
Taylor C: 1227
Taylor C R: 1972
Taylor G A: 399, 986, 1510, 1866, 1867, 1878, 1879, 1880, 2323, 3149, 4009
Taylor K J: 1758, 2418, 3355
Taylor R: 4010
Taylor S B: 4011
Taylor W K: 3852
Tazioli P R: 107
Te Strake L: 2185
Teal J S: 1567, 4027, 4028
Teasdale E: 3702
Teefey S: 2516, 2626
Teefey S A: 1264, 1331, 1338, 1881
Tegtmeyer C J: 1364
Tehranzadeh J: 2646, 2647, 3150, 3151
Teifke A: 380
Teigen C: 750
Teitcher J: 3834
Teitelbaum G P: 3264, 3342
Teixeira W R: 3864, 3865
Telander R L: 1388
Tellis C J: 601
Tempesta P: 1460
Templeton A W: 3347, 3681, 3682
Templeton P A: 912
Ten Haken G B: 1721
Ten Hove W: 428
Teng S S: 2027, 2258
Teplick J G: 429, 678, 3152, 3153, 3154, 3155, 3156
Teplick S K: 282, 283, 429, 678, 1545, 3152, 3154
Tepper J E: 1511
Terada Y: 3164
Teramo M: 3774
Terasaki K K: 4012

Terhorst L L: 4013
Terjesen T: 2673
Termote J L: 2537
Terpstra O T: 1270
Terrier F: 1266, 1339
Terriff B: 131
Terry B: 35
Teruel Agustin J J: 3157
Terwey B: 3499
Terwinghe G: 2552, 2681
Teteris N J: 2402
Tetickovic E: 2645
Thaete F L: 1875
Thaler M: 1963
Thane T T: 3565
Theissen P: 353
Thelen M: 473, 572, 576, 1090, 1215, 1216, 1255, 2125, 3908
Thickman D: 258, 2296
Thiebot J: 3359, 3670
Thiede G: 3158
Thiene G: 1698
Thierman D: 2149
Thies E: 1391
Thijssen H O: 2541
Thoden U: 3102
Thoeni R F: 337, 338, 1615, 1656, 1882
Thoma G: 2564
Thomaides S: 3827
Thomalla J V: 2010
Thomas D G: 3238
Thomas D J: 3845
Thomas D S: 1254
Thomas F: 433
Thomas F D: 872
Thomas J H: 3955
Thomas J L: 154, 773, 972, 1340, 2329, 2554, 3261, 3277, 4014
Thomas R J: 2807
Thomas S R: 858
Thomas W H: 3107
Thompson J R: 2838, 3159, 3553, 3690, 3752, 4015
Thompson W M: 294, 1049, 1050, 1458, 1477, 1573, 1655, 1657, 1658, 1694, 1749, 3860
Thompson W R: 2194
Thorbjarnarson B: 2532
Thornbury J R: 2397
Thornhill B A: 1517, 2330
Thornton R S: 3195
Thorsen K: 1023
Thorsen M K: 225, 238, 430, 431, 432, 990, 1022, 1315, 1341, 1689, 1939, 2225, 3230
Thron A: 3922
Thun F: 4093
Thurer R L: 239
Thurlbeck W M: 815
Thurn P: 509, 531, 537, 538, 539, 758, 1090, 3304
Thurnher S: 1134
Tichy P: 3485
Ticket L: 2680
Tierney L M Jr: 1600
Tievsky A L: 676, 2753
Tilak S: 3225
Tilak S P: 3266
Tillisch J: 3352
Tillmann B: 2484
Tillmann U: 445
Timmerman H: 853
Timmermans G: 1596
Tindall G T: 2710
Tines S C: 3683
Tipaldi L: 1459
Tisdal R G: 2239
Tishler J M: 1701
Tisnado J: 1883, 2234, 2339, 2419, 2420
Titelbaum D S: 1234, 4016
Tobben P J: 4017
Tobias J: 3945
Tobin K D: 330
Tocino I M: 433
Todo G: 821
Togashi K: 82, 1618, 2409, 2410, 2411
Tohdo G: 1618

Tokiguchi S: 4018
Tokuda M: 1076
Tolentino C S: 1091, 1763
Tolly E: 4019
Tominaga K: 808
Tomita S: 3612
Tomita T: 3768
Tomiyama N: 425
Tompkins R: 2485
Tonon C: 3106, 3812
Toombs B D: 1235, 1337, 1342, 1471, 3160
Toomes H: 735
Torizuka K: 82, 821, 822, 1618, 2409, 2410
Torrent O: 3074, 3880
Torres W E: 405, 434, 1101, 1199, 1236, 2173
Torricelli P: 3161
Tosch U: 3162
Totty W G: 2150, 2538, 2583, 2836, 3121, 3199, 3603
Touei H: 657
Towbin R: 1229, 1771, 3828
Towbin R B: 113, 2712
Towers M J: 2539
Towfigh H: 3899
Toyonaga Y: 1066
Tracey P: 2043
Trafton O: 3202
Traill T: 4090
Train J S: 2478
Trattnig S: 4020, 4021
Traupe H: 4022
Trautmann M: 2851
Traverso L W: 1385
Travis W D: 638, 2179
Traxler M: 1067, 1726
Trebo S: 3545
Trecco F: 3021, 3022, 3023
Trede M: 2189
Trefler M: 4023
Treisch J: 3163, 3186, 3187, 3188
Tremmel K: 1473
Tress B M: 4024
Treu E B: 2648
Treugut R: 2096, 2151, 2152, 2153, 2164, 2202
Trevor R P: 3312
Triebel H J: 869, 913, 2649, 3014, 4025
Trigaux J P: 435, 1659
Triller J: 436, 437, 914, 1296, 1343, 1474, 1884, 1885, 1886, 1973, 2331, 2332, 2412, 2615
Triller J K: 1339
Trinkwalter W: 3430
Triolo P: 3019
Trommer B L: 4026
Troup B R: 613
Troup P J: 3494
Troupin R H: 3658
Truc J B: 2346
Truss C D: 1329
Trygstad O: 1868
Tsai C C: 841
Tsai F Y: 3211, 4027, 4028
Tschakert C: 1887, 2413, 4029
Tschappeler H: 2650
Tscholakoff D: 704, 882
Tso W K: 1686
Tsuchida T: 4003
Tsuchiya F: 573
Tsuchiya S: 1179
Tsuji H: 3164
Tsuji K: 1612
Tsuji M: 1250
Tsuji R: 2998
Tsujiuchi J: 3458
Tsukamoto Y: 350, 1174, 2870
Tsukioka M: 2408
Tsukune Y: 1075
Tsuru M: 2991
Tuchmann A: 307
Tucker W: 1691
Tuckman G A: 971
Tuengerthal S: 661
Tully R J: 3165
Tumeh S S: 2540
Tunn U W: 2302

Turner D A: 569, 1171, 1172, 2519
Turner M A: 1883
Turner R J: 189, 1888
Turner R M: 3033, 4030
Turney S Z: 516
Turski P: 4071
Turski P A: 2806
Turto H: 2041
Twickler D M: 2414, 3924
Twomey B P: 2000
Tylen U: 484, 915
Tyminski L J: 1897
Tyrrel R T: 1237, 1889, 1890, 2415
Tyson R: 2925
Tzavaras N: 3222

Uchida H: 844, 1344
Uchino A: 1249, 3518
Uchiyama M: 1333
Udelsman R: 1812, 1835
Uden P: 2253
Udis D S: 2294
Ueda J: 1344, 2154
Uetani M: 1163
Uhl H: 635
Uhlenbrock D: 2155
Uhlich F: 231
Uji T: 553
Ulbricht D: 2558
Ullrich C G: 3013, 3166
Umali C B: 448
Umer M A: 2343
Umezu Y: 3781
Umlas S L: 1974
Unayama S: 2468
Ungeheuer E: 292
Unger E: 873, 3467
Unger E C: 1238
Unger G F: 1689, 1939
Unger J M: 438, 3350
Ungersbock K: 4020, 4021
Unverferth L J: 3271
Updike M L: 3214
Urban M: 307
Urich V: 1258
Usselman J A: 444
Utsunomiya J: 1177
Utz R: 3557

Vachon L A: 1328
Vadala G: 1711, 3167
Vadrot D: 656, 2345
Vainwright J R: 1159
Valavanis A: 2588, 3098, 3099, 3100, 4031, 4065
Valdivieso M: 773
Valencak E: 2829
Valentine A: 3621
Valentini A L: 242
Valk J: 2648
Vallancien G: 2317
Vallee D: 933
Valsecchi F: 3106
Valvassori G E: 3703, 3704
Van Beers B: 435, 1143, 1659
Van Besien R: 2469
Van Bockel S R: 2542
Van Dalsem V: 1379
Van Damme B: 998, 2726
Van de Velde E: 3172
Van den Bergh R: 2740
Van den Burg W: 186
Van der Laan R T: 1975
Van der Vliet A M: 2541
Van der Voorde F: 643
Van Dongen K J: 3091, 4032
Van Dyk J: 783
Van Dyke J: 2340
Van Dyke J A: 916, 3650
Van Engelshoven J M: 932, 1187, 2333
Van Eys J: 3684
Van Gansbeke D: 3910
Van Gijn J: 3611, 4032
Van Gijsegem D: 1196
Van Hasselt A: 3962
Van Heerden J A: 1388, 2236
Van Heesewijk H P: 2416

Van Kaick G: 284, 318, 356, 464, 518, 607, 661, 681, 682, 683, 735, 736, 763, 811, 906, 907, 917, 941, 1106, 1746, 2052, 2996, 3281, 3497
Van Kuijk C: 3168
Van Natta F: 1160
Van Nieuwenhuizen O: 3495, 3501
Van Roost W: 4068
Van Russelt J: 4068
Van Schaik F D: 3169
Van Schaik J J: 3169
Van Schaik H J P: 428
Van Steenbergen W: 998
Van Tassel P: 2947, 2948, 3685, 4033
Van Waes P F: 114, 115, 116, 1660, 1721, 1743, 2354, 2444, 2487, 3757, 4106
Van Zanten T E: 1892, 2648
Vanarthos W: 3151
Vanarthos W J: 1661
Vandaele L: 1909
Vandekerckhove T: 3172
Vandeman F: 1872
Vandergriend R A: 2868
Vanderslice L: 903
Vanderstigel M: 1954
Vandyke J A: 1926
Vannier M: 2504
Vannier M W: 117, 2475, 2538, 4034
Vansonnenberg E: 351, 439, 440, 441, 918, 1817, 1891, 4072
Vanzandt T F: 976
Vanzulli A: 1372
Varma R R: 1023
Varnell R M: 1122
Varney R R: 441, 918
Vas W: 919, 1893
Vas W G: 112, 1917, 3170
Vasile N: 442, 761, 790, 1136, 1137, 1138, 1139, 1140, 1141, 1142, 1143, 1239, 1954, 2023, 2935, 2936
Vassal J: 2671
Vassallo P: 465
Vassiliadis A: 2514
Vassallo P: 465
Vassilopoulos P: 3607
Vassilouthis J: 3973
Vazquez P M: 2297
Vedal S: 815, 901
Vega A: 1190
Veillon B: 2317
Velitschkov L: 2754
Vellody D: 4046
Venable D D: 3476
Venjakob K: 2503
Verbeeten B Jr: 466, 1975
Verbiest H: 3169
Vercruyssen J: 1596
Vereycken H: 1196
Vermess M: 180, 181, 182, 804, 1006, 1154, 1155, 1156, 1936
Vernacchia F S: 218, 1475
Verschakelen J A: 717
Verstraete K L: 3172
Veseth Rogers J: 3494
Vestring T: 574
Viamonte M Jr: 3945
Vibhakar S D: 1782, 1976
Vick C W: 2038, 2401, 2417
Vignaud J: 2677
Vigo M: 1698, 1894, 3283
Vigorito R D: 3472
Vijayamohan G: 3053
Vijungco J G: 2796
Vilgrain V: 443
Villacin A: 3354
Villacorta L: 1325
Villforth J C: 4035
Vincent L M: 1806
Vincenzoni M: 242
Vint V C: 444
Vinuela F: 2892, 3974
Vinuela F V: 2620, 4036

Violi L: 873
Virapongse C: 1848, 2627, 3897, 4037
Virtama P: 167
Vital J M: 2818
Vix V A: 496
Vlachos L: 3607
Vlahos L: 285, 2235, 2814, 3034, 3805
Vock P: 58, 143, 316, 445, 446, 530, 674, 843, 920, 921
Voegeli E: 1895
Vogel H: 73
Vogel H J: 575
Vogel J: 1847, 1896, 2062, 3913
Vogel W: 1095
Vogelsang H: 3265
Vogelzang R: 3400
Vogelzang R L: 118, 183, 198, 233, 447, 1240, 1550, 1757, 2456, 3173, 3496, 4038
Vogl G: 4039, 4040
Vogl T: 3431
Vogler J B: 3174
Vogt Moykopf I: 318, 683, 736, 811, 941
Voigt K: 3922, 4039
Voisin C: 865
Voisin M C: 3317
Volberding P: 3747
Volberg F M: 2902
Voldby B: 2903
Volle E: 3175
Vollhaber H H: 464, 907
Vollrath T: 3176
Volle E: 3175
Volpato S: 639
Volpe R J: 1795
Volta S: 1813, 2446, 3460
Von Einsiedel H G: 3867
Von Gumppenberg S: 2615
Von Heyden D: 3499
Von Krogh J: 3691
Von Kummer R: 4041
Von Mittelstaedt G: 2189, 2190
Von Rottkay P: 2543
Von Schulthess G K: 1008, 1134, 2473
Von Schweinitz D: 2437
Von Uexkull Guldenband V: 768, 3011, 3913
Von Uexkull V: 3286
Vonofakos D: 4042
Voorhees R L: 3600
Vouge M: 4043
Vowinckel M: 2450
Vrla R F: 118
Vrlenich L: 2065
Vu D N: 1169
Vu L H: 3752
Vucich J: 3426, 3427
Vucich J J: 3552
Vuitton D: 1000
Vujic I: 669, 1205, 1241, 1897
Vukanovic S: 4044
Vymazal J: 1118

Wackenheim A: 2715, 3392, 3394
Wackerle B: 1767
Wada A: 1246
Wada Y: 1176
Wade C T: 3967
Wade K C: 3873
Wadsworth D E: 2084
Waer M: 1910
Wagener D J: 1970
Wagener J: 262
Waggenspack G A: 4045
Wagle V: 3506
Wagner A G: 1809
Wagner B: 2285
Wagner D P: 3638
Wagner L K: 119
Wagner M: 2369
Wagner Manslau C: 1898, 3177
Wagner P K: 1281
Wagner R B: 922
Wagner S: 505
Wagner T: 2192
Wahl R L: 2611

Wahlers B: 574
Wahn U: 356
Waigand J: 231
Waite R: 1772
Waite R J: 448
Wakao F: 1152
Wakuta Y: 3518
Walden C: 236
Waldron R L: 4046
Walgenbach S: 740
Waligore M P: 1899
Walker M D: 3178
Walker P S: 101, 3861
Walker R: 2913
Walkey M M: 1900, 4047
Wall S: 1302, 1571
Wall S D: 449, 1475, 1600, 1762
Wallace J R: 1247
Wallace S: 161, 993, 1036, 1504, 1741, 2360, 2479, 3111, 3277, 3684
Wallesch C: 3696
Wallman J: 3730
Wallner B: 1209, 1847
Walsh J: 1373
Walsh J W: 937, 1883, 2038, 2339, 2401, 2417, 2418, 2419, 2420, 2421, 2422
Walsh P C: 2193
Walshe J M: 1001
Walter E: 450, 756, 1422, 1901
Walter G F: 3912
Walter K: 2605, 2915
Walter P: 899
Walther M M: 2173
Waltman A C: 1831
Waluch V: 2704
Wang A M: 451, 3072, 3088, 3179, 3180, 3181, 3528, 4048, 4049, 4050, 4051
Wang H: 2694, 2984, 3214, 3488, 4105
Wang K P: 320, 349, 695, 746
Wannenmacher M: 45, 3960
Wanner K: 1312
Wappenschmidt J: 3095
Ward A: 3536
Ward B A: 1157
Ward E M: 1376, 1432
Ward M P: 4052
Ward R E: 3608
Wareham G: 3981
Warhit J M: 463, 1531
Warmath M A: 444
Warmuth Metz M: 2604, 2637, 3182, 3183
Warner M A: 3779
Warner R M: 2102
Warren L P: 1345
Warren R C: 120
Warshaw A L: 1476
Warsof S L: 3620
Warwick W J: 243
Wasenko J J: 2651
Wass J L: 2010, 2359
Wasserman T H: 952
Wassipaul M: 1067
Watanabe A S: 4053
Watanabe A T: 4054
Watanabe H: 1174, 1612
Watanabe K: 355, 2161
Watanabe T: 2409
Watanabe T J: 3671
Watanabe Y: 423, 452
Watkins T: 3036
Watschinger B: 2123
Watson A J: 4090
Watson J T: 3808
Watson R A: 1872
Watson R C: 701, 2582, 3532
Watters D H: 2394
Watts R W: 1902
Watzinger F: 1527
Way L W: 1320, 1437
Wayne K S: 743
Weatherbee L: 2471
Webb W R: 21, 247, 279, 360, 415, 416, 453, 454, 455, 456, 457, 458, 508, 532, 670, 671, 720, 722, 780, 781, 792, 813,

814, 902, 908, 923, 924, 925, 926, 953, 954, 955, 2652, 3576, 3983
Weber A L: 2621
Weber F: 4066
Weber M: 1215, 2124
Wechsler R J: 420, 421, 459, 1184, 1242, 1560, 2544, 3740
Weekes R G: 2653
Weese J L: 2623
Weetman R: 627
Wegener O H: 121, 138, 460, 776, 927, 1727, 2683, 3259
Wegenke J D: 1740
Weh H J: 2649
Wehunt W D: 2939
Weiand G: 949, 1593, 1903
Weibull H: 2152
Weich Y: 1581
Weidenmaier W: 122
Weider D J: 3344
Weigel J: 2067
Weigel J W: 2068
Weigelbaum K: 518
Weigert F: 1904, 2706
Weiler S: 1000
Weill A: 2654
Weill F: 1000, 1708
Wein A J: 1347, 2315
Weinberg D S: 3180
Weinberg J: 930
Weinberg P E: 3305
Weinberg S M: 60
Weinberger E: 2156
Weinberger G: 2655
Weiner M: 2586
Weiner S N: 1346
Weinerman P M: 1347
Weinerth J L: 2679
Weingarten K: 3192
Weinmann H J: 138
Weinreb J C: 836, 1695, 2118, 2973, 3184
Weinstein A J: 1046
Weinstein B J: 2470
Weinstein J B: 461
Weinstein M A: 3065, 3360, 3745
Weinstein P R: 3127
Weinstein R: 2823
Weinstein Z R: 2822
Weir I H: 928
Weis L D: 3271
Weis R R: 3272
Weisberg L A: 3185, 4055
Weisbrod G L: 650, 857, 862
Weiske R: 291, 691, 2859
Weiss C: 462
Weiss C A: 1411
Weiss H: 2190
Weiss H D: 1390, 2051, 2192, 3212, 3217
Weiss K L: 2618
Weiss L M: 463
Weiss M A: 1444
Weiss P: 2786
Weiss P J: 101, 3861
Weiss S L: 2397
Weiss S M: 1959
Weiss S W: 2573
Weiss T: 943, 1993, 3186, 3187, 3188
Weissleder R: 1033
Weissman B N: 3107
Weissman J L: 4056
Weitzman S S: 2595
Weitzner I Jr: 3147
Weksberg A P: 2382
Welch K: 4057
Welch T J: 13, 1113, 1414, 2236, 4058
Welke M: 729
Welker H: 2463, 4059
Wellenstein D E: 872
Wells R G: 3921, 4060
Wells T H Jr: 86
Wells T Jr: 3792
Wenda K: 2910
Wende S: 184, 3700, 4061, 4062
Wendling L: 3290
Wendt F C: 2505

Wener L: 3666
Wenk M: 2845
Wentworth W: 14
Wentz K U: 464
Wenz W: 635, 3960
Wenzel E: 2843
Wernecke K: 465, 1243, 3853
Werner P H: 238
Werner W R: 3112
Wertman D: 2629
Wesbey G 3d: 227
Westbury G: 3269
Westcott J: 703
Westcott J W: 701
Wester K: 4063
Westerman B R: 2012
Westra D: 466
Wetherbee J N: 3494
Wettstein P: 1399, 1625, 4044
Wetzel E: 725
Wetzel L H: 1787, 2075
Wexler J A: 590, 1295
Wexler L: 387, 475, 522
Weyman P J: 1059, 1238, 1261, 1329, 1429, 1457, 1488, 2107, 2191, 2340
Whalen E: 1244
Whalen J P: 256, 966, 1210, 1672, 1852, 1922, 2056, 3248, 3249
Whaley D: 2237
Whaley R A: 3901, 3959
Wharam M D: 478
Wharam M D Jr: 2506
Wheat R: 3420
Wheeler D E: 3924
Wheeler P S: 711, 712, 866, 867, 3445, 3851
Wheeler P S,: 868
Wheelock J B: 2417
Whelan C A: 480, 1495
Whelan M A: 3189, 3190, 3191, 3192, 4064
Whelchel J: 1358
Whelchel J D: 2141
Whitacre M: 467, 806
White E A: 2210
White E M: 1476
White M: 1206
White P: 1212
White R I Jr: 973
White S J: 3838
White T J: 3341
White W: 1842
Whitelaw G: 2793
Whitlatch S: 1844
Whitley J: 1053
Whitley J E: 467, 806
Whitley N O: 327, 328, 329, 467, 806, 1053, 1159, 1316, 1751, 1905, 1906, 1957
Whitman G J: 468
Whitmire L F: 1236
Wholahan J D: 3769
Whyte M K: 579
Wichman R D: 347
Wichmann W: 4065
Wicks J D: 3
Widlus D M: 1907
Widmann W D: 313
Wiedenmann S D: 963
Wiederkehr P: 290
Wiens C W: 2954
Wiese H: 1131
Wiesel S: 3029
Wiesen E: 36
Wiesen E J: 3193
Wietholter H: 4040
Wilbur A C: 123, 483, 2318, 2334, 2545, 3145
Wilder W M: 2047
Will A: 2979
Will A D: 3690
Will C H: 1887
Willeit J: 4066
Willemse J: 3501
William R: 1781
Williams A G Jr: 1636
Williams A L: 1753, 2225, 2675, 2688, 2689, 2722, 2724, 2748,

2819, 3194, 3195, 3196, 3378, 3379, 3380, 3381, 3521, 3522, 3901
Williams C D: 1936
Williams D: 533
Williams D M: 1952
Williams E: 2103
Williams H C: 1542
Williams J J: 2166, 2532
Williams J L: 2245
Williams M P: 302, 469, 1908, 2260
Williams R A: 470
Williams S: 2470
Williamson B Jr: 2165, 2467
Williamson B R: 400, 554, 805, 1364, 2106
Williamson M R: 1860, 2232
Williford M E: 471, 1477, 1657
Willing S J: 1505
Willis J J: 2805
Willis M: 804, 1154, 1155, 1156
Wills J S: 1207, 2486
Wills K: 141
Wilmink J T: 185, 186, 3197, 3198
Wilmouth R J: 1853
Wilms G: 968, 1486, 1703, 1800, 1909, 1910, 1980, 2238, 2460, 2740, 4068
Wilms G E: 219, 1132
Wilms W: 1459
Wilner H I: 2901
Wilson A J: 3199
Wilson C: 3524
Wilson C R: 14, 1287
Wilson D A: 2239
Wilson D M: 4069
Wilson J A: 1410
Wilson J D: 3301
Wilson J S: 2546
Wilson M A: 2982
Wilson R: 1428
Wilson S R: 2184
Wilson T E: 1478
Wimbish K J: 472, 951
Wimmer B: 462, 635, 1056, 1245, 1348, 1361, 1554, 1911, 1912, 2791, 2792, 2794, 3200, 3201, 3932
Winer Muram H T: 929
Winfield A C: 2157
Wing S D: 3237, 3797
Wing V W: 1293, 1303, 1475, 1500, 1762, 1913, 3202
Winkler M: 3127
Winkler R: 1551, 1552
Winkler S: 4071
Winquist R A: 2837, 2961, 2962
Winter J: 124, 2327, 3329, 3512
Winzelberg G G: 930
Wirguin I: 3493
Wirth R L: 606, 3203
Wise A: 3239
Wise D J: 487
Wise R H Jr: 1914
Wismer G L: 2631
Wisoff J H: 2908
Wiss D A: 2861
Witanowski L S: 2266
Witcofski R L: 3675
Witt H: 3162
Witt W S: 3542
Witte G: 125
Witte J: 342
Witten R M: 3967
Wittenberg J: 1033, 1230, 1380, 1470, 1476, 1511, 1816, 1831, 2619, 3440, 4072
Wittich G R: 441, 918
Wittkowski W: 3461
Wobbes T: 1970
Wodarz R: 4073, 4074
Woerner H: 1349, 2423
Woerther J P: 3296
Wofsy C B: 1824
Wojtowicz J: 1915, 2656
Wojtowycz M M: 1662

Wojtys E: 3027
Wold L E: 2660
Wolf A P: 3385
Wolf B S: 3002
Wolf E J: 1537
Wolf K J: 1051, 2366, 3430
Wolfe P: 3373
Wolfe S A: 3232
Wolff H: 1129, 1424, 2459
Wolff M: 313
Wolff P: 473, 572, 576
Wolfram N T: 204, 975, 1479, 1515
Wolfram Gabel R: 3394
Wolfson J J: 1037
Wolfson R J: 3996, 3999
Wolfson S K Jr: 4086
Wolpert S M: 126, 130
Wolverson M: 298, 1893
Wolverson M K: 112, 297, 300, 301, 1916, 1917, 2199, 2335, 2336, 2657, 3170, 3533
Wondergem J: 135
Wondergem J H: 575
Wong L C: 1686
Wong R: 55
Wong V: 904
Wong W: 2143
Wong W S: 261, 2158, 4075
Woo E: 4076
Wood B P: 1873, 2658
Wood G W: 2662
Wood L P: 187
Woodhurst W B: 3847
Woodring J H: 188, 931
Woodruff W: 2805
Woolfitt R A: 4077
Wouters E F: 932
Wrba F: 704
Wroblewski H: 73
Wulff K: 2840, 2841
Wunschik F: 2190, 2276, 2316, 4078
Wurche K D: 933
Wurtzebach L R: 2186
Wussow W: 3137
Wustner Hofmann M: 2587
Wuttke V: 3540, 3914
Wycoff R R: 2704, 3775
Wynchank S: 983

Xu G L: 4079

Yadley R A: 2704
Yagan R: 3204
Yaghoobian J: 1322
Yakes W F: 3561
Yale Loehr A J: 2159
Yamada I: 4071
Yamada K: 3662
Yamada T: 474, 1736
Yamaguchi A: 1146
Yamaguchi H: 50
Yamaguchi N: 379
Yamaguchi T: 475, 2998
Yamamoto K: 1057
Yamamoto M: 1246, 2616, 4080
Yamamoto R: 1246
Yamamoto S: 582, 583, 584, 585, 1246
Yamamoto T: 716, 3580
Yamaoka Y: 1057
Yamasaki H: 1070
Yamato M: 4081, 4082
Yamauchi T: 1084, 1085
Yamawaki Y: 1069
Yamazaki H: 1299
Yana C: 3456
Yanagi T: 1333
Yandow D R: 2799
Yang C F: 3109
Yang N C: 1247
Yang P J: 1248, 3205, 3469, 3601, 4083
Yang S L: 1242
Yang W C: 4084
Yankaskas B: 1760
Yankelevitz D F: 634
Yao J S: 4038

Yashiro N: 1078, 1086, 1089, 1300, 1301, 2160
Yasuda A: 3164
Yasumitsu T: 309
Yasumori K: 1249, 3518
Yeager V L: 2796
Yeates A: 2842
Yedlicka J: 2077
Yeh H C: 476, 1350, 1663, 1664, 1918, 1919, 3206
Yeoh J L: 856
Yeoman L J: 477
Yeon K M: 310, 718
Yester M V: 12
Yeung H P: 2184
Yi J G: 1276
Yip C K: 365
Yock D H Jr: 4085
Yokoi K: 808
Yokoyama K: 583, 584, 585
Yokoyama M: 2161
Yonas H: 4086
Yoneda M: 1333
Yonekura Y: 822
Yong Hing K: 2795
Yoo H W: 3349
Yoo K S: 1784
Yoon J W: 3683
Yoon Y: 721
Yoshida H: 1088, 1089, 1439, 2160
Yoshida M: 3771
Yoshii F: 4080
Yoshikai T: 1480
Yoshikawa J: 934, 1250, 1251
Yoshikawa K: 1300, 1439, 2674, 3645
Yoshimatsu H: 839
Yoshimatsu S: 1252
Yoshimitsu K: 1665
Yoshimura H: 844
Yoshimura T: 3207
Yoshino K: 3573, 3574
Yoshioka H: 2383
Yoshy C: 2547
Yoshy C S: 3952
Youker J E: 431, 432
Young H H: 2337
Young I R: 3845, 3863
Young J W: 3062, 4087
Young R: 1920
Young R G: 3635
Young S C: 4088
Young S W: 88, 89, 127, 189, 220, 386, 1003, 1186, 1888, 3336, 3942, 4089
Young W: 3894
Yousem D: 3208, 4090
Yousem D M: 1666
Yrjana J: 737
Ytterbergh C: 39, 2995, 3274, 3543, 3755, 3756
Yu A C: 1283
Yu B F: 1602
Yu E J: 721
Yu E S: 1275, 3353
Yu R H: 3769
Yu S W: 3447
Yu V L: 3881
Yu W S: 4091
Yu Y L: 190, 3209, 4076
Yuan H A: 3013
Yueh N: 128
Yulish B S: 281
Yurberg E: 4103, 4104
Yuri T: 1072
Yust Y: 3251
Yuzuriha H: 3781

Z Nedden D: 341
Zabel J: 736
Zacharias C E: 2519
Zafaranloo S: 1290
Zafrani E S: 1239
Zagoria R J: 2162, 2337
Zajko A B: 1094, 1947, 4017
Zamani A: 451, 3687, 4051
Zamani A A: 3179, 3180, 3181, 3528

Zamenhof R G: 130
Zanella F E: 4092, 4093
Zankovich R: 1599
Zaontz M: 2081
Zaparackas Z G: 3465
Zapf S: 2424, 2910
Zappasodi F: 2220
Zappoli F: 153
Zaret C R: 3305
Zarro V J: 738
Zatz L M: 3203, 3210
Zaunbauer W: 290, 935, 1296, 1360, 1398, 1678
Zeanah W R: 2659
Zeck O F: 119
Zee C S: 958, 3211, 3245, 3330, 4012, 4027, 4094
Zegel H G: 6
Zehnder R: 2772
Zeifer B: 3490
Zeiss J: 1096

Zelaya B: 2675
Zelch M G: 2188
Zelenik M E: 191
Zeman R K: 226, 1198, 1222, 1253, 1254, 1465, 1481, 2001, 2081, 2163, 3342, 3435, 3620
Zerbi A: 1372
Zerhouni E A: 129, 478, 711, 744, 745, 746, 747, 782, 866, 867, 891, 892, 926, 936, 937, 945, 965, 973, 1149, 1151, 1269, 1605, 1649, 1960, 2187, 2472, 2787, 3128, 4095
Zeumer H: 104
Zhu X P: 624, 4096
Zick R: 1387
Zieger M: 42, 2164
Ziegler G: 2801
Ziegler K: 479
Ziegler M: 2006, 2304

Ziegler U: 1034
Ziegler V M: 3212
Ziessman H A: 2180
Zikman J M: 2270
Zilkha A: 3213, 4097
Zilkha K J: 3405
Zimmer P: 1473
Zimmer W D: 2165, 2660
Zimmerman J B: 93
Zimmerman R A: 3492, 3575, 3801, 4016, 4088, 4098, 4099, 4100
Zimmerman R D: 3078, 3299, 3389, 4101, 4102, 4103, 4104
Zingas A P: 2039, 2297
Zingg E: 2196
Zinn W L: 480, 833
Zinreich E S: 3876, 3900
Zinreich S J: 2785, 2984, 3214, 3666, 3848, 4105

Ziprkowski M: 766
Zirinsky K: 966, 1672, 1852, 1921, 1922, 2056, 2166, 2167, 2312, 2532
Zirn J R: 634
Zissin R: 481, 2168
Zito J L: 3384
Ziv N: 2602
Zlatkin M B: 2691, 2826, 3215
Zlotogorski A: 3493
Zobel B B: 3021, 3022
Zocholl G: 1255, 1653
Zoffmann E: 3323
Zoller A: 1332
Zollikofer C: 1674
Zonneveld F W: 114, 115, 3376, 4106
Zorn G L: 889
Zornoza J: 1256, 1808, 2554, 3046, 3111
Zucker Pinchoff B: 3216

Zuelzer W: 3271
Zulch K J: 4022
Zum Winkel K: 1103, 1104, 1482, 2209, 3064
Zuna I: 284, 518, 683
Zur Nedden D: 339, 340, 2829
Zuurbier R: 3342
Zuurbier R A: 3264
Zwaan M: 3217
Zwanger Mendelsohn S: 800, 2338
Zweig G: 2956
Zwergel T: 2304
Zwicker C: 1257, 1258, 1923
Zwicker R D: 130
Zwillenberg S: 3993, 3994, 4000
Zwirewich C V: 131, 938, 939
Zylak C J: 547, 919
Zyroff J: 3925

Subject Index

Abdomen
–, anatomical relationships of   315
–, anatomy of   341–343
–, perforation of   324
Abscess   484
–, attenuation value of   89
–, development of   88
–, diagnosis of   89
–, Douglas   448
–, drainage of   117
–, gravitation   167
– –, gas deposits   167
– –, phlegmonous permation   167
–, hematogenous   466
–, (of) liver   269 f.
– –, amebic   269 f.
– –, fungal   269 f.
– –, pyogenic   269 f.
–, (of) pancreas   310 f.
–, perirenal   462
–, (of) peritoneal cavity   350
–, psoas   466 f.
–, pulmonary   200, 228
– –, abscess cavity   201
– –, abscess membrane   203
– –, empyema   201
– –, pneumatocele   201
– –, scar   201
–, renal   386, 388–390
– –, attenuation value   390
– –, gas formation   390
– –, membrane   390
–, tubo-ovarian   448
Absorption of X-rays   565
Acetabulum   553, 555
–, roof   553
Acromegaly   404
Addison's disease   412
Addition of image sections   565
Adenocarcinoma
–, (of) biliary tract   286
–, (of) peritoneal cavity   350
–, (of) stomach   325
Adenoma   212 f.
–, adrenocortical   404–406
– –, hyperadrenalism in   404
– –, inactive   406
– –, tissue density of   405
–, bilateral   404
–, bronchial   212 f.
– –, carcinoid   213
– –, CT of   213
– –, cylindroma   213
–, Conn's   404 f.
– –, calcification of   404
–, Cushing's   404 f.

–, cystadenoma   296
– –, serous   296
–, (of) gallbladder   282
–, hepatic   252
– –, biliary   252
– –, cystadenoma   252
–, (of) liver   254
–, macrocystic   296 f.
–, microcystic   296 f.
–, nonfunctioning   406
–, (of) pancreas   296 f.
–, parathyroid   159
– –, hemorrhage of   159
– –, necrosis of   159
–, pituitary   404
–, prostatic   414, 426, 429
– –, enlargement of
    the prostate   426
– –, enucleation of   426
– –, infravesical
    obstruction by   426
– –, trabeculated bladder   414
–, renal   379
Adenomyomatosis   282, 437
–, uterine   441
Adnexes   435
Adnexitis   449
Adrenal
–, carcinoma   487
–, cortex   404
–, cyst   410 f.
– –, calcification of   410
– –, endothelial   410
– –, parasitic   410
– –, pseudo-   410
–, glands   401–412
– –, adenoma of   404
– –, anatomy of   403
– –, atrophy of   412
– –, configuration of   402
– –, cortical tumor of   404
– – –, hormonal activity of   404
– – –, suppression test   404
– –, enlargement of   412
– –, false tumor of   403
– –, hyperplasia of   404
– –, metastases into   409
– – –, hemorrhage   410
– – –, necrosis   410
– –, size of   402
–, hematoma (pseudocyst)   411
–, hemorrhage   410, 412
– –, etiology of   410
– –, septicemia   411
–, hypoplasia   412
–, inflammation   411

– –, calcification in   412
– –, enlargement of
    the adrenals   412
– –, etiology of   411
– –, fibrosis in   412
– –, mycosis   412
– –, necrosis in   411
–, insufficiency   409
–, medullary tumors   407
– –, myelolipoma   407
– – –, attenuation value of   407
– – –, calcification of   407
– –, neuroblastoma   408
– – –, calcification of   408 f.
– – –, cystic degeneration   408
– – –, hemorrhage in   408
– – –, location of   408
– – –, lymph node
       enlargement in   409
– – –, metastases of   409
– – –, metastatic spread of   408
– – –, necrosis of   408
– – –, tumor conglomerate   409
– –, pheochromoblastoma   408
– – –, hormonal activity of   408
– – –, metastatic spread of   408
– –, pheochromocytoma   407
– – –, calcification of   407
– – –, cystic degeneration of   407
– – –, fibrisis of   407
– – –, hemorrhage in   407
–, pituitary insufficiency   412
Adrenocortical
–, adenoma   404–406
– –, hyperadrenalism in   404
– –, inactive   406
– –, tissue density of   405
–, carcinoma   405
– –, adrenogenital syndrome   405
– –, calcification of   406
– –, Cushing's syndrome   405
– –, hemorrhage in   406
– –, necrosis in   406
–, hyperplasia   404
AHCT see CT, arterial hepato-
    graphic
Algorithm   565
Amebiasis   334
Amyloidosis   477
Anemia
–, sickle cell   364
Aneurysm   481
–, abdominal   372
–, complications   485
– –, anastomosis   485
– –, infection of prothesis   485

– –, stitch 485
–, aortic 162f., 179, 398, 480
– –, dissecting 164
– –, infrarenal 480
– –, traumatic 165
–, cerebral 372
–, chronic 170
–, dissecting 165, 481, 483f.
– –, arteriosclerosis 165
– –, cystic medial necrosis 165
– –, intramural hematoma 165
– – –, thrombosis of 165
– –, laceration of intima wall 165
– –, lumina 165, 484
– – –, false 165
– – –, true 165
– –, membrane 166, 484
– –, pericardial effusion 166
– –, thrombosis of 165, 484
– –, types of 165
–, (of) heart 175
–, hemorrhage in 483
–, infection of 483
–, inflammatory aortic 481
–, mycotic 484
– –, gas 484
– –, inflammation 484
– – –, abscess 484
– – –, empyema 484
– – –, osteomyelitis 484
–, Pseudo- 483
–, rupture of 483
–, ruptured aortic 482f.
–, saccular 165
–, spurious 169, 482f.
–, stitch 485
–, suture 483
Angiogram sign 219
Angiomyolipoma 380f.
–, aneurysmal deformation 381
–, diagnostic sign 381
–, hemorrhage 381
Angiosarcoma
–, (of) spleen 361
Angle
–, measurement 565
–, pericardiophrenic 160
Anulus
–, fibrosus 518f., 521
– –, bulging 518
– –, calcification 518
– –, dehydration 518
– –, gas 518
Aorta 137, 144, 162
–, abdominal 453, 481
– –, aneurysm 481
– – –, calcification 481
– – –, types 481
–, root of 144
–, thoracic 162
– –, aneurysm of 162
– – –, arteriosclerotic 162
– – –, diameter of 162

– – –, intima degeneration of 162
– – –, mediastinal hematoma
       in 163
– – –, mycotic 162
– – –, rupture of 162
– – –, sclerosis of 163
– – –, thrombotic deposits of 162
– – –, types of 162
Aplasia 178
Apophyse
–, anular 519
Appendicitis 335, 449, 469
Appendix
–, abscess of 335
– –, after appendectomy 335
–, retrocecal 336
Arch, vertebral
–, aortic 162, 170
– –, anomalies 162
– –, double 162
– –, right 162
–, azygos 140
–, root (of) 517, 523
–, spinous 536
– –, dislocation 536
Archives 565
Arrhenoblastoma 447
Artery
–, brachiocephalic 170
–, common hepatic 453
–, common iliac 480
– –, aneurysm of 480
–, gastric 344
–, hepatic 251
–, inferior mesenteric 455
–, pulmonary 138, 166f., 185, 189
– –, ectasia of 166f.
–, renal 398, 455
–, splenic 364, 455
– –, occlusion of 364
–, subclavian 137
–, superior mesenteric 455
Arthritis
–, rheumatoid 203
Arthrosis
–, intervertebral 518
–, Spondyl- 526, 529
–, uncovertebral 521
Articulation 535
–, intervertebral 515, 518, 535
– –, subluxation 535
Artifact 521, 565
–, beam-hardening 86
–, high-contrast 86
–, motion 85
Asbestosis 207, 230f.
–, CT of 207f., 231
–, development of 207
–, pleural plaques due to 230
Ascites 372
–, biliary 350
– –, in peritoneal cavity 350
–, (of) peritoneal cavity 344–348

Asplenia 366
Atelectasis 188–192
Atrium 138
Attenuation of X-rays 565
Attenuation value 85–91
–, (of) abscess 88f.
–, (of) blood 87f.
–, (of) boundary surfaces 87
–, (of) cysts 87
–, (of) exsudate 87
–, (of) hematoma 87f.
–, (of) solid tissue 89
– –, bony tissue 89
– –, fatty tissue 89
– –, lung tissue 89
– –, mixed tissue 89
–, (of) transsudate 87
Axis 541
–, arch of 541
– –, fracture of 541
– – –, classification of 541

Back projection 565
Bifurcation
–, aortic 453
–, tracheal 141, 144
Bile duct
–, common 279, 285f., 297f.
– –, air in 285
– –, congenital anomalies of 286f.
– –, CT of 279
– –, dilatation of 283f., 298, 300
– –, obstruction of 297
–, dilatation of 283f.
–, hepatocholedochal 284
–, intrahepatic 279, 282
– –, dilatation of 282
Bilharziosis 416f.
Biliary tract 277–287
–, anatomy of 278f.
–, bile fluid 280f.
– –, attenuation value of 280f.
– – –, vacuum phenomena
        and 281
–, Caroli's disease 287
–, cholangiopancreatography 283
– –, endoscopic retrograde
       (ERCP) 283
–, cholecystolithiasis 281
–, congenital anomalies of 286f.
–, dilatation of 300
–, ERCP 283
–, gallbladder 279, 281–283
– –, acromegaly, effects of 279
– –, calcification of 279
– –, calculi of 281
– –, cholecystitis 279f.
– –, cholecystogram 279
– –, cholelithiasis 279, 281
– –, diabetes mellitus,
       effects of 279
– –, empyema of 279f.
– –, enlargement of 279

– –, inflammatory changes of   279
– –, porcelain   280
– –, thickening of   280 f.
– –, tumors of   282
–, infection of   284–286
–, Klatskin's tumor   286
–, obstruction of   282–284
–, pericholecystic abscess   280
–, porta hepatis   282, 286
–, tumors of   286
Biloma   351
–, of peritoneal cavity   348
Bladder see Urinary bladder
Blastoma
–, sympathetic   160
Bone
–, chondrification of   503
–, compact   542
– –, islands of   542
–, cyst of   237 f.
–, tumor of   501–509
– –, aneurysmal bone cyst   509
– –, calcification of   503
– –, chondrogenous   503
– – –, attenuation value of   504
– – –, benign   503
– – –, malignant   503 f.
– –, chondrosarcoma   503 f.
– –, classification of   503
– –, CT of   503
– –, enchondroma   503
– –, Ewing's sarcoma   505 f.
– –, fibrocytoma   505
– –, fibrous   505
– –, giant cell   509
– –, hemangioma   509
– –, histiocytoma   505
– –, "ivory whorl" sign   507
– –, lipoma   505
– –, lymphoma   507
– – –, Hodgkin's   507
– – –, non-Hodgkin's   507
– –, lytic lesions in   507
– –, medullary infiltration in   507
– –, metastases   508
– –, myelogenic   505–507
– –, ossification   509
– –, osteogenic   505 f.
– –, osteolysis in   507, 509
– –, osteoma   504
– – –, osteoid   504
– –, osteomyelitis in   507
– –, osteoporosis in   509
– –, osteosarcoma   502, 504
– – –, CT diagnosis of   504 f.
– – –, juxtacortical   505
– – –, pelvic   502
– –, parosteal   507
– –, plasmocytoma   506 f.
– –, sarcoma   507
– – –, Ewing's   505, 507
– – –, reticulum cell   507
– –, sclerosis in   507, 509

– –, X-ray of   503
Bourneville-Pringle syndrome
    370, 380
Bowel
–, small see Intestine, small
Bronchi
–, obstruction of   188
–, segmental   185
Bronchiectasis   197
–, cylindrical   199
–, cystic   197
–, saccular   199
–, varicose   196, 199
Bronchogram
–, air   192, 219
Bronchus
–, intermediate   138
Brucellosis   362
Budd-Chiari syndrome   275
Bursa
–, omental   307, 311, 344
Bypass
–, aortocoronary   175 f.

Calcification   393
Calculi
–, biliary   284
–, (of) gallbladder   281
–, prostatic   429
Canal
–, inguinal   434
–, vertebral   161
Capsule
–, renal   379, 387, 399
– –, cord formation   379
– –, cortical "rim" sign   399
– –, scar tissue   399
– –, superinfection   399
Carbuncle
–, renal   390
– –, superinfection   390
Carcinoid
–, (of) small bowel   327
Carcinoma   213, 215,
    219–221, 426
–, adeno   148
–, adrenal   487
–, adrenocortical   404
–, bladder   475
– –, metastases of   475
–, (of) breast   239 f.
–, bronchial   150, 191, 213–215,
    219–221, 262, 385
– –, angiogram sign with   219
– –, classification of   215
– –, CT of   215–221
– –, lymphatic spread   220
– –, metastases of   221
– –, poststenotic pneumonia
        with   220
– –, pulmonary infiltrates   219
– –, staging of   213
– –, types of   215

–, bronchio-alveolar   219
–, cervical   436, 438 f., 475
– –, infection   439
– –, infiltration   437 f.
– –, irradiation of   439
– –, metastases of   437, 475
– –, radiotherapy of   437
– –, staging of   436
–, (of) colon   262, 327–332, 474
– –, metastatic, to liver   262 f.
–, colorectal   328–332
–, embryonal testicular   476
– –, metastases of   476
–, (of) esophagus   150, 317
– –, metastases from   317
–, (of) gallbladder   282 f.
–, hepatocellular   256–258, 487
– –, cirrhosis with   256–258
– –, CT of   258
–, ovarian   440, 444 f., 474
– –, staging of   444
–, (of) pancreas   286, 297–302
–, (of) peritoneal cavity   354
–, prostatic   427
– –, metastases of   427
– –, protrusion of prostate   427
–, renal cell   240, 374 f., 377–379,
    386, 475, 486
– –, attenuation   377
– –, calcification   375, 378
– –, cystic   378
– –, differential diagnosis   379
– –, hematoma   377
– –, hemorrhage   377
– –, metastases of   475
– –, protrusion   377
– –, staging   374
– –, vascularization   377
–, renal pelvis   382
–, sigmoid   475
– –, metastases   475
–, squamous cell   219
– –, necrosis with   219
–, (of) stomach   321–324
–, testicular   474
–, thyroid   158, 239
–, tonsillar   262
–, tracheal   159
–, tubal   440
–, urothelial   383
– –, calcification   383
– –, macrohematuria   383
– –, metastases   383
–, uterine   474
– –, body   439–441
– –, abscesses in   442
– –, hematoma in   442
– –, postoperative scars   442
– –, radiation fibrosis   442
– –, recurrences   441
– –, staging of   439
– –, tumor expansion   442
– –, vaginal stump   441

Carcinomatosis
–, (of) peritoneal cavity   345, 349, 352–354
Cardiac computed tomography
–, Cine-CT, ultra fast   173, 176
–, ECG-gated   173
Cardiomyopathy   174f.
Caroli's disease   287
–, medullary sponge disease   287
Cartilage   526
–, degeneration   526
– –, vacuum phenomena   526
Castleman's disease   301
Cauda equina   515, 517, 519, 521
Cavity
–, joint   526
–, perirenal   381
–, pleural   203, 228
–, retroperitoneal   453, 465f., 470, 477
–, sino-auricular   517
–, subperitoneal   435
–, subpleural   203
–, uterine   438, 448
– –, dilated   438
Center   565
Cervix   436, 449, 459
Chest
–, trauma   242
–, wall of   235–242
– –, abscess   241
– –, anatomy of   236f.
– –, bone destruction   239
– –, cartilage destruction   239
– –, CT of   237
– –, inflammation   240f.
– –, invasion of   239
– –, metastatic involvement of   239f.
– –, neoplasms of   237–241
– – –, CT of   238–241
– –, phlegmon   241
– –, sclerosis   241
– –, sternoclavicular dislocation   242
– –, surgery   237
– – –, thoracic   237
– –, trauma   242
– –, tumor of   237
Cholangiectasis   272
Cholangiopancreatography   259, 297, 310
–, endoscopic retrograde (ERCP)   259, 297
Cholangitis   285
Cholecystectomy   284
Cholecystitis   279, 281
Choledochectasia   371
Cholesterosis   282
Chondroma
–, (of) chest wall   237
Chondrosarcoma   220, 222, 494
–, (of) chest wall   237

–, pulmonary metastases   220
Chordoma   543
Chorionepithelioma   156
Cine-CT   565
Cirrhosis
–, (of) liver   267f.
– –, CT of   267f.
– –, types of   267
Coarctation   162
Colitis
–, granulomatous   335
–, ischemic   335
–, radiation   335
–, ulcerative   285, 334f., 469
Collecting structures
–, renal   397
– –, attenuation value   397
– –, inflammation   397
Collection system
–, renal   396
– –, dilatation   396
– –, layering phenomena   396
Collimation   565
Colon   329, 336
–, abscess of   331–333, 335–337
–, adenocarcinoma of   328
–, adenoma   329
– –, villous   329
–, carcinoma of   328f.
– –, anal   329
– –, colorectal   328
– –, CT detection of   328
– –, metastases from   328f.
– –, recurrence of   329
–, colitis   335
– –, granulomatous   335
– –, ischemic   335
– –, radiation   335
– –, ulcerative   334f.
– – –, CT diagnosis of   334f.
–, contrast medium administration   329
–, Crohn's disease   335
–, CT of   328–332
–, diverticulitis of   328, 336
–, "double halo" sign   332
–, fibrosis of   331f., 334
–, fistulae in   331–333, 335–337
–, granulomatous   335
– –, ischemic   335
–, "halo" sign   335
–, inflammation of   332, 334, 336f.
–, lymph nodes of   332f., 335
– –, enlargement of   329, 332f., 335
–, lymph vessels of   332
– –, sclerosis of   332
–, mesocolon   345
– –, transverse   345
–, perforation of   336, 347
–, polyps of   334
– –, pseudopolyps   334

–, proctectomy   330
– –, tumor recurrence after   330–332
–, radiotherapy in   331
–, scar tissue in   331
–, sigmoid   329, 336
– –, carcinoma of   329
–, "target" sign   332
–, yersiniosis in   333
Column
–, pubic   553
– –, ilioischial   553
– –, iliopubic   553
–, renal   395
Compartment
–, pararenal   457
– –, anterior   457
– –, posterior   457
–, perirenal   457, 459, 464
– –, abscess   464
– –, fibrosis   464
– –, hematomas   464
– – –, attenuation value of   464
–, (of) peritoneum see Peritoneal cavity
–, prevesical   459
–, retroperitoneal   459
–, syndrome   494
Conn's syndrome   404
Contraceptives
–, (in) hepatic adenoma   252
Contrast medium   97–110
–, administration of   93f.
– –, bolus injection   93f.
– – –, intravascular enhancement   93
– – –, parenchymatous enhancement   93f.
– –, vascularization   94
– – –, effects of   94
–, barium suspension   106
–, biliary   105
–, bolus injection of   99, 293, 316
– –, bolus geometry   101
– –, circulation time   102f.
– –, controlled   103
– –, duration of   103
– –, intravenous   102
– –, peak-time   100
– –, protracted   103
– –, scan sequence time   103
– –, time-density curve   99
–, Gastrografin®   316
–, infusion of   104
– –, distribution   104
– –, intravenous   104
–, injection   105
– –, intra-arterial   105
– –, intravascular distribution of   98
–, opacification   106
– –, intestinal   106
– – –, colon contrast   109

– – – –, oral   109
– – – –, rectal   109
– – –, complete bowel
        contrast   109
– – –, partial bowel contrast   108
– –, intracavitary   106
–, principles of enhancement   99
– –, angiography   99
– –, blood-brain barrier   99
– –, choledochography   99
– –, parenchymal enhancement   99
– –, renography   99
– –, urography   99
–, urographic   100
Contrast resolution   565
Convolution   565
Coordinates   565
Cortex
–, adrenal   404
–, renal   387
Coxitis   559f.
–, arthritis   560
–, causes of infection   560
– –, tuberculous   560
– – –, osteoporosis   560
–, chronic   559
–, demineralization   560
–, hemarthrosis   560
–, hydrarthrosis   560
Crohn's disease   326, 332f.,
    335, 469f.
–, esophageal stricture   319
CT
–, arterial hepatographic
    (AHCT)   105
–, -assisted myelography   110, 547
–, -assisted peritoneography   109
–, Cine-   565
–. Osteo-   573
–, portography   105, 263
– –, (of) liver   248, 263
–, -postmyelographic   517
–, signs
– –, "double halo"   332
– –, "double-ring"   332
– –, "ivory whorl"   507
– –, "rim"   365
– –, "target" (board)   332
–, Spiral-   580
Cushing's syndrome   404
Cyst
–, (of) biliary tract   372
–, bone   237f.
–, bronchogenic   159f., 162
– –, attenuation value of   160
– –, avascularity of   160
–, calyceal   371
–, chocolate   443
–, choledochal   249, 283, 286f.
–, complex   370f.
–, dermoid   156, 443, 448, 481
– –, attenuation value of   156
– –, calcification of   156, 444

– –, calcified lesion of skin   156
– –, contents of   443
– – –, sebaceous material   156
– –, ectodermal vestigia of   444
– –, hemorrhage   156
– –, local invasion   156
– –, sebaceous material   156
–, duplication   319
–, dysontogenetic   249, 293f.
–, echinococcal   358
–, echinococcus   249
–, epidermoid   359
–, (of) esophagus   319
–, hepatic   249, 273
–, lime milk   370
–, (of) liver   372
–, (of) mesentery   326f.
–, Müllerian   426
–, neuro-enteric   162
– –, location of   162
–, neurogenic   161
–, ovarian   442
–, (of) pancreas   249, 293–296, 372
–, parasitic   359
–, paro-ophoron   443
–, parovarian   443
–, pericardial   178
–, peripelvic   393
–, pleuropericardial   160
–, prostatic   426
–, Pseudo-   462f.
–, renal   249, 369f.
– –, differential diagnosis   370
– –, multiple   370
– – –, dialysis therapy   370
–, (of) small bowel   326
– –, duplication   326
– –, mesenteric   326
–, (of) spleen   359
–, superinfection   390
–, synovial   526
–, thymic   155
–, tubo-ovarian   448
Cystadenocarcinoma   443
–, of pancreas   301
Cystadenoma   442f.
Cystitis
–, candidial   417
–, cystica   416f.
Cystography   470
–, bladder deformity   470
–, retrograde   416

Densitometry
–, of bone   91f.
Density
–, profile   565
–, resolution   565
DEQCT see Dual-energy quantita-
    tive computed tomography
Derangement
–, internal   519
Detector   565, 568

Diaphragm   454f.
–, anatomical relationships of   315
–, anatomy of   341, 454
Diastematomyelia   545
Digital image   568
Directory   568
Disc
–, degeneration   518, 521, 526
–, fragment of   519, 521f.
– –, free   519, 521f.
– –, sequestered   519
–, herniation of   518–525
– –, cervical   521
– –, characteristic sign   521
– –, extraforaminal   523
– –, lateral   520–523
– –, localization   519
– –, lumbosacral   521
– –, medial   519, 522
– –, mediolateral   520–522
– –, pathogenesis of   519
– –, recurrent   524f.
– –, subligamental   521
– –, transligamental   519, 521
–, intervertebral   513, 518, 522f.
– –, anulus fibrosus   513
– –, attenuation value of   513, 523
– –, configuration of   522
– –, degeneration of   518
– –, nucleus pulposus   513
– –, prolapse of   522
– –, protrusion   522
–, perforation   519
–, prolapse   519, 524f.
– –, recurring   524f.
–, protrusion   518
–, segment   524
– –, free   524
–, sequester   522
– –, free   522
–, sequestration   521
Discitis
–, Spondylo-   548f.
Disease
–, Addison's   412
–, Caroli's   287
–, Castleman's   301
–, Crohn's   326, 332f., 335, 469f.
–, Hodgkin's   145, 148
–, hydatid   271f.
–, Paget's   237, 542f., 561
–, renal   371f.
– –, polycystic   371f.
– – –, (in) adults   371
– – –, (in) children   371
– – –, enhancement pattern   372
– – –, hemorrhage   372
–, Whipple's   333, 335, 477
Disk
–, magnetic   573
Dissection
–, aortic   170
Display

–, device   568
–, (of) images   568 f.
Distance
–, measurement of   569
Diverticulitis   328
Diverticulum
–, calyceal   371
–, (of) pericardium   178
Documentation of images   569
Dose   569
"Double halo" sign   332
Dressler's syndrome   179
Dual-energy quantitative computed
    tomography (DEQCT)   92, 565
Duct
–, false pancreatic   292
–, mesonephric   430
–, (of) Santorini   292
–, thoracic   141, 455
–, (of) Wirsung   292
–, Wolffian   443
Dysplasia
–, fibrous   542, 561
–, multicystic renal   372
Dysrhaphism   162
Dystrophy
–, muscular   491 f.

Ectasis
–, (of) kidney   287
Ectopia
–, renal   403
Effusion
–, pleural   225–227
Ehlers-Danlos' syndrome   165
Embolism
–, arterial   338
Emphysema
–, mediastinal   169
–, pulmonary   140
Empyema   279, 484
–, pleural   226–229
Enchondroma
–, (of) chest wall   237
Endometriosis   442
Endostoma   237
Eosinophilic granuloma   206
Epididymis   430
Epithelial body   158
–, adenoma of   158
–, attenuation value of   158
–, ectopia of   158
–, hyperfunction of   158
–, hyperplasia of   158
Epithelium
–, germinal   444
ERCP see Cholangiopancreato-
    graphy, endoscopic retrograde
Esophagus   140 f., 144, 169
–, anatomic relationships of   315
–, esophagitis   319
– –, candidial   319
– –, reflux   319

– –, vs. tuberculosis
    and syphilis   319
–, inflammation of   319
–, metastatic involvement
    of   317 f.
–, sclerosis of   320
–, stricture of   319
–, tumor of   317, 319
– –, benign   319
– –, pseudodiverticulosis   319
–, varices of   320
– –, portal hypertension and   320
– –, "downhill"   320
–, wall thickening   320
Ewing's sarcoma   237, 499,
    505–507
Excrescenses
–, osseus   521
Extravasation
–, lymphatic   466

Facet   515
–, articular   526
– –, fracture of   526
–, naked   535
Fallopian tube   434 f., 444, 446
Fan beam   569
Fascia
–, Gerota   386 f., 391
–, perivisceral   141
–, prevertebral   141
–, renal   377
–, retroperitoneal   457
–, subperitoneal   458 f.
Female genital organs   431–449
Femur
–, neck of   554
Fenestration
–, interlaminar   524
Fibroepithelioma
–, (of) esophagus   319
Fibrolipomatosis   393
–, pelvic   470
–, renal   393
– –, chronic pyelonephritis
    in   393
– –, nephrolithiasis in   393
– –, prostatic adenoma in   393
Fibroma   153 f., 381
–, (of) soft tissue   496 f.
–, (of) stomach   326
Fibromyosarcoma   441
Fibrosarcoma
–, (of) chest wall   239
–, (of) pericardium   177
–, (of) soft tissue   496, 499
Fibrosis   214
–, (of) lung   203–206
–, (of) pleura   229
–, post-radiotherapeutic   239
–, pulmonary   214
– –, radiogenic pneumonitis
    in   214

–, retroperitoneal   168, 285,
    467–470
– –, constipation of   470
– –, cystitis of   470
– –, dysuria of   470
– –, idiopathic   467–469
– – –, calcification of   468
– – –, fibrotic plate of   468
– – –, inflammation of   468
– – –, localized enhancement   469
– – –, stenosis of ureter   468
– – –, urinary obstruction   468 f.
– –, primary   468
– –, radiogenic   468 f.
– –, secondary   467, 469
– – –, carcinoma   467, 469
– – –, collagenosis   469
– – –, infection   467, 469
– – –, irridiation   467
– – –, retroperitoneal tumor   469
– – –, trauma   467, 469
– – –, vasculitis   467
–, sclerosing   168
Fibrothorax   229
Filter   569
Filtered back projection   569
Filtration   569 f.
Filum
–, terminale   516
Fissure
–, hepatic   245
– –, hemangioma on   255
–, symphyseal   554
Fistula
–, bronchopleural   228
–, colovesical   416
Fluid
–, pericardial   178–180
FNH see Hyperplasia, focal nodular
Fold
–, peritoneal   434
Foramen
–, intervertebral   517, 523
–, neural   513, 515 f., 521
Foramina   553
–, sacral   553
Fossa
–, acetabular   554
–, ischiorectal   435
–, ovarian   435, 442
–, supraclavicular   376
Fracture
–, acetabular   555, 557 f.
– –, classification of   557
– –, dislocation in   558
– –, osteoporosis in   557
–, pelvic   559
– –, hemarthrosis   559
– –, hemorrhage   559
– –, soft-tissue   559
–, (of) ribs   242

Gallbladder
–, adenomyomatosis   282
–, anatomy of   278f.
–, bile fluid   280, 282
–, calcification of   279
–, calculi of   281
–, carcinoma of   282
–, cholecystogram   282
–, cholesterosis   282
–, CT of   279–283
–, empyema of   279f.
–, enlargement of   279
–, inflammation of   279
– –, cholecystitis   279f.
– –, cholelithiasis   279, 281
–, porcelain   280
–, tumor of   282f.
–, wall of thickening of   280
Gallstones   281, 285, 287, 304
Gantry   570
Ganglion
–, spinal   517
Gardner's syndrome   479
Gastrinoma
–, (of) pancreas   302
Gastrointestinal tract   313–338
–, anatomy of   315f.
–, CT of   315f.
– –, patient positioning   316
–, esophagus   317
– –, abnormalities   319f.
– – –, inflammatory   319f.
– –, tumor of   317–319
– –, varices of   320f.
–, lymph nodes of   314
–, perforation in   347
–, small intestine
      and colon   326, 331
– –, appendicitis   335f.
– –, carcinoma of   328
– – –, colorectal   328–331
– –, colitis   334f.
– – –, ulcerative   334f.
– –, cysts of   326
– –, diverticulitis   336f.
– –, functional diseases of   338
– –, inflammation of   332–334
– –, lymphoma and
      myosarcoma   327
– – –, malignant   327
– –, malignant tumors of   327
– –, protectomy   331f.
– – –, tumor recurrence
         after   331f.
– –, solid tumor of   327
–, stomach   321
– –, carcinoma of   321–324
– –, inflammation of   326
– –, sarcoma of   324
– –, tumor of   325
– – –, benign   325f.
–, tumor of   327
Germ cell   156, 447

Gerota's fascia   386f., 391
Girdle   555f.
–, pelvic   555f.
– –, fracture of   555f.
Gland
–, adrenal   144, 401–412
–, thyroid   140, 157f.
– –, attenuation value of   141
– –, calcification of   159
– –, cyst   159
– –, normal   140
– –, vascularisation of   141
Glisson's capsule   403
Goiter
–, cervicothoracic   157
–, colloid   157
–, cystic change of   157
–, ectopic   157
–, hyperplasia of   157
–, inflammation of   157
–, retrosternal   157
–, substernal   157
–, tissue density of   157
Gonadal dose   570
Gonadoblastoma   447
Granuloma
–, eosinophilic   206
Gutter
–, paracolic   342, 345

Hamartoma   380
–, mesenchymal   256
Hamartosis   249, 372
Heart   171–180
–, anatomy of   173
–, aneurysm   175
– –, (of) heart wall   175
–, bypass   175f.
– –, aortocoronary   176
– – –, occlusion of   176
– – –, patency of   176
– –, aortocoronary   175
–, cardiomyopathy   175, 180
–, chambers of   173
–, coronal arteries of   173
–, coronary heart disease   175
– –, myocardial infarction   175f.
–, CT of   173f.
– –, applications   174
– –, Cine-CT, ultra-fast   173
– –, ECG-gating   173
– –, functional conditions of   174
– –, pressure stress   174
– – –, hypertension   174
– –, volume stress   174
–, interventricular septum
– –, rotation of   174f.
–, intracavitary masses   176
– –, myxoma   176
– –, rhabdomyoma   176
– –, sarcoma   176
–, left-to-right shunt   174
–, mitral stenosis of   174, 176

–, myocardial infarction of   179
–, sclerosis   174
– –, coronary   174
–, topography of   172
–, valvular defects   176
– –, mitral stenosis   176
Hemangioma   381, 481
–, (of) chest   237
–, (of) esophagus   319
–, (of) liver   254–256
–, (of) soft tissue   496, 498
–, (of) spleen   359, 361
–, (of) stomach   326
Hemangiopericytoma   479, 481
Hemangiothelioma
–, (of) spleen   361
Hematoma   466, 525
–, (of) chest   242
–, intrarenal   395
– –, attenuation value of   395
– –, sedimentation
         phenomena   395
–, mediastinal   168–170
– –, attenuation value of   170
– –, rupture of aneurysm   169
– –, trauma   169
– –, whiplash injury of   169
–, para-aortic   482
–, perirenal   463f., 482
– –, aneurysm ruptures   464
–, (of) peritoneal cavity   349
–, (of) retroperitoneum   311
Hematometra   441
Hemochromatosis
–, secondary   412
Hemothorax   227, 229
Hepatitis   267
Hernia
–, abdominal   338
–, inguinal   338
Hiatus
–, aortic   455
High-contrast resolution   570
Highlighting   570
High resolution computed tomo-
      graphy (HRCT)   570
Hilum
–, pulmonary   138
–, splenic   455
Histiocytoma
–, (of) soft tissue   496, 499
Histiocytosis X   151, 206
–, fibrosis in   206
–, pneumothorax   206
Histoplasmosis   362
Hodgkin's disease   145, 148
Horner's syndrome   220
Hounsfield unit (HU)   570f.
HRCT see High resolution com-
      puted tomography
HU see Hounsfield unit
Hydatid disease
–, (of) liver   271f.

– –, Echinococcus alveolaris   272
– –, Echinococcus
        granulosus   271 f.
Hydronephrosis   391, 395, 441
Hydrosalpinx   448 f.
Hygroma   154, 550
Hyperaldosteronism
–, primary   404
Hypernephroma   374, 464
Hyperplasia
–, angiofollicular   151
–, focal nodular (FNH)   252–254
–, non-specific   153
– –, calcification of   153
–, prostatic   426 f.
–, thymic   153, 155
Hypertension
–, portal   287, 320
– –, esophageal varices   320
Hyperthyroidism   447
Hysterectomy   441

Iliopubic eminence   554
Image analysis   79–97, 571 f.
–, attenuation value   86 f.
– –, (of) boundary surfaces   87
–, contrast enhanced images   95
– –, differential diagnosis of   95
–, contrast medium   93 f.
– –, bolus injection of   93 f.
– – –, effects of vascularization   94
– – –, flow phenomena   93
– – –, intravascular
            enhancement   93
– – –, parenchymatous enhance-
            ment   93
–, densitometry   85–92
– –, artifacts   85–87
– – –, beam-hardening   86
– – –, high-contrast   86
– – –, motion   85
– –, attenuation value   85
– –, (of) bone   91 f.
– – –, DEQCT   92
– – –, SEQCT   92
– –, falsification of
            measurement   85
– –, region of interest (ROI)   85
–, morphological   83–85
– –, boundary surfaces   83
– – –, evaluation of   83
– –, infiltrating processes   84
– –, nodular structures   83
– –, space-occupying processes   84
– –, tubular structures   83
–, pathomorphological
            variation   87
– –, abscess   88
– –, blood   87 f.
– –, exudate   87
– –, fluid-filled formations   87
– –, hematoma   87 f.
– –, regressive change   89–91

– – –, amyloidosis   91
– – –, calcification   89
– – –, necrosis   91
– –, solid tissue   89
– – –, bony tissue   89
– – –, fatty   89
– – –, lung tissue   89
– – –, mixed   89
– –, transudate   87
–, structural   81–83
– –, interpretation of images   81
– – –, horizontal masking   81
– – –, partial volume
            averaging   81
– – –, vertical tangential scanning
            phenomena   81
– – –, volume element (voxel)   81
– –, window setting   81–83
Image reconstruction   572
Imaging system   572 f.
Immunocytoma   147
Infarction
–, myocardial   175 f., 398
–, renal   398 f.
– –, embolism   398
– –, occlusion   398
Infection
–, fungal   241
–, renal   387
Inflammation
–, adnexal   448
–, parametrial   449
– –, abscess   449
– –, exudation   449
–, uterine   448
– –, empyema   448
– –, pyometra   448
Inlet
–, pelvic   463, 468
Insufficiency
–, mitral valvular   398
–, pituitary   412
Insulinoma
–, (of) pancreas   302
Interactive display functions   573
Intestine, small and colon
–, abscess of   331–333, 335
–, amebiasis and   334
–, anatomical
        relationships of   315 f.
–, colitis   335, 338
– –, granulomatous   335
– –, ischemic   335
– –, ulcerative   333–335
–, Crohn's disease   332 f., 335
–, CT of   315 f.
–, cysts of   326
– –, duplication   326
– –, mesenteric   326 f.
– –, duodenum   326
– –, paraganglioma of   326
–, enteritis   338
–, enterocyclis of   332

–, fissures of   332
–, fistulae in   331–333, 335, 348
–, functional diseases of   338
– –, herniation   338
– –, obstruction   338
–, granulomatous diseases of   332
–, "halo" sign   335
–, hernia   338
–, herniation   338
–, ileus   338
–, infarction of   338
–, inflammation of   332
–, ischemia of   337
–, lymph nodes of   333, 335
– –, enlargement of   333, 335
–, mesenteric ischemia   338
–, mesenteric vein occlusion   338
–, mesentery   342, 345 f.
–, obstruction of   338
–, pneumatosis of   338
–, shigellosis and   334
–, tumor
– –, solid   327
– – –, benign   327
– – –, carcinoids   327
– – –, carcinoma, colorectal   328
– – –, lymphoma, malignant   327
– – –, malignant   327
– – –, myosarcoma   327
– – –, recurrence of after
            proctectomy   331
–, wall thickening in   332 f.
–, Whipple's disease   333
–, yersiniosis   333
Ischemia
–, (of) small bowel   337

Jefferson fracture   539
Joint
–, cavity   526
–, facet   536
– –, dislocation   536
– –, fracture dislocation   536
– –, stratified fracture   536
– –, subluxation   536
–, hip   553 f.
– –, capsule of   554
–, sacro-iliac   553 f., 556, 559
– –, dislocation of   556
– –, rupture of   556
– –, vacuum phenomena in   556
–, sternoclavicular   237, 242
– –, dislocation of   242
Jones-Thompson quotient   528

Kaposi's sarcoma   477
Kerckring's folds   316
Kidney   367–400
–, anatomy of   369
– –, cortex   369
– –, papilla   369
– –, pelvis   369
– –, pyramid   369

– –, segment   369
– –, sinus   369
– –, tubule   369
–, angiomyolipoma of   381
–, anomalies of   399 f.
– –, absence of kidney   399
– –, agenesis of kidney   399
– –, aplasia of kidney   399
– –, crossed dystopia   400
– –, fetal lobulation   400
– –, horseshoe kidney   400
– – –, bridge formation   400
– – –, renal malrotation   400
– –, lobar dysmorphism   399 f.
– –, malposition   400
–, atrophic   400
– –, pyelonephrotic   400
–, attenuation   369
–, cystic   371 f.
–, ectasis   287
–, fibroma of   381
–, hemangioma of   381
–, horseshoe   399
–, hypoplastic   400
–, leiomyoma of   381
–, lipoma of   381
–, medullary sponge kidney   287
–, time-density curve   369
Klatskin's tumor   258, 286
Kupffer cell   253

Lamina   513
Laminectomy   524
Leiomyoma   381
–, (of) esophagus   319
–, (of) soft tissue   496, 498
–, (of) stomach   325
–, uterine   436
– –, calcification of   436
– –, degeneration of   436
– –, fibromyomatas   436
– –, infection of   436
– –, necrosis of   436
– –, transformation of   436
Leiomyosarcoma   487
–, (of) esophagus   317
–, prostatic   427
–, (of) small bowel   327
–, (of) soft tissue   496, 498
–, (of) stomach   324
–, uterine   441
Leukemia
–, chronic lymphatic   471
–, peritoneal neoplasms   351
Ligament(um)
–, arteriosum   169
–, broad   438
–, cardinal   434
–, coronary   341
–, falciform   245, 341, 344
–, flavum   515, 517, 526, 529
–, gastrocolic   307, 344
–, gastrohepatic   307, 315, 341

–, gastrosplenic   307, 341, 344, 357
–, hepatoduodenal   282, 321,
      341, 344
–, longitudinal   515 f., 518 f., 521
– –, dorsal   521
– –, posterior   519, 521
–, ovarian   435
–, phrenico-esophageal   315
–, pulmonary   185
–, round   434
–, sacrouterine   438
–, splenorenal   341, 357
–, uterosacral   434, 439
– –, thickening of   439
–, venosum   245
Linear attenuation coefficient   573
Lipo-fibrosarcoma   153
Lipoma   153 f., 381
–, attenuation value of   480
–, calcification   479
–, (of) chest wall   238 f.
–, (of) liver   253 f.
–, retroperitoneal   470
–, (of) soft tissue   496–498
–, (of) stomach   326
–, thymic   155
Lipomatosis   153 f.
–, pancreatic   292, 312
Liposarcoma
–, attenuation value of   480
–, calicification   479
–, (of) chest wall   239
–, (of) soft tissue   496–500
–, types of   480
– –, mixed   480
– –, pseudocystic   480
– –, solid   480
Lithiasis   309
Lithotripsy   398
Liver   243–275
–, abscess of   269 f.
– –, amebic   269 f.
– –, cryptogenic   269
– –, "double target" sign   270
– –, fungal   269 f.
– –, gas in   270
– –, pyogenic   269 f.
–, anatomy of   245
– –, segmental   246 f.
–, attenuation value of   248
–, Budd-Chiari syndrome   275
–, cholangiocarcinoma   258 f.
– –, CT of   259
– –, development of   258
– –, ERCP of   259
– –, Klatskin's tumor with   258
–, cirrhosis of   267 f., 358
– –, CT of   268
– –, types of   267
–, contrast enhancement   248
–, CT of   248
– –, contrast enhancement   248
– –, delayed scan   248

– –, portography   248, 263
–, cystic disease of   248 f.
– –, dysontogenetic cyst   249
– –, solitary hepatic cyst   249
–, echinococcosis
      (hydatid disease)   271
–, enlargement of   357
–, fatty infiltration of   265 f.
– –, CT of   266
– –, diseases causing   266
– –, due to cirrhosis   266
–, focal nodular hyperplasia
      (FNH) of   252–254
– –, adenomatous   252
– – –, contraceptives in   252
– – –, development of   252
– –, CT of   253
– –, scintigraphy   253
–, hamartosis   248
–, hemangioma   254–256
– –, cavernous   254, 256
– –, CT of   256
– – –, "iris" phenomenon   256
– –, hemangio-endothelioma   254
–, hemochromatosis   268
– –, CT of   269
– –, differential diagnosis   269
– –, types of   268
–, hepatitis   266 f.
–, hepatocellular carcinoma
      256–258, 260
– –, cirrhosis with   256, 258
– –, differential diagnosis of   258
– –, fibrolamellar   260
– –, regenerating nodules   258
– –, types of   257
–, hydatid disease   272
– –, Echinococcus alveolaris   272
– –, Echinococcus
      granulosus   271 f.
–, hyperplasia
– –, focal nodular (FNH)   252–254
–, lobe   247
– –, caudate   247
– –, quadrate   247
–, lymphoma   264–266
– –, CT of   265
– –, non-Hodgkin's   265
–, mesenchymal hamartoma   256
–, metastases   260–264
– –, (from) carcinoid   260
– –, (from) carcinoma of colon
      260, 262
– –, CT of   264
– – –, window setting   264
– –, (from) gastrinoma   261
– –, (from) hypernephroma   261
– –, (from) malignant schwanno-
      ma   260
– –, regressive changes due to   262
– –, (from) tonsillar
      carcionoma   262
–, porta hepatis   244, 315, 341

– –, anatomy of   245, 247, 341
– –, CT of   248
– –, topography of   244
–, portal structures   245
–, portal venous thrombosis   275
–, scintigraphy   253f.
–, segmental anatomy of   246f.
–, solid tumors of   250–252
– –, CT portography   251
– –, delayed CT scan   251
– –, enhancement pattern   251
– –, hypervascularized   250f.
– –, hypovascularized   250
– –, hypovascular   251
– –, isovascular   250f.
–, trauma to   272–275
–, vascular processes   275
– –, Budd-Chiari syndrome   275
– –, portal venous thrombosis   275
Low-contrast resolution   573
Lung   181–222
–, abscess   200
–, alveolitis   198
– –, extrinsic allergic   198
–, anatomy of   183
– –, bronchial tree   182
– –, bronchopulmonary
        segments   185
– – –, boundaries   185
– –, lobule(s)   186
– – –, primary   186
– – – –, structure of   186
– – –, secondary   186
– –, lymph nodes   185
– –, pulmonary ligaments   182
– –, septa   182
– –, visceral pleura   186
–, asbestosis   207f.
–, atelectasis   189, 197
– –, exudation   189
– –, mediastinal displacement   189
– –, patterns of   189
– –, round   192
– – –, visceral pleura   192
–, bronchiectasis   196f.
– –, cystic   197
– –, varicose   196
–, bronchopulmonary
        segments   185
–, bronchus   185, 212
– –, bronchial adenoma   212f.
– – –, carcinoid tumor   213
– – –, cylindroma   213
– –, bronchial carcinoma   191
– –, bronchial obstruction   188
– –, segmental   185
–, bullae   195
–, carcinoma   213, 215
– –, bronchial   213–221
– – –, adenocarcinoma   215
– – –, bronchial stenosis in   217
– – –, bronchial occlusion in   217
– – –, classification of   215

– – –, CT appearance of   217
– – – –, Rigler's sign   218
– – – –, "radiating corona"
           sign   217
– – –, CT of   215–217
– – –, large-cell   215
– – –, signs of malignancy   218
– – –, small-cell (oat cell)   215
– – –, squamous cell   215
– – –, staging of   213
–, collagen disease of   203
–, density gradient   187
–, dystelectasis   188
–, embolism and infarction of   210
– –, CT of   210
– –, development of   210
– –, differential diagnosis   211
– – –, vascular sign   211
–, emphysema   193, 195
– –, bullous   195
– –, centrilobular   194f.
– – –, hyperinflation   194
– –, cicatricial   195f.
– –, destructive   195
– –, interstitial edema   193
– – –, Kerley B lines   195
– – –, patterns   195
– – – –, nodular   195
– – – –, reticulonodular   195
– – – –, reticular   195
– –, panlobar   196
– – –, alpha-1-antitrypsin
           deficiency   196
– –, panlobular   194f.
– –, peribronchial signs   196
– –, periseptal   195
–, fibrosis   198, 202f.
– –, idiopathic   203
– – –, desquamative alveolitis
           (DIP)   203
– – –, differential diagnosis   203
– – – –, collagen diseases   203
– – – –, rheumatoid arthritis   203
– – – –, scleroderma   203
– – –, "honeycomb" pattern   203
– – –, structural
           transformation   203
– – –, subpleural cavity   203
– –, post-pneumonic   198
–, hilum of   140, 185
–, imaging   183
– –, high-resolution CT   186
– –, penumbra formation   183
– –, pulmonary histogram   187
– –, spiral CT   187
– –, thin-slice CT   183
– –, window setting   183, 191f.
–, infiltration   192f., 198
– –, air bronchogram   192
– –, broncho-alveolar   192f.
– – –, air bronchogram   193
– – –, CT patterns   193
– –, bronchopneumonic   198

– –, interstitial   193
– – –, lymphatic   193
– – –, perivascular   193
– –, subpleural space   192
– – –, window setting   192
–, inflammation of   199f.
–, injury   211f.
– –, contusion   211
– – –, hematoma in   211
– – –, pneumothorax in   211
– –, laceration   211
– –, pneumothorax   211f.
– – –, traumatic   211f.
– –, trauma   211
–, interstitial disease   203–206
–, interstitial tissue   210
– –, infiltration of   210
–, lymphangiomyomatosis   206f.
– –, accompaniments   207
– – –, chylous effusion   207
– – –, lymph node
           enlargement   207
– – –, pneumothorax   207
–, lymphangitis   208
– –, carcinomatous   208
– –, CT of   201, 209
– –, Kerley B lines   209
–, neoplasm   212
– –, atelectasis in   212
– –, chondroma   212
– –, CT of   212
– –, hamartoma   212
– – –, "popcorn-like"
           calcification   212
– –, lipoma   212
– –, osteoma   212
–, nodules   186f.
– –, pulmonary   186f.
– – –, air inclusions   187
– – –, attenuation value of   187
– – –, calcification of   187
– –, solitary   222
–, pleura   192
– –, visceral   192
–, pneumonia   198–200
–, pulmonary inflammation   196
–, respiration defects   188
– –, lung collapse   188
– – –, atelectasis   188f.
– – –, dystelectasis   188
– –, ventilation   187f.
– – –, overventilation   188
– – –, underventilation   188
–, sarcoidosis   203–205
– –, CT appearance of   205f.
– –, disseminated   204
– –, fibrosis   206
– –, nodular   204
– –, pattern of spread   205
–, sequestration   196f.
– –, calcification   197
– –, cystic transformation   197
– –, extralobular   197

– –, hemoptysis   197
– –, infection   197
– –, intralobular   197
–, silicosis   208 f.
–, "honeycomb" pattern of   202 f.
Lymph node(s)   459, 462
–, attenuation value of   474
–, bronchopulmonary   144
–, conglomerates   462, 474
–, drainage   474
–, enlargement of   145, 474
–, (of) gastrointestinal tract   314
–, iliac   474
–, intercostal   143
–, mediastinal   143 f.
– –, classification of   143
– –, diameter of   144
–, mesenteric   461, 474
–, metastases   150, 474, 477
– –, calcification of   150
– –, conglomerate   150
– –, drainage zones   150
– –, inflammation   150
– –, micro-   150
– –, transverse diameter   150
–, para-aortic   474
–, paracardiac   148
–, parasternal   241
–, paratracheal   148
–, parietal   143
–, pelvic   461
–, presacral   474
–, prevascular   143
–, retroperitoneal   460, 474
–, sternal   143
–, tuberculosis   151, 477
– –, calcification of   151
–, visceral   143
Lymphadenitis   477
Lymphadenopathie
–, benign   477
Lymphangioma   154
–, (of) spleen   359
Lymphangiomyomatosis   206 f.
Lymphangitis
–, carcinomatous   208–210
Lymphoblastoma
–, lymphatic   145
Lymphocele   349, 462, 464–466
Lymphography   461 f.
Lymphoma
–, attenuation value of   148
–, calcification of   148
–, conglomerate   481
–, Hodgkin's   147, 237, 351,
      360 f., 471 f.
– –, attenuation value of   471
– –, fibrosis   473
– –, involvement   473
– – –, gastrointestinal   473
– – –, intestine   473
– – –, liver   473
– – –, lymph nodes   473

– – –, spleen   473
– –, (of) peritoneal cavity   351
–, (of) liver   264–266
– –, non-Hodgkin's   265
–, malignant   145, 151, 234, 286,
      301, 327, 470, 477
– –, displacement of adjacent
        organs   470
– –, lymph nodes   470
– –, metastatic spread from   301
– –, pattern of involvement of   145
– –, (of) small bowel   327
– –, spleen   470
– –, staging   470
–, nodular structures in   148
– –, pericardium   148
– –, pleura   148
– –, retrosternal space   148
–, non-Hodgkin's   145, 147, 351,
      360 f., 470–473
– –, attenuation value of   471
– –, diffuse   470
– –, displacement of adjacent
        organs   470
– –, fibrosis   473
– –, involvement   473
– – –, gastrointestinal   473
– – –, liver   473
– – –, lymph node   473
– – –, spleen   473
– –, lymph node   470
– –, nodular   470
– –, (of) peritoneal cavity   351
– –, splenomegaly   470
–, (of) peritoneal cavity   354
–, (of) pleura   234
–, renal   384 f.
– –, attenuation value of   385
– –, CT manifestation of   384
– –, primary   384
– –, secondary   384
– – –, non-Hodgkin's
          lymphoma   384
–, (of) spleen   359

Magnetic disk   573
Magnetic resonance imaging (MRI)
–, (of) soft tissue tumors   500
Malacoplakia   416
Marfan's syndrome   165
Masses
–, intraspinal   544–546
– –, acquired   544–546
– – –, astrocytoma   544
– – –, ependymoma   544
– – –, glioma   544
– – –, meningioma   545
– – –, neurofibroma   545
– – –, paraglioma   544
– – –, syringohydromyelia   544
– –, congenital   544, 546
– – –, dermoid cyst   544
– – –, epidermoid cyst   544

– – –, lipoma   544
– – –, meningocele   544
– – –, teratoma   544
–, lateral   513
–, lipoferous   152
Mastocytosis   477
Matrix   573
Mediastinitis
–, acute   167 f.
– –, abscess   168
– –, exudation   168
– –, injuries   168
– –, perforation   168
– –, phlegmon   168
– –, pleural effusion   168
–, chronic   168
– –, calcification   168
– –, etiology of   168
– –, infection   168
– –, lymph node enlargement   168
–, granulomatous   168
–, idiopathic fibrous   168
Mediastinum   135–170
–, anatomy of   137
– –, anterior   137, 143
– –, middle   137, 143
– –, posterior   137, 140, 143
Medulla
–, renal   387
Melanoma   148
–, metastases from   361
– –, (to) spleen   361
–, metastatic spread   282
– –, (to) gallbladder   282
Membrane
–, abscess   560
–, synovial   560
– –, inflammation of   560
Memory   573
Meningioma   546
–, calcification   546
Meningiosis carcinomatosa   546
Meningocele
–, herniation of leptomeninges   161
–, Pseudo-   525
–, thoracic   545
Mesentery
–, abscess of   345
–, anatomy of   342
–, CT of   345 f.
–, cysts of   326 f.
–, inflammation of   345
–, inflammatory disease of   332
–, ischemia of   338
– –, CT diagnosis of   338
–, lymph nodes of   327
– –, enlargement of   327
–, mesenteric vein   338
– –, occlusion of   338
Mesocolon
–, sigmoid   346
– –, fluid in   346
–, transverse   345

Mesothelioma
–, benign   231 f.
–, (of) chest wall   239
–, malignant   232 f.
–, (of) pericardium   180
–, (of) peritoneal cavity   351
Metastases   221
–, (from) carcinoma of the
  breast   240
–, pulmonary   221 f.
– –, CT of   221 f.
– –, necrosis and calcification
  with   222
–, renal   385
–, (from) renal cell carcinoma   240
Mirizzi's syndrome   284
Modulation transfer function
  (MTF)   573
Monitor   573
Mononucleosis   363
Morrison's pouch   343
Mouse   573
MRI see Magnetic resonance
  imaging
MTF see Modulation transfer
  function
Müllerian cyst   426
Muscle
–, iliopsoas   466, 554
– –, abscess of   466
– –, hematoma of   466
– –, rhabdomyosarcoma of   466
–, obturator   439
– –, internus   554
–, psoas   467, 479
– –, hematoma of   467
– –, neoplastic infiltration
    of   467
Muscular tissue   489–494
–, abscess of   492 f.
–, atrophy of   491 f.
– –, Duchenne   491
– –, limb girdle   491
–, calcification of   493 f.
–, dystrophy of   491
– –, fatty metaplasia in   492
– –, necrosis in   491
– –, pattern of involvement in   492
– –, progressive   491 f.
– – –, pelvic girdle involvement
      in   491
–, hematoma of   492–494
– –, CT of   494
–, hypertrophy of   491
–, inflammatory disease of   492
– –, myositis   492
– – –, pyogenic   492
– –, polymyositis   493
– –, sarcoidosis   493
–, liposclerotic metaplasia of   493
–, myositis   492–494
– –, ossificans   494
– – –, CT of   494

– – –, etiology of   494
– –, pelvic girdle involvement
    in   492
– –, pyogenic   492 f.
–, necrosis of   492 f.
–, ossification of   494
–, phlegmons in   492
–, polymyositis of   493
–, pseudohypertrophy of   491
–, sarcoidosis   493
–, trauma to   492 f.
Myasthenia gravis   155
Myelofibrosis   542
Myelography   517
–, CT-assisted   547
Myeloma   542
–, tracheal   159
Myocardial infarction   175 f., 398
Myoma   436
–, uterine   435, 437, 440
– –, deformation of uterus   440
– –, dilatation of uterus   440
Myometrium   440, 448
Myosarcoma
–, (of) colon   327
–, (of) small bowel   327
Myositis
–, dermato-   493
–, poly-   493
–, pyogenic   492 f.
Myxoma   176
–, atrial   398

Neoplasm see also Carcinoma see
  also Tumor
–, chondroma   212
–, hamartoma   212
– –, "popcorn-like" calcification
    of   212
–, hourglass   161
–, lipoma   212
–, osteoma   212
Nephradenoma   379 f.
–, calcification in   380
–, (in) dialysis patients   379
–, nephrosclerosis and   379
–, pyelonephritis and   379
Nephritis   387–391
–, focal   389
– –, bacterial   387, 389
– – –, microabscess   387, 389
– –, enhancement pattern   389
–, Glomerulo-   387
–, interstitial   387
–, Peri-   388
–, Pyelo-   387, 389–391, 464
– –, chronic   391
– – –, nodules in   391
– – –, radiologic features in   391
– – –, scarred indentation   391
– –, emphysematous   390
– – –, clinical symptoms   390
– – –, diabetic patients with   390

– –, xanthogranulomatous   390
– – –, fistulae   390
– – –, hydronephrosis   391
– – –, renal pelvic stone   391
Nephroblastoma   386
–, attenuation value of   386
–, cystic degeneration   386
–, filling defect   386
–, hemorrhage   386
–, necrosis   386
Nephrogram   396
–, obstructive   396
Nephroma   373, 379
–, multilocular cystic   373
– –, clinical symptoms   373
Nephrosis   392, 396 f.
–, Hydro-   371, 395–397
–, Pyo-   371, 390, 392, 396 f.
– –, calcification in   392, 396
– –, inflammation in   396
– –, obliteration in   396
– –, obstruction in   396
– –, tuberculous   392
– –, ulcerative cavernous form
      of   392
– – –, attenuation value   392
– – –, hydrocalices in   392
Neurinoma   160, 523, 547
–, (of) stomach   326
Neurofibroma   160, 480
–, (of) stomach   326
Neuroforamen
–, dilatation of   162
–, dilated   161
Nodule
–, pulmonary   186 f., 222
– –, solitary   222
– – –, benign neoplasm   222
– – –, bronchial carcinoma   222
– – –, evaluation of   222
– – –, granuloma   222
Noise   573
Nucleus
–, pulposus   518 f., 524
– –, calcification of   519
– –, dehydration of   518
– –, tissue of   519, 524
– –, vacuum phenomena   519

Obstruction
–, renal   468
–, urinary   395 f.
– –, compression   395
– –, lithiasis   395
– –, neurogenic reflux   395
– –, trauma   395
– –, tumor   395
– –, ureterovesical reflux   395
Omentum
–, lesser   341, 344
Oncocytoma   379 f.
–, spoke wheel configuration   380
–, stellate scar   380

Osteo-CT   573
Osteoblastoma
–, (of) chest wall   237
Osteochondroma   494
–, (of) chest wall   237
Osteomyelitis   484
Osteosarcoma   222
Ovary
–, carcinoma of   447
–, cysts in   442
– –, chocolate   442
– –, functional   442
– –, neoplastic   442
– –, polycystic changes   442
– –, retention   442
–, cystadenocarcinoma of   444
–, cystadenoma of   442, 444
– –, calcification of   442
– –, cilial glandular serous   442
– –, pseudomucinous   442
– –, simple serous   442
–, fossa   442
–, metastases to   447
–, stroma to   447
– –, tumor of   447
– – –, arrhenoblastoma   447
– – –, dysgerminoma   447
– – –, gonadoblastoma   447
– – –, granulosa cell   447
– – –, hypernephroid   447
– – –, malignant teratoma   447
– – –, thecal cell   447
–, tumors   446

Paget's disease   237, 542f., 561
Pancoast's tumor   220
Pancreas   289–312, 455
–, abscess of   295, 307, 310f.
–, anatomy of   290–294
–, atrophy of   312
–, carcinoma of   297–302, 359
– –, metastases from   359
–, cholangiopancreatography   297
–, contrast enhancement of   293
–, cystadenocarcinoma of   301
–, cysts of   294, 310
– –, dysontogenetic   294
– –, pseudo-   294f., 298, 310, 349
– –, retention   294f.
–, dimensions of   293
–, divided   293
–, ducts of   292, 298
– –, accessory
        (duct of Santorini)   292
– –, false duct   292
– –, main pancreatic   292f.,
        298, 309f.
– – –, dilatation of   298, 310
– – –, occlusion of   312
– –, main (duct of Wirsung)   292
–, enlargement of   306
–, ERCP   297, 310
–, fatty infiltration of   292

–, gas in   307
–, lipomatosis of   310, 312
– –, atrophy and   312
– –, sclero-   310, 312
–, lipomatosis of   292, 298
–, metastatic spread to   301
–, metastatic tumors of   303
–, pancreatectomy   300
–, pancreatitis   298, 300, 306f., 311
– –, acute   304–307
– – –, necrotizing   306f.
– –, chronic   300, 307–310
– – –, atrophy due to   309
– – –, calcification due to   309
– – –, swelling due to   310
– –, edematous   302f., 306, 311
– –, hemorrhagic necrotizing   306
– –, serous exudative   306
– –, suppurative   307
–, pseudocyst of   294f., 298,
        310, 349
–, sclerolipomatosis of   309f., 312
–, trauma to   311
–, tumors of   296–303
– –, adenoma   296
– – –, macrocystic   296f.
– – –, microcystic   296f.
– –, insulinoma   302
– –, islet cell   302
–, uncinate process   291–293, 298
Pancreatitis   345, 469
–, acute   304–307
–, alcoholism and   304, 307
–, ascites due to   304
–, chronic   307–310
–, edematous   311
–, gallstones and   304
–, gastric wall thickening
        due to   326
–, suppurative   307
Papilloma
–, (of) gallbladder   282
Paraganglioma   161
–, calcification of   161
–, (of) duodenum   326
–, (of) soft tissue   496, 500
Parametritis   449
Parametrium   435, 438
–, broad   434
Paraproctitis   449
Pararenal space   397
Pelvic girdle   555
–, destabilization of   555
–, dislocation of   555
–, fracture of   555
–, rupture of   555
–, stability of   555
Pelvis
–, bony   551–562
– –, anatomy of   553
– –, axes of   553
– –, ligamental structures   554
– –, osseous destruction in   562

– – –, lymphoma   562
– – –, metastases   562
– – –, patterns of   562
–, female   432
– –, topography of   432
–, male   424
– –, topography of   424
–, renal   381, 390, 395f.
– –, carcinoma of   381
– – –, transitional cell   381
– –, papillary tumor   381
Penumbra   140
Pericarditis   178
–, bacterial   178
–, neoplastic   178
–, non-specific   178
–, rheumatic   178
–, tuberculous   179
Pericardium
–, absence of   178
–, anatomy of   177f.
–, calcification of   180
–, congenital anomalies of   178
–, CT of   177f.
–, cysts of   178
–, effusion of   178f.
– –, causes of   179
– –, CT of   179f.
–, fibrosarcoma of   180
–, fibrosis of   180
–, fluid   178
–, hemato-   178, 180
–, mesothelioma of   180
–, pericarditis   178, 180
– –, bacterial   178
– –, chronic constrictive   180
– –, non-specific   178
– –, rheumatic   178
–, tamponade
– –, cardiac   178
–, thickening of   154, 180
–, tumor of   180
Periostitis
–, reactive   494
Perirenal space   390, 394, 397,
        399, 462
Perisalpingitis   448
Peritoneal cavity   339–354
–, abdominal cavity   341, 349
– –, compartments of   341f.
– –, hemorrhage in   349f.
–, abdominal wall   341
– –, anatomy of   341
–, abscess of   247, 347f., 350
– –, development of   247
– –, intraperitoneal   245, 347–350
–, anatomy of   340f., 343f.
–, ascites in   344, 346, 350, 353
– –, biliary   350
– –, bloody   347
– –, CT of   346
– –, diseases accompanied
        by   346

– –, peritoneal carcinomatosis
    with   346
– –, protein content of   346f.
–, biloma of   348
–, calcification of   351, 353
–, carcinomatosis of   246, 349,
    352–354
–, fluid   345, 350
– –, intraperitoneal   345, 350
–, hematoma of   348, 350
–, hemoperitoneum   349
–, hemorrhage in   349f.
–, inflammation of   345, 350
–, infracolic space   345
–, inframesocolic compartment
    341, 345
– –, anatomy of   341, 345
–, intraperitoneal abscess of   245,
    347f., 350
–, lesser omentum   341
–, lesser sac   341
–, lymphoma of   351
–, mesentery   342, 345, 349
– –, anatomy of   342
– –, hematoma of   349
– –, inflammation of   345f.
–, mesothelioma of   351
–, metastases in   351–354
–, Morrison's pouch   347
–, neoplasm of   351
– –, primary and metastatic
    351–354
–, paracolic gutter   345
–, peritoneal folds   345
–, peritonitis   347f.
– –, CT diagnosis of   348f.
–, pouch of Douglas   342,
    345, 347f.
– –, abscess of   347
– –, fluid in   345
–, pseudocyst of   348
–, pseudomyxoma of   350
–, subhepatic space   245, 343
– –, anatomy of   343
– –, fluid in   345
– –, Morrison's pouch   343
–, subphrenic compartment   343
– –, anatomy of   343
–, subphrenic space   345
– –, fluid in   345
–, supramesocolic
    compartment   341
– –, anatomy of   341
Peritoneum
–, metastases to   446
Peritonitis   365
–, pelvic   448
Pheochromoblastoma   149, 408
Pheochromocytoma   161, 410,
    420, 481
–, calcification of   161
–, (of) chest wall   239
–, hypertonic crisis   161

Picture element   574
Pixel   5, 574
Plasmocytoma   147, 301
–, anaplastic   146
Pleura   223–234
–, anatomy of   225
–, asbestosis   230f.
–, benign neoplasm of   231
– –, fibroma   231
– –, hyaloserositis   231
– – –, "iced" pleura   231
– –, lipoma   231
– –, mesothelioma   231
–, calcification of   229f.
–, callosity of   229
–, carcinomatosis of   234
–, costoparietal   237
–, drainage   229
–, effusion of   225–227, 234
– –, causes of   225
– –, CT of   227
– – –, artifacts   227
– –, dry pleuritis in   227
– –, empyema in   227
–, empyema   226–229
– –, CT of   228
–, enhancement of   227
–, extrapleural tissue layers   224
–, exudate of   234
–, malignant mesothelioma   232f.
– –, CT of   232
–, mediastinal   141, 154
–, metastases to   233f.
– –, lymphoma   234
– –, pleural carcinosis in   233
–, plaques   230
–, pleural processes   224
– –, differentiation of   224
–, thickening   229f.
– –, causes of   229
– –, CT of   230
–, visceral   186, 192, 228
–, window setting   225
Pleuritis
–, dry   227
–, fibrinous deposits   227
Plexus
–, basivertebral   517
–, venous   455, 516, 521
– –, interspinal   521
–, vertebral   516f.
– –, external   516
– –, internal   516f.
Pneumoconiosis
–, calcification   151
Pneumomediastinum   169
–, accumulation of air   169
–, drainage of   169
Pneumonectomy
–, pleural thickening after   229
Pneumonia   198f., 203, 220
–, bronchopneumonia   200
–, gangrenous   203

–, interstitial   200
– –, infiltration   200
– – –, perivascular and
        lymphatic   200
– –, septal thickening   200
–, lobar   200
– –, air bronchogram   200
–, Pneumocystis carinii   199
–, poststenotic   220
– –, suppurative   200
Pneumonitis   203
–, necrotizing   203
Pneumothorax   169
Polysplenia   366
Porta
–, hepatis   453, 461
Portal vein see Vein, portal
Post-thoracotomy syndrome   179
Pouch of Douglas   345, 446
–, fluid in   345
Process
–, articular   513
–, spinous   513, 515, 536
– –, dislocation of   536
– –, distraction of   536
Promontory   553
–, sacral   553
Prostate   423–430
–, anatomy of   425
–, calcification of   425
–, capsule of   427
–, density of   425
–, infection   429
– –, abscesses
        of prostate   429
– –, atrophy of prostate   429
– –, phlegmons of prostate   429
–, tumor of   427
– –, carcinoma   427
– –, infracapsular   428
– –, leiomyosarcoma   427
– –, rhabdomyosarcoma   427
– –, sarcoma   427
–, volume artifacts of   425
Prostatitis   426, 429
–, acute   429
–, chronic   429
Pseudocyst
–, pancreatogenic   162
Pseudodiverticulosis   319
Pseudomyxoma
–, peritoneal   350f., 442
Pyometra   440f., 448
Pyosalpinx   448f.
Pyothorax   229
Pyramid
–, renal   395

QCT (Quantitative computed to-
    mography)   574
Quotient
–, Jones-Thompson   528

Radiation dose   574f.
Radiography
–, Pelvio-   553
– –, volume artifacts in   553
Recess
–, azygo-esophageal   140, 144
–, lateral   517, 523f., 526
– –, obstruction of   526
–, recto-uterine   433
–, supraazygeal   140
–, vesico-uterine   433
Rectum   433
Reformatted (secondary) images
    576, 578
Region
–, paralumbar   439
–, presacral   439
–, vesico-uterine   414
Region of interest (ROI)   85, 578
Reiter's syndrome   560
Renal capsule   387
Renal cell carcinoma   240, 374f.,
    377–379, 386, 475, 486
Renal cyst   249, 369f.
Renal pelvis carcinoma   382
Renal transplant   392f.
–, postoperative complications   393
– –, abscess   393
– –, gas collection   393
– –, hematoma   393
– –, lymphocele   393
– –, rejection   393
– – –, acute   393
– – –, chronic   393
Retrocrural space   455
Retroperitoneal cavity   451–487
–, anatomy of   453
Retroperitoneum   457
–, hematoma into   311
Rhabdomyolysis   494
Rhabdomyoma
–, (of) heart   176
Rhabdomyosarcoma   466
–, prostatic   427
–, (of) soft tissue   496f., 499
Riedel's struma   168, 285
ROI see Region of interest
Root
–, mesenteric   470
–, nerve   521, 523f.
– –, displacement of   521
– –, retraction of   524
Rupture
–, aortic   482
–, symphyseal   555

Sacroiliitis   560f.
–, chronic   561
– –, abscess in   561
– –, ankylosis in   561
– –, bony bridging in   561
– –, erosion in   561
– –, osteomyelitis in   561

– –, sclerosis in   561
–, Reiter's syndrome   560
–, rheumatic diseases   560
Sacrum   435, 554
–, fracture   556
– –, fatigue   556
Salpinx   448
Sarcoidosis   150, 326, 477
–, calcification of   151
–, pulmonary   203
Sarcoma   150, 481
–, (of) chest wall   237
–, (of) esophagus   317
–, Ewing's   237, 499, 505–507
–, (of) gallbladder   282
–, (of) heart   176
–, Kaposi's   477
–, neurogenic   479
–, (of) peritoneal cavity   351
–, prostatic   427, 429
–, retroperitoneal   479
–, (of) stomach   324
–, uterine   437, 441
Scan
–, high-resolution   513
Scanner
–, computed tomography
– –, multiple detector   4
– –, rotation   4
– – –, (with) movable detectors   4
– – –, (with) stationary detectors   4
– –, single detector   4
Scanning   578f.
–, thin-section   521
Scar
–, tissue   524f.
– –, epidural   524
Schwannoma
–, (of) soft tissue   496, 500
–, (of) stomach   326
Scintigraphy
–, (of) liver   253f.
Scleroderma   203
Sclerolipomatosis   310, 312
Sclerosis
–, Arterio-   398
–, (of) chest wall   241
–, subchondral   526
–, tuberous   370, 380
–, vascular   398
– –, renal   398
Scoutview   579
SD (Standard deviation)   579
Seminal vesicles   423–430, 459
–, abscesses of   430
–, agenesis   430
–, anatomy of   425
–, aplasia of   430
–, cyst of   430
–, deferent canals of   425
–, dilatation of   428
–, dysplasia of   430
–, mesonephric duct   430

–, mobility of   425
–, tumor invasion of   428
–, tumor of   430
Seminoma   156
–, embryonal testicular   476
– –, metastases of   476
Septicemia
–, meningococcal   411
SEQCT see Single-energy quantita-
    tive computed tomography
Sheehan's syndrome   412
Shigellosis   334
Shrinkage   393
Silicosis   207f.
–, CT of   208
–, development of   208
–, egg-shell   151
– –, calcification of   151
–, pulmonary fibrosis in   208
Single-energy quantitative com-
    puted tomography (SEQCT)
    92, 580
Sipple's syndrome   407
Slice (section)   579f.
–, geometry   579
Space
–, infracolic   345
–, medullary   503
–, para-aortic   406
–, pararenal   397, 465
– –, anterior   465
– – –, abscess   465
– – –, extraperitoneal
        perforation   465
– – –, gas   465
– – –, hemorrhagic effusion   465
– – –, injuries   465
– – –, trauma   465
– –, posterior   465
– – –, hemorrhage   465
– – –, spondylitis   465
–, perirenal   390, 394, 397,
    399, 462
–, presacral   556
–, retrocrural   455
–, retroperitoneal   144
–, retrosacral   556
–, subarachnoidal   516
–, subhepatic   345
–, subperitoneal   467
– –, fascial   458f.
–, subphrenic   247, 341, 344f.
–, subpleural   192
Spinal canal   513–515, 522, 526,
    542, 546
–, enlargement of   546
–, obstruction of   533
–, protrusion of   526
–, soft-tissue tumor   542
Spinal column   466, 479, 518
–, kyphosis   536
–, segment   518
Spinal cord   515f., 519

Spinal deformity   530
Spinal degeneration   518
Spinal dehydration   518
Spinal dislocation
–, atlanto-occipital   537
–, rotatory atlantoaxial   537
Spinal fracture   531–535,
     538–540, 542
– –, atlas   538 f.
– –, incomplete closure   538
– –, Jefferson fracture   539
– –, oblique fracture   538
–, chance fracture   535
–, classification of   531
–, complete burst fracture   534 f.
–, dens fracture   539 f.
–, impacted compression
        fracture   532 f.
– –, etiology   533
–, incomplete burst fracture   532 f.
–, Jefferson fracture   538
–, laminar fracture   542
Spinal injury   530, 536
–, pathogenesis   530
– –, compression   530
– –, hyperextension   530
– –, hyperflexion   530
– –, rotation   530
–, translation injuries   536 f.
– –, rotary   537
Spinal instability   530
Spinal stenosis   521, 527 f.
–, aquired   527
–, cervical   529
– –, absolute   529
– –, central   529
– –, foraminal   529
– –, relative   529
–, congenital   527
–, developmental   527
–, focal   529
–, lumbar   529
Spinal subluxation   530
–, atlanto-odontoid   537
Spinal trauma   536
–, flexion-distraction   536
Spine   511–550
–, anatomy of   513
–, lumbar   513, 553
– –, lordosis   553
Spiral CT   580
Spleen   355–366, 470
–, abscess of   362 f.
– –, attenuation value of   362
–, accessory   366
–, anatomy of   341, 356 f.
–, angiosarcoma of   361
–, artery
– –, splenic   364
– – –, occlusion of   364
–, asplenia   366
–, attenuation value of   357,
        361, 364

–, benign tumors of   359
–, calcification of   358, 365
– –, "rim" sign   365
–, compression of   364
–, congenital anomalies of   366
–, contrast enhancement of   357
–, CT of   357, 363 f.
–, cysts of   358 f.
– –, attenuation value of   359
– –, calcification of   359
– –, epidermoid   359
– –, pseudo-   363
–, deformity of   364
–, dimensions of   357
–, echinococcal cyst in   358
–, enlargement of   357 f.,
        362 f., 365
– –, causes of   358
–, hemangioma of   359, 361
–, hemangiothelioma of   361
–, hematoma of   363 f.
–, index
– –, splenic   356 f.
–, infarction of   364 f.
–, infection of   362 f.
– –, fungal   363
– –, granulomatous   362
–, inflammation of   363
–, laceration of   363 f.
–, lymphangiomatosis   359
–, lymphoma of   359, 361
– –, malignant   361 f.
– – –, calcification of   362
– – –, metastases of   362
– – –, phleboliths of   362
–, metastases to   359–361
–, plasmocytoma of   359
–, pneumocystosis   366
–, polysplenia   366
–, pseudocysts of   363
–, rupture of   364
–, splenomegaly   357
–, trabeculation of   361
–, trauma to   363
–, vein, splenic   365
– –, thrombosis of   365 f.
Spondylarthrosis   526, 529
Spondylitis   465, 549
–, abscess   549 f.
– –, epidural   550
– –, paravertebral   549
–, fungal infection   549
–, tuberculosis   549
Spondylodiscitis   548 f.
Spondylolisthesis
–, Pseudo-   526 f., 529
–, true   527
Spondylophyte   518
Spondylosis   527
–, intervertebral   518
Standard deviation (SD)   580
Stein-Leventhal syndrome   442
Stenosis

–, artery   398
– –, renal   398
Stomach
–, adenocarcinoma   325
–, adenoma of   326
–, carcinoma of   321 f.
– –, cardia   321, 323
– –, leiomyosarcoma   324
– –, of antrum   323
– –, recurrence of   322
–, CT of   316, 322
–, inflammation of   326
– –, wall thickening in   326
–, leiomyoma of   325
–, leiomyosarcoma of   324 f.
–, lymph nodes of   322
– –, CT of   322
–, lymphoma of   324 f.
– –, Hodgkin's   324
– –, leiomyosarcoma   324
– –, non-Hodgkin's   324
– –, wall thickening in   325
–, malignant lymphoma of   324 f.
–, metastatic involvement of   321
–, polyps of   326
–, sarcoma of   324
– –, lymphadenopathy and   324
–, tumors of   322, 325
– –, benign   325
– –, recurrence of   322
–, ulcer of   326
–, varices of   320
–, wall thickening   325
Struma
–, Riedel's   168, 285
Superimposition of edges   580
Supraclavicular fossa   376
Surface
–, articular   526
– –, fracture of   526
Syndrome   220
–, adrenogenital   404
–, Bourneville-Pringle   370, 380
–, Budd-Chiari   275
–, Conn's   404
–, compartment   494
–, Cushing's   404
–, Dressler's   179
–, Ehlers-Danlos'   165
–, Gardner's   479
–, Horner's   220
–, Marfan's   165
–, Mirizzi's   284
–, post-thoracotomy   179
–, Reiter's   560
–, Sheehan's   412
–, Sipple's   407
–, Stein-Leventhal   442
–, Tietze's   239
–, Verner-Morrison   302
–, von Hippel-Lindau   370, 374
–, Waterhouse-Friderichsen   411
–, Werner's   407

–, Zollinger-Ellison   302
Synovioma   233
Syringomyelia   545

"Target" sign   332
Table increment   580
Tendon
–, psoas major   554
– –, bursa of   554
Teratoblastoma   156
Teratocarcinoma   156
Teratoma   155 f.
–, attenuation value of   156
–, calcification of   156
–, calcified lesions of the skin   156
–, hemorrhage   156
–, local invasion of   156
–, malignant   447 f.
Thecal sac   515–517, 521, 524
–, compression   521
Thecoma   447
Thorax
–, CT of   237
–, inlet of   137
–, musculature of   237
–, surgery of   237
Thorotrast   358, 361
Three-column model   530
–, anterior   530
–, middle   530
–, posterior   530
Thrombus
–, parietal cardiac   176
Thymic
–, cyst   155
–, hyperplasia   155
–, lipoma   155
Thymoma   154
–, attenuation value of   155
–, calcification of   155
–, cystic   153, 155
–, effusion fluid   155
–, tumor invasion   155
Thymus   144
–, configuration of   144
–, physiological
      enlargement of   155
–, shape of   145
–, tissue density of   145
Thyroid gland
–, anatomical relationships of   315
Thyrotoxicosis   404
Tietze's syndrome   239
Tissue
–, solid   89
– –, bony tissue   89
– –, fatty   89
– –, lung tissue   89
– –, mixed   89
Tomography
–, computed
– –, attenuation value   7
– –, biopsy

– – –, CT-guided   116 f.
– – – –, contraindications to   117
– –, Cine-CT
– – –, ultra fast   173, 176
– –, contrast medium administra-
      tion   93, 113, 115
– – –, antiperistaltic
         agents in   113
– – –, bolus injection   93–95, 115
– – –, flow phenomena.   93
– – –, oral   113
– –, densitometry   7
– –, diagnostic procedures   113
– –, dual-energy quantitative CT
      (DEQCT)   92
– –, ECG-gated   175
– –, examination strategies   115
– – –, evaluation
– – – –, of spread   115
– – – –, of adjacent
            structures   115
– – –, organ-oriented   115
– – –, screening (orientational
         scan)   116
– –, gantry angulation   113
– –, Hounsfield density scale   7
– –, image
– – –, reconstruction   5
– – –, variation   8
– – – –, window setting   8 f.
– – – – –, bone window   8
– – – – –, level   9
– – – – –, lung window   9
– – – – –, pleural window   9
– – – – –, soft-tissue window   8
– – – – –, width   9
– –, interscan time   113
– –, interventional   116 f.
– – –, abscess drainage
– – – –, CT-guided   117
– – –, biopsy
– – – –, CT-guided   116 f.
– – –, masking
– – –, horizontal   81
– –, partial volume errors in   81
– –, patient preparation   113
– –, picture element (pixel)   5
– –, principles
– – –, mathematical   3
– – – –, absorption   3
– – – –, picture element   3
– – – –, spatial resolution   3
– –, radiation dose   114
– –, scan
– – –, interval   113 f.
– – –, sequence   113
– – –, time   114
– –, scanner   4
– – –, multiple detector rotate-
         translate   4
– – –, rotation
– – – –, (with) movable
            detectors   4

– – – –, (with) stationary detec-
         tors   4
– – –, single detector rotate-trans-
         late   4
– –, Serio-CT   114
– –, single-energy quantitative CT
      (SEQCT)   92
– –, slice thickness   113
– –, table increment   113
– –, tangential scanning phenomena
      in   81
– –, technical parameters for
      113–115
– –, technical realization   4
– –, techniques and strategies of
      1–9, 111–117
– –, volume element (voxel)   5
Topogram   580
Trachea   141, 144, 157
–, anatomical relationships of   315
–, carcinoma of   159
–, myeloma of   159
Trauma
–, aortic   485
– –, laceration   485
– –, puncture   485
–, (to) liver   272–275
–, pelvic   555
–, renal   393 f.
– –, contusion   393 f.
– – –, enhancement pattern   394
– – –, hemorrhage   394
– – –, laceration   394
– – –, urine accumulation   394
– – –, vascular constriction   394
– –, hematoma   393 f.
– – –, etiology   394
– –, laceration   393
– –, pedicle injuries   394
– – –, laceration   394
– – –, retroperitoneal
         hematoma   394
– – –, thrombotic occlusion   394
– –, rupture   393
– –, thrombosis   393
– –, transection   393
– –, urine extravasation   393
Trunk
–, brachiocephalic   166
– –, ectasia of   166 f.
–, celiac   453
–, pulmonary   138, 144, 154
Tube
–, Fallopian   434 f., 444, 446
–, uterine   434
Tuberculosis   241, 326, 362, 416 f.,
      466, 477
–, genital   429
–, renal   391 f.
– –, calyceal destruction   392
– –, florid   391
– –, strictures in   392
– –, ulcero-cavernous form   391

Tumor   219
–, biliary   286
–, (of) bone   501–509
–, carcinoid   327
– –, (of) small bowel   327
–, (of) chest wall   237–241
–, chondrogenic   237
– –, chondroma   237
– –, chondrosarcoma   237
– –, enchondroma   237
– –, osteochondroma   237
–, (of) colon   327
–, cystic   296, 480
– –, lympangiomas   480
– –, (of) pancreas   296
– – –, mucinous   296
– – –, serous   296
–, endometrioid   444
–, infracapsular   428
– –, prostatic   428
–, insulinoma   302
–, islet cell   296, 302
– –, (of) pancreas   302f.
–, Klatskin's   258, 286
–, Krukenberg   447
–, (of) liver   250–252
–, mesenchymal   153
– –, fibroma   153f.
– – –, phlebolith   154
– –, hemangioma   154
– –, hygroma   154
– –, lipo-fibrosarcoma   153
– –, lipoma   153f.
– –, lymphangioma   154
–, neurogenic   160, 326
– –, (of) stomach   326
–, osteogenic   237
– –, endostoma   237
– –, osteoblastoma   237
– –, sarcoma   237
–, ovarian   446, 449
– –, ascites   446
– –, calcification of   446
– –, cystic-solid   446
– –, lymphatic
        micrometastases   446
– –, nodules   446
– –, peritoneal seedings   446
– –, solid   446
–, Pancoast's   220
–, parathyroid   158
–, retroperitoneal   478
– –, frequency of   478
– –, benign   478
– – –, ganglioneuroma   478
– – –, leiomyoma   478
– – –, lipoma   478
– – –, myxoma   478
– – –, neurofibroma   478
– – –, pheochromocytoma   478
– – –, teratoma
– –, malign   478
– – –, liposarcoma   478

– – –, mesenchymoma   478
– – –, myosarcoma   478
– – –, neuroblastoma   478
–, (of) small bowel   327
–, (of) soft tissue   495–500
– –, attenuation value of   498f.
– –, classification of   496
– –, CT of   498
– –, cystic changes due to   497
– –, Ewing's sarcoma   499
– –, fibroma   497
– –, fibrosarcoma   497, 499
– –, hemangioma   498
– –, hemorrhage due to   497
– –, histiocytoma   499
– –, leiomyoma   498
– –, leiomyosarcoma   498
– –, lipoma   497f.
– –, liposarcoma   497–499
– –, MRI diagnosis of   500
– –, necrosis due to   497
– –, paraganglioma   500
– –, phleboliths and   498
– –, rhabdomyosarcoma   497, 499
– –, schwannoma   500
– –, signs of malignancy in   499f.
–, (of) stomach   321–325
– –, benign   325f.
–, vertebral   542
– –, hemangioma   542
–, Wilm's   386, 409

Urachus
–, persistent   416
Uremia   371
Ureter   395f., 428, 435, 438, 468
Urethra   433
Urinary bladder   381, 395,
    413–421, 425, 428, 433, 435
–, anatomy of   415
–, anomalies of   416
–, cancer of   417
– –, staging of   417
–, carcinoma of   417, 419, 421
– –, diverticular   420
– –, papillary   417
– – –, staging of   418
– –, urachal   420
–, configuration of   415
–, cystectomy of   419
–, displacement of   415
–, diverticulum of   415f.
–, duplication of   415
–, fistula of   417
– –, enterocolic   417
–, infection of   416
– –, acute   416
– –, bilharziosis   416
– –, chronic   417
– –, cystitis cystica   416
– –, dysuria   416
– –, polypoid filling defects   416
– –, scar tissue   416

–, leiomyoma of   420
–, leiomyosarcoma of   420
–, papilloma of   417f.
– –, incrustation in   418
–, pheochromocytoma of   420
–, rhabdomyoma of   420
–, rhabdomyosarcoma of   420
– –, embryonal   420
–, trigone of   425, 435
–, wall infiltration of   428
–, wall of   416f.
– –, calcification of   416
– –, thickening of   417
Urinoma   349, 463
Urography   391, 415
Urolithiasis   397
–, attenuation value   397
Urothelial carcinoma   383
Uterus   414, 434
–, cavity of   433
–, cervix of   433f.
–, corpus of   433
–, fornix of   433
–, fundus of   435
–, supporting apparatus of   434
Utriculocele   426
Utriculus
–, mega-   426

Vagina   433f., 449
Vein
–, axillary   138
–, azygos   140, 166f., 486
– –, continuation of   486
– –, continuity syndrome in   166f.
– –, dilation of   486
– –, ectasia of   167
–, basivertebral   517
–, brachiocephalic   137
–, hemiazygos   486
– –, continuation of   486
– –, dilation of   486
–, mesenteric   338
– –, occlusion of   338
–, portal   247f., 251, 284, 287, 453
– –, contrast enhencement   248
– –, thrombosis of   284
–, pulmonary   140, 185
–, renal   379, 399
– –, occlusion   399
– – –, incomplete   399
– –, patency of   379
– –, thrombosis of   399
– – –, complete obstruction   399
–, splenic   364f.
– –, occlusion of   364
– –, thrombosis of   365
–, subclavian   138
–, vena cava   487
– –, inferior   245, 248, 453, 485f.
– – –, anomalies   485f.
– – –, duplication   485
– – –, thrombosis   486

– –, leiomyosarcoma   487
– –, partial obstruction   487
– –, occlusion syndrome
        of   168
– –, superior   137
– –, thrombosis   487
– – –, septic   487
Verner-Morrison syndrome   302
Vertebral arch   515
Vertebral body   513, 515
Vertebral canal   161
Vesicle *see* Seminal vesicles
von Hippel-Lindau syndrome
    370, 374
Voxel   81, 580

Waterhouse-Friderichsen syn-
    drome   411
Werner's syndrome   407
Whipple's disease   333, 335, 477
Wilm's tumor   237–241, 327, 386,
    409, 496–509
Window   580
–, aortopulmonary   140, 144
Window setting   580
–, (for) bone   8, 513
–, (for) lung   9, 183, 191 f., 231
–, (for) pleura   9, 231
–, pulmonary   231
–, (for) soft tissue   8
Wolffian duct   443

X-ray scatter   580
x-, y-coordinates   580

z-axis   580
Zollinger-Ellison syndrome   302